W9-BWB-729

Alert icon highlights high-alert drugs and critical considerations

Easily confused drug names located beneath the header

Special doses included throughout

Black Box Warnings identify serious and life-threatening adverse effects

Pharmacokinetic information presented in a box format

DAUNOrubicin

High Alert

*DAUNOrubicin (℞)

...w-noe-roo'bi-sin)
...ubidine

...UNOrubicin
...ate liposomal (℞)

...noXome

...*class.:* Antineoplastic, antibi-

Chem. class.: Anthracycline glycoside

Do not confuse:
DAUNOrubicin/DOXOrubicin

Action: Inhibits DNA synthesis, primarily; derived from *Streptomyces coerulorubidus;* replication is decreased by binding to DNA, which causes strand splitting; cell cycle specific (S phase); a vesicant

Uses: Acute lymphocytic leukemia (ALL), acute myelogenous leukemia (AML); *liposomal:* Karposi's sarcoma

Unlabeled uses: *Liposomal:* Multiple myeloma, AML, breast cancer, non-Hodgkin's lymphoma

DOSAGE AND ROUTES

Use decreased dose for those >60 yr of age

...bicin
...45 mg/m²/day × 3 days, then
...sequent courses in combina-

...25-60 mg/m² depending on
cycle

DAUNOrubicin citrate liposomal
- *Adult:* **IV** 40 mg/m² q2wk

Renal dose
- *Adult:* **IV** Serum CCr >3 mg/dl reduce dose by 50%

Hepatic dose
- *Adult:* **IV** Serum bilirubin 1.2-3 mg/dl reduce dose by 25%; bilirubin >3 mg/dl reduce dose by 50%

Available forms: Inj 20 mg powder/vial, sol for inj 5 mg/ml (DaunoXome); *liposomal:* dispersion for inj 2 mg/ml

SIDE EFFECTS

DAUNOrubicin

CNS: Fever, chills
CV: **Dysrhythmias, CHF, pericarditis, myocarditis,** peripheral edema
GI: Nausea, vomiting, anorexia, mucositis, **hepatotoxicity**
GU: Impotence, sterility, amenorrhea, gynecomastia, hyperuricemia
HEMA: **Thrombocytopenia, leukopenia, anemia**
INTEG: Rash, **extravasation,** dermatitis, reversible alopecia, cellulitis, thrombophlebitis at inj site
SYST: **Anaphylaxis**

DAUNOrubicin citrate liposomal

CNS: Fatigue, headache, depression, insomnia, dizziness, *malaise, neuropathy*
CV: Chest pain, edema
GI: Abdominal pain, stomatitis, *nausea, vomiting, diarrhea,* constipation
INTEG: Alopecia, pruritus, sweating
MISC: Allergic reactions, chest pain, fever, edema, flulike symptoms
MS: Rigors, arthralgia, back pain
RESP: Cough, dyspn... tis

Contraindication... breastfeeding, hypers... infections, cardiac dis... depression

Precautions: Tumor l... infection, thrombocytopenia, renal/hepatic disease; gout

Black Box Warning: Bone marrow suppression, cardiac disease, extravasation, renal failure

PHARMACOKINETICS

Half-life 18½ hr, liposome 55½ hr; metabolized by liver; crosses placenta; excreted in breast milk, urine, bile

INTERACTIONS

Increase: bleeding risk—NSAI... licylates
Increase: toxicity—other antin... tics, radiation, cyclophosphamide
Decrease: antibody reaction—liv... vaccines

⚠ Safety alert *"Tall Man" lettering

Formulas

Surface area rule:

$$\text{Child dose} = \frac{\text{Surface area (m}^2\text{)}}{1.73 \text{ m}^2} \times \text{Adult dose}$$

Calculating strength of a solution:

Solution Strength: *Desired Solution:*

$$\frac{x}{100} = \frac{\text{Amount of drug desired}}{\text{Amount of finished solution}}$$

Calculating flow rate for IV:

$$\text{Rate of flow} = \frac{\text{Amount of fluid} \times \text{Administration set calibration}}{\text{Running time}}$$

$$\frac{x}{1} = \frac{\text{(ml) (gtt/min)}}{\text{min}}$$

Calculation of medication dosages:

Formula method:

$$\frac{\text{Amount ordered}}{\text{Amount on hand}} \times \text{Vehicle} = \text{Number of tablets, capsules, or amount of liquid}$$

Vehicle is the drug form or amount of liquid containing the dosage. Amounts used in calculation by formula must be in same system.

Ratio–proportion method:

1 tablet:tablet in mg on hand: :x tablet order in mg

Know or have: :Want to know or order

Multiply means and extremes, divide both sides by known amount to get x. Amounts used in equation must be in same system.

Dimensional analysis method:

$$\text{Order in mg} \times \frac{\text{1 tablet or capsule}}{\text{What 1 tablet or capsule is in mg}} = \text{Tablets or capsules to be given}$$

If amounts are in different systems:

$$\text{Order in mg} \times \frac{\text{1 tablet or capsule}}{\text{What 1 tablet or capsule is in g}} \times \frac{1}{\text{1000 mg}}$$

$$= \text{Tablets or capsules to be given}$$

Temperature conversion:

$F = C \times 9/5 + 32$

$C = 5/9\ (F - 32)$

Nomogram for calculation of body surface area

Place a straight edge from the patients hei ght in the left column to the patient's weight in the right column. The point of intersection on the body surface area column indicates the body surface area (BSA). (Reproduced in Behrman RE, Kliegman RM, Jenson HB: *Nelson textbook of pediatrics,* ed 18, Philadelphia, 2007, WB Saunders; Nomogram modified from data of E. Boyd by CD West.)

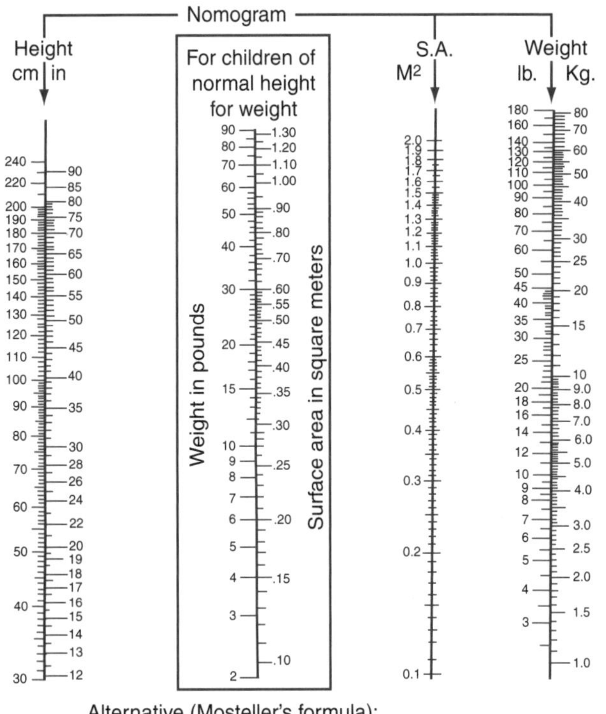

Alternative (Mosteller's formula):

$$\text{Surface area (m}^2\text{)} = \sqrt{\frac{\text{Height (cm)} \times \text{Weight (kg)}}{3600}}$$

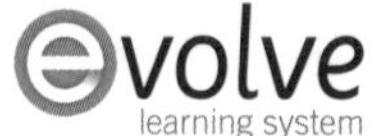

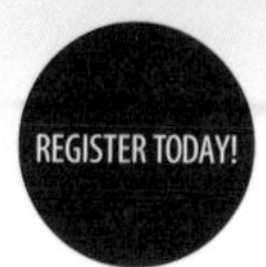

To access your Online Resources, visit:

http://evolve.elsevier.com/nursingdrugupdates/Skidmore/NDR

Register today and gain access to:

- **Drug Monographs**
  Includes full monographs for drugs new to this edition.
- **FDA Alerts**
  Provides updates on drug recalls, labeling changes, new interactions, and safety warnings.
- **Recently Approved Drugs**
  Offers a table of drugs approved by the FDA after publication of the book, including links to approved product inserts.
- **Drug Name Safety Information**
  Links to organizations and resources involved in reducing medication errors caused by drug name confusion.
- **Selected Prescription Drugs with Potential for Abuse**
  Features a table of drugs that can be addictive or dangerous when misused, provided by the National Institute on Drug Abuse.
- **Color Pill Atlas**
  Provides full-color photographs identifying the most commonly prescribed medications and dosages.
- **English-to-Spanish Translation**
  Provides Spanish translations and pronunciations for common drug phrases and terms.

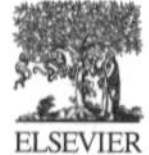

2011

Mosby's NURSING DRUG REFERENCE

24th Edition

Be in the know on the go!

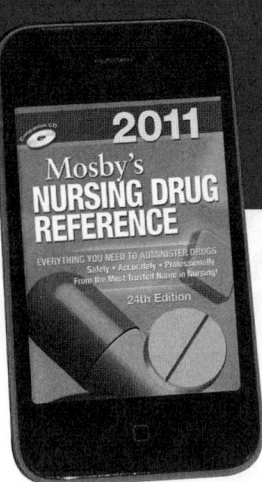

powered by skyscape!

Mosby's 2011 Nursing Drug Reference

Linda Skidmore-Roth, RN, MSN, NP

Available via Skyscape:
www.skyscape.com

Take drug information with you on the job! Powered by Skyscape, this PDA software offers **instant access to all of the content found in Mosby's 2011 Nursing Drug Reference** – with key information on more than 1,300 generic and 4,500 trade-name drugs, thousands of new drug facts, and approximately 25 drugs recently approved by the FDA.

Bonus material includes:

- Nursing drug dosage calculations
- A database of similar drug names – combining more than 1,200 pairs of easily confused drug names
- Extensive cross-linking and search capabilities
- And more!

ELSEVIER

Order your copy today!

Available formats:

- iPhone®/iPod Touch®
- Blackberry®/SmartPhone®
- Palm®
- Pocket PC®
- Android™

Download it directly to your device!
Visit www.skyscape.com

SL100191

2011

Mosby's NURSING DRUG REFERENCE

24th Edition

Linda Skidmore-Roth, RN, MSN, NP

Consultant

Littleton, Colorado

Formerly, Nursing Faculty

New Mexico State University

Las Cruces, New Mexico;

El Paso Community College

El Paso, Texas

ELSEVIER

MOSBY

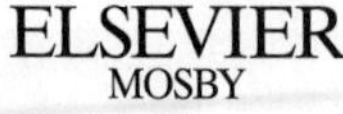

3251 Riverport Lane
St. Louis, Missouri 63043

MOSBY'S 2011 NURSING DRUG REFERENCE,
TWENTY-FOURTH EDITION

ISBN: 978-0-323-06918-2
ISSN: 1044-8470

Copyright © 2011 by Mosby, Inc., an affiliate of Elsevier Inc. All rights reserved.

No part of this publication may be reproduced or transmitted in any form or by any means, electronic or mechanical, including photocopying, recording, or any information storage and retrieval system, without permission in writing from the publisher. Details on how to seek permission, further information about the Publisher's permissions policies and our arrangements with organizations such as the Copyright Clearance Center and the Copyright Licensing Agency, can be found at our website: www.elsevier.com/permissions.

This book and the individual contributions contained in it are protected under copyright by the Publisher (other than as may be noted herein).

Notices

Knowledge and best practice in this field are constantly changing. As new research and experience broaden our understanding, changes in research methods, professional practices, or medical treatment may become necessary.

Practitioners and researchers must always rely on their own experience and knowledge in evaluating and using any information, methods, compounds, or experiments described herein. In using such information or methods they should be mindful of their own safety and the safety of others, including parties for whom they have a professional responsibility.

With respect to any drug or pharmaceutical products identified, readers are advised to check the most current information provided (i) on procedures featured or (ii) by the manufacturer of each product to be administered, to verify the recommended dose or formula, the method and duration of administration, and contraindications. It is the responsibility of practitioners, relying on their own experience and knowledge of their patients, to make diagnoses, to determine dosages and the best treatment for each individual patient, and to take all appropriate safety precautions.

To the fullest extent of the law, neither the Publisher nor the authors, contributors, or editors, assume any liability for any injury and/or damage to persons or property arising as a matter of products liability, negligence or otherwise, or from any use or operation of any methods, products, instructions, or ideas contained in the material herein.

ISBN: 978-0-323-06918-2

Acquisitions Editor: Nancy O'Brien
Associate Developmental Editor: Angela Perdue
Publishing Services Manager: Pat Joiner-Myers
Senior Project Manager: Joy Moore
Designer: Teresa McBryan

Printed in the United States of America

Last digit is the print number:
9 8 7 6 5 4 3 2

Working together to grow
libraries in developing countries

www.elsevier.com | www.bookaid.org | www.sabre.org

ELSEVIER BOOK AID International Sabre Foundation

Consultants

Timothy L. Brenner, PharmD, BCOP
Clinical Pharmacy Specialist
UPMC Cancer Centers
Pittsburgh, Pennsylvania

Claudia Chiesa, PhD
Marana, Arizona

David S. Chun, PharmD, BCPS
Richmond Heights, Missouri

Jeffrey J. Fong, PharmD, BCPS
Assistant Professor of Pharmacy Practice
Massachusetts College of Pharmacy and Health Sciences
Worcester, Massachusetts

Amanda Gross, RPh
Clinical Pharmacist
University of Colorado Hospital
Aurora, Colorado

Dana H. Hamamura, PharmD
Clinical Pharmacist, Emergency Department
University of Colorado Hospital
Aurora, Colorado

Rose Knapp, DNP, RN, APRN-C
Assistant Professor of Nursing/Pharmacology
New York University
New York, New York

Michael J. Koronkowski, PharmD, CGP
Clinical Assistant Professor, Geriatrics
University of Illinois, College of Pharmacy
Chicago, Illinois

Shalini S. Lynch, PharmD
Assistant Clinical Professor of Pharmacy
University of California, San Francisco School of Pharmacy
San Francisco, California

Michele Matthews, PharmD
Assistant Professor
Massachusetts College of Pharmacy
Clinical Pharmacist
Brigham and Women's Hospital
Boston, Massachusetts

Sandra Meeker, MSN, RN
Assistant Professor
University of Mary Hardin Baylor
Belton, Texas

Joshua J. Neumiller, PharmD, CDE, CGP, FASCP
Assistant Professor
Washington State University
Spokane, Washington

Christopher T. Owens, PharmD, BCPS
Associate Professor and Chair
Idaho State University College of Pharmacy
Pocatello, Idaho

Brenda Pavill, PhD, RN, FNP, IBCLC
Associate Professor
University of North Carolina at Wilmington
Wilmington, North Carolina

Adam B. Pesaturo, PharmD, BCPS
Critical Care Pharmacist
Baystate Medical Center
Springfield, Massachusetts

Kimberly A. Pesaturo, PharmD, BCPS
Assistant Professor of Pharmacy Practice
Massachusetts College of Pharmacy and Health Sciences
Worcester, Massachusetts

Sarah Reidunn Pool, MS, RN
Nurse Manager
Mayo Clinic
Rochester, Minnesota

Randolph Eldon Regal, BS, PharmD, RPh
Clinical Associate Professor
Adult Internal Medicine
University of Michigan
Ann Arbor, Michigan

Sheila M. Seed, PharmD, RPh, MPH
Assistant Professor of Pharmacy Practice
Massachusetts College of Pharmacy and Health Sciences
Worcester, Massachusetts

Stephen M. Setter, PharmD, DVM, CDE, CGP, FASCP
Associate Professor of Pharmacotherapy
Elder Services/Visiting Nurses Association
Washington State University
Spokane, Washington

Travis E. Sonnett, PharmD
Clinical Assistant Professor
Washington State University
Pullman, Washington

Patricia R. Teasley, MSN, RN
Nursing Programs Coordinator
Professor
Central Texas College
Killeen, Texas

Juanita C. Widener, MAEd, BSN, RN
Instructor of Nursing
Bainbridge College
Bainbridge, Georgia

Preface

Since the first publication of *Mosby's Nursing Drug Reference* in 1988, more than 100 U.S. and Canadian pharmacists and consultants have reviewed the book's content closely. Today, *Mosby's 2011 Nursing Drug Reference* is more up to date than ever—with features that make it easy to find critical information fast!

New Features

- Twenty-five recent FDA-approved drugs located throughout the book and in Appendix A (see Table of Contents for a complete list). Included are monographs for:
  - asenapine (Saphris)—used for schizophrenia
  - dronedarone (Multaq)—used for atrial fibrillation or atrial flutter
  - everolimus (Affinitor)—used for advanced renal cell carcinoma
  - pitavastatin (Livalo)—used for hypercholesterolemia
  - telavancin (Vibatin)—used for complicated gram-positive infections
- A companion CD-ROM that offers complete and printable monographs for 100 of the most commonly prescribed drugs in the United States, numerous patient teaching guides in English and Spanish for these same drugs, hundreds of normal laboratory values, an English-to-Spanish guide for drug phrases and terms, 30 calculators, and Canadian resources

New Facts

This edition features more than 2000 new drug facts, including:

- New drugs and new dosage information
- Newly researched side effects and adverse reactions
- New Black Box Warnings
- The latest precautions, interactions, and contraindications
- IV therapy updates
- Revised nursing considerations
- Updated patient/family teaching guidelines

Organization

This reference is organized into four main sections:

- Drug categories
- Full-color insert
- Individual drug monographs (in alphabetical order by generic name)
- Appendixes (identified by the wide, dark blue thumb tabs on the edge)

The guiding principle behind this book is to provide fast, easy access to drug information and nursing considerations. Every detail—from the paper, typeface, cover, binding, use of color, and appendixes—has been carefully chosen with the user in mind.

Color Insert

This insert features 14 detailed, four-color illustrations to help enhance the understanding of the mechanism or site of action for the following select drugs and drug classes:

- ACE inhibitors
- Adrenocortical steroids
- Antidepressants
- Antidiabetic agents
- Antifungal agents
- Antiinfective agents
- Antiplatelet agents
- Antiretroviral agents
- Benzodiazepines
- Diuretics
- Drugs used to treat GERD
- Narcotic agonist-antagonist analgesics
- Narcotic analgesics
- Sympatholytics

Also included in the color insert are the 2010 recommended childhood and adolescent immunization schedules for the United States.

Individual Drug Monographs

This book contains monographs for more than 1300 generic and 4500 trade medications. Common trade names are given for all drugs regularly used in the United States and Canada, with drugs available only in Canada identified by a maple leaf 🍁.

The following information is provided, whenever possible, for safe, effective administration of each drug:

High-alert status: Identifies high-alert drugs with a label and icon. Visit the Institute for Safe Medication Practices (ISMP) at http://www.ismp.org/tools/highalertmedications.pdf for a list of medications and drug classes with the greatest potential for patient harm if they are used in error.

"Tall Man" lettering: Uses the capitalization of distinguishing letters to avoid medication errors and is required by the FDA for drug manufacturers.

Pronunciation: Helps the nurse master complex generic names.

℞/OTC: Identifies prescription or over-the-counter drugs.

Functional and chemical classifications: Allows the nurse to see similarities and dissimilarities among drugs in the same functional but different chemical classes.

Controlled-substance schedule: Includes schedules for the United States and Canada.

Do not confuse: Presents drug names that might easily be confused, within each appropriate monograph.

Action: Describes pharmacologic properties concisely.

Uses: Lists the conditions the drug is used to treat.

Unlabeled uses: Describes drug uses that may be encountered in practice but are not yet FDA-approved.

Dosages and routes: Lists all available and approved dosages and routes for adult, pediatric, and geriatric patients.

Available forms: Includes tablets, capsules, extended-release, injectables (IV, IM, SUBCUT), solutions, creams, ointments, lotions, gels, shampoos, elixirs, suspensions, suppositories, sprays, aerosols, and lozenges.

Side effects: Groups these reactions by alphabetical body system, with common side effects *italicized* and life-threatening reactions (those that are potentially fatal and/or permanently disabling) in **bold type** for emphasis.

Contraindications: Lists conditions under which the drug absolutely should not be given, including FDA pregnancy safety categories D or X.

Precautions: Lists conditions that require special consideration when the drug is prescribed, including FDA pregnancy safety categories A, B, or C.

Black box warnings: Identifies FDA warnings that highlight serious and life-threatening adverse effects.

Pharmacokinetics: Outlines metabolism, distribution, and elimination.

Interactions: Includes confirmed drug interactions, followed by the drug or nutrient causing that interaction, when applicable.

Drug/herb: Highlights more than 400 potential interactions between herbal products and prescription or OTC drugs.

Drug/food: Identifies many common drug interactions with foods.

Drug/lab test: Identifies how the drug may affect lab test results.

Nursing considerations: Identifies key nursing considerations for each step of the nursing process: Assess, Administer, Perform/Provide, Evaluate, and Teach Patient/Family. Instructions for giving drugs by various routes (e.g., PO, IM, IV) are included, with route subheadings in bold.

Compatibilities: Lists syringe, Y-site, and additive compatibilities and incompatibilities. If no compatibilities are listed for a drug, the necessary compatibility testing has not been done and that compatibility information is unknown. To ensure safety, assume that the drug may not be mixed with other drugs unless specifically stated.

"Nursing Alert" icon ⚠: Highlights a critical consideration.

Treatment of overdose: Provides drugs and treatment for overdoses where appropriate.

Appendixes

Selected new drugs: Includes comprehensive information on 22 key drugs approved by the FDA during the last 12 months.

Ophthalmic, otic, nasal, and topical products: Provides essential information for more than 140 ophthalmic, otic, nasal, and topical products commonly used today, grouped by chemical drug class.

Vaccines and toxoids: Features an easy-to-use table with generic and trade names, uses, dosages and routes, and contraindications for 39 key vaccines and toxoids.

Antitoxins and antivenins: Provides names, uses, dosages, and contraindications.

Combination products: Provides details on the forms and uses of more than 550 combination products.

FDA pregnancy categories: Explains the five FDA pregnancy categories.

Abbreviations: Lists abbreviations alphabetically with their meanings.

I am indebted to the nursing and pharmacology consultants who reviewed the manuscript and thank them for their criticism and encouragement. I would also like to thank Nancy O'Brien and Angela Perdue, my editors, whose active encouragement and enthusiasm have made this book better than it might otherwise have been. I am likewise grateful to Joy Moore and Graphic World Inc. for the coordination of the production process and assistance with the development of the new edition.

Linda Skidmore-Roth

Contents

Drug categories, 1

Color insert

Individual drugs, 77

Continued

α-ADRENERGIC BLOCKERS

Action: α-Adrenergic blockers act by binding to α-adrenergic receptors, causing dilation of peripheral blood vessels. Lowers peripheral resistance, resulting in decreased B/P.

Uses: α-adrenergic blockers are used for benign prostatic hyperplasia, pheochromocytoma, prevention of tissue necrosis and sloughing associated with extravasation of IV vasopressors.

Side effects: The most common side effects are hypotension, tachycardia, nasal stuffiness, nausea, vomiting, and diarrhea.

Contraindications: Hypersensitive reactions may occur, and allergies should be identified before these products are given. Patients with MI, coronary insufficiency, angina, or other evidence of CAD should not use these products.

Pharmacokinetics: Onset, peak, and duration vary among products.

Interactions: Vasoconstrictive and hypertensive effects of epinephrine are antagonized by α-adrenergic blockers.

Possible nursing diagnoses:
- Risk for injury *[adverse reactions]*
- Sleep deprivation *[adverse reactions]*
- Ineffective tissue perfusion *[uses]*
- Impaired urinary elimination *[uses]*

Nursing Considerations

Assess:
- Electrolytes: K, Na, Cl, CO_2
- Weight daily, I&O
- B/P lying, standing before starting treatment, q4hr thereafter
- Nausea, vomiting, diarrhea
- Skin turgor, dryness of mucous membranes for hydration status

Administer:
- Starting with low dose, gradually increasing to prevent side effects
- With food or milk for GI symptoms

Evaluate:
- Therapeutic response: decreased B/P, increased peripheral pulses

Teach patient/family:
- To avoid alcoholic beverages
- To report dizziness, palpitations, fainting
- To change position slowly or fainting may occur
- To take product exactly as prescribed
- To avoid all OTC products (cough, cold, allergy) unless directed by prescriber

Selected Generic Names

phentolamine

α 1 blockers

silodosin

tamsulosin

ANESTHETICS—GENERAL/LOCAL

Action: Anesthetics (general) act on the CNS to produce tranquilization and sleep before invasive procedures. Anesthetics (local) inhibit conduction of nerve impulses from sensory nerves.

Uses: General anesthetics are used to premedicate for surgery, induction and maintenance in general anesthesia. For local anesthetics, refer to individual product listing for indications.

Side effects: The most common side effects are dystonia, akathisia, flexion of arms, fine tremors, drowsiness, restlessness, and hypotension. Also common are chills, respiratory depression, and laryngospasm.

Contraindications: Persons with cerebrovascular accident, increased intracranial pressure, severe hypertension, cardiac decompensation should not use these products since severe adverse reactions can occur.

Precautions: Anesthetics (general) should be used with caution in the geriatric, CVD (hypotension, bradydysrhythmias), renal/hepatic disease, Parkinson's disease, children <2 yr. The precaution for anesthetics (local) is pregnancy.

Pharmacokinetics: Onset, peak, and duration vary widely among products. Most products are metabolized in the liver and excreted in urine.

Interactions: MAOIs, tricyclics, phenothiazines may cause severe hypotension or hypertension when used with local anesthetics. CNS depressants will potentiate general and local anesthetics.

Possible nursing diagnoses:

General:

- Risk for injury *[adverse reactions]*
- Deficient knowledge *[teaching]*

Local:

- Deficient knowledge *[teaching]*
- Acute pain *[uses]*

Nursing Considerations

Assess:

- VS q10min during IV administration, q30min after IM dose

Administer:

- Anticholinergic preoperatively to decrease secretions
- Only with crash cart, resuscitative equipment nearby

Perform/provide:

- Quiet environment for recovery to decrease psychotic symptoms

Evaluate:

- Therapeutic response: maintenance of anesthesia, decreased pain

Selected Generic Names (Injectables Only)

General anesthetics

droperidol
etomidate
fentanyl
fentanyl/droperidol
fentanyl transdermal
fospropofol
midazolam
propofol
thiopental

Local anesthetics

lidocaine
procaine
ropivacaine
tetracaine

ANTACIDS

Action: Antacids are basic compounds that neutralize gastric acidity and decrease the rate of gastric emptying. Products are divided into those containing aluminum, magnesium, calcium, or a combination of these.

Uses: Antacids decrease hyperacidity in conditions such as peptic ulcer disease, reflux esophagitis, gastritis, and hiatal hernia.

Side effects: The most common side effect caused by aluminum-containing antacids is constipation, which may lead to fecal impaction and bowel obstruction. Diarrhea occurs often when magnesium products are given. Alkalosis may occur when systemic products are used. Constipation occurs more frequently than laxation with calcium carbonate. The release of CO_2 from carbonate-containing antacids causes belching, abdominal distention, and flatulence. Sodium bicarbonate may act as a systemic antacid and produce systemic electrolyte disturbances and alkalosis. Calcium carbonate and sodium bicarbonate may cause rebound hyperacidity and milk-alkali syndrome. Alkaluria may occur when products are used on a long-term basis, particularly in persons with abnormal renal function.

Contraindications: Sensitivity to aluminum or magnesium products may cause hypersensitive reactions. Aluminum products should not be used by persons sensitive to aluminum; magnesium products should not be used by persons sensitive to magnesium. Check for sensitivity before administering.

Precautions: Magnesium products should be given cautiously to patients with renal insufficiency, and during pregnancy and breastfeeding. Sodium content of antacids may be significant; use with caution for patients with hypertension, congestive heart failure, or those on a low-sodium diet.

Pharmacokinetics: Duration is 20-40 min. If ingested 1 hr after meals, acidity is reduced for at least 3 hr.

Interactions: Products whose effects may be increased by some antacids: quinidine, amphetamines, pseudoephedrine, levodopa, valproic acid, dicumarol. Products whose effects may be decreased by some antacids: cimetidine, corticosteroids, ranitidine, iron salts, phenothiazines, phenytoin, digoxin, tetracyclines, ketoconazole, salicylates, isoniazid.

Possible nursing diagnoses:
- Constipation *[adverse reactions]*
- Diarrhea *[adverse reactions]*
- Chronic pain *[uses]*

Nursing Considerations

Assess:
- Aggravating and alleviating factors of epigastric pain or hyperacidity; identify the location, duration, and characteristics of epigastric pain
- GI symptoms, including constipation, diarrhea, abdominal pain; if severe abdominal pain with fever occurs, these products should not be given
- Renal symptoms, including increasing urinary pH, electrolytes

Administer:
- Not to take other products within 1-2 hr of antacid administration, since antacids may impair absorption of other products
- All products with an 8-oz glass of water to ensure absorption in the stomach
- Another antacid if constipation occurs with aluminum products

Evaluate:
- Therapeutic response: absence of epigastric pain, and decreased acidity

Selected Generic Names

aluminum hydroxide
bismuth subsalicylate
calcium carbonate
magaldrate
magnesium oxide
sodium bicarbonate

ANTI-ALZHEIMER AGENTS

Action: Anti-Alzheimer agents improve cognitive functioning by increasing acetylcholine and inhibiting cholinesterase in the CNS. Do not cure condition, but improve symptoms.

Uses: Anti-Alzheimer agents are used for the treatment of Alzheimer's symptoms.

Side effects: The most common side effects are nausea, vomiting, diarrhea, dry mouth, insomnia, dizziness, as well as urinary frequency, incontinence, and rash. The most serious side effects are seizures and dysrhythmias.

Contraindications: Persons with hypersensitivity reactions should not use these products.

Precautions: Anti-Alzheimer agents should be used cautiously in pregnancy (C), breastfeeding, sick sinus syndrome, GI bleeding, bladder obstruction, and seizures.

Pharmacokinetics: Onset, peak, and duration vary widely among products. Most products are metabolized in the liver and excreted by the kidneys.

Interactions: Increased synergistic reactions may occur with succinylcholine, cholinesterase inhibitors, and cholinergic agonists. There may be a decrease in the action of anticholinergics, and there may be additive effects when used with cholinergic agents.

Possible nursing diagnoses:

- Chronic confusion *[uses]*
- Deficient knowledge *[teaching]*
- Noncompliance *[teaching]*

Nursing Considerations

Assess:

- B/P, hypotension, hypertension
- Mental status: affect, mood, behavioral changes, depression, confusion
- GI status: nausea, vomiting, anorexia, diarrhea
- GU status: urinary frequency, incontinence

Administer:

- Lowest possible dose for therapeutic result; adjust dose to response

Perform/provide:

- Assistance with ambulation during beginning therapy if dizziness, ataxia occur

Evaluate:

- Therapeutic response: decrease in confusion, improved mood

Teach patient/family:

- To report side effects, adverse reactions to health care provider
- To use exactly as prescribed, at regular intervals
- Not to increase or abruptly decrease dose; serious consequences may result
- That product is not a cure, but relieves symptoms

Selected Generic Names

donepezil
galanthamine
memantine
rivastigmine

ANTIANGINALS

Action: Antianginals are divided into the nitrates, calcium channel blockers, and β-adrenergic blockers. The nitrates dilate coronary arteries, causing decreased preload, and dilate systemic arteries, causing decreased afterload. Calcium channel blockers dilate coronary arteries and decrease SA/AV node conduction. β-Adrenergic blockers decrease heart rate so that myocardial O_2 use is decreased. Dipyridamole selectively dilates coronary arteries to increase coronary blood flow.

Uses: Antianginals are used in chronic stable angina pectoris, unstable angina, vasospastic angina. Some (i.e., calcium channel blockers and β-blockers) may be used for dysrhythmias and in hypertension.

Side effects: The most common side effects are postural hypotension, headache, flushing, dizziness, nausea, edema, and drowsiness. Also common are rash, dysrhythmias, and fatigue.

Contraindications: Persons with known hypersensitivity, increased intracranial pressure, or cerebral hemorrhage should not use some of these products.

Precautions: Antianginals should be used with caution in postural hypotension, pregnancy, breastfeeding, children, renal disease, and hepatic injury.

Pharmacokinetics: Onset, peak, and duration vary widely among coronary products. Most products are metabolized in the liver and excreted in urine.

Interactions: Interactions vary widely among products. Check individual monographs for specific information.

Possible nursing diagnoses:

- Decreased cardiac output *[adverse reactions]*
- Risk for injury *[uses]*
- Deficient knowledge *[teaching]*
- Acute pain *[uses]*
- Ineffective tissue perfusion *[uses]*

Nursing Considerations

Assess:

- Orthostatic B/P, pulse
- Pain: duration, time started, activity being performed, character
- Tolerance if taken over long period
- Headache, light-headedness, decreased B/P; may indicate a need for decreased dosage

Perform/provide:

- Storage protected from light, moisture; place in cool environment

Evaluate:

- Therapeutic response: decrease, prevention of anginal pain

Teach patient/family:

- To keep tabs in original container
- Not to use OTC products unless directed by prescriber
- To report bradycardia, dizziness, confusion, depression, fever
- To take pulse at home, advise when to notify prescriber
- To avoid alcohol, smoking, sodium intake
- To comply with weight control, dietary adjustments, modified exercise program
- To carry emergency ID to identify product that you are taking, allergies
- To make position changes slowly to prevent fainting

Selected Generic Names

Nitrates

amyl nitrite
isosorbide
nitroglycerin

β-Adrenergic blockers

atenolol
dipyridamole
metoprolol
nadolol
propranolol

Calcium channel blockers
amlodipine
bepridil
diltiazem
niCARdipine
NIFEdipine
verapamil
Miscellaneous
ranolazine

ANTIANXIETY AGENTS

Action: Benzodiazepines potentiate the action of GABA, including any other inhibitory transmitters in the CNS resulting in decreased anxiety. Most agents cause a decrease in CNS excitability.
Uses: Anxiety is relieved in conditions such as generalized anxiety disorder and phobic disorders. Benzodiazepines are also used for acute alcohol withdrawal to prevent delirium tremens, and some products are used for relaxation before surgery.
Side effects: The most common side effects are dizziness, drowsiness, blurred vision, and orthostatic hypotension. Most adverse reactions are mediated through the CNS. There is the potential for abuse and physical dependence with some products.
Contraindications: These products are contraindicated in hypersensitivity, acute closed-angle glaucoma, children <6 mo, hepatic disease (clonazepam), and breastfeeding (diazepam).
Precautions: Antianxiety agents should be used cautiously in geriatric or debilitated patients. Usually smaller doses are needed since metabolism is slowed. Persons with renal/hepatic disease may show delayed excretion. Clonazepam may increase the incidence of seizures.
Pharmacokinetics: Most of these agents are metabolized by the liver and excreted via the kidneys.
Interactions: Increased CNS depression may occur when given with other CNS depressants. These products should be used together cautiously. Alcohol should not be used, as fatal reactions have occurred. The serum concentration and toxicity may be increased when used with benzodiazepines.
Possible nursing diagnoses:
- Anxiety *[uses]*
- Risk for injury *[adverse reactions]*
- Deficient knowledge *[teaching]*

Nursing Considerations

Assess:
- B/P (lying and standing), pulse; if systolic B/P drops 20 mm Hg, hold product and notify prescriber; orthostatic hypotension can be severe
- Hepatic/renal studies: AST, ALT, bilirubin, creatinine, LDH, alk phos
- Physical dependency and withdrawal with some products, including headache, nausea, vomiting, muscle pain, and weakness after long-term use

Administer:
- With food or milk for GI symptoms; may give crushed if patient is unable to swallow whole (tabs only, no controlled- or sustained-release products)

Evaluate:
- Therapeutic response: decreased anxiety, increased relaxation

Teach patient/family:
- That product should not be used for everyday stress or long-term use; not to take more than prescribed

amount since product is habit forming

- To avoid driving and activities that require alertness since drowsiness and dizziness may occur
- To abstain from alcohol, other psychotropic medications unless directed by prescriber
- Not to discontinue abruptly; after extended periods, withdrawal symptoms may occur

Selected Generic Names

Benzodiazepines
alprazolam
chlordiazepoxide
clonazepam
diazepam
lorazepam
midazolam
oxazepine
temazepine
triazolam

Miscellaneous
busPIRone
doxepin
hydrOXYzine
meprobamate
paroxetine
venlafaxine

ANTIASTHMATICS

Action: Bronchodilators are divided into anticholinergics, α/β-adrenergic agonists, β-adrenergic agonists, and phosphodiesterase inhibitors. Also included in antiasthmatic agents are corticosteroids, leukotriene antagonists, mast cell stabilizers, and monoclonal antibodies. Anticholinergics act by inhibiting interaction of acetylcholine at receptor sites on bronchial smooth muscle. α/β-Adrenergic agonists act by relaxing bronchial smooth muscle and increasing diameter of nasal passages. β-Adrenergic agonists act by action on β_2-receptors, which relaxes bronchial smooth muscle. Phosphodiesterase inhibitors act by blocking phosphodiesterase and increasing cAMP, which mediates smooth muscle relaxation in the respiratory system. Corticosteroids act by decreasing inflammation in the bronchial system. Leukotriene receptor antagonists decrease leukotrienes, and mast cell stabilizers decrease histamine; both act to decrease bronchospasm.

Uses: Antiasthmatics are used for bronchial asthma; bronchospasm associated with bronchitis, emphysema, or other obstructive pulmonary diseases; Cheyne-Stokes respirations; and prevention of exercise-induced asthma. Some products are used for rhinitis and other allergic reactions.

Side effects: The most common side effects are tremors, anxiety, nausea, vomiting, and irritation in the throat. The most serious adverse reactions are bronchospasm and dyspnea.

Contraindications: Persons with hypersensitivity, closed-angle glaucoma, tachydysrhythmias, and severe cardiac disease should not use some of these products.

Precautions: Antiasthmatics should be used with caution in breastfeeding, pregnancy, hyperthyroidism, hypertension, prostatic hypertrophy, and seizure disorders.

Pharmacokinetics: Onset, peak, and duration vary widely among products. Most products are metabolized by the liver and excreted in urine.

Interactions: Interactions vary widely among products. Check individual monographs for specific information.

Possible nursing diagnoses:

- Activity intolerance *[uses]*
- Ineffective airway clearance *[uses]*
- Risk for injury *[adverse reactions]*
- Deficient knowledge *[teaching]*
- Noncompliance *[teaching]*

Nursing Considerations

Assess:

- Respiratory function: vital capacity, forced expiratory volume, ABGs, lung sounds, heart rate and rhythm, aggravating and alleviating factors

Administer:

- Inhaled product after shaking; exhale, place mouthpiece in mouth, inhale slowly, hold breath, remove, exhale slowly
- PO product with meals to decrease gastric irritation

Perform/provide:

- Storage of inhaled product in light-resistant container; do not expose to temps over 86° F (30° C)
- Gum, small sips of water for dry mouth

Evaluate:

- Therapeutic response: decrease severity and number of asthma attacks; absence of dyspnea, wheezing

Teach patient/family:

- To avoid hazardous activities; drowsiness or dizziness may occur with some products
- To obtain blood work as required; some products require blood levels to be drawn
- Avoid all OTC medications unless approved by provider
- To report side effects, including insomnia, heart palpitations, lightheadedness; these side effects may occur with some products

Selected Generic Names

Bronchodilators

albuterol
arformoterol
atropine
bitolterol
dyphylline
formoterol
ipratropium
isoproterenol
levalbuterol
metaproterenol
pirbuterol
terbutaline
theophylline
tiotropium

Adrenergics

epinephrine

Corticosteroids

beclomethasone
betamethasone
budesonide
cortisone
dexamethasone
flunisolide
fluticasone
hydrocortisone
methylPREDNISolone
predniSONE
trimicinolone

Leukotriene antagonists

zafirlukast

Mast cell stabilizers

cromolyn
nedocromil

Monoclonal antibodies

omalizumab

ANTICHOLINERGICS

Action: Anticholinergics inhibit the muscarinic actions of acetylcholine at receptor sites in the autonomic nervous system. Anticholinergics are also known as antimuscarinic products.

Uses: Anticholinergics are used for a variety of conditions: decreasing involuntary movements in parkinsonism (benztropine, trihexyphenidyl); bradydysrhythmias (atropine); nausea and vomiting (scopolamine); and as cycloplegic mydriatics (atropine, homatropine, scopolamine, cyclopentolate, tropicamide). Gastrointestinal anticholinergics are used to decrease motility (smooth muscle tone) in the GI, biliary, and urinary tracts and for their ability to decrease gastric secretions (propantheline, glycopyrrolate).

Side effects: The most common side effects are dry mouth, constipation, urinary retention, urinary hesitancy, headache, and dizziness. Also common is paralytic ileus.

Contraindications: Persons with closed-angle glaucoma, myasthenia gravis, or GI/GU obstruction should not use some of these products.

Precautions: Anticholinergics should be used with caution in patients who are geriatric, pregnant, or breastfeeding or in those with prostatic hypertrophy, congestive heart failure, or hypertension; use with caution in presence of high environmental temperature.

Pharmacokinetics: Onset, peak, and duration vary widely among products. Most products are metabolized in the liver and excreted in urine.

Interactions: Increased anticholinergic effects may occur when used with MAOIs and tricyclics and amantadine. Anticholinergics may cause a decreased effect of phenothiazines and levodopa.

Possible nursing diagnoses:

- Decreased cardiac output *[uses]*
- Constipation *[adverse reactions]*
- Deficient knowledge *[teaching]*

Nursing Considerations

Assess:

- I&O ratio; retention commonly causes decreased urinary output
- Urinary hesitancy, retention; palpate bladder if retention occurs
- Constipation; increase fluids, bulk, exercise if this occurs
- For tolerance over long-term therapy, dose may need to be increased or changed
- Mental status: affect, mood, CNS depression, worsening of mental symptoms during early therapy

Administer:

- Parenteral dose with patient recumbent to prevent postural hypotension
- With or after meals to prevent GI upset; may give with fluids other than water
- Parenteral dose slowly; keep in bed for at least 1 hr after dose; monitor vital signs
- After checking dose carefully; even slight overdose can lead to toxicity

Perform/provide:

- Storage at room temperature
- Hard candy, frequent drinks, sugarless gum to relieve dry mouth

Evaluate:

- Therapeutic response: decreased secretions, absence of nausea and vomiting

Teach patient/family:

- To avoid driving or other hazardous activities; drowsiness may occur

• To avoid OTC medication: cough, cold preparations with alcohol, antihistamines unless directed by prescriber

Selected Generic Names

atropine
benztropine
biperiden
dicyclomine
glycopyrrolate
hyoscyamine
propantheline
scopolamine (transdermal)
solifenacin
trihexyphenidyl

ANTICOAGULANTS

Action: Anticoagulants interfere with blood clotting by preventing clot formation.

Uses: Anticoagulants are used for deep vein thrombosis, PE, MI, open-heart surgery, disseminated intravascular clotting syndrome; atrial fibrillation with embolization, transfusion, and dialysis.

Side effects: The most serious adverse reactions are hemorrhage, agranulocytosis, leukopenia, eosinophilia, and thrombocytopenia, depending on the specific product. The most common side effects are diarrhea, rash, and fever.

Contraindications: Persons with hemophilia and related disorders, leukemia with bleeding, peptic ulcer disease, thrombocytopenic purpura, blood dyscrasias, acute nephritis, and subacute bacterial endocarditis should not use these products.

Precautions: Anticoagulants should be used with caution in alcoholism, geriatric patients, and pregnancy.

Pharmacokinetics: Onset, peak, and duration vary widely among products. Most products are metabolized in the liver and excreted in urine.

Interactions: Salicylates, steroids, and nonsteroidal antiinflammatories will potentiate the action of anticoagulants. Anticoagulants may cause serious effects; check individual monographs.

Possible nursing diagnoses:

- Risk for injury *[side effects]*
- Deficient knowledge *[teaching]*
- Ineffective tissue perfusion *[uses]*

Nursing Considerations

Assess:

- Blood studies (Hct, platelets, occult blood in stools) q3mo
- Partial PT, which should be 1½-2 × control PPT daily, also APTT, ACT
- B/P; watch for increasing signs of hypertension
- Bleeding gums, petechiae, ecchymosis; black, tarry stools; hematuria
- Fever, skin rash, urticaria
- Needed dosage change q1-2wk

Administer:

- At same time each day to maintain steady blood levels
- In abdomen between pelvic bone, rotate sites; do not massage area or aspirate when giving SUBCUT injection; do not pull back on plunger, leave in for 10 sec, apply gentle pressure for 1 min
- Without changing needles
- Avoiding all IM inj that may cause bleeding

Perform/provide:

- Storage in tight container

Evaluate:

• Therapeutic response: decrease of DVT

Teach patient/family:

• To avoid OTC preparations that may cause serious product interactions unless directed by prescriber

• That product may be held during active bleeding (menstruation), depending on condition

• To use soft-bristle toothbrush to avoid bleeding gums; avoid contact sports, use electric razor

• To carry emergency ID identifying product taken

• To report any signs of bleeding: gums, under skin, urine, stools

Selected Generic Names

ardeparin
argatroban
dalteparin
danaparoid
desirudin
enoxaparin
fondaparinux
heparin
lepirudin
tinzaparin
warfarin

ANTICONVULSANTS

Action: Anticonvulsants are divided into the barbiturates, benzodiazepines, hydantoins, succinimides, and miscellaneous products. Barbiturates and benzodiazepines are discussed in separate sections. Hydantoins act by inhibiting the spread of seizure activity in the motor cortex. Succinimides act by inhibiting spike and wave formation; they also decrease amplitude, frequency, duration, and spread of discharge in seizures.

Uses: Hydantoins are used in generalized tonic-clonic seizures, status epilepticus, and psychomotor seizures. Succinimides are used for absence (petit mal) seizures. Barbiturates are used in generalized tonic-clonic and cortical focal seizures.

Side effects: Bone marrow depression is the most life-threatening adverse reaction associated with hydantoins or succinimides. The most common side effects are GI symptoms. Other common side effects for hydantoins are gingival hyperplasia and CNS effects such as nystagmus, ataxia, slurred speech, and mental confusion.

Contraindications: Hypersensitive reactions may occur, and allergies should be identified before these products are given.

Precautions: Persons with renal/hepatic disease should be watched closely.

Pharmacokinetics: Onset, peak, and duration vary widely among products. Most products are metabolized in the liver and excreted in urine, bile, and feces.

Interactions: Decreased effects of estrogens, oral contraceptives (hydantoins).

Possible nursing diagnoses:

• Injury, risk for *[uses]*

• Noncompliance *[teaching]*

• Sleep deprivation *[adverse reactions]*

Nursing Considerations

Assess:

• Renal studies, including BUN, creatinine, serum uric acid, urine creatinine clearance before and during therapy
• Blood studies: RBC, Hct, Hgb, reticulocyte counts q wk for 4 wk then q mo
• Hepatic studies: AST, ALT, bilirubin, creatinine
• Mental status, including mood, sensorium, affect, behavorial changes; if mental status changes, notify prescriber
• Eye problems, including need for ophthalmic exam before, during, and after treatment (slit lamp, funduscopy, tonometry)
• Allergic reactions, including red, raised rash; if this occurs, product should be discontinued
• Blood dyscrasia, including fever, sore throat, bruising, rash, jaundice
• Toxicity, including bone marrow depression, nausea, vomiting, ataxia, diplopia, CV collapse, Stevens-Johnson syndrome

Administer:

• With food, milk to decrease GI symptoms

Perform/provide:

• Good oral hygiene as it is important for hydantoins

Evaluate:

• Therapeutic response: decreased seizure activity; document on patient's chart

Teach patient/family:

• To carry emergency ID stating products taken, condition, prescriber's name, phone number
• To avoid driving, other activities that require alertness

Selected Generic Names

Barbiturates
phenobarbital
primidone
thiopental

Hydantoins
fosphenytoin
phenytoin

Succinimides
ethosuximide

Miscellaneous
acetaZOLAMIDE
carbamazepine
clonazepam
diazepam
felbamate
gabapentin
lacosamide
lamotrigine
magnesium sulfate
paraldehyde
paramethadione
phenacemide
rufinamide
tiagabine
topiramate
valproate/valproic acid, divalproex sodium
vigabatrin
zonisamide

ANTIDEPRESSANTS

Action: Antidepressants are divided into the tricyclics, MAOIs, and miscellaneous antidepressants (SSRIs). The tricyclics work by blocking reuptake of norepinephrine and serotonin into nerve endings and increasing action of norepinephrine and serotonin in nerve cells. MAOIs act by increasing concentrations of endogenous epinephrine, norepinephrine, serotonin, DOPamine in storage sites in CNS by inhibition of MAO; increased concentration reduces depression.

Uses: Antidepressants are used for depression and, in some cases, enuresis in children.

Side effects: The most serious adverse reactions are paralytic ileus, acute renal failure, hypertension, and hypertensive crisis, depending on the specific product. Common side effects are dizziness, drowsiness, diarrhea, dry mouth, urinary retention, and orthostatic hypotension.

Contraindications: The contraindications to antidepressants are seizure disorders, prostatic hypertrophy and severe renal/hepatic/cardiac disease depending on the type of medication.

Precautions: Antidepressants should be used cautiously in suicidal patients, severe depression, schizophrenia, hyperactivity, diabetes mellitus, pregnancy, and geriatric patients.

Pharmacokinetics: Onset, peak, and duration vary widely among products. Most products are metabolized in the liver and excreted in urine.

Interactions: Interactions vary widely among products. Check individual monographs for specific information.

Possible nursing diagnoses:

- Ineffective coping *[uses]*
- Risk for injury *[uses/adverse reactions]*
- Deficient knowledge *[teaching]*

Nursing Considerations

Assess:

- B/P (lying, standing), pulse q4hr; if systolic B/P drops 20 mm Hg, hold product, notify prescriber; take VS q4hr in patients with cardiovascular disease
- Blood studies: CBC, leukocytes, differential, cardiac enzymes if patient is receiving long-term therapy
- Hepatic studies: AST, ALT, bilirubin, creatinine
- Weight q wk; appetite may increase with product
- EPS, primarily in geriatric patients: rigidity, dystonia, akathisia
- Mental status: mood, sensorium, affect, suicidal tendencies, increase in psychiatric symptoms: depression, panic
- Urinary retention, constipation; constipation is more likely to occur in children, geriatric patients
- Withdrawal symptoms: headache, nausea, vomiting, muscle pain, weakness; do not usually occur unless product was discontinued abruptly
- Alcohol consumption; if alcohol is consumed, hold dose until morning

Administer:

- Increased fluids if urinary retention occurs, bulk in diet, if constipation occurs
- With food or milk for GI symptoms

Perform/provide:

- Storage in tight container at room temperature; do not freeze
- Assistance with ambulation during beginning therapy since drowsiness, dizziness occur
- Safety measures including side rails primarily in geriatric patients
- Checking to see PO medication swallowed
- Gum, hard candy, or frequent sips of water for dry mouth

Evaluate:

- Therapeutic response: decreased depression

Teach patient/family:

- That therapeutic effects may take 2-3 wk

• To use caution in driving, other activities requiring alertness because of drowsiness, dizziness, blurred vision
• To avoid alcohol ingestion, other CNS depressants
• Not to discontinue medication quickly after long-term use; may cause nausea, headache, malaise
• To wear sunscreen or wide-brimmed hat since photosensitivity may occur

Selected Generic Names

Tetracyclics
mirtazapine
Tricyclics
amitriptyline
amoxapine
clomiPRAMINE
desipramine
doxepin
imipramine
nortriptyline
trimipramine
Miscellaneous
buPROPion
duloxetine
trazodone
venlafaxine
MAOIs
phenelzine
tranylcypromine
SSRIs
citalopram
escitalopram
fluoxetine
fluvoxamine
paroxetine
sertraline

ANTIDIABETICS

Action: Antidiabetics are divided into the insulins that decrease blood glucose, phosphate, and potassium and increase blood pyruvate and lactate; and oral antidiabetics that cause functioning β-cells in the pancreas to release insulin, improve the effect of endogenous and exogenous insulin.

Uses: Insulins are used for ketoacidosis and diabetes mellitus types 1 and 2; oral antidiabetics are used for stable adult-onset diabetes mellitus type 2.

Side effects: The most common side effect of insulin and oral antidiabetics is hypoglycemia. Other adverse reactions to oral antidiabetics include blood dyscrasias, hepatotoxicity, and rarely, cholestatic jaundice. Adverse reactions to insulin products include allergic responses and, more rarely, anaphylaxis.

Contraindications: Hypersensitive reactions may occur, and allergies should be identified before these products are given. Oral antidiabetics should not be used in juvenile or brittle diabetes, diabetic ketoacidosis, or severe renal/hepatic disease.

Precautions: Oral antidiabetics should be used with caution in the geriatric patient, in cardiac disease, pregnancy, breastfeeding, and in the presence of alcohol.

Pharmacokinetics: Onset, peak, and duration vary widely among products. Oral antidiabetics are metabolized in the liver, with metabolites excreted in urine, bile, and feces.

Interactions: Interactions vary widely among products. Check individual monographs for specific information.

Possible nursing diagnoses:
• Imbalanced nutrition: more than body requirements *[uses]*

Nursing Considerations

Assess:

- Blood, urine glucose levels during treatment to determine diabetes control (oral products)
- Fasting blood glucose, 2 hr PP (60-100 mg/dl normal fasting level) (70-130 mg/dl normal 2-hr level)
- Hypoglycemic reaction that can occur during peak time

Administer:

- Insulin after warming to room temperature by rotating in palms to prevent lipodystrophy from injecting cold insulin
- Human insulin to those allergic to beef or pork
- Oral antidiabetic 30 min before meals

Perform/provide:

- Rotation of inj sites when giving insulin; use abdomen, upper back, thighs, upper arm, buttocks; rotate sites within one of these regions; keep a record of sites

Evaluate:

- Therapeutic response: decrease in polyuria, polydipsia, polyphagia, clear sensorium; absence of dizziness; stable gait

Teach patient/family:

- To avoid alcohol and salicylates except on advice of prescriber
- Symptoms of ketoacidosis: nausea, thirst, polyuria, dry mouth, decreased B/P; dry, flushed skin; acetone breath, drowsiness, Kussmaul respiration
- Symptoms of hypoglycemia: headache, tremors, fatigue, weakness; that candy or sugar should be carried to treat hypoglycemia
- To test urine for glucose/ketones tid if this product is replacing insulin
- To continue weight control, dietary restrictions, exercise, hygiene
- Obtain yearly eye exams

Selected Generic Names

chlorproPAMIDE
glipiZIDE
glyBURIDE
insulin aspart
insulin detemir
insulin glargine
insulin glulisine
insulin lispro
insulin, regular
insulin, regular concentrated
insulin, zinc suspension (Lente)
insulin, zinc suspension extended (Ultralente)
metformin
miglitol
nateglinide
pioglitazone
repaglinide
rosiglitazone
saxagliptan
sitagliptin

ANTIDIARRHEALS

Action: Antidiarrheals work by various actions, including direct action on intestinal muscles to decrease GI peristalsis; by inhibiting prostaglandin synthesis responsible for GI hypermotility; by acting on mucosal receptors responsible for peristalsis; or by decreasing water content of stools.

Uses: Antidiarrheals are used for diarrhea of undetermined causes.

Side effects: The most serious adverse reactions of some products are paralytic ileus, toxic megacolon, and angioneurotic edema. The most common side effects are constipation, nausea, dry mouth, and abdominal pain.

Contraindications: Persons with severe ulcerative colitis, pseudomembranous colitis with some products.

Precautions: Antidiarrheals should be used with caution in the geriatric patient, pregnancy, breastfeeding, children, dehydration.

Pharmacokinetics: Onset, peak, and duration vary widely among products. Most products are metabolized in the liver and excreted in urine.

Interactions: Interactions vary widely among products. Check individual monographs for specific information.

Possible nursing diagnoses:

- Constipation *[adverse reactions]*
- Diarrhea *[uses]*
- Deficient fluid volume *[adverse reactions]*
- Deficient knowledge *[teaching]*

Nursing Considerations

Assess:

- Electrolytes (K, Na, Cl) if on long-term therapy
- Bowel pattern before; for rebound constipation after termination of medication
- Response after 48 hr; if no response, product should be discontinued
- Dehydration in children

Administer:

- For 48 hr only

Evaluate:

- Therapeutic response: decreased diarrhea

Teach patient/family:

- To avoid OTC products
- Not to exceed recommended dose

Selected Generic Names

bismuth subsalicylate
kaolin/pectin
loperamide

ANTIDYSRHYTHMICS

Action: Antidysrhythmics are divided into four classes and miscellaneous antidysrhythmics:

- Class I increases the duration of action potential and effective refractory period and reduces disparity in the refractory period between a normal and infarcted myocardium; further subclasses include Ia, Ib, Ic
- Class II decreases the rate of SA node discharge, increases recovery time, slows conduction through the AV node, and decreases heart rate, which decreases O_2 consumption in the myocardium
- Class III increases the duration of action potential and the effective refractory period
- Class IV inhibits calcium ion influx across the cell membrane during cardiac depolarization; decreases SA node discharge; decreases conduction velocity through the AV node
- Miscellaneous antidysrhythmics include those such as adenosine, which slows conduction through the AV node, and digoxin, which decreases conduction velocity and prolongs the effective refractory period in the AV node

Uses: Antidysrhythmics are used for PVCs, tachycardia, hypertension, atrial fibrillation, angina pectoris.

Side effects: Side effects and adverse reactions vary widely among products.

Contraindications: Contraindications vary widely among products.

Precautions: Precautions vary widely among products.

Pharmacokinetics: Onset, peak, and duration vary widely among products.

Interactions: Interactions vary widely among products. Check individual monographs for specific information.

Possible nursing diagnoses:

- Decreased cardiac output *[uses]*
- Diarrhea *[adverse reactions]*
- Impaired gas exchange *[adverse reactions]*
- Ineffective tissue perfusion *[uses]*

Nursing Considerations

Assess:

- ECG continuously to determine product effectiveness, premature ventricular contractions, or other dysrhythmias
- IV inf rate to avoid causing nausea, vomiting
- For dehydration or hypovolemia
- B/P continuously for hypotension, hypertension
- I&O ratio
- Serum potassium
- Edema in feet and legs daily

Evaluate:

- Therapeutic response: decrease in B/P in hypertension; decreased B/P, edema, moist crackles in congestive heart failure

Teach patient/family:

- To comply with dosage schedule, even if patient is feeling better
- To report bradycardia, dizziness, confusion, depression, fever

Selected Generic Names

Class I
moricizine

Class Ia
disopyramide
procainamide
quinidine

Class Ib
lidocaine
mexiletine
phenytoin
tocainide

Class Ic
flecainide
propafenone

Class II
acebutolol
esmolol
propranolol
sotalol

Class III
amiodarone
dronedarone
ibutilide

Class IV
verapamil

Miscellaneous
adenosine
atropine
digoxin

ANTIEMETICS

Action: The antiemetics are divided into the 5-HT3 receptor antagonists, the phenothiazines, and the miscellaneous products. The 5HT3 receptor antagonists work by blocking serotonin peripherally, centrally, and in the small intestine. The phenothiazines act by blocking the chemoreceptor trigger zone in the brain. The miscellaneous products work by either decreasing motion sickness or delaying gastric emptying.

Uses: Antiemetics are used to prevent nausea and vomiting due to cancer chemotherapy, radiotherapy, and surgery (5-HT3 receptor antagonists); some of the miscellaneous products (antihistamines) work by decreasing motion sickness. Most other products are used for many types of nausea and vomiting.

Side effects: The most common side effects are headache, dizziness, fatigue, and diarrhea.

Contraindications: Persons developing hypersensitive reactions should not use these products.

Precautions: Antiemetics should be used cautiously in pregnancy, breast-feeding, hepatic disease, and some GI disorders.

Pharmacokinetics: Onset, peak, and duration vary widely among products. Most products are metabolized by the liver and excreted by the kidneys.

Interactions: Interactions vary widely among products. Check individual monographs for specific information. Other CNS depressants increase CNS depression.

Possible nursing diagnoses:

- Deficient fluid volume *[uses]*
- Risk for injury *[uses, adverse reactions]*
- Deficient knowledge *[teaching]*
- Imbalanced nutrition: less than body requirements *[uses]*

Nursing Considerations

Assess:

- For reason for nausea, vomiting; absence of nausea and vomiting after giving product
- For hypersensitivity reactions: rash, bronchospasm with some products

Administer:

- Prophylactically, before nausea and vomiting occur, in cancer chemotherapy

Perform/provide:

- Storage at room temperature vial/ampules, oral products

Evaluate:

- Therapeutic response: absence or decreasing nausea and vomiting after use

Teach patient/family:

- To avoid hazardous activities if dizziness occurs; ask for assistance if hospitalized
- To rise slowly to prevent orthostatic hypotension
- To teach all aspects of product usage
- Conservative methods to control nausea and vomiting such as sips of water or other fluids and dry crackers

Selected Generic Names

5-HT3 antagonists

dolasetron
granisetron
ondansetron
palonosetron

Phenothiazines

chlorproMAZINE
prochlorperazine
promethazine
thiethylperazine

Miscellaneous

aprepitant
dimenhyDRINATE
fosaprepitant
meclizine
metoclopramide
scopolamine
trimethobenzamide

ANTIFUNGALS (SYSTEMIC)

Action: Antifungals act by increasing cell membrane permeability in susceptible organisms by binding sterols and decreasing potassium, sodium, and nutrients in the cell.

Uses: Antifungals are used for infections of histoplasmosis, blastomycosis, coccidioidomycosis, cryptococcosis, aspergillosis, phycomycosis, candidiasis, sporotrichosis causing severe meningitis, septicemia, and skin infections.

Side effects: The most serious adverse reactions include renal tubular acidosis, permanent renal impairment, anuria, oliguria, hemorrhagic gastroenteritis, acute hepatic failure, and blood dyscrasias. Some common side effects include hypokalemia, nausea, vomiting, anorexia, headache, fever, and chills.

Contraindications: Persons with severe bone depression or hypersensitivity should not use these products.

Precautions: Antifungals should be used with caution in renal/hepatic disease and pregnancy.

Pharmacokinetics: Onset, peak, and duration vary widely among products. Most products are metabolized in the liver and excreted in urine.

Interactions: Interactions vary widely among products. Check individual monographs for specific information.

Possible nursing diagnoses:

- Risk for infection *[uses]*
- Risk for injury *[adverse reactions]*
- Deficient knowledge *[teaching]*

Nursing Considerations

Assess:

- VS q15-30min during first infusion; note changes in pulse, B/P
- I&O ratio; watch for decreasing urinary output, change in specific gravity; discontinue product to prevent permanent damage to renal tubules
- Blood studies: CBC, K, Na, Ca, Mg q2wk
- Weight weekly; if weight increases over 2 lb/wk, edema is present; renal damage should be considered
- For renal toxicity: increasing BUN, if >40 mg/dl or if serum creatinine >3 mg/dl; product may be discontinued or dosage reduced
- For hepatotoxicity: increasing AST, ALT, alk phos, bilirubin
- For allergic reaction: dermatitis, rash; product should be discontinued, antihistamines (mild reaction) or epinephrine (severe reaction) administered
- For hypokalemia: anorexia, drowsiness, weakness, decreased reflexes, dizziness, increased urinary output, increased thirst, paresthesias
- For ototoxicity: tinnitus (ringing, roaring in ears), vertigo, loss of hearing (rare)

Administer:

- IV using in-line filter (mean pore diameter >1 μm) using distal veins; check for extravasation, necrosis q8hr
- Product only after C&S confirms organism; make sure product is used in life-threatening infections

Perform/provide:

- Protection from light during inf, cover with foil
- Symptomatic treatment as ordered for adverse reactions: aspirin, antihistamines, antiemetics, antispasmodics
- Storage protected from moisture and light; diluted sol is stable for 24 hr

Evaluate:

• Therapeutic response: decreased fever, malaise, rash, negative C&S for infecting organism

Teach patient/family:

• That long-term therapy may be needed to clear infection (2 wk-3 mo depending on type of infection)

Selected Generic Names

amphotericin B
anidulafungin
caspofungin
fluconazole
griseofulvin
itraconazole
ketoconazole
micafungin
nystatin
posaconazole
voriconazole

ANTIHISTAMINES

Action: Antihistamines compete with histamines for H_1-receptor sites. They antagonize in varying degrees most of the pharmacologic effects of histamines.

Uses: Antihistamines are used to control the symptoms of allergies, rhinitis, and pruritus.

Side effects: Most products cause drowsiness; however, fexofenadine and loratadine produce little, if any, drowsiness. Other common side effects are headache and thickening of bronchial secretions. Serious blood dyscrasias may occur, but are rare. Urinary retention, GI effects occur with many of these products.

Contraindications: Hypersensitivity to H_1-receptor antagonists occurs rarely. Patients with acute asthma and lower respiratory tract disease should not use these products since thick secretions may result. Other contraindications include closed-angle glaucoma, bladder neck obstruction, stenosing peptic ulcer, symptomatic prostatic hypertrophy, newborns, and breastfeeding.

Precautions: Antihistamines must be used cautiously in conjunction with intraocular pressure since they increase intraocular pressure. Caution should also be used in geriatric patients, those with renal/cardiac disease, hypertension, seizure disorders, pregnancy, and those breastfeeding.

Pharmacokinetics: Onset varies from 20-60 min, with duration lasting 4-24 hr. In general, pharmacokinetics vary widely among products.

Interactions: Barbiturates, opioids, hypnotics, tricyclics, or alcohol can increase CNS depression when taken with antihistamines.

Possible nursing diagnoses:

• Ineffective airway clearance *[uses]*

Nursing Considerations

Assess:

• I&O ratio; be alert for urinary retention, frequency, dysuria; product should be discontinued if these occur

• CBC during long-term therapy since hemolytic anemia, although rare, may occur

• Blood dyscrasias: thrombocytopenia, agranulocytosis (rare)

• Respiratory status: rate, rhythm, increase in bronchial secretions, wheezing, chest tightness

• Cardiac status: palpitations, increased pulse, hypotension

Administer:

- With food or milk to decrease GI symptoms; absorption may be decreased slightly
- Whole (sustained-release tabs)

Perform/provide:

- Hard candy, gum; frequent rinsing of mouth for dryness

Evaluate:

- Therapeutic response: absence of allergy symptoms, itching

Teach patient/family:

- To notify prescriber if confusion, sedation, hypotension occur
- To avoid driving, other hazardous activity if drowsiness occurs
- To avoid concurrent use of alcohol, other CNS depressants
- To discontinue a few days before skin testing

Selected Generic Names

brompheniramine
budesonide
cetirizine
chlorpheniramine
cyproheptadine
desloratadine
diphenhydrAMINE
fexofenadine
levocetirizine
loratadine
promethazine

ANTIHYPERTENSIVES

Action: Antihypertensives are divided into angiotensin-converting enzyme (ACE) inhibitors, β-adrenergic blockers, calcium channel blockers, centrally acting adrenergics, diuretics, peripherally acting antiadrenergics, and vasodilators. β-Blockers, calcium channel blockers, and diuretics are discussed in separate sections. Angiotensin-converting enzyme inhibitors act by selectively suppressing renin-angiotensin I to angiotensin II; dilation of arterial and venous vessels occurs. Centrally acting adrenergics act by inhibiting the sympathetic vasomotor center in the CNS that reduces impulses in the sympathetic nervous system; B/P, pulse rate, and cardiac output decrease. Peripherally acting antiadrenergics inhibit sympathetic vasoconstriction by inhibiting release of norepinephrine and/or depleting norepinephrine stores in adrenergic nerve endings. Vasodilators act on arteriolar smooth muscle by producing direct relaxation or vasodilation; a reduction in B/P, with concomitant increases in heart rate and cardiac output, occurs.

Uses: Antihypertensives are used for hypertension. Some products are used for heart failure not responsive to conventional therapy. Some products are used in hypertensive crisis, angina, and for some cardiac dysrhythmias.

Side effects: The most common side effects are hypotension, bradycardia, tachycardia, headache, nausea, and vomiting. Side effects and adverse reactions may vary widely between classes and specific products.

Contraindications: Hypersensitive reactions may occur, and allergies should be identified before these products are given. Antihypertensives should not be used in children or in patients with heart block.

Precautions: Antihypertensives should be used with caution in geriatric and dialysis patients, and in the presence of hypovolemia, leukemia, and electrolyte imbalances.

Pharmacokinetics: Onset, peak, and duration vary widely among products. Most products are metabolized in the liver, with metabolites excreted in urine, bile, and feces.

Interactions: Interactions vary widely among products. Check individual monographs for specific information.

Possible nursing diagnoses:
- Decreased cardiac output *[uses]*
- Diarrhea *[adverse reactions]*
- Impaired gas exchange *[adverse reactions]*
- Ineffective tissue perfusion *[uses]*

Nursing Considerations

Assess:
- Blood studies: neutrophil; decreased platelets occur with many of the products
- Renal studies: protein, BUN, creatinine; watch for increased levels that may indicate nephrotic syndrome; obtain baselines in renal and hepatic function studies before beginning treatment
- Edema in feet and legs daily
- Allergic reaction, including rash, fever, pruritus, urticaria: product should be discontinued if antihistamines fail to help
- Symptoms of congestive heart failure: edema, dyspnea, wet crackles, B/P
- Renal symptoms: polyuria, oliguria, frequency

Perform/provide:
- Supine or Trendelenburg position for severe hypotension

Evaluate:
- Therapeutic response: decrease in B/P in hypotension; decreased B/P, edema, moist crackles in congestive heart failure

Teach patient/family:
- To comply with dosage schedule, even if feeling better
- To rise slowly to sitting or standing position to minimize orthostatic hypotension

Selected Generic Names

Aldosterone receptor antagonist
eplerenone

Angiotensin-converting enzyme inhibitors
benazepril
enalapril
fosinopril
lisinipril
quinapril
ramipril
trandolapril

Angiotensin II receptor blockers
candesartan
eprosartan
irbesartan
losartan
olmesartan
telmisartan
valsartan

Centrally acting adrenergics
clonidine
guanfacine
methyldopa

Peripherally acting antiadrenergics
doxazosin
prazosin
reserpine
terazosin

Vasodilators
ambrisentan
diazoxide
fenoldopam
hydrALAZINE
minoxidil
nitroprusside

Antiadrenergic combined α-/β-blocker
labetalol
Direct renin inhibitors
aliskiren

ANTIINFECTIVES

Action: Antiinfectives are divided into several groups, which include but are not limited to penicillins, cephalosporins, aminoglycosides, sulfonamides, tetracyclines, monobactam, erythromycins, and quinolones. These products act by inhibiting the growth and replication of susceptible bacterial organisms.

Uses: Antiinfectives are used for infections of susceptible organisms. These products are effective against bacterial, rickettsial, and spirochetal infections.

Side effects: The most common side effects are nausea, vomiting, and diarrhea. Adverse reactions include bone marrow depression and anaphylaxis.

Contraindications: Hypersensitivity reactions may occur. Allergies should be identified before these products are given. Cross-sensitivity can occur between products of different classes (penicillins and cephalosporins). Many persons allergic to penicillins are also allergic to cephalosporins.

Precautions: Antiinfectives should be used with caution in persons with renal/hepatic disease.

Pharmacokinetics: Onset, peak, and duration vary widely among products. Most products are metabolized in the liver. Metabolites are excreted in urine, bile, and feces.

Interactions: Interactions vary widely among products. Check individual monographs for specific information.

Possible nursing diagnoses:
- Diarrhea *[adverse reactions]*
- Risk for infection *[uses]*

Nursing Considerations

Assess:
- Nephrotoxicity: increased BUN, creatinine
- Blood studies: AST, ALT, CBC, Hct, bilirubin; test monthly if patient is on long-term therapy
- Bowel pattern daily; if severe diarrhea occurs, product should be discontinued
- Urine output; if decreasing, notify prescriber; may indicate nephrotoxicity
- Allergic reaction: rash, fever, pruritus, urticaria; product should be discontinued
- Bleeding: ecchymosis, bleeding gums, hematuria, stool guaiac daily
- Overgrowth of infection: perineal itching, fever, malaise, redness, pain, swelling, drainage, rash, diarrhea, change in cough, sputum

Administer:
- For 10-14 days to ensure organism death, prevention of superinfection
- Product after C&S completed; product may be taken as soon as C&S is drawn

Evaluate:
- Therapeutic response, including absence of fever, fatigue, malaise, draining wounds

Teach patient/family:
- To comply with dosage schedule, even if feeling better
- To report sore throat, bruising, bleeding, joint pain; may indicate blood dyscrasias (rare)

Selected Generic Names

Aminoglycosides
amikacin
azithromycin
clarithromycin
gentamicin
kanamycin
neomycin
streptomycin
tobramycin

Cephalosporins
cefaclor
cefadroxil
cefazolin
cefdinir
cefditoren
cefepime
cefixime
cefonicid
cefoperazone
cefotaxime
cefprozil
ceftibuten
cefuroxime
cephalexin
cephapirin
cephradine

Fluoroquinolones
alatrofloxacin/trovafloxacin
ciprofloxacin
enoxacin
gemifloxacin
levofloxacin
lomefloxacin
norfloxacin
ofloxacin
sparfloxacin

Ketolides
telithromycin

Miscellaneous
adefovir dipivoxil
daptomycin
doripenem
ertapenem
meropenem
peginterferon alfa-2a
telavancin
vancomycin

Penicillins
amoxicillin/clavulanate
ampicillin/sulbactam
cloxacillin
dicloxacillin
imipenem/cilastatin
mezlocillin
nafcillin
oxacillin
penicillin G benzathine
penicillin G
penicillin G procaine
penicillin V
piperacillin
ticarcillin
ticarcillin/clavulanate

Sulfonamides
sulfasalazine
sulfiSOXAZOLE

Tetracyclines
demeclocycline
doxycycline
minocycline
tetracycline

ANTILIPIDEMICS

Action: Antilipidemics are divided into three categories or subclassifications; HMG-CoA reductase inhibitors (statins), bile acid sequestrants, and miscellaneous products. The HMG-CoA reductase inhibitors work by reduction of an enzyme that is responsible for the beginning step in cholesterol production. Bile acid sequestrants work by binding cholesterol in the GI system. The miscellaneous products work by various actions.

Uses: Primary hypercholesterolemia in individuals as an adjunct with other lifestyle changes.

Side effects: The most common side effects are headache, dizziness, fatigue, insomnia, peripheral edema, dysrhythmias, sinusitis, pharyngitis, abdominal pain, diarrhea, constipation, flatulence, and back pain.

Contraindications: Persons breastfeeding (some products) or those with hypersensitivity to any product or severe hepatic disease should not take these products. Antilipidemics are identified as pregnancy category X on some products.

Precautions: Some products are identified as pregnancy category C.

Pharmacokinetics: Pharmacokinetics and pharmacodynamics vary with each product.

Interactions: Interactions vary widely among products. Check individual monographs for specific information.

Possible nursing diagnoses:

- Constipation *[adverse reactions]*
- Diarrhea *[adverse reactions]*
- Deficient knowledge *[teaching]*
- Noncompliance *[teaching]*

Nursing Considerations

Assess:

- Obtain a diet and lifestyle history, including exercise, smoking, alcohol, and stress-related activities

Administer:

- As directed by health care provider; times will vary with medication used

Perform/provide:

- Protection from sunlight and heat

Evaluate:

- Therapeutic response: decrease in triglycerides and LDL cholesterol levels

Teach patient/family:

- All aspects of medication use
- To combine medication with lifestyle changes, including low-cholesterol diet, decreasing LDL in diet; avoid smoking, alcohol, and sedentary daily routine

Selected Generic Names

HMG-CoA reductase inhibitors

atorvastatin
fluvastatin
lovastatin
pitavastatin
pravastatin
rosovastatin
simvastatin

Bile acid sequestrants

cholestyramine
colesevelam
colestipol

Miscellaneous

ezetimibe
fenofibrate
fenofibric acid
gemfibrozil
niacin
niacinamide

ANTINEOPLASTICS

Action: Antineoplastics are divided into alkylating agents, antimetabolites, antibiotic agents, hormonal agents, and miscellaneous agents. Alkylating agents act by cross-linking strands of DNA. Antimetabolites act by inhibiting DNA synthesis. Antibiotic agents act by inhibiting RNA synthesis and by delaying or inhibiting mitosis. Hormones alter the effects of androgens, luteinizing hormone, follicle-stimulating hormone, and estrogen by changing the hormonal environment.

Uses: Antineoplastics uses vary widely among products and classes of products. They are used to treat leukemia, Hodgkin's disease, lymphomas, and other tumors throughout the body.

Side effects: Most products cause thrombocytopenia, leukopenia, and anemia. If these reactions occur, the product may have to be stopped until the problem is corrected. Other side effects include nausea, vomiting, glossitis, and hair loss. Some products also cause hepatotoxicity, nephrotoxicity, and cardiotoxicity.

Contraindications: Hypersensitive reactions may occur, and allergies should be identified before these products are given. Also, persons with severe hepatic/renal disease should not use these products unless the benefits outweigh the risks.

Precautions: Persons with bleeding, severe bone marrow depression, or renal/hepatic disease should be watched closely.

Pharmacokinetics: Onset, peak, and duration vary widely among products. Most products cross the placenta and are excreted in breast milk and in urine.

Interactions: Toxicity may occur when used with other antineoplastics or radiation.

Possible nursing diagnoses:

- Risk for infection *[adverse reactions]*
- Imbalanced nutrition: less than body requirements *[adverse reactions]*
- Impaired oral mucous membrane *[adverse reactions]*

Nursing Considerations

Assess:

- CBC, differential, platelet count weekly; withhold product if WBC is <4000/mm^3 or platelet count is <75,000/mm^3; notify prescriber of results
- Renal function studies: BUN, creatinine, serum uric acid, and urine CCr before and during therapy
- I&O ratio; report fall in urine output of 30 ml/hr
- Monitor temp q4hr (may indicate beginning infection)
- LFTs before and during therapy (bilirubin, AST, ALT, LDH) monthly or as needed
- Bleeding, including hematuria, guaiac, bruising or petechiae, mucosa, or orifices q8hr; obtain prescription for viscous Xylocaine (lidocaine)
- Yellowing of skin, sclera, dark urine, clay-colored stools, itchy skin, abdominal pain, fever, diarrhea
- Edema in feet, joint pain, stomach pain, shaking
- Inflammation of mucosa, breaks in skin

Administer:

- Checking IV site for irritation; phlebitis
- Epinephrine for hypersensitivity reaction
- Antibiotics for prophylaxis of infection

Perform/provide:

- Strict asepsis, protective isolation if WBC levels are low
- Comprehensive oral hygiene, using careful technique and soft-bristle brush

Evaluate:

- Therapeutic response: decreased tumor size

Teach patient/family:

- To report signs of infection, including increased temp, sore throat, malaise
- To report signs of anemia, including fatigue, headache, faintness, SOB, irritability
- To report bleeding and avoid use of razors or commercial mouthwash

Selected Generic Names

Alkylating agents
bendamustine
busulfan
carboplatin
carmustine
chlorambucil
cisplatin
cyclophosphamide
dacarbazine
lomustine
mechlorethamine
melphalan
oxaliplatin
thiotepa

Antimetabolites
capecitabine
cytarabine
decitabine
etoposide
fludarabine
fluorouracil
mercaptopurine
methotrexate
pemetrexed
pralatrexate
thioguanine (6-TG)

Antibiotic agents
bleomycin
dactinomycin
DAUNOrubicin
DOXOrubicin
epirubicin
mitomycin
mitoxantrone
plicamycin

Hormonal agents
aminoglutethimide
estramustine
flutamide
fulvestrant
goserelin
irinotecan
leuprolide
megestrol
mitotane
nilutamide
tamoxifen
testolactone
topotecan

Miscellaneous
alemtuzumab
anastrozole
arsenic trioxide
asparaginase
azacitidine
bortezomib
cetuximab
cladribine
dasatinib
erlotinib
gefitinib
gemcitabine
ibritumomab
imatinib
interferon alfa-2a
interferon alfa-2b
irinotecan
ixabepilone
lapatinib
nilotinib
panitumumab
pentostatin
porfimer
procarbazine
ranibizumab
rituximab
sunitinib
vinBLAStine
vinCRIStine
vinorelbine

ANTIPARKINSON AGENTS

Action: Antiparkinson agents are divided into cholinergics, DOPamine, and monoamine oxidase type B agonists. Cholinergics work by blocking or competing at central acetylcholine receptors. DOPamine agonists work by decarboxylation to DOPamine or by activation of DOPamine receptors. Monoamine oxidase type B inhibitors work by increasing DOPamine activity by inhibiting MAO type B activity.

Uses: Antiparkinson agents are used alone or in combination for patients with Parkinson's disease.

Side effects: Side effects and adverse reactions vary widely among products. The most common side effects include involuntary movements, headache, numbness, insomnia, nightmares, nausea, vomiting, dry mouth, and orthostatic hypotension.

Contraindications: Persons with hypersensitivity, closed-angle glaucoma, and undiagnosed skin lesions should not use these products.

Precautions: Antiparkinson agents should be used with caution in pregnancy, breastfeeding, children, renal/cardiac/hepatic disease, and affective disorder.

Pharmacokinetics: Onset, peak, and duration vary widely among products. Most products are metabolized in the liver and excreted in urine.

Interactions: Interactions vary widely among products. Check individual monographs for specific information.

Possible nursing diagnoses:
- Risk for injury *[uses]*
- Deficient knowledge *[teaching]*
- Impaired physical mobility *[uses]*

Nursing Considerations

Assess:
- B/P, respiration
- Mental status: affect, mood, behavioral changes, depression, complete suicide assessment

Administer:
- Product up until NPO before surgery
- Dosage adjustment depending on patient response
- With meals; limit protein taken with drug
- Only after MAOIs have been discontinued for 2 wk

Perform/provide:
- Assistance with ambulation, during beginning therapy
- Testing for diabetes mellitus, acromegaly if on long-term therapy

Evaluate:
- Therapeutic response: decrease in akathisia, increased mood

Teach patient/family:
- To change positions slowly to prevent orthostatic hypotension
- To report side effects: twitching, eye spasm; indicate overdose
- To use product exactly as prescribed; if product is discontinued abruptly, parkinsonian crisis may occur

Selected Generic Names

amantadine
apomorphine
benztropine
bromocriptine
cabergoline
carbidopa-levodopa
pramipexole
rasagiline
selegiline
tolcapone
trihexyphenidyl

ANTIPLATELETS

Action: The antiplatelets are divided into the platelet aggregation inhibitors, platelet adhesion inhibitors, and the glycoprotein IIb, IIIa inhibitors. The platelet aggregation inhibitors work by action on thrombin; the platelet adhesion inhibitors work by inhibition of phosphodiesterase; and the glycoprotein IIb, IIIa inhibitors work by preventing fibrin from binding to glycoprotein IIb, IIIa receptors.

Uses: Antiplatelets are used to prevent MI and stroke; other products are used for coronary syndromes.

Side effects: The most common side effects are headache, dizziness, bleeding, and diarrhea.

Contraindications: Persons developing hypersensitive reactions should not use these products.

Precautions: Antiplatelets should be used cautiously in pregnancy, breastfeeding, and bleeding disorders.

Pharmacokinetics: Onset, peak, and duration vary widely among products. Most products are metabolized by the liver and excreted by the kidneys.

Interactions: Interactions vary widely among products. Check individual monographs for specific information.

Possible nursing diagnoses:
- Risk for injury *[uses, adverse reactions]*
- Deficient knowledge *[teaching]*

Nursing Considerations

Assess:
- For reason for use of these products
- For hypersensitivity reactions with some products
- For bleeding from orifices, in stool, urine
- Blood studies: platelets, Hgb, Hct, PT/APTT, and INR

Administer:
- With heparin or other aspirin (some products)

Perform/provide:
- Storage at room temperature vial/ampules, oral products

Evaluate:
- Therapeutic response: absence of MI, stroke or other coronary syndromes

Teach patient/family:
- To avoid hazardous activities if drowsiness, dizziness occurs; ask for assistance if hospitalized
- To teach all aspects of product usage

Selected Generic Names

Platelet aggregation inhibitors
cilostazol
clopidogrel
ticlopidine

Platelet adhesion inhibitors
dipyridamole

Glycoprotein IIb, IIIa inhibitors
eptifibatide
tirofiban

ANTIPSYCHOTICS

Action: Antipsychotics/neuroleptics are divided into several subgroups: phenothiazines, thioxanthenes, butyrophenones, dibenzoxazepines, dibenzodiazepines, and indolones and other heterocyclic compounds. Although chemically different, these subgroups share many pharmacologic and clinical properties. All antipsychotics work to block postsynaptic DOPamine receptors in the brain that are responsible for psychotic behavior, including hallucinations, delusions, and paranoia.

Uses: Antipsychotic behavior is decreased in conditions such as schizophrenia, paranoia, and mania. These agents are also effective for severe anxiety, intractable hiccups, nausea, vomiting, behavioral problems in children, and for relaxation before surgery.

Side effects: The most common side effects include EPS such as pseudoparkinsonism, akathisia, dystonia, and tardive dyskinesia, which may be controlled by use of antiparkinson agents. Serious adverse reactions such as hypotension, agranulocytosis, cardiac arrest, and laryngospasm have occurred. Other common side effects include dry mouth and photosensitivity.

Contraindications: Persons with hepatic damage, severe hypertension or coronary disease, cerebral arteriosclerosis, blood dyscrasias, bone marrow depression, parkinsonism, severe depression, closed-angle glaucoma, children <12 yr, or persons withdrawing from alcohol or barbiturates should not use antipsychotics until these conditions are corrected.

Precautions: Caution must be used when antipsychotics are given to the geriatric patient since metabolism is slowed and adverse reactions can occur rapidly. Hepatic/renal disease may cause poor metabolism and excretion of the product. Seizure threshold is decreased with these products; increases in the dose of anticonvulsants may be required. Persons with diabetes mellitus, prostatic hypertrophy, chronic respiratory disease, and peptic ulcer disease should be monitored closely.

Pharmacokinetics: Onset, peak, and duration vary widely with different products and routes. Products are metabolized by the liver, are excreted in urine as metabolites, are highly bound to plasma proteins, cross the placenta, and enter breast milk. Half-life can be extended over 3 days.

Interactions: Because other CNS depressants can cause oversedation, these combinations should be used carefully. Anticholinergics may decrease the therapeutic actions of phenothiazines and also cause increased anticholinergic effects.

Possible nursing diagnoses:
- Chronic confusion *[uses]*
- Disturbed sensory perception *[uses]*

Nursing Considerations

Assess:
- Bilirubin, CBC, hepatic studies q mo since these products are metabolized in the liver and excreted in urine
- I&O ratio: palpate bladder if low urinary output occurs, since urinary retention occurs with many of these products
- Affect, orientation, LOC, reflexes, gait, coordination, sleep pattern disturbances
- Dizziness, faintness, palpitations, tachycardia on rising
- B/P (lying and standing); wide fluctuations between lying and standing B/P may require dosage or product change since orthostatic hypotension is occurring
- EPS, including akathisia, tardive dyskinesia, pseudoparkinsonism

Administer:

- Antiparkinson agent if EPS occur
- Liquid concentrates mixed in glass of juice or cola since taste is unpleasant; avoid contact with skin when preparing liquid concentrate or parenteral medications
- Patient should remain lying down for at least 30 min after IM inj

Perform/provide:

- Supervised ambulation until stabilized on medication; do not involve in strenuous exercise program because fainting is possible; patient should not stand still for long periods
- Increased fluids to prevent constipation
- Sips of water, candy, gum for dry mouth

Evaluate:

- Therapeutic response: decrease in excitement, hallucinations, delusions, paranoia; reorganization of thought patterns, speech

Teach patient/family:

- To rise from sitting or lying position gradually since fainting may occur
- To avoid hot tubs, hot showers, or tub baths since hypotension may occur
- To wear a sunscreen or protective clothing to prevent burns
- To take extra precautions during hot weather to stay cool; heat stroke can occur
- To avoid driving, other activities requiring alertness until response to medication is known
- That drowsiness or impaired mental/motor activity is evident the first 2 wk, but tends to decrease over time

Selected Generic Names

Phenothiazines
chlorproMAZINE
fluphenazine
perphenazine
prochlorperazine
thioridazine
thiothixene
trifluoperazine

Butyrophenone
haloperidol

Miscellaneous
aripiprazole
asenapine
iloperidone
loxapine
olanzapine
paliperidone
quetiapine
risperidone
ziprasidone

ANTIPYRETICS

Action: Antipyretics act on the CNS to control fever and also inhibit prostaglandin production.

Uses: Antipyretics are used to decrease fever.

Side effects: The most common side effects are nausea, vomiting, and rash.

Contraindications: Persons developing hypersensitive reactions should not use these products.

Precautions: Antipyretics should be used cautiously in pregnancy, breastfeeding, hepatic disease, geriatric patients, and those with certain GI disorders.

Pharmacokinetics: Onset, peak, and duration vary widely among products. Most products are metabolized by the liver and excreted by the kidneys.

Interactions: Interactions vary widely among products. Check individual monographs for specific information.

Possible nursing diagnoses:

- Risk for injury *[uses, adverse reactions]*
- Deficient knowledge *[teaching]*

Nursing Considerations

Assess:

- Temperature frequently
- For reason for use and expected outcome
- For hypersensitivity reactions: rash, bronchospasm with some products

Administer:

- Around the clock to keep fever reduced

Perform/provide:

- Storage at room temperature

Evaluate:

- Therapeutic response: absence or decreasing fever after use

Teach patient/family:

- All aspects of product usage

Selected Generic Names

acetaminophen
aspirin
choline/magnesium salicylates
choline salicylate
ibuprofen
ketoprofen
magnesium salicylate
naproxen
salsalate

ANTIRETROVIRALS

Action: Antiretrovirals act by blocking DNA synthesis.

Uses: Antiretrovirals are used for HIV infections to slow the progression of the disease.

Side effects: The most common side effects are nausea, vomiting, anorexia, headache, and diarrhea. The most serious adverse reactions are nephrotoxicity and blood dyscrasias.

Contraindications: Persons with hypersensitivity should not use these products.

Precautions: Antiretrovirals should be used cautiously in renal/hepatic disease, pregnancy, and breastfeeding. Protease inhibitors should be used cautiously in diabetes.

Pharmacokinetics: Onset, peak, and duration vary widely among products. Most products are metabolized by the liver and excreted by the kidneys.

Interactions: Interactions vary widely among products. Check individual monographs for specific information.

Possible nursing diagnoses:

- Risk for infection *[uses]*
- Risk for injury *[adverse reactions]*
- Deficient knowledge *[teaching]*
- Noncompliance *[teaching]*

Nursing Considerations

Assess:

- For signs of HIV infection: increased CD4 counts, decreased viral load
- Patients with compromised renal system; since product is excreted slowly in poor renal system function, toxicity may occur rapidly

Administer:

- In equal intervals around the clock

Perform/provide:

- Storage at room temperature

Evaluate:

- Therapeutic response: decreased viral load, increased CD4 count, improvement in the symptoms of HIV/AIDS

Teach patient/family:

- To report sore throat, fever, fatigue; may indicate superinfection
- That medication does not cure condition or prevent infecting others but controls symptoms
- That product must be taken around the clock, in equal intervals to maintain blood levels for duration of therapy
- To notify prescriber of side effects such as bruising, bleeding, fatigue, malaise; may indicate blood dyscrasias

Selected Generic Names

Nonnucleoside reverse transcriptase inhibitors

delavirdine
efavirenz
etravirine
nevirapine

Nucleoside reverse transcriptase inhibitors

abacavir
didanosine
emtricitabine
lamivudine
stavudine
tenofovir
zalcitabine
zidovudine

Protease inhibitors

amprenavir
atazanavir
fosamprenavir
indinavir
nelfinavir
ritonavir
saquinavir
tipranavir

Fusion inhibitors

enfuvirtide

Miscellaneous

raltegravir

ANTITUBERCULARS

Action: Antituberculars act by inhibiting RNA or DNA, or interfering with lipid and protein synthesis, thereby decreasing tubercle bacilli replication.

Uses: Antituberculars are used for pulmonary tuberculosis.

Side effects: They vary widely among products. Most products can cause nausea, vomiting, anorexia, and rash. Serious adverse reactions include renal failure, nephrotoxicity, ototoxicity, and hepatic necrosis.

Contraindications: Persons with severe renal disease or hypersensitivity should not use these products.

Precautions: Antituberculars should be used with caution with pregnancy, breastfeeding, and hepatic disease.

Pharmacokinetics: Onset, peak, and duration vary widely among products. Most products are metabolized in the liver and excreted in urine.

Interactions: Interactions vary widely among products. Check individual monographs for specific information.

Possible nursing diagnoses:

- Risk for infection *[uses]*
- Risk for injury *[adverse reactions]*
- Deficient knowledge *[teaching]*
- Noncompliance *[teaching]*

Nursing Considerations

Assess:

• Signs of anemia: Hct, Hgb, fatigue

• Hepatic studies q wk: ALT, AST, bilirubin

• Renal status before, q mo: BUN, creatinine, output, specific gravity, urinalysis

• Hepatic status: decreased appetite, jaundice, dark urine, fatigue

Administer:

• For some of these agents on empty stomach, 1 hr before meals (only for isoniazid and rifampin) or 2 hr after meals

• Antiemetic if vomiting occurs

• After C&S is completed; q mo to detect resistance

Evaluate:

• Therapeutic response: decreased symptoms of TB, culture negative

Teach patient/family:

• That compliance with dosage schedule, duration is necessary

• That scheduled appointments must be kept; relapse may occur

• To avoid alcohol while taking product

• To report flulike symptoms: excessive fatigue, anorexia, vomiting, sore throat; unusual bleeding, yellowish discoloration of skin/eyes

Selected Generic Names

ethambutol
isoniazid
pyrazinamide
rifabutin
rifampin
streptomycin

ANTITUSSIVES/EXPECTORANTS

Action: Antitussives act by suppressing the cough reflex by direct action on the cough center in the medulla. Expectorants act by liquefying and reducing the viscosity of thick, tenacious secretions.

Uses: Antitussives/expectorants are used to treat cough occurring in pneumonia, bronchitis, TB, cystic fibrosis, and emphysema; as an adjunct in atelectasis (expectorants); and nonproductive cough (antitussives).

Side effects: The most common side effects are drowsiness, dizziness, and nausea.

Contraindications: Some products are contraindicated in hypothyroidism, pregnancy, and breastfeeding.

Precautions: Some products should be used cautiously in asthmatic, geriatric, and debilitated patients.

Pharmacokinetics: Onset, peak, and duration vary widely among products. Some products are metabolized in the liver and excreted in urine.

Interactions: Interactions vary widely among products. Check individual monographs for specific information.

Possible nursing diagnoses:

• Ineffective airway clearance *[uses]*

• Ineffective breathing pattern *[uses]*

• Deficient knowledge *[teaching]*

Nursing Considerations

Assess:

• Cough: type, frequency, character (including sputum)

Administer:

• Decreased dose to geriatric patients; their metabolism may be slowed

Perform/provide:

- Increased fluids to liquefy secretions
- Humidification of patient's room

Evaluate:

- Therapeutic response: absence of cough

Teach patient/family:

- To avoid driving, other hazardous activities until patient is stabilized on this medication
- To avoid smoking, smoke-filled rooms, perfumes, dust, environmental pollutants, cleaners that increase cough

Selected Generic Names

acetylcysteine
ammonium chloride
benzonatate
codeine
dextromethorphan
diphenhydrAMINE
guaifenesin
hydrocodone

ANTIVIRALS

Action: Antivirals act by interfering with DNA synthesis that is needed for viral replication.

Uses: Antivirals are used for mucocutaneous herpes simplex virus, herpes genitalis (HSV-1, HSV-2), varicella infections, herpes zoster, and herpes simplex encephalitis.

Side effects: The most common side effects are nausea, vomiting, anorexia, headache, and diarrhea. The most serious adverse reactions are nephrotoxicity and blood dyscrasias.

Contraindications: Persons with hypersensitivity or immunosuppressed individuals should not use these products.

Precautions: Antivirals should be used cautiously in renal/hepatic disease, pregnancy, and breastfeeding.

Pharmacokinetics: Onset, peak, and duration vary widely among products. Most products are metabolized by the liver and excreted by the kidneys.

Interactions: Interactions vary widely among products. Check individual monographs for specific information.

Possible nursing diagnoses:

- Risk for infection *[uses]*
- Risk for injury *[adverse reactions]*
- Deficient knowledge *[teaching]*

Nursing Considerations

Assess:

- For signs of infection, anemia
- Patients with a compromised renal system; since product is excreted slowly in poor renal system function, toxicity may occur rapidly
- Renal studies: urinalysis, BUN, serum creatinine or decreased CCr may indicate nephrotoxicity; I&O ratio; report hematuria, oliguria, fatigue, weakness; check for protein in the urine during treatment
- C&S before treatment, agent may be taken as soon as culture is taken; repeat C&S after treatment
- Bowel pattern before, during treatment; if severe abdominal pain with bleeding occurs, agent should be discontinued
- Skin reactions: rash, urticaria, itching
- Hepatic studies: AST, ALT
- Blood studies: WBC, RBC, Hct, Hgb, bleeding time; blood dyscrasias

Administer:

- Increased fluids to 3 L/day to decrease crystalluria when given IV

Perform/provide:

- Storage at room temperature for up to 12 hr after reconstitution

Evaluate:

- Therapeutic response: absence or control of infection

Teach patient/family:

- To report sore throat, fever, fatigue; may indicate superinfection
- That medication does not prevent infecting others or cure condition but controls symptoms
- That product must be taken around the clock in equal intervals to maintain blood levels for duration of therapy
- To notify prescriber of side effects such as bruising, bleeding, fatigue, malaise; may indicate blood dyscrasias

Selected Generic Names

acyclovir
amantadine
cidofovir
docosanol
entecavir
famciclovir
foscarnet
ganciclovir
lamivudine
maraviroc
oseltamivir
penciclovir
ribavirin
valacyclovir
valganciclovir
zanamivir

β-ADRENERGIC BLOCKERS

Action: β-Blockers are divided into selective and nonselective blockers. Selective β-blockers competitively block stimulation of β_1-receptors in cardiac smooth muscle; these products produce chronotropic and inotropic effects. Nonselective blockers produce a fall in blood pressure without reflex tachycardia or reduction in heart rate through a mixture of β-blocking effects; elevated plasma renins are reduced.

Uses: β-Blockers are used for hypertension, ventricular dysrhythmias, and prophylaxis of angina pectoris.

Side effects: The most common side effects are orthostatic hypotension, bradycardia, diarrhea, nausea, and vomiting. Serious adverse reactions include blood dyscrasias, bronchospasm, and congestive heart failure.

Contraindications: Hypersensitive reactions may occur, and allergies should be identified before these products are given. β-Adrenergic blockers should not be used in heart block, congestive heart failure, or cardiogenic shock.

Precautions: β-Blockers should be used with caution in the geriatric patient, or in renal/thyroid disease, COPD, coronary artery disease, diabetes mellitus, pregnancy, and asthma.

Pharmacokinetics: Onset, peak, and duration vary widely among products. Most products are metabolized in the liver, with metabolites excreted in urine, bile, and feces.

Interactions: Interactions vary widely among products. Check individual monographs for specific information.

Possible nursing diagnoses:
• Decreased cardiac output *[uses]*
• Diarrhea *[adverse reactions]*
• Impaired gas exchange *[adverse reactions]*
• Ineffective tissue perfusion *[uses]*

Nursing Considerations

Assess:
• Renal studies: protein, BUN, creatinine; watch for increased levels that may indicate nephrotic syndrome; obtain baselines in renal/hepatic function studies before beginning treatment
• I&O, weight daily
• B/P during beginning treatment and periodically thereafter; pulse q4hr, note rate, rhythm, quality
• Apical/radial pulse before administration; notify prescriber of significant changes
• Edema in feet and legs daily

Administer:
• PO before meals and at bedtime; tabs may be crushed or swallowed whole
• Reduced dosage in renal dysfunction

Evaluate:
• Therapeutic response: decrease in B/P in hypertension; decreased B/P, edema, moist crackles in congestive heart failure

Teach patient/family:
• To comply with dosage schedule even if feeling better
• To rise slowly to sitting or standing position to minimize orthostatic hypotension
• To report bradycardia, dizziness, confusion, depression, and fever
• To take pulse at home; advise when to notify prescriber
• To comply with weight control, dietary adjustment, modified exercise program
• To wear support hose to minimize effects of orthostatic hypotension
• Not to discontinue product abruptly; taper over 2 wk; may precipitate angina

Selected Generic Names

Selective β_1-receptor blockers
acebutolol
atenolol
esmolol
metoprolol
nebibolol
Combined α_1-, β_1-, and β_2-receptor blocker
labetalol
Nonselective β_1- and β_2-blockers
carteolol
nadolol
pindolol
propranolol
timolol

BONE RESORPTION INHIBITORS

Action: Bone resorption inhibitors are divided into biphosphonates and selective estrogen receptor modulators. Biphosphonates act by absorbing calcium phosphate crystals in bone and may directly block dissolution of hydroxyapatite crystals of bone, inhibiting normal and abnormal bone resorption and mineralization. Selective estrogen receptor modulators act by reducing resorption of bone and decreasing bone turnover; medicated through estrogen receptor binding.

Uses: Bone resorption inhibitors are used for prevention and treatment of osteoporosis in postmenopausal women, treatment of Paget's disease and treatment of osteoporosis in men.

Side effects: The most common side effects are nausea, vomiting, headache, bone pain, and rash.

Contraindications: Persons developing hypersensitive reactions or those with hypocalcemia should not use these products.

Precautions: Bone resorption inhibitors should be used cautiously in pregnancy, breastfeeding, hepatic/renal disease, the geriatric patient, and some GI disorders.

Pharmacokinetics: Onset, peak, and duration vary widely among products. Most products are taken up by the bones and excreted by the kidneys.

Interactions: Interactions vary widely among products. Check individual monographs for specific information.

Possible nursing diagnoses:

- Risk for injury *[uses, adverse reactions]*
- Deficient knowledge *[teaching]*

Nursing Considerations

Assess:

- For reason for use and expected outcome
- For bone density test; hormonal status (women) before starting treatment and thereafter
- For hypercalcemia: paresthesia, twitching, laryngospasm; Chvostek's, Trousseau's signs

Administer:

- For 6 months or more in Paget's disease

Perform/provide:

- Storage at room temperature

Evaluate:

- Therapeutic response: increase in bone mass, absence of fractures

Teach patient/family:

- To remain upright for at least 30 min after taking, to prevent esophageal irritation
- To teach all aspects of product usage
- To use weight-bearing exercise to increase bone density

Selected Generic Names

Bisphosphonates

alendronate
etidronate
ibandronate
pamidronate
risedronate

Selective estrogen receptor modulators

raloxifene

CALCIUM CHANNEL BLOCKERS

Action: Calcium channel blockers act by inhibiting calcium ion influx across the cell membrane in cardiac and vascular smooth muscle. This action produces relaxation of coronary vascular smooth muscle, dilates coronary arteries, slows SA/AV node conduction, and dilates peripheral arteries.

Uses: Calcium channel blockers are used for chronic stable angina pectoris, vasospastic angina, dysrhythmias, hypertension, and unstable angina.

Side effects: The most common side effects are dysrhythmias and edema. Also common are headache, fatigue, drowsiness, and flushing.

Contraindications: Persons with 2nd-/3rd-degree heart block, sick sinus syndrome, hypotension of <90 mm Hg systolic, Wolff-Parkinson-White syndrome, or cardiogenic shock should not use these products since worsening of those conditions may occur.

Precautions: Congestive heart failure since edema may be increased. Hypotension may worsen since B/P is decreased. Patients with renal/hepatic disease should use these products cautiously since they are metabolized in the liver and excreted by the kidneys.

Pharmacokinetics: Onset, peak, and duration vary widely with route of administration. Products are metabolized by the liver and excreted in the urine primarily as metabolites.

Interactions: Increased levels of digoxin and theophylline may occur when used with these products. Increased effects of β-blockers and antihypertensives may occur with calcium channel blockers.

Possible nursing diagnoses:

- Decreased cardiac output *[adverse reactions]*
- Ineffective tissue perfusion *[uses]*

Nursing Considerations

Assess:

- Cardiac system: B/P, pulse, respirations, ECG intervals (PR, QRS, QT)

Administer:

- PO before meals and at bedtime

Evaluate:

- Therapeutic response: decreased anginal pain; decreased B/P, dysrhythmias

Teach patient/family:

- How to take pulse before taking product; patient should record or graph pulses to identify changes
- To avoid hazardous activities until stabilized on this product since dizziness commonly occurs
- The need for compliance in all areas of medical regimen, including diet, exercise, stress reduction, and product therapy

Selected Generic Names

amlodipine
clevidipine
diltiazem
felodipine
isradipine
niCARdipine
NIFEdipine
verapamil

CARDIAC GLYCOSIDES

Action: Cardiac glycosides act by inhibiting sodium and potassium ATPase and then making more calcium available to activate contracted proteins. Cardiac contractility and cardiac output are increased.

Uses: Cardiac glycosides are used for congestive heart failure, atrial fibrillation, atrial flutter, atrial tachycardia, and rapid digitalization in these disorders.

Side effects: The most common side effects are cardiac disturbances, headache, hypotension, and GI symptoms. Also common are blurred vision and yellow-green halos.

Contraindications: Hypersensitive reactions may occur, and allergies should be identified before these products are given. Also, persons with ventricular tachycardia, ventricular fibrillation, and carotid sinus syndrome should not use these products.

Precautions: Persons with acute MI and those who have or may develop serum potassium, calcium, or magnesium imbalances should use these products cautiously. Also, geriatric patients and those with AV block, severe respiratory disease, hypothyroidism, or renal/hepatic disease should exercise caution when these products are prescribed.

Pharmacokinetics: Onset, peak, and duration vary widely with the route of administration. Digitoxin is inactivated by the liver, and inactive metabolites are excreted in urine. Digoxin is excreted in urine mainly as the parent product and metabolites.

Interactions: Toxicity may occur when used with diuretics, succinylcholine, quinidine, and thioamines. Increased blood levels may occur with propantheline bromide, spironolactone, quinidine, verapamil, aminoglycosides (PO), amiodarone, anticholinergics, and quinine. Diuretics may increase toxicity.

Possible nursing diagnoses:

- Decreased cardiac output *[adverse reactions]*
- Ineffective tissue perfusion *[uses]*

Nursing Considerations

Assess:

- Cardiac system: B/P, pulse, respirations, and increased urine output
- Apical pulse for 1 min before giving product; if pulse <60 bpm, take again in 1 hr; if still <60 bpm, notify prescriber
- Electrolytes: K, Na, Cl, Mg; renal function studies, including BUN and creatinine; and blood studies, including AST, ALT, bilirubin
- I&O ratio, daily weights
- Monitor therapeutic product levels

Administer:

- K supplements if ordered for K levels <3 mg/dl

Evaluate:

- Therapeutic response: decreased weight, edema, pulse, respiration; increased urine output

Teach patient/family:

- How to take pulse before taking product; patient should record or graph pulse to identify changes
- To avoid hazardous activities until stabilized on this product, since dizziness commonly occurs
- The need for compliance in all areas of medical regimen, including diet, exercise, stress reduction, product therapy

Selected Generic Name

digoxin

CHOLINERGICS

Action: Cholinergics act by preventing destruction of acetylcholine, which increases concentration at sites where acetylcholine is released. This exaggerates the effects of acetylcholine and facilitates transmission of impulses across the myoneural junction. Cholinergics may also act by stimulating receptors for acetylcholine.

Uses: Cholinergics are used for myasthenia gravis, as antagonists of nondepolarizing neuromuscular blockade, postoperative bladder distention and urinary distention, and postoperative ileus.

Side effects: The most serious adverse reactions are respiratory depression, bronchospasm, constriction, laryngospasm, respiratory arrest, seizures, and paralysis. The most common side effects are nausea, diarrhea, and vomiting.

Contraindications: Persons with obstruction of the intestine or renal system should not use these products.

Precautions: Caution should be used in patients with bradycardia, hypotension, seizure disorders, bronchial asthma, coronary occlusion, hyperthyroidism, breastfeeding, and in children.

Pharmacokinetics: Onset, peak, and duration vary widely among products. Most products are metabolized in the liver and excreted in urine.

Interactions: Interactions vary widely among products. Check individual monographs for specific information.

Possible nursing diagnoses:

- Ineffective breathing pattern *[uses]*
- Deficient knowledge *[teaching]*
- Noncompliance *[teaching]*
- Impaired urinary elimination *[uses]*

Nursing Considerations

Assess:

- VS, respiration q8hr
- I&O ratio; check for urinary retention or incontinence
- Bradycardia, hypotension, bronchospasm, headache, dizziness, seizures, respiratory depression; product should be discontinued if toxicity occurs

Administer:

- Only with atropine sulfate available for cholinergic crisis
- Only after all other cholinergics have been discontinued
- Increased doses if tolerance occurs
- Larger doses after exercise or fatigue
- On empty stomach for better absorption

Perform/provide:

- Storage at room temperature

Evaluate:

- Therapeutic response: increased muscle strength, hand grasp; improved muscle gait; absence of labored breathing (if severe)

Teach patient/family:

- That product is not a cure; it only relieves symptoms (myasthenia gravis)
- To carry emergency ID specifying myasthenia gravis, products taken

Selected Generic Names

bethanechol
neostigmine
physostigmine
pyridostigmine

CHOLINERGIC BLOCKERS

Action: Cholinergic blockers inhibit or block acetylcholine at receptor sites in the autonomic nervous system.

Uses: Many cholinergic blockers are used to decrease secretions before surgery, to reverse neuromuscular blockade, and to decrease motility of GI, biliary, urinary tracts. Other products are used for parkinsonian symptoms, including dystonia associated with neuroleptic products.

Side effects: The most common side effects are dryness of the mouth and constipation, which can be prevented by frequent rinsing of the mouth and by increasing water and bulk in the diet.

Contraindications: Hypersensitivity can occur, and allergies should be identified before administering these products. Persons with GI and GU obstruction should not use these products since constipation and urinary retention may occur. They are also contraindicated in closed-angle glaucoma and myasthenia gravis.
Precautions: Caution must be used when these products are given to the geriatric patient since metabolism is slowed. Also, persons with tachycardia or prostatic hypertrophy should use these products with caution.
Pharmacokinetics: Onset, peak, and duration vary with route.
Interactions: Increase in anticholinergic effect occurs when used with opioids, barbiturates, antihistamines, MAOIs, phenothiazines, and amantadine.
Possible nursing diagnoses:
- Impaired physical mobility *[uses]*
- Chronic pain *[uses]*

Nursing Considerations

Assess:
- I&O ratio; be alert for urinary retention, frequency, dysuria; product should be discontinued if these occur
- Urinary hesitancy, retention; palpate bladder if retention occurs
- Constipation; increase fluids, bulk, exercise
- For tolerance over long-term therapy; dose may have to be increased or changed
- Mental status: affect, mood, CNS depression, worsening of mental symptoms during early therapy

Administer:
- With food or milk to decrease GI symptoms
- Parenteral dose with patient recumbent to prevent postural hypotension; give parenteral dose slowly, monitoring vital signs

Perform/provide:
- Hard candy, gum, frequent rinsing of mouth for dryness

Evaluate:
- Therapeutic response: absence of cramps and EPS

Teach patient/family:
- To avoid driving, other hazardous activities if drowsiness occurs
- To avoid concurrent use of cough, cold preparations with alcohol, antihistamines unless directed by prescriber
- To use with caution in hot weather since medication may increase susceptibility to heat stroke

Selected Generic Names

atropine
benztropine
biperiden
glycopyrrolate
scopolamine
trihexyphenidyl

CORTICOSTEROIDS

Action: Corticosteroids are divided into glucocorticoids and mineralocorticoids. Glucocorticoids decrease inflammation by the suppression of migration of polymorphonuclear leukocytes, fibroblasts, increased capillary permeability, and lysosomal stabilization. They also have varied metabolic effects and modify the body's immune responses to many stimuli. Mineralocorticoids act by increasing resorption of sodium by increasing hydrogen and potassium excretion in the distal tubule.

Uses: Glucocorticoids are used to decrease inflammation and for immunosuppression. In addition, some products may be given for allergy, adrenal insufficiency, or cerebral edema. Mineralocorticoids are given for adrenal insufficiency or adrenogenital syndrome.

Side effects: The most common side effects include change in behavior, including insomnia and euphoria; GI irritation, including peptic ulcer; metabolic reactions, including hypokalemia, hyperglycemia, and carbohydrate intolerance; and sodium and fluid retention. Most adverse reactions are dose dependent.

Contraindications: Hypersensitivity may occur and should be identified before administering. Since these products mask infection, they should not be used in systemic fungal infections or amebiasis. Mothers taking pharmacologic doses of corticosteroids should not breastfeed.

Precautions: Caution must be used when these products are prescribed for diabetic patients since hyperglycemia may occur. Also, patients with glaucoma, seizure disorders, peptic ulcer, impaired renal function, congestive heart failure, hypertension, ulcerative colitis, or myasthenia gravis should be monitored closely if corticosteroids are given. Use with caution in children, the geriatric patients, and during pregnancy.

Pharmacokinetics: For oral preparations, the onset of action occurs between 1 and 2 hr, and duration can be up to 2 days, with a half-life of 2-4 days. Pharmacokinetics vary widely among products. These products cross the placenta and appear in breast milk.

Interactions: Decreased corticosteroid effect may occur with barbiturates, rifampin, and phenytoin; corticosteroid dose may have to be increased. There is a possibility of GI bleeding when used with salicylates and indomethacin. Steroids may reduce salicylate levels. When using with digoxin, glycosides, potassium-depleting diuretics, and amphotericin, serum potassium levels should be monitored.

Possible nursing diagnoses:

- Disturbed body image *[adverse reactions]*
- Risk for infection *[adverse reactions]*
- Risk for suicide *[adverse reactions]*

Nursing Considerations

Assess:

- Potassium, blood glucose, urine glucose while on long-term therapy; hypokalemia and hyperglycemia are common
- Weight daily; notify prescriber of weekly gain >5 lb since these products alter fluid and electrolyte balance
- I&O ratio; be alert for decreasing urinary output and increasing edema
- Plasma cortisol levels during long-term therapy (normal level is 138-635 nmol/L SI units when drawn at 8 AM)
- Infection: increased temp, WBC, even after withdrawal of medication; product masks symptoms of infection
- Adrenal insufficiency: nausea, anorexia, fatigue, dizziness, dyspnea, weakness, joint pain

• Potassium depletion: paresthesias, fatigue, nausea, vomiting, depression, polyuria, dysrhythmias, weakness
• Mental status: affect, mood, behavioral changes, aggression; if severe personality changes occur, including depression, product may have to be tapered and then discontinued

Administer:

• With food or milk to decrease GI symptoms
• Take single daily or alternate-day doses in the morning before 9 AM (for replacement therapy)

Evaluate:

• Therapeutic response: decreased inflammation

Teach patient/family:

• That emergency ID as steroid user should be carried
• Not to discontinue this medication abruptly; adrenal crisis can result
• All aspects of product use, including cushingoid symptoms
• To take with meals or a snack
• To avoid exposure to chickenpox or measles if taking immunosuppressives

Selected Generic Names

Glucocorticoids

beclomethasone
betamethasone
cortisone
dexamethasone
hydrocortisone
hydrocortisone sodium phosphate
methylPREDNISolone
prednisoLONE
predniSONE
triamcinolone

Mineralocorticoid

fludrocortisone

DIURETICS

Action: Diuretics are divided into subgroups: thiazides and thiazide-like diuretics, loop diuretics, carbonic anhydrase inhibitors, osmotic diuretics, and potassium-sparing diuretics. Each one of these subgroups has its own mechanism of action. Thiazides and thiazide-like diuretics increase excretion of water and sodium by inhibiting resorption in the early distal tubule. Loop diuretics inhibit resorption of sodium and chloride in the thick ascending limb of the loop of Henle. Carbonic anhydrase inhibitors increase sodium excretion by decreasing sodium-hydrogen ion exchange throughout the renal tubule. Carbonic anhydrase inhibitors also decrease secretion of aqueous humor in the eye and thus decrease intraocular pressure. Osmotic diuretics increase the osmotic pressure of glomerular filtrate, thus decreasing net absorption of sodium. The potassium-sparing diuretics interfere with sodium resorption at the distal tubule, thus decreasing potassium excretion.

Uses: B/P is reduced in hypertension; edema is reduced in congestive heart failure; intraocular pressure is decreased in glaucoma.

Side effects: Hypokalemia, hyperuricemia, and hyperglycemia occur most frequently with thiazide diuretics. Aplastic anemia, blood dyscrasias, volume depletion, and dehydration may occur when thiazide-like diuretics, loop diuretics, or carbonic anhydrase inhibitors are given. Side effects and adverse reactions vary widely for the miscellaneous products.

Contraindications: Persons with electrolyte imbalances (Na, Cl, K), dehydration, or anuria should not be given these products until the problem is corrected.

Precautions: Caution must be used when diuretics are given to the geriatric patient since electrolyte disturbances and dehydration can occur rapidly. Hepatic/renal disease may cause poor metabolism and excretion of the product.

Pharmacokinetics: Onset, peak, and duration vary widely among the different subgroups of these products.

Interactions: Cholestyramine and colestipol will decrease the absorption of thiazide diuretics. Concurrent use of thiazides with diazoxide may increase hyperuricemia, hyperglycemia, and antihypertensive effects of thiazides. Ototoxicity may occur when loop diuretics are used with aminoglycosides. Thiazide and loop diuretics may increase therapeutic and toxic effects of lithium.

Possible nursing diagnoses:

- Decreased cardiac output *[adverse reactions]*
- Excess fluid volume *[uses]*

Nursing Considerations

Assess:

- Weight, I&O daily to determine fluid loss; check skin turgor for dehydration
- Electrolytes: K, Na, Cl; include BUN, blood glucose, CBC, serum creatinine, blood pH, ABGs, uric acid, Ca; electrolyte imbalances may occur quickly
- B/P (lying and standing); postural hypotension may occur since fluid loss occurs first from intravascular spaces
- Signs of metabolic alkalosis, including drowsiness and restlessness
- Signs of hypokalemia with some products: postural hypotension, malaise, fatigue, tachycardia, leg cramps, weakness

Administer:

- In AM to avoid interference with sleep if using product as a diuretic
- K replacement if K is <3 mg/dl

Evaluate:

- Therapeutic response: improvement in edema of feet, legs, sacral area daily if medication is being used in congestive heart failure; improvement in B/P if medication is being used as a diuretic; improvement in intraocular pressure if medication is being used to decrease aqueous humor in the eye

Teach patient/family:

- To take product early in the day (diuretic) to prevent nocturia

Selected Generic Names

Thiazides
chlorothiazide
hydrochlorothiazide

Thiazide-like
chlorthalidone
indapamide
metolazone

Loop
bumetanide
furosemide
torsemide

Carbonic anhydrase inhibitor
acetaZOLAMIDE

Potassium-sparing
amiloride
spironolactone
triamterene

Osmotics
mannitol
urea

HISTAMINE H_2 ANTAGONISTS

Action: Histamine H_2 antagonists act by inhibiting histamine at the H_2-receptor site in parietal cells, which inhibits gastric acid secretion.

Uses: Histamine H_2 antagonists are used for short-term treatment of duodenal and gastric ulcers and maintenance therapy for duodenal ulcer; gastroesophageal reflux disease.

Side effects: The most serious adverse reactions are agranulocytosis, thrombocytopenia, neutropenia, aplastic anemia, and exfoliative dermatitis. The most common side effects are confusion (not with ranitidine), headache, and diarrhea.

Contraindications: Persons with hypersensitivity should not use these products.

Precautions: Caution should be used in pregnancy, breastfeeding, child <16 yr, organic brain syndrome, hepatic/renal disease.

Pharmacokinetics: Onset, peak, and duration vary widely among products. Most products are metabolized in the liver and excreted in urine.

Interactions: Antacids interfere with absorption of histamine H_2 antagonists. Check individual monographs for specific information.

Possible nursing diagnoses:
- Risk for injury *[bleeding]*
- Deficient knowledge *[teaching]*
- Chronic pain *[uses]*

Nursing Considerations

Assess:
- Gastric pH (>5 should be maintained)
- I&O ratio, BUN, creatinine

Administer:
- With meals for prolonged product effect
- Antacids 1 hr before or 1 hr after cimetidine
- IV slowly; bradycardia may occur; give over 30 min

Perform/provide:
- Storage of diluted sol at room temperature for up to 48 hr

Evaluate:
- Therapeutic response: decreased pain in abdomen

Teach patient/family:
- That gynecomastia, impotence may occur but are reversible
- To avoid driving, other hazardous activities until patient is stabilized on this medication
- To avoid black pepper, caffeine, alcohol, harsh spices, extremes in temperature of food
- To avoid OTC preparations: aspirin, cough, cold preparations
- That product must be continued for prescribed time to be effective
- To report bruising, fatigue, malaise; blood dyscrasias may occur

Selected Generic Names

cimetidine
famotidine
ranitidine

IMMUNOSUPPRESSANTS

Action: Immunosuppressants act by inhibiting lymphocytes (T).

Uses: Most immunosuppressants are used for organ transplants to prevent rejection.

Side effects: The most serious adverse reactions are albuminuria, hematuria, proteinuria, renal failure, and hepatotoxicity. The most common side effects are overgrowth of oral *Candida,* gum hyperplasia, tremors, and headache. The most serious adverse reactions for azathioprine are hematologic (leukopenia and thrombocytopenia) and GI (nausea and vomiting). There is a risk of secondary infection.

Contraindications: Products are contraindicated in hypersensitivity.

Precautions: Caution should be used in severe renal/hepatic disease and pregnancy.

Pharmacokinetics: Onset, peak, and duration vary widely among products. Most products are metabolized in the liver and excreted in urine.

Interactions: Interactions vary widely among products. Check individual monographs for specific information.

Possible nursing diagnoses:

- Risk for infection *[adverse reactions]*
- Risk for injury *[uses]*
- Deficient knowledge *[teaching]*

Nursing Considerations

Assess:

- Renal studies: BUN, creatinine at least q mo during treatment, 3 mo after treatment
- Hepatic studies: alk phos, AST (SGOT), ALT (SGPT), bilirubin
- Product blood levels during treatment
- Hepatotoxicity: dark urine, jaundice, itching, light-colored stools; product should be discontinued

Administer:

- For several days before transplant surgery
- With meals for GI upset or product mixed with chocolate milk
- With oral antifungal for *Candida* infections

Evaluate:

- Therapeutic response: absence of rejection

Teach patient/family:

- To report fever, chills, sore throat, fatigue since serious infections may occur
- To use contraceptive measures during treatment and for 12 wk after ending therapy

Selected Generic Names

azathioprine
basiliximab
cycloSPORINE
everolimus
muromonab-CD3
sirolimus
tacrolimus

LAXATIVES

Action: Laxatives are divided into bulk products, lubricants, osmotics, saline laxative stimulants, and stool softeners. Bulk laxatives work by absorbing water and expanding to increase moisture content and bulk in the stool. Lubricants increase water retention in the stool causing reabsorption of water in the bowel. Osmotics increase distention and promote peristalsis. Saline draws water into the intestinal lumen. Stimulants act by increasing peristalsis by direct effect on the intestine. Stool softeners reduce surface tension of liquids of the bowel.

Uses: Laxatives are used as a preparation for bowel and rectal exam, constipation, and stool softener.

Side effects: The most common side effects are nausea, abdominal cramps, and diarrhea.
Contraindications: Persons with GI obstruction, perforation, gastric retention, toxic colitis, megacolon, abdominal pain, nausea, vomiting, or fecal impaction should not use these products.
Precautions: Caution should be used in rectal bleeding, large hemorrhoids, and anal excoriation.
Pharmacokinetics: Onset, peak, and duration vary among products.
Interactions: Interactions vary widely among products. Check individual monographs for specific information.
Possible nursing diagnoses:
- Constipation *[uses]*
- Diarrhea *[adverse reactions]*
- Deficient knowledge *[teaching]*

Nursing Considerations

Assess:
- Blood, urine electrolytes if product is used often by patient
- I&O ratio to identify fluid loss
- Cause of constipation: identify whether fluids, bulk, or exercise missing from lifestyle
- Cramping, rectal bleeding, nausea, vomiting; if these symptoms occur, product should be discontinued

Administer:
- Swallow tabs whole; do not break, crush, or chew
- Alone only with water for better absorption; do not take within 1 hr of antacids, milk, or cimetidine

Evaluate:
- Therapeutic response: decrease in constipation

Teach patient/family:
- Not to use laxatives for long-term therapy; bowel tone will be lost
- That normal bowel movements do not always occur daily
- Not to use in presence of abdominal pain, nausea, vomiting
- To notify prescriber of abdominal pain, nausea, vomiting
- To notify prescriber if constipation is unrelieved or if symptoms of electrolyte imbalance: muscle cramps, pain, weakness, dizziness

Selected Generic Names

Bulk laxatives
calcium polycarbophil
methylcellulose
psyllium
Osmotic agents
glycerin
lactulose
Saline laxatives
magnesium salts
sodium biphosphate/phosphate
Stimulants
bisacodyl
cascara sagrada
senna
Stool softener
docusate

NEUROMUSCULAR BLOCKING AGENTS

Action: Neuromuscular blocking agents are divided into depolarizing and nondepolarizing blockers. They act by inhibiting transmission of nerve impulses by binding with cholinergic receptor sites.
Uses: Neuromuscular blocking agents are used to facilitate endotracheal intubation and skeletal muscle relaxation during mechanical ventilation, surgery, or general anesthesia.

Side effects: The most serious adverse reactions are prolonged apnea, bronchospasm, cyanosis, respiratory depression, and malignant hyperthermia. The most common side effects are bradycardia and decreased motility.

Contraindications: Persons who are hypersensitive should not be given this product.

Precautions: Caution should be used in pregnancy, thyroid disease, collagen disease, cardiac disease, breastfeeding, children <2 yr, electrolyte imbalances, dehydration, neuromuscular disease (myasthenia gravis), and respiratory disease.

Pharmacokinetics: Onset, peak, and duration vary widely among products. Most products are metabolized in the liver and excreted in urine.

Interactions: Aminoglycosides potentiate neuromuscular blockade. Check individual monographs for specific information.

Possible nursing diagnoses:

- Ineffective breathing pattern *[uses]*
- Risk for injury *[adverse reactions]*
- Deficient knowledge *[teaching]*

Nursing Considerations

Assess:

- For electrolyte imbalances (K, Mg); may lead to increased action of this product
- VS (B/P, pulse, respirations, airway) q15min until fully recovered; rate, depth, pattern of respirations, strength of hand grip
- I&O ratio; check for urinary retention, frequency, hesitancy
- Recovery: decreased paralysis of face, diaphragm, leg, arm, rest of body
- Allergic reactions: rash, fever, respiratory distress, pruritus; product should be discontinued

Administer:

- Using nerve stimulator by anesthesia provider to determine neuromuscular blockade
- Anticholinesterase to reverse neuromuscular blockade
- IV undiluted over 1-2 min (only by qualified person, usually an anesthesiologist)

Perform/provide:

- Storage in light-resistant container, cool area
- Reassurance if communication is difficult during recovery from neuromuscular blockade

Evaluate:

- Therapeutic response: paralysis of jaw, eyelid, head, neck, rest of body

Selected Generic Names

atracurium
doxacurium
gallamine
mivacurium
pancuronium
pipecuronium
rocuronium
succinylcholine
vecuronium

NONSTEROIDAL ANTIINFLAMMATORIES

Action: Nonsteroidal antiinflammatories decrease prostaglandin synthesis by inhibiting an enzyme needed for biosynthesis.

Uses: Nonsteroidal antiinflammatories are used to treat mild to moderate pain, osteoarthritis, rheumatoid arthritis, and dysmenorrhea.

Side effects: The most serious adverse reactions are nephrotoxicity (dysuria, hematuria, oliguria, azotemia), blood dyscrasias, and cholestatic hepatitis. The most common side effects are nausea, abdominal pain, anorexia, dizziness, and drowsiness.

Contraindications: Persons with hypersensitivity, asthma, severe renal/hepatic disease should not use these products.

Precautions: Caution should be used in pregnancy, breastfeeding, children, geriatric patients, bleeding/GI/cardiac disorders, and hypersensitivity to other antiinflammatory agents.

Pharmacokinetics: Onset, peak, and duration vary widely among products. Most products are metabolized in the liver and excreted in urine.

Interactions: Interactions vary widely among products. Check individual monographs for specific information.

Possible nursing diagnoses:
- Deficient knowledge *[teaching]*
- Impaired physical mobility *[uses]*
- Noncompliance *[teaching]*
- Chronic pain *[uses]*

Nursing Considerations

Assess:
- Renal, hepatic, blood studies: BUN, creatinine, AST, ALT, Hgb, before treatment, periodically thereafter
- Audiometric, ophthalmic examination before, during, and after treatment
- For eye, ear problems: blurred vision, tinnitus; may indicate toxicity

Administer:
- With food to decrease GI symptoms; however, best to take on empty stomach to facilitate absorption

Perform/provide:
- Storage at room temperature

Evaluate:
- Therapeutic response: decreased pain, stiffness in joints; decreased swelling in joints; ability to move more easily

Teach patient/family:
- To report blurred vision, ringing, roaring in ears; may indicate toxicity
- To avoid driving, other hazardous activities if dizziness, drowsiness occur, especially in geriatric patients
- To report change in urine pattern, increased weight, edema, increased pain in joints, fever, blood in urine; indicate nephrotoxicity
- That therapeutic effects may take up to 1 mo

Selected Generic Names

celecoxib
diclofenac
etodolac
fenoprofen
ibuprofen
indomethacin
ketoprofen
ketorolac
nabumetone
naproxen
piroxicam
sulindac

OPIOID ANALGESICS

Action: Opioid analgesics act by depressing pain impulse transmission at the spinal cord level by interacting with opioid receptors. Products are divided into opiates and nonopiates.

Uses: Most opioid analgesics are used to control moderate to severe pain and are used before and after surgery.

Side effects: GI symptoms, including nausea, vomiting, anorexia, constipation, and cramps, are the most common side effects. Other common side effects include light-headedness, dizziness, and sedation. Serious adverse reactions such as respiratory depression, respiratory arrest, circulatory depression, and increased intracranial pressure may result but are less common and usually dose dependent.

Contraindications: Hypersensitive reactions occur frequently. Check for sensitivity before administering. These products should be used cautiously if opiate addiction is suspected.

Precautions: Caution must be used when these products are given to a person with an addictive personality since the possibility of addiction is so great. Also, they may worsen intracranial pressure. Persons with severe heart disease, hepatic/renal disease, respiratory conditions, or seizure disorders should be monitored closely for worsening condition.

Pharmacokinetics: Onset of action is immediate by IV route and rapid by IM and PO routes. Peak occurs from 1-2 hr, depending on route, with a duration of 2-8 hr. These agents cross the placenta and appear in breast milk.

Interactions: Barbiturates, other opioids, hypnotics, antipsychotics, or alcohol can increase CNS depression when taken with opioids.

Possible nursing diagnoses:

- Impaired gas exchange *[adverse reactions]*
- Acute pain *[uses]*

Nursing Considerations

Assess:

- I&O ratio; be alert for urinary retention, frequency, and dysuria; product should be discontinued if these occur
- Respiratory dysfunction: respiratory depression, rate, rhythm, character; notify prescriber if respirations are <12/min
- CNS changes: dizziness, drowsiness, hallucinations, euphoria, LOC, pupil reaction
- Allergic reactions: rash, urticaria
- Need for pain medication; use pain scoring

Administer:

- With antiemetic if nausea or vomiting occurs
- When pain is beginning to return; determine dosage interval by response

Perform/provide:

- Assistance with ambulation; patient should not be ambulating during product peak

Evaluate:

- Therapeutic response: decrease in pain

Teach patient/family:

- To report any symptoms of CNS changes, allergic reactions, or SOB
- That physical dependency may result when used for extended periods
- That withdrawal symptoms may occur, including nausea, vomiting, cramps, fever, faintness, anorexia
- To avoid alcohol and other CNS depressants

Selected Generic Names

alfentanil
buprenorphine
butorphanol
codeine
fentanyl
fentanyl transdermal
hydromorphone
meperidine
methadone
morphine
nalbuphine
oxycodone
oxymorphone
pentazocine
propoxyphene
remifentanil

SALICYLATES

Action: Salicylates have analgesic, antipyretic, and antiinflammatory effects. The analgesic and antiinflammatory activities may be mediated through the inhibition of prostaglandin synthesis. Antipyretic action results from inhibition of the hypothalamic heat-regulating center.

Uses: The primary uses of salicylates are relief of mild to moderate pain and fever and in inflammatory conditions such as arthritis, thromboembolic disorders, and rheumatic fever.

Side effects: The most common side effects are GI symptoms and rash. Serious blood dyscrasias and hepatotoxicity may result when used for long periods at high doses. Tinnitus or impaired hearing may indicate that blood salicylate levels are reaching or exceeding the upper limit of the therapeutic range.

Contraindications: Hypersensitivity to salicylates is common. Check for sensitivity before administering. Persons with bleeding disorders, GI bleeding, and vit K deficiency should not use these products since salicylates increase PT. Children should not use these products since salicylates have been associated with Reye's syndrome.

Precautions: Caution is needed when salicylates are given to patients with anemia, hepatic/renal disease, and Hodgkin's disease. Caution should also be exercised in pregnancy and breastfeeding.

Pharmacokinetics: Onset of action occurs in 15-30 min, with a peak of 1-2 hr and a duration up to 6 hr. These products are metabolized by the liver and excreted by the kidneys.

Interactions: Increased effects of anticoagulants, insulin, methotrexate, heparin, valproic acid, and oral sulfonylureas may occur when used with salicylates. Aspirin may decrease serum concentrations of nonsteroidal antiinflammatory agents.

Possible nursing diagnoses:
- Activity intolerance *[uses]*
- Impaired physical mobility *[uses]*
- Acute pain *[uses]*
- Chronic pain *[uses]*
- Disturbed sensory perception, auditory *[adverse reactions]*
- Ineffective thermoregulation *[uses]*

Nursing Considerations

Assess:
- Hepatic/renal studies: AST, ALT, bilirubin, creatinine, LDH, alk phos, BUN if patient is on long-term therapy since these products are metabolized and excreted by the liver and kidney

• Blood studies: CBC, hematocrit, hemoglobin, and PT if patient is on long-term therapy since these products increase the possibility of bleeding and blood dyscrasias
• Hepatotoxicity: dark urine, clay-colored stools; yellowing of skin, sclera; itching, abdominal pain, fever, diarrhea, which may occur with long-term use
• Ototoxicity: tinnitus; ringing, roaring in ears; audiometric testing is needed before and after long-term therapy

Administer:

• With food or milk to decrease gastric irritation; give 30 min before or 1 hr after meals with a full glass of water

Evaluate:

• Therapeutic response: decreased pain, fever

Teach patient/family:

• That blood glucose levels should be monitored closely if patient is diabetic
• Not to exceed recommended dosage; acute poisoning may result
• That therapeutic response takes 2 wk in arthritis
• To avoid use of alcohol since GI bleeding may result
• To notify prescriber of ringing in the ears or persistent GI pain
• To take with full glass of water to reduce risk of lodging in esophagus

Selected Generic Names

aspirin
choline salicylate
magnesium salicylate
salsalate

SEDATIVES/HYPNOTICS

Action: Sedatives/hypnotics depress the CNS; some products at the cerebral cortex, others inhibit transmitters in the CNS.

Uses: Sedatives/hypnotics are used for the treatment of sleep disorders, seizures, muscle spasms, and alcohol withdrawal.

Side effects: The most common side effects are nausea and drowsiness. The most serious side effects are Stevens-Johnson syndrome, blood dyscrasias, and risk of dependency.

Contraindications: Persons with hypersensitivity reactions should not use these products.

Precautions: Sedatives/hypnotics should be used cautiously in pregnancy (C) and breastfeeding.

Pharmacokinetics: Onset, peak, and duration vary widely among products. Most products are metabolized in the liver and excreted by the kidneys.

Interactions: Increased CNS depression may occur with other CNS depressants such as alcohol, opiates, antipsychotics, and antidepressants.

Possible nursing diagnoses:

• Deficient knowledge *[teaching]*
• Noncompliance *[teaching]*
• Sleep deprivation *[uses]*

Nursing Considerations

Assess:

• Mental status: affect, mood, behavioral changes, depression, confusion; seizure activity

Administer:

• Lowest possible dose for therapeutic result; adjust dose to response

Perform/provide:

• Assistance with ambulation during beginning therapy if dizziness, ataxia occur

Evaluate:

• Therapeutic response: ability to sleep throughout the night; absence or decreasing seizure activity

Teach patient/family:

• That these products should only be used for short-term insomnia
• Not to drive or engage in other hazardous activities while taking these products
• To avoid breastfeeding while taking these products
• To avoid alcohol or other CNS depressants since drowsiness will increase
• That some of the products take 2 nights to be effective
• To report side effects, adverse reactions to health care provider
• To use exactly as prescribed, at regular intervals

Selected Generic Names

Barbiturates
phenobarbital
Benzodiazepines
chlordiazepoxide
clorazepate
diazepam
flurazepam
lorazepam
midazolam
oxazepam
temazepam
triazolam
Miscellaneous products
chloral hydrate
dexmedetomidine
droperidol
eszopiclone
hydrOXYzine
promethazine
ramelteon
zaleplon
zolpidem

SKELETAL MUSCLE RELAXANTS

Action: Most skeletal muscle relaxants inhibit synaptic responses in the CNS by stimulating receptors and decreasing neurotransmission, decreasing pain and spasticity.
Uses: Skeletal muscle relaxants are used for musculoskeletal disorders with pain or spasticity related to spinal cord injuries.
Side effects: The most common side effects are dizziness, weakness, fatigue, drowsiness, and headache. Some products can cause seizures, CV collapse, and severe CNS depression.
Contraindications: Persons with hypersensitivity should not use these products.
Precautions: Skeletal muscle relaxants should be used cautiously in pregnancy (C), peptic ulcer, renal/hepatic disease, stroke, seizure disorder, diabetes, breastfeeding, and the geriatric patient.
Pharmacokinetics: Pharmacokinetics varies widely among products. Check individual monographs for specific information.
Interactions: CNS depressants used with skeletal muscle relaxants may lead to increased CNS depression.
Possible nursing diagnoses:

• Risk for injury *[adverse reactions]*
• Deficient knowledge *[teaching]*
• Impaired physical mobility *[uses]*
• Acute pain *[uses]*
• Chronic pain *[uses]*

Nursing Considerations

Assess:

- Pain: character, location, duration, alleviating/aggravating factors

Administer:

- When pain is beginning to return, not after pain is severe

Perform/provide:

- Storage in dry area, away from heat and sunlight

Evaluate:

- Therapeutic response: decrease pain or spasticity

Teach patient/family:

- Not to use with other CNS depressant unless prescriber approved
- That many products require 1-2 mo of treatment for full effect
- To avoid hazardous activities until response to medication is known
- That most products should not be discontinued quickly, but tapered over 1-2 wk

Selected Generic Names

Centrally acting

baclofen
carisoprodol
chlorzoxazone
cyclobenzaprine
diazepam
metaxalone
methocarbamol
orphenadrine

Direct-acting

dantrolene

THROMBOLYTICS

Action: Thrombolytics act by activating conversion of plasminogen to plasmin (fibrinolysin). Plasmin is able to break down clots (fibrin).

Uses: Thrombolytics are used to treat DVT, PE, arterial thrombosis, arterial embolism, arteriovenous cannula occlusion, lysis of coronary artery thrombi after MI, and acute, evolving transmural MI.

Side effects: Serious adverse reactions include GI, GU, intracranial retroperitoneal bleeding, and anaphylaxis. The most common side effects are decreased Hct, urticaria, headache, and nausea.

Contraindications: Persons with hypersensitivity, active bleeding, intraspinal surgery, neoplasms of the CNS, ulcerative colitis/enteritis, severe hypertension, renal/hepatic disease, hypocoagulation, COPD, subacute bacterial endocarditis, rheumatic valvular disease, cerebral embolism/thrombosis/hemorrhage, recent intraarterial diagnostic procedure or surgery (10 days), and recent major surgery should not use these products.

Precautions: Caution should be used in arterial emboli from left side of heart and pregnancy.

Pharmacokinetics: Onset, peak, and duration vary widely among products. Most products are metabolized in the liver and excreted in urine.

Interactions: Interactions vary widely among products. Check individual monographs for specific information.

Possible nursing diagnoses:

- Risk for injury *[uses]*

Nursing Considerations

Assess:

- VS, B/P, pulse, resp, neurologic signs, temp at least q4hr; temp >104° F (40° C) indicator of internal bleeding; cardiac rhythm following intracoronary administration; systolic pressure increase of >25 mm Hg should be reported to prescriber

• For neurologic changes that may indicate intracranial bleeding

• Retroperitoneal bleeding: back pain, leg weakness, diminished pulses

• Allergy: fever, rash, itching, chill; mild reaction may be treated with antihistamines

• For bleeding during 1st hr of treatment: hematuria, hematemesis, bleeding from mucous membranes, epistaxis, ecchymosis

• Blood studies (Hct, platelets, PTT, PT, TT, aPTT) before starting therapy; PT or APTT must be <2× control before starting therapy or PT q3-4hr during treatment

Administer:

• As soon as thrombi identified; not useful for thrombi over 1 wk old

• Cryoprecipitate or fresh, frozen plasma if bleeding occurs

• Loading dose at beginning of therapy; may require increased loading doses

• Heparin after fibrinogen level is over 100 mg/dl; heparin inf to increase PTT to 1.5-2 × baseline for 3-7 days

• About 10% of patients have high streptococcal antibody titers requiring increased loading doses

• IV therapy using 0.8 μm filter

Perform/provide:

• Storage of reconstituted product in refrigerator; discard after 24 hr

• Bed rest during entire course of treatment

Evaluate:

• Therapeutic response: resolution of thrombosis, embolism

Teach patient/family:

• To avoid venous or arterial puncture, inj, rectal temp

• To treat fever with acetaminophen or aspirin

• To apply pressure for 30 sec to minor bleeding sites; inform prescriber if this does not attain hemostasis; apply pressure dressing

Selected Generic Names

alteplase
anistreplase
drotrecogin alfa
streptokinase
tenecteplase
urokinase

THYROID HORMONES

Action: Thyroid hormones act by increasing metabolic rates resulting in increased cardiac output, O_2 consumption, body temp, blood volume, growth, development at cellular level, respiratory rate, and enzyme system activity.

Uses: Thyroid hormones are used for thyroid replacement.

Side effects: The most common side effects include insomnia, tremors, tachycardia, palpitations, angina, dysrhythmias, weight loss, and changes in appetite. Serious adverse reactions include thyroid storm.

Contraindications: Persons with adrenal insufficiency, MI, or thyrotoxicosis should not use these products.

Precautions: Geriatric patients and those with angina pectoris, hypertension, ischemia, cardiac disease, diabetes mellitus or insipidus should be watched closely when using these products. Caution should be used in pregnancy (A) and breast-feeding.

Pharmacokinetics: Pharmacokinetics vary widely among products. Check individual monographs for specific information.

Interactions:

• Impaired absorption of thyroid products may occur when administered with cholestyramine, iron products (separate by 4-5 hr)

• Increased effects of anticoagulants, sympathomimetics, tricyclics, catecholamines may occur

• Decreased effects of digoxin, glycosides, insulin, hypoglycemics may occur

• Decreased effects of thyroid products may occur with estrogens

Possible nursing diagnoses:

• Disturbed body image *[adverse reactions]*

• Deficient knowledge *[teaching]*

• Noncompliance *[teaching]*

Nursing Considerations

Assess:

• B/P, pulse before each dose

• I&O ratio

• Weight daily in same clothing, using same scale, at same time of day

• PT should be closely monitored and dosage of anticoagulant therapy may need adjustment

• Height, growth rate if given to a child

• T_3, T_4, which are decreased; radioimmunoassay of TSH, which is increased; ratio uptake, which is decreased if patient is on too low a dosage of medication

• Increased nervousness, excitability, irritability; may indicate overdosage, usually after 1-3 wk of treatment

• Cardiac status: angina, palpitation, chest pain, change in VS

Administer:

• At same time each day to maintain product level

• Only for hormone imbalances; not to be used for obesity, male infertility, menstrual conditions, lethargy

Perform/provide:

• Removal of medication 4 wk before RAIU test

Evaluate:

• Therapeutic response: absence of depression; increased weight loss; diuresis; pulse; appetite; absence of constipation; peripheral edema; cold intolerance; pale, cool, dry skin; brittle nails; alopecia; coarse hair; menorrhagia; night blindness; paresthesias; syncope; stupor; coma; rosy cheeks

Teach patient/family:

• That hair loss will occur in child and is temporary

• To report excitability, irritability, anxiety, chest pain, palpitations, increased pulse, excessive sweating, heat intolerance; indicates overdose

• Not to switch brands unless directed by prescriber

• That hypothyroid child will show almost immediate behavior/personality change

• That treatment product is not to be taken to reduce weight

• To avoid OTC preparations with iodine; read labels

• To avoid iodine in food: iodinized salt, soybeans, tofu, turnips, some seafood, some bread

Selected Generic Names

levothyroxine (T_4)
liothyronine (T_3)
liotrix
thyroid USP

VASODILATORS

Action: Vasodilators have various modes of action. Check individual monographs for specific action.

Uses: Vasodilators are used to treat intermittent claudication, arteriosclerosis obliterans, vasospasm and muscular ischemia, ischemic cerebral vascular disease, hypertension, and angina.

Side effects: The most common side effects are headache, nausea, hypotension, hypertension, and ECG changes.

Contraindications: Some products are contraindicated in acute MI, paroxysmal tachycardia, and thyrotoxicosis.

Precautions: Caution should be used in uncompensated heart disease or peptic ulcer disease.

Pharmacokinetics: Onset, peak, and duration vary widely among products. Most products are metabolized in the liver and excreted in urine.

Interactions: Interactions vary widely among products. Check individual monographs for specific information.

Possible nursing diagnoses:

- Decreased cardiac output *[uses]*
- Deficient knowledge *[teaching]*
- Ineffective tissue perfusion *[uses]*

Nursing Considerations

Assess:

- Bleeding time in individuals with bleeding disorders
- Cardiac status: B/P, pulse, rate, rhythm, character; watch for increasing pulse

Administer:

- With meals to reduce GI symptoms

Perform/provide:

- Storage in tight container at room temperature

Evaluate:

- Therapeutic response: ability to walk without pain, increased temp in extremities, increased pulse volume

Teach patient/family:

- That medication is not a cure; may need to be taken continuously
- That it is necessary to quit smoking to prevent excessive vasoconstriction
- That improvement may be sudden, but usually occurs gradually over several weeks
- To report headache, weakness, increased pulse, as product may have to be decreased or discontinued
- To avoid hazardous activities until stabilized on medication; dizziness may occur

Selected Generic Names

amyl nitrite
bosentan
dipyridamole
hydrALAZINE
isoxsuprine
midodrine
minoxidil
nesiritide
papaverine

VITAMINS

Action: The action of vitamins varies widely among products and classes. Check individual monographs for specific information.

Uses: Vitamins are used to correct and prevent vitamin deficiencies.

Side effects: There are no side effects or adverse reactions with the water-soluble vitamins (C, B). However, fat-soluble vitamins (A, D, E, K) may accumulate in the body and cause adverse reactions (see individual monographs).

Contraindications: Hypersensitive reactions may occur, and allergies should be identified before these products are given.

Pharmacokinetics: Onset, peak, and duration vary widely among products. Check individual monographs for specific information.

Possible nursing diagnoses:

- Imbalanced nutrition: less than body requirements *[uses]*

Nursing Considerations

Administer:

- PO with food for better absorption

Perform/provide:

- Storage in tight, light-resistant container

Evaluate:

- Therapeutic response: no vitamin deficiency

Teach patient/family:

- Not to take more than prescribed amount

Selected Generic Names

Fat-soluble

phytonadione (vitamin K_1)
vitamin A
vitamin D
vitamin E

Water-soluble

ascorbic acid (C)
cyanocobalamin (B_{12})
pyridoxine (B_6)
riboflavin (B_2)
thiamine (B_1)

Miscellaneous

multivitamins

MECHANISMS AND SITES OF ACTION

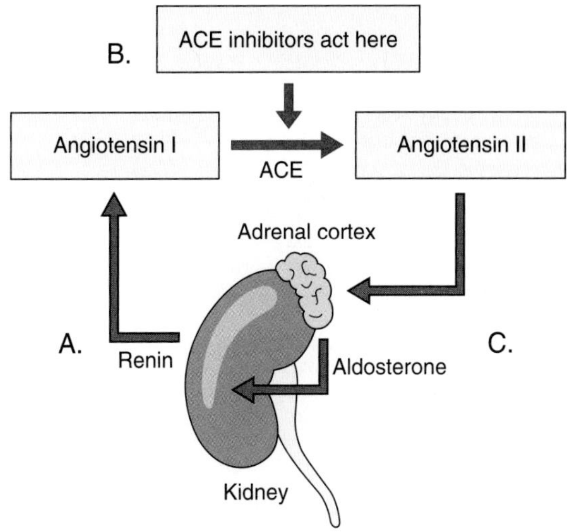

Plate 1: Sites of Action – ACE Inhibitors

The renin-angiotensin-aldosterone system plays a major role in regulating B/P. Any condition that decreases renal blood flow, reduces B/P, or stimulates beta$_1$-adrenergic receptors prompts the kidneys to release renin **(A).** Renin acts on angiotensinogen, which is converted to angiotensin I, a weak vasoconstrictor. Angiotensin-converting enzyme (ACE) converts angiotensin I to angiotensin II, which causes systemic and renal blood vessels to constrict **(B).** Systemic vasoconstriction increases peripheral vascular resistance, raising the B/P. Renal vasoconstriction decreases glomerular filtration, resulting in sodium and water retention and increasing blood volume and B/P. In addition, angiotensin II also acts on the adrenal cortex causing it to release aldosterone **(C).** This makes the kidneys retain additional sodium and water, which further increases the B/P.

ACE inhibitors, such as captopril, enalapril, and lisinopril, block the action of ACE. As a result, angiotensin II cannot form, which prevents systemic and renal vasoconstriction and the release of aldosterone. (From Prosser S, Worster B, Dewar K: *Applied Pharmacology for Nurses and Other Health Care Professionals*, St. Louis, 2000, Mosby.)

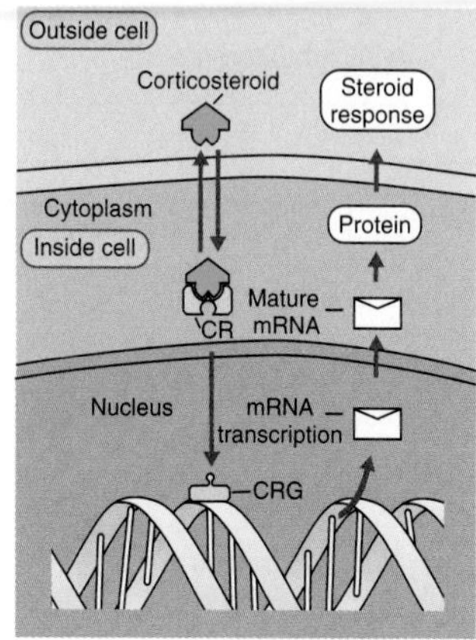

Plate 2: Mechanisms of Action – Adrenocortical Steroids
Adrenocortical steroids (also called corticosteroids) are available in many forms, such as predniSONE, and produce a wide range of effects, such as immunosuppression and antiinflammation. Here's how these products work at the cellular level.

Corticosteroids are hormones that are naturally produced by the body (endogenous hormones). Synthetic corticosteroids work much the same as the endogenous hormones. When a corticosteroid enters a cell, it binds to corticosteroid receptors (CRs) in the cell's cytoplasm, forming a complex. The complex moves to the nucleus, where it causes the transcription of corticosteroid responsive genes (CRGs) to messenger ribonucleic acid (mRNA), eventually translating to a protein that produces a steroid response in target tissues. (From Taylor: *Mosby's Crash Course Pharmacology*, St. Louis, 1998, Mosby.)

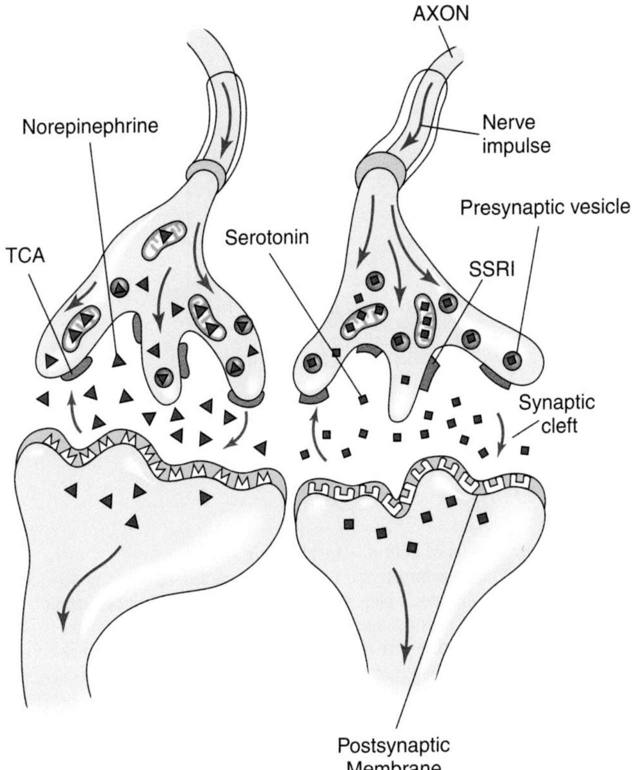

Plate 3: Mechanisms of Action – Antidepressants

Depression is thought to occur when levels of neurotransmitters, such as norepinephrine and serotonin, are reduced at postsynaptic receptor sites. These neurotransmitters affect a wide array of functions, including mood, obsessions, appetite, and anxiety. Antidepressants work by increasing the availability of these neurotransmitters at postsynaptic membranes and by enhancing and prolonging their effects. As a result, these agents improve mood, reduce anxiety, and minimize obsessions.

Antidepressants typically are classified as tricyclic antidepressants (TCAs), monoamine oxidase inhibitors (not shown), selective serotonin reuptake inhibitors (SSRIs), and atypical antidepressants (not shown). TCAs, such as amitriptyline and desipramine, primarily block norepinephrine reuptake at presynaptic membranes, thereby increasing the norepinephrine concentration at synapses and making more available at postsynaptic receptors.

SSRIs, such as fluoxetine and paroxetine, selectively inhibit serotonin uptake at presynaptic membranes. This action leads to increased serotonin availability at postsynaptic receptors. (From Gutierrez K: *Pharmacotherapeutics: Clinical Decision Making in Nursing*, Philadelphia, 1999, Saunders.)

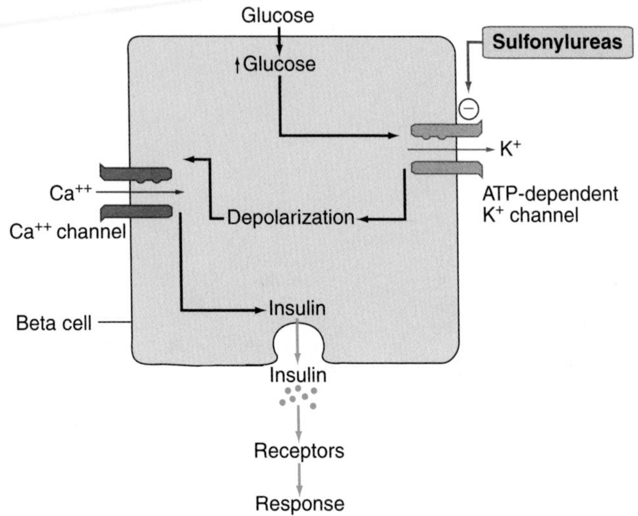

Plate 4: Mechanisms of Action – Antidiabetic Agents

Diabetes mellitus takes two forms: type 1 diabetes, characterized by a complete lack of insulin, and type 2 diabetes, which is marked by insufficient insulin secretion, insulin resistance in peripheral tissues, or both. Normally, the beta cells in the pancreatic islets of Langerhans are responsible for secreting insulin. When glucose levels rise in the beta cell, it triggers adenosine triphosphate (ATP)–dependent potassium (K^+) channels in the membranes of beta cells to close. Then the beta cells depolarize and calcium (Ca^{++}) enters the cell through Ca^{++} channel, and insulin is released from the cell. When circulating insulin engages with insulin receptors on cell membranes, it facilitates the movement of glucose into the cell, among other actions.

Type 1 diabetes is treated with the use of exogenous insulin, which mimics natural insulin in the body. Insulin takes many forms with varying degrees of onset, peak, and duration, including rapid, regular, intermediate, and long-acting.

Type 2 diabetes is usually treated with oral agents. Sulfonylureas, such as glyburide, block ATP-dependent K^+ channels in the cell membranes of beta cells, ultimately resulting in the release of insulin. (From Taylor M: *Mosby's Crash Course Pharmacology*, St. Louis, 1998, Mosby.)

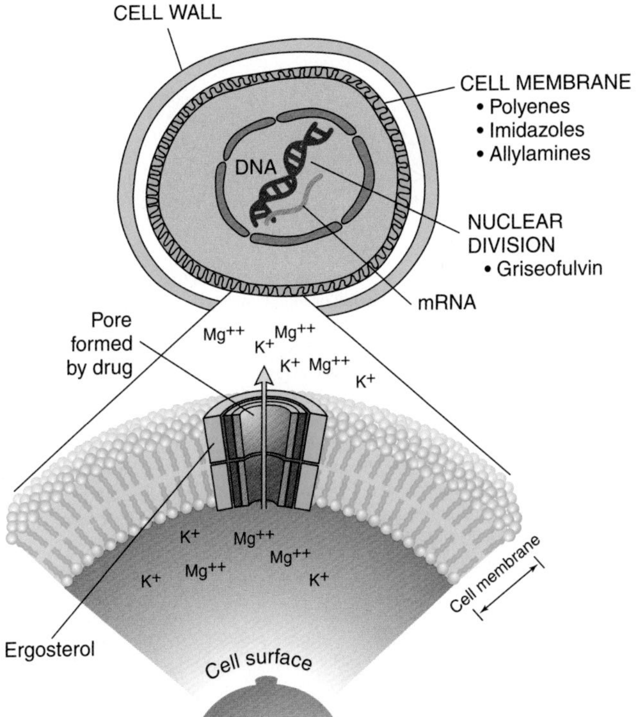

Plate 5: Sites and Mechanisms of Action – Antifungal Agents

Antifungal agents primarily affect fungi at one of two sites: the cell membrane or the cell nucleus. Most of these agents, such as polyene, imidazole, and allylamine antifungals, act on the fungal cell membrane. Polyene antifungals, such as amphotericin B, bind to ergosterol and increase cell membrane permeability. Imidazole antifungals, such as fluconazole and ketoconazole, interfere with ergosterol synthesis by inhibiting the cytochrome P450 enzyme system, altering the cell membrane, and inhibiting fungal growth. Allylamine antifungals, such as terbinafine, inhibit the enzyme squaline epoxidase, which disrupts ergosterol production—and cell membrane integrity. When cell membrane permeability increases, cellular components, including potassium (K^+) and magnesium (Mg^{++}), leak out. Loss of these cellular components leads to cell death.

Another antifungal agent, griseofulvin, directly affects the fungal nucleus, interfering with mitosis. By binding to structures in the mitotic spindle, it prevents cells from dividing, which eventually leads to their death. (From Gutierrez K: *Pharmacotherapeutics: Clinical Decision Making in Nursing*, Philadelphia, 1999, Saunders.)

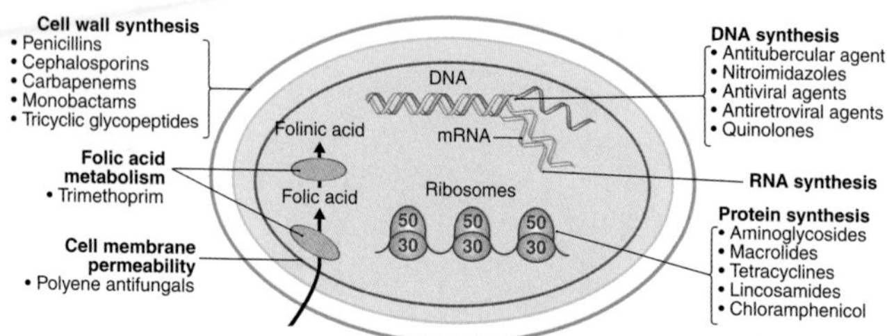

Plate 6: Sites and Mechanisms of Action – Antiinfective Agents
The goal of antiinfective therapy is to kill or inhibit the growth of microorganisms, such as bacteria, viruses, and fungi. To achieve this goal, antiinfective agents must reach their targets, which usually occurs through absorption and distribution by the circulatory system. When the target is reached, a drug can kill or suppress microorganisms by:

- Inhibiting cell wall synthesis or activating enzymes that disrupt the cell wall, which leads to cellular weakening, lysis, and death. Penicillins (ampicillin), cephalosporins (cefazolin), carbapenems (imipenem), monobactams (aztreonam), and tricyclic glycopeptides (vancomycin) act in this way.
- Altering cell membrane permeability through direct action on the cell wall, which allows intracellular substances to leak out and destabilizes the cell. Polyene antifungals (amphotericin) work by this mechanism.
- Altering protein synthesis by binding to bacterial ribosomes (50/30) or affecting ribosomal function, which leads to cell death or slowed growth, respectively. Aminoglycosides (gentamicin), macrolides (erythromycin), tetracyclines (doxycycline), lincosamides (clindamycin), and the miscellaneous antiinfective chloramphenicol act in this way.
- Inhibiting DNA or RNA, including messenger RNA (mRNA), by synthesis by binding to nucleic acids or interacting with enzymes required for their synthesis. Antitubercular agents (rifampin), nitroimidazoles (metronidazole), antiviral agents (acyclovir), antiretroviral agents (stavudine), and quinolones (ciprofloxacin) act like this.
- Inhibiting the metabolism of folic acid and folinic acid or other cellular components that are essential for bacterial cell growth. The miscellaneous anti-infective trimethoprim employs this mechanism of action. (From Page C, et al: *Integrated Pharmacology*, ed 2, St. Louis, 2002, Mosby.)

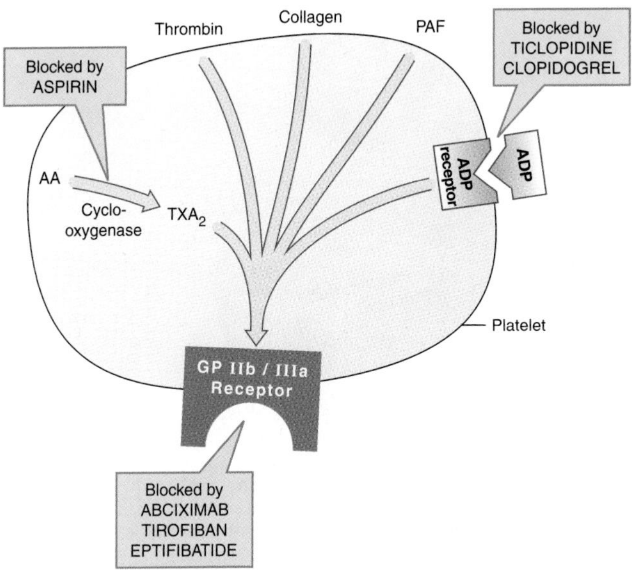

Plate 7: Sites and Mechanisms of Action – Antiplatelet Agents
Antiplatelet products are prescribed to prevent arterial thrombosis because they prevent platelet aggregation. These products include aspirin, adenosine diphosphate (ADP) receptor antagonists, or glycoprotein (GP) receptor IIb/IIIa antagonists. The degree of antiplatelet activity exerted by each product or product class depends on where the product acts in the platelet activation pathway.

Aspirin suppresses platelet aggregation and vasoconstriction by inhibiting cyclooxygenase, an enzyme that's needed to create thromboxane A_2 (TXA_2) from arachidonic acid (AA). TXA_2 is responsible for platelet activation and vasoconstriction.

ADP receptor antagonists, such as ticlopidine and clopidogrel, block ADP receptors on the surface of platelets, preventing platelet aggregation.

GP receptor IIb/IIIa inhibitors, such as abciximab, tirofiban, and eptifibatide, are powerful antiplatelet agents because they prevent platelet aggregation in the common pathway, whether aggregation is triggered by thromboxane, ADP, or another factor. These products block GP IIb/IIIa receptors from the effects of fibrinogen, thrombin, platelet activating factor (PAF), collagen, and other adhesive molecules. (From Lehne RA: *Pharmacology for Nursing Care*, ed 5, St. Louis, 2004, Saunders.)

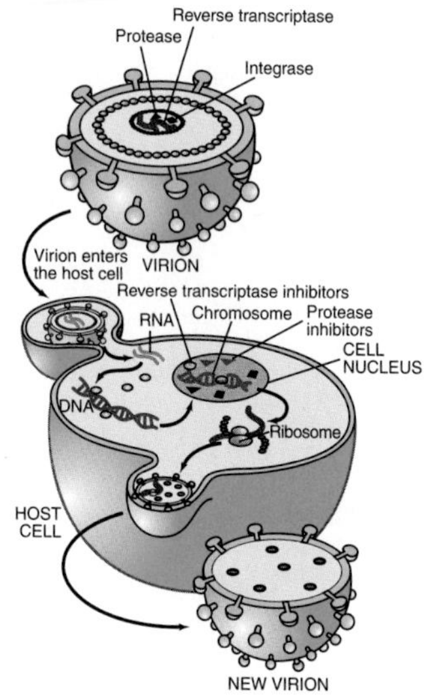

Plate 8: Mechanisms and Sites of Action – Antiretroviral Agents

To understand how antiretroviral agents work, you need to know how viruses reproduce. First, the infectious viral particle or virion enters the host cell. The virion attaches to the cell's surface and then inserts itself into the host cell. Once inside, the virion uncoats, and the enzyme reverse transcriptase makes two copies of the viral RNA: one copy is identical; the other is a mirror image. These two copies merge to form double-stranded viral DNA. This newly formed viral DNA enters the host cell's nucleus, where it inserts itself into the host cell's DNA with the help of the enzyme integrase. Then viral DNA reprograms the host cell to produce additional viral RNA, which begins the process of forming new viruses. Specifically, messenger RNA (mRNA) instructs ribosomal RNA (rRNA) to produce a new chain of proteins and enzymes that are used to form new viruses. Protease, another enzyme, cuts the chains of proteins, creating individual proteins. These individual proteins combine with new RNA to create new virions, which bud and are then released from the host cell.

Antiretroviral agents target specific enzymes during viral reproduction. Many of them work to inhibit reverse transcriptase. Nucleoside reverse transcriptase inhibitors, such as stavudine, interfere with the action of reverse transcriptase by mimicking naturally occurring nucleosides. Nucleotide reverse transcriptase inhibitors, such as tenofovir, block reverse transcriptase by competing with the natural substrate deoxyadenosine triphosphate and by causing DNA chain termination. Nonnucleoside reverse transcriptase inhibitors, such as delavirdine, work by directly binding to reverse transcriptase. All of these actions block the conversion of single-stranded viral RNA into double-stranded DNA. As a result, no viral DNA is available to insert itself into the host cell's DNA. Protease inhibitors, such as indinavir, bind to and interefere with the action of protease. By blocking protease, the new chain of proteins formed by rRNA cannot be cut into individual proteins to make new viruses. (From Gutierrez K: *Pharmacotherapeutics: Clinical Decision Making in Nursing*, Philadelphia, 1999, Saunders.)

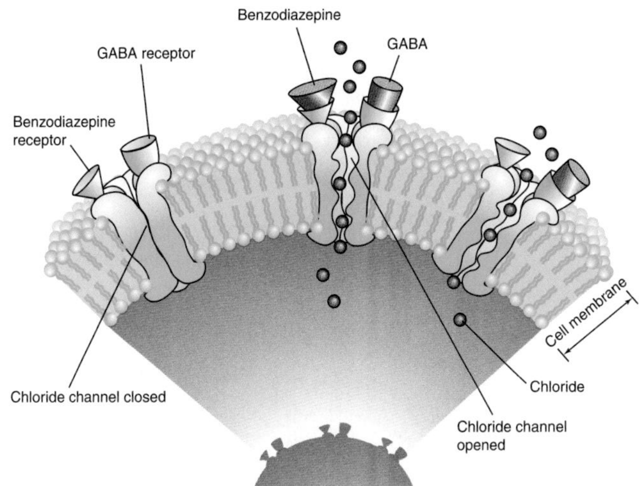

Plate 9: Mechanisms of Action – Benzodiazepines
Benzodiazepines reduce anxiety by stimulating the action of the inhibitory neurotransmitter, gamma-aminobutyric acid (GABA), in the limbic system. The limbic system plays an important role in the regulation of human behavior. Dysfunction of GABA neurotransmission in the limbic system may be linked to the development of certain anxiety disorders.

The limbic system contains a highly dense area of benzodiazepine receptors that may be linked to the antianxiety effects of benzodiazepines. These benzodiazepine receptors are located on the surface of neuronal cell membranes and are adjacent to GABA receptors. The binding of a benzodiazepine to its receptor enhances the affinity of a GABA receptor for GABA. In the absence of a benzodiazepine, the binding of GABA to its receptor causes the chloride channel in the cell membrane to open, which increases the influx of chloride into the cell. This influx of chloride results in hyperpolarization of the neuronal cell membrane and reduces the neuron's ability to fire, which is why GABA is considered an inhibitory neurotransmitter.

A benzodiazepine acts only in the presence of GABA. When it binds to a benzodiazepine receptor, it prolongs the time that the chloride channel remains open. This results in greater depression of neuronal function and a reduction in anxiety. (From Gutierrez K: *Pharmacotherapeutics: Clinical Decision Making in Nursing*, Philadelphia, 1999, Saunders.)

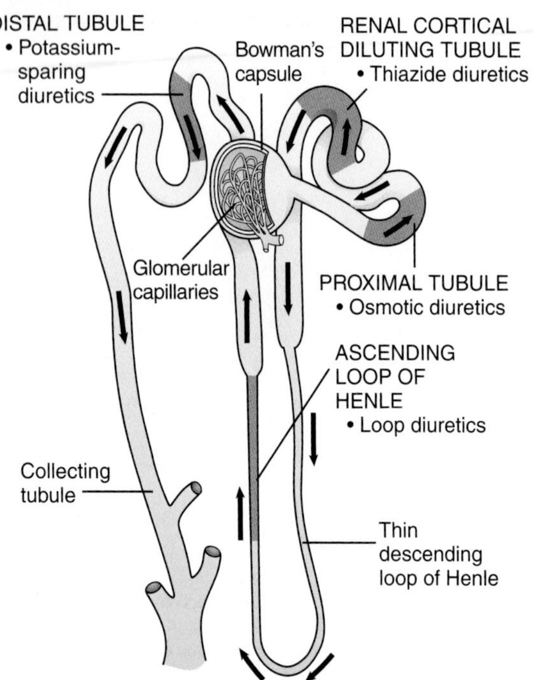

Plate 10: Sites of Action – Diuretics

Diuretics act primarily to increase water and sodium excretion by the kidneys, thereby increasing urine output. In the process, chloride, potassium, and other electrolytes may also be excreted. Most diuretics act by blocking sodium, water, and chloride reabsorption by peritubular capillaries in the nephrons. Water and electrolytes remain in the convoluted tubules to be excreted as urine. The increased water and electrolyte excretion reduces blood volume—and ultimately blood pressure.

Diuretics belong to four major subclasses:

1. Thiazide diuretics, such as hydrochlorothiazide, act in the cortical diluting segment. These products block sodium, chloride, and water reabsorption and promote their excretion along with potassium.

2. Loop diuretics, such as furosemide, act primarily in the thick ascending limb of the loop of Henle, blocking sodium, water, and chloride reabsorption. Then these substances are excreted along with potassium.

3. Potassium-sparing diuretics, such as spironolactone, act in the late portion of the distal convoluted tubule and collecting tubule. Here, they inhibit the action of aldosterone, leading to sodium excretion and potassium retention. Although triamterene and amiloride act at the same site, they do not affect aldosterone. Instead, these products directly block the exchange of sodium and potassium, leading to decreased sodium reabsorption and decreased potassium excretion.

4. Osmotic diuretics, such as mannitol, work in the proximal convoluted tubule. As their name implies, these diuretics increase the osmotic pressure of the glomerular filtrate, inhibiting the passive reabsorption of water, sodium, and chloride. (From Gutierrez K: *Pharmacotherapeutics: Clinical Decision Making in Nursing*, Philadelphia, 1999, Saunders.)

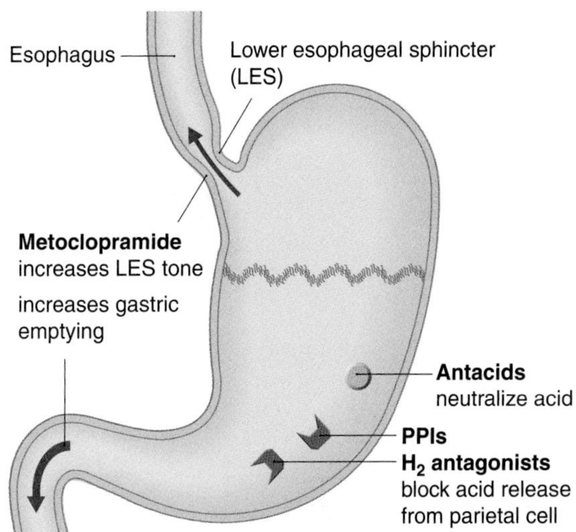

Plate 11: Sites of Action – Drugs Used to Treat GERD

Gastroesophageal reflux disease (GERD) occurs when acidic stomach contents regurgitate into the esophagus, causing heartburn. The disorder may result from a weakness or incompetence of the lower esophageal sphincter (LES). Because the malfunctioning LES makes the reflux leave the stomach and reenter the esophagus slowly, the esophageal mucosa is exposed to the acid for a long time. Because the enzymatic action of parietal cells in the stomach makes the reflux highly acidic, GERD causes irritation and possible erosion of the esophageal mucosa.

Treatment of GERD can employ drugs from several classes: histamine (H_2) antagonists, proton pump inhibitors (PPIs), the miscellaneous GI agent metoclopramide, and antacids. H_2 antagonists, such as cimetidine, act in parietal cells of the stomach. Normally, H_2-receptor stimulation results in gastric acid secretion. By blocking these receptors, H_2 antagonists decrease the amount and acidity of gastric secretion, including secretion that occurs with fasting, food consumption at night, and stomach distention.

PPIs, such as esomeprazole, also suppress gastric acid secretion. However, they do it by inhibiting the hydrogen-potassium-adenosine triphosphatase enzyme system, which is located on the surface of parietal cells and controls their gastric acid secretion. PPIs block acid secretion that results from fasting or abdominal distention caused by food ingestion.

Metoclopramide increases the tone and motility of the upper GI tract. It works by stimulating the release of acetylcholine from GI nerve endings, which improves LES tone and leads to decreased reflux. The drug also stimulates gastric emptying, which reduces gastric contents.

Antacids, such as aluminum hydroxide, act primarily in the stomach by chemically combining with the hydrogen ions (H^+) in gastric acid and raising the pH of gastric contents. They do not prevent reflux. However, they make the reflux less acidic, so it causes less damage to the esophageal mucosa. (From Page C, et al: *Integrated Pharmacology*, ed 2, St. Louis, 2002, Mosby.)

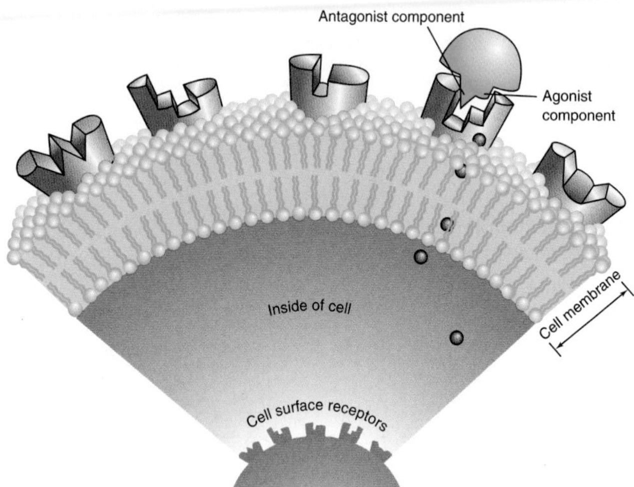

Plate 12: Mechanisms of Action – Narcotic Agonist-Antagonist Analgesics Cell membranes have different types of opioid receptors, such as mu, kappa, and delta receptors. Opioid agonist-antagonists work by stimulating one type of receptor, while simultaneously blocking another type. As agonists, they work primarily by activating kappa receptors to produce analgesia and such other effects as CNS and respiratory depression, decreased GI motility, and euphoria. As antagonists, they compete with opioids at mu receptors, helping to reverse or block some of the other effects of agonists. (From Gutierrez K: *Pharmacotherapeutics: Clinical Decision Making in Nursing*, Philadelphia, 1999, Saunders.)

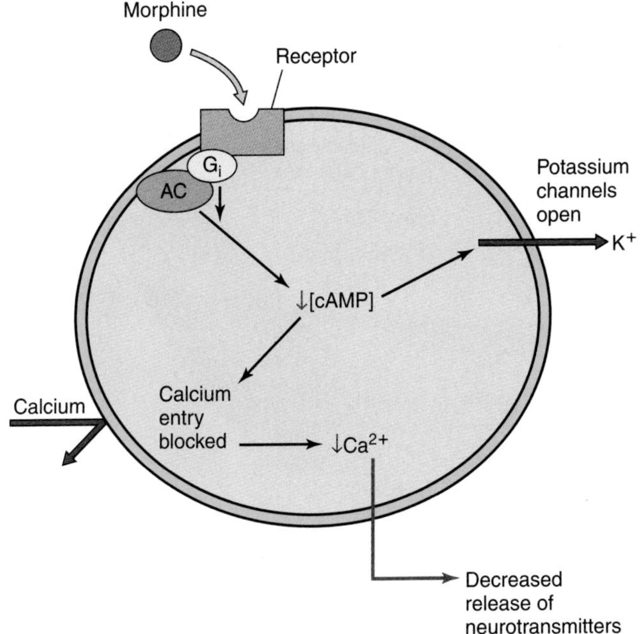

Plate 13: Mechanisms of Action – Narcotic Analgesics
Narcotic analgesics bind to three types of opioid receptors: mu, kappa, and delta receptors. They produce analgesia primarily by activating mu receptors. However, they also engage with and activate kappa and delta receptors, producing other effects, such as sedation and vasomotor stimulation.

When morphine or another narcotic analgesic binds to opioid receptors, activation occurs. The receptors send signals to the enzyme adenyl cyclase (AC) to slow activity by way of G proteins (G_i). Decreased adenyl cyclase activity causes less cyclic adenosine monophosphate (cAMP) to be produced. A secondary messenger substance, cAMP is important for regulating cell membrane channels. A reduced cAMP level allows fewer potassium ions to leave the cell and blocks calcium ions from entering the cell. This ion imbalance—especially the reduced intracellular calcium level—ultimately decreases the release of neurotransmitters from the cell, thereby blocking or reducing pain impulse transmission. (From Brody TM, Larner J, Minneman KP: *Human Pharmacology: Molecular to Clinical*, ed 3, St. Louis, 1998, Mosby.)

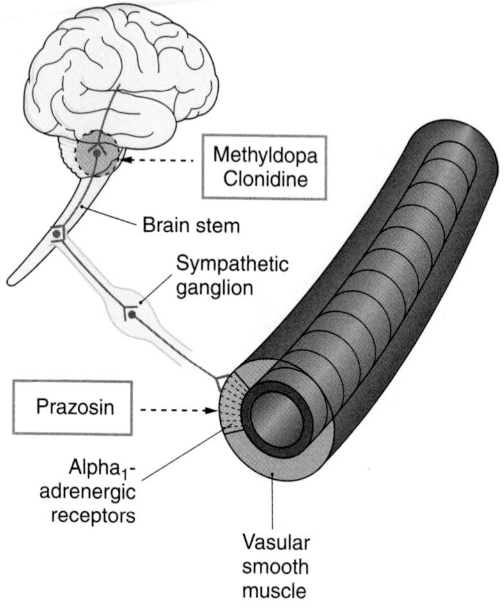

Plate 14: Sites of Action – Sympatholytics
Sympatholytics inhibit sympathetic nervous system (SNS) activity, which plays a major role in regulating BP. Normally when the SNS is stimulated, nerve impulses travel from the cardiovascular center of the CNS to the sympathetic ganglia. From there, the impulses travel along postganglionic fibers to specific effector organs, such as the heart and blood vessels. SNS stimulation also triggers the release of norepinephrine, which acts primarily at alpha-adrenergic receptors.

Sympatholytics fall into two subclasses: central-acting alpha$_2$ agonists and peripheral-acting alpha$_1$-adrenergic antagonists. Central-acting alpha$_2$ agonists, such as methyldopa and clonidine, stimulate alpha$_2$-adrenergic receptors in the cardiovascular center of the CNS and reduce activity in the vasomotor center of the brain, interfering with sympathetic stimulation of the heart and blood vessels. This causes blood vessel dilation and decreased cardiac output, which leads to reduced B/P.

Peripheral-acting alpha$_1$-adrenergic antagonists, such as prazosin, inhibit the stimulation of alpha$_1$-adrenergic receptors by norepinephrine in vascular smooth muscle, interfering with SNS-induced vasoconstriction. As a result, the blood vessels dilate, reducing peripheral vascular resistance and venous return to the heart. These effects, in turn, lead to decreased B/P. (From Prosser S, Worster B, Dewar K: *Applied Pharmacology for Nurses and Other Health Care Professionals*, St. Louis, 2000, Mosby.)

Recommended 2010 United States Immunization Schedule for Persons Aged 0 Through 6 Years

Vaccine ▼ Age ▶	Birth	1 month	2 months	4 months	6 months	12 months	15 months	18 months	19–23 months	2–3 years	4–6 years
Hepatitis B*	HepB	HepB				HepB					
Rotavirus*			RV	RV	RV*						
Diphtheria, Tetanus, Pertussis*			DTaP	DTaP	DTaP	*	DTaP				DTaP
Haemophilus influenzae type b*			Hib	Hib	Hib*	Hib					
Pneumococcal*			PCV	PCV	PCV	PCV				PPSV	
Inactivated Poliovirus*			IPV	IPV		IPV					IPV
Influenza*								Influenza (Yearly)			
Measles, Mumps, Rubella*						MMR			*		MMR
Varicella*						Varicella			*		Varicella
Hepatitis A*							HepA (2 doses)			HepA Series	
Meningococcal*										MCV	

Light shading: Range of recommended ages for all children except certain high-risk groups

Dark shading: Range of recommended ages for certain high-risk groups

This schedule includes recommendations in effect as of December 15, 2009. Any dose not administered at the recommended age should be administered at a subsequent visit, when indicated and feasible. The use of a combination vaccine generally is preferred over separate injections of its equivalent component vaccines. Considerations should include provider assessment, patient preference, and the potential for adverse events. Providers should consult the relevant Advisory Committee on Immunization Practices statement for detailed recommendations: **http://www.cdc.gov/vaccines/pubs/acip-list.htm**. Clinically significant adverse events that follow immunization should be reported to the Vaccine Adverse Event Reporting System (VAERS) at **http://www.vaers.hhs.gov** or by telephone, **800-822-7967.**

*For complete information go to **http://www.cdc.gov/vaccines/recs/schedules/child-schedule.htm.**

Recommended 2010 United States Immunization Schedule for Persons Aged 7 Through 18 Years

Vaccine ▼ Age ▶	7–10 years	11–12 years	13–18 years
Tetanus, Diphtheria, Pertussis*		Tdap	Tdap
Human Papillomavirus*	*	HPV (3 doses)	HPV series
Meningococcal*	MCV	MCV	MCV
Influenza*	Influenza (Yearly)		
Pneumococcal*	PPSV		
Hepatitis A*	HepA Series		
Hepatitis B*	Hep B Series		
Inactivated Poliovirus*	IPV Series		
Measles, Mumps, Rubella*	MMR Series		
Varicella*	Varicella Series		

Range of recommended ages for all children except certain high-risk groups

Range of recommended ages for catch-up immunization

Range of recommended ages for certain high-risk groups

This schedule includes recommendations in effect as of December 15, 2009. Any dose not administered at the recommended age should be administered at a subsequent visit, when indicated and feasible. The use of a combination vaccine generally is preferred over separate injections of its equivalent component vaccines. Considerations should include provider assessment, patient preference, and the potential for adverse events. Providers should consult the relevant Advisory Committee on Immunization Practices statement for detailed recommendations: **http://www.cdc.gov/vaccines/pubs/acip-list.htm.** Clinically significant adverse events that follow immunization should be reported to the Vaccine Adverse Event Reporting System (VAERS) at **http://www.vaers.hhs.gov** or by telephone, **800-822-7967.**

*For complete information go to **http://www.cdc.gov/vaccines/recs/schedules/child-schedule.htm**.

abacavir (℞)
(ah-bak'ah-veer)
Ziagen
Func. class.: Antiretroviral
Chem. class.: Nucleoside reverse transcriptase inhibitor (NRTI)

Action: A synthetic nucleoside analog with inhibitory action against HIV-1; inhibits replication of the virus by incorporating into cellular DNA by viral reverse transcriptase, thereby terminating the cellular DNA chain

Uses: In combination with other antiretroviral agents for HIV-1 infection (not to be used with lamivudine or tenofovir)

Unlabeled uses: HIV prophylaxis following occupational exposure

DOSAGE AND ROUTES

- *Adult:* **PO** 300 mg bid or 600 mg/day with other antiretrovirals
- *Adolescents and child ≥3 mo:* **PO** 8 mg/kg bid, max 300 mg bid with other antiretrovirals

Hepatic dose

- *Adult:* **PO** (Child-Pugh 5-6) (oral sol) 200 mg bid

HIV prophylaxis (unlabeled)

- *Adult:* **PO** 300 mg bid to be added to the basic 2-drug regimen ×4wk

Available forms: Tabs 300 mg; oral sol 20 mg/ml

SIDE EFFECTS

CNS: Fever, headache, malaise, insomnia, paresthesia

GI: Nausea, vomiting, diarrhea, anorexia, cramps, abdominal pain, increased AST, ALT, **hepatotoxicity**

HEMA: **Granulocytopenia, anemia, lymphopenia**

INTEG: Rash, urticaria, hypersensitivity reactions

META: **Lactic acidosis**

OTHER: Increased CPK, **fatal hypersensitivity reactions**

RESP: Dyspnea

Contraindications:

Black Box Warning: Hypersensitivity, lactic acidosis, moderate severe hepatic disease

Precautions: Pregnancy (C), breastfeeding, children <3 mo, granulocyte count <1000/mm^3 or Hgb <9.5 g/dl, severe renal disease, impaired hepatic function

PHARMACOKINETICS

Rapid/extensive absorption, distributed to extravascular space then erythrocytes; 50% plasma protein binding; extensively metabolized to inactive metabolites; half-life 1½ hr; excreted in urine, feces (unchanged)

INTERACTIONS

Increase: possible lactic acidosis—ribavirin

Increase: abacavir levels—alcohol

Decrease: abacavir levels—tipranavir

Decrease: levels of methadose

Drug/Lab Test

Increase: glucose, triglycerides

NURSING CONSIDERATIONS

Assess:

- For symptoms of HIV and for possible infections; increased temp

⚠ For lactic acidosis (elevated lactate levels, increased LFTs), severe hepatomegaly with steatosis, discontinue treatment and do not restart; may have large liver, elevated AST, ALT, lactate levels

⚠ For fatal hypersensitivity reactions: fever, rash, nausea, vomiting, fatigue, cough, dyspnea, diarrhea, abdominal discomfort; treatment should be discontinued and not restarted

- For blood dyscrasias (anemia, granulocytopenia): bruising, fatigue, bleeding, poor healing
- Renal studies: BUN, serum uric acid, CCr before, during therapy; these may be elevated throughout treatment
- Hepatic studies before and during therapy: bilirubin, AST, ALT, amylase, alk phos, creatine phosphokinase, creatinine, q mo

• Blood counts q2wk; monitor viral load and CD4 counts during treatment; watch for decreasing granulocytes, Hgb; if low, therapy may have to be discontinued and restarted after hematologic recovery; blood transfusions may be required

Administer:

• Give in combination with other antiretrovirals with or without food

• Reduce dose in hepatic disease, use oral sol

Perform/provide:

• Storage in cool environment; protect from light; oral sol stored at room temperature; do not freeze

Evaluate:

• Therapeutic response: increased CD4 count, decrease viral load

Teach patient/family:

• That product is not a cure but will control symptoms; patient is still infective, may pass AIDS virus on to others

• To notify prescriber of sore throat, swollen lymph nodes, malaise, fever; other infections may occur; to stop product if skin rash, fever, cough, shortness of breath, GI symptoms, notify prescriber immediately; advise all health care providers that allergic reaction has occurred with abacavir

• That follow-up visits must be continued since serious toxicity may occur; blood counts must be done

• To use contraception during treatment

• Give patient Medication Guide and Warning Card, discuss points on guide

• That other products may be necessary to prevent other infections

• Do not drink alcohol while taking this product

abatacept (℞)

(ab-a-ta′sept)

Orencia

Func. class.: Antirheumatic agent (disease modifying); biologic response modifier

Action: A selective costimulation modulator, inhibits T-lymphocytes, inhibits tumor necrosis factor (TNF-α), interferon-γ, interleukin-2, which are involved in immune and inflammatory reactions

Uses: Polyarticular juvenile rheumatoid arthritis; acute, chronic rheumatoid arthritis that has not responded to other disease-modifying agents, may use in combination with DMARDs; do not use with TNF antagonists (adalimumab, etanercept, infliximab), anakinra

DOSAGE AND ROUTES

• Give at 2, 4 wk after first inf, then q4wk

• *Adult >100 kg:* **IV INF** 1 g

• *Adult 60-100 kg:* **IV INF** 750 mg

• *Adult <60 kg:* **IV INF** 500 mg

Juvenile rheumatoid arthritis (JRA)/juvenile idiopathic arthritis (JIA)

• *Child ≥6 yr/adolescent >100 kg:* **IV INF** 1000 mg over 30 min q2wk × 2 doses, then 1000 mg over 30 min q4wk starting at wk 8

• *Child ≥6 yr/adolescent >75 kg:* **IV INF** 750 mg over 30 min q2wk × 2 doses, then 750 mg over 30 min q4wk starting at wk 8

Available forms: Lyophilized powder, single use vials 250 mg

SIDE EFFECTS

CNS: Headache, asthenia, dizziness

CV: Hypo/hypertension

GI: Abdominal pain, dyspepsia, nausea

INTEG: Rash, *inj site reaction,* flushing, urticaria, pruritus

RESP: Pharyngitis, cough, URI, non-URI, *rhinitis,* wheezing

SYST: **Anaphylaxis, malignancies, angioedema**

Contraindications: Hypersensitivity, TB, viral hepatitis

Precautions: Pregnancy (C), breastfeeding, children, geriatric patients, recurrent infections, COPD

PHARMACOKINETICS

Terminal half-life 13-16 days, steady state 60 days

INTERACTIONS

• Do not give concurrently with vaccines; immunizations should be brought up to date before treatment
• Do not use with TNF antagonists: (adalimumab, etanercept, infliximab); anakinra
• Do not use with corticosteroids, immunosuppressives

NURSING CONSIDERATIONS

Assess:

• For latent/active TB, viral hepatitis before beginning treatment
• Pain, stiffness, ROM, swelling of joints during treatment
• For inj site pain, swelling
• Patient's overall health on each visit; product should not be given with active infections

Administer:

• To reconstitute, remove plastic flip top from vial and wipe the top with alcohol wipe; insert syringe needle into vial and direct stream of sterile water for inj on the wall of vial; rotate vial until mixed; vent with needle to rid foam after reconstitution 25 mg/ml; further dilute in 100 ml from a 100-ml inf bag/bottle; withdraw the needed volume (2 vials remove 20 mg; 3 vials remove 30 ml, 4 vials remove 40 ml); slowly add the reconstituted Orencia sol from each vial into the inf bag/bottle using the same disposable syringe supplied; mix gently, discard unused portions of vials; do not use if particulate is present or discolored; give over 30 min; use non–protein binding filter (0.2-1.2 mcg)
• Do not admix with other sol or medications

Perform/provide:

• Storage in refrigerator; do not use expired vials

Evaluate:

• Therapeutic response: decreased inflammation, pain in joints

Teach patient/family:

• That product must be continued for prescribed time to be effective
• To use caution when driving; dizziness may occur
• Not to have vaccinations while taking this product
• Regarding patient information included in packaging

Rarely Used ⚠ High Alert

abciximab (℞)

(ab-six′i-mab)
ReoPro
Func. class.: Platelet aggregation inhibitor

Uses: Used with heparin and aspirin to prevent acute cardiac ischemia following percutaneous transluminal coronary angioplasty (PTCA) in patients at high risk for reclosure of affected arteries
Unlabeled uses: Acute MI, Kawasaki disease (child)

DOSAGE AND ROUTES

Percutaneous coronary intervention (PCI)

• *Adult:* **IV BOL** 250 mcg (0.25 mg)/kg 10-60 min prior to PCI, followed by 0.125 mcg/kg/min **CONT INF** for 12 hr

MI

• *Adult:* **IV BOL** 0.25 mg/kg over 5 min, then 0.125 mcg/kg/min, max 10 mcg/min; **IV INF** for 12 hr unless complications

Contraindications: Hypersensitivity to this product or murine protein; GI, GU bleeding; CVA within 2 yr, bleeding disorders, intracranial neoplasm, intracranial arteriovenous malformations, intracranial aneurysm, platelet count <100,000/mm^3, recent surgery, aneurysm, uncontrolled severe hypertension, vasculitis, coagulopathy

Rarely Used

abobotulinumtoxinA

(ay-boh-bot'yoo-li-num-tox'in-A)

Dysport

Func. class.: Skeletal muscle relaxant

Uses: Cervical dystonia, facial wrinkles

DOSAGE AND ROUTES

Cervical dystonia

• *Adult:* **IM** 500 units divided among affected muscles and repeated q12wk or longer

Facial wrinkles

• *Adult <65 yr:* **IM** 50 units administered in 5 equal aliquots of 10 units each, may last up to 4 months

Contraindications: Hypersensitivity to this product or bovine products, infection

acarbose (℞)

(ay-car'bose)

Precose

Func. class.: Oral antidiabetic

Chem. class.: α-Glucosidase inhibitor

Do not confuse:

Precose/preCare

Action: Delays digestion/absorption of ingested carbohydrates by inhibiting α glucosidase, results in smaller rise in postprandial blood glucose after meals; does not increase insulin production

Uses: Type 2 diabetes mellitus, alone or in combination with a sulfonylurea, metformin

Unlabeled uses: Adjunct in type 1 diabetes mellitus

DOSAGE AND ROUTES

• *Adult >60 kg:* **PO** 25 mg tid initially, with first bite of meal; maintenance dose may be increased to 50-100 mg tid; dosage adjustment at 4-8 wk intervals

• *Adult <60 kg:* **PO** max 50 mg tid

Type 1 diabetes mellitus (unlabeled)

• *Adult:* **PO** 50 mg tid with meals × 2 wk, then 100 mg tid with meals

Available forms: Tabs 25, 50, 100 mg

SIDE EFFECTS

GI: Abdominal pain, diarrhea, flatulence, increased serum transaminase level

Contraindications: Breastfeeding, hypersensitivity, diabetic ketoacidosis, cirrhosis, inflammatory bowel disease, ileus, colonic ulceration, partial intestinal obstruction, chronic intestinal disease, serum creatinine >2 mg/dl

Precautions: Pregnancy (B), children, renal/hepatic disease

PHARMACOKINETICS

Poor systemic absorption, peak 1 hr, metabolized in GI tract, excreted as intact product in urine, half-life 2 hr

INTERACTIONS

Increase: hypoglycemia—sulfonylureas, insulin

Decrease: effect, increase hyperglycemia—digestive enzymes, intestinal absorbents, thiazide diuretics, loop diuretics, corticosteroids, estrogen, progestins, oral contraceptives, sympathomimetics, calcium channel blockers, isoniazid, phenothiazines, digoxin

Drug/Herb

Increase: hypoglycemia—alfalfa, aloe, basil, bay, bilberry, bitter melon, black cohosh, buchu, burdock, chromium, coenzyme Q10, coriander, eyebright (PO), fenugreek, garlic, ginseng *(Panax),* glucomannan, glucosamine, goat's rue, gymnema, horehound, horse chestnut, jambul, myrrh, myrtle, raspberry, Siberian ginseng

Decrease: hypoglycemia—bee pollen, blue cohosh, broom, chromium, elecampane, eucalyptus, gotu kola, senega

Drug/Lab Test

Increase: AST, bilirubin

Decrease: calcium, vit B_6

NURSING CONSIDERATIONS

Assess:

- Hypoglycemia (weakness, hunger, dizziness, tremors, anxiety, tachycardia, sweating), hyperglycemia; even though product does not cause hypoglycemia, if patient is on sulfonylureas or insulin, hypoglycemia may be additive; if hypoglycemia occurs, treat with dextrose, or if severe, IV glucose or glucagon
- 1 hr postprandial glucose for establishing effectiveness, then A1c q3mo
- Monitor AST, ALT q3mo × 1 yr and periodically thereafter; if elevated, dose may need to be reduced or discontinued; obtain A1c periodically
- For stress, surgery, or other trauma that may require change in dose
- GI side effects for tolerability/compliance

Administer:

PO route

- Tid with first bite of each meal 3×/day

Perform/provide:

- Storage in tight container in cool environment

Evaluate:

- Therapeutic response: improved signs/symptoms of diabetes mellitus (decreased polyuria, polydipsia, polyphagia; clear sensorium, absence of dizziness, stable gait)

Teach patient/family:

- The symptoms of hypo/hyperglycemia, what to do about each
- That medication must be taken as prescribed; explain consequences of discontinuing medication abruptly; that insulin may need to be used for stress, including trauma, surgery, fever
- To avoid OTC medications, herbal supplements unless approved by health care provider
- That diabetes is lifelong illness; diet and exercise regimen must be followed; that this product is not a cure
- To carry emergency ID for emergency purposes; carry glucagon kit, sugar source
- That blood glucose monitoring required to assess product effect
- Not to breastfeed
- That GI side effects may occur

acebutolol (℞)

(a-se-byoo′toe-lole)

Monitan ♣, Sectral

Func. class.: Antihypertensive, antidysrhythmic (II)

Chem. class.: β_1 Blocker

Action: Competitively blocks stimulation of β-adrenergic receptors within vascular smooth muscle; decreases rate of SA node discharge, increases recovery time, slows conduction of AV node resulting in decreased heart rate (negative chronotropic effect), which decreases O_2 consumption in myocardium due to β_1-receptor antagonism; also decreases renin-aldosterone-angiotensin system at high doses, inhibits β_2-receptors in bronchial system (high doses)

Uses: Mild to moderate hypertension, management of PVCs

DOSAGE AND ROUTES

Hypertension

- *Adult:* **PO** 400 mg/day or in 2 divided doses; may be increased to desired response; maintenance 200-1200 mg/day in 2 divided doses
- *Geriatric:* **PO** Max 800 mg/day; not to exceed 800 mg/day

Ventricular dysrhythmia

- *Adult:* **PO** 200 mg bid, may increase gradually; usual range 600-1200 mg/day; should be tapered over 2 wk before discontinuing
- *Geriatric:* Not to exceed 800 mg/day

PVC management

- *Adult:* **PO** 200 mg bid, may increase gradually; usual range 600-1200 mg/day in divided doses
- *Geriatric:* Not to exceed 800 mg/day

Renal dose

- *Adult:* **PO** CCr 25-50 ml/min, reduce dose by 50%; if <25 ml/min reduce dose by 75%

Available forms: Caps 200, 400 mg; tabs 100, 200, 400 mg ♣

SIDE EFFECTS

CNS: *Insomnia, fatigue, dizziness, mental changes,* memory loss, hallucinations, depression, lethargy, drowsiness, strange dreams, catatonia, headache

CV: **Profound hypotension, bradycardia, CHF,** *cold extremities, postural hypotension,* **2nd-/3rd-degree heart block,** edema

EENT: Sore throat; dry, burning eyes

ENDO: Increased hypoglycemic response to insulin

GI: *Nausea, diarrhea,* vomiting, **mesenteric arterial thrombosis, ischemic colitis, flatulence**

GU: *Impotence,* decreased libido, dysuria, nocturia, polyuria

HEMA: **Agranulocytosis, thrombocytopenia, purpura**

INTEG: Rash, flushing, pruritus, sweating, alopecia, dry skin

MISC: Facial swelling, weight gain, decreased exercise tolerance

MS: Joint pain, cramping

RESP: **Bronchospasm,** dyspnea, wheezing, cough

Contraindications: Hypersensitivity to this agent or β-blockers; cardiogenic shock, heart block (2nd, 3rd degree), sinus bradycardia, CHF, cardiac failure

Precautions: Pregnancy (B), breastfeeding, children, major surgery, peripheral vascular disease, diabetes mellitus, COPD, asthma, well-compensated heart failure, thyroid/renal/hepatic disease

Black Box Warning: Abrupt discontinuation

PHARMACOKINETICS

Rapid absorption, onset 1-1½ hr, peak 2-4 hr, duration 10-12 hr, half-life 3-4 hr, metabolized in liver, 30%-40% excreted in urine, protein binding 10%-26%, crosses placenta, enters breast milk (small amounts)

INTERACTIONS

- Attenuated effects: oral sulfonylureas
- Peripheral ischemia: ergots

Increase: hypotension, bradycardia—reserpine, hydrALAZINE, methyldopa, prazosin, anticholinergics, cardiac glycosides, diltiazem, verapamil, diuretics, other antihypertensives, calcium channel blockers, cimetidine

Increase: hypoglycemic effect—insulin

Decrease: antihypertensive effects—NSAIDs, calcium, cholestyramine, colestipol

Decrease: bronchodilation—theophyllines, β_2-agonists

Drug/Herb

- May increase acebutolol effect—aloe, betel palm, buckthorn bark/berry, butterbur, cascara sagrada bark, cola tree, figwort, fumitory, guarana, hawthorn, lily of the valley, motherwort, plantain, rhubarb root, senna leaf/fruits
- Toxicity/death: aconite

Decrease: acebutolol effect—St. John's wort

Decrease: antihypertensive effect—coenzyme Q10, yohimbe

Drug/Lab Test

Increase: serum lipoprotein levels, BUN, potassium, triglyceride, uric acid, LDH, AST, ALT, blood glucose, alk phos

Positive: ANA titer

NURSING CONSIDERATIONS

Assess:

- B/P during beginning treatment, periodically thereafter; pulse q4hr; note rate, rhythm, quality
- Apical/radial pulse before administration; notify prescriber of any significant changes (pulse <50 bpm); signs of CHF (dyspnea, crackles, weight gain, jugular vein distention)
- Baselines in renal, hepatic studies before therapy begins
- Edema in feet, legs daily: monitor I&O
- Skin turgor, dryness of mucous membranes for hydration status, especially geriatric patient

Administer:

PO route

- Product before meals, at bedtime, tab may be crushed or swallowed whole; give with food to prevent GI upset

Perform/provide:

- Storage protected from light, moisture; place in cool environment

Evaluate:

- Therapeutic response: decreased B/P after 1-2 wk; decreased dysrhythmias

Teach patient/family:

⚠ Not to discontinue product abruptly, severe cardiac reactions may occur, taper over 2 wk; do not double dose; if a dose is missed, take as soon as remembered up to 4 hr before next dose

- Drug may mask signs of hypoglycemia or alter blood glucose levels
- Not to use OTC products containing α-adrenergic stimulants (such as nasal decongestants, OTC cold preparations) unless directed by prescriber
- To report low pulse, dizziness, confusion, depression, fever
- To take pulse, B/P at home, advise when to notify prescriber
- To comply with weight control, dietary adjustments, modified exercise program
- To carry emergency ID to identify product, allergies
- To avoid hazardous activities if dizziness, drowsiness is present
- To report symptoms of CHF: difficult breathing, especially on exertion or when lying down, night cough, swelling of extremities
- To continue with required lifestyle changes (exercise, diet, weight loss, stress reduction)

Treatment of overdose: Lavage, IV atropine for bradycardia, IV theophylline for bronchospasm, digoxin, O_2, diuretic for cardiac failure, IV glucose for hypoglycemia, IV diazepam (or phenytoin) for seizures

acetaminophen (OTC)

(a-seat-a-mee′noe-fen)

Abenol ♣, Acephen, Aceta, APAP, Apo-Acetaminophen ♣, Apra, Atasol ♣, Children's Feverall, Equaline Children's Pain Relief, Equaline Infant's Pain Relief, Exdol ♣, Genapap, Genebs, GoodSense Acetaminophen, GoodSense Children's Pain Relief, Infantaire, Leader Children's Pain Reliever, Mapap, Panadol, Q-Pap, Q-Pap Children's, Redutemp, Robigesic ♣, Rounax ♣, Silapap, T-Painol, Tylenol, Walgreen's Non-Aspirin, XS pain reliever, Walgreen's Acetaminophen

Func. class.: Nonopioid analgesic, antipyretic

Chem. class.: Nonsalicylate, paraaminophenol derivative

Action: May block pain impulses peripherally that occur in response to inhibition of prostaglandin synthesis; does not possess antiinflammatory properties; antipyretic action results from inhibition of prostaglandins in the CNS (hypothalamic heat-regulating center)

Uses: Mild to moderate pain or fever, arthralgia, dental pain, dysmenorrhea, headache, myalgia, osteoarthritis

Unlabeled uses: Migraine

DOSAGE AND ROUTES

- *Adult and child >12 yr:* **PO/RECT** 325-650 mg q4-6hr prn, max 4 g/day
- *Child 1-12 yr:* **PO** 10-15 mg/kg q4-6hr, max 5 doses/24 hr
- *Child 1-12 yr:* **RECT** 10-20 mg/kg/dose q4-6hr
- *Neonate:* **RECT** 10-15 mg/kg/dose q6-8hr

Migraine (unlabeled)

• *Adult and adolescent:* **PO** 500-1000 mg, max 1 g/dose or max 4 g/day

Available forms: Rect supp 80, 120, 125, 325, 600, 650 mg; soft chew tabs 80, 160 mg; caps 500 mg; elix 120, 160, 325 mg/5 ml; liq 160 mg/5 ml, 500 mg/15 ml; sol 100 mg/1 ml, 120 mg/2.5 ml; granules 80 mg/packet, 80 mg/cap; tabs 160, 325, 500, 650 mg

SIDE EFFECTS

CNS: Stimulation, drowsiness

GI: Nausea, vomiting, abdominal pain; **hepatotoxicity, hepatic seizure (overdose), GI bleeding**

GU: **Renal failure (high, prolonged doses)**

HEMA: **Leukopenia, neutropenia, hemolytic anemia (long-term use), thrombocytopenia, pancytopenia**

INTEG: Rash, urticaria

SYST: Hypersensitivity

TOXICITY: **Cyanosis, anemia, neutropenia, jaundice, pancytopenia, CNS stimulation, delirium followed by vascular collapse, seizures, coma, death**

Contraindications: Hypersensitivity, intolerance to tartrazine (yellow dye #5), alcohol, table sugar, saccharin, depending on product

Precautions: Pregnancy (B), breastfeeding, geriatric patients, anemia, renal/hepatic disease, chronic alcoholism

PHARMACOKINETICS

85%-90% metabolized by liver, excreted by kidneys; metabolites may be toxic if overdose occurs; widely distributed; crosses placenta in low concentrations; excreted in breast milk; half-life 1-4 hr

PO: Onset 10-30 min, peak ½-2 hr, duration 4-6 hr, well absorbed

RECT: Onset slow, peak 1-2 hr, duration 4-6 hr, absorption varies

INTERACTIONS

• Hypoprothrombinemia: warfarin, long-term use, high doses of acetaminophen

• Bone marrow suppression: zidovudine

• Renal adverse reactions: NSAIDs, salicylates

Decrease: effect, increase hepatotoxicity—barbiturates, alcohol, carbamazepine, hydantoins, rifampin, rifabutin, isoniazid, diflunisal, sulfinpyrazone

Decrease: absorption—colestipol, cholestyramine

Drug/Herb

Decrease: acetaminophen effect—St. John's wort

Drug/Lab Test

Interference: chemstrip G, Dextrostix, Visidex II, 5-HIAA

NURSING CONSIDERATIONS

Assess:

• Hepatic studies: AST, ALT, bilirubin, creatinine prior to therapy if long-term therapy is anticipated; may cause hepatic toxicity at doses >4 g/day with chronic use

• Renal studies: BUN, urine creatinine, occult blood, albumin, if patient is on long-term therapy; presence of blood or albumin indicates nephritis

• Blood studies: CBC, PT if patient is on long-term therapy

• I&O ratio; decreasing output may indicate renal failure (long-term therapy)

• For fever and pain: type of pain, location, intensity, duration

• For chronic poisoning: rapid, weak pulse; dyspnea; cold, clammy extremities; report immediately to prescriber

• Hepatotoxicity: dark urine; clay-colored stools; yellowing of skin, sclera; itching, abdominal pain; fever; diarrhea if patient is on long-term therapy

• Allergic reactions: rash, urticaria; if these occur, product may have to be discontinued

Administer:

PO route

• Crushed or whole; chewable tabs may be chewed; give with full glass of water

• With food or milk to decrease gastric symptoms if needed

• Suspension after shaken well

Perform/provide:

- Storage of suppositories <80° F (27° C)

Evaluate:

- Therapeutic response: absence of pain using pain scoring; fever

Teach patient/family:

⚠ Not to exceed recommended dosage; acute poisoning with liver damage may result

⚠ That acute toxicity includes symptoms of nausea, vomiting, abdominal pain; prescriber should be notified immediately

- That toxicity may occur when used with other combination products
- Not to use with alcohol, herbals without approval of prescriber
- To recognize signs of chronic overdose: bleeding, bruising, malaise, fever, sore throat
- To notify prescriber of pain or fever lasting over 3 days

Treatment of overdose: Product level, gastric lavage, activated charcoal; administer oral acetylcysteine to prevent hepatic damage *(see acetylcysteine monograph)*, monitor for bleeding

*acetaZOLAMIDE (℞)

(a-set-a-zole'a-mide)

acetaZOLAMIDE, Apo-Acetazolamide ♣, Dazamide, Diamox, Diamox Sequels

Func. class.: Diuretic, carbonic anhydrase inhibitor, antiglaucoma agent, antiepileptic

Chem. class.: Sulfonamide derivative

Do not confuse:

acetaZOLAMIDE/acetoHEXAMIDE

Diamox/Trimox/Dobutrex

Action: Inhibits carbonic anhydrase activity in proximal renal tubules to decrease reabsorption of water, sodium, potassium, bicarbonate resulting in increased urine volume and alkalinization of urine; decreases carbonic anhydrase in CNS, increasing seizure threshold; able to decrease secretion of aqueous humor in eye, which lowers intraocular pressure

Uses: Open-angle glaucoma, closed-angle glaucoma (preoperatively, if surgery delayed), epilepsy (petit mal, grand mal, mixed), edema in CHF, product-induced edema, acute altitude sickness

Unlabeled uses: Urine alkalinization, metabolic alkalosis in mechanical ventilation, decrease CSF production in infants with hydrocephalus, familial periodic paralysis, nystagmus

DOSAGE AND ROUTES

Closed-angle glaucoma

- *Adult:* **PO/IV** 250 mg q4hr or 250 mg bid, to be used for short-term therapy

Open-angle glaucoma

- *Adult:* **PO/IV** 250 mg-1 g/day in divided doses for amounts over 250 mg or 500 mg SR bid

Edema in CHF

- *Adult:* **IV** 250-375 mg/day in AM
- *Child:* **IV** 5 mg/kg/day in AM

Seizures

- *Adult:* **PO/IV** 8-30 mg/kg/day, in 1-4 divided doses, usual range 375-1000 mg/day; **ER** not recommended in seizures
- *Child:* **PO/IV** 8-30 mg/kg/day in divided doses tid or qid, or 300-900 mg/m^2/day, not to exceed 1 g/day

Altitude sickness

- *Adult:* **PO** 250 mg q8-12hr; **EXT REL** 500 mg q12-24hr, start therapy 24-48hr prior to ascent and for ≥48 hr after arrival at high altitude

Renal dose

- *Adult:* **PO/IV** CCr 10-50 ml/min give dose q12hr; CCr <10 ml/min, avoid use
- *Geriatric:* **PO** 250 mg bid, use lowest effective dose

Infants with hydrocephalus (unlabeled)

- *Infant:* **PO/IV** 5 mg/kg q6hr, may increase by 25 mg/kg/day; max 100 mg/kg/day

Urine alkalinization (unlabeled)

- *Adult:* **PO** 5 mg/kg/dose, repeat 2-3× over 24 hr

Familial periodic paralysis (unlabeled)
- *Adult:* **PO** 250-375 mg/day in divided doses

Metabolic alkalosis in mechanical ventilation (unlabeled)
- *Adult:* **IV** 500 mg as a single dose or 250 mg q6hr × 4 doses

Vestibular nystagmus (unlabeled)
- *Adult:* **PO** 250 mg, increase by 250 mg q3days; max 3 g/day in divided doses

Available forms: Tabs 125, 250 mg; ext rel caps 500 mg; inj 500 mg

SIDE EFFECTS

CNS: Anxiety, confusion, **seizures,** depression, dizziness, *drowsiness,* fatigue, headache, *paresthesia,* stimulation
EENT: Myopia, tinnitus
ENDO: Hyperglycemia
GI: Nausea, vomiting, anorexia, diarrhea, melena, weight loss, **hepatic insufficiency, cholestatic jaundice, fulminant hepatic necrosis,** *taste alterations,* **bleeding**
GU: Frequency, polyuria, **uremia,** glucosuria, hematuria, dysuria, crystalluria, renal calculi
HEMA: **Aplastic anemia, hemolytic anemia, leukopenia, thrombocytopenia, purpura, pancytopenia**
INTEG: Rash, pruritus, urticaria, fever, **Stevens-Johnson syndrome,** photosensitivity, flushing
META: Hypokalemia, hyperchloremic acidosis, hyponatremia, sulfonamide-like reactions

Contraindications: Hypersensitivity to sulfonamides, severe renal/hepatic disease, electrolyte imbalances (hyponatremia, hypokalemia), hyperchloremic acidosis, Addison's disease, long-term use in closed-angle glaucoma, adrenalcortical insufficiency

Precautions: Pregnancy (C), breastfeeding, hypercalciuria, respiratory acidosis, COPD

PHARMACOKINETICS

65% absorbed if fasting (oral), 75% absorbed if given with food; half-life 2½-5½ hr; excreted unchanged by kidneys (80% within 24 hr), crosses placenta
PO: Onset 1-1½ hr, peak 2-4 hr, duration 8-12 hr
PO-SUS REL: Onset 2 hr, peak 3-6 hr, duration 18-24 hr
IV: Onset 2 min, peak 15 min, duration 4-5 hr

INTERACTIONS

Increase: action of amphetamines, flecainide, memantine, phenytoin, procainamide, quinidine, anticholinergics
Increase: excretion of lithium, primidone
Increase: toxicity—salicylates, cycloSPORINE
Increase: side effects—diflunisal
Decrease: acetaZOLAMIDE effect—methenamine
Decrease: primidone levels

Drug/Lab Test
Decrease: thyroid iodine uptake
False positive: urinary protein, 17 hydroxysteroid

NURSING CONSIDERATIONS

Assess:
- Weight daily, I&O daily to determine fluid loss; effect of product may be decreased if used daily; monitor geriatric patients for dehydration
- For cross-sensitivity between other sulfonamides and this product
- B/P lying, standing; postural hypotension may occur
- Electrolytes: K, Na, Cl; also BUN, blood glucose, CBC, serum creatinine, blood pH, ABGs, LFTs; I&O, glucose, patient may need to be on a high-potassium diet

Administer:
- In AM to avoid interference with sleep if using product as diuretic
- Potassium replacement if potassium level is <3 mg/dl

PO route

- Do not break, crush, or chew sus rel caps
- With food if nausea occurs; absorption may be decreased slightly

IV route

- After diluting 500 mg in >5 ml sterile H_2O for injection; direct IV—give at 100-500 mg/min; may be diluted further in LR, D_5W, $D_{10}W$, 0.45% NaCl, 0.9% NaCl, or Ringer's sol and infused over 4-8 hr; use within 24 hr of dilution

Additive compatibilities: Cimetidine, ranitidine

Perform/provide:

- Storage in dark, cool area; use reconstituted solution within 24 hr

Evaluate:

- Therapeutic response: improvement in edema of feet, legs, sacral area daily if medication is being used in CHF; or decrease in aqueous humor if medication is being used in glaucoma

Teach patient/family:

- To take exactly as prescribed; if dose is missed, take as soon as remembered; do not double dose
- To notify prescriber if sore throat, unusual bleeding, bruising, paresthesias, tremors, flank pain, or skin rash occurs
- To use sunscreen to prevent photosensitivity; to monitor blood glucose and urine for sugar
- To avoid hazardous activities if drowsiness occurs
- Increase fluids to 2-3 L/day if not contraindicated
- Report nausea, vertigo, rapid weight gain, change in stools

Treatment of overdose: Lavage if taken orally; monitor electrolytes; administer dextrose in saline; monitor hydration, CV, renal status

acetylcholine ophthalmic

See Appendix B

acetylcysteine (℞)

(a-se-teel-sis′tay-een)

Acetadote, Mucomyst ✦, Parvolex ✦

Func. class.: Mucolytic; antidote—acetaminophen

Chem. class.: Amino acid L-cysteine

Action: Decreases viscosity of secretions by breaking disulfide links of mucoproteins; serves as a substrate in place of glutathione, which is necessary to inactivate toxic metabolites in acetaminophen overdose

Uses: Acetaminophen toxicity; bronchitis; cystic fibrosis; COPD; atelectasis

Unlabeled uses: Prevention of contrast medium nephrotoxicity, distal intestinal obstruction, giant papillary conjunctivitis (GPC)

DOSAGE AND ROUTES

Mucolytic

- *Adult and child:* **INSTILL** 1-20 ml (10%-20% sol) q2-6hr prn or 3-5 ml (20% sol) or 6-10 ml (10% sol) tid or qid; nebulization (face mask, mouthpiece, tracheostomy) 1-10 ml of a 20% sol, or 2-20 ml of a 10% sol, q2-6hr; nebulization (tent, croupette) may require large dose, up to 300 ml/treatment

Acetaminophen toxicity

- *Adult and child:* **PO** 140 mg/kg, then 70 mg/kg q4hr × 17 doses to total of 1330 mg/kg; **IV** loading dose 150 mg/kg over 60 min (dilution 150 mg/kg in 200 ml of D_5); maintenance dose 1: 50 mg/kg over 4 hr (dilution 50 mg/kg in 500 ml D_5): maintenance dose 2: 100 mg/kg over 16 hr (dilution 100 mg/kg in 1000 ml D_5)

Nephrotoxicity prophylaxis (unlabeled)

- *Adult:* **PO** 600 mg bid, given day prior to and day of administration of contrast media or in acute MI, **IV** BOL 1200 mg before contrast medium and 1200 mg **PO** bid × 48 hr

Giant papillary conjunctivitis (GPC) (unlabeled)

• *Adult:* **OPHTHALMIC** 1%-2% sol prepared by mixing in artificial tears, administer topically 4-6 ×/day

Meconium ileus (unlabeled)

• *Child:* **PO/RECT** 5-30 ml of 10% sol, 3-6 ×/day

Available forms: Oral sol 10%, 20%; inj 20% (200 mg/ml)

SIDE EFFECTS

CNS: *Dizziness, drowsiness,* headache, fever, chills

CV: Hypotension, flushing tachycardia

EENT: *Rhinorrhea,* tooth damage

GI: *Nausea,* stomatitis, constipation, vomiting, anorexia, **hepatotoxicity,** diarrhea

INTEG: Urticaria, rash, fever, clamminess, pruritus

RESP: **Bronchospasm,** burning, **hemoptysis,** chest tightness, cough

Contraindications: Hypersensitivity, increased intracranial pressure, status asthmaticus

Precautions: Pregnancy (B), breastfeeding, hypothyroidism, Addison's disease, CNS depression, brain tumor, asthma, renal/hepatic disease, COPD, psychosis, alcoholism, seizure disorders, bronchospasms, asthma, anaphylactoid reactions, fluid restriction, weight <40 kg

PHARMACOKINETICS

INH/INSTILL: Onset 5-10 min, duration 1 hr, metabolized by liver, excreted in urine, half-life 5.6 hr (adult), 11 hr (newborn)

IV: Protein binding 83%

INTERACTIONS

• Do not use with iron, copper, rubber

• Do not mix with antibiotics: tetracycline, chlortetracycline, oxytetracycline, erythromycin lactobionate, amphotericin B, sodium ampicillin; iodized oil, chymotrypsin, trypsin, hydrogen peroxide

Increase: effect—nitrates

NURSING CONSIDERATIONS

Assess:

• Cough: type, frequency, character, including sputum

• Rate, rhythm of respirations, increased dyspnea; sputum; discontinue if bronchospasm occurs

• VS, cardiac status including checking for dysrhythmias, increased rate, palpitations

• ABGs for increased CO_2 retention in asthma patients

• Antidotal use: LFTs, PT, BUN, glucose, electrolytes, acetaminophen levels; inform prescriber if dose is vomited or vomiting is persistent

• Nausea, vomiting, rash; notify prescriber if these occur

Administer:

PO route

• Antidotal use: give within 24 hr; give with cola or soft drink to disguise taste; can be given with H_2O through tubes; use within 1 hr

Direct intratracheal instill route

• By syringe 1-2 ml of 10%-20% up to q1hr

• Decreased dose to geriatric patients; their metabolisms may be slowed

• Only if suction machine is available

• Before meals ½-1 hr for better absorption, to decrease nausea

• 20% solutions diluted with NS or water for inj; may give 10% solution undiluted

• Only after patient clears airway by deep breathing, coughing

IV route

• Dilute with D_5, 0.45% NaCl

Incompatibilities: Rubber, metals, stability with other products not known

Perform/provide:

• Storage in refrigerator; use within 96 hr of opening

• Assistance with inhaled dose: bronchodilator if bronchospasm occurs

• Mechanical suction if cough insufficient to remove excess bronchial secretions

• Gum, hard candy, frequent rinsing of mouth for dryness of oral cavity

Evaluate:

- Therapeutic response: absence of purulent secretions when coughing; absence of hepatic damage in acetaminophen toxicity

Teach patient/family:

- About mucolytic use
- That unpleasant odor will decrease after repeated use
- That discoloration of solution after bottle is opened does not impair its effectiveness
- To report vomiting since dose may need to be repeated

acyclovir (℞)

(ay-sye′kloe-veer)

Avirax ✤, Zovirax

Func. class.: Antiviral

Chem. class.: Acyclic purine nucleoside analog

Action: Interferes with DNA synthesis by conversion to acyclovir triphosphate, causing decreased viral replication, time of lesional healing

Uses: Mucocutaneous herpes simplex virus, herpes genitalis (HSV-1, HSV-2), varicella infections, herpes zoster, herpes simplex encephalitis

Unlabeled uses: Bells palsy, prevention/treatment of CMV, Epstein-Barr, esophagitis, hairy leukoplakia, prevention of herpes labialis, herpes simplex, herpes simplex ocular, keratoconjunctivitis, pharyngitis, pneumonitis, prevention of postherpetic neuralgia, proctitis, stomatitis, tracheobronchitis, varicella prophylaxis

DOSAGE AND ROUTES

Renal dose

- *Adult and child:* **PO/IV** CCr >50 ml/min 100% dose q8hr, CCr 25-50 ml/min 100% dose q12hr, CCr 10-25 ml/min 100% dose q24hr, CCr 0-10 ml/min 50% dose q24hr

Herpes simplex

- *Adult:* **PO** 200 mg q4hr
- *Adult and child >12 yr:* **IV INF** 5 mg/kg over 1 hr q8hr × 7 days
- *Child <12 yr:* **IV INF** 250 mg/m^2 or 30 mg/kg/day divided q8hr over 1 hr × 5 days
- *Neonate (unlabeled):* **IV INF** 10 mg/kg q8hr × 10 days

Genital herpes

- *Adult:* **PO** 200 mg q4hr (5×/day while awake) for 5 days to 6 mo depending on whether initial, recurrent, or chronic; **IV** 5 mg/kg q8hr × 5 days

Herpes simplex encephalitis

- *Adult:* **IV** 10 mg/kg over 1 hr q8hr × 10 days
- *Child 3 mo-12 yr:* **IV** 20 mg/kg q8hr × 10 days
- *Child birth-3 mo:* **IV** 10 mg/kg q8hr × 10 days

Herpes zoster

- *Adult:* **PO** 800 mg q4hr while awake × 7-10 days; **IV** 10 mg/kg q8hr × 7 days

Varicella-zoster

- *Adult and child >40 kg:* **PO** 800 mg qid × 5 days; **IV** (unlabeled) 20 mg/kg/day q8hr × 5 days (immunocompetent); 10 mg/kg/dose q8hr × 7-10 days (immunocompromised)
- *Child ≥2 yr, <40 kg:* **PO** 20 mg/kg qid × 5 days

Mucosal/cutaneous herpes simplex infections in immunosuppressed patients

- *Adult and child >12 yr:* **IV** 5 mg/kg q8hr × 7 days
- *Child <12:* **IV** 10 mg/kg q8hr × 7 days

Bell's palsy (unlabeled)

- *Adult:* **PO** 400-800 mg 5×/day × 7 days, given with predniSONE

Hairy leukoplakia in HIV (unlabeled)

- *Adult:* **PO** 800 mg q6hr × 20 days

CMV infection (unlabeled)

- *Adult:* **IV** 500 mg/m^2 q8hr

Herpes simplex in pneumonitis/ esophagitis/tracheobronchitis/ proctitis/stomatitis/pharyngitis (unlabeled)

• *Adult and adolescent:* **IV** 5-10 mg/kg q8hr × 2-7 days or **PO** 400 mg 3-5×/day × 10 or more days

• *Child 6 mo-12 yr:* **IV** 250-500 mg/m^2 or 5-10 mg/kg q8hr × 5-7 days

Herpes simplex prophylaxis for chronic suppression therapy (unlabeled)

• *Adult and adolescent:* **PO** 400 mg bid up to 12 mo

• *Child:* **PO** 800-1000 mg/day in 2-5 divided doses, max 80 mg/kg/day

Available forms: Caps 200 mg; inj 500 mg, oral susp, tabs 400, 800 mg

SIDE EFFECTS

CNS: Tremors, confusion, lethargy, hallucinations, **seizures,** dizziness, *headache,* encephalopathic changes

EENT: Gingival hyperplasia

GI: Nausea, vomiting, diarrhea, increased ALT, AST, abdominal pain, glossitis, colitis

GU: **Oliguria, proteinuria, hematuria,** vaginitis, moniliasis, **glomerulonephritis, acute renal failure,** changes in menses, polydipsia

HEMA: **Thrombotic thrombocytopenia purpura, hemolytic uremic syndrome** (immunocompromised patients)

INTEG: Rash, urticaria, pruritus, pain or phlebitis at IV site, unusual sweating, alopecia

MS: Joint pain, leg pain, muscle cramps

Contraindications: Hypersensitivity to this product or famciclovir, ganciclovir, penciclovir, valacyclovir, valganciclovir

Precautions: Pregnancy (B), breastfeeding, renal/hepatic disease, electrolyte imbalance, dehydration, neurologic disease

PHARMACOKINETICS

Distributed widely; crosses placenta; CSF concentrations are 50% plasma; protein binding 9%-33%

PO: Absorbed minimally, onset unknown, peak 1½-2 hr, terminal half-life 3½ hr

IV: Onset immediate, peak immediate, duration unknown, half-life 20 min-3 hr (terminal); metabolized by liver, excreted by kidneys as unchanged product (95%)

INTERACTIONS

• Synergistic effect: interferon

• CNS side effects: zidovudine

Increase: levels, toxicity—probenecid, mycophenolate

• Zoster vaccine: avoid use

NURSING CONSIDERATIONS

Assess:

• Signs of infection, anemia

⚠ Any patient with compromised renal system since product is excreted slowly in poor renal system function; toxicity may occur rapidly

• Hepatic, renal studies: AST, ALT; BUN, creatinine before and during treatment

• Blood studies: WBC, RBC, Hct, Hgb, bleeding time; blood dyscrasias may occur; product should be discontinued

• Renal studies: urinalysis, protein, BUN, creatinine, CCr, watch for increasing BUN and serum creatinine or decreased CCr, may indicate nephrotoxicity; I&O ratio; report hematuria, oliguria, fatigue, weakness; may indicate nephrotoxicity; check for protein in urine during treatment

• C&S before product therapy; product may be taken as soon as culture is taken; repeat C&S after treatment; determine the presence of other infections

• Bowel pattern before, during treatment; if severe abdominal pain with bleeding occurs, product should be discontinued

• Skin eruptions: rash, urticaria, itching

• Allergies before treatment, reaction of each medication; place allergies on chart in bright red letters

• Neurologic status in herpes encephalitis

Administer:

PO route

- Do not break, crush, or chew caps
- May give without regard to meals, with 8 oz of water
- Shake suspension before use
- Lower dose in acute or chronic renal failure

IV route

- Increased fluids to 3 L/day to decrease crystalluria
- After reconstituting with 10 ml compatible sol/500 mg of product, concentration of 50 mg/ml, shake, further dilute in 50-100 ml compatible sol; use within 12 hr; give over at least 1 hr (constant rate) by infusion pump to prevent nephrotoxicity; do not reconstitute with sol containing benzyl alcohol in neonates

Additive compatibilities: Fluconazole

Solution compatibilities: D_5W, LR, or NaCl (D_5 0.9% NaCl, 0.9% NaCl) solutions

Y-site compatibilities: Allopurinol, amikacin, ampicillin, amphotericin B, cefazolin, cefonicid, cefoperazone, cefotaxime, cefoxitin, ceftazidime, ceftizoxime, ceftriaxone, cefuroxime, cephapirin, chloramphenicol, cholesteryl sulfate complex, cimetidine, clindamycin, dexamethasone sodium phosphate, dimenhyDRINATE, diphenhydrAMINE, DOXOrubicin, doxycycline, erythromycin, famotidine, filgrastim, fluconazole, gallium, gentamicin, granisetron, heparin, hydrocortisone sodium succinate, hydromorphone, imipenem/cilastatin, lorazepam, magnesium sulfate, melphalan, methylPREDNISolone sodium succinate, metoclopramide, metronidazole, multivitamin, nafcillin, oxacillin, paclitaxel, penicillin G potassium, pentobarbital, perphenazine, piperacillin, potassium chloride, propofol, ranitidine, remifentanil, sodium bicarbonate, tacrolimus, teniposide, theophylline, thiotepa, ticarcillin, tobramycin, trimethoprim-sulfamethoxazole, vancomycin, zidovudine

Perform/provide:

- Storage at room temperature for up to 12 hr after reconstitution; if refrigerated, sol may show a precipitate that clears at room temperature, yellow discoloration does not affect potency
- Adequate intake of fluids (2 L) to prevent deposit in kidneys

Evaluate:

- Therapeutic response: absence of itching, painful lesions; crusting and healed lesions; decreased symptoms of chickenpox

Teach patient/family:

- To take as prescribed; if dose is missed, take as soon as remembered up to 1 hr before next dose; do not double dose; that product does not cure the condition
- That product may be taken orally before infection occurs; product should be taken when itching or pain occurs, usually before eruptions
- That sexual partners need to be told that patient has herpes; they can become infected; condoms must be worn to prevent reinfections
- Not to touch lesions to avoid spreading infection to new sites
- That product does not cure infection, just controls symptoms and does not prevent infecting others
- ⚠ To report sore throat, fever, fatigue (may indicate superinfection)
- That product must be taken in equal intervals around the clock to maintain blood levels for duration of therapy
- To notify prescriber of side effects of bruising, bleeding, fatigue, malaise; may indicate blood dyscrasias
- To seek dental care during treatment to prevent gingival hyperplasia
- That women with genital herpes are more likely to develop cervical cancer; to keep all gynecologic appointments

Treatment of overdose: Discontinue product, hemodialysis, resuscitate if needed

acyclovir topical

See Appendix B

adalimumab (℞)

(add-a-lim′yu-mab)

Humira

Func. class.: Antirheumatic agent (disease modifying), immunomodulator

Chem. class.: Recombinant human IgG1 monoclonal antibody, DMARDs

Action: A form of human IgG1 monoclonal antibody specific for human tumor necrosis factor (TNF); elevated levels of TNF are found in patients with rheumatoid arthritis

Uses: Reduction in signs and symptoms and inhibiting progression of structural damage in patients with moderate to severe active rheumatoid arthritis in patients ≥18 years of age who have not responded to other disease-modifying agents, juvenile rheumatoid arthritis (JRA), psoriatic arthritis, Crohn's disease, moderate-severe plaque psoriasis

DOSAGE AND ROUTES

Rheumatoid arthritis/ankylosing spondylitis/psoriatic arthritis

• *Adult:* **SUBCUT** 40 mg every other wk

JRA

• *Child ≥4 yr/adolescent ≥30 kg:* **SUBCUT** 40 mg every other wk

• *Child ≥4 yr/adolescent ≥15 kg to <30 kg:* **SUBCUT** 20 mg every other wk

Crohn's disease

• *Adult:* **SUBCUT** 160 mg given as 4 inj on day 1, or 2 inj each on days 1 and 2; then 80 mg at wk 2, and 40 mg every other wk, starting at wk 4

Plaque psoriasis

• *Adult:* **SUBCUT** 80 mg baseline as 2 inj, then 40 mg every other wk starting 1 wk after dose × 16 wk

Available form: Inj 40 mg/0.8 ml

SIDE EFFECTS

CNS: Headache

CV: Hypertension

EENT: Sinusitis

GI: Abdominal pain, nausea, hepatic damage

INTEG: Rash, *inj site reaction*

MISC: Flulike symptoms, UTI, hypertension, back pain, lupuslike syndrome, **increased cancer risk,** antibody development to this drug; **risk of infection (TB, invasive fungal infections, other opportunistic infections), may be fatal**

RESP: URI, **pulmonary fibrosis**

Contraindications: Hypersensitivity

Black Box Warning: Active infections

Precautions: Pregnancy (B), breastfeeding, children, geriatric patients, CNS demyelinating disease, lymphoma, latent TB, CHF, hepatitis B carriers

PHARMACOKINETICS

Terminal half-life 2 wk, lower clearance with advancing age 40-75 yr, high RA factor

INTERACTIONS

• Do not give concurrently with vaccines; immunizations should be brought up to date before treatment

NURSING CONSIDERATIONS

Assess:

• Pain, stiffness, ROM, swelling of joints during treatment

• For inj site pain, swelling; usually occur after 2 inj (4-5 days)

⚠ For infections (fever, flulike symptoms, dyspnea, change in urination, redness/swelling around any wounds), stop treatment if present; some serious infections including sepsis may occur, may be fatal; patients with active infections should not be started on this product

Administer:

SUBCUT route

• Do not admix with other sol or medications; do not use filter; protect from light; give at 45-degree angle using abdomen, thighs; rotate inj sites; discard unused portions

- Other DMARDs should be continued during this therapy

Evaluate:

- Therapeutic response: decreased inflammation, pain in joints, decreased joint destruction

Teach patient/family:

- About self-administration if appropriate: inj should be made in thigh, abdomen, upper arm; rotate sites at least 1 inch from old site, do not inject in areas that are bruised, red, hard
- That if medication is not taken when due, inject next dose as soon as remembered and inject next dose as scheduled
- Not to take any live virus vaccines during treatment
- To report signs of infection, allergic reaction, or lupus-like syndrome

adefovir (℞)

(add-ee-foh′veer)

Hepsera

Func. class.: Antiviral

Chem. class.: Adenosine monophosphate analog

Action: Inhibits hepatitis B virus DNA polymerase by competing with natural substrates and by causing DNA termination after its incorporation into viral DNA; causes viral DNA death

Uses: Chronic hepatitis B

DOSAGE AND ROUTES

- *Adult:* **PO** 10 mg/day, optimal duration unknown

Renal dose

- *Adult:* **PO** CCr ≥50 ml/min 10 mg q24hr; CCr 30-49 ml/min 10 mg q48hr; CCr 10-29 ml/min 10 mg q72hr; hemodialysis 10 mg q7 days following dialysis

Available forms: Tabs 10 mg

SIDE EFFECTS

CNS: Headache

GI: Dyspepsia, abdominal pain, nausea, vomiting, diarrhea, hepatomegaly

GU: Hematuria, glycosuria, **nephrotoxicity**

MISC: Fever, rash, weight loss

Contraindications: Hypersensitivity

Precautions: Pregnancy (C), breastfeeding, children, geriatric patients

Black Box Warning: Severe renal disease, impaired hepatic function, lactic acidosis, HIV

PHARMACOKINETICS

PO: Rapidly absorbed from GI tract, peak 1¾ hr, excreted by kidneys 45%, terminal half-life 7.48 hr

INTERACTIONS

- Granulocytopenia: acetaminophen, aspirin, indomethacin

Increase: serum concentration and possible toxicity—amphotericin B, dapsone, flucytosine, adriamycin, interferon, vinCRIStine, vinBLAStine, pentamidine, probenecid, experimental nucleoside analogs, benzodiazepines, cimetidine, morphine, sulfonamides, acyclovir, ganciclovir, DOXOrubicin, acetaminophen, indomethacin, fluconazole, phenytoin, trimethoprim

Black Box Warning: *Increase:* NNRTIs, NRTIs

Drug/Lab Test

Increase: ALT, AST, amylase, creatine kinase

NURSING CONSIDERATIONS

Assess:

- ⚠ For nephrotoxicity: increasing CCr, BUN
- For HIV before beginning treatment, because HIV resistance may occur in chronic hepatitis B patients
- ⚠ For lactic acidosis, severe hepatomegaly with stenosis
- Geriatric patients more carefully; may develop renal, cardiac symptoms more rapidly
- For exacerbations of hepatitis after discontinuing treatment, monitor LFTs

Administer:

- By mouth without regard to food

Perform/provide:

- Storage in cool environment; protect from light

Evaluate:

- Therapeutic response: decreased symptoms of chronic hepatitis B, improving LFTs

Teach patient/family:

- That optimal duration of treatment is unknown, that product is not a cure; transmission may still occur
- To avoid use with other medications unless approved by prescriber
- To notify prescriber of decreased urinary output
- To avoid breastfeeding

⚠ High Alert

adenosine (℞)

(a-den′oh-seen)

Adenocard, Adeno-jec, Adenoscan

Func. class.: Antidysrhythmic

Chem. class.: Endogenous nucleoside

Do not confuse:

Adenocard/adenosine phosphate

Action: Slows conduction through AV node, can interrupt reentry pathways through AV node, and can restore normal sinus rhythm in patients with paroxysmal supraventricular tachycardia (PSVT)

Uses: SVT, as a diagnostic aid to assess myocardial perfusion defects in CAD, Wolff-Parkinson-White (WPW) syndrome

Unlabeled uses: Wide-complex tachycardia diagnosis

DOSAGE AND ROUTES

Antidysrhythmic

- *Adult and child >50 kg:* **IV BOL** 6 mg; if conversion to normal sinus rhythm does not occur within 1-2 min, give 12 mg by rapid **IV BOL;** may repeat 12 mg dose again in 1-2 min
- *Infant and child <50 kg:* **IV BOL** 0.05 mg/kg; if not effective, increase dose by 0.05 mg/kg q2min to a max of 0.3 mg/kg/dose or 12 mg

Diagnostic use

- *Adult:* **IV INF** 140 mcg/kg/min × 6 min

Wolff-Parkinson-White (WPW) syndrome

- *Adult/adolescent/child ≥50 kg:* Rapid **IV BOL** 6 mg, follow with saline flush; then **IV BOL** 12 mg if needed

Wide-complex tachycardia diagnosis (unlabeled)

- *Adult/adolescent/child ≥50 kg:* Rapid **IV BOL** 6 mg, follow with saline flush; then **IV BOL** 12 mg if needed

Available forms: Inj 3-mg/ml vial, 6 mg/2-ml vial

SIDE EFFECTS

CNS: Light-headedness, dizziness, arm tingling, numbness, apprehension, blurred vision, headache

CV: Chest pain, pressure, **atrial tachydysrhythmias,** sweating, palpitations, hypotension, *facial flushing*

GI: Nausea, metallic taste, throat tightness, groin pressure

RESP: Dyspnea, chest pressure, hyperventilation, **bronchospasm (asthmatics)**

Contraindications: Hypersensitivity, 2nd- or 3rd-degree heart block, AV block, sick sinus syndrome, atrial flutter, atrial fibrillation, ventricular tachycardia

Precautions: Pregnancy (C), breastfeeding, children, geriatric patients, asthma

PHARMACOKINETICS

Cleared from plasma in <30 sec, half-life 10 sec

INTERACTIONS

- Higher degree of heart block: carbamazepine
- Possible ventricular fibrillation: digoxin
- Smoking: increase tachycardia

Increase: effects of adenosine—dipyridamole

A

Decrease: activity of adenosine—theophylline or other methylxanthines (caffeine)

Drug/Herb

Increase: toxicity/death—aconite

Increase: adenosine effect—aloe, broom, buckthorn, cascara sagrada (chronic use), figwort, fumitory, goldenseal, kudzu, licorice, rhubarb, senna

Increase: serotonin effect—horehound

Decrease: adenosine effect—coltsfoot, guarana

NURSING CONSIDERATIONS

Assess:

- I&O ratio, electrolytes (K, Na, Cl)
- Cardiopulmonary status: B/P, pulse, respiration, ECG intervals (PR, QRS, QT); check for transient dysrhythmias (PVCs, PACs, sinus tachycardia, AV block)
- Respiratory status: rate, rhythm, lung fields for crackles, watch for respiratory depression; bilateral crackles may occur in CHF patient; increased respiration, increased pulse, product should be discontinued
- CNS effects: dizziness, confusion, psychosis, paresthesias, seizures; product should be discontinued

Administer:

IV, direct route

- Undiluted; give 6 mg or less by rapid inj over 1-2 sec; if using an IV line, use port near insertion site, flush with NS (50 ml)

Intermittent INF (diagnostic testing)

- Use 30 ml vial, undiluted, by peripheral vein at a rate of 140 mcg/kg/min over 6 min for a total dose of 0.84 mg/kg, inject Thalium 201 as close to venous access as possible after 3 min of infusion

Y-site compatibilities: abciximab

Solution compatibilities: D_5LR, D_5W, LR, 0.9% NaCl

Perform/provide:

- Storage at room temperature; sol should be clear; discard unused product

Evaluate:

- Therapeutic response: normal sinus rhythm or diagnosis of perfusion defect

Teach patient/family:

- To report facial flushing, dizziness, sweating, palpitations, chest pain
- To rise from sitting or standing slowly to prevent orthostatic hypotension

Treatment of overdose: Defibrillation, vasopressor for hypotension

albumin, normal serum 5%/25% (℞)

(al-byoo′min)

Albuminar 5%, Albuminar 25%, Albutein 5%, Albutein 25%, Buminate 5%, Buminate 25%, Flexbumin 25%, Plasbumin 5%, Plasbumin 25%

Func. class.: Plasma volume expander

Chem. class.: Placental human plasma

Action: Exerts oncotic pressure, which expands volume of circulating blood and maintains cardiac output

Uses: Restores plasma volume in burns, hyperbilirubinemia, shock, hypoproteinemia, prevention of cerebral edema, cardiopulmonary bypass procedures, ARDS, nephrotic syndrome

DOSAGE AND ROUTES

Burns

- *Adult:* **IV** dose to maintain plasma albumin at 30-50 g/L, use 5% sol initially, then 25% sol after 24 hr

Shock

- *Adult:* **IV** 500 ml of 5% sol q30min, as needed
- *Child:* **IV** 0.5-1 g/kg/dose 5% sol, may repeat as needed, max 6 g/kg/day

Hypoproteinemia

- *Adult:* **IV** 25 g, may repeat in 15-30 min, or 50-75 g of 25% albumin infused at ≤2 ml/min
- *Child and infant:* **IV** 0.5-1 g/kg/dose over 2-4 hr, may repeat q1-2days

Hyperbilirubinemia/ erythroblastosis fetalis

• *Infant:* **IV** 1 g of 25% sol/kg 1-2 hr before transfusion

Available forms: Inj 50, 250 mg/ml (5%, 25%)

SIDE EFFECTS

CNS: Fever, chills, flushing, headache

CV: Fluid overload, hypotension, erratic pulse, tachycardia

GI: Nausea, vomiting, increased salivation

INTEG: Rash, urticaria

RESP: Altered respirations, **pulmonary edema**

Contraindications: Hypersensitivity, CHF, severe anemia, renal insufficiency, pulmonary edema

Precautions: Pregnancy (C), decreased salt intake, decreased cardiac reserve, lack of albumin deficiency, renal/hepatic disease, chronic anemia

PHARMACOKINETICS

In hyponutrition states, metabolized as protein/energy source, terminal half-life 21 days

INTERACTIONS

Drug/Lab Test

False increase: alk phos

NURSING CONSIDERATIONS

Assess:

• Blood studies Hct, Hgb; if serum protein declines, dyspnea, hypoxemia can result

• Decreased B/P, erratic pulse, respiration

• I&O ratio: urinary output may decrease

⚠ CVP, pulmonary wedge pressure will increase if overload occurs

• Allergy: fever, rash, itching, chills, flushing, urticaria, nausea, vomiting, hypotension, requires discontinuation of inf, use of new lot if therapy reinstituted; premedicate with diphenhydrAMINE

• CVP reading: distended neck veins indicate circulatory overload; shortness of breath, anxiety, insomnia, expiratory crackles, frothy blood-tinged cough, cyanosis indicate pulmonary overload

Administer:

IV route

• Slowly, to prevent fluid overload; dilute with NS for injection or D_5W; 5% may be given undiluted; 25% may be given diluted or undiluted, give over 4 hr, use infusion pump

• 5% solution may be used in hypovolemic/intravascular depletion

• 25% solution may be used in sodium/fluid restrictions

Solution compatibilities: LR, NaCl, Ringer's, D_5W, $D_{10}W$, $D_{2½}W$, dextrose/saline, $dextran_6$ D_5, $dextran_6$ NaCl 0.9%, dextrose/Ringer's, dextrose/LR

Y-site compatibilities: Diltiazem

Perform/provide:

• Adequate hydration before, during administration

• Check type of albumin; some stored at room temperature, some need to be refrigerated, use within 4 hr of opening

Evaluate:

• Therapeutic response: increased B/P, decreased edema, increased serum albumin levels, increased plasma protein

albuterol (℞)

(al-byoo′ter-ole)

Accuneb, albuterol, Gen-Salbutamol ✷, Novo-Salmol ✷, Proair HFA, Proventil, Proventil HFA, Ventodisk, Ventolin HFA, Vospire ER

Func. class.: Adrenergic β_2-agonist, sympathomimetic, bronchodilator

Do not confuse:

albuterol/atenolol

Ventolin/Vantin

Proventil/Prinivil

Salbutamol/salmeterol

Action: Causes bronchodilation by action on β_2 (pulmonary) receptors by increasing levels of cAMP, which relaxes smooth muscle; produces bronchodilation, CNS, cardiac stimulation, as well as

increased diuresis and gastric acid secretion; longer acting than isoproterenol
Uses: Prevention of exercise-induced asthma, acute bronchospasm, bronchitis, emphysema, bronchiectasis, or other reversible airway obstruction
Unlabeled uses: Hyperkalemia in dialysis patients

DOSAGE AND ROUTES

To prevent exercise-induced bronchospasm
- *Adult:* **INH** (metered dose inhaler) 2 puffs 15 min before exercising

Other respiratory conditions
- *Adult and child ≥12 yr:* **INH** (metered dose inhaler) 2 puffs q4hr; **PO** 2-4 mg tid-qid, not to exceed 8 mg; **NEB/IPPB** 2.5 mg tid-qid
- *Geriatric:* **PO** 2 mg tid-qid, may increase gradually to 8 mg tid-qid
- *Child 2-12 yr:* **INH** (metered dose inhaler) 0.1 mg/kg tid (max 2.5 mg tid-qid); **NEB/IPPB** 0.1-0.15 mg/kg/dose tid-qid or 1.25 mg tid-qid for child 10-15 kg or 2.5 mg tid-qid >15 kg

Hyperkalemia (unlabeled)
- *Adult:* **ORAL INH** (Albuterol nebulizer sol) 10-20 mg

Available forms: Aerosol 90 mcg/actuation; oral sol 2 mg/5 ml; tabs 2, 4 mg; ext rel 4, 8 mg; INH sol 0.5, 0.83, 1, 2, 5 mg/ml; powder for INH (Ventodisk) 200, 400 mcg; INH cap 200 mcg; 100 mcg/spray, 80 INH/canister, 200 INH/canister

SIDE EFFECTS

CNS: Tremors, anxiety, insomnia, headache, dizziness, stimulation, *restlessness,* hallucinations, flushing, irritability
CV: Palpitations, tachycardia, angina, hypo/hypertension, dysrhythmias
EENT: Dry nose, irritation of nose and throat
GI: Heartburn, nausea, vomiting
MISC: Flushing, sweating, anorexia, bad taste/smell changes, hypokalemia
MS: Muscle cramps
RESP: Cough, wheezing, dyspnea, **bronchospasm**, dry throat

Contraindications: Hypersensitivity to sympathomimetics, tachydysrhythmias, severe cardiac disease, heart block
Precautions: Pregnancy (C), breastfeeding, cardiac/renal disease, hyperthyroidism, diabetes mellitus, hypertension, prostatic hypertrophy, angle-closure glaucoma, seizures, exercise-induced bronchospasm (aerosol) in children <12 yr, hypoglycemia

PHARMACOKINETICS

Extensively metabolized in the liver and tissues, crosses placenta, breast milk, blood-brain barrier
PO: Onset ½ hr, peak 2-3 hr, duration 4-6 hr, half-life 2.7-6 hr, well absorbed
PO-ER: Onset ½ hr; peak 2-3 hr; duration 8-12 hr
INH: Onset 5-15 min, peak 0.5-2 hr, duration 2-6 hr, half-life 4 hr

INTERACTIONS

- ECG changes/hypokalemia: potassium-losing diuretics

Increase: severe hypotension—oxytocics
Increase: toxicity—theophylline
Increase: action of aerosol bronchodilators
Increase: action of albuterol—tricyclics, MAOIs, other adrenergics; do not use together
Increase: CV effects—atomoxetine, selegiline
Decrease: albuterol—other β-blockers
Drug/Herb
Increase: stimulation—caffeine (cola nut, green/black tea, guarana, yerba maté, coffee, chocolate)

NURSING CONSIDERATIONS

Assess:
- Respiratory function: vital capacity, forced expiratory volume, ABGs; lung sounds, heart rate and rhythm, B/P, sputum (baseline and peak)
- That patient has not received theophylline therapy before giving dose
- Patient's ability to self-medicate

- For evidence of allergic reactions
- Paradoxical bronchospasm, hold medication, notify prescriber if bronchospasm occurs

Administer:

PO route

- Do not break, crush, or chew ext rel tabs
- With meals to decrease gastric irritation
- Oral solution to children (no alcohol, sugar)

Inhalation route

- In geriatric patients and children, a spacing device is advised
- After shaking metered dose inhaler, exhale, place mouthpiece in mouth, inhale slowly, while depressing inhaler, hold breath, remove, exhale slowly; give INH at least 1 min apart
- NEB/IPPB diluting 5 mg/ml sol/2.5 ml 0.9% NaCl for INH; other sol do not require dilution; for neb O_2 flow or compressed air 6-10 L/min
- Gum, sips of water for dry mouth

Perform/provide:

- Storage in light-resistant container, do not expose to temperatures over 86° F (30° C)

Evaluate:

- Therapeutic response: absence of dyspnea, wheezing after 1 hr, improved airway exchange, improved ABGs

Teach patient/family:

- To use exactly as prescribed; take missed dose when remembered, alter dosing schedule
- Not to use OTC medications; excess stimulation may occur
- Use of inhaler; review package insert with patient; use demonstration, return demonstration
- To avoid getting aerosol in eyes; blurring of vision may result; or using near flames or source of heat
- To wash inhaler in warm water daily and dry
- To track number of inhalations used and discard when labeled inhalations have been used
- To avoid smoking, smoke-filled rooms, persons with respiratory infections

⚠ That paradoxic bronchospasm may occur and to stop product immediately, call prescriber

- To limit caffeine products such as chocolate, coffee, tea, and colas

Treatment of overdose: Administer a β_1-adrenergic blocker, IV fluids

⚠ High Alert

aldesleukin, IL-2 (℞)

(al-dess-loo′ken)

Proleukin

Func. class.: Antineoplastic—miscellaneous

Chem. class.: Interleukin-2, human recombinant (cytokine)

Do not confuse:

aldesleukin/oprelvekin

Proleukin/oprelvekin/Prokine

Action: Enhancement of lymphocyte mitogenesis and stimulation of IL-2–dependent cell lines; enhancement of lymphocyte cytotoxicity; induction of killer cell activity; induction of interferon-γ production; results in activation of cellular immunity, production of cytokines, and inhibition of tumor growth

Uses: Metastatic renal cell carcinoma in adults, phase II for HIV in combination with zidovudine; melanoma (metastatic)

Unlabeled uses: Acute myelogenous leukemia (AML), cutaneous T-cell lymphoma (CTCL), HIV, Hansen's disease (leprosy), mycosis fungoides, non-Hodgkin's lymphoma

DOSAGE AND ROUTES

Renal cell cancer/malignant melanoma

- *Adult:* **IV INF** 600,000 international units/kg (0.037 mg/kg) over 15 min q8hr × 14 doses; off 9 days, repeat schedule for another 14 doses, for a max of 28 doses/course

Hansen's disease (leprosy) (unlabeled)
• *Adult:* **INTRADERMAL** 180,000 international units inj into each lesion bid × 8 days

Acute myelogenous leukemia (AML) (unlabeled)
• *Adult:* **IV** 9 million international units/m^2/day over 1 hr on days 1-5 and 8-12 q6wk, max 4 cycles (patients who have had 2nd remission after standard treatment)

Refractory non-Hodgkin's lymphoma/cutaneous T-cell lymphoma (CTCL) (mycosis fungoides) (unlabeled)
• *Adult:* **CONT IV INF** 20 million international units/m^2/day for 3 courses of 5, 4, 3 days on weeks 1, 3, 5, respectively

HIV (unlabeled)
• *Adult:* **IV** 18 million international units/m^2/day × 5 days q2mo × 6 cycles; **SUBCUT** 3-18 million international units/m^2/day

Available forms: Powder for inj 22 million international units/vial

SIDE EFFECTS

CNS: Mental status changes, dizziness, sensory dysfunction, syncope, motor dysfunction, *fever, chills,* headache, impaired memory, depression, sleep disturbances, hallucinations, rigors, neuropathy
CV: Hypotension, sinus tachycardia, dysrhythmias, bradycardia, PVCs, PACs, myocardial ischemia, **myocardial infarction, cardiac arrest, capillary leak syndrome, CVA**
EENT: Reversible visual changes
GI: Nausea, vomiting, diarrhea, stomatitis, anorexia, GI bleeding, dyspepsia, constipation, **intestinal perforation**/ileus, jaundice, ascites
GU: **Oliguria/anuria, proteinuria, hematuria,** dysuria, **renal failure**
HEMA: Anemia, **thrombocytopenia, leukopenia, coagulation disorders, leukocytosis, eosinophilia**
INTEG: Pruritus, erythema, rash, dry skin, **exfoliative dermatitis,** purpura, petechiae, urticaria
MS: Arthralgia, myalgia
RESP: Pulmonary congestion, *dyspnea,* **pulmonary edema, respiratory failure, apnea,** tachypnea, pleural effusion, wheezing
SYST: Infection

Contraindications: Hypersensitivity, abnormal thallium stress test or pulmonary function tests, organ allografts

Black Box Warning: Cardiac/pulmonary disease, coma

Precautions: Pregnancy (C), breastfeeding, children, CNS metastases, bacterial infections, renal/hepatic disease, anemia, thrombocytopenia

Black Box Warning: Capillary leak syndrome, infection

PHARMACOKINETICS

Renal elimination half-life 85 min; onset 4 wk, duration, variable

INTERACTIONS

• Potentiate hypotension: antihypertensives
• Reduced antitumor effectiveness: glucocorticoids
• Unpredictable reactions: psychotropics

Increase: toxicity—aminoglycosides, indomethacin, cytotoxic chemotherapy, methotrexate, asparaginase, DOXOrubicin

Drug/Lab Test

Increase: bilirubin, BUN, serum creatinine, transaminase, alk phos; hypomagnesemia, acidosis hypocalcemia, hypophosphatemia, hypokalemia, hyperuricemia, hypoalbuminemia, hypoproteinemia, hyponatremia, hyperkalemia, alkalosis (toxic effect of product)

NURSING CONSIDERATIONS

Assess:

• CBC, differential, platelet count weekly; withhold product if WBC is <2000/mm^3 or platelet count is <75,000/mm^3; notify prescriber of these results
⚠ Capillary leak syndrome including a drop in mean arterial pressure (2-12 hr after initiating therapy); hypotension and

hypoperfusion will occur; if B/P <90 mm Hg, use CVP, ECG, VS

• Renal studies: BUN, serum uric acid, urine CCr, electrolytes before, during therapy; I&O ratio; report fall in urine output to <30 ml/hr

• Monitor temp q4hr

• Hepatic studies before, during therapy: bilirubin, AST, ALT, alk phos, LDH as needed or monthly

• ECG; ST-T wave changes, low QRS and T, possible dysrhythmias (sinus tachycardia, PVCs)

⚠ Baselines in pulmonary function; document FEV >2 L or ≥75% prior to therapy; check VS q4hr, monitor temp q4hr, pulse oximetry, dyspnea, crackles, ABGs; watch for respiratory failure, intubate if necessary

• Stress thallium study prior to therapy; document normal ejection fraction, unimpaired wall motion

• Bleeding: hematuria, guaiac, bruising petechiae, mucosa or orifices q8hr

• Buccal cavity q8hr for dryness, sores, ulceration, white patches, oral pain, bleeding, dysphagia

• Local irritation, pain, burning at inj site

• GI symptoms: frequency of stools, cramping; acidosis, signs of dehydration: rapid respirations, poor skin turgor, decreased urine output, dry skin, restlessness, weakness

Administer:

Intermittent IV INF route

• Hydrocortisone, dexamethasone, or sodium bicarbonate (1 mEq/1 ml) for extravasation, apply ice compresses

• Antiemetic 30-60 min before giving product to prevent vomiting

• IV after diluting 22 million international units (1.3 mg)/1.2 ml sterile H_2O for inj at site of vial and swirl, do not shake; dilute dose with 50 ml D_5W and give over 15 min; use plastic bag; do not use an in-line filter, give through Y-tube or 3-way stopcock

• DOPamine 1-5 kg/min before onset of hypotension; decreased dose preserves kidney output

Y-site compatibilities: Amikacin, amphotericin B, calcium gluconate, diphenhydrAMINE, DOPamine, fluconazole, foscarnet, gentamicin, heparin, IV fat emulsion, magnesium sulfate, metoclopramide, morphine, ondansetron, piperacillin, potassium chloride, ranitidine, ticarcillin, tobramycin, TPN #145, trimethoprim-sulfamethoxazole

Perform/provide:

• Liquid diet: carbonated beverage, gelatin (Jell-O) may be added if patient is not nauseated or vomiting

• Rinsing of mouth tid-qid with water, club soda; brushing of teeth bid-tid with soft brush or cotton-tipped applicators for stomatitis; use unwaxed dental floss

• Increased fluid when able to reduce renal problems

• Storage in refrigerator of diluted product; protect from light, do not freeze; administer within 48 hr; bring to room temperature before infusing; discard unused portion

Evaluate:

• Therapeutic response: decreased tumor size, spread of malignancy

Teach patient/family:

• To use a nonhormonal contraceptive method during therapy

• To report any complaints, side effects to nurse or prescriber

• To avoid foods with citric acid, hot or rough texture

• To avoid alcohol, NSAIDs, salicylates, vaccinations; GI bleeding may occur

• To report any bleeding, white spots, ulcerations in mouth to prescriber; tell patient to examine mouth daily

• To avoid crowds and persons with infections when granulocyte count is low

• Visual problems may occur, but are reversible

Rarely Used

alefacept (℞)

(ah-leh'fa-cept)

Amevive

Func. class.: Immunosuppressive

Uses: Adults with moderate to severe plaque psoriasis

DOSAGE AND ROUTES

• *Adult:* **IV BOL** 7.5 mg q wk or IM 15 mg q wk, for 12 wk

Contraindications: Hypersensitivity

alemtuzumab (℞)

(al-em-tuz'uh-mab)

Campath

Func. class.: Antineoplastic—miscellaneous

Chem. class.: Monoclonal antibody

Action: Composed of recombinant DNA-derived humanized monoclonal antibody (campath-1H), binds to CD52 antigen that is present on surface of B and T lymphocytes, causes lysis of leukemic cells

Uses: B-cell chronic lymphocytic leukemia that has been treated with alkylating agents and that has failed fludarabine therapy, graft-versus-host disease (GVHD)

Unlabeled uses: Cutaneous T-cell lymphoma (CTCL) (mycosis fungoides), prophylaxis of GVHD, non-Hodgkin's lymphoma (NHL), stem cell transplant

DOSAGE AND ROUTES

Chronic lymphocytic leukemia (CLL)

• *Adult:* **IV** 3 mg over 2 hr/day; when tolerated, increase to 10 mg; when 10 mg tolerated increase to 30 mg/day, maintenance is 30 mg/day 3×/wk on alternate days for 12 wk, titration usually takes 3-7 days, max single dose 30 mg; max weekly dose 90 mg

Cutaneous T-cell lymphoma (CTCL) (mycosis fungoides)/non-Hodgkin's lymphoma (unlabeled)

• *Adult:* **IV** 3 mg over 2 hr/day; when tolerated, increase to 10 mg; when 10 mg tolerated, increase to 30 mg/day, maintenance is 30 mg/day 3×/wk on alternate days for 12 wk, titration usually takes 3-7 days, max single dose 30 mg; max weekly dose 90 mg

Graft-versus-host disease prophylaxis (unlabeled)

• *Adult:* **IV** 20 mg/day given over 8 hr with cycloSPORINE

Available forms: Sol for inj 30 mg/ml

SIDE EFFECTS

CNS: Dizziness, insomnia, depression, headache, tremor, somnolence, fatigue, drowsiness, weakness

CV: Hypo/hypertension, tachycardia, edema, chest pain, supraventricular tachycardia

GI: Anorexia, diarrhea, constipation, *nausea, stomatitis, vomiting, abdominal pain, dyspepsia*

HEMA: **Anemia, neutropenia, thrombocytopenia, pancytopenia,** purpura, epistaxis

INTEG: Rash, local reaction, pruritus

MISC: Rigors, fever, *infusion reactions,* **sepsis, risk for fatal infection**

MS: Back pain

RESP: Cough, pneumonia, rhinitis, **bronchospasm,** dyspnea, pharyngitis

Contraindications: Hypersensitivity

Black Box Warning: Active systemic infection, immunodeficiency

Precautions: Pregnancy (C), breastfeeding, children

Black Box Warning: Infusion-related reactions

PHARMACOKINETICS

Complete bioavailability, half-life 12 days, steady state 6 wk

INTERACTIONS

Increase: bone marrow depression—radiation, other antineoplastics

Decrease: antibody reaction—live virus vaccines

Drug/Lab Test

Interference: diagnostic tests using antibodies

NURSING CONSIDERATIONS

Assess:

- CBC, platelets q wk or more often if myelosuppression occurs; CD4+ after therapy until recovery of >200 cells/μl; irradiate blood if transfusions are required to prevent GVHD
- For symptoms of infection; chills, fever, headache, may be masked by product fever; do not administer product if infection is present
- CNS reaction: LOC, mental status, dizziness, confusion
- Cardiac status: lung sounds; ECG before and during treatment, especially in those with cardiac disease; monitor B/P hypotensive effect during administration
- Bone marrow depression: bruising, bleeding, blood in stools, urine, sputum, emesis

Administer:

IV route

- Do not give IV push or bolus
- Withdraw amount needed, use 5-micron filter before dilution, check for particulate matter and discoloration; dilute with 100 ml sterile 0.9% NaCl or D_5W, gently invert to mix; do not add other products or infuse in same IV tubing
- Do not shake ampule
- Give diphenhydrAMINE 50 mg and acetaminophen 650 mg ½ hr prior to infusion; give hydrocortisone 200 mg to decrease severe infusion reactions; give trimethoprim-sulfamethoxazole DS bid 3×/wk and famciclovir 250 mg bid; continue for 2 mo or until CD4+ ≥200 cells/mm^3, whichever is later

Perform/provide:

- Storage of reconstituted sol for ≤8 hr at room temperature, do not freeze; protect from light

Evaluate:

- Therapeutic response: decrease in production of malignant lymphocytes

Teach patient/family:

- To take acetaminophen for fever
- To avoid hazardous tasks, because confusion, dizziness may occur
- To report signs of infection: sore throat, fever, diarrhea, vomiting
- To avoid breastfeeding, effects are unknown, do not resume for ≥3 mo after last dose
- To use contraception during treatment

alendronate (℞)

(al-en-drone′ate)

Fosamax

Func. class.: Bone-resorption inhibitor

Chem. class.: Bisphosphonate

Do not confuse:

Fosamax/Flomax

Action: Decreases rate of bone resorption and may directly block dissolution of hydroxyapatite crystals of bone, inhibits osteoclast activity

Uses: Treatment and prevention of osteoporosis in postmenopausal women, treatment of osteoporosis in men, Paget's disease, treatment of corticosteroid-induced osteoporosis in postmenopausal women not receiving estrogen and men who are on continuing corticosteroid treatment with low bone mass

DOSAGE AND ROUTES

Osteoporosis in postmenopausal women

- *Adult and geriatic:* **PO** 10 mg/day or 70 mg q wk

Osteoporosis in men

- *Adult:* **PO** 10 mg/day or 70 mg q wk

Paget's disease

- *Adult and geriatric:* **PO** 40 mg/day × 6 mo, consider retreatment for relapse

Prevention of osteoporosis

- *Adult:* **PO** 5 mg/day or 35 mg q wk

Corticosteroid-induced osteoporosis in postmenopausal women (not receiving estrogen)

- *Adult:* **PO** 10 mg/day

Corticosteroid-induced osteoporosis in men or premenopausal women

• *Adult:* **PO** 5 mg/day

Renal dose

• *Adult:* **PO** CCr ≤35 ml/min, not recommended

Available forms: Tabs 5, 10, 35, 40, 70 mg; oral sol 70 mg/75 ml

SIDE EFFECTS

CNS: Headache

CV: **Atrial fibrillation**

GI: Abdominal pain, constipation, nausea, vomiting, esophageal ulceration, acid reflux, dyspepsia, **esophageal perforation,** diarrhea

META: Hypophosphatemia, hypocalcemia

MS: Bone pain, osteonecrosis of the jaw

SYST: **Angioedema, Stevens-Johnson syndrome, toxic epidermal necrolysis**

Contraindications: Hypersensitivity to bisphosphonates, delayed esophageal emptying, inability to sit or stand for 30 min, hypocalcemia

Precautions: Pregnancy (C), breastfeeding, children, CCr <35 ml/min, esophageal disease, ulcers, gastritis, poor dental health

PHARMACOKINETICS

Bioavailability 60%, protein binding 78%, rapidly cleared from circulation, taken up mainly by bones, eliminated primarily through kidneys, after bound to bone, half-life >10 yr

INTERACTIONS

• Possible GI adverse reactions: NSAIDs, salicylates, H_2 blockers, proton pump inhibitors (PPIs), gastric mucosal agents

Decrease: absorption—antacids, calcium supplements, aminoglycosides

Drug/Food

Decrease: absorption when used with caffeine, orange juice

NURSING CONSIDERATIONS

Assess:

⚠ Serious reactions: angioedema, Stevens-Johnson syndrome, toxic epidermal necrolysis, atrial fibrillation

• Hormonal status if a woman, before treatment

• For osteoporosis: bone density test before and during treatment

• For Paget's disease: increased skull size, bone pain, headache; decreased vision, hearing

• Electrolytes; renal function studies; Ca, P, Mg, K

• For hypercalcemia: paresthesia, twitching, laryngospasm, Chvostek's, Trousseau's signs

• Alk phos levels, baseline and periodically, 2 × upper limit of normal is indicative of Paget's disease

• Dental status: regular dental exams should be done; dental extractions (cover with antiinfectives before procedure)

Administer:

• For 6 months to be effective in Paget's disease; take with 8 oz of water 30 min before 1st food, beverage, or medication of the day

Perform/provide:

• Storage in cool environment, out of direct sunlight

Evaluate:

• Therapeutic response: increased bone mass, absence of fractures

Teach patient/family:

• To remain upright for 30 min after dose to prevent esophageal irritation, if dose is missed, skip dose, do not double doses or take later in day

• To take in AM before food, other meds, take with 6-8 oz of water only (no mineral water)

• To take calcium, vit D if instructed by health care provider

• To use weight-bearing exercise to increase bone density

• To let health care provider know if pregnant or if pregnancy is planned or if breastfeeding

• To maintain good oral hygiene

Rarely Used

alfentanil (℞)

(al-fen'ta-nil)

Alfenta, Rapifen ♣

Func. class.: Opioid analgesic

Controlled Substance Schedule II

Uses: In combination with other products in general anesthesia, as a primary anesthetic in general surgery, monitored anesthesia care (MAC)

DOSAGE AND ROUTES

Anesthesia <30 min

Combination

• *Adult:* **IV** 8-50 mcg/kg, may increase by 3-15 mcg/kg

Anesthetic induction

• *Adult:* **IV** 3-5 mcg/kg, then 0.5-1.5 mcg/kg/min; total dose is 8-40 mcg/kg

Anesthesia 30-60 min

Induction

• *Adult:* **IV** 20-50 mcg/kg

Maintenance

• *Adult:* **IV** 5-15 mcg/kg; may give up to 75 mcg/kg total dose

Continuous anesthesia >45 min

Induction

• *Adult:* **IV** 50-75 mcg/kg

Maintenance

• *Adult:* **IV** 0.5-3.0 mcg/kg/min; rate should be decreased by 30%-50% after 1 hr maintenance **INF;** may be increased to 4 mcg/kg/min or **BOL** doses of 7 mcg/kg

Induction of anesthesia >45 min

• *Adult:* **IV** 130-245 mcg/kg, then 0.5-1.5 mcg/kg/min

MAC

Induction

• *Adult:* **IV** Duration ≤½ hr 3-8 mcg/kg

Maintenance

• *Adult:* **IV** 3-5 mcg/kg q5-20min to 1 mcg/kg/min, total dose 3-40 mcg/kg

Contraindications: Children <12 yr, hypersensitivity

alfuzosin (℞)

(al-fyoo'zoe-sin)

Uroxatral

Func. class.: Urinary tract, antispasmodic, α_1-agonist

Chem. class.: Quinazolone

Action: Binds to α_{1A}-adrenoceptor subtype located mainly in the prostate, relaxing smooth muscles

Uses: Symptoms of benign prostatic hyperplasia

Unlabeled uses: Lower urinary tract symptoms, erectile dysfunction with sildenafil

DOSAGE AND ROUTES

• *Adult:* **PO** ext rel 10 mg/day, taken after same meal each day

Available forms: Ext rel tabs 10 mg

SIDE EFFECTS

CNS: Dizziness, headache, fatigue, flushing

CV: Postural hypotension (dizziness, lightheadedness, fainting) within a few hours of administration, chest pain, tachycardia, angina

GI: Nausea, abdominal pain, dyspepsia, constipation, diarrhea, liver injury, jaundice

INTEG: Rash, urticaria, **angioedema,** pruritus

GU: Impotence, priaprism

MISC: Body pain in general, xerostomia, rhinitis

RESP: Upper respiratory infection, pharyngitis, bronchitis, sinusitis

Contraindications: Hypersensitivity, moderate to severe hepatic impairment, not indicated for use in women or children, breastfeeding

Precautions: Pregnancy (B) but not used in females, geriatric patients; CAD, coronary insufficiency, mild hepatic disease, mild/moderate/severe renal disease, history of QT prolongation or coadministration with meds known to prolong QT interval, prostate cancer, torsade de pointes, syncope, surgery, prostate cancer, orthostatic hypotension, ocular surgery, CAD, dysrhythmias, angina

PHARMACOKINETICS

Peak 8 hr, elimination half-life 10 hr, extensively metabolized in liver by CYP3A4 enzyme, excreted via urine (11% unchanged), moderately protein binding (82%-90%)

INTERACTIONS

• Not to be taken with: prazosin, terazosin, doxazosin

Increase: effects of alfuzosin—alcohol

Increase: effects—CYP3A4 inhibitors (ketoconazole, itraconazole, and ritonavir); do not use together

Increase: hypotension—β-blockers, phosphodiesterase 5 inhibitors, nitrates

NURSING CONSIDERATIONS

Assess:

• Prostatic hyperplasia: change in urinary patterns (hesitancy, dribbling, dysuria, urgency), baseline and throughout treatment

• CBC with diff and LFTs; B/P and heart rate; monitor for orthostatic hypotension; B/P lying and standing; QT prolongation

• BUN, uric acid, urodynamic studies (urinary flow rates, residual volume)

• I&O ratios, weight daily, edema, report weight gain or edema

Administer:

PO route

• Do not break, crush, or chew tabs; give with food; take at same time of day

Perform/provide:

• Storage in tight container in cool environment

Evaluate:

• Therapeutic response: decreased symptoms of benign prostatic hyperplasia

Teach patient/family:

• To take at same time of day with food; do not double doses

• Not to drive or operate machinery for 4 hr after first dose or after dosage increase, dizziness may occur

• About orthostatic hypotension; to rise slowly from sitting or lying

aliskiren (℞)

(a-lis'kir-en)

Tekturna

Func. class.: Antihypertensive

Chem. class.: Direct renin inhibitor

Action: Renin inhibitor that acts on the renin-angiotensin system (RAS)

Uses: Hypertension, alone or in combination with other antihypertensives

DOSAGE AND ROUTES

• *Adult:* **PO** 150 mg/day, may increase to 300 mg/day if needed, max 300 mg/day

Available forms: Tabs 150, 300 mg

SIDE EFFECTS

CV: Orthostatic hypotension, hypotension

CNS: Headache, dizziness

GI: Diarrhea

GU: Renal stones, increased uric acid

INTEG: Rash

META: Hyperkalemia

MISC: **Angioedema**

Contraindications: Hypersensitivity

Black Box Warning: Pregnancy (D) 2nd/3rd trimester

Precautions: Pregnancy (C) 1st trimester, breastfeeding, children, geriatric patients, angioedema, aortic/renal artery stenosis, cirrhosis, CAD, dialysis, hyper/hypokalemia, hyponatremia, hypotension, hypovolemia, renal/hepatic disease, surgery, diabetes, seizures

PHARMACOKINETICS

Poorly absorbed, bioavailability 2.3%, peak 1-3 hr, steady state 7-8 days, 91% excreted unchanged in the feces

INTERACTIONS

Increase: potassium levels—ACE inhibitors, angiotensin receptor antagonists
Increase: hypotension—other antihypertensives, diuretics
Increase: aliskiren levels—atorvastatin, ketoconazole
Decrease: levels of warfarin

Drug/Food

Decrease: absorption—high-fat meal

Drug/Lab Test

Increase: uric acid, CPK, BUN, serum creatinine
Decrease: Hct, Hgb

NURSING CONSIDERATIONS

Assess:

- Blood studies: CBC with differential; Hct, Hgb may be decreased; uric acid, serum creatinine, BUN may be increased; potassium, hyperkalemia may occur
- Allergic reactions: angioedema may occur
- Daily dependent edema in feet, legs; weight, B/P, orthostatic hypotension

Administer:

- PO; do not use with a high-fat meal
- Daily with a full glass of water, titrate up to achieve correct dose
- Do not discontinue abruptly

Perform/provide:

- Storage in tight container at room temperature

Evaluate:

- Therapeutic response: decrease in B/P

Teach patient/family:

- The importance of complying with dosage schedule even if feeling better
- To notify if pregnancy is planned or suspected; if pregnant, product will need to be discontinued
- How to take B/P and normal reading for age-group
- That if dose is missed, take as soon as possible; if it is almost time for the next dose, take only that dose; do not double dose
- Not to use OTC products including herbs, supplements unless approved by prescriber
- To report to prescriber immediately: dizziness, faintness, chest pain, palpitations, uneven or rapid heart beat, headache, severe diarrhea, swelling of tongue or lips, trouble breathing, difficulty swallowing, tightening of the throat
- Not to operate machinery or perform hazardous tasks if dizziness occurs
- To avoid faintness; do not get up or stand up rapidly

alitretinoin (℞)

(a-li-tret′i-noyn)

Panretin

Func. class.: Retinoid, 2nd generation, topical antineoplastic

Action: Controls cellular differentiation and proliferation of neoplastic and healthy cells by binding to retinoid receptors

Uses: AIDS-related Kaposi's sarcoma

DOSAGE AND ROUTES

- *Adult:* **TOP** Apply enough gel to cover lesions bid with a generous coating; allow to dry for 3-5 min before covering with clothing; do not apply near mucosal areas; do not rub gel into the lesion

Available forms: Gel 0.1%

SIDE EFFECTS

*INTEG: **Rash***, stinging, warmth, redness, erythema, blistering, crusting, peeling, contact dermatitis, ***pain***

Contraindications: Pregnancy (D), hypersensitivity to retinoids

Precautions: Breastfeeding, geriatric patients, eczema, sunburn, cutaneous T-cell lymphoma

PHARMACOKINETICS

Poor systemic absorption

INTERACTIONS

- Do not use around DEET (an insect repellant agent)

NURSING CONSIDERATIONS

Assess:

- Area of body involved, what helps or aggravates condition; cysts, dryness, itching; lesions may worsen at beginning of treatment
- Dermal toxicity that may start as erythema, then edema, may need to be discontinued and restarted

Administer:

- Bid initially to lesions, can be increased to tid-qid according to tolerance

Perform/provide:

- Storage at room temperature
- Hand washing after application

Evaluate:

- Therapeutic response: decrease in size and number of lesions

Teach patient/family:

- To avoid application on normal skin; getting cream in eyes, nose, other mucous membranes; not to rub into lesion; do not use occlusive dressing; wait 20 min after bath, shower to apply; wait at least 3 hr after using to shower, bathe, swim
- To avoid sunlight, sunlamps, or use protective clothing, sunscreen
- That treatment may cause warmth, stinging, dryness, peeling will occur
- That product does not cure condition; only relieves symptoms
- That therapeutic results may be seen in 2-3 wk but may not be optimal until after 6 wk

allopurinol (℞)

(al-oh-pure'i-nole)

Aloprim, allopurinol, Apo-Allopurinol ✤, Zyloprim

Func. class.: Antigout drug, antihyperuricemic

Chem. class.: Xanthene oxidase inhibitor

Do not confuse:

allopurinol/Apresoline

Zyloprim/Zovirax

Action: Inhibits the enzyme xanthine oxidase, reducing uric acid synthesis

Uses: Chronic gout, hyperuricemia associated with malignancies, recurrent calcium oxalate calculi, uric acid calculi

DOSAGE AND ROUTES

Increased uric acid levels in malignancies

- *Adult:* **PO** 600-800 mg/day in divided doses for 2-3 days; start up to 1-2 days prior to chemotherapy; **IV INF** 200-400 mg/m^2/day, max 600 mg/day 24-48 hr prior to chemotherapy, may be divided at 6, 8, 12 hr intervals
- *Child 6-10 yr:* **PO** 300 mg/day, adjust dose after 48 hr
- *Child <6 yr:* **PO** 150 mg/day, adjust dose after 48 hr
- *Child:* **IV INF** 200 mg/m^2/day, initially as a single dose or divided q6-12hr

Recurrent calculi

- *Adult:* **PO** 200-300 mg/day in a single dose or divided bid-tid, max 300 mg/dose, 800 mg/day

Uric acid nephropathy prevention

- *Adult and child >10 yr:* **PO** 600-800 mg/day × 2-3 days

Gout (mild)

- *Adult:* **PO** 100-300 mg/day, increase q wk based on uric acid levels, max 800 mg/day; maintenance dose 100-200 mg bid-tid

Gout (moderate-severe)

- *Adult:* **PO** 400-600 mg/day in a single dose or divided bid-tid, max 800 mg/day, doses >300 mg should be given in divided doses

Renal dose

- *Adult:* **PO/IV** CCr 10-20 ml/min 100-200 mg/day; CCr 3-9 ml/min 100 mg/day or 100 mg every other day; CCr 3 ml/min 100 mg q24hr or longer or 100 mg every third day

Available forms: Tabs, scored 100, 300 mg; inj 500 mg/vial

SIDE EFFECTS

CNS: Headache, drowsiness, neuritis, paresthesia

EENT: Retinopathy, cataracts, epistaxis
GI: *Nausea, vomiting, anorexia, malaise,* metallic taste, cramps, peptic ulcer, diarrhea, stomatitis
HEMA: **Agranulocytosis, thrombocytopenia, aplastic anemia, pancytopenia, leukopenia, bone marrow suppression, eosinophilia**
INTEG: Fever, chills, dermatitis, pruritus, purpura, erythema, ecchymosis, alopecia, rash, **Stevens-Johnson syndrome**
MISC: Myopathy, arthralgia, hepatomegaly, **cholestatic jaundice, renal failure, exfoliative dermatitis**
Contraindications: Hypersensitivity
Precautions: Pregnancy (C), breastfeeding, children, renal/hepatic disease

PHARMACOKINETICS

PO: Peak 1.5 hr; excreted in feces, urine; half-life 1-2 hr
IV: Peak up to 30 min

INTERACTIONS

Increase: kidney stone formation—ammonium chloride, vit C, potassium/sodium phosphate
Increase: rash—ampicillin, amoxicillin
Increase: action of oral anticoagulants, oral antidiabetics, theophylline
Increase: hypersensitivity—ACE inhibitors, thiazides
Increase: bone marrow depression—antineoplastics (mercaptopurine, azathioprine)
Increase: xanthine nephropathy, calculi—rasburicase

NURSING CONSIDERATIONS

Assess:
- Uric acid levels q2wk; uric acid levels should be 6 mg/dl or less
- CBC, AST, BUN, creatinine before starting treatment, periodically
- I&O ratio; increase fluids to 2 L/day to prevent stone formation and toxicity
- For rash, hypersensitivity reactions, discontinue allopurinol
- For gout: joint pain, swelling; may use with NSAIDs for acute gouty attacks

Administer:

PO route
- With meals to prevent GI symptoms; may crush and add to foods or fluids
- A few days before antineoplastic therapy

Intermittent IV INF route
- Reconstitute 30-ml vial with 25 ml of sterile water for inj; dilute to desired conc with 0.9% NaCl for inj or D_5 for inj, begin inf within 10 hr

Solution incompatibilities: Amikacin, amphotericin B, carmustine, cefotaxime, chlorproMAZINE, cimetidine, clindamycin, cytarabine, dacarbazine, DAUNOrubicin, diphenhydrAMINE, DOXOrubicin, doxycycline, droperidol, floxuridine, gentamicin, haloperidol, hydrOXYzine, idarubicin, imipenem, cilastatin, mechlorethamine, meperidine, metoclopramide, methylPREDNISolone, minocycline, nalbuphine, netilmicin, ondansetron, prochlorperazine, promethazine, sodium bicarbonate, streptozocin, tobramycin, vinorelbine

Evaluate:
- Therapeutic response: decreased pain in joints, decreased stone formation in kidneys, decreased uric acid levels

Teach patient/family:
- That tabs may be crushed
- To take as prescribed; if dose is missed, take as soon as remembered; do not double dose
- To increase fluid intake to 2 L/day
- To report skin rash, stomatitis, malaise, fever, aching; product should be discontinued
- To avoid hazardous activities if drowsiness or dizziness occurs
- To avoid alcohol, caffeine; will increase uric acid levels
- To avoid large doses of vit C; kidney stone formation may occur
- To reduce dairy products, refined sugars, sodium, meat if taking for calcium oxalate stones

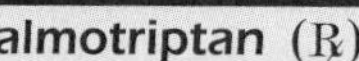

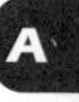

almotriptan (℞)

(al-moh-trip′tan)

Axert

Func. class.: Antimigraine agent, abortive

Chem. class.: 5-HT_1-receptor agonist, triptan

Action: Binds selectively to the vascular $5\text{-HT}_{1B/1D/1F}$-receptors, exerts antimigraine effect

Uses: Acute treatment of migraine with or without aura (adult/adolescent/child ≥12 yr)

DOSAGE AND ROUTES

Adult, adolescent, and child ≥12 yr: **PO** 6.25-12.5 mg; may repeat dose after 2 hr; do not give more than 2 doses/24 hr, 25 mg/day or 4 treatment cycles within any 30-day period

Hepatic/renal dose

• *Adult:* **PO** 6.25 mg initially, max 12.5 mg

Available forms: Tabs 6.25, 12.5 mg

SIDE EFFECTS

CNS: Tingling, hot sensation, burning, feeling of pressure, tightness, numbness, dizziness, sedation, headache, anxiety, fatigue, cold sensation, **seizures**

CV: Flushing, palpitations, tachycardia, **coronary artery vasospasm, MI, ventricular fibrillation, ventricular tachycardia**

EENT: Throat, mouth, nasal discomfort; vision changes

GI: Nausea, xerostomia

INTEG: Sweating

MS: Weakness, neck stiffness, myalgia

RESP: Chest tightness, pressure

Contraindications: Hypersensitivity, cluster headache, hemiplegia, vascular migraine, ischemic heart disease or risk for, peripheral vascular syndrome, concurrent use of ergotamine-containing preparations, uncontrolled hypertension, basilar or hemiplegic migraine; concurrent MAOI therapy or within 2 wk

Precautions: Pregnancy (C), postmenopausal women, men >40 yr, breastfeeding, children <18 yr, geriatric patients, risk factors for CAD, MI; hypercholesterolemia, obesity, diabetes, impaired renal/hepatic function, sulfonamide hypersensitivity

PHARMACOKINETICS

Onset of pain relief 2 hr; peak 1-3 hr; duration 3-4 hr; bioavailability 70%; protein binding 35%; metabolized in the liver (metabolite), metabolized by MAO-A, CYP2D6, CYP3A4; excreted in urine (40%), feces (13%); half-life 3-4 hr

INTERACTIONS

Increase: vasospastic effects—ergot, ergot derivatives, other 5-HT_1 agonists; avoid concurrent use

⚠ ***Increase:*** almotriptan effect—MAOIs, CYP2D6 inhibitors; do not use together

Increase: plasma concentration of almotriptan—ketoconazole

Drug/Herb

Increase: almotriptan effect—butterbur, feverfew

NURSING CONSIDERATIONS

Assess:

• Migraine: pain location, aura, duration, intensity, nausea, vomiting

• B/P; signs/symptoms of coronary vasospasms

• Tingling, hot sensation, burning, feeling of pressure, numbness, flushing

• For stress level, activity, recreation, coping mechanisms

• Neurologic status: LOC, blurring vision, nausea, vomiting, tingling in extremities preceding headache

• Ingestion of tyramine foods (pickled products, beer, wine, aged cheese), food additives, preservatives, colorings, artificial sweeteners, chocolate, caffeine, which may precipitate these types of headaches

Administer:

- Avoid using more than 2× per wk, rebound headache may occur
- Swallow tabs whole; do not break, crush, or chew

Perform/provide:

- Quiet, calm environment with decreased stimulation from noise, bright light, excessive talking

Evaluate:

- Therapeutic response: decrease in severity of migraine

Teach patient/family:

- To report chest pain, drowsiness, dizziness, tingling, flushing, pressure
- To use contraception while taking product, notify prescriber if pregnancy is planned or suspected, avoid breastfeeding
- That if one dose does not relieve migraine to take another after 2 hr
- To provide dark, quiet environment
- That product does not prevent or reduce number of migraine attacks; use to relieve attack only

alprazolam (℞)

(al-pray′zoe-lam)
Apo-Alpraz ✦, Niravam, Novo-Alprazol ✦, Nu-Alpraz ✦, Xanax, Xanax XR

Func. class.: Antianxiety
Chem. class.: Benzodiazepine (short/intermediate acting)

Controlled Substance Schedule IV

Do not confuse:

alprazolam/lorazepam
Xanax/Lanoxin/Tylox/Zantac

Action: Depresses subcortical levels of CNS, including limbic system, reticular formation

Uses: Anxiety, panic disorders with or without agoraphobia, anxiety with depressive symptoms

Unlabeled uses: Premenstrual dysphoric disorders, insomnia, PMS, alcohol withdrawal syndrome

DOSAGE AND ROUTES

Anxiety disorder

- *Adult:* **PO** 0.25-0.5 mg tid, may increase q3-4days if needed, max 4 mg/day in divided doses
- *Geriatric:* **PO** 0.125-0.25 mg bid; increase by 0.125 as needed

Panic disorder

- *Adult:* **PO** 0.5 mg tid, may increase up to 1 mg/day q3-4days, max 10 mg/day; **EXT REL** (Xanax XR) give daily in AM 0.5-1 mg initially, maintenance 1-10 mg/day

Hepatic dose

- Reduce dose by 50%

Premenstrual dysphoric disorders/ PMS (unlabeled)

- *Adult:* **PO** 0.25 mg bid-qid, starting on day 16-18 of menses, taper over 2-3 days when menses occurs

Insomnia (unlabeled)

- *Adult:* **PO** 0.25-0.5 mg at bedtime

Available forms: Tabs 0.25, 0.5, 1, 2 mg; ext rel tabs (Xanax XR) 0.5, 1, 2, 3 mg; orally disintegrating tabs 0.25, 0.5, 1, 2 mg; oral solution 1 mg/ml

SIDE EFFECTS

CNS: *Dizziness, drowsiness,* confusion, headache, anxiety, tremors, stimulation, fatigue, depression, insomnia, hallucinations, memory impairment, poor coordination

CV: *Orthostatic hypotension,* **ECG changes, tachycardia,** hypotension

EENT: *Blurred vision,* tinnitus, mydriasis

GI: Constipation, dry mouth, nausea, vomiting, anorexia, diarrhea, weight gain/loss, increased appetite

GU: Decreased libido

INTEG: Rash, dermatitis, itching

Contraindications: Pregnancy (D), breastfeeding, hypersensitivity to benzodiazepines, closed-angle glaucoma, psychosis, addiction

Precautions: Geriatric patients, debilitated, hepatic disease, obesity, severe pulmonary disease

PHARMACOKINETICS

PO: Well absorbed; widely distributed; onset 30 min; peak 1-2 hr; duration 4-6 hr; oral disintegrating tab peak 1.5-2 hr; therapeutic response 2-3 days; metabolized by liver (CYP3A4), excreted by kidneys; crosses placenta, breast milk; half-life 12-15 hr, protein binding 80%

INTERACTIONS

Increase: alprazolam action—CYP3A4 inhibitors (cimetidine, disulfiram, erythromycin, fluoxetine, isoniazid, itraconazole, ketoconazole, metoprolol, propoxyphene, propanolol, valproic acid)

Increase: CNS depression—anticonvulsants, alcohol, antihistamines, sedative/hypnotics, opioids

Decrease: sedation—xanthines

Decrease: alprazolam action—CYP3A4 inducers (barbiturates, rifampin)

Decrease: action of levodopa

Decrease: product level—cigarette smoking

Drug/Herb

Increase: CNS depression—cat's claw, chamomile, cowslip, echinacea, goldenseal, hops, kava, licorice, Queen Anne's lace, skullcap, St. John's wort, valerian, wild cherry

Drug/Food

Increase: product level—grapefruit juice

Drug/Lab Test

Increase: AST/ALT, alk phos

NURSING CONSIDERATIONS

Assess:

- Mental status: anxiety, mood, sensorium, affect, sleeping pattern, drowsiness, dizziness, especially in geriatric patients
- B/P lying, standing; pulse; if systolic B/P drops 20 mm Hg, hold product, notify prescriber
- Hepatic, blood studies: AST, ALT, bilirubin, creatinine, LDH, alk phos, CBC; may cause neutropenia, decreased Hct, increased LFTs
- For indications of increasing tolerance and abuse

⚠ Physical dependency, withdrawal symptoms: anxiety, panic attacks, agitation, seizures, headache, nausea, vomiting, muscle pain, weakness; withdrawal seizures may occur after rapid decrease in dose or abrupt discontinuation; since duration of action is short, considered to be the product of choice in the geriatric patient

Administer:

- Tabs may be crushed, mixed with food or fluids if patient is unable to swallow medication whole; do not break, crush, or chew ext rel (XR)
- With food or milk for GI symptoms; high-fat meal will decrease absorption
- Give ext rel tab in AM
- To discontinue, decrease by 0.5 mg q3days
- May divide total daily doses into more times/day, if anxiety occurs between doses
- Orally disintegrating tabs on tongue to dissolve and swallow

Evaluate:

- Therapeutic response: decreased anxiety, restlessness, sleeplessness

Teach patient/family:

- Not to double doses; take exactly as prescribed; if dose is missed, take within 1 hr as scheduled
- That product may be taken with food
- Not to use for everyday stress or longer than 4 mo unless directed by prescriber; not to take more than prescribed amount; may be habit forming; memory impairment is a sign of long-term use
- To avoid OTC preparations unless approved by prescriber
- To avoid driving, activities that require alertness, since drowsiness may occur
- To avoid alcohol ingestion or other psychotropic medications unless directed by prescriber
- Not to discontinue medication abruptly after long-term use

- To rise slowly or fainting may occur, especially geriatric patients
- That drowsiness may worsen at beginning of treatment

Treatment of overdose: Lavage, VS, supportive care, flumazenil

Rarely Used

alprostadil (℞)

(al-pros′ta-dil)
Caverject, Edex, Muse, prostaglandin E_1, Prostin VR ✦, Prostin VR Pediatric
Func. class.: Hormone

Uses: To maintain patent ductus arteriosus (temporary treatment), erectile dysfunction

DOSAGE AND ROUTES

Patent ductus arteriosus

- *Infant:* **IV INF** 0.1 mcg/kg/min, until desired response, then reduce to lowest effective amount, 0.4 mcg/kg/min not likely to produce greater beneficial effects

Erectile dysfunction of vasculogenic or mixed etiology, psychogenic

- *Men:* **INTRACAVERNOSAL** 2.5 mcg may increase by 2.5 mcg; may then increase by 5-10 mcg until adequate response occurs; **INTRAURETHRAL** administer as needed to achieve erection

Contraindications: Hypersensitivity, respiratory distress syndrome, those at risk for priapism

⚠ High Alert

alteplase (℞)

(al-ti-plaze′)
Activase, Activase rt-PA ✦, Cathflo, Lysatec-rt-PA ✦, tissue plasminogen activator, t-PA
Func. class.: Thrombolytic enzyme
Chem. class.: Tissue plasminogen activator (TPA)

Do not confuse:
alteplase/**Altace**

Action: Produces fibrin conversion of plasminogen to plasmin; able to bind to fibrin, convert plasminogen in thrombus to plasmin, which leads to local fibrinolysis, limited systemic proteolysis

Uses: Lysis of obstructing thrombi associated with acute MI, ischemic conditions requiring thrombolysis (i.e., PE, unclotting arteriovenous shunts, acute ischemic CVA), central venous catheter occlusion

Unlabeled uses: Arterial thromboembolism, deep vein thrombosis (DVT), occlusion prophylaxis, percutaneous coronary intervention (PCI), subarachnoid hemorrhage

DOSAGE AND ROUTES

MI (standard infusion)

- *Adult >65 kg:* 100 mg total given over 3 hr as: 6-10 mg IV bolus over 1-2 min; then the remaining 50-54 mg over the remainder of the hr, during 2nd, 3rd hr 20 mg is given by **CONT IV INF** (20 mg/hr)
- *Adult <65 kg:* 1.25 mg/kg over 3 hr: 60% in 1st hr (6%-10% as a bolus); remaining 50-54 mg over remainder of hr; during the 2nd hr, 20% of dose is given by CONT IV INF, and 20% during 3rd hr by CONT IV INF

MI (accelerated infusion)

- *Adult >67 kg:* 100 mg total dose: give 15 mg IV bolus, then 50 mg over 30 min, then 35 mg over 60 min
- *Adult <67 kg:* 15 mg IV bolus: then 0.75 mg/kg (max 50 mg) over 30 min;

0.5 mg/kg (max 35 mg) over the next 60 min

Pulmonary embolism

• *Adult:* **IV** 100 mg over 2 hr, then heparin

Acute ischemic stroke

• *Adult:* **IV** 0.9 mg/kg, max 90 mg; give as **INF** over 1 hr, give 10% of dose **IV BOL** over 1st min

Arterial thromboembolism (unlabeled)

• *Adult:* **IV** 2 mg/hr for up to 5 hr

Deep venous thrombosis (DVT) (unlabeled)

• *Adult:* **IV** 4 mcg/kg/min as a 2 hr inf, then 1 mcg/kg/min × 33 hr

Percutaneous coronary intervention (PCI) (unlabeled)

• *Adult:* **INTRACARDIAC** 20 mg over 5 min, then 50 mg over the next 60 min

Occlusion prophylaxis (unlabeled)

• *Adult >30 kg:* Do not exceed 2 mg in 2 ml; may use up to 2 doses (120 min apart)

Available forms: Powder for inj 50 mg (29 million international units/vial), 100 mg (58 million international units/vial); lyophilized powder for inj 2 mg

SIDE EFFECTS

CV: **Sinus bradycardia, ventricular tachycardia, accelerated idioventricular rhythm, bradycardia, recurrent ischemic stroke**, hypotension

INTEG: Urticaria, rash

SYST: **GI, GU, intracranial, retroperitoneal bleeding,** *surface bleeding,* **anaphylaxis,** fever

Contraindications: Hypersensitivity, active internal bleeding, history of CVA, severe uncontrolled hypertension, intracranial/intraspinal surgery/trauma (within 3 mo), aneurysm, brain tumor, seizures, platelets <100,000 mm^3

Precautions: Pregnancy (C), breastfeeding, children, geriatric patients, neurologic deficits, mitral stenosis, recent GI/GU bleeding, diabetic retinopathy, subacute bacterial endocarditis, arrhythmias, diabetic hemorrhage retinopathy

PHARMACOKINETICS

Cleared by liver, 80% cleared within 10 min of product termination, onset immediate, peak 45 min, duration 4 hr, half-life 35 min

INTERACTIONS

Increase: bleeding—anticoagulants, salicylates, dipyridamole, other NSAIDs, abciximab, eptifibatide, tirofiban, clopidogrel, ticlopidine, some cephalosporins, plicamycin, valproic acid

Decrease: effect—nitroglycerin

Drug/Herb

Increase: risk of bleeding—agrimony, alfalfa, angelica, anise, basil, bay, bilberry, black haw, bogbean, bromelain, buchu, cat's claw, chondroitin, cinchona bark, dong quai, evening primrose, fenugreek, feverfew, garlic, ginger, ginkgo, ginseng, green tea, horse chestnut, Irish moss, kelp, kelpware, khella, lovage, lungwort, meadowsweet, mother wort, mugwort, nettle, papaya, parsley (large amts), pau d'arco, pineapple, poplar, prickly ash, safflower, saw palmetto, tonka bean, tumeric, wintergreen, yarrow

Decrease: anticoagulant effect—chamomile, coenzyme Q10, flax, glucomannan, goldenseal, guar gum

Drug/Lab Test

Increase: PT, APTT, TT

NURSING CONSIDERATIONS

Assess:

• VS, B/P, pulse, respirations, neurologic signs, temp at least q4hr; temp >104° F (40° C) indicates internal bleeding; monitor rhythm closely; ventricular dysrhythmias may occur with hyperfusion; monitor heart, breath sounds, neurologic status, peripheral pulses; assess neurologic status, neurologic change may indicate intracranial bleeding

⚠ For bleeding during first hour of treatment and 24 hr after procedure: hematuria, hematemesis, bleeding from mucous membranes, epistaxis, ecchymosis; guaiac all body fluids, stools. Do not use 150 mg or more total dose; intracranial bleeding may occur

⚠ Hypersensitivity: fever, rash, itching, chills, facial swelling, dyspnea, notify prescriber immediately; stop product, keep resuscitative equipment nearby; mild reaction may be treated with antihistamines

- Blood studies (Hct, platelets, PTT, PT, TT, APTT) before starting therapy; PT or APTT must be less than 2 × control before starting therapy TT or PT q3-4hr during treatment
- ECG continuously, cardiac enzymes, radionuclide myocardial scanning/coronary angiography

Administer:

Intermittent IV INF route

- After reconstituting with provided diluent, add appropriate amount of sterile water for inj (no preservatives) 20-mg vial/20 ml or 50-mg vial/50 ml to make 1 mg/ml, mix by slow inversion or dilute with NaCl, D_5W to a concentration of 0.5 mg/ml; 1.5 to <0.5 mg/ml may result in precipitation of product; use 18G needle; flush line with NaCl after administration, give over 3 hr for MI, 2 hr for PE
- Heparin therapy after thrombolytic therapy is discontinued, TT, ACT, or APTT less than 2 × control (about 3-4 hr)
- Reconstituted IV solution within 8 hr or discard
- Within 6 hr of coronary occlusion for best results

Additive compatibilities: Lidocaine, morphine, nitroglycerin

Y-site compatibilities: Lidocaine, metoprolol, propranolol

Perform/provide:

- Avoidance of invasive procedures, inj, rectal temp
- Pressure for 30 sec to minor bleeding sites; 30 min to sites of atrial puncture, followed by pressure dressing; inform prescriber if this does not attain hemostasis; apply pressure dressing
- Storage of powder at room temperature or refrigerate; protect from excessive light

Evaluate:

- Therapeutic response: lysis of thrombi

Teach patient/family:

- The purpose and expected results of the treatment; to report adverse reactions

aluminum hydroxide (OTC)

AlternaGEL, Alugel ✱, aluminum hydroxide, Alu-Tab, Amphojel, Basaljel ✱, Dialume

Func. class.: Antacid, hypophosphatemic

Chem. class.: Aluminum product, phosphate binder

Action: Neutralizes gastric acidity, binds phosphates in GI tract; these phosphates are excreted

Uses: Antacid, hyperphosphatemia in chronic renal failure; adjunct in gastric, peptic, duodenal ulcers; hyperacidity, reflux esophagitis, heartburn, stress ulcer prevention in critically ill, GERD

Unlabeled uses: GI bleeding

DOSAGE AND ROUTES

Antacid

- *Adult:* **PO** 600 mg 1 hr after meals, at bedtime, chewed; max 6 doses/day

Hyperphosphatemia

- *Adult:* **PO** 300-600 mg tid
- *Child:* **PO** 50-150 mg/kg/day in 4-6 divided doses

GI bleeding

- *Infant:* **PO** 2-5 ml/dose q1-2hr
- *Child:* **PO** 5-15 ml/dose q1-2hr

Available forms: Caps 500 mg; tabs 600 mg; susp 320 mg/5 ml, 450 mg/5 ml, 600 mg/5 ml, 675 mg/5 ml

SIDE EFFECTS

GI: Constipation, anorexia, **obstruction,** fecal impaction

META: Hypophosphatemia, hypercalciuria

Contraindications: Hypersensitivity to this product or aluminum products

Precautions: Pregnancy (C), breastfeeding, geriatric patients, fluid restriction, decreased GI motility, GI obstruction, dehydration, renal disease, sodium-restricted diets

PHARMACOKINETICS

PO: Onset 20-40 min, duration 1-3 hr, excreted in feces

INTERACTIONS

Decrease: effectiveness of allopurinol, amprenavir, cephalosporins, corticosteroids, delavirdine, digoxin, gabapentin, gatifloxacin, H_2-antagonists, iron salts, isoniazid, ketoconazole, penicillamine, phenothiazines, phenytoin, quinidine, quinolones, tetracyclines, thyroid hormones, ticlopidine, anticholinergics; separate by at least 4-6 hr

Drug/Herb

Decrease: action of buckthorn, cascara sagrada, castor, Chinese rhubarb

Drug/Food

Decrease: product effect—high protein meal

NURSING CONSIDERATIONS

Assess:

- Pain: location, intensity, duration, character
- Phosphate levels, since product is bound in GI system
- Hypophosphatemia: anorexia, weakness, fatigue, bone pain, hyporeflexia
- Constipation; increase bulk in diet if needed
- Urinary pH, Ca^{++}, electrolytes

Administer:

- 2 tsp (10 ml) will neutralize 20 mEq of acid; 2 tabs will neutralize 16 mEq of acid

PO route

- Give with 8 oz water/meals for hyperphosphatemia, unless contraindicated
- Tablets must be chewed well, then give 8 oz water
- Laxatives or stool softeners if constipation occurs, especially geriatric patients
- After shaking susp
- With small amount of water or milk

NG route

- By nasogastric tube if patient unable to swallow

Evaluate:

- Therapeutic response: absence of pain, decreased acidity, healed ulcers, decreased phosphate levels

Teach patient/family:

- To increase fluids to 2 L/day unless contraindicated; measures to prevent constipation
- To avoid phosphate foods (most dairy products, eggs, fruits, carbonated beverages) during product therapy for hyperphosphatemia
- Not to use for prolonged periods in patients with low serum phosphate or if on a low-sodium diet
- To add cheese, corn, pasta, plums, prunes, lentils after product is discontinued
- That stools may appear white or speckled
- To check with prescriber after 2 wk of self-prescribed antacid use
- To separate other medications by 2 hr

alvimopan (℞)

(al-vi′moe-pan)

Entereg

Func. class.: Functional GI disorder agent

Chem. class.: Peripheral μ-opioid receptor antagonist

Action: Acts within the GI tract, antagonizes opioid-induced GI dysfunction

Uses: Ileus, postoperative

Unlabeled uses: Opiate-induced constipation

DOSAGE AND ROUTES

Ileus, postoperative

- *Adult:* **PO** 12 mg given ½-5 hr before surgery, then 12 mg bid the day after surgery, max 7 days (15 doses)

Opiate-induced constipation (unlabeled)

- *Adult:* **PO** 0.5-1 mg/day

Available forms: Caps 12 mg

SIDE EFFECTS

CV: **MI**
GI: Dyspepsia, flatulence, constipation
GU: Urinary retention
MISC: **Anemia,** hypokalemia
MS: Back pain

Contraindications: Hypersensitivity

Black Box Warning: No more than 15 doses

Precautions: Pregnancy (B), breastfeeding, children, renal/hepatic disease, GI obstruction, MI, complete GI obstruction surgery

PHARMACOKINETICS

Excreted by kidneys (35%), terminal half-life 10-18 hr, protein binding 80%-94%, high-fat meal decreases absorption

INTERACTIONS

- Duplicate therapy: opiate antagonists, methylnaltrexone

Increase: alvimopan effect—amiodarone, bepridil, cycloSPORINE, diltiazem, itraconazole, quinidine, quinine, spironolactone, verapamil

Increase: GI adverse reactions—opiate agonists; do not give if opiate agonists were taken for ≥7 days

NURSING CONSIDERATIONS

Assess:

- Hgb/Hct, serum potassium

Administer:

- Use in hospital only; therapeutic doses of opiates should not be used for >7 consecutive days
- Give without regard to food
- Must register in EASE program
- Do not give >15 doses (short-term hospital use only)

Perform/provide:

- Storage at room temperature

Evaluate:

- Therapeutic response: resolution of ileus

Teach patient/family:

- The reason for the product

amantadine (℞)

(a-man'ta-deen)
amantadine HCl, Symmetrel
Func. class.: Antiviral, antiparkinsonian agent
Chem. class.: Tricyclic amine

Do not confuse:
amantadine/ranitidine/rimantidine
Symmetrel/Synthroid

Action: Prevents uncoating of nucleic acid in viral cell, preventing penetration of virus to host; causes release of DOPamine from neurons

Uses: Prophylaxis or treatment of influenza type A, EPS, parkinsonism, Parkinson's disease

Unlabeled uses: Neuroleptic malignant syndrome, MS-associated fatigue

DOSAGE AND ROUTES

Influenza type A

- *Adult and child >12 yr:* **PO** 200 mg/day in single dose or divided bid, max 400 mg/day
- *Geriatric:* **PO** No more than 100 mg/day
- *Child 9-12 yr:* **PO** 100 mg bid
- *Child 1-9 yr:* **PO** 5 mg/kg/day divided bid-tid, not to exceed 150 mg/day

Extrapyramidal reaction/parkinsonism

Adult: **PO** 100 mg bid, up to 400 mg/day in EPS; give for 1 wk, then 100 mg as needed up to 400 mg in parkinsonism

Renal dose

- *Adult:* **PO** CCr 30-50 ml/min 200 mg first day, then 100 mg/day; CCr 15-29 ml/min 100 mg first day, then 100 mg on alternate days; CCr 15 ml/min reduce dose and interval to 200 mg q7days

MS-associated fatigue (unlabeled)

- *Adult:* **PO** 200 mg/day or 100 mg bid

Neuroleptic malignant syndrome (unlabeled)

- *Adult:* **PO** 100 mg bid × 3 wk

Available forms: Caps 100 mg; syr 50 mg/5 ml

A

SIDE EFFECTS

CNS: Headache, dizziness, drowsiness, fatigue, *anxiety*, psychosis, *depression, hallucinations*, tremors, **seizures**, confusion, *insomnia*
CV: Orthostatic hypotension, **CHF**
EENT: Blurred vision
GI: Nausea, vomiting, constipation, dry mouth, anorexia
GU: Frequency, retention
HEMA: **Leukopenia, agranulocytosis**
INTEG: Photosensitivity, dermatitis, livedo reticularis
Contraindications: Hypersensitivity, breastfeeding, children <1 yr, eczematic rash
Precautions: Pregnancy (C), geriatric patients, epilepsy, CHF, orthostatic hypotension, psychiatric disorders, renal/hepatic disease, peripheral edema

PHARMACOKINETICS

PO: Onset 48 hr, peak 2-4 hr, half-life 11-15 hr, not metabolized, excreted in urine (90%) unchanged, crosses placenta, excreted in breast milk

INTERACTIONS

Increase: anticholinergic response—atropine, other anticholinergics
Increase: CNS stimulation—CNS stimulants
Decrease: amantadine effect—metoclopramide, phenothiazines
Decrease: renal excretion of amantadine—triamterene, hydrochlorothiazide
Decrease: effect—intranasal influenza vaccine, avoid use 2 wk before or 48 hr after amantadine

Drug/Herb

Increase: anticholinergic effect—belladonna, henbane
Increase: action/side effects—pheasant's eye, quinine, scopolia root
Decrease: effect—kava

NURSING CONSIDERATIONS

Assess:

- I&O ratio; report frequency, hesitancy; serum BUN, creatinine baseline
- Hematologic status for leukopenia, agranulocytosis
- CHF (weight gain, jugular venous distention, dyspnea, crackles)
- Bowel pattern before, during treatment
- Skin eruptions, photosensitivity after administration of product
- Respiratory status: rate, character, wheezing, tightness in chest
- Allergies before initiation of treatment, reaction of each medication
- Signs of infection
- Livedo reticularis: mottling of the skin, usually red, edema, itching in lower extremities
- Parkinson's disease: gait, tremors, akinesia, rigidity
- Toxicity: confusion, behavioral changes, hypotension, seizures

Administer:

- Before exposure to influenza; continue for 10 days after contact
- At least 4 hr before bedtime to prevent insomnia
- After meals for better absorption, to decrease GI symptoms
- In divided doses to prevent CNS disturbances: headache, dizziness, fatigue, drowsiness

Perform/provide:

- Storage in tight, dry container

Evaluate:

- Therapeutic response: absence of fever, malaise, cough, dyspnea in infection; tremors, shuffling gait in Parkinson's disease

Teach patient/family:

- To change body position slowly to prevent orthostatic hypotension
- About aspects of product therapy: need to report dyspnea, weight gain, dizziness, poor concentration, dysuria, behavioral changes
- To avoid hazardous activities if dizziness, blurred vision occurs
- To take product exactly as prescribed; parkinsonian crisis may occur if product is discontinued abruptly; do not double dose; if a dose is missed, do not take within 4 hr of next dose; caps may be opened and mixed with food

- To avoid alcohol
- Not to breastfeed

Treatment of overdose: Withdraw product, maintain airway, administer epinephrine, aminophylline, O_2, IV corticosteroids, physostigmine

ambrisentan (℞)

(am-bri-sen'tan)

Letairis, Volibris ♣

Func. class.: Antihypertensive

Chem class.: Vasodilator/endothelin receptor antagonist

Action: Endothelin–1 receptor antagonist; endothelin-1 is vasoconstrictor

Uses: Pulmonary arterial hypertension, alone or in combination with other antihypertensives

DOSAGE AND ROUTES

- *Adult:* **PO** 5 mg/day; may increase to 10 mg if needed

Available forms: Tabs 5, 10 mg

SIDE EFFECTS

CNS: Headache, fever, flushing

CV: Orthostatic hypotension, hypotension, peripheral edema

EENT: Sinusitis, rhinitis

GI: Abdominal pain, constipation

GU: Decreased sperm counts

HEMA: Anemia

INTEG: Rash

RESP: Pharyngitis, dyspnea

Contraindications: Breastfeeding, hypersensitivity

Black Box Warning: Pregnancy (X)

Precautions: Children, females, geriatric patients, hepatitis, anemia, heart failure, jaundice, peripheral edema

Black Box Warning: Hepatic disease

PHARMACOKINETICS

Rapidly absorbed, peak 2 hr, protein binding 99%, metabolized by CYP3A4, CYP2C19, terminal half-life 15 hr

INTERACTIONS

- Possibly increase ambrisentan: cimetidine, clopidogrel, efavirenz, felbamate, fluoxetine, modafinil, oxcarbazepine, ticlopidine
- Need for ambrisentan dosage change: barbiturates, fosphenytoin, griseofulvin, nevirapine, phenytoin, rifabutin, rifampin, rifapentine

Increase: hypotension—other antihypertensives, diuretics, MAOIs

Increase: ambrisentan—CYP3A4 inhibitors (amprenavir, aprepitant, atazanavir, clarithromycin, conivaptan, cycloSPORINE, dalfopristin, danazol, darunavir, erythromycin, estradiol, imatinib, itraconazole, ketoconazole, nefazodone, nelfinavir, propoxyphene, quinupristin, ritonavir, RU-486, saquinavir, tamoxifen, telithromycin, troleandomycin, zafirlukast); CYP2C19/CYP3A4 (chloramphenicol, delavirdine, fluconazole, fluvoxamine, isoniazid, voriconazole)

Decrease: ambrisentan absorption—mefloquine, nicardipine, propafenone, quinidine, ranolazine, tacrolimus, testosterone

Drug/Herb

- Need for ambrisentan dosage change: St. John's wort

Drug/Food

- Avoid use with grapefruit products

Drug/Lab Test

Increase: LFTs

Decrease: Hct, Hgb

NURSING CONSIDERATIONS

Assess:

- Blood studies: CBC with differential; Hct, Hgb may be decreased
- Daily edema in feet, legs; weight, B/P, orthostatic hypotension
- Liver function tests: AST, ALT, bilirubin
- Assess pregnancy status before giving this product; pregnancy category X

Administer:

- Do not break, crush, or chew tabs
- Daily with a full glass of water without regard to food
- Do not discontinue abruptly

• Only those facilities enrolled in the LEAP program may administer this product

Perform/provide:

• Storage in tight container at room temperature

Evaluate:

• Therapeutic response: decrease in B/P; decreased shortness of breath

Teach patient/family:

• The importance of complying with dosage schedule even if feeling better

• To notify if pregnancy is planned or suspected; if pregnant, product will need to be discontinued

• If a dose is missed, take as soon as possible; if it is almost time for the next dose, take only that dose; do not double dose

• Not to use OTC products including herbs, supplements unless approved by prescriber

• To report to prescriber immediately: dizziness, faintness, chest pain, palpitations, uneven or rapid heart rate, headache

• Not to operate machinery or perform hazardous tasks if dizziness occurs

• To avoid faintness; do not get up or stand up rapidly

amifostine (℞)

(a-mi-foss′teen)

Ethyol

Func. class.: Cytoprotective agent for cisplatin/radiation

Action: Binds and detoxifies damaging metabolites of cisplatin, alkylating agents, DNA-reactive agents, and ionizing radiation by converting this product by alk phos in tissue to an active free thiol compound

Uses: Used to reduce renal toxicity when cisplatin is given repeatedly in ovarian cancer, non–small cell lung cancer; reduces xerostomia (dry mouth) in radiation therapy for head, neck cancer

Unlabeled uses: To prevent or reduce cisplatin-induced neurotoxicity, cyclophosphamide-induced granulocytopenia; prevent or reduce toxicity of radiation therapy; reduce toxicity of paclitaxel, myelodysplastic syndrome (MDS)

DOSAGE AND ROUTES

Reduction of renal damage with cisplatin

• *Adult:* **IV** 910 mg/m²/day, within ½ hr before chemotherapy, give over 15 min; may reduce dose to 740 mg/m² if higher dose is poorly tolerated

Xerostomia

• *Adult:* **IV** 200 mg/m²/day over 3 min as an infusion 15-30 min before radiation therapy

Bone marrow suppression prophylaxis/nephrotoxicity prophylaxis/neurotoxicity prophylasis (unlabeled)

• *Adult:* **IV** 100-340 mg/m²/day over 15 min prior to each dose of chemotherapy/radiation

Myelodysplastic syndrome (MDS) (unlabeled)

• *Adult:* **IV** 100 mg/m² 3×/wk, max 300 mg/m² 3×/wk

Available forms: Powder for inj, lyophilized 500 mg/vial

SIDE EFFECTS

CNS: Dizziness, somnolence, loss of consciousness

CV: Hypotension

EENT: Sneezing

GI: Nausea, vomiting, hiccups, diarrhea

INTEG: Flushing, feeling of warmth

MISC: Hypocalcemia, rash, chills, **anaphylaxis, toxic epidermal necrolysis, Stevens-Johnson syndrome, exfoliative dermatitis,** *erythema multiforme*

Contraindications: Breastfeeding, hypersensitivity to mannitol, aminothiol; hypotension, dehydration

Precautions: Pregnancy (C), children, geriatric patients, CV disease

PHARMACOKINETICS

Metabolized to free thiol compound, half-life 8 min, onset 5-8 min

INTERACTIONS

Increase: hypotension—antihypertensives

NURSING CONSIDERATIONS

Assess:

- For xerostomia: mouth lesions, dry mouth during therapy
- Fluid status before administration; administer antiemetic prior to administration to prevent severe nausea and vomiting; also, dexamethasone 20 mg IV and a serotonin antagonist such as ondansetron, dolasetron, or granisetron
- Calcium levels before and during treatment, may cause hypocalcemia; calcium supplements may be given for hypocalcemia
- B/P prior to and q5min during infusion; antihypertensive should be discontinued 24 hr prior to inf if severe hypotension occurs, give IV 0.9% NaCl to expand fluid volume, place in modified Trendelenburg position

Administer:

Intermittent IV INF route

- Intermittent inf after reconstituting with 9.7 ml of sterile 0.9% NaCl, further dilute with 0.9% NaCl to a concentration of 5-40 mg/ml, give over 15 min within ½ hr of chemotherapy
- Supine position during infusion

Y-site compatibilities: Amikacin, aminophylline, ampicillin, ampicillin/sulbactam, aztreonam, bleomycin, bumetanide, buprenorphine, butorphanol, calcium gluconate, carboplatin, carmustine, cefazolin, cefonicid, cefotaxime, cefotetan, cefoxitin, ceftazidime, ceftizoxime, ceftriaxone, cefuroxime, cimetidine, ciprofloxacin, clindamycin, cyclophosphamide, cytarabine, dacarbazine, dactinomycin, DAUNOrubicin, dexamethasone, diphenhydrAMINE, DOBUTamine, DOPamine, DOXOrubicin, doxycycline, droperidol, enalaprilat, etoposide, famotidine, floxuridine, fluconazole, fludarabine, fluorouracil, furosemide, gallium, gentamicin, granisetron, haloperidol, heparin, hydrocortisone, hydromorphone, idarubicin, ifosfamide, imipenem-cilastatin, leucovorin, lorazepam, magnesium sulfate, mannitol, mechlorethamine, meperidine, mesna, methotrexate, methylPREDNISolone, metoclopramide, metronidazole, mezlocillin, mitomycin, mitoxantrone, morphine, nalbuphine, netilmicin, ondansetron, piperacillin, plicamycin, potassium chloride, promethazine, ranitidine, sodium bicarbonate, streptozocin, teniposide, thiotepa, ticarcillin, ticarcillin/clavulanate, tobramycin, trimethoprim-sulfamethoxazole, trimetrexate, vancomycin, vinBLAStine, vinCRIStine, zidovudine

Solution compatibility: 0.9% NaCl

Additive incompatibilities: Do not mix with other products

Evaluate:

- Therapeutic response: prevention of renal toxicity associated with cisplatin therapy; decreased xerostomia associated with radiation therapy of head, neck cancer

Teach patient/family:

- The reason for the medication and expected results
- That side effects may cause severe nausea, vomiting, decreased B/P, chills, dizziness, somnolence, hiccups, sneezing
- Do not breastfeed

amikacin (℞)

(am-i-kay′sin)

amikacin sulfate, Amikin

Func. class.: Antiinfective

Chem. class.: Aminoglycoside

Do not confuse:

Amikin/Amicar

Action: Interferes with protein synthesis in bacterial cell by binding to ribosomal subunit, which causes misreading of genetic code; inaccurate peptide sequence forms in protein chain, causing bacterial death

Uses: Severe systemic infections of CNS, respiratory, GI, urinary tract, bone, skin, soft tissues caused by *Staphylococcus aureus (MSSA), Pseudomonas aeruginosa, Escherichia coli, Enterobacter, Acinetobacter, Providencia, Citrobacter, Serratia, Proteus, Klebsiella pneumoniae*
Unlabeled uses: *Mycobacterium avium* complex (intrathecal or intraventricular) in combination; aerosolization, actinomycotic mycetoma

DOSAGE AND ROUTES

Severe systemic infections

- *Adult and child:* **IV INF** 15 mg/kg/day in 2-3 divided doses q8-12hr in 100-200 ml D_5W over 30-60 min, max 1.5 g; use for 7-10 days; decreased doses are needed in poor renal function as determined by blood levels, renal studies; pulse dosing (once-daily dosing) may be used with some infections; **IM** 15 mg/kg/day in divided doses q8-12hr; daily or extended interval dosing as an alternative dosing regimen
- *Infant:* **IV/IM** 10 mg/kg initially; then 7.5 mg/kg q12hr
- *Neonate:* **IV/IM** 10 mg/kg, initially, 7.5 mg/kg q12hr
- *Premature neonate:* 10 mg/kg initially, then 7.5 mg/kg q8-12hr

Severe urinary tract infections

- *Adult:* **IM** 15 mg/kg/day divided q8-12hr

Hemodialysis

- *Adult:* **IM/IV** 7.5 mg/kg followed by 5 mg/kg 3×/week after each dialysis session (for TIW dialysis)

TB or other mycobacterial infection

- *Adult and adolescent:* **IV** 7.5-15 mg/kg divided q12-24hr as part of multiple-drug regimen
- *Child:* **IV** 15-30 mg/kg/day divided q12-24hr as part of multiple-drug regimen, max 1.5 g/day

Renal dose

- *Adult:* **IV/IM** 7.5 mg/kg initially, then increased as determined by blood levels, renal function studies

Mycobacterium avium complex (MAC) (unlabeled)

- *Adult and adolescent:* **IV** 7.5-15 mg/kg divided q12-24hr as part of multiple-drug regimen
- *Child:* **IV** 15-30 mg/kg/day divided q12-24hr as part of multiple-drug regimen, max 1.5 g/day

Actinomycotic mycetoma (unlabeled)

- *Adult:* **IM/IV** 15 mg/kg/day in 2 divided doses × 3 wk with co-trimoxazole for 5 wk; repeat cycle once, may be repeated 2×

Available forms: Inj 50, 250 mg/ml

SIDE EFFECTS

CNS: Confusion, depression, numbness, tremors, **seizures,** muscle twitching, **neurotoxicity,** dizziness, vertigo, tinnitus, **neuromuscular blockade with respiratory paralysis**

CV: Hypo/hypertension, palpitations

EENT: *Ototoxicity,* deafness, visual disturbances

GI: *Nausea, vomiting, anorexia;* increased ALT, AST, bilirubin; hepatomegaly, **hepatic necrosis,** splenomegaly

GU: **Oliguria, hematuria, renal damage, azotemia, renal failure, nephrotoxicity**

HEMA: **Agranulocytosis, thrombocytopenia, leukopenia, eosinophilia, anemia**

INTEG: *Rash,* burning, urticaria, dermatitis, alopecia

Contraindications: Pregnancy (D), mild to moderate infections, hypersensitivity to aminoglycosides, sulfites

Precautions: Breastfeeding, neonates, geriatric patients, myasthenia gravis, Parkinson's disease

Black Box Warning: Hearing impairment, renal/neuromuscular disease

PHARMACOKINETICS

IM: Onset rapid, peak 1-2 hr, leads to unpredictable concentrations, IV preferred

IV: Onset immediate, peak 15-30 min; plasma half-life 2-3 hr, prolonged up to 7 hr in infants; not metabolized; excreted unchanged in urine; crosses placental barrier; poor penetration into CSF; removed by hemodialysis

INTERACTIONS

• May increase serum trough and peak: indomethacin

• Mask ototoxicity: dimenhyDRINATE, ethacrynic acid

• Nephrotoxicity: cephalosporins, acyclovir, vancomycin, amphotericin B, cycloSPORINE

• Do not use with cidofovir

Increase: neuromuscular blockade, respiratory depression—anesthetics, nondepolarizing neuromuscular blockers

Drug/Herb

• Do not use acidophilus with antiinfectives; separate by several hours

• Toxicity: lysine (large amounts)

Drug/Lab Test

Increase: BUN, ALT, AST, bilirubin, LDH, alk phos, creatinine

Decrease: Ca, Na, K, Mg

NURSING CONSIDERATIONS

Assess:

• Weight before treatment; calculation of dosage is usually based on ideal body weight but may be calculated on actual body weight

• I&O ratio; urinalysis daily for proteinuria, cells, casts; report sudden change in urine output

• VS during infusion; watch for hypotension, change in pulse

• IV site for thrombophlebitis including pain, redness, swelling q30 min; change site if needed; apply warm compresses to discontinued site

• Serum aminoglycoside concentration; serum peak, drawn at 30-60 min after IV infusion or 60 min after IM inj, trough level drawn just before next dose; peak 20-30 mcg/ml, trough 4-8 mcg/ml; adjust dosage per levels

• Urine pH if product is used for UTI; urine should be kept alkaline

• Renal impairment by securing urine for CCr, BUN, serum creatinine; lower dosage should be given in renal impairment (CCr <80 ml/min); nephrotoxicity may be reversible if product stopped at first sign

⚠ Deafness by audiometric testing, ringing, roaring in ears, vertigo; assess hearing before, during, after treatment

• Dehydration: high specific gravity, decrease in skin turgor, dry mucous membranes, dark urine

• Overgrowth of infection, including increased temp, malaise, redness, pain, swelling, perineal itching, diarrhea, stomatitis, change in cough, sputum

• C&S before starting treatment to identify organism

• Vestibular dysfunction: nausea, vomiting, dizziness, headache; product should be discontinued if severe

• Inj sites for redness, swelling, abscesses; use warm compresses at site

Administer:

IM route

• Inj in large muscle mass; rotate inj sites

• Bicarbonate to alkalinize urine if ordered for UTI because product is most active in alkaline environment

Intermittent IV INF route

• Dilute 500 mg of product/100-200 ml of IV D_5W, D_5RL, D_5NaCl, or 0.9% NaCl and give over ½-1 hr; flush after administration with D_5W or 0.9% NaCl; solution is clear or pale yellow; discard if precipitate or dark color develops

• In evenly spaced doses to maintain blood level

Additive compatibilities: Avoid admixing

Syringe compatibilities: Clindamycin, doxapram

Y-site compatibilities: Acyclovir, alatrofloxacin, aldesleukin, amifostine, aminophylline, amiodarone, amsacrine, anidulafungin, aztreonam, cefepime, cisatracurium, cyclophosphamide, dexamethasone, diltiazem, enalaprilat, esmolol, filgrastim, fluconazole, fludarabine, foscarnet, furosemide, granisetron, idarubicin, IL-2, labetalol, lorazepam, magnesium sulfate, melphalan, midazolam, morphine, ondansetron, paclitaxel, perphenazine, remifentanil, sargramostim, teniposide, thiotepa, TPN #54, #61, #91, #203, #204, #212, vinorelbine, warfarin, zidovudine

Perform/provide:

- Adequate fluids of 2-3 L/day, unless contraindicated, to prevent irritation of tubules
- Flush of IV line with NS or D_5W after infusion
- Supervised ambulation, other safety measures with vestibular dysfunction

Evaluate:

- Therapeutic response: absence of fever, draining wounds, negative C&S after treatment

Teach patient/family:

- To report headache, dizziness, symptoms for overgrowth of infection, renal impairment

⚠ To report loss of hearing, ringing, roaring in ears or feeling of fullness in head

- To report hypersensitivity: rash, itching, trouble breathing, facial edema; notify health care provider

Treatment of hypersensitivity: Hemodialysis, exchange transfusion in the newborn, monitor serum levels of product, may give ticarcillin or carbenicillin

amiloride (℞)

(a-mill'oh-ride)

amiloride HCl, Midamor

Func. class.: Potassium-sparing diuretic

Chem. class.: Pyrazine

Do not confuse:
amiloride/amlodipine

Action: Inhibits sodium, potassium ATPase in the distal tubule, cortical collecting duct resulting in inhibition of sodium reabsorption and decreasing potassium secretion

Uses: Edema in CHF in combination with other diuretics, for hypertension, adjunct with other diuretics to maintain potassium, polyuria due to lithium administration

Unlabeled uses: Ascites

DOSAGE AND ROUTES

- *Adult:* **PO** 5-10 mg/day in 1-2 divided doses; may be increased to 10-20 mg/day if needed

Ascites (unlabeled)

- *Adult:* **PO** 10 mg/day, max 40 mg

Available forms: Tabs 5 mg

SIDE EFFECTS

CNS: Headache, dizziness, fatigue, weakness, paresthesias, tremor, depression, anxiety

CV: Orthostatic hypotension, dysrhythmias, chest pain

EENT: Blurred vision, increased intraocular pressure

ELECT: **Hyperkalemia,** dehydration

GI: Nausea, diarrhea, dry mouth, *vomiting, anorexia,* cramps, constipation, abdominal pain, jaundice

GU: Polyuria, dysuria, urinary frequency, impotence

HEMA: **Aplastic anemia, neutropenia**

INTEG: Rash, pruritus, alopecia, urticaria

MS: Cramps

RESP: Cough, dyspnea, shortness of breath

Contraindications: Anuria, hypersensitivity, impaired renal function

Black Box Warning: Hyperkalemia

Precautions: Pregnancy (B), breastfeeding, geriatric patients, dehydration, diabetes, acidosis

PHARMACOKINETICS

15%-25% absorbed from GI tract; widely distributed; onset 2 hr; peak 6-10 hr; duration 24 hr; excreted in urine, feces; half-life 6-9 hr

INTERACTIONS

- Hyperkalemia: other potassium-sparing diuretics, potassium products, ACE inhibitors, salt substitutes, cycloSPORINE, tacrolimus
- Lithium toxicity: lithium

Increase: action of antihypertensives
Decrease: effect of amiloride—NSAIDs
Drug/Herb
• Fatal hypokalemia: arginine
• Hypokalemia: bearberry, gossypol, licorice
• Severe photosensitivity: St. John's wort
Increase: effect—cucumber, dandelion, horsetail, licorice, nettle, pumpkin, Queen Anne's lace
Increase: hypotension—khella
Drug/Food
• Possible hyperkalemia: foods high in potassium
Drug/Lab Test
Interference: GTT

NURSING CONSIDERATIONS

Assess:
• Weight, I&O daily to determine fluid loss; effect of product may be decreased if used daily
• B/P lying, standing; postural hypotension may occur
• Electrolytes: K, Na, Cl; glucose (serum), BUN, CBC, serum creatinine, blood pH, ABGs
Administer:
• In AM to avoid interference with sleep if using product as a diuretic; if second daily dose is needed, give in late afternoon
• With food; if nausea occurs, absorption may be decreased slightly
Evaluate:
• Therapeutic response: improvement in edema of feet, legs, sacral area daily if medication is being used in CHF
Teach patient/family:
• To take as prescribed; if dose is missed, take when remembered within 1 hr of next dose
• About adverse reactions: muscle cramps, weakness, nausea, dizziness, blurred vision
• To take with food or milk for GI symptoms
• To take early in day to prevent nocturia
• To avoid potassium-rich foods: oranges, bananas; salt substitutes, dried fruits
Treatment of overdose: Lavage if taken orally, monitor electrolytes, administer sodium bicarbonate for potassium >6.5 mEq/L, IV glucose, kayoxalate as needed; monitor hydration, CV, renal status

amino acid injection (℞)

(a-mee'noe)
FreAmine, HepatAmine
Func. class.: Nitrogen product

Action: Needed for anabolism to maintain structure, decrease catabolism, promote healing
Uses: Hepatic encephalopathy, cirrhosis, hepatitis, nutritional support in cancer; to prevent nitrogen loss when adequate nutrition by mouth, gastric, or duodenal tube cannot be used

DOSAGE AND ROUTES

• *Adult:* **IV** 80-120 g/day; 500 ml of amino acids/500 ml D_{50} given over 24 hr
Available forms: Inj; many strengths, types

SIDE EFFECTS

CNS: *Dizziness, headache,* confusion, **loss of consciousness**
CV: Hypertension, **CHF, pulmonary edema**
ENDO: *Hyperglycemia, rebound hypoglycemia, electrolyte imbalances, hyperosmolar syndrome, hyperosmolar hyperglycemic nonketotic syndrome,* alkalosis, acidosis, hypophosphatemia, hyperammonemia, dehydration, hypocalcemia
GI: Nausea, vomiting, liver fat deposits, abdominal pain
GU: Glycosuria, osmotic diuresis
INTEG: Chills, flushing, warm feeling, rash, urticaria, extravasation necrosis, phlebitis at inj site
Contraindications: Hypersensitivity, severe electrolyte imbalances, anuria, severe liver damage, maple syrup urine disease, PKU
Precautions: Pregnancy (C), breastfeeding, children, renal disease, diabetes mellitus, CHF

INTERACTIONS

Decrease: protein sparing effects—tetracycline

NURSING CONSIDERATIONS

Assess:

- Electrolytes (K, Na, Ca, Cl, Mg), blood glucose, ammonia, phosphate, ketones
- Renal, hepatic studies: BUN, creatinine, ALT, AST, bilirubin
- Inj site for extravasation: redness along vein, edema at site, necrosis, pain, hard tender area; site should be changed immediately
- Respiratory function q4hr: auscultate lung fields bilaterally for crackles, respirations, quality, rate, rhythm
- Temp q4hr for increased fever, indicating infection; if infection suspected, inf is discontinued, tubing and solution cultured

⚠ For impending hepatic coma: asterixis, confusion, uremic fetor, lethargy

- Hyperammonemia: nausea, vomiting, malaise, tremors, anorexia, seizures

Administer:

CONT IV INF route

- Up to 40% protein and dextrose (up to 12.5%) via peripheral vein; stronger solutions require central IV administration
- TPN only mixed with dextrose to promote protein synthesis
- Immediately after mixing under strict aseptic technique, use infusion pump, in-line filter (0.22 μm) unless mixed with fat emulsion and dextrose (3 in 1)

⚠ Using careful monitoring technique; do not speed up infusion; pulmonary edema, glucose overload will result

Additive compatibilities: Amikacin, aminophylline, aztreonam, calcium gluconate, cefazolin, cefepime, cefotaxime, cefoxitin, cefsulodin, ceftazidime, ceftriaxone, cefuroxime, cimetidine, clindamycin, cyanocobalamin, cyclophosphamide, cycloSPORINE, cytarabine, DOPamine, epoetin, erythromycin, famotidine, folic acid, fosphenytoin, furosemide, heparin, insulin (regular), isoproterenol, lidocaine, meperidine, metaraminol, methicillin, methotrexate, methyldopate, methylPREDNISolone, metoclopramide, morphine, nafcillin, netilmicin, nizatidine, norepinephrine, ondansetron, oxacillin, penicillin G potassium, penicillin G sodium, phytonadione, polymyxin B, sodium bicarbonate, tacrolimus, tobramycin, vancomycin

Y-site compatibilities: Amikacin, aminophylline, amoxicillin, ampicillin, ascorbic acid inj, atracurium, azlocillin, aztreonam, bumetanide, buprenorphine, calcium gluconate, carboplatin, cefonicid, cefoperazone, cefotaxime, cefotetan, cefoxitin, ceftazidime, ceftizoxime, ceftriaxone, cefuroxime, cephalothin, cephapirin, chloramphenicol, chlorproMAZINE, cimetidine, clindamycin, clonazepam, dexamethasone, diazepam, digoxin, diphenhydrAMINE, DOBUTamine, DOPamine, doxycycline, droperidol, enalaprilat, epinephrine, erythromycin, famotidine, fentanyl, flucloxacillin, fluconazole, folic acid, foscarnet, gentamicin, granisetron, haloperidol, heparin, hydrocortisone, hydromorphone, hydrOXYzine, idarubicin, ifosfamide, IL-2, imipenem/cilastatin, insulin (regular), isoproterenol, kanamycin, leucovorin, levorphanol, lidocaine, lorazepam, magnesium sulfate, mannitol, meperidine, mesna, methicillin, metronidazole, mezlocillin, miconazole, morphine, moxalactam, multivitamins, nafcillin, netilmicin, nitroglycerin, nitroprusside, norepinephrine, octreotide, ofloxacin, ondansetron, oxacillin, paclitaxel, penicillin G, penicillin G potassium, pentobarbital, phenobarbital, piperacillin, potassium chloride, prochlorperazine, ranitidine, salbutamol, sargramostim, tacrolimus, thiotepa, ticarcillin, ticarcillin/clavulanate, tobramycin, trimethoprim-sulfamethoxazole, urokinase, vancomycin, vecuronium, zidovudine

Perform/provide:

- Storage depends on type of solution; consult manufacturer
- Changing dressing and IV tubing to prevent infection q24-48hr

Evaluate:
- Therapeutic response: weight gain, decrease in jaundice in liver disorders, increased LOC

Teach patient/family:
- The reason for use of TPN
- If chills, sweating are experienced, report at once
- About infusion pump and blood glucose monitoring

amino acid solution (℞)

Aminees, Aminosyn, Branch Amin, FreAmine III, NephrAmine, Novamine, ProcalAmine, Ren Amin, Travasol, Troph Amine

Func. class.: Nitrogen product

Action: Needed for anabolism to maintain structure, decrease catabolism, promote healing

Uses: Nutritional support in cancer, trauma, intestinal obstruction, short bowel syndrome, severe malabsorption

DOSAGE AND ROUTES

- *Adult:* **IV** 1-1.5 g/kg/day titrated to patient's needs
- *Child:* **IV** 2-3 g/kg/day titrated to patient's needs

Available forms: Inj, many types, strengths

SIDE EFFECTS

CNS: Dizziness, headache, confusion, **loss of consciousness**

CV: Hypertension, **CHF, pulmonary edema**

ENDO: *Hyperglycemia, rebound hypoglycemia, electrolyte imbalances, hyperosmolar syndrome, hyperosmolar hyperglycemic nonketotic syndrome,* alkalosis, acidosis, hypophosphatemia, hyperammonemia, dehydration, hypocalcemia

GI: Nausea, vomiting, liver fat deposits, abdominal pain, jaundice

GU: Glycosuria, osmotic diuresis

INTEG: Chills, flushing, warm feeling, rash, urticaria, extravasation necrosis, phlebitis at inj site

Contraindications: Hypersensitivity, severe electrolyte imbalances, anuria, severe liver damage, maple syrup urine disease, PKU

Precautions: Pregnancy (C), breastfeeding, children, renal disease, diabetes mellitus, CHF

NURSING CONSIDERATIONS

Assess:
- Electrolytes (K, Na, Ca, Cl, Mg), blood glucose, ammonia, phosphate
- Renal, hepatic studies: BUN, creatinine, ALT, AST, bilirubin
- Inj site for extravasation: redness along vein, edema at site, necrosis, pain, hard tender area; site should be changed immediately
- Monitor respiratory function q4hr: auscultate lung fields bilaterally for crackles, respirations, quality, rate, rhythm
- Monitor temp q4hr for increased fever, indicating infection; if infection suspected, discontinue infusion, culture tubing, bottle
- Urine glucose q6hr using Tes-Tape, Clinistix, which are not affected by infusion substances; blood glucose is preferred testing method
- Hyperammonemia: nausea, vomiting, malaise, tremors, anorexia, seizures

Administer:

CONT IV INF route
- Up to 40% protein and dextrose (up to 12.5%) via peripheral vein; stronger solutions require central IV administration, use infusion pump
- TPN only mixed with dextrose to promote protein synthesis
- Immediately after mixing in pharmacy under strict aseptic technique using laminar flow hood, use infusion pump, in-line filter (0.22 μm) unless mixed with fat emulsion and dextrose (3 in 1)

⚠ Using careful monitoring technique; do not speed up infusion; pulmonary edema, glucose overload will result

Y-site compatibilities: Cefazolin, cefoperazone, cefotaxime, cefoxitin, cephalothin, cephapirin, chloramphenicol, clindamycin, digoxin, DOBUTamine, DOPamine, doxycycline, erythromycin lactobionate, fat emulsion, foscarnet, furosemide, gentamicin, isoproterenol, kanamycin, lidocaine, meperidine, methicillin, mezlocillin, miconazole, morphine, nafcillin, netilmicin, norepinephrine, oxacillin, penicillin G potassium, piperacillin, sargramostim, ticarcillin, tobramycin, urokinase, vancomycin

Perform/provide:

- Storage depends on type of solution; consult label
- Dressing and IV tubing change q24-48hr to prevent infection

Evaluate:

- Therapeutic response: weight gain, decrease in jaundice in liver disorders, increased serum albumin

Teach patient/family:

- The reason for use of TPN
- That any chills, sweating should be reported at once
- About infusion pump and blood glucose monitoring

aminophylline (theophylline ethylenediamine) (℞)

(am-in-off'i-lin)

Phyllocontin, Truphylline

Func. class.: Bronchodilator, spasmolytic

Chem. class.: Methylxanthine

Action: Exact mechanism unknown, relaxes smooth muscle of respiratory system by blocking phosphodiesterase, which increases cAMP; increased cAMP alters intracellular calcium ion movements; produces bronchodilation, increased pulmonary blood flow, relaxation of respiratory tract

Uses: Bronchial asthma, bronchospasm associated with chronic bronchitis, emphysema, bradycardia, apnea in infancy for respiratory/myocardial stimulation

Unlabeled uses: Methotrexate toxicity, sleep apnea, status asthmaticus

DOSAGE AND ROUTES

- *Adult:* **PO** 6 mg/kg, then 3 mg/kg q6hr × 2 doses, then 3 mg/kg q8hr maintenance, max 900 mg/day or 13 mg/kg; **PO** in CHF 6 mg/kg, then 2 mg/kg q8hr × 2 doses, then 1-2 mg/kg q12hr maintenance; **IV** 4.7 mg/kg, then 0.55 mg/kg/hr × 12 hr, then 0.36/kg/hr maintenance; **IV** in CHF 4.7 mg/kg, then 0.39 mg/kg/hr × 12 hr, then 0.08-0.16 mg/kg/hr maintenance
- *Geriatric and in cor pulmonale:* **PO** 6 mg/kg, then 2 mg/kg q6hr × 2 doses, then 2 mg/kg q8hr maintenance; **IV** 4.7 mg/kg, then 0.47 mg/kg/hr × 12 hr, then 0.24 mg/kg/hr maintenance
- *Child 9-16 yr:* **PO** 6 mg/kg, then 3 mg/kg q4hr × 3 doses, then 3 mg/kg q6hr maintenance, max 18 mg/kg/day for 12-16 yr old, or 20 mg/kg/day for 9-12 yr old; **IV** 4.7 mg/kg, then 0.79 mg/kg/hr × 12 hr, then 0.63 mg/kg/hr maintenance
- *Child 6 mo-9 yr:* **PO** 4 mg/kg q4hr × 3 doses, then 4 mg/kg q6hr maintenance, max 24 mg/kg/day; **IV** 4.7 mg/kg, then 0.95 mg/kg/hr × 12 hr, then 0.79 mg/kg/hr maintenance
- *Infant 6-52 wk:* Dose (0.2 × age in wk) ÷ 5 × kg = 24 hr dose in mg
- *Neonate—up to 40 wk premature postconception age:* **PO/IV** 1 mg/kg q12hr
- *Neonate at birth or 40 wk postconception age:* **PO/IV** over 8 wk postnatal 1-3 mg/kg q6hr; 4-8 wk postnatal 1-2 mg/kg q8hr; up to 4 wk postnatal 1-2 mg/kg q12hr

Hepatic disease

- *Adult:* **PO** 6 mg/kg then 2 mg/kg q8hr × 2 doses, then 1-2 mg/kg q12hr maintenance; **IV** 4.7 mg/kg, then 0.39 mg/kg/hr × 12 hr, then 0.08-0.16 mg/kg/hr maintenance

Methotrexate toxicity (unlabeled)

- *Adult and child 3-16 yr:* **IV** 2.5 mg/kg over 45-60 min

Sleep apnea in CHF-induced systolic dysfunction (unlabeled)

• *Adult:* **PO** 3.3 mg/kg bid × 5 days

Status asthmaticus (unlabeled)

• *Adult and child:* **IV** 5 mg/kg over 20-30 min; **PO** 5 mg/kg

Available forms: Inj 250 mg/10 ml, 500 mg/20 ml, 100 mg/100 ml in 0.45% NaCl, 200 mg/100 ml in 0.45% NaCl; rect supp 250, 500 mg; oral liq 105 mg/5 ml; tabs 100, 200 mg; con rel tabs 225, 350 mg

SIDE EFFECTS

CNS: Anxiety, restlessness, insomnia, *dizziness,* **seizures,** headache, lightheadedness, muscle twitching, tremors

CV: Palpitations, sinus tachycardia, hypotension, flushing, **dysrhythmias,** edema

GI: Nausea, vomiting, diarrhea, dyspepsia, anal irritation (suppositories), epigastric pain, reflux, anorexia

GU: Urinary frequency, SIADH

INTEG: Flushing, urticaria

MISC: Hyperglycemia

RESP: Tachypnea, increased respiratory rate

Contraindications: Hypersensitivity to xanthines, tachydysrhythmias

Precautions: Pregnancy (C), breastfeeding, children, geriatric patients, CHF, cor pulmonale, hepatic disease, diabetes mellitus, hyperthyroidism, hypertension, seizure disorder, irritation of the rectum or lower colon, alcoholism, active peptic ulcer disease

PHARMACOKINETICS

Metabolized by liver (caffeine); excreted in urine; crosses placenta; appears in breast milk; half-life 6.5-10.5 hr; half-life increased in geriatric patients, hepatic disease, CHF, neonates, premature infants; protein binding 40%

PO: Onset ¼ hr, peak 1-2 hr, duration 6-8 hr, well absorbed

PO-ER: Onset unknown, peak 4-7 hr, duration 8-12 hr, well absorbed slowly

IV: Onset rapid, duration 6-8 hr

RECT: Onset erratic, peak 1-2 hr, duration 6-8 hr, supp absorbed erratically, sol absorbed quickly

INTERACTIONS

• Dose-dependent reversal of neuromuscular blockade

• Dysrhythmias: halothane

• May increase or decrease aminophylline levels: carbamazepine, loop diuretics, isoniazid

Increase: action of aminophylline, toxicity—cimetidine, nonselective β-blockers, erythromycin, clarithromycin, oral contraceptives, corticosteroids, interferons, fluoroquinolones, disulfiram, mexiletine, fluvoxamine, high doses of allopurinol, influenza vaccines, interferon, benzodiazepines

Increase: adverse reactions—tetracyclines

Increase: elimination—smoking

Decrease: effects of lithium

Decrease: effect of aminophylline—nicotine products, adrenergics, barbiturates, phenytoin, ketoconazole, rifampin

Drug/Herb

Increase: effects—cola tree, guarana, yerba maté, tea (black, green), horsetail, ginseng, Siberian ginseng

Decrease: effects—St. John's wort

Drug/Food

Increase: effect—xanthines

Increase: elimination by low-carbohydrate, high-protein diet; charcoal-broiled beef

Decrease: elimination by high-carbohydrate and low-protein diet

Drug/Lab Test

Increase: plasma-free fatty acids

NURSING CONSIDERATIONS

Assess:

• Theophylline blood levels (therapeutic level is 10-20 mcg/ml); toxicity may occur with small increase above 20 mcg/ml, especially in geriatric patients

- Monitor I&O; diuresis occurs; dehydration may occur in geriatric patients or children
- Whether theophylline was given recently (24 hr)
- Respiratory rate, rhythm, depth; auscultate lung fields bilaterally; notify prescriber of abnormalities
- Allergic reactions: rash, urticaria; if these occur, product should be discontinued

Administer:

- Avoid IM inj; pain and tissue damage may occur

PO route

- Do not break, crush, or chew enteric-coated or cont rel tabs
- Avoid giving with food

Rectal route

- If patient is unable to take PO, retain rectal dose for ½ hr
- Remain in bed 15-20 min after rect supp is inserted to avoid removal

IV route

- Only clear sol; flush IV line before dose
- May be diluted for IV INF in 100-200 ml in D_5W, $D_{10}W$, $D_{20}W$, 0.9% NaCl, 0.45% NaCl, LR
- Give loading dose over ½ hr; max rate of inf 25 mg/min, use infusion pump; after loading dose give by cont inf

Additive compatibilities: Amobarbital, bretylium, calcium gluconate, chloramphenicol, cibenzoline, cimetidine, dexamethasone, diphenhydrAMINE, DOPamine, erythromycin lactobionate, esmolol, floxacillin, flumazenil, furosemide, heparin, hydrocortisone, lidocaine, mephentermine, meropenem, methyldopate, metronidazole/sodium bicarbonate, nitroglycerin, pentobarbital, phenobarbital, potassium chloride, ranitidine, secobarbital, sodium bicarbonate, terbutaline

Syringe compatibilities: Heparin, metoclopramide, pentobarbital, thiopental

Y-site compatibilities: Allopurinol, amifostine, amphotericin B, amrinone, aztreonam, ceftazidime, cholesteryl sulfate complex, cimetidine, cladribine, DOXOrubicin liposome, enalaprilat, esmolol, famotidine, filgrastim, fluconazole, fludarabine, foscarnet, gallium, granisetron, heparin sodium with hydrocortisone sodium succinate, labetalol, melphalan, meropenem, netilmicin, paclitaxel, pancuronium, piperacillin/tazobactam, potassium chloride, propofol, ranitidine, remifentanil, sargramostim, tacrolimus, teniposide, thiotepa, tolazoline, vecuronium

Perform/provide:

- Storage of diluted solution for 24 hr if refrigerated

Evaluate:

- Therapeutic response: decreased dyspnea, respiratory stimulation in infancy, clear lung fields bilaterally

Teach patient/family:

- To take doses as prescribed, not to skip dose, not to double dose
- To check OTC medications, current prescription medications for ephedrine; will increase CNS stimulation; not to drink alcohol or caffeine products (tea, coffee, chocolate, colas)
- To avoid hazardous activities; dizziness may occur
- If GI upset occurs, to take product with 8 oz water; avoid food, since absorption may be decreased
- ⚠ To notify prescriber of toxicity: insomnia, anxiety, nausea, vomiting, rapid pulse, seizures, flushing, headache, diarrhea; notify prescriber immediately
- To notify prescriber of change in smoking habit; a change in dose may be required
- To increase fluids to 2 L/day to decrease secretion viscosity
- To avoid smoking; decreases blood levels and terminal half-life

⚠ High Alert

amiodarone (℞)

(a-mee-oh'da-rone)

Cordarone, Pacerone

Func. class.: Antidysrhythmic (class III)

Chem. class.: Iodinated benzofuran derivative

Do not confuse:
amiodarone/Inamrinone
Cordarone/Inocor

Action: Prolongs duration of action potential and effective refractory period, noncompetitive α- and β-adrenergic inhibition; increases PR and QT intervals, decreases sinus rate, decreases peripheral vascular resistance

Uses: Severe ventricular tachycardia, supraventricular tachycardia, ventricular fibrillation not controlled by first-line agents

Unlabeled uses: Atrial fibrillation treatment/prophylaxis, atrial flutter, cardiac arrest, cardiac surgery, CPR, heart failure, PSVT, Wolff-Parkinson-White (WPW) syndrome

DOSAGE AND ROUTES

Ventricular dysrhythmias

• *Adult:* **PO** Loading dose 800-1600 mg/day for 1-3 wk; then 600-800 mg/day × 1 mo; maintenance 400 mg/day; **IV** loading dose (first rapid) 150 mg over the first 10 min then slow 360 mg over the next 6 hr; maintenance 540 mg given over the remaining 18 hr, decrease rate of the slow inf to 0.5 mg/min

• *Child:* **PO** Loading dose 10-15 mg/kg/day in 1-2 divided doses for 4-14 days then 5 mg/kg/day (not recommended in children)

• *Child and infant:* **IV/INTRAOSSEOUS** 5 mg/kg as a bolus (PALS guidelines)

Perfusion tachycardia

• *Adult:* **IV** 5 mg/kg loading dose given over 20-60 min

Supraventricular tachycardia

• *Adult:* **PO** 600-800 mg/day × 7 days or until desired response, then 400 mg/day × 21 days, then 200-400 mg/day maintenance

• *Child:* **PO** 10 mg/kg/day (800 mg/1.72 m^2/day) × 10 days or until desired response, then 5 mg/kg/day (400 mg/1.72 m^2/day) × 21-28 days, then 2.5 mg/kg/day (200 mg/1.72 m^2/day) (not recommended in children)

Supraventricular dysrhythmias (atrial fibrillation, atrial flutter, PSVT, WPW syndrome) (unlabeled)

• *Adult:* **PO** 1.2-1.8 g/day divided until a total of 10 g has been given, then 200-400 mg/day (class IIa recommendation); **IV** 5-7 mg/kg over 30-60 min, then 1.2-1.8 g as **CONT IV INF** or in divided PO doses until 10 g, then 200-400 mg/day (class IIa recommendation)

• *Child and infant:* **PO** 10-20 mg/kg/day in divided doses for 7-10 days, then 5-10 mg/kg/day once daily

Available forms: Tabs 100, 200, 400 mg; inj 50 mg/ml

SIDE EFFECTS

CNS: Headache, dizziness, involuntary movement, tremors, peripheral neuropathy, malaise, fatigue, ataxia, paresthesias, insomnia

CV: Hypotension, bradycardia, **sinus arrest, CHF, dysrhythmias, SA node dysfunction**

EENT: Blurred vision, halos, photophobia, **corneal microdeposits,** dry eyes

ENDO: Hypo/hyperthyroidism

GI: Nausea, vomiting, diarrhea, abdominal pain, anorexia, constipation, **hepatotoxicity**

INTEG: Rash, photosensitivity, blue-gray skin discoloration, alopecia, spontaneous ecchymosis, **toxic epidermal necrolysis,** urticaria

MISC: Flushing, abnormal taste or smell, edema, abnormal salivation, coagulation abnormalities

MS: Weakness, pain in extremities

RESP: **Pulmonary fibrosis,** pulmonary inflammation, **ARDS; gasping syndrome if used in neonates**

Contraindications: Pregnancy (D), breastfeeding, neonates, infants, severe sinus node dysfunction, hypersensitivity, cardiogenic shock

Black Box Warning: 2nd-3rd degree AV block, bradycardia

Precautions: Children, goiter, Hashimoto's thyroiditis, electrolyte imbalances, CHF, respiratory disease

Black Box Warning: Severe hepatic disease, cardiac arrhythmias, pneumonitis, pulmonary fibrosis

PHARMACOKINETICS

PO: Onset 1-3 wk, peak 2-7 hr, half-life 15-100 days, metabolized by liver, excreted by kidneys

INTERACTIONS

Increase: bradycardia—β-blockers, calcium channel blockers

Increase: levels of cycloSPORINE, dextromethorphan, digoxin, disopyramide, flecainide, methotrexate, phenytoin, procainamide, quinidine, theophylline

Increase: anticoagulant effects—warfarin

Drug/Herb

Increase: serotonin effect—horehound

Increase: toxicity/death—aconite

Increase: amiodarone effect—aloe, broom, buckthorn, cascara sagrada, Chinese rhubarb, figwort, fumitory, goldenseal, kudzu, licorice, rhubarb, senna

Decrease: amiodarone effect—coltsfoot

Drug/Food

- Toxicity: grapefruit juice

Drug/Lab Test

Increase: T_4

NURSING CONSIDERATIONS

Assess:

⚠ Pulmonary toxicity: dyspnea, fatigue, cough, fever, chest pain; product should be discontinued

- ECG continuously to determine product effectiveness; measure PR, QRS, QT intervals; check for PVCs, other dysrhythmias, B/P continuously for hypo/hypertension; report dysrhythmias, slowing heart rate
- I&O ratio; electrolytes (K, Na, Cl); hepatic studies: AST, ALT, bilirubin, alk phos
- Chest x-ray, thyroid function tests
- For dehydration or hypovolemia
- For rebound hypertension after 1-2 hr
- For ARDS, pulmonary fibrosis, crackles, dyspnea, tachypnea
- CNS symptoms: confusion, psychosis, numbness, depression, involuntary movements; if these occur, product should be discontinued
- Hypothyroidism: lethargy; dizziness; constipation; enlarged thyroid gland; edema of extremities; cool, pale skin
- Hyperthyroidism: restlessness; tachycardia; eyelid puffiness; weight loss; frequent urination; menstrual irregularities; dyspnea; warm, moist skin
- Ophthalmic exams baseline and periodically (PO)
- Cardiac rate, respiration: rate, rhythm, character, chest pain; start with patient hospitalized and monitored up to 1 wk

Administer:

PO route

- Loading dose with food to decrease nausea

IV, direct route

- Peripheral: Max 2 mg/ml for longer than 1 hr; preferred through central venous line with in-line filter; concentration greater than 2 ml should be given by central line
- Give 300 bol; may repeat 150 mg after 3-5 min; used for cardiac arrest

Intermittent IV INF route

- 1000 mg/24 hr during loading/maintenance
- Initial loading: add 3 ml (150 mg), 100 ml D_5W (1.5 mg/ml), give over 10 min
- Loading inf: add 18 ml (900 mg), 500 ml D_5W (1.8 mg/ml), give over next 6 hr
- Maintenance inf: give remainder of loading inf 540 mg over 18 hr (0.5 mg/min)

CONT IV INF route

- After 24 hr, give 1-6 mg/ml at 0.5 mg/min, max 30 mg/min

Additive compatibilities: DOBUTamine, lidocaine, potassium chloride, procainamide, verapamil

Y-site compatibilities: Amikacin, bretylium, clindamycin, DOBUTamine, DOPamine, doxycycline, erythromycin, esmolol, gentamicin, insulin, isoproterenol, labetalol, lidocaine, metaraminol, metronidazole, midazolam, morphine, nitroglycerin, norepinephrine, penicillin G potassium, phentolamine, phenylephrine, potassium chloride, procainamide, tobramycin, vancomycin

Solution compatibility: D_5W, 0.9% NaCl

Evaluate:

- Therapeutic response: decrease in ventricular tachycardia, supraventricular tachycardia or fibrillation

Teach patient/family:

- To take this product as directed; avoid missed doses; do not use with grapefruit juice
- To use sunscreen or stay out of sun to prevent burns
- To report side effects immediately
- That skin discoloration is usually reversible
- That dark glasses may be needed for photophobia

Treatment of overdose: O_2, artificial ventilation, ECG, administer DOPamine for circulatory depression, administer diazepam or thiopental for seizures, isoproterenol

amitriptyline (℞)

(a-mee-trip′ti-leen)

amitriptyline HCl,

Apo-Amitriptyline ♣

Func. class.: Antidepressant—tricyclic

Chem. class.: Tertiary amine

Do not confuse:
amitriptyline/nortriptyline

Action: Blocks reuptake of norepinephrine, serotonin into nerve endings, increasing action of norepinephrine, serotonin in nerve cells

Uses: Major depression

Unlabeled uses: Neuropathic pain, prevention of cluster/migraine headaches, fibromyalgia, ADHD, bulimia nervosa, diabetic neuropathy, enuresis, insomnia, panic disorder, postherpetic neuralgia, hiccups, social phobia

DOSAGE AND ROUTES

Depression

- *Adult:* **PO** 25-75 mg/day in divided doses, may increase to 150 mg/day, max 300 mg/day
- *Geriatric and adolescent:* **PO** 10-25 mg at bedtime, may be increased to 100 mg/day

Cluster/migraine headache (unlabeled)

- *Adult:* **PO** 10-300 mg/day

Pain (unlabeled)

- *Adult:* **PO** 75-300 mg/day

Fibromyalgia/insomnia (unlabeled)

- *Adult:* **PO** 10-50 mg nightly

Enuresis (unlabeled)

- *Child 11-14 yr:* **PO** 50 mg at bedtime
- *Child 6-10 yr:* **PO** 25 mg at bedtime

ADHD/bulimia nervosa (unlabeled)

- *Adult:* **PO** 25 mg tid, titrate to 200 mg/day by 25-50 mg at weekly intervals
- *Child 6-12 yr:* **PO** 10-30 mg/day or 1-5 mg/kg/day in divided doses

Available forms: Tabs 10, 25, 50, 75, 100, 150 mg

SIDE EFFECTS

CNS: Dizziness, drowsiness, confusion, headache, anxiety, tremors, stimulation, weakness, insomnia, nightmares, EPS (geriatric patients), increased psychiatric symptoms, **seizures**

CV: Orthostatic hypotension, **ECG changes, tachycardia, hypertension,** palpitations, **dysrhythmias**

EENT: Blurred vision, tinnitus, mydriasis, ophthalmoplegia

GI: Constipation, dry mouth, weight gain, nausea, vomiting, **paralytic ileus,** increased appetite, cramps, epigastric distress, jaundice, **hepatitis,** stomatitis

GU: Urinary retention

HEMA: **Agranulocytosis, thrombocytopenia, eosinophilia, leukopenia, aplastic anemia**
INTEG: Rash, urticaria, sweating, pruritus, photosensitivity
Contraindications: Hypersensitivity to tricyclics, recovery phase of myocardial infarction
Precautions: Pregnancy (C), breastfeeding, geriatric patients, seizure disorders, prostatic hypertrophy, schizophrenia, psychosis, severe depression, increased intraocular pressure, closed-angle glaucoma, urinary retention, renal/hepatic/cardiac disease, hyperthyroidism, electroshock therapy, elective surgery

Black Box Warning: Children <12 yr, suicidal patients

PHARMACOKINETICS

Onset 45 min; peak 2-12 hr; therapeutic response 4-10 days; metabolized by liver; excreted in urine, feces; crosses placenta; excreted in breast milk; half-life 10-46 hr

INTERACTIONS

⚠ Hyperpyretic crisis, seizures, hypertensive episode: MAOIs
Increase: risk of agranulocytosis—antithyroid agents
Increase: QT prolongation—procainamide, quinidine, amiodarone, tricyclics, class IA, III antidysrhythmics
Increase: amitriptyline levels, toxicity—cimetidine, fluoxetine, phenothiazines, oral contraceptives, antidepressants, carbamazepine, class IC antidysrhythmics
Increase: effects of direct-acting sympathomimetics (epinephrine), alcohol, barbiturates, benzodiazepines, CNS depressants, opioids, sedative/hypnotics
Decrease: effects of guanethidine, clonidine, indirect-acting sympathomimetics (ephedrine)

Drug/Herb

Increase: serotonin syndrome—SAM-e, St. John's wort
Increase: CNS depression—kava, skullcap, hops, chamomile, lavender, valerian
Increase: anticholinergic effect—belladonna leaf/root, henbane leaf, jimsonweed, scopolia
Increase: action of amitriptyline—jimsonweed, scopolia root
Increase: hypertension—yohimbe

Drug/Lab Test

Increase: serum bilirubin, blood glucose, alk phos

NURSING CONSIDERATIONS

Assess:

- B/P lying, standing; pulse q4hr; if systolic B/P drops 20 mm Hg, hold product, notify prescriber; take vital signs q4hr in patients with CV disease
- Blood studies: CBC, leukocytes, differential, cardiac enzymes if patient is receiving long-term therapy
- Hepatic studies: AST, ALT, bilirubin
- Weight q wk; appetite may increase with product
- ECG for flattening of T wave, prolongation of QTc interval, bundle branch block, AV block, dysrhythmias in cardiac patients
- EPS primarily in geriatric: rigidity, dystonia, akathisia
- Mental status: mood, sensorium, affect, suicidal tendencies; increase in psychiatric symptoms: depression, panic
- Urinary retention, constipation; constipation is most likely to occur in children and geriatric patients
- Withdrawal symptoms: headache, nausea, vomiting, muscle pain, weakness; do not usually occur unless product was discontinued abruptly
- Alcohol consumption; if alcohol is consumed, hold dose until morning

Administer:

- Increased fluids, bulk in diet if constipation, urinary retention occur, especially geriatric patients
- With food or milk for GI symptoms
- Crushed if patient is unable to swallow medication whole
- Dosage at bedtime if oversedation occurs during day; may take entire dose at bedtime; geriatric patients may not tolerate once/day dosing

Perform/provide:

• Storage at room temperature; do not freeze

• Assistance with ambulation during beginning therapy, since drowsiness/dizziness occurs

• Gum; hard, sugarless candy; or frequent sips of water for dry mouth

Evaluate:

• Therapeutic response: decrease in depression, absence of suicidal thoughts

Teach patient/family:

• To take medication as directed; do not double dose; that therapeutic effects may take 2-3 wk

• To use caution in driving, other activities requiring alertness because of drowsiness, dizziness, blurred vision; to avoid rising quickly from sitting to standing, especially geriatric patients; management of anticholinergic effects

• To avoid alcohol ingestion, other CNS depressants

• Not to discontinue medication quickly after long-term use: may cause nausea, headache, malaise

• To wear sunscreen or large hat, since photosensitivity occurs

• That contraception is recommended during treatment

Treatment of overdose: ECG monitoring, lavage, administer anticonvulsant, sodium bicarbonate

amlodipine (℞)

(am-loe'di-peen)

Norvasc

Func. class.: Antianginal, antihypertensive, calcium channel blocker

Chem. class.: Dihydropyridine

Do not confuse:

amlodipine/amiloride

Norvasc/Navane/Norvir/Nascor

Action: Inhibits calcium ion influx across cell membrane during cardiac depolarization; produces relaxation of coronary vascular smooth muscle and peripheral vascular smooth muscle; dilates coronary vascular arteries; increases myocardial O_2 delivery in patients with vasospastic angina

Uses: Chronic stable angina pectoris, hypertension, variant angina (Prinzmetal's angina); may coadminister with other antihypertensives, antianginals

Unlabeled uses: Hypertension (pediatric patients)

DOSAGE AND ROUTES

Coronary artery disease

• *Adult:* **PO** 5-10 mg/day

• *Geriatric:* **PO** 5 mg/day, may increase max 10 mg/day

Hypertension

• *Adult:* **PO** 2.5-5 mg/day initially, max 10 mg/day

• *Geriatric:* **PO** 2.5 mg/day, may increase to 5 mg/day, max 10 mg/day

• *Child 6-16 yr (unlabeled):* **PO** 2.5-5 mg/day

• *Child <6 yr (unlabeled):* **PO** 0.05-0.2 mg/kg/day in 1-2 divided doses

Hepatic dose

• *Adult:* **PO** 2.5 mg/day; may increase up to 10 mg/day (antihypertensive); 5 mg/day, may increase up to 10 mg/day (antianginal)

Available forms: Tabs 2.5, 5, 10 mg

SIDE EFFECTS

CNS: Headache, fatigue, dizziness, asthenia, anxiety, depression, insomnia, paresthesia, somnolence

CV: Peripheral edema, bradycardia, hypotension, palpitations, syncope, chest pain

GI: Nausea, vomiting, diarrhea, gastric upset, constipation, flatulence, anorexia, gingival hyperplasia, dyspepsia, dysphagia

GU: Nocturia, polyuria, sexual difficulties

INTEG: Rash, pruritus, urticaria, hair loss

OTHER: Flushing, muscle cramps, cough, weight gain, tinnitus, epistaxis

Contraindications: Hypersensitivity to this product, severe aortic stenosis, severe obstructive CAD

Black Box Warning: Hypersensitivity to dihydropyridine

Precautions: Pregnancy (C), breastfeeding, children, geriatric patients, CHF, hypotension, hepatic injury

PHARMACOKINETICS

Onset not determined; peak 6-12 hr; half-life 30-50 hr; increased in geriatric patients, hepatic disease; metabolized by liver; excreted in urine (90% as metabolites); protein binding >95%

INTERACTIONS

Increase: neurotoxicity—lithium
Increase: hypotension—alcohol, antihypertensives, nitrates, fentanyl, quinidine
Increase: amlodipine level—diltiazem
Decrease: antihypertensive effect—NSAIDs

Drug/Herb

Increase: effects—barberry, betel palm, burdock, goldenseal, khat, khella, lily of the valley, plantain
Decrease: effect—yohimbe

Drug/Food

Increase: hypotensive effect—grapefruit juice

NURSING CONSIDERATIONS

Assess:

- Cardiac status: B/P, pulse, respiration, ECG; some patients have developed severe angina, acute MI after calcium channel blockers if obstructive CAD is severe
- I&O ratio, weight daily; CHF: peripheral edema, dyspnea, jugular vein distention, crackles
- Angina: intensity, location, duration of pain

Administer:

- Once a day, without regard to meals

Evaluate:

- Therapeutic response: decreased anginal pain, decreased B/P, increased exercise tolerance

Teach patient/family:

- To take product as prescribed, do not double or skip dose
- To avoid hazardous activities until stabilized on product, dizziness is no longer a problem
- To avoid OTC products, grapefruit juice unless directed by prescriber
- To comply in all areas of medical regimen: diet, exercise, stress reduction, product therapy, smoking cessation
- To notify prescriber of irregular heartbeat; SOB; swelling of feet, face and hands; severe dizziness; constipation; nausea; hypotension
- To use correct technique in monitoring pulse, to contact prescriber if pulse <50 bpm
- To avoid large amounts of grapefruit juice or alcohol
- To change positions slowly, to prevent orthostatic hypotension
- To continue with good oral hygiene to prevent gingival disease
- To notify all health care providers of this product use

Treatment of overdose: Defibrillation, β-agonists, IV calcium inotropic agents, diuretics, atropine for AV block, vasopressor for hypotension

amoxapine (℞)

(a-mox'a-peen)
amoxapine, Asendin
Func. class.: Antidepressant
Chem. class.: Dibenzoxazepine derivative—secondary amine

Do not confuse:
amoxapine/amoxicillin/Amoxil

Action: Blocks reuptake of norepinephrine, serotonin into nerve endings, increasing action of norepinephrine, serotonin in nerve cells

Uses: Depression with anxiety or agitation

DOSAGE AND ROUTES

- *Adult:* **PO** 50 mg bid-tid, may increase to 100 mg tid on 3rd day of therapy; not to exceed 300 mg/day unless lower doses have been given for at least 2 wk, may be given daily dose at bedtime, not to exceed 600 mg/day in hospitalized patients

• *Geriatric:* **PO** 25 mg bid-tid, may increase by 25 mg/wk, up to 300 mg/day in divided doses

Available forms: Tabs 25, 50, 100, 150 mg

SIDE EFFECTS

CNS: Dizziness, drowsiness, confusion, headache, anxiety, tremors, stimulation, weakness, insomnia, nightmares, EPS (geriatric patients), increased psychiatric symptoms, paresthesia, **neuroleptic malignant syndrome,** impairment of sexual functioning, **seizures**

CV: Orthostatic hypotension, ECG changes, tachycardia, hypertension, palpitations, **dysrhythmias**

EENT: Blurred vision, tinnitus, mydriasis, ophthalmoplegia

GI: Dry mouth, weight gain, *constipation,* nausea, vomiting, **paralytic ileus,** increased appetite, cramps, epigastric distress, jaundice, **hepatitis,** stomatitis

GU: Urinary retention, **acute renal failure**

HEMA: **Agranulocytosis, thrombocytopenia, eosinophilia, leukopenia**

INTEG: Rash, urticaria, sweating, pruritus, photosensitivity

META: Increased prolactin levels

Contraindications: Hypersensitivity to tricyclics, recovery phase of myocardial infarction, seizure disorders, prostatic hypertrophy, angle-closure glaucoma

Precautions: Pregnancy (C), geriatric patients, severe depression, increased intraocular pressure, urinary retention, hepatic/cardiac disease, hyperthyroidism, electroshock therapy, elective surgery, schizophrenia, urinary retention

Black Box Warning: Children, suicidal patients

PHARMACOKINETICS

Peak 90 min, steady state 2-7 days, metabolized by liver, excreted by kidneys, crosses placenta, half-life 8 hr, metabolite 30 hr

INTERACTIONS

⚠ Hyperpyretic crisis, seizures, hypertensive episode: MAOIs

Increase: QT prolongation—tricyclics, phenothiazines, class IA/III antidysrhythmics, mibefradil, bepridil, flecainide, probucol, propafenone, ranolazine

Increase: CNS depression—CNS depressants

Increase: amoxapine level—cimetidine, fluoxetine, fluvoxamine, paroxetine, sertraline

Increase: toxicity—SSRIs

Increase: hypertensive effect—clonidine, epinephrine, norepinephrine

Decrease: amoxapine effect—barbiturates

Drug/Herb

Increase: CNS depression—chamomile, hops, kava, lavender, skullcap, St. John's wort, valerian

Increase: anticholinergic effects—belladonna, corkwood, henbane, jimsonweed

Increase: action of amoxapine—SAM-e, scopolia root

Drug/Lab Test

Increase: LFTs, blood glucose

Decrease: WBC, blood glucose

NURSING CONSIDERATIONS

Assess:

• B/P lying, standing; pulse q4hr; if systolic B/P drops 20 mm Hg, hold product, notify prescriber; take vital signs q4hr in patients with CV disease

• ECG for flattening of T wave, bundle branch block, AV block, dysrhythmias in cardiac patients

• Blood studies: CBC, leukocytes, differential, cardiac enzymes LFTs, thyroid function tests patient if receiving long-term therapy

• Blood level: therapeutic 20-100 ng/ml

• Hepatic studies: AST, ALT, bilirubin

• Weight q wk, appetite may increase with product

• EPS primarily in geriatric patients: rigidity, dystonia, akathisia

- Mental status: mood, sensorium, affect, suicidal tendencies; increase in psychiatric symptoms: depression, panic; confusion (geriatric patients)
- Urinary retention, constipation; constipation is more likely to occur in children, geriatric patients
- Withdrawal symptoms: headache, nausea, vomiting, muscle pain, weakness; do not usually occur unless product is discontinued abruptly
- Alcohol consumption; if alcohol is consumed, hold dose until morning

Administer:

- Increased fluids, bulk in diet if constipation, urinary retention occur, especially in geriatric patients
- Crushed if patient is unable to swallow medication whole, with food or milk for GI symptoms
- Dosage at bedtime if oversedation occurs during day; may take entire dose at bedtime; geriatric patients may not tolerate once/day dosing

Perform/provide:

- Storage at room temperature; do not freeze
- Check to see PO medication swallowed
- Gum, hard candy, or frequent sips of water for dry mouth

Evaluate:

- Therapeutic response: decreased depression, absence of suicidal thoughts

Teach patient/family:

- To take as directed, not to double dose
- That therapeutic effects may take 4-6 wk
- To use caution in driving or other activities requiring alertness because of drowsiness, dizziness, blurred vision
- To avoid alcohol ingestion, other CNS depressants, may potentiate effects
- Not to discontinue medication quickly after long-term use; may cause nausea, headache, malaise
- To wear sunscreen or large hat, since photosensitivity occurs

Treatment of overdose: ECG monitoring, induce emesis, lavage, activated charcoal, administer anticonvulsant

amoxicillin (℞)

(a-mox-i-sill'in)

amoxicillin, Amoxil, Apo-Amoxi ♣, DisperMox, Novamoxin ♣, Nu-Amoxi ♣, Trimox, Wymox

Func. class.: Antiinfective, antiulcer

Chem. class.: Aminopenicillin

Do not confuse:

amoxicillin/**amoxapine/Amoxil**

Trimox/**Diamox/Tylox**

Wymox/**Tylox**

Action: Interferes with cell wall replication of susceptible organisms; the cell wall, rendered osmotically unstable, swells and bursts from osmotic pressure; bactericidal, lysis mediated by bacterial cell wall autolysins

Uses: Treatment of skin, respiratory, GI, GU infections; otitis media, gonorrhea. For gram-positive cocci *(Staphylococcus aureus, Streptococcus pyogenes, Streptococcus faecalis, Streptococcus pneumoniae)*, gram-negative cocci *(Neisseria gonorrhoeae, Neisseria meningitidis)*, gram-positive bacilli *(Corynebacterium diphtheriae, Listeria monocytogenes)*, gram-negative bacilli *(Haemophilus influenzae, Escherichia coli, Proteus mirabilis, Salmonella)*; prophylaxis of bacterial endocarditis; in combination with other products used for treatment of *Helicobacter pylori*

Unlabeled uses: Lyme disease, anthrax treatment and prophylaxis, cervicitis, *Chlamydia trachomatis,* dental abscess/infection, dyspepsia, gastric ulcer, nongonococcal urethritis (NGU), periodontitis, typhoid fever

DOSAGE AND ROUTES

Systemic infections

- *Adult:* **PO** 750 mg-1.75 g/day in divided doses q8hr or q12hr
- *Child:* **PO** 20-50 mg/kg/day in divided doses q8hr

Renal disease

• *Adult:* **PO** CCr 10-30 ml/min 250-500 mg q12hr; CCr <10 ml/min 250-500 mg q24hr; do not use 875 mg strength if CCr <50 ml/min

Gonorrhea/urinary tract infections

• *Adult:* **PO** 3 g given with 1 g probenecid as a single dose; followed by tetracycline or erythromycin therapy

Chlamydia trachomatis

• *Adult:* **PO** 500 mg/tid × 1 wk

Bacterial endocarditis prophylaxis

• *Adult:* **PO** 2 g 1 hr prior to procedure

• *Child:* **PO** 50 mg/kg/hr 1 hr prior to procedure; max 2 g

Helicobacter pylori

• *Adult:* **PO** 1000 mg bid, given with lansoprazole 30 mg bid, clarithromycin 500 mg bid × 2 wk or 1000 mg bid given with omeprazole 20 mg bid, clarithromycin 500 mg bid × 2 wk, or 1000 mg tid given with lansoprazole 30 mg tid × 2 wk

Lyme disease (unlabeled)

• *Adult:* **PO** 250-500 mg tid × 10-30 days

• *Child:* **PO** 20-50 mg/kg/day in divided doses q8hr × 10-30 days

Duodenal/gastric ulcer/dyspepsia from* H. pylori *infection (unlabeled)

• *Adult:* **PO** 1000 mg bid with lansoprazole or clarithromycin/omeprazole

Anthrax treatment/prophylaxis (unlabeled)

• *Adult and child >20 kg:* **PO** 500 mg q8hr × 10-14 days (prophylaxis), 60 days (treatment)

Available forms: Caps 250, 500 mg; chew tabs 125, 200, 250, 400 mg; tabs 500, 875 mg; susp pediatric drops 50 mg/ml; susp 125, 200, 250, 400 mg/5 ml

SIDE EFFECTS

CNS: Headache, **seizures,** agitation, confusion, dizziness

GI: Nausea, vomiting, diarrhea, increased AST, ALT, abdominal pain, glossitis, colitis, **pseudomembranous colitis**

HEMA: Anemia, increased bleeding time, **bone marrow depression, granulocytopenia, hemolytic anemia**

INTEG: Urticaria, rash

SYST: **Anaphylaxis, respiratory distress, serum sickness, Stevens-Johnson syndrome**

Contraindications: Hypersensitivity to penicillins

Precautions: Pregnancy (B), breastfeeding, neonates, hypersensitivity to cephalosporins, severe renal disease, acute lymphocytic leukemia

PHARMACOKINETICS

PO: Peak 2 hr, duration 6-8 hr, half-life 1-1⅓ hr, metabolized in liver, excreted in urine, crosses placenta, enters breast milk

INTERACTIONS

Increase: amoxicillin level—probenecid

Increase: anticoagulant action—warfarin

Increase: methotrexate levels—methotrexate

Decrease: effectiveness of oral contraceptives

Drug/Herb

• Do not use acidophilus with antiinfectives; separate by several hours

Decrease: absorption—khat; separate by 2 hr

Drug/Lab Test

False positive: urine glucose, urine protein, direct Coombs' test

NURSING CONSIDERATIONS

Assess:

• I&O ratio; report hematuria, oliguria, since penicillin in high doses is nephrotoxic

• Any patient with a compromised renal system, since product is excreted slowly in poor renal system function; toxicity may occur rapidly

• Hepatic studies: AST, ALT

• Blood studies: WBC, RBC, Hgb and Hct, bleeding time

• Renal studies: urinalysis, protein, blood, BUN, creatinine

A

- C&S before product therapy; product may be given as soon as culture is taken
- Bowel pattern before, during treatment; diarrhea, cramping, blood in stools, report to prescriber; pseudomembranous colitis may occur
- Skin eruptions after administration of penicillin to 1 wk after discontinuing product
- Respiratory status: rate, character, wheezing, tightness in the chest
- Anaphylaxis: rash, itching, dyspnea, facial/laryngeal edema

Administer:

PO route

- Shake suspension well before each dose; may be used alone or mixed in drinks; use immediately; discard unused portion of susp after 14 days
- Give around the clock, caps may be emptied and mixed with liquids if needed

Perform/provide:

- Adrenaline, suction, tracheostomy set, endotracheal intubation equipment on unit
- Adequate intake of fluids (2 L) during diarrhea episodes
- Scratch test to assess allergy after securing order from prescriber; usually done when penicillin is only product of choice
- Storage in tight container; after reconstituting, oral suspension refrigerated for 14 days

Evaluate:

- Therapeutic response: absence of infection; prevention of endocarditis, resolution of ulcer symptoms

Teach patient/family:

- That caps may be opened and contents taken with fluids; chewable form is available
- To take as prescribed, not to double dose
- All aspects of product therapy: need to complete entire course of medication to ensure organism death (10-14 days); culture may be taken after completed course of medication
- ⚠ To report sore throat, fever, fatigue, diarrhea (may indicate superinfection or agranulocytopenia)
- That product must be taken in equal intervals around the clock to maintain blood levels; take without regard to food
- To wear or carry emergency ID if allergic to penicillins

Treatment of anaphylaxis: Withdraw product, maintain airway, administer epinephrine, aminophylline, O_2, IV corticosteroids

amoxicillin/clavulanate potassium (℞)

(a-mox-i-sill′in)

Augmentin, Augmentin ES-600, Augmentin XR, Clavulin ✤

Func. class.: Broad-spectrum antiinfective

Chem. class.: Aminopenicillin β-lactamase inhibitor

Action: Bacteriocidal, interferes with cell wall replication of susceptible organisms; the cell wall, rendered osmotically unstable, swells and bursts from osmotic pressure; lysis mediated by bacterial cell wall autolytic enzymes, combination increases spectrum of activity against β-lactamase–resistant organisms

Uses: Sinus infections, pneumonia, otitis media, skin infection, UTI; effective for strains of *Escherichia coli, Proteus mirabilis, Haemophilus influenzae, Streptococcus faecalis, Streptococcus pneumoniae,* and some β-lactamase–producing organisms

DOSAGE AND ROUTES

- *Adult:* **PO** 250-500 mg q8hr or 500-875 mg q12hr depending on severity of infection
- *Child ≤40 kg:* **PO** 20-90 mg/kg/day in divided doses q8-12hr

Renal disease

- *Adult:* **PO** CCr 10-30 ml/min dose q12hr; CCr <10 ml/min dose q24hr; do not use 875 mg strength or ext rel if CCr

<30 ml/min; Augmentin XR is contraindicated in renal disease

Available forms: Tabs 250, 500, 875 mg/125 mg clavulanate; chew tabs 125, 200, 250, 400 mg; powder for oral susp 125, 200, 250, 400 mg/5 ml; ext rel tabs (XR) 1000 mg amoxicillin, 62.5 mg clavulanate; powder for oral susp (ES) 600 mg amoxicillin, 42.9 mg clavulanate

SIDE EFFECTS

CNS: Headache, fever, **seizures**

GI: Nausea, diarrhea, vomiting, increased AST, ALT, abdominal pain, glossitis, colitis, black tongue, **pseudomembranous colitis**

GU: Oliguria, proteinuria, hematuria, *vaginitis, moniliasis,* **glomerulonephritis**

HEMA: Anemia, **bone marrow depression, granulocytopenia, leukopenia, eosinophilia,** thrombocytopenic purpura

INTEG: Rash, urticaria, dermatitis, **toxic epidermal necrolysis**

META: Hypo/hyperkalemia, alkalosis, hypernatremia

SYST: **Anaphylaxis, respiratory distress, serum sickness, superinfection, Stevens-Johnson syndrome**

Contraindications: Hypersensitivity to penicillins

Precautions: Pregnancy (B), breastfeeding, neonates, hypersensitivity to cephalosporins; renal/GI disease

PHARMACOKINETICS

PO: Peak 2 hr, duration 6-8 hr, half-life 1-1⅓ hr, metabolized in liver, excreted in urine, crosses placenta, excreted in breast milk, removed by hemodialysis

INTERACTIONS

Increase: amoxicillin levels—probenecid

Increase: anticoagulant effect—warfarin

Increase: skin rash—allopurinol

Decrease: action of oral contraceptives

Drug/Herb

• Delayed/reduced absorption: khat; separate by 2 hr

• Do not use acidophilus with antiinfectives; separate by several hours

Drug/Lab Test

False positive: Urine glucose, urine protein, direct Coombs' test

NURSING CONSIDERATIONS

Assess:

• I&O ratio; report hematuria, oliguria since penicillin in high doses is nephrotoxic

• Any patient with a compromised renal system since product is excreted slowly in poor renal system function; toxicity may occur

• Hepatic studies: AST, ALT

• Blood studies: WBC, RBC, Hgb and Hct, bleeding time

• Renal studies: urinalysis, protein, blood, BUN, creatinine

• C&S before product therapy; product may be given as soon as culture is taken

• Bowel pattern before, during treatment; diarrhea, cramping, blood in stools, report to prescriber, pseudomembranous colitis may occur

• Skin eruptions after administration of penicillin to 1 wk after discontinuing product

• Respiratory status: rate, character, wheezing, tightness in chest

• Anaphylaxis: rash, itching, dyspnea, facial/laryngeal edema

Administer:

PO route

• Do not break, crush, or chew XR (ext rel) product

⚠ Only as directed, 2 (250 mg tab) not equivalent to 1 (500 mg tab) due to strength of clavulanate

• Shake suspension well before each dose, may be used alone or mixed in drinks, use immediately, discard unusual portion of susp after 14 days

• Give around the clock

Perform/provide:

• Adrenaline, suction, tracheostomy set, endotracheal intubation equipment on unit

• Adequate intake of fluids (2 L) during diarrhea episodes

• Scratch test to assess allergy after securing order from prescriber; usually done when penicillin is only product of choice

• Storage refrigerated for 10 days

Evaluate:

• Therapeutic response: absence of infection

Teach patient/family:

• To take as prescribed, not to double dose

• All aspects of product therapy: need to complete entire course of medication to ensure organism death (10-14 days); culture may be taken after completed course of medication

⚠ To report sore throat, fever, fatigue (may indicate superinfection or agranulocytosis)

• That product must be taken in equal intervals around the clock to maintain blood levels

• To wear or carry emergency ID if allergic to penicillins

• To notify prescriber of diarrhea, cramping, blood in stools; pseudomembranous colitis may occur

• To use alternative contraceptive measures, if using oral contraceptives

Treatment of hypersensitivity: Withdraw product, maintain airway, administer epinephrine, aminophylline, O_2, IV corticosteroids for anaphylaxis

AMPHOTERICIN B

amphotericin B desoxycholate (℞)
(am-foe-ter′i-sin)
Fungizone
amphotericin B cholesteryl sulfate (℞)
Amphotec
amphotericin B lipid based (℞)
Abelcet
amphotericin B liposome (℞)
AmBisome
Func. class.: Antifungal
Chem. class.: Amphoteric polyene

Action: Increases cell membrane permeability in susceptible fungi by binding sterols; alters cell membrane, causing leakage of cell components and cell death

Uses: Histoplasmosis, blastomycosis, coccidioidomycosis, cryptococcosis, aspergillosis, zygomycosis, candidiasis, sporotrichosis, cryptococcal meningitis; mucomycosis caused by mucormycosis, *Rhizopus, Absidia, Entomorphthora, Basidiobolus*

Unlabeled uses: Candiduria (bladder irrigation), funguria, *Acremonium* sp., coccidioidomycosis prophylaxis, histoplasmosis/cryptococcosis prophylaxis, *Fusarium* sp., sinusitis

DOSAGE AND ROUTES

Fungizone

• *Adult:* **IV** Give test dose of 1 mg (not required); then 0.25 mg/kg, increase daily slowly to 0.5 mg/kg, may give 1 mg/kg/day or 1.5 mg/kg/day, alternate-day dosing may be used

• *Child:* **IV** 0.25 mg/kg infused initially, increase by 0.25 mg/kg every other day to max of 1 mg/kg/day

• *Adult and child:* **TOP** Apply 2-4 ×/day

• *Adult and child:* **PO** 1 ml (100 mg) qid

Amphotec
• *Adult and child:* **IV** 3-4 mg/kg/day, max 7.5 mg/kg/day
Abelcet
• *Adult and child:* **IV** 5 mg/kg/day as a 1 mg/ml inf given 2.5 mg/kg/hr
AmBisome
Fungal infections
• *Adult and child:* **IV** 3-5 mg/kg q24hr
Visceral leishmaniasis
• *Adult:* **IV** 3-4 mg/kg q24hr days 1-5
Fungal/histoplasmosis/ coccidioidomycosis/cryptococcosis (unlabeled)
• *Adult:* **IV** 1 mg/kg q wk

Available forms: *Desoxycholate:* inj 50-mg vial; oral susp 100 mg/ml; cream, ointment, lotion 3%; *cholesteryl:* powder for inj 50 mg/20 ml, 100 mg/50 ml; *lipid complex:* susp for inj 100 mg/20-ml vial; *liposome:* powder for inj 50-mg vial

SIDE EFFECTS

CNS: Headache, fever, chills, peripheral nerve pain, paresthesias, peripheral neuropathy, **seizures,** dizziness
EENT: Tinnitus, deafness, diplopia, blurred vision
GI: Nausea, vomiting, anorexia, diarrhea, cramps, **hemorrhagic gastroenteritis, acute liver failure**
GU: Hypokalemia, azotemia, hyposthenuria, **renal tubular acidosis,** nephrocalcinosis, **permanent renal impairment, anuria, oliguria**
HEMA: Normochromic, normocytic anemia, **thrombocytopenia, agranulocytosis, leukopenia, eosinophilia,** hypokalemia, hyponatremia, hypomagnesemia
INTEG: Burning, irritation, pain, necrosis at inj site with extravasation, flushing, dermatitis, skin rash (topical route)
MS: Arthralgia, myalgia, generalized pain, weakness, weight loss
SYST: **Stevens-Johnson syndrome, toxic epidermal neurolysis, exfoliative dermatitis**

Contraindications: Hypersensitivity, severe bone marrow depression

Precautions: Pregnancy (B), breastfeeding, children, renal disease, anemia, hypokalemia, hypomagnesemia, infections

Black Box Warning: Fungal infections

PHARMACOKINETICS

IV: Peak 1-2 hr; initial half-life 24 hr; metabolized in liver; excreted in urine (metabolites), breast milk; protein binding 90%; penetrates poorly CSF, bronchial secretions, aqueous humor, muscle, bone

INTERACTIONS

Increase: nephrotoxicity—other nephrotoxic antibiotics (aminoglycosides, cisplatin, vancomycin, cycloSPORINE, polymyxin B)
Increase: hypokalemia—corticosteroids, digoxin, skeletal muscle relaxants, thiazides

Drug/Herb
• Do not use acidophilus with antiinfectives; separate by several hours
Increase: possibility of nephrotoxicity—gossypol

NURSING CONSIDERATIONS

Assess:
• VS q15-30min during first infusion; note changes in pulse, B/P
• I&O ratio; watch for decreasing urinary output, change in specific gravity; discontinue product to prevent permanent damage to renal tubules
• Blood studies: CBC, K, Na, Ca, Mg q2wk, BUN, creatinine weekly
• Weight weekly; if weight increases over 2 lb/wk, edema is present; renal damage should be considered
⚠ For renal toxicity: increasing BUN, serum creatinine; if BUN is >40 mg/dl or if serum creatinine >3 mg/dl, product may be discontinued or dosage reduced
⚠ For hepatotoxicity: increasing AST, ALT, alk phos, bilirubin
• For allergic reaction: dermatitis, rash; product should be discontinued, antihis-

tamines (mild reaction) or epinephrine (severe reaction) administered

- For hypokalemia: anorexia, drowsiness, weakness, decreased reflexes, dizziness, increased urinary output, increased thirst, paresthesias
- For ototoxicity: tinnitus (ringing, roaring in ears) vertigo, loss of hearing (rare)

Administer:

- Do not confuse four different types; these are not interchangeable: conventional amphotericin B, amphotericin B cholesteryl, amphotericin B lipid complex, amphotericin B liposome

IV route

- Product only after C&S confirms organism, product needed to treat condition; make sure product is used in life-threatening infections

Desoxycholate

- After diluting 50 mg/10 ml sterile water (no preservatives) (5 mg per 1 ml), shake, dilute with 500 ml of D_5W to concentration of 0.1 mg/ml
- Test dose of 1 mg/20 ml D_5W; give over 10-30 min

Intermittent IV INF route

- IV using in-line filter (mean pore diameter >1 micron) using distal veins; check for extravasation, necrosis q8hr; use an infusion pump; infuse over 2-6 hr; rapid infusion may result in circulation collapse; use central line if possible

Additive compatibilities: Heparin, hydrocortisone, sodium bicarbonate

Syringe compatibilities: Heparin

Y-site compatibilities: Aldesleukin, diltiazem, DOXOrubicin liposome, famotidine, remifentanil, tacrolimus, teniposide, thiotepa, zidovudine

Solution compatibilities: D_5W

Cholesteryl

IV route

- Reconstitute 50-mg vial/10 ml, 100-mg vial/20 ml sterile water for inj (5 mg/5 ml); swirl or shake gently until dissolved, further dilute with D_5W (0.6 mg/ml); wear gloves while preparing
- Test dose 10 ml of final solution (1.6-8.3 mg) over ½ hr, observe for next ½ hr for reactions
- Give 1 mg/kg/hr using infusion pump, do not give rapidly, may increase infusion, if tolerated

Additive compatibilities: Heparin

Liposomal complex

IV route

- Reconstitute with 12 ml sterile water/50-ml vial (4 mg/ml), shake, use 5-micron filter, dilute in D_5W (1-2 mg/ml), give over 2 hr
- Do not admix

Lipid complex

IV route

- Shake vial until dissolved, withdraw dose using 18G needle, replace needle from syringe with product using 5 micron filter needle (use needle for 4 vials or less), empty contents in IV of D_5W (1 mg/ml), give at 2.5 mg/kg/hr, use infusion pump
- Do not admix

Perform/provide:

- Acetaminophen and diphenhydrAMINE 30 min prior to infusion to reduce fever, chills, headache
- Storage protected from moisture and light; diluted solution is stable for 24 hr at room temperature

Evaluate:

- Therapeutic response: decreased fever, malaise, rash, negative C&S for infecting organism

Teach patient/family:

- That long-term therapy may be needed to clear infection (2 wk-3 mo depending on type of infection)
- To notify prescriber of bleeding, bruising, or soft tissue swelling

ampicillin (℞)

(am-pi-sill'in)

Ampicin ♣, Apo-Ampi ♣, NovoAmpicillin ♣, Nu-Ampi ♣, Omnipen, Penbritin ♣, Principen

Func. class.: Antiinfective—broad-spectrum

Chem. class.: Aminopenicillin

Do not confuse:
Omnipen/imipenem

Action: Interferes with cell wall replication of susceptible organisms; the cell wall, rendered osmotically unstable, swells, bursts from osmotic pressure, lysis mediated by cell wall autolysins

Uses: Effective for gram-positive cocci *(Staphylococcus aureus, Streptococcus pyogenes, Streptococcus faecalis, Streptococcus pneumoniae)*, gram-negative cocci *(Neisseria meningitidis)*, gram-negative bacilli *(Haemophilus influenzae, Proteus mirabilis, Salmonella, Shigella, Listeria monocytogenes)*, gram-positive bacilli

Unlabeled uses: Biliary tract infection, shigellosis, typhoid fever

DOSAGE AND ROUTES

Systemic infections

- *Adult and child ≥40 kg:* **PO** 250-500 mg q6hr; **IV/IM** 2-8 g/day in divided doses q4-6hr
- *Child <40 kg:* **PO** 50-100 mg/kg/day in divided doses q6-8hr; **IV/IM** 100-200 mg/kg/day in divided doses q6-8hr

Bacterial meningitis

- *Adult:* **IM/IV** 500 mg-3 g q6hr, max 14 g/day
- *Child:* **IM/IV** 200-400 mg/kg/day in divided doses q6hr, max 12 g/day

Gonorrhea (urethritis)

- *Adult and child ≥45 kg:* **PO** 3.5 g given with 1 g probenecid as a single dose

Prevention of bacterial endocarditis

- *Adult:* **IM/IV** 2 g 30 min before procedure
- *Child:* **IM/IV** 50 mg/kg 30 min prior to procedure, max 2 g

***GI/GU infections other than caused by* N. gonorrhoeae**

- *Adult and child >20 kg:* **PO** 250-500 mg q6hr, may use larger dose for more serious infections
- *Child ≤20 kg:* **PO** 50-100 mg/kg/day in divided doses q6hr

Renal disease

- *Adult and child:* CCr 30-50 ml/min q6-8hr; CCr 10-30 ml/min dose q8-12hr; CCr <10 ml/min dose q12hr

Biliary tract infection (unlabeled)

- *Adult/adolescent/child ≥20 kg:* **IM/IV** 200 mg/kg/day in equally divided doses q3-4hr, max 14 g/day

Shigellosis in AIDS patients (unlabeled)

- *Adult:* **PO** 500 mg qid × 5 days

Typhoid fever (unlabeled)

- *Adult/adolescent/child:* **IV** 100 mg/kg/day divided q6hr × 14 days or more

Available forms: Powder for inj 125, 250, 500 mg, 1, 2, 10 g; IV inj 500 mg, 1, 2 g; caps 250, 500 mg; powder for oral susp 125, 250/5 ml

SIDE EFFECTS

CNS: Lethargy, hallucinations, anxiety, depression, twitching, **coma, seizures**

GI: Nausea, vomiting, diarrhea, **pseudomembranous colitis,** stomatitis

GU: Oliguria, proteinuria, hematuria, *vaginitis, moniliasis,* **glomerulonephritis**

HEMA: Anemia, increased bleeding time, **bone marrow depression, granulocytopenia,** leukopenia, eosinophilia

INTEG: Rash, urticaria

MISC: **Anaphylaxis, serum sickness, Stevens-Johnson syndrome, toxic epidermal necrolysis**

Contraindications: Hypersensitivity to penicillins

Precautions: Pregnancy (B), breastfeeding, neonates, hypersensitivity to cephalosporins; renal disease

PHARMACOKINETICS

Half-life 50-110 min; metabolized in liver; excreted in urine, bile, breast milk; crosses placenta; removed by dialysis

PO: Peak 2 hr, duration 6-8 hr

IM: Peak 1 hr

IV: Peak 5 min

INTERACTIONS

Increase: ampicillin concentrations—probenecid

Increase: ampicillin-induced skin rash—allopurinol

Decrease: effectiveness of oral contraceptives

Drug/Herb

- Delayed/reduced absorption—khat; separate by 2 hr
- Do not use acidophilus with antiinfectives; separate by several hours

Drug/Lab Test

Increase: AST, ALT

Decrease: conjugated estrone in pregnancy, conjugated estriol

False positive: urine glucose, urine protein, direct Coombs'

NURSING CONSIDERATIONS

Assess:

- I&O ratio; report hematuria, oliguria, since penicillin in high doses is nephrotoxic

⚠ Any patient with compromised renal system, since product is excreted slowly in poor renal system function; toxicity may occur

- Hepatic studies: AST, ALT
- Blood studies: WBC, RBC, Hgb and Hct, bleeding time
- Renal studies: urinalysis, protein, blood, BUN, creatinine
- C&S before product therapy; product may be taken as soon as culture is taken
- Bowel pattern before, during treatment
- Skin eruptions after administration of penicillin to 1 wk after discontinuing product
- Respiratory status: rate, character, wheezing, tightness in chest
- Anaphylaxis: rash, itching, dyspnea, facial swelling; stop product, notify prescriber, have emergency equipment available

Administer:

PO route

- On empty stomach, with plenty of water for best absorption (1-2 hr before meals or 2-3 hr after meals)
- Shake suspension well before each dose

IM route

- Reconstitute by adding 0.9-1.2 ml/125-mg vial; 0.9-1.9 ml/250-mg vial; 1.2-1.8 ml/500-mg vial; 2.4-7.4 ml/1-g vial; 6.8 ml/2-g vial

IV route

- After diluting with sterile H_2O 0.9-1.2 ml/125 mg product, administer over 3-5 min (up to 500 mg), 10-15 min (>500 mg) by direct IV; may be diluted in 50 ml or more of D_5W, D_5 0.45% NaCl to a concentration of 30 mg/ml or less; IV sol is stable for 1 hr; give at prescribed rate

Additive compatibilities: Clindamycin, erythromycin, floxacillin, furosemide

Syringe compatibilities: Chloramphenicol, heparin, procaine

Y-site compatibilities: Acyclovir, allopurinol, amifostine, aztreonam, cyclophosphamide, DOXOrubicin liposome, enalaprilat, esmolol, famotidine, filgrastim, fludarabine, foscarnet, granisetron, heparin, insulin (regular), labetalol, magnesium sulfate, melphalan, meperidine, morphine, multivitamins, ofloxacin, perphenazine, phytonadione, potassium chloride, propofol, remifentanil, tacrolimus, teniposide, theophylline, thiotepa, tolazoline, vit B/C

Perform/provide:

- Adequate intake of fluids (2 L) during diarrhea episodes
- Scratch test to assess allergy after securing order from prescriber; usually done when penicillin is only product of choice
- Storage in tight container; after reconstituting, oral suspension refrigerated for 2 wk or stored at room temperature for 1 wk

Evaluate:

- Therapeutic response: absence of temp, draining wounds, other symptoms of infections

Teach patient/family:

- That tabs may be crushed; caps may be opened and mixed with water
- To take oral ampicillin on empty stomach with full glass of water
- All aspects of product therapy: need to complete entire course of medication to ensure organism death (10-14 days); culture may be taken after completed course of medication
- ⚠ To report sore throat, fever, fatigue, diarrhea (may indicate superinfection); report rash or other signs of allergy
- That product must be taken in equal intervals around the clock to maintain blood levels
- To wear or carry emergency ID if allergic to penicillins

Treatment of anaphylaxis: Withdraw product, maintain airway, administer epinephrine, aminophylline, O_2, IV corticosteroids

ampicillin, sulbactam (℞)

Unasyn

Func. class.: Antiinfective—broad-spectrum

Chem. class.: Aminopenicillin with β-lactamase inhibitor

Action: Interferes with cell wall replication of susceptible organisms; the cell wall, rendered osmotically unstable, swells, bursts from osmotic pressure; lysis due to cell wall autolytic enzymes; combination extends spectrum of activity by β-lactamase inhibition

Uses: Skin infections, intraabdominal infections, pneumonia *(Staphylococcus aureus, Escherichia coli, Klebsiella, Proteus mirabilis, Bacteroides fragilis, Haemophilus influenzae, Enterobacter, Acinetobacter calcoaceticus)*, intraabdominal infections *(Enterobacter, Klebsiella, Bacteroides, E. coli)*, gynecologic infections *(E. coli, Bacteroides)*, meningitis, septicemia

DOSAGE AND ROUTES

- *Adult and child ≥40 kg:* **IM/IV** 1 g ampicillin, 0.5 g sulbactam to 2 g ampicillin and 1 g sulbactam q6hr, not to exceed 4 g/day sulbactam
- *Child ≤40 kg:* **IV** 100-200 mg/kg/day (ampicillin component) divided q6hr, max 8 g/day

Renal disease

- *Adult ≥40 kg:* **IM/IV** CCr 15-29 ml/min dose q12hr; CCr 5-14 ml/min dose q24hr

Available forms: Powder for inj 1.5 g (1 g ampicillin, 0.5 g sulbactam), 3 g (2 g ampicillin, 1 g sulbactam), 10 g (10 g ampicillin, 5 g sulbactam)

SIDE EFFECTS

CNS: Lethargy, hallucinations, anxiety, depression, twitching, **coma, seizures**

GI: *Nausea, vomiting, diarrhea,* increased AST, ALT, abdominal pain, glossitis, colitis, **pseudomembranous colitis, hepatic necrosis/failure**

GU: Oliguria, proteinuria, hematuria, *vaginitis, moniliasis,* **glomerulonephritis,** dysuria

HEMA: Anemia, increased bleeding time, **bone marrow depression, granulocytopenia, leukopenia, eosinophilia**

MISC: **Anaphylaxis, serum sickness, toxic epidermal necrolysis, Stevens-Johnson syndrome**

Contraindications: Hypersensitivity to penicillins, ampicillin, or sulbactam

Precautions: Pregnancy (B), breastfeeding, neonates, hypersensitivity to cephalosporins, renal disease

PHARMACOKINETICS

IV: Peak 5 min, half-life 50-110 min, little metabolized in liver, 75%-85% of both products excreted in urine, diffuses to breast milk, crosses placenta

INTERACTIONS

Increase: ampicillin-induced skin rash—allopurinol
Increase: ampicillin level—probenecid, disulfiram
Increase: methotrexate level—methotrexate
Decrease: oral contraceptive effect

Drug/Herb

- Do not use acidophilus with antiinfectives; separate by several hours

Decrease: absorption—khat; separate by 2 hr

Drug/Lab Test

False positive: urine glucose, urine protein

NURSING CONSIDERATIONS

Assess:

- Bowel pattern before, during treatment
- Respiratory status: rate, character, wheezing, tightness in chest
- I&O ratio; report hematuria, oliguria, since penicillin in high doses is nephrotoxic

⚠ Any patient with compromised renal system, since product is excreted slowly in poor renal system function; toxicity may occur rapidly

- Hepatic studies: AST, ALT if on long-term therapy
- Blood studies: WBC, RBC, Hct, Hgb, bleeding time
- Renal studies: urinalysis, protein, blood, BUN, creatinine
- C&S before product therapy; product may be given as soon as culture is taken
- Skin eruptions after administration of ampicillin to 1 wk after discontinuing product
- Allergies before initiation of treatment; reaction of each medication; report allergies

Administer:

IM route

- Reconstitute by adding 3.2 ml sterile water/1.5-g vial; 6.4 ml/3-g vial, give deep in large muscle

IV route

- After diluting 1.5 g/3.2 ml sterile H_2O for inj or 3 g/6.4 ml (250 mg ampicillin/125 mg sulbactam); allow to stand until foaming stops; may give over 15 min as direct IV; dilute further in 50 ml or more of D_5W, NaCl, administer within 1 hr after reconstitution; give as an intermittent infusion over 15-30 min

Additive compatibilities: Aztreonam

Y-site compatibilities: Amifostine, aztreonam, cefepime, enalaprilat, famotidine, filgrastim, fluconazole, fludarabine, gallium, granisetron, heparin, insulin (regular), meperidine, morphine, paclitaxel, remifentanil, tacrolimus, teniposide, theophylline, thiotepa

Perform/provide:

- Adrenaline, suction, tracheostomy set, endotracheal intubation equipment on unit for possible anaphylaxis
- Adequate intake of fluids (2 L) during diarrhea episodes
- Scratch test to assess allergy after securing order from prescriber; usually done when penicillin is only product choice
- Storage in tight container, out of light

Evaluate:

- Therapeutic response: absence of fever, draining wounds, negative C&S

Teach patient/family:

- That oral contraceptives may be reduced and a nonhormonal contraceptive should be taken while on this product if pregnancy is to be prevented
- To report superinfection: vaginal itching, loose, foul-smelling stools, black furry tongue

⚠ To report immediately pseudomembranous colitis: fever, diarrhea with pus, blood, or mucus; may occur up to 4 wk after treatment

- To wear or carry emergency ID if allergic to penicillin products

Treatment of anaphylaxis: Withdraw product, maintain airway, administer epinephrine, aminophylline, O_2, IV corticosteroids

anagrelide (℞)

(a-na'gre-lide)

Agrylin

Func. class.: Antiplatelet

Chem. class.: Imidazo-quinazolinone

Action: Reduces platelet count and prevents early platelet shape changes in response to aggregating agents thus inhibiting platelet aggregation

Uses: Chronic myelogenous leukemia (CML), polycythemia vera, thrombocytosis

DOSAGE AND ROUTES

• *Adult:* **PO** 0.5 mg qid or 1 mg bid, may be adjusted after 1 wk, max 10 mg/day or 2.5 mg single dose; maintenance: titrate to lowest dose to maintain platelets <600,000/mcL; dosage range 1.5-3 mg/day

Available forms: Caps 0.5, 1 mg

SIDE EFFECTS

CNS: Headache, dizziness, **seizures,** *paresthesia,* **CVA,** *fever*

CV: Postural hypotension, tachycardia, palpitations, **CHF, MI, cardiomyopathy, cardiomegaly, complete heart block, atrial fibrillation,** dysrhythmia, **chest pain**

EENT: Amblyopia, diplopia, tinnitus

GI: Diarrhea, abdominal pain, nausea, flatulence, vomiting, anorexia, constipation, pancreatitis

GU: Dysuria

HEMA: **Anemia, thrombocytopenia, ecchymosis, lymphadenoma**

INTEG: Rash, photosensitivity

MISC: Edema, pain,

MS: Asthenia, back pain

RESP: Dyspnea

Contraindications: Hypersensitivity

Precautions: Pregnancy (C), breastfeeding, children <16 yr, renal/hepatic/cardiac disease, hypotension, abrupt discontinuation, females

PHARMACOKINETICS

Peak 1 hr, duration >24 hr, metabolized in liver, excreted in feces/urine, terminal half-life 3-4 days

INTERACTIONS

Increase: bleeding risk—abciximab, anticoagulants, aspirin, ciprofloxacin, cimetidine, eptifibatide, NSAIDs, thrombolytics, ticlopidine, tirofiban, SSRIs

Decrease: absorption—sucralfate

Drug/Herb

• Gastric irritation: arginine

Increase: effect—bogbean, dong quai

Increase: bleeding risk; green tea, feverfew, ginger, ginkgo

Decrease: effect—bilberry, saw palmetto

Drug/Food

• Avoid grapefruit or juice

Decrease: bioavailability, plasma concentrations

NURSING CONSIDERATIONS

Assess:

• Platelet counts q2day × 1 wk, and q wk thereafter, response should begin after 1-2 wk; Hgb, WBC, LFTs, renal function studies

• B/P, pulse during treatment until stable; take B/P lying, standing; orthostatic hypotension is common

• Cardiac status: chest pain, what aggravates or ameliorates condition

Administer:

• May give with food, monitor closely for dosage adjustment, there is better absorption on empty stomach

Perform/provide:

• Storage at room temperature

Evaluate:

• Therapeutic response: decreased platelet count

Teach patient/family:

• That medication is not a cure: may have to be taken continuously in evenly spaced doses only as directed

• That it is necessary to quit smoking to prevent excessive vasoconstriction
• To avoid hazardous activities until stabilized on medication; dizziness may occur
• To rise slowly from sitting or lying to prevent orthostatic hypotension
• Not to use alcohol or OTC medications unless approved by prescriber; to use sunscreen, protective clothing to prevent burns; avoid grapefruit or juice
• To report cardiac reactions, increased bruising, bleeding
• To use contraception (female, childbearing age), fetal harm may occur
• To report medicine use, if having any surgery
• Do not double doses; if dose is missed, take as soon as remembered; if close to next dose, omit dose

anakinra (℞)

(an-ah-kin'rah)
Kineret
Func. class.: Antirheumatic (DMARD), immunomodulator
Chem. class.: Recombinant form of human interleukin-1 receptor antagonist (IL-1Ra)

Action: A form of human interleukin-1 receptor antagonist (IL-1Ra) produced by DNA technology; blocks activity of IL-1, resulting in decreased cartilage degradation and decreased bone resorption
Uses: Reduction in signs and symptoms of moderate to severe active rheumatoid arthritis in patients ≥18 years of age who have not responded to other disease-modifying agents
Unlabeled uses: Cryopyrin-associated periodic syndromes

DOSAGE AND ROUTES

• *Adult:* **SUBCUT** 100 mg/day

Renal dose

• *Adult:* **SUBCUT** 100 mg every other day

Available form: Inj 100 mg/0.67 ml prefilled glass syringe

SIDE EFFECTS

CNS: Headache
EENT: Sinusitis
GI: Abdominal pain, nausea, diarrhea
HEMA: **Neutropenia**
INTEG: Rash, *inj site reaction,* allergic reaction
MISC: Flulike symptoms
MS: Worsening of RA, arthralgia
RESP: URI

Contraindications: Hypersensitivity to *Escherichia coli*–derived proteins or this product, sepsis
Precautions: Pregnancy (B), breastfeeding, children, geriatric patients, renal impairment, active infections

PHARMACOKINETICS

Terminal half-life 4-6 hr

INTERACTIONS

• Do not give concurrently with vaccines, immunizations should be brought up to date before treatment

Increase: risk of severe infection—TNF blocking agents (etanercept)
Decrease: antibody reactions

NURSING CONSIDERATIONS

Assess:

• Pain, stiffness, ROM, swelling of joints, baseline periodically during treatment
• For inj site pain, swelling; usually occur after 2 inj (4-5 days)
• For infections (increased WBC, fever, flulike symptoms); stop treatment if present
• Neutrophil counts prior to treatment and monthly × 3 mo and quarterly for up to 1 yr thereafter
• For allergic reactions (rash, dyspnea); discontinue if severe

Administer:

• Do not use if cloudy or discolored or if particulate is present, protect from light
• Do not admix with other sol or medications, do not use filter
• At same time each day

Evaluate:

- Therapeutic response: decreased inflammation, pain in joints

Teach patient/family:

- Not to receive vaccines while taking this product
- About self-administration if appropriate: inj should be made in thigh, abdomen, upper arm; rotate sites at least 1 inch from old site, give at same time of day
- To notify prescriber if pregnancy is planned or suspected, avoid breastfeeding
- To notify prescriber of allergic reaction

anastrozole (℞)

(an-a-stroh'zole)

Arimidex

Func. class.: Antineoplastic

Chem. class.: Aromatase inhibitor

Action: Highly selective nonsteroidal aromatase inhibitor that lowers serum estradiol concentrations; many breast cancers have strong estrogen receptors

Uses: Advanced breast carcinoma not responsive to other therapy in estrogen-receptor–positive patients (usually postmenopausal); patients with advanced disease on tamoxifen, adjunct therapy in early breast cancer

Unlabeled uses: Uterine leiomyomata, breast cancer (in those who have received tamoxifen for 2-3 yr)

DOSAGE AND ROUTES

- *Adult:* **PO** 1 mg/day

Available forms: Tabs 1 mg

SIDE EFFECTS

CNS: Hot flashes, headache, lightheadedness, depression, dizziness, confusion, insomnia, anxiety

CV: Chest pain, hypertension, thrombophlebitis, edema, angina, **MI, cerebral infarct, CVA**

GI: Nausea, vomiting, altered taste leading to anorexia, diarrhea, constipation, abdominal pain, dry mouth

GU: Vaginal bleeding, vaginal dryness, pelvic pain, pruritus vulvae, UTI

HEMA: **Leukopenia**

INTEG: Rash, **Stevens-Johnson syndrome**

MS: Bone pain, myalgia, *asthenia,* bone loss/osteoporosis, arthralgia, fractures

RESP: Cough, sinusitis, dyspnea, **pulmonary embolism**

Contraindications: Pregnancy (X), breastfeeding, hypersensitivity

Precautions: Children, geriatric patients, females, osteoporosis, hepatic/cardiac disease

PHARMACOKINETICS

Peak 4-7 hr; half-life 50 hr; excreted in feces, urine

INTERACTIONS

Drug/Lab Test

Increase: GGT, AST, ALT, alk phos, cholesterol, LDL

NURSING CONSIDERATIONS

Assess:

- For side effects during treatment

Administer:

- Give with food

Perform/provide:

- Storage in light-resistant container at room temperature

Evaluate:

- Therapeutic response: decreased tumor size, spread of malignancy

Teach patient/family:

- To report any complaints, side effects to prescriber
- That vaginal bleeding, pruritus, hot flashes are reversible after discontinuing treatment
- To report vaginal bleeding immediately
- If premenopausal, do not breastfeed; use reliable barrier contraception
- That tumor flare—increase in size of tumor, increased bone pain—may occur

and will subside rapidly; may take analgesics for pain

- To take adequate calcium and vitamin D due to risk for bone loss

anidulafungin (℞)

(a-nid-yoo-luh-fun′jin)

Eraxis

Func. class.: Antifungal, systemic

Chem. class.: Echinocandin

Action: Inhibits fungal enzyme synthesis; causes direct damage to fungal cell wall

Uses: Esophageal candidiasis, *Candida albicans, C. glabrata, C. parapsilosis, C. tropicalis*

Unlabeled uses: Fungal prophylaxis

DOSAGE AND ROUTES

Candidemia and other candida infections

- *Adult*: **IV** Loading dose 200 mg on day 1, then 100 mg/day until 14 days or more until last positive culture

Esophageal candidiasis

- *Adult*: **IV** Loading dose 100 mg on day 1, then 50 mg/day for at least 14 days and for at least 7 days after symptoms are resolved

Fungal prophylaxis (unlabeled)

- *Adolescent and child 2-17 yr:* **IV** 1.5 mg/kg over 90 min, then 0.75 mg/kg/day over 45 min over 5-28 days

Available forms: Powder for inj, lyophilized 50, 100 mg

SIDE EFFECTS

Candidemia/other Candida infections

CNS: **Seizures,** dizziness, *headache*

CV: DVT, **atrial fibrillation, right bundle branch block**, hypotension, **sinus arrhythmia, thrombophlebitis superficial, ventricular extrasystoles (rare)**

GI: Nausea, anorexia, vomiting, diarrhea, increased AST, ALT

META: Hypokalemia

Esophageal candidiasis

CNS: Headache

GI: Nausea, anorexia, vomiting, diarrhea, **hepatic necrosis**

HEMA: **Neutropenia, thrombocytopenia, leukopenia, coagulopathy**

INTEG: Rash

META: Hypocalcemia, hyperglycemia, hyperkalemia, hypernatremia, hypomagnesium (rare)

MS: Back pain, rigors

Contraindications: Hypersensitivity to this product, or other echinocandins

Precautions: Pregnancy (C), breastfeeding, children, severe hepatic disease

PHARMACOKINETICS

Steady state after loading dose, distribution half-life 0.5-1 hr, terminal half-life 40-50 hr, protein binding 99%

INTERACTIONS

Increase: plasma concentrations—cycloSPORINE

Drug/Lab Test

Increase: amylase, bilirubin, CPK, creatinine, ECG, QT prolongation, lipase

Decrease: platelets, magnesium, potassium, transferase, urea

NURSING CONSIDERATIONS

Assess:

- For infection, clearing of cultures during treatment; obtain culture baseline and throughout; product may be started as soon as culture is taken
- CBC (RBC, Hct, Hgb), differential, platelet count periodically; notify prescriber of results
- Renal studies: BUN, serum uric acid, urine CCr, electrolytes before and during therapy
- Hepatic studies before and during treatment: bilirubin, AST, ALT, alk phos, as needed
- Bleeding: hematuria, heme-positive stools, bruising or petechiae, mucosa or orifices; blood dyscrasias can occur

• GI symptoms: frequency of stools, cramping, if severe diarrhea occurs, electrolytes may need to be given

Administer:

IV route

• Reconstitute with provided dilutent 50-mg vial/5 ml (3.33 mg/ml), dilute with D_5 of 0.9% NaCl, only to a concentration of 0.5 mg/ml, run at no more than 1.1 mg/ml

• Rate of inf max 1.1 mg/min

• Give only as IV inf, not for IV bolus

• Do not use if cloudy or precipitated; do not admix

Perform/provide:

• Storage at room temperature, away from light, do not freeze; diluted sol must be used within 24 hr

Evaluate:

• Therapeutic response: decreased symptoms of *Candida* infection, negative culture

Teach patient/family:

• To notify prescriber if pregnancy is suspected or planned; use nonhormonal form of contraception while taking this product

• To avoid breastfeeding while taking this product

• To inform prescriber of renal/hepatic disease

• To report bleeding

• To report signs of infection: increased temp, sore throat, flulike symptoms

• To notify prescriber of nausea, vomiting, diarrhea, jaundice, anorexia, clay-colored stools, dark urine; hepatotoxicity may occur

⚠ High Alert

anistreplase (℞)

(ah-nis'tre-place)

anisoylated plasminogen, APSAC, Eminase

Func. class.: Thrombolytic enzyme

Chem. class.: Plasminogen activator

Action: Promotes thrombolysis by promoting conversion of plasminogen to plasmin

Uses: Acute MI for lysis of coronary artery thrombi; ST-elevation MI (STEMI) for lysis of coronary artery thrombi as soon as possible or within 12 hr of symptoms or within 24 hr if ischemia symptoms persist

DOSAGE AND ROUTES

• *Adult:* **IV** 30 units over 2-5 min as soon as possible after onset of symptoms

Available forms: Powder, lyophilized 30 units/vial

SIDE EFFECTS

CNS: Headache, fever, sweating, agitation, dizziness, paresthesia, tremor, vertigo, **intracranial hemorrhage, stroke**

CV: Hypotension, **dysrhythmias,** conduction disorders

GI: Nausea, vomiting

HEMA: Decreased Hct; **GI, GU, intracranial, retroperitoneal,** surface bleeding; **thrombocytopenia**

INTEG: Rash, urticaria, phlebitis at inj site, itching, flushing

MS: Low back pain, arthralgia, myalgia

RESP: Altered respirations, dyspnea, **bronchospasm, lung edema, pulmonary bleeding**

SYST: **Anaphylaxis (rare), bleeding**

Contraindications: Hypersensitivity to anistreplase, streptokinase; active internal bleeding, intraspinal or intracranial surgery, neoplasms of CNS, severe, uncontrolled hypertension, cerebral embolism/thrombosis/hemorrhage, previous hemorrhagic stroke, recent trauma/history of CVA

Precautions: Pregnancy (C), breastfeeding, geriatric patients, arterial emboli from left side of heart, ulcerative colitis/enteritis, hepatic/renal disease, hypocoagulation, COPD, subacute bacterial endocarditis, rheumatic valvular disease, intraarterial diagnostic procedure or surgery (10 days), recent major surgery, previous streptokinase/anistreplase in last 12 mo

PHARMACOKINETICS

Inactivated by binding to plasma activators, half-life 70-120 min

INTERACTIONS

Increase: bleeding potential—aspirin, other NSAIDs, heparin, antiplatelets, abciximab, eptifibatide, tirofiban, clopidogrel, ticlopidine, some cephalosporins, plicamycin, valproic acid, anticoagulants, dipyridamole

Decrease: action of anistreplase—aminocaproic acid, aprotinin, tranexamic acid

Drug/Herb

Increase: risk of bleeding—agrimony, alfalfa, angelica, anise, basil, bay, bilberry, black currant, black haw, bladderwrack, bogbean, boldo, borage, bromelain, buchu, capsaicin, cat's claw, chaparral, chondroitin, cinchona bark, clove oil, curcumin, dandelion, dong quai, evening primrose, fenugreek, feverfew, garlic, ginger, ginkgo, ginseng, guggul, horse chestnut, Irish moss, kava, kelp, kelpware, khella, licorice, lovage, lungwort, meadowsweet, motherwort, mugwort, nettle, papaya, parsley (large amts), pau d'arco, pineapple, poplar, prickly ash, red clover, safflower, saw palmetto, skullcap, tanshen, tonka bean, tumeric, wintergreen, yarrow

Decrease: anticoagulant effect—chamomile, coenzyme Q10, flax, glucomannan, goldenseal, guar gum

Drug/Lab Test

Increase: PT, APTT, TT

Decrease: fibrinogen, plasminogen

NURSING CONSIDERATIONS

Assess:

- VS, B/P, pulse, respirations, neurologic signs, temp at least q4hr, temp >104° F (40° C) or indicators of internal bleeding, treat bradycardia, ventricular changes; assess neurologic status, neurologic change may indicate intracranial bleeding; ECG continuously, cardiac enzymes, radionuclide, myocardial scanning/coronary angiography
- Hypersensitivity: fever, rash, itching, chills, facial swelling, dyspnea; notify prescriber immediately, stop product, keep resuscitative equipment nearby; mild reaction may be treated with antihistamines

⚠ Bleeding during first hr of treatment (hematuria, hematemesis, bleeding from mucous membranes, epistaxis, ecchymosis), continue to monitor for 24 hr after treatment

- Blood studies (Hct, platelets, PTT, PT, TT, APTT) before starting therapy; PT or APTT must be less than 2 × control before starting therapy; TT or PT q3-4hr during treatment

Administer:

IV, direct route

- Reconstitute single-dose vial/5 ml sterile water for inj (not bacteriostatic water), and roll (not shake) to enhance reconstitution; give over 2-5 min by direct IV, give within ½ hr of reconstitution or discard, do not add other meds to vial or syringe; give within 6 hr of thrombi identification for best results
- Pressure of 30 sec to minor bleeding sites, 30 min to sites of arterial puncture followed by dressing; inform prescriber if hemostasis not attained; apply pressure dressing
- Use powder within 30 min after reconstitution
- Cryoprecipitate or fresh frozen plasma if bleeding occurs
- Heparin therapy after thrombolytic therapy is discontinued, TT or APTT <2 × control (about 3-4 hr)

• About 10% of patients have high streptococcal antibody titers, requiring increased loading doses

Perform/provide:

• Bed rest during entire course of treatment; handle patient as little as possible during therapy

• Storage of powder in refrigerator

• Avoid invasive procedures: inj, rectal temp

• Treat fever with acetaminophen

Evaluate:

• Therapeutic response: absence of thrombi formation in MI, improved ventricular function, chest pain resolution

Teach patient/family:

• Reason for product and expected results

⚠ High Alert

antihemophilic factor VIII (AHF) (℞)

(an-tee-hee-moe-fill'ik)

antihemophilic factor, Alphanate, Bioclate, Helixate FS, Hemofil M, Humate-P, Hyate C, Koate-DVI, Kogenate, Kogenate FS, Monoclate-P, Recombinate, ReFacto

Func. class.: Hemostatic

Chem. class.: Factor VIII

Do not confuse:

Kogenate/Kogenate-2

Action: Necessary for clotting; activates factor X in conjunction with activated factor IX; transforms prothrombin to thrombin

Uses: Prevention/treatment of hemophilia A, patients with acquired circulating factor VIII inhibitors, factor VIII deficiency; prevention of surgical bleeding, risk of thrombosis (von Willebrand disease)

DOSAGE AND ROUTES

Massive hemorrhage

• *Adult and child:* **IV** 40-50 units/kg, then 20-25 units/kg q8-12hr

Overt bleeding

• *Adult and child:* **IV** 15-25 units/kg, then 8-15 units/kg q8-12hr × 4 days

Hemorrhage near vital organs

• *Adult and child:* **IV** 25 units/kg, then 15 units/kg q8hr × 2 days, then 4 units/kg q8hr × 2 days

Minor hemorrhage

• *Adult and child:* **IV** 8-10 units/kg q24hr × 2-3 days or 8 units/kg q12hr × 2 days, then q24hr × 2 days

Joint bleeding

• *Adult and child:* **IV** 15 units/kg q8-12hr × 1-2 days

Available forms: Inj 250, 500, 1000, 1500 units/vial (number of units noted on label)

SIDE EFFECTS

CNS: Headache, *lethargy, chills, fever, flushing,* LOC

CV: Hypotension, tachycardia

GI: Nausea, vomiting, abdominal cramps, constipation, diarrhea, anorexia, jaundice, **viral hepatitis**

HEMA: **Thrombosis, hemolysis, risk of hepatitis B, risk of HIV**

INTEG: Rash, flushing, *urticaria,* stinging at inj site

MISC: **Anaphylaxis,** blurred vision, back pain

RESP: **Bronchospasm,** rhinitis, dyspnea, nosebleeds, wheezing

Contraindications: Hypersensitivity; mouse, hamster, bovine, porcine protein, lactation, HIV

Precautions: Pregnancy (C), neonates/infants, hepatic disease; blood types A, B, AB; factor VIII inhibitor, viral infection

PHARMACOKINETICS

IV: Half-life 4 hr, terminal 15 hr

INTERACTIONS

Increase: bleeding—anticoagulants, NSAIDs, salicylates

NURSING CONSIDERATIONS

Assess:

- Blood studies (coagulation factors assay by % normal: 5% prevents spontaneous hemorrhage, 30%-50% for surgery, 80%-100% for severe hemorrhage)
- I&O, urine color; notify prescriber if urine becomes orange, red
- Pulse: discontinue infusion if significant increase
- Hct, Coombs' test with blood types A, B, AB
- Test for factor VIII inhibitors before starting treatment, may require concomitant antiinhibitor coagulant complex therapy
- Allergy: fever, rash, itching, jaundice; give diphenhydrAMINE HCl (Benadryl), continue therapy if reaction is mild
- Blood group of patient, donors (if applicable; most factor VIII not from specific blood group donors)

⚠ Bleeding: ankles, knees, elbows, other joints

Administer:

- Hepatitis A/B vaccination at birth, if diagnosed with hemophilia

IV route

- To prepare, administer factor VIII concentrates at first sign of danger
- After rotating gently to mix
- Warm to room temperature using plastic syringe to reconstitute and administer; adheres to glass; use another needle as a vent when reconstituting
- After dilution with warm NS, D_5W, LR, give within 3 hr; complete dissolution may take up to 10 min

IV INF route

- Give at ≤2 ml/min if concentration exceeds 34 units/ml or over 3 min if concentration is <34 units/ml, filter before use

Perform/provide:

- Storage in refrigerator; do not freeze; after reconstitution, do not refrigerate; give within 3 hr

Evaluate:

- Therapeutic response: absence of bleeding

Teach patient/family:

- To report any signs of bleeding: gums, under skin, urine, stools, emesis; review methods to prevent bleeding
- To avoid salicylates, NSAIDs (increase bleeding tendencies)
- To advise health professionals of treatment for hemophilia
- The signs of viral hepatitis, AIDS
- That immunization for hepatitis B may be given first
- To report hives, urticaria, chest tightness, hypotension; may be monoclonal antibody–derived factor VIII
- To be checked q2-3mo for HIV screen
- To carry emergency ID describing disease process
- To report suspected transmission of infection to respective manufacturers

⚠ High Alert

antithrombin III, human (℞)

(an'tee-throm-bin)

ATryn, Thrombate III

Func. class.: Antithrombin

Chem. class.: Pooled human plasma

Action: Inactivates thrombin and the activated forms of factors IX, X, XI, XII, resulting in inhibition of coagulation

Uses: During surgical or obstetric procedures, or for thromboembolism in patients with known antithrombin III deficiency

Unlabeled uses: Disseminated intravascular coagulation (DIC)

DOSAGE AND ROUTES

Dosage is individualized

- Expect a 1.4% rise from baseline for every 1 international unit/kg administered

Units required =

$$\frac{\text{(Desired level} - \text{Baseline)} \times \text{Weight in kg}}{1.4\%}$$

DIC (unlabeled)

- *Adult:* **IV** Target at III at >100%-120%

Available forms: 500 units in 10 ml; 1000 units in 20 ml; powder for inj 1750 units

SIDE EFFECTS

CNS: Dizziness, chills, severe lightheadedness

GI: Nausea, cramps, bowel fullness

RESP: Shortness of breath

SYST: **Bleeding,** surface bleeding, **anaphylaxis,** vasodilatory effects

Contraindications: Goat milk hypersensitivity

Precautions: Pregnancy (B), breastfeeding, children

PHARMACOKINETICS

Biologic half-life 2.5 days, peak 15-30 min

INTERACTIONS

• Do not administer with other products in syringe or solutions

Increase: bleeding risk—anticoagulants, thrombolytics, pentosan, NSAIDs, salicylates, low-molecular-weight heparins (LMWHs), platelet inhibitors, antineoplastics, antithymocyte globulin, strontium-89

Drug/Food

Increase: bleeding risk—fish oil, omega-3 fatty acids

Drug/Herb

Increase: bleeding risk—garlic, ginger, ginkgo, green tea, horse chestnut

NURSING CONSIDERATIONS

Assess:

• AT-III levels q12hr, maintain at >80% of normal activity until stabilized, then daily before dose

• VS, B/P, pulse, respirations, neurologic signs, temp at least q4hr, temp 104° F (40° C) or platelet count, thromboplastin time, aPI, pro-time, fibrinogen levels, cardiac rhythm

⚠ For child born of parents with hereditary AT-III deficiency, obtain AT-III levels immediately after birth

⚠ For neurologic changes that may indicate intracranial bleeding

⚠ Retroperitoneal bleeding: back pain, leg weakness, diminished pulses

Administer:

• ATryn is not indicated for treatment of thromboembolic events in hereditary antithrombin deficiency

• Heparin after fibrinogen level is over 100 mg/dl; heparin infusion to increase PTT to 1.5-2 × baseline for 3-7 days

IV route

• Only by IV route over 10-20 min (Thrombate III)

• After reconstituting 500 international units/10 ml of NS or D_5W; do not shake; rotate to dissolve; allow to warm to room temperature; use within 3 hr of reconstitution; give 50 international units or less/min; do not exceed 100 international units/min using 0.22 or 0.45 microfilter

Perform/provide:

• Storage in refrigerator

Evaluate:

• Therapeutic response: absence of thrombi formation

Teach patient/family:

• About product use and expected results

• To report adverse reactions; bleeding, bruising

• That maintenance dosing not usually required

• That there are many drug and herb interactions, obtain approval from provider before taking

antithymocyte

See lymphocyte immune globulin

apraclonidine ophthalmic

See Appendix B

A

aprepitant (℞)

(ap-re'pi-tant)
Emend
Func. class.: Antiemetic
Chem. class.: Miscellaneous

Action: A selective antagonist of human substance P/neurokinin 1 (NK_1) receptors decreasing emetic reflex

Uses: Prevention of nausea/vomiting associated with cancer chemotherapy (highly emetogenic/moderately emetogenic) including high-dose cisplatin, used in combination with other antiemetics; postoperative nausea/vomiting

DOSAGE AND ROUTES

Highly emetogenic

• *Adult:* **PO** Day 1 (1 hour prior to chemotherapy) aprepitant 125 mg with 12 mg dexamethasone **PO,** with 32 mg ondansetron IV; day 2 aprepitant 80 mg with 8 mg dexamethasone **PO;** day 3 aprepitant 80 mg with 8 mg dexamethasone **PO;** day 4 only dexamethasone 8 mg **PO**

Moderately emetogenic

• *Adult:* **PO** Day 1 125 mg aprepitant with dexamethasone 12 mg **PO,** with ondansetron 8 mg **PO** × 2; days 2 and 3 80 mg aprepitant only

Prevention of postoperative nausea/vomiting

• *Adult:* **PO** 40 mg within 3 hr of induction of anesthesia

Available forms: Caps 40, 80, 125 mg

SIDE EFFECTS

CNS: Headache, dizziness, insomnia, anxiety, depression, confusion, peripheral neuropathy

CV: Bradycardia, tachycardia, DVT, hypo/hypertension

GI: Diarrhea, constipation, abdominal pain, anorexia, gastritis, increased AST, ALT, *nausea,* vomiting, heartburn

GU: Increased BUN, serum creatine, proteinuria, dysuria

HEMA: Anemia, **thrombocytopenia, neutropenia**

INTEG: Pruritus, rash, urticaria

MISC: Asthenia, fatigue, dehydration, fever, hiccups, tinnitus, alopecia

SYST: **Anaphylaxis**

Contraindications: Hypersensitivity

Precautions: Pregnancy (B), breastfeeding, children, geriatric patients, hepatic disease

PHARMACOKINETICS

Absorption 60%-65%, peak 4 hr, metabolized in liver by CYP3A4 enzymes to an active metabolite, half-life 9-12 hr, 95% protein bound, not excreted in kidneys, crosses blood-brain barrier

INTERACTIONS

Increase: aprepitant action—CYP3A4 inhibitors (ketoconazole, itraconazole, nefazodone, troleandomycin, clarithromycin, ritonavir, nelfinavir, diltiazem)

Increase: action of CYP3A4 substrates (pimozide, cisapride, dexamethasone, methylPREDNISolone, midazolam, alprazolam, triazolam, docetaxel, paclitaxel, etoposide, irinotecan, imatinib, ifosfamide, vinorelbine, vinBLAStine, vinCRIStine)

Decrease: aprepitant action—CYP3A4 inducers (rifampin, carbamazepine, phenytoin)

Decrease: action of CYP2C9 substrates (warfarin, tolbutamide, phenytoin), oral contraceptives

Decrease: action of both products—paroxetine

Drug/Food

Decrease: effect—grapefruit juice

NURSING CONSIDERATIONS

Assess:

⚠ For hypersensitive reactions: pruritus, rash, urticaria, anaphylaxis

• CV status: hypo/hypertension, bradycardia, tachycardia, DVT

• For absence of nausea, vomiting during chemotherapy

Administer:

- Do not break, crush, or chew
- PO on 3-day schedule, give with full glass of water 1 hr before chemotherapy, with or without food

Perform/provide:

- Storage at room temperature; keep in original bottles, blisters

Evaluate:

- Therapeutic response: absence of nausea, vomiting during cancer chemotherapy

Teach patient/family:

- To report diarrhea, constipation
- To take only as prescribed, take 1st dose 1 hr prior to chemotherapy
- To report all medications and herbals to prescriber prior to taking this medication
- Advise to use nonhormonal form of contraception while taking this agent and for 1 mo thereafter; oral contraceptive effect may be decreased
- Advise those on warfarin to have clotting monitored closely during 2-wk period following administration of aprepitant
- To avoid breastfeeding

arformoterol (℞)

(ar-for-moe'ter-ole)

Brovana

Func. class.: Long–acting adrenergic β_2-agonist, sympathomimetic, bronchodilator

Action: Causes bronchodilation by action on β_2 (pulmonary) receptors by increasing levels of cAMP, which relaxes smooth muscle; produces bronchodilation and CNS, cardiac stimulation, as well as increased diuresis and gastric acid secretion; longer acting than isoproterenol

Uses: COPD, including chronic bronchitis, emphysema

DOSAGE AND ROUTES

COPD

- *Adult:* **NEB** 15 mcg, bid, AM, PM

Available forms: Inh sol 15 mcg/2 ml

SIDE EFFECTS

CNS: ***Tremors, anxiety,*** insomnia, headache, dizziness, stimulation, ***restlessness,*** hallucinations, flushing, irritability

CV: Palpitations, tachycardia, hypertension, angina, hypotension, dysrhythmias

EENT: Dry nose, irritation of nose and throat

GI: Heartburn, nausea, vomiting

MISC: Flushing, sweating, anorexia, bad taste/smell changes, hypokalemia, **anaphylaxis**

MS: Muscle cramps

RESP: Cough, wheezing, dyspnea, **bronchospasm,** dry throat

Contraindications: Hypersensitivity to sympathomimetics, this product, or racemic formoterol; tachydysrhyhmias, severe cardiac disease, heart block, children

Black Box Warning: Actively deteriorating COPD

Precautions: Pregnancy (C), breastfeeding, cardiac disorders, hyperthyroidism, diabetes mellitus, hypertension, prostatic hypertrophy, angle-closure glaucoma, seizures, hypoglycemia

PHARMACOKINETICS

Onset 5 min; peak 1-1½ hr; duration 4-6 hr; terminal half-life (COPD) 26 hr; extensively metabolized by direct conjugation by CYP2D6, CYP2C19; crosses placenta; protein binding 52%-65%; excreted in urine 63%, feces 11%

INTERACTIONS

Increase: severe hypotension—oxytocics

Increase: toxicity—theophylline

Increase: ECG changes/hypokalemia—potassium-losing diuretics

Increase: action of nebulized bronchodilators

Increase: action of arformoterol—tricyclics, MAOIs, other adrenergics; do not use together

Decrease: arformoterol action—other β-blockers

Drug/Herb

Increase: stimulation—caffeine (cola nut, green/black tea, guarana, yerba maté, coffee, chocolate)

NURSING CONSIDERATIONS

Assess:

- Respiratory function: vital capacity, forced expiratory volume, ABGs; lung sounds, heart rate and rhythm, B/P, sputum (baseline and peak)
- That patient has not received theophylline therapy or other bronchodilators before giving dose
- Patient's ability to self-medicate
- For evidence of allergic reactions; anaphylaxis may occur
- Paradoxical bronchospasm; hold medication, notify prescriber if bronchospasm occurs

Administer:

- Must be used by nebulization

Perform/provide:

- Storage in refrigerator

Evaluate:

- Therapeutic response: absence of dyspnea, wheezing after 1 hr, improved airway exchange, improved ABGs

Teach patient/family:

- To use exactly as prescribed; that death has resulted from asthma with products similar to this one
- Not to use OTC medications; excess stimulation may occur

⚠ High Alert

argatroban (℞)

(are-ga-troe'ban)

Argatroban

Func. class.: Anticoagulant

Chem. class.: Thrombin inhibitor

Do not confuse:

argatroban/Aggrastat

Action: Direct inhibitor of thrombin, it reversibly binds to the thrombin active site

Uses: Anticoagulation prevention/treatment of thrombosis in heparin-induced thrombocytopenia or adjunct to percutaneous coronary intervention (PCI) in those with a history of HIT

Unlabeled uses: Acute MI, DIC, use in infants/children/adolescents

DOSAGE AND ROUTES

Heparin-induced thrombocytopenia/thrombosis syndrome (HIT or HITTS)

- *Adult:* **CONT IV INF** 2 mcg/kg/min (1 mg/ml); adjust dose until steady-state aPTT is 1.5-3× initial baseline, not to exceed 100 sec, max dose 10 mcg/kg/min
- *Infant/child/adolescent (unlabeled):* **CONT IV INF** 0.75 mcg/kg/min, monitor aPTT q2hr

Hepatic dose

- *Adult:* **CONT INF** 0.5 mcg/kg/min, adjust rate based on aPTT

Percutaneous coronary intervention (PCI) in HIT

- *Adult:* **IV INF** 25 mcg/kg/min and a bolus of 350 mcg/kg given over 3-5 min, check ACT 5-10 min after bolus is completed; proceed if ACT >300 sec if ACT <300 sec, give another 150 mcg/kg **BOL** and increase inf rate to 30 mcg/kg/min, recheck ACT in 5-10 min; if ACT >450 sec, decrease inf rate to 15 mcg/kg/min, recheck ACT in 5-10 min; once ACT is therapeutic, continue for duration of procedure

Acute MI (unlabeled)

- *Adult:* **IV** 1-3 mcg/kg/min

DIC (unlabeled)

- *Adult:* **CONT IV** 0.7 mcg/kg/min

Available forms: Inj 100 mg/ml (2.5 ml) (must dilute 100-fold)

SIDE EFFECTS

CNS: *Fever,* **intracranial bleeding,** headache

CV: **Atrial fibrillation, coronary thrombosis, MI, myocardial ischemia, coronary occlusion, ventricular tachycardia, bradycardia,** *chest pain, hypotension*

GI: Nausea, vomiting, abdominal pain, diarrhea, **GI bleeding**

GU: **Hematuria,** abnormal kidney function, UTI

HEMA: **Hemorrhage**
MISC: ***Back pain, headache,*** infection
RESP: Pneumonia, dyspnea, coughing, hemoptysis
SYST: **Sepsis**

Contraindications: Hypersensitivity, overt major bleeding

Precautions: Pregnancy (B), breastfeeding, children, intracranial bleeding, renal function impairment, hepatic disease, severe hypertension, after lumbar puncture, spinal anesthesia, major surgery, congenital or acquired bleeding, GI ulcers

PHARMACOKINETICS

Metabolized in the liver by P450 CYP3A 4/5, distributed to extracellular fluid, 54% plasma protein binding, half-life 39-51 min, excreted in feces, steady state 1-3 hr

INTERACTIONS

Increase: bleeding risk—antiplatelets, NSAIDs, salicylates, dipyridamole, clopidogrel, ticlopidine, heparin, warfarin, glycoprotein IIb/IIIa antagonists (abciximab, tirofiban, eptifibatide), thrombolytics (streptokinase, alteplase, reteplase, urokinase, tenecteplase), other anticoagulants

Drug/Herb

Increase: bleeding risk—agrimony, alfalfa, angelica, anise, bilberry, black currant, black haw, bogbean, buchu, cat's claw, chondroitin, dong quai, fenugreek, feverfew, fish oils, garlic, ginger, ginkgo, ginseng, horse chestnut, Irish moss, kava, kelp, kelpware, khella, licorice, lovage, lungwort, meadowsweet, motherwort, mugwort, nettle, papaya, parsley, pau d'arco, pineapple, poplar, prickly ash, safflower, saw palmetto, senega, skullcap, turmeric, wintergreen

Decrease: argatroban effect—chamomile, coenzyme Q10, flax, glucomannan, goldenseal, guar gum

NURSING CONSIDERATIONS

Assess:

- Obtain baseline in aPTT before treatment; do not start treatment if aPTT ratio ≥2.5, then aPTT 2 hr after initiation of treatment and at least daily thereafter
- aPTT, which should be 1.5-3 × control

⚠ Bleeding gums; petechiae; ecchymosis; black, tarry stools; hematuria/epistaxis; B/P; vaginal bleeding and possible hemorrhage

⚠ Anaphylaxis: dyspnea, rash during treatment

- Fever, skin rash, urticaria

Administer:

- Avoiding all IM inj that may cause bleeding

IV, direct route

- For PCI: 350 mg/kg bol, then continuous inf of 25 mcg/kg/min

Intermittent IV INF route

- Dilute in 0.9% NaCl, D_5, LR to a final conc 1 mg/ml; dilute each 2.5-ml vial 100-fold by mixing with 250 ml of diluent, mix by repeated inversion of the diluent bag for 1 min; may be slightly hazy briefly
- Dosage adjustment may be made after review of aPTT, not to exceed 10 mcg/kg/min

Evaluate:

- Therapeutic response: absence or decrease of thrombosis

Teach patient/family:

- To use soft-bristle toothbrush to avoid bleeding gums, avoid contact sports, use electric razor, avoid IM inj
- To report any signs of bleeding: gums, under skin, urine, stools
- To notify prescriber if planning to become pregnant or breastfeeding

aripiprazole (℞)

(a-rip-ip-pra′zol)
Abilify, Abilify Dismelt
Func. class.: Antipsychotic
Chem. class.: Quinolinone

Action: Exact mechanism unknown; may be mediated through both DOPamine type

2 (D_2, D_3) and serotonin type 2 ($5\text{-}HT_{1A}$, $5\text{-}HT_{2A}$) antagonism

Uses: Schizophrenia and bipolar disorder (adults and adolescents), agitation, mania, major depressive disorder, short-term mania or mixed episodes of bipolar disorder

Unlabeled uses: Psychosis in dementia

DOSAGE AND ROUTES

Major depressive disorder

- *Adult:* **PO** 2-5 mg/day as an adjunct to other antidepressant treatment; adjust by 5 mg at ≥1 wk (range 2-15 mg/day)

Schizophrenia

- *Adult:* **PO** 10-15 mg/day; if needed, dosage may be increased to 30 mg/day after 2 wk; maintenance 15 mg/day, periodically reassess

Bipolar disorder

- *Adult:* **PO** 30 mg/day, may reduce to 15 mg if needed

Agitation in bipolar disorder/ schizophrenia

- *Adult:* **IM** 9.75 mg as a single dose, may start with a lower dose

Available forms: Tabs 2, 5, 10, 15, 20, 30 mg; inj 9.75 mg/1.3 ml; orally disintegrating tab 10, 15 mg; oral sol 1 mg/ml

SIDE EFFECTS

CNS: Drowsiness, insomnia, agitation, anxiety, headache, **seizures, neuroleptic malignant syndrome,** *lightheadedness, akathisia, asthenia, tremor,* **stroke, suicidal ideation,** dystonia

CV: Orthostatic hypotension, **tachycardia**

EENT: Blurred vision, rhinitis

GI: Constipation, nausea, vomiting, jaundice, *weight gain*

INTEG: Rash

META: Hypoglycemia

RESP: Cough

SYST: **Death in geriatric patients with dementia**

Contraindications: Breastfeeding, hypersensitivity, seizure disorders

Precautions: Pregnancy (C), geriatric patients, renal/hepatic/cardiac disease

Black Box Warning: Children, dementia, suicidal ideation

PHARMACOKINETICS

PO: Absorption 87%; extensively metabolized by liver to a major active metabolite; plasma protein binding >99%; terminal half-life 75-146 hr; excretion urine 25%, feces 55%; clearance decreased in geriatric patients

INTERACTIONS

Increase: effects of aripiprazole—CYP3A4 inhibitors (ketoconazole, erythromycin), CYP2D6 inhibitors (quinidine, fluoxetine, paroxetine); reduce dose of aripiprazole

Increase: sedation—other CNS depressants, alcohol

Increase: EPS—other antipsychotics, lithium

Decrease: aripiprazole level—famotidine, valproate

Decrease: effects of aripiprazole—CYP3A4 inducers (carbamazepine)

Drug/Herb

Increase: EPS—betel palm, kava

Increase: neuroleptic effect—cola tree, hops, nettle, nutmeg

NURSING CONSIDERATIONS

Assess:

- Mental status before initial administration
- Swallowing of PO medication; check for hoarding or giving of medication to other patients
- I&O ratio; palpate bladder if urinary output is low
- Bilirubin, CBC, LFTs q mo
- Affect, orientation, LOC, reflexes, gait, coordination, sleep pattern disturbances
- B/P standing and lying; also pulse, respirations; take q4hr during initial treatment; establish baseline before starting treatment; report drops of 30 mm Hg; watch for ECG changes
- Dizziness, faintness, palpitations, tachycardia on rising

• EPS, including akathisia (inability to sit still, no pattern to movements), tardive dyskinesia (bizarre movements of the jaw, mouth, tongue, extremities), pseudoparkinsonism (rigidity, tremors, pill rolling, shuffling gait)

⚠ For neuroleptic malignant syndrome: hyperthermia, increased CPK, altered mental status, muscle rigidity; notify prescriber immediately

• Constipation, urinary retention daily; if these occur, increase bulk and water in diet; stool softeners, laxatives may be needed

Administer:

• Reduced dose in geriatric patients

Perform/provide:

• Supervised ambulation until patient is stabilized on medication; do not involve in strenuous exercise program because fainting is possible; patient should not stand still for a long time

• Storage in tight, light-resistant container

Evaluate:

• Therapeutic response: decrease in emotional excitement, hallucinations, delusions, paranoia; reorganization of patterns of thought, speech

Teach patient/family:

• That orthostatic hypotension may occur and to rise from sitting or lying position gradually

• To avoid hot tubs, hot showers, tub baths; hypotension may occur

• To avoid abrupt withdrawal of this product; EPS may result; product should be withdrawn slowly

• To avoid OTC preparations (cough, hay fever, cold) unless approved by prescriber, serious product interactions may occur; avoid use with alcohol, CNS depressants; increased drowsiness may occur

• To avoid hazardous activities if drowsy or dizzy

• Compliance with product regimen

• To report impaired vision, tremors, muscle twitching, urinary retention

• In hot weather, that heat stroke may occur; take extra precautions to stay cool

• To notify prescriber if pregnant or intend to become pregnant; not to breastfeed

Treatment of overdose: Lavage if orally ingested; provide airway; *do not induce vomiting*

Rarely Used

armodafinil (℞)

(ar-moe-daf′in-il)

Nuvigil

Controlled Substance Schedule IV

Uses: Narcolepsy, obstructive sleep apnea/hypoapnea syndrome, circadian rhythm disruption (shift work sleep problems)

DOSAGE AND ROUTES

Narcolepsy, obstructive sleep apnea/hypoapnea syndrome

• *Adult and adolescent ≥17 yr:* **PO** 150-250 mg in AM

Circadian rhythm disruption (shift work sleep problems)

• *Adult and adolescent ≥17 yr:* **PO** 150 mg at start of shift

Contraindications: Hypersensitivity to this product or modafinil

ascorbic acid (vit C) (OTC, ℞)

(a-skor′bic)

Apo-C ♣, ascorbic acid, Ascorbicap, Cebid, Cecon, Cecore-500, Cemill, Cenolate, Cetane, Cevalin, Cevi-Bid, Ce-Vi-Sol, C-Span, Flavorcee, Mega-C/A Plus, Ortho/CS, Sunkist

Func. class.: Vit C—water-soluble vitamin

Action: Needed for wound healing, collagen synthesis, antioxidant, carbohydrate metabolism

Uses: Vit C deficiency, scurvy, delayed wound and bone healing, chronic disease, urine acidification, before gastrectomy, dietary supplement

Unlabeled uses: Common cold prevention

DOSAGE AND ROUTES

Dietary supplementation

- *Adult:* 50-500 mg/day
- *Child 14-18 yr:* **PO** 65 mg (female), 75 mg (male)
- *Child 11-14 yr:* **PO** 50 mg/day
- *Child 4-10 yr:* **PO** 45 mg/day
- *Child 1-3 yr:* **PO** 40 mg/day
- *Child 6 mo-1 yr:* **PO** 35 mg/day
- *Child <6 mo:* **PO** 30 mg/day

Scurvy

- *Adult:* **PO/SUBCUT/IM/IV** 100 mg-250 mg/day × 2 wk, then 50 mg or more daily
- *Child:* **PO/SUBCUT/IM/IV** 100-300 mg/day × 2 wk, then 35 mg or more daily

Wound healing/chronic disease/ fracture (may be given with zinc)

- *Adult:* **SUBCUT/IM/IV/PO** 200-500 mg/day for 1-2 mo
- *Child:* **SUBCUT/IM/IV/PO** 100-200 mg added doses for 1-2 mo

Urine acidification

- *Adult:* 4-12 g/day in divided doses
- *Child:* 500 mg q6-8hr

Available forms: Tabs 25, 50, 100, 250, 500, 1000, 1500 mg; effervescent tabs 1000 mg; chewable tabs 100, 250, 500 mg; timed-release tabs 500, 750, 1000, 1500 mg; timed-release caps 500 mg; crys 4 g/tsp; powder 4 g/tsp; liq 35 mg/0.6 ml; sol 100 mg/ml; syr 20 mg/ml, 500 mg/5 ml; inj SUBCUT, IM, IV 100, 250, 500 mg/ml

SIDE EFFECTS

CNS: Headache, insomnia, dizziness, fatigue, flushing

GI: Nausea, vomiting, diarrhea, anorexia, heartburn, cramps

GU: Polyuria, urine acidification, oxalate or urate renal stones, dysuria

HEMA: **Hemolytic anemia in patients with G6PD**

INTEG: Inflammation at inj site

Contraindications: Tartrazine, sulfite sensitivity; G6PD deficiency

Precautions: Pregnancy (C), gout, diabetes, renal calculi (large doses)

PHARMACOKINETICS

PO/INJ: Readily absorbed PO, metabolized in liver, unused amounts excreted in urine (unchanged) and metabolites, crosses placenta, breast milk

INTERACTIONS

Drug/Lab Test

False positive: negatives in glucose tests

False negative: occult blood, urine bilirubin, leukocyte determination

NURSING CONSIDERATIONS

Assess:

- I&O ratio; urine pH (acidification)
- Ascorbic acid levels throughout treatment if continued deficiency is suspected
- Nutritional status: citrus fruits, vegetables
- Inj sites for inflammation
- Thrombophlebitis, if on large dose

Administer:

PO route

- Do not crush or chew ext rel tab or caps
- That caps may be opened and contents mixed with jelly

IV, direct route

- Undiluted by direct IV 100 mg over at least 1 min, rapid inf may cause fainting

Intermittent IV INF route

- Diluted with D_5W, D_5NaCl, NS, LR, Ringer's, sodium lactate and given over 15 min

Additive compatibilities: Amikacin, calcium chloride, calcium gluceptate, calcium gluconate, cephalothin, chloramphenicol, chlorproMAZINE, colistimethate, cyanocobalamin, diphenhydrAMINE, heparin, kanamycin, methicillin, methyldopate, penicillin G potassium, polymyxin B, prednisolone, procaine, prochlorperazine, promethazine, verapamil

Syringe compatibilities: Metoclopramide, aminophylline, theophylline
Y-site compatibilities: Warfarin
Evaluate:
• Therapeutic response: absence of anorexia, irritability, pallor, joint pain, hyperkeratosis, petechiae, poor wound healing
Teach patient/family:
• The necessary foods in diet, such as citrus fruits
• That smoking decreases vit C levels, not to exceed prescribed dose; increases will be excreted in urine, except timed release

asenapine (℞)
(a-sen'a-peen)
Saphris
Func. class.: Antipsychotic, atypical
Chem. class.: Benzisoxazole derivative

Action: Unknown; may be mediated through both DOPamine type 2 (D2) and serotonin type 2 (5-HT2A) antagonism
Uses: Bipolar 1 disorder, schizophrenia

DOSAGE AND ROUTES
Schizophrenia
• *Adult:* **SL** 5 mg bid, max 20 mg/day
Bipolar 1 disorder
• *Adult:* **SL** 10 mg bid, may decrease to 5 mg bid as needed, max 20 mg/day
Available forms: SL tab 5, 10 mg

SIDE EFFECTS
CNS: EPS, pseudoparkinsonism, akathisia, dystonia, tardive dyskinesia; drowsiness, insomnia, agitation, anxiety, headache, **seizures, neuroleptic malignant syndrome,** dizziness
CV: Orthostatic hypotension, **sinus tachycardia; heart failure, QT prolongation, stroke, bundle branch block**
GI: Nausea, vomiting, *constipation,* weight gain, increased appetite
GU: Hyperprolactinemia, hyperglycemia, hyponatremia
HEMA: **Thrombocytopenia**

Contraindications: Breastfeeding, hypersensitivity
Precautions: Pregnancy (C), children, geriatric patients, cardiac/renal/hepatic disease, breast cancer, Parkinson's disease, dementia, seizure disorder, CNS depression, agranulocytosis, QT prolongation, torsade de pointes, suicidal ideation, substance abuse

PHARMACOKINETICS
Extensively metabolized by liver, protein binding 95%, peak 0.5-1.5 hr, terminal half-life 24 hr

INTERACTIONS
Increase: sedation—other CNS depressants, alcohol
Increase: EPS—CYP2D6 inhibitors/ substrates (SSRIs)
Increase: EPS—other antipsychotics
Increase: asenapine excretion—carbamazepine
Increase: QT prolongation—class IA/ III antidysrhythmics, some phenothiazines, β-agonists, local anesthetics, tricyclics, bepridil, haloperidol, methadone, chloroquine, clarithromycin, droperidol, erythromycin, grepafloxacin, halofantrine, pentamidine, probucol, sparfloxacin
Decrease: asenapine action—CYP2D6 inducers (carbamazepine, barbiturates, phenytoins, rifampin)
Drug/Herb
Increase: CNS depression—kava
Increase: EPS—betel palm, kava
Drug/Lab Test
Increase: prolactin levels

NURSING CONSIDERATIONS
Assess:
⚠ Mental status before initial administration, watch for suicidal thoughts and behaviors
• Affect, orientation, LOC, reflexes, gait, coordination, sleep pattern disturbances
• B/P standing and lying; also pulse, respirations; take these q4hr during initial treatment; establish baseline before starting treatment; report drops of 30 mm Hg;

watch for ECG changes; QT prolongation may occur
- Dizziness, faintness, palpitations, tachycardia on rising
- EPS, including akathisia, tardive dyskinesia (bizarre movements of the jaw, mouth, tongue, extremities), pseudoparkinsonism (rigidity, tremors, pill rolling, shuffling gait)
- For neuroleptic malignant syndrome: hyperthermia, increased CPK, altered mental status, muscle rigidity
- For serious reactions in geriatric patients: heart failure, sudden death
- Constipation daily; increase bulk and water in diet if needed
- Weight gain, hyperglycemia, metabolic changes in diabetes

Administer:
- Reduced dose in geriatric patients
- Anticholinergic agent on order from prescriber, to be used for EPS
- Avoid use with CNS depressants
- SL tab: remove tab; place tab under tongue; after it dissolves, swallow; advise not to chew, crush, or swallow tabs; not to eat or drink for 10 min

Perform/provide:
- Supervised ambulation until patient is stabilized on medication; do not involve in strenuous exercise program because fainting is possible; patient should not stand still for a long time
- Increased fluids to prevent constipation
- Storage in tight, light-resistant container

Evaluate:
- Therapeutic response: decrease in emotional excitement, hallucinations, delusions, paranoia; reorganization of patterns of thought, speech

Teach patient/family:
- That orthostatic hypotension may occur and to rise from sitting or lying position gradually
- To avoid hot tubs, hot showers, tub baths; hypotension may occur
- To avoid abrupt withdrawal of this product; EPS may result; product should be withdrawn slowly
- To avoid OTC preparations (cough, hay fever, cold) unless approved by prescriber; serious product interactions may occur; avoid use of alcohol; increased drowsiness may occur
- To avoid hazardous activities if drowsy or dizzy
- Compliance with product regimen
- That heat stroke may occur in hot weather; take extra precautions to stay cool
- To use contraception, inform prescriber if pregnancy is planned or suspected

Treatment of overdose: Lavage if orally ingested; provide airway; *do not induce vomiting*

Rarely Used ⚠ High Alert

asparaginase (℞)

(a-spare'a-gi-nase)

Elspar, Kidrolase ♣

Func. class.: Antineoplastic

Chem. class.: Escherichia coli enzyme

Uses: Acute lymphocytic leukemia in combination with other antineoplastics

DOSAGE AND ROUTES

In combination
- *Adult and child:* **IM/IV** 25,000 international units/m^2/wk × 2 wk or 6000 international units/m^2 every other day × 3-4 wk or 1000-20,000 international units/m^2 for 10-12 days

Contraindications: Hypersensitivity to this product or *E. coli* protein, thromboembolic disease, infants, breastfeeding, pancreatitis

aspirin (OTC)

(as'pir-in)

acetylsalicylic acid, Acuprin, Apo-ASA ♣, Apo-Asen ♣, Arthrinol ♣, Arthrisin ♣, Artria S.R., A.S.A., Aspergum, Aspirin ♣, Aspir-Low, Aspirtab, Astrin ♣, Bayer Aspirin, Coryphen ♣, Easprin, Ecotrin, 8-Hour Bayer Timed Release, Empirin, Entrophen ♣, Halfprin, Norwich Extra-Strength, Novasen ♣, PMS-ASA ♣, Sloprin, St. Joseph Children's, Supasa ♣, Therapy Bayer, ZORprin

Func. class.: Nonopioid analgesic, nonsteroidal antiinflammatory, antipyretic, antiplatelet

Chem. class.: Salicylate

Action: Blocks pain impulses in CNS, reduces inflammation by inhibition of prostaglandin synthesis; antipyretic action results from vasodilation of peripheral vessels; decreases platelet aggregation

Uses: Mild to moderate pain or fever including RA, osteoarthritis, thromboembolic disorders; TIAs, rheumatic fever, postmyocardial infarction, prophylaxis of MI, ischemic stroke, angina, acute MI

Unlabeled uses: Prevention of cataracts (long-term use), prevention of pregnancy loss in women with clotting disorders, bone pain, claudication, colorectal cancer prophylaxis, Kawasaki disease, PCI, preeclampsia/thrombosis prophylaxis, vernal keratoconjunctivitis, pericarditis

DOSAGE AND ROUTES

Arthritis

- *Adult:* **PO** 3 g/day in divided doses q4-6hr
- *Child >25 kg (55 lb):* **PO** 90-130 mg/kg/day in divided doses

Pain/fever

- *Adult:* **PO/RECT** 325-650 mg q4hr prn, max 4 g/day
- *Child 2-11 yr:* **PO** 10-15 mg/kg/dose q4hr, max 4 g/day

Thromboembolic disorders

- *Adult:* **PO** 325-650 mg/day or bid

Transient ischemic attacks (risk)

- *Adult:* **PO** 50-325 mg/day (grade 1A)

Evolving MI with ST segment elevation (STEMI)

- *Adult:* **PO** 160-325 mg nonenteric, chewed and swallowed immediately, maintenance 75-162 mg daily

MI, stroke prophylaxis

- *Adult:* **PO** 160-325 mg/day

Prevention of recurrent MI

- *Adult:* **PO** 75-162 mg/day

CABG

- *Adult:* **PO** 325 mg/day starting 6 hr postprocedure, continue for 1 yr

PTCA

- *Adult:* **PO** 325 mg 2 hr presurgery

Thrombosis prophylaxis in ACS (unlabeled)

- *Adult:* **PO** 160-325 mg non–enteric coated, chew/swallow immediately

Idiopathic/viral pericarditis (unlabeled)

- *Adult:* **PO** 800 mg tid-qid × 7-10 days with gradual tapering to 800 mg/day q wk for additional 2-3 wk

Colorectal cancer prophylaxis (unlabeled)

- *Adult:* **PO** 325 mg every other day

Kawasaki disease (unlabeled)

- *Child:* **PO** 80-100 mg/kg/day in 4 divided doses, maintenance 3-5 mg/kg/day

Available forms: Tabs 81, 325, 500, 650, 800 mg; chewable tabs 81 mg; supp 300, 600 mg; gum 227 mg; enteric coated tabs 81, 325, 500, 975 mg; ext rel tabs 800 mg; del rel tabs 325, 500 mg

SIDE EFFECTS

CNS: Stimulation, drowsiness, dizziness, confusion, **seizures,** headache, flushing, hallucinations, **coma**

CV: Rapid pulse, pulmonary edema

EENT: Tinnitus, hearing loss

ENDO: Hypoglycemia, hyponatremia, hypokalemia

GI: Nausea, vomiting, **GI bleeding,** diarrhea, heartburn, anorexia, **hepatitis**

HEMA: **Thrombocytopenia, agranulocytosis, leukopenia, neutropenia, hemolytic anemia,** increased PT, APTT, bleeding time
INTEG: *Rash,* urticaria, bruising
RESP: Wheezing, hyperpnea
SYST: **Reye's syndrome (children), anaphylaxis, laryngeal edema**

Contraindications: Pregnancy (D) 3rd trimester, breastfeeding, children <12 yr, children with flulike symptoms, hypersensitivity to salicylates, tartrazine (FDC yellow dye #5), GI bleeding, bleeding disorders, vit K deficiency, peptic ulcer, acute bronchospasm, agranulocytosis, increased intracranial pressure, intracranial bleeding, nasal polyps, urticaria

Precautions: Abrupt discontinuation, acetaminophen/NSAIDs hypersensitivity, acid/base imbalance, alcoholism, ascites, asthma, bone marrow suppression elderly, dehydration, G6PD deficiency, gout, heart failure, anemia, renal/hepatic disease, pre/postoperatively, gastritis

PHARMACOKINETICS

Enteric metabolized by liver; inactive metabolites excreted by kidneys; crosses placenta; excreted in breast milk; half-life 15-20 min, up to 9 hr in large dose; rectal products may be erratic, protein binding 90%

PO: Onset 15-30 min, peak 1-2 hr, duration 4-6 hr, well absorbed

RECT: Onset slow, duration 4-6 hr

INTERACTIONS

• Gastric ulcer: steroids, antiinflammatories, NSAIDs, alcohol

Increase: bleeding—alcohol, plicamycin, cefamandole, thrombolytics, ticlopidine, clopidogrel, tirofiban, eptifibatide, anticoagulants

Increase: effects of warfarin, insulin, methotrexate, thrombolytic agents, penicillins, phenytoin, valproic acid, oral hypoglycemics, sulfonamides

Increase: salicylate levels—urinary acidifiers, ammonium chloride, nizatidine

Increase: hypotension—nitroglycerin

Decrease: effects of aspirin—antacids (high doses), urinary alkalizers, corticosteroids

Decrease: antihypertensive effect—ACE inhibitors

Decrease: effects of probenecid, spironolactone, sulfinpyrazone, sulfonylamides, NSAIDs, β-blockers, loop diuretics

Drug/Herb

• Gastric irritation: arginine, gossypol

Increase: risk of bleeding—anise, arnica, bilberry, bogbean, chamomile, chondroitin, clove, dong quai, fenugreek, feverfew, garlic, ginger, ginkgo, ginseng *(Panax),* horse chestnut, Irish moss, kelpware, licorice, pansy, red clover

Drug/Food

• Foods acidifying urine may increase aspirin level

Drug/Lab Test

Increase: coagulation studies, LFTs, serum uric acid, amylase, CO_2, urinary protein

Decrease: serum potassium, cholesterol

Interference: VMA, 5-HIAA, xylose tolerance test, TSH, pregnancy test

NURSING CONSIDERATIONS

Assess:

• Pain: character, location, intensity; ROM before and 1 hr after administration
• Fever: temperature before and 1 hr after administration
• Hepatic studies: AST, ALT, bilirubin, creatinine if patient is on long-term therapy
• Renal studies: BUN, urine creatinine; I&O ratio; decreasing output may indicate renal failure (long-term therapy)
• Blood studies: CBC, Hct, Hgb, PT if patient is on long-term therapy
⚠ Hepatotoxicity: dark urine, clay-colored stools, yellowing of skin, sclera, itching, abdominal pain, fever, diarrhea if patient is on long-term therapy
• Allergic reactions: rash, urticaria; if these occur, product may have to be discontinued; patients with asthma, nasal polyps, allergies: severe allergic reaction may occur

• Ototoxicity: tinnitus, ringing, roaring in ears; audiometric testing needed before, after long-term therapy
• Salicylate level: therapeutic level 150-300 mcg/ml for chronic inflammation
• Edema in feet, ankles, legs
• Products history; many product interactions

Administer:

PO route

• Do not break, crush, or chew enteric product
• Crushed or whole; chewable tablets may be chewed
• ½ hr before planned exercise
• With food or milk to decrease gastric symptoms; separate by 2 hr of enteric product
• With 8 oz H_2O and sit upright for ½ hr after dose to facilitate product passing into the stomach

Evaluate:

• Therapeutic response: decreased pain, inflammation, fever

Teach patient/family:

• To report any symptoms of hepatotoxicity, renal toxicity, visual changes, ototoxicity, allergic reactions, bleeding (long-term therapy)
• To avoid if allergic to tartrazine
• Not to exceed recommended dosage; acute poisoning may result
• To read label on other OTC products; many contain aspirin or salicylates
• That the therapeutic response takes 2 wk (arthritis)
• To report tinnitus, confusion, diarrhea, sweating, hyperventilation
• To avoid alcohol ingestion; GI bleeding may occur
• That patients who have allergies, nasal polyps, asthma may develop allergic reactions
• To discard tabs if vinegar-like smell is detected
• That medication is not to be given to children or teens with flulike symptoms or chickenpox; Reye's syndrome may develop

Treatment of overdose: Lavage, activated charcoal, monitor electrolytes, VS

atazanavir (℞)

(at-a-za-na'veer)
Reyataz
Func. class.: Antiretroviral
Chem. class.: Protease inhibitor

Action: Inhibits human immunodeficiency virus (HIV-1) protease, which prevents maturation of the infectious virus

Uses: HIV-1 infection in combination with other antiretroviral agents

DOSAGE AND ROUTES

Antiretroviral-naive patients

• *Adult:* **PO** 400 mg/day
• *Child ≥6 yr/adolescent ≥39 kg:* **PO** 300 mg with ritonavir 100 mg daily
• *Child ≥6 yr/adolescent 32-39 kg:* **PO** 250 mg with ritonavir 100 mg daily
• *Child ≥6 yr/adolescent 25-32 kg:* **PO** 200 mg with ritonavir 100 mg daily

Antiretroviral-experienced patients

• *Adult:* **PO** 300 mg/day and ritonavir 100 mg/day
• *Child ≥6 yr/adolescent ≥39 kg:* **PO** 300 mg with ritonavir 100 mg daily
• *Child ≥6 yr/adolescent 32-39 kg:* **PO** 250 mg with ritonavir 100 mg daily
• *Child ≥6 yr/adolescent 25-32 kg:* **PO** 200 mg with ritonavir 100 mg daily

Hepatic dose

• *Adult:* **PO** (Child-Pugh B) 300 mg/day; (Child-Pugh C) do not use

Available forms: Caps 100, 150, 200, 300 mg

SIDE EFFECTS

CNS: Headache, depression, dizziness, insomnia, peripheral neurologic symptoms
GI: Vomiting, *diarrhea, abdominal pain, nausea,* **hepatotoxicity**
INTEG: *Rash,* **Stevens-Johnson syndrome,** *photosensitivity*
MISC: Fatigue, fever, arthralgia, back pain, cough, lipodystrophy, pain, gynecomastia, nephrolithiasis

Contraindications: Hypersensitivity

Precautions: Pregnancy (B), breastfeeding, children, geriatric patients, hepatic disease, alcoholism, drug resistance, AV block, diabetes, dialysis, elderly, females, hemophilia, hypercholesterolemia, immune reconstitution syndrome, lactic acidosis, pancreatitis

PHARMACOKINETICS

Rapidly absorbed, absorption increased with food, peak 2½ hr, 86% protein bound, extensively metabolized in liver by CYP3A4, 27% excreted unchanged in urine/feces (minimal), half-life 7 hr

INTERACTIONS

⚠ ***Increase:*** levels, increased toxicity of immunosuppressants (cycloSPORINE, sirolimus, tacrolimus, sildenafil), tricylic antidepressants, warfarin, calcium channel blockers, clarithromycin, chlorazepate, diazepam, irinotecan, HMG-CoA reductase inhibitors, antidysrhythmics, midazolam, triazolam, ergots, pimozide

Increase: effects of estrogens, oral contraceptives

Increase: atazanavir levels—CYP3A4 substrates, CYP3A4 inhibitors

Increase: hyperbilirubinemia—indinavir

Decrease: atazanavir levels—CYP3A4 inducers, rifampin, antacids, didanosine, efavirenz, proton pump inhibitors, H_2-receptor antagonists

Drug/Herb

Decrease: atazanavir levels—St. John's wort

Drug/Lab Test

Increase: AST, ALT, total bilirubin, amylase, lipase, CK

Decrease: Hgb, neurophils, platelets

NURSING CONSIDERATIONS

Assess:

⚠ For hepatic failure; hepatic studies: ALT, AST, bilirubin

- Signs of infection, anemia
- Bowel pattern before, during treatment; if severe abdominal pain with bleeding occurs, product should be discontinued; monitor hydration
- Viral load, CD4 count throughout treatment
- Skin eruptions, rash, urticaria, itching
- Allergies before treatment, reaction of each medication; place allergies on chart

Administer:

- With food 2 hr before or 1 hr after antacid or didanosine

Evaluate:

- Therapeutic response: increasing CD4 counts; decreased viral load, resolution of symptoms of HIV-1 infection

Teach patient/family:

- To take as prescribed with other antiretrovirals as prescribed, if dose is missed, take as soon as remembered up to 1 hr before next dose; do not double dose, do not share with others
- That product must be taken daily to maintain blood levels for duration of therapy
- May cause photosensitivity, use protective clothing, or stay out of the sun
- To notify prescriber if diarrhea, nausea, vomiting, rash occurs; dizziness, light-headedness, ECG may be altered
- That product interacts with many products and St. John's wort, advise prescriber of all products, herbal products used
- That redistribution of body fat may occur, the effect is not known
- That product does not cure HIV-1 infection or prevent transmission to others, only controls symptoms
- That if taking phosphodiesterase type 5 inhibitor with atazanavir, there may be an increased risk of phosphodiesterase type 5 inhibitor-associated adverse events, including hypotension and prolonged penile erection; notify physician promptly of these symptoms

atenolol (℞)

(a-ten′oh-lole)

Apo-Atenol ♣, atenolol ♣, Novo-Atenol ♣, Tenormin

Func. class.: Antihypertensive, antianginal

Chem. class.: β-Blocker, β_1-, β_2-blocker (high doses)

Do not confuse:
atenolol/albuterol
Tenormin/thiamine/Imuran

Action: Competitively blocks stimulation of β-adrenergic receptor within vascular smooth muscle; produces negative chronotropic activity (decreases rate of SA node discharge, increases recovery time), slows conduction of AV node, decreases heart rate, negative inotropic activity decreases O_2 consumption in myocardium; also decreases renin-aldosterone-angiotensin system at high doses, inhibits β_2 receptors in bronchial system at higher doses

Uses: Mild to moderate hypertension, prophylaxis of angina pectoris; suspected or known myocardial infarction (IV use)

Unlabeled uses: Migraine prophylaxis, supraventricular tachycardia prophylaxis (PSVT), unstable angina, alcohol withdrawal

DOSAGE AND ROUTES

- *Adult:* **PO** 25-50 mg/day, increasing q1-2wk to 100 mg/day; may increase to 200 mg/day for angina or up to 100 mg for hypertension
- *Child:* **PO** 0.8-1 mg/kg/dose initially, range 0.8-1.5 mg/kg/day, max 2 mg/kg/day
- *Geriatric:* **PO** 25 mg/day initially

Renal disease

- *Adult:* **PO** CCr 15-35 ml/min, max 50 mg/day; CCr <15 ml/min max dose 25 mg/day; hemodialysis 25-50 mg after dialysis

PSVT prophylaxis (unlabeled)

- *Child:* **PO** 0.3-1.3 mg/kg/day

Ethanol withdrawal prevention (unlabeled)

- *Adult:* **PO** 50-100 mg/day

Migraine prophylaxis (unlabeled)

- *Adult:* **PO** 50-150 mg/day, titrate to response

Available forms: Tabs 25, 50, 100 mg

SIDE EFFECTS

CNS: Insomnia, fatigue, dizziness, mental changes, memory loss, hallucinations, depression, lethargy, drowsiness, strange dreams, catatonia

CV: **Profound hypotension, bradycardia, CHF,** *cold extremities, postural hypotension, 2nd- or 3rd-degree heart block*

EENT: Sore throat, dry burning eyes, blurred vision, stuffy nose

ENDO: Increased hypoglycemic response to insulin

GI: Nausea, diarrhea, vomiting, **mesenteric arterial thrombosis, ischemic colitis**

GU: Impotence, decreased libido

HEMA: **Agranulocytosis, thrombocytopenia purpura**

INTEG: Rash, fever, alopecia

RESP: **Bronchospasm,** dyspnea, wheezing, pulmonary edema

Contraindications: Pregnancy (D), hypersensitivity to β-blockers, cardiogenic shock, 2nd- or 3rd-degree heart block, sinus bradycardia, cardiac failure, Raynaud's disease, pulmonary edema

Precautions: Breastfeeding, major surgery, diabetes mellitus, thyroid/renal disease, CHF, COPD, asthma, well-compensated heart failure, dialysis, myasthenia gravis

Black Box Warning: Abrupt discontinuation

PHARMACOKINETICS

PO: Peak 2-4 hr; onset 1 hr; duration 24 hr; half-life 6-9 hr; excreted unchanged in urine, feces (50%); protein binding 5%-15%

IV: Onset rapid, peak 5 min, duration unknown

A

INTERACTIONS

• Mutual inhibition: sympathomimetics (cough, cold preparations)

Increase: hypotension, bradycardia—reserpine, hydrALAZINE, methyldopa, prazosin, anticholinergics, digoxin, diltiazem, verapamil, cardiac glycosides, antihypertensives

Increase: hypertension amphetamines, ephedrine, pseudoephedrine

Decrease: effect—insulin, oral antidiabetic agents, theophylline, DOPamine, MAOIs

Drug/Herb

Increase: atenolol effect—betel palm, butterbur, cola tree, figwort, fumitory, guarana, hawthorn, jaborandi tree, lily of the valley, motherwort, plantain

Decrease: atenolol effect—coenzyme Q10, yohimbe

Drug/Lab Test

Increase: blood glucose, BUN, K, triglycerides, uric acid, ANA titer

NURSING CONSIDERATIONS

Assess:

• I&O, weight daily; watch for CHF (rales/crackles, jugular vein distention, weight gain, edema)

• B/P, pulse q4hr; note rate, rhythm, quality; apical/radial pulse before administration; notify prescriber of any significant changes (<50 bpm); ECG

• Baselines in renal/hepatic studies before therapy begins

Administer:

PO route

• Product before meals, at bedtime; tab may be crushed or swallowed whole

• Reduced dosage in renal dysfunction

IV, direct route

• Undiluted over 5 min

Intermittent IV INF route

• Diluted in 10-50 ml of D_5W, D_5/NaCl, or NS and give as an infusion at prescribed rate

Y-site compatibilities: Acyclovir, amphotericin B liposome, daptomycin, diltiazem, ertapenem, granisetron, hydromorphone, linezolid, lorazepam, meperidine, meropenem, morphine, ondansetron, palonosetron, piperacillin/tazobactam, tacrolimus, tirofiban, voriconazole

Perform/provide:

• Storage protected from light, moisture; place in cool environment

Evaluate:

• Therapeutic response: decreased B/P after 1-2 wk, increased activity tolerance, decreased anginal pain

Teach patient/family:

⚠ Not to discontinue product abruptly, taper over 2 wk (angina), take at same time each day as directed

• Not to use OTC products unless directed by prescriber

• To report bradycardia, dizziness, confusion, depression, fever

• To take pulse at home; advise when to notify prescriber

• To limit alcohol, smoking, sodium intake

• To comply with weight control, dietary adjustments, modified exercise program

• To carry emergency ID to identify product, allergies, conditions being treated

• To avoid hazardous activities if dizziness is present

• To change position slowly

• That product may mask symptoms of hypoglycemia in diabetic patients

• To use contraception while taking this product, pregnancy category (D)

Treatment of overdose: Lavage, IV atropine for bradycardia, IV theophylline for bronchospasm, dextrose for hypoglycemia, digoxin, O_2, diuretic for cardiac failure, hemodialysis

atomoxetine (℞)

(at-o-mox′eh-teen)

Strattera

Func. class.: Psychotherapeutic—miscellaneous

Chem. class.: Selective norepinephrine reuptake inhibitor

Action: A selective norepinephrine reuptake inhibitor; may inhibit the presynaptic norepinephrine transporter.

Uses: Attention deficit hyperactivity disorder

DOSAGE AND ROUTES

• *Child ≤70 kg:* **PO** 0.5 mg/kg, increase after 3 days to a target daily dose of 1.2 mg/kg in AM or evenly divided doses AM, late afternoon; max 1.4 mg/kg/day or 100 mg/day, whichever is less

• *Adult and child >70 kg:* **PO** 40 mg/day, increase after 3 days to a target daily dose of 80 mg in AM or evenly divided doses AM, late afternoon; max 100 mg/day

Maintenance

• *Adolescent ≤15 yr and child ≥6 yr:* **PO** 1.2-1.8 mg/kg/day

Initial dose titration with strong CYP2D6 inhibitors

• *Adult and child >6 yr weighing >70 kg:* **PO** 40 mg/day each AM or 2 evenly divided doses, titrate to target of 80 mg/day if symptoms do not improve after 4 wk and dose is well tolerated

Hepatic dose

• (Child-Pugh B) reduce dose by 50%; (Child-Pugh C) reduce dose by 75%

Available forms: Caps 10, 18, 25, 40, 60, 80, 100 mg

SIDE EFFECTS

CNS: Insomnia, dizziness, headache, irritability, crying, mood swings, fatigue, hypoesthesia, lethargy, paresthesia

CV: Palpitations, hot flushes, tachycardia, increased B/P

ENDO: Growth retardation

GI: Dyspepsia, nausea, anorexia, dry mouth, weight loss, vomiting, diarrhea, constipation, **hepatic injury**

GU: Urinary hesitancy, retention, dysmenorrhea, erectile disturbance, ejaculation failure, impotence, prostatis, orgasm abnormal, male pelvic pain

INTEG: **Exfoliative dermatitis,** sweating, rash

MISC: Cough, rhinorrhea, dermatitis, ear infection

Contraindications: Hypersensitivity, angle-closure glaucoma, arteriosclerosis, cardiac disease, cardiomyopathy, heart failure, jaundice, MAOI therapy

Precautions: Pregnancy (C), breastfeeding, hepatic disease, angioedema, bipolar disorder, dysrhythmias, CAD, hypo/hypertension

Black Box Warning: Children <6 yr, suicidal ideation

PHARMACOKINETICS

Peak 1-2 hr, metabolized by liver, excreted by kidneys, 98% protein binding

INTERACTIONS

Increase: hypertensive crisis—MAOIs or within 14 days of MAOIs, vasopressors

Increase: cardiovascular effects of albuterol, pressor agents

Increase: effects of atomoxetine—CYP 2D6 inhibitors (amiodarone, cimetidine [weak], clomipramine, delavirdine, gefitinib, imatinib, propafenone, quinidine [potent], ritonavir, citalopram, escitalopram, fluoxetine, sertraline, paroxetine, thioridazine, venlafaxine)

NURSING CONSIDERATIONS

Assess:

• VS, B/P; check patients with cardiac disease more often for increased B/P

• Height, growth rate q3mo in children; growth rate may be decreased

⚠ Mental status: mood, sensorium, affect, stimulation, insomnia, aggressiveness, suicidal ideation

- Appetite, sleep, speech patterns
- For attention span, decreased hyperactivity in ADHD persons

Administer:

- Whole; do not break, crush, or chew
- Gum, hard candy, frequent sips of water for dry mouth
- Without regard to food

Evaluate:

- Therapeutic response: decreased hyperactivity (ADHD)

Teach patient/family:

- To avoid OTC preparations unless approved by prescriber
- To avoid alcohol ingestion
- To avoid hazardous activities until stabilized on medication
- To get needed rest; patients will feel more tired at end of day; not to take dose late in day, insomnia may occur
- To report suicidal ideation

atorvastatin (℞)

(a-tore′va-stat-in)

Lipitor

Func. class.: Antilipidemic

Chem. class.: HMG-CoA reductase inhibitor

Action: Inhibits HMG-CoA reductase enzyme, which reduces cholesterol synthesis; high doses lead to plaque regression

Uses: As an adjunct in primary hypercholesterolemia (types Ia, Ib), dysbetalipoproteinemia, elevated triglyceride levels, prevention of CV disease by reduction of heart risk in those with mildly elevated cholesterol

Unlabeled uses: Atherosclerosis

DOSAGE AND ROUTES

- *Adult:* **PO** 10-20 mg/day, usual range 10-80, dosage adjustments may be made in 2-4 wk intervals, max 80 mg/day; patients requiring >45% reduction in LDL may be started at 40 mg/day

Atherosclerosis (unlabeled)

- *Adult:* **PO** 80 mg/day

Available forms: Tabs 10, 20, 40, 80 mg

SIDE EFFECTS

CNS: Headache, asthenia, **ALS (Lou Gehrig's disease)**

EENT: Lens opacities

GI: Abdominal cramps, constipation, diarrhea, flatus, heartburn, dyspepsia, **liver dysfunction,** pancreatitis, nausea, increased serum transaminase

GU: Impotence

INTEG: Rash, pruritus, alopecia

MISC: Hypersensitivity

MS: Arthralgia, myalgia, **rhabdomyolysis**

RESP: Pharyngitis, sinusitis

Contraindications: Pregnancy (X), breastfeeding, hypersensitivity, active hepatic disease

Precautions: Past hepatic disease, alcoholism, severe acute infections, trauma, severe metabolic disorders, electrolyte imbalance

PHARMACOKINETICS

Metabolized in liver, highly protein bound, excreted primarily in urine, half-life 14 hr; protein binding 98%

INTERACTIONS

- Risk of possible rhabdomyolysis: azole antifungals, cycloSPORINE, erythromycin, niacin, gemfibrozil, clofibrate

Increase: serum level of digoxin

Increase: levels of oral contraceptives

Increase: levels of atorvastatin—erythromycin

Increase: effects of warfarin

Decrease: atorvastatin levels—colestipol

Drug/Herb

Increase: effect—glucomannan

Decrease: effect—gotu kola, St. John's wort

Drug/Food

- Possible toxicity when used with grapefruit juice; oat bran may reduce effectiveness

Drug/Lab Test
Increase: bilirubin, alk phos
Interference: thyroid function tests

NURSING CONSIDERATIONS

Assess:

- Diet, obtain diet history including fat, cholesterol in diet
- Cholesterol triglyceride levels periodically during treatment; check lipid panel 6 wk after changing dose
- Hepatic studies q1-2mo during the first 1½ yr of treatment; AST, ALT, LFTs may be increased
- Renal studies in patients with compromised renal system: BUN, I&O ratio, creatinine

⚠ For muscle pain, tenderness, obtain CPK baseline and if markedly increased, product may need to be discontinued

Administer:

- Total daily dose any time of day without regard to meals

Perform/provide:

- Storage in cool environment in tight container protected from light

Evaluate:

- Therapeutic response: decrease in cholesterol to desired level after 6 wk

Teach patient/family:

- That blood work and eye exam will be necessary during treatment
- To report blurred vision, severe GI symptoms, headache, muscle pain, weakness
- That previously prescribed regimen will continue: low-cholesterol diet, exercise program, smoking cessation
- Not to take product if pregnant
- To stay out of the sun, or use sunscreen, protective clothing to prevent photosensitivity (rare)

atovaquone (℞)

(a-toe'va-kwon)
Mepron
Func. class.: Antiprotozoal
Chem. class.: Aromatic diamide derivative, analog of ubiquinone

Action: Interferes with DNA/RNA synthesis in protozoa

Uses: *Pneumocystis jiroveci* infections in patients intolerant of trimethoprim-sulfamethoxazole, prophylaxis, *Toxoplasma gondii,* toxoplasmosis

Unlabeled uses: Babesiosis, malaria treatment/prophylaxis, toxoplasmosis prophylaxis, *Plasmodium* sp.

DOSAGE AND ROUTES

Acute, mild, moderate* Pneumocystis jiroveci *pneumonia

- *Adult and adolescent 13-16 yr:* **PO** 750 mg with food bid for 21 days

Pneumocystis jiroveci *pneumonia, prophylaxis*

- *Adult and adolescent:* **PO** 1500 mg/day with meal

Babesiosis (unlabeled)

- *Adult:* **PO** 750 mg q12hr with azithromycin (500-1000 mg on day 1, then 250 mg/day × 7-14 days)

Toxoplasmosis prophylaxis in AIDS (unlabeled)

- *Adult:* **PO** 1500 mg alone or in combination

Plasmodium falciparum *(unlabeled)*

- *Adult:* **PO** 250 mg with proguanil daily
- *Child:* **PO** 17 mg/kg/day with proguanil daily

Available forms: Susp 750 mg/5 ml

SIDE EFFECTS

CNS: Dizziness, headache, anxiety, insomnia, asthenia, fever
CV: Hypotension
GI: Nausea, vomiting, diarrhea, anorexia, increased AST and ALT, **acute pancreatitis,** constipation, abdominal pain

HEMA: Anemia, **leukopenia, neutropenia, thrombocytopenia, methemoglobinemia**
INTEG: Pruritus, urticaria, *rash*, oral monilia, sweating, **angioedema, Stevens-Johnson syndrome**
META: Hyperkalemia, hypoglycemia, hyponatremia
OTHER: Cough, dyspnea
Contraindications: Hypersensitivity or history of developing life-threatening allergic reactions to any component of the formulation, benzyl alcohol sensitivity
Precautions: Pregnancy (C), breastfeeding, neonates, hepatic disease, GI disease, respiratory insufficiency

PHARMACOKINETICS

Excreted unchanged in feces (94%), highly protein bound (99%)

INTERACTIONS

• Use caution when administering concurrently with other highly plasma protein–bound products with narrow therapeutic indices
Decrease: effect of atovaquone—rifampin, rifabutin, tetracycline

NURSING CONSIDERATIONS

Assess:
• Signs of infection, anemia
• Bowel pattern before, during treatment
• Respiratory status: rate, character, wheezing, dyspnea; ABGs, chest films
• Allergies before treatment, reaction of each medication
Administer:
• With high-fat food because of increased absorption of the product and higher plasma concentrations
• Oral susp, shake before using
• All contents of foil pouch
Evaluate:
• Therapeutic response: decreased temp, ability to breathe
Teach patient/family:
• To take with food to increase plasma concentrations

Rarely Used

atracurium (℞)

(a-tra-kyoor′ee-um)
Func. class.: Neuromuscular blocker (nondepolarizing)

Uses: Facilitation of endotracheal intubation, skeletal muscle relaxation during mechanical ventilation, surgery, or general anesthesia

DOSAGE AND ROUTES

• *Adult and child >2 yr:* **IV BOL** 0.4-0.5 mg/kg, then 0.08-0.1 mg/kg 20-45 min after first dose if needed for prolonged procedures; give smaller doses with halothane
• *Child 1 mo-2 yr:* **IV BOL** 0.3-0.4 mg/kg
Contraindications: Hypersensitivity
Black Box Warning: Respiratory insufficiency

⚠ High Alert

atropine (℞)

(a′troe-peen)
Atreza, atropine sulfate, AtroPen, Sal-Tropine
Func. class.: Antidysrhythmic, anticholinergic parasympatholytic, antimuscarinic
Chem. class.: Belladonna alkaloid

Do not confuse:
atropine/Akarpine
Action: Blocks acetylcholine at parasympathetic neuroeffector sites; increases cardiac output, heart rate by blocking vagal stimulation in heart; dries secretions by blocking vagus
Uses: Bradycardia <40-50 bpm, bradydysrhythmia, reversal of anticholinesterase agents, insecticide poisoning, blocking cardiac vagal reflexes, decreasing secretions before surgery, antispasmodic with GU, biliary surgery, bronchodilator, AV heart block

Unlabeled uses: Cardiac arrest, CPR, diarrhea, pulseless electrical activity, ventricular asystole, asthma

DOSAGE AND ROUTES

Bradycardia/bradydysrhythmia

- *Adult:* **IV BOL** 0.5-1 mg given q3-5min, max 2 mg
- *Child:* **IV BOL** 0.01-0.03 mg/kg up to 0.4 mg or 0.3 mg/m^2; may repeat q4-6hr; min dose 0.1 mg to avoid paradoxical reaction

Organophosphate poisoning

- *Adult and child:* **IM/IV** 2 mg q hr until muscarinic symptoms disappear, may need 6 mg q hr
- *Adult and child 90 lb, usually >10 yr:* **Atro-pen** 2 mg
- *Child 40-90 lb, usually 4-10 yr:* **Atro-pen** 1 mg
- *Child 15-40 lb, 6 mo-4 yr:* **Atro-pen** 0.05 mg

Presurgery

- *Adult and child >20 kg:* **SUBCUT/IM/IV** 0.4-0.6 mg before anesthesia
- *Child <20 kg:* **IM/SUBCUT** 0.01 mg/kg up to 0.4 mg ½-1 hr preop, max 0.6 mg/dose

Available forms: Inj 0.05, 0.1, 0.3, 0.4, 0.5, 0.8, 1 mg/ml; tabs 0.4 mg; Atropen 0.5, 1, 2 mg inj prefilled autoinjectors

SIDE EFFECTS

CNS: Headache, dizziness, involuntary movement, confusion, psychosis, anxiety, **coma,** flushing, drowsiness, insomnia, weakness; delirium (geriatric patients)

CV: Hypotension, paradoxical bradycardia, angina, PVCs, hypertension, **tachycardia,** ectopic ventricular beats

EENT: Blurred vision, photophobia, glaucoma, eye pain, pupil dilation, nasal congestion

GI: Dry mouth, nausea, vomiting, abdominal pain, anorexia, constipation, **paralytic ileus,** abdominal distention, altered taste

GU: Retention, hesitancy, impotence, dysuria

INTEG: Rash, urticaria, contact dermatitis, dry skin, flushing

MISC: Suppression of lactation, decreased sweating

Contraindications: Hypersensitivity to belladonna alkaloids, closed-angle glaucoma, GI obstructions, myasthenia gravis, thyrotoxicosis, ulcerative colitis, prostatic hypertrophy, tachycardia/tachydysrhythmias, asthma, acute hemorrhage, severe hepatic disease, myocardial ischemia

Precautions: Pregnancy (C), breastfeeding, children <6 yr, geriatric patients, renal disease, CHF, hyperthyroidism, COPD, hypertension, intraabdominal infection, Down syndrome, spastic paralysis, gastric ulcer

PHARMACOKINETICS

Half-life 13-40 hr, excreted by kidneys unchanged (70%-90% in 24 hr), metabolized in liver, 40%-50% crosses placenta, excreted in breast milk

PO: Onset ½ hr, peak ½-1 hr, duration 4-6 hr, well absorbed

IM/SUBCUT: Onset 15-50 min, peak 30 min, duration 4-6 hr, well absorbed

IV: Peak 2-4 min, duration 4-6 hr

INTERACTIONS

- Mucosal lesions: potassium chloride tab

Increase: anticholinergic effects, tricyclics, amantadine, antiparkinson agents

Decrease: absorption—ketoconazole, levodopa

Decrease: effect of atropine—antacids

Drug/Herb

- Forms insoluble complex: black root
- Serotonin effect: horehound

Increase: atropine effect—aloe, buckthorn, cascara sagrada, figwort, fumitory, goldenseal, jimsonweed, kudzu, licorice, rhubarb, senna, scopolia

Increase: toxicity/death—aconite

Decrease: effect—coltsfoot

NURSING CONSIDERATIONS

Assess:

- I&O ratio; check for urinary retention, daily output

- ECG for ectopic ventricular beats, PVC, tachycardia, in cardiac patients
- For bowel sounds; check for constipation
- Respiratory status: rate, rhythm, cyanosis, wheezing, dyspnea, engorged neck veins
- Increased intraocular pressure: eye pain, nausea, vomiting, blurred vision, increased tearing
- Cardiac rate: rhythm, character, B/P continuously
- Allergic reaction: rash, urticaria

Administer:

PO route

- Increased bulk, water in diet if constipation occurs
- ½ hr before meals

IM route

- Atropine flush may occur in children and is not harmful

Atro-Pen

- Use no more than 3 Atro-Pen inj unless under the supervision of trained medical provider
- Use as soon as symptoms appear (tearing, wheezing, muscle fasciculations, excessive oral secretions)

IV route

- Undiluted or diluted with 10 ml sterile H_2O, give at 0.6 mg/min, give through Y-tube or 3-way stopcock; do not add to IV sol; may cause paradoxical bradycardia lasting 2 min

Additive compatibilities: DOBUTamine, furosemide, meropenem, netilmicin, sodium bicarbonate, verapamil

Syringe compatibilities: Benzquinamide, butorphanol, chlorproMAZINE, cimetidine, dimenhyDRINATE, diphenhydrAMINE, droperidol, fentanyl, glycopyrrolate, heparin, hydromorphone, hydrOXYzine, meperidine, metoclopramide, midazolam, milrinone, morphine, nalbuphine, pentazocine, perphenazine, prochlorperazine, promazine, promethazine, propiomazine, ranitidine, scopolamine, sufentanil

Y-site compatibilities: Amrinone, etomidate, famotidine, heparin, hydrocortisone, meropenem, nafcillin, potassium chloride, sufentanil, vit B/C

Perform/provide:

- Sugarless hard candy, gum, frequent rinsing of mouth for dryness

Evaluate:

- Therapeutic response: decreased dysrhythmias, increased heart rate, secretions; GI, GU spasms; bronchodilation

Teach patient/family:

- To report blurred vision, chest pain, allergic reactions, constipation, urinary retention
- Not to perform strenuous activity in high temperatures; heat stroke may result
- To take as prescribed; not to skip or double doses
- Not to operate machinery if drowsiness occurs
- Not to take OTC products without approval of prescriber

Treatment of overdose: O_2, artificial ventilation, ECG; administer DOPamine for circulatory depression; administer diazepam or thiopental for seizures; assess need for antidysrhythmics

atropine ophthalmic

See Appendix B

Rarely Used

auranofin (℞)

(au-rane′oh-fin)

Ridaura

Func. class.: Antiinflammatory

Do not confuse:

Ridaura/Cardura

Uses: RA; not for first-line therapy

Unlabeled uses: SLE, psoriatic arthritis, pemphigus

DOSAGE AND ROUTES

- *Adult:* **PO** 6 mg/day or 3 mg bid; may increase to 9 mg/day after 3 mo

Contraindications: Breastfeeding, children <6 yr, hypersensitivity to gold, necrotizing enterocolitis, pulmonary fibrosis, exfoliative dermatitis, recent radiation therapy, renal/hepatic disease, marked hypertension, uncontrolled CHF

Black Box Warning: Bone marrow suppression, blood dyscrasias, hematuria, anemia, diarrhea

⚠ High Alert

azacitidine (℞)

(a-za-sie-ti′deen)

Vidaza

Func. class.: Antineoplastic hormone

Chem. class.: DNA demethylation agent

Do not confuse:
azacitidine/azathioprine

Action: Cytotoxic by producing damage to double-strand DNA during DNA synthesis

Uses: Myelodysplastic syndrome (MDS)

Unlabeled uses: Acute myelogenous leukemia (AML), chronic myelogenous leukemia (CML)

DOSAGE AND ROUTES

• *Adult:* **SUBCUT** 75 mg/m^2/day × 7 days, q4wk, premedicate with antiemetic; dose may be increased to 100 mg/m^2 if no response is seen after 2 treatment cycles, minimum treatment 4 cycles

Available forms: Powdered for inj, lyophilized 100 mg

SIDE EFFECTS

CNS: Anxiety, depression, dizziness, fatigue, headache

CV: Cardiac murmur, hypotension, tachycardia, peripheral edema

GI: Diarrhea, nausea, vomiting, anorexia, constipation, abdominal pain, distention, tenderness, hemorrhoids, mouth hemorrhage, tongue ulceration, stomatitis, dyspepsia, **hepatotoxicity, hepatic coma**

GU: **Renal failure, renal tubular acidosis**, dysuria, UTI

HEMA: **Leukopenia, anemia, thrombocytopenia, neutropenia**, ecchymosis

INTEG: Irritation at site, rash, sweating, pyrexia

META: Hypokalemia

Contraindications: Pregnancy (D), hypersensitivity to this product or mannitol, advanced malignant hepatic tumors

Precautions: Breastfeeding, children, geriatric patients, renal/hepatic disease, baseline albumin <30 g/L; a man should not father a child while taking this product

PHARMACOKINETICS

Rapidly absorbed, peak ½ hr, metabolized in the liver, half-life 35-49 min, excreted in urine

INTERACTIONS

Increase: bone marrow depression—other antineoplastics

NURSING CONSIDERATIONS

Assess:

• For CNS symptoms: fever, headache, chills, dizziness

• Hematologic response: with baseline WBC ≥3000/mm^3, absolute neutrophil count (ANC) ≥1500/mm^3, and platelets >7500/mm^3, adjust dose; ANC <500/mm^3, platelets <25,000/mm^3, give 50% dose next course; ANC 500-1500/mm^3, platelets 25,000-50,000/mm^3, give 67% next course

• Buccal cavity q8hr for dryness, sores, or ulceration, white patches, oral pain, bleeding, dysphagia

• Bone marrow depression: bruising, bleeding, blood in stools, urine, sputum, emesis

Administer:

• Antiemetics and dexamethasone 10 mg at least ½ hr before antineoplastics

SUBCUT route

• Reconstitute with 10 ml sterile water for inj (25 mg/ml), inject diluents slowly into vial, invert vial 2-3 times and gently rotate; sol will be cloudy, use immediately; divide doses >4 ml into two syringes; resuspend the contents 2-3 times

and gently roll syringe between the palms for 30 sec immediately before administration
- Rotate inj site

Perform/provide:
- Increased fluid intake to 2-3 L/day to prevent dehydration, unless contraindicated
- Rinsing of mouth tid-qid with water, club soda; brushing of teeth bid-tid with soft brush or cotton-tipped applicator for stomatitis; use unwaxed dental floss
- Nutritious diet with iron, vitamin supplement, low fiber, few dairy products

Evaluate:
- Therapeutic response: improvement in blood counts in refractory anemia, or refractory anemia with excess blasts

Teach patient/family:
- To avoid crowds, persons with known infections; not to receive immunizations
- To avoid foods with citric acid or hot or rough texture if stomatitis is present; to drink adequate fluids
- To report stomatitis; any bleeding, white spots, ulcerations in mouth; tell patient to examine mouth daily, report symptoms
- To use contraception during therapy; not to breastfeed
- Not to father a child while receiving this product

azathioprine (℞)

(ay-za-thye'oh-preen)

Azasan, Imuran

Func. class.: Immunosuppressant

Chem. class.: Purine antagonist

Do not confuse:
Imuran/Imferon/Elmiron/IMDUR/Enduron/Tenormin

Action: Produces immunosuppression by inhibiting purine synthesis in cells

Uses: Renal transplants to prevent graft rejection, refractory rheumatoid arthritis, glomerulonephritis, nephrotic syndrome, bone marrow transplant

Unlabeled uses: Myasthenia gravis, chronic ulcerative colitis, Crohn's disease, Behçet's disease, autoimmune hepatitis, dermatomyositis, thrombocytopenic purpura, lupus nephritis, polymyositis, pulmonary fibrosis, systemic lupus erythematosus (SLE), Wegener's granulomatosis, vasculitis, atopic dermatitis

DOSAGE AND ROUTES

Prevention of rejection
- *Adult and child:* **IV** 3-5 mg/kg/day, then maintenance **(PO)** of at least 1-3 mg/kg/day

Refractory rheumatoid arthritis
- *Adult:* **PO** 1 mg/kg/day, may increase dose after 2 mo by 0.5 mg/kg/day, not to exceed 2.5 mg/kg/day

Renal disease
- CCr 10-50 ml/min 75% of dose; CCr <10 ml/min 50% of dose

Lupus nephritis/SLE/Wegener's granulomatosis/idiopathic pulmonary fibrosis (unlabeled)
- *Adult:* **PO** 2.3 mg/kg/day

Atopic dermatitis (unlabeled)
- *Adult/adolescent ≥16 yr:* **PO** 2.5 mg/kg/day

Available forms: Tabs 50, 75, 100 mg; inj 100 mg

SIDE EFFECTS

GI: Nausea, vomiting, stomatitis, esophagitis, **pancreatitis, hepatotoxicity, jaundice**

HEMA: **Leukopenia, thrombocytopenia, anemia, pancytopenia, bleeding**

INTEG: Rash, alopecia

MISC: **Serum sickness,** Raynaud's symptoms

MS: Arthralgia, muscle wasting

Contraindications: Pregnancy (D), hypersensitivity, breastfeeding

Precautions: Severe renal/hepatic disease, geriatric patients, thiopurine methyltransferase deficiency

Black Box Warning: Bone marrow suppression, neoplastic disease

PHARMACOKINETICS

Metabolized in liver, excreted in urine (active metabolite), crosses placenta, half-life 5 hr

INTERACTIONS

• Leukopenia: ACE inhibitors; co-trimoxazole

• Do not admix with other products

Increase: myelosuppression—cycloSPORINE, antineoplastics

Increase: action of azathioprine—allopurinol

Decrease: immune response—vaccines

Decrease: action of warfarin—warfarin

Drug/Herb

Increase: immunosuppression—astragalus, echinacea, melatonin, safflower

Decrease: immunosuppression—ginseng, maitake, mistletoe, schisandra, St. John's wort, tumeric

Drug/Lab Test

Increase: LFTs

Decrease: uric acid

Interference: CBC, differential count

NURSING CONSIDERATIONS

Assess:

• For infection: increased temp, WBC; sputum, urine

• For rheumatoid arthritis, pain, mobility, ROM

• I&O, weight daily, report decreasing urine output; toxicity may occur

• Blood studies: Hgb, WBC, platelets during treatment monthly; if leukocytes are <3000/mm^3 or platelets <100,000/mm^3, product should be discontinued

⚠ Hepatotoxicity: dark urine, jaundice, itching, light-colored stools, increased LFTs; product should be discontinued; hepatic studies: alk phos, AST, ALT, bilirubin

• Arthritis: pain; location, ROM, swelling, before and during treatment

Administer:

• All medications PO if possible, avoiding IM inj, since bleeding may occur

PO route

• With meals to reduce GI upset

IV route

• Prepare in biologic cabinet using gown, gloves, mask

• After diluting 100 mg/10 ml of sterile H_2O for inj; rotate to dissolve; may further dilute with 50 ml or more saline or glucose in saline, give over ½-1 hr

• For several days before transplant surgery

Solution compatibilities: D_5W, NaCl 0.9%, NaCl 0.45%

Evaluate:

• Therapeutic response: absence of graft rejection, immunosuppression in autoimmune disorders

Teach patient/family:

• To take as prescribed, do not miss doses, if dose is missed on daily regimen, skip dose; if on multiple dosing/day, take as soon as remembered

• That therapeutic response may take 3-4 mo in RA; to continue with prescribed exercise, rest, other medications

• To report fever, rash, severe diarrhea, chills, sore throat, fatigue, since serious infections may occur; report unusual bleeding or bruising

• To use contraceptive measures during treatment, for 16 wk after ending therapy; to avoid vaccinations

• To avoid crowds to reduce risk for infection

• To use soft-bristled toothbrush to prevent bleeding

• That treatment is ongoing to prevent transplant rejection

azelaic acid topical

See Appendix B

azelastine nasal agent

See Appendix B

azelastine ophthalmic

See Appendix B

azithromycin (℞)

(ay-zi-thro-my′sin)
Zithromax, Zmax
Func. class.: Antiinfective
Chem. class.: Macrolide (azalide)

Do not confuse:
azithromycin/erythromycin
Zithromax/Zinacef

Action: Binds to 50S ribosomal subunits of susceptible bacteria and suppresses protein synthesis; much greater spectrum of activity than erythromycin; more effective against gram-negative organisms

Uses: Mild to moderate infections of the upper respiratory tract, lower respiratory tract, uncomplicated skin and skin structure infections caused by *Moraxella catarrhalis, Streptococcus pneumoniae, Streptococcus pyogenes, Staphylococcus aureus, Streptococcus agalactiae, Mycoplasma pneumoniae, Haemophilus influenzae, Clostridium, Legionella pneumophila;* NGU or cervicitis due to *Chlamydia trachomatis;* in children: acute otitis media *(H. influenzae, M. catarrhalis, S. pneumoniae)* **PO;** acute pharyngitis/tonsillitis (group A streptococcal) **PO;** acute skin/soft tissue infections **(PO);** community-acquired pneumonia *(Chlamydia pneumoniae, H. influenzae, M. pneumoniae, S. pneumoniae)* **PO;** pharyngitis/tonsillitis *(S. pyogenes);* prophylaxis of disseminated *Mycobacterium avium* complex (MAC)

Unlabeled uses: Babesiosis, cholera, cystic fibrosis, dental abscess/infection, endocarditis prophylaxis, granuloma inguinale, *Helicobacter pylori, Klebsiella granulomatis,* Legionnaire's disease, Lyme disease, lymphogranuloma venereum, MAC, *Mycoplasma hominis,* periodontitis, pertussis, prostatitis, *Rickettsia tsutsugamushi, Salmonella typhi,* shigellosis, syphilis, toxoplasmosis, typhoid fever

DOSAGE AND ROUTES

Most infections
- *Adult:* **PO** 500 mg on day 1, then 250 mg/day on days 2-5 for a total dose of 1.5 g
- *Child 2-15 yr:* **PO** 10 mg/kg on day 1, then 5 mg/kg × 4 days

Disseminated MAC infections
- *Adult:* **PO** 600 mg/day in combination with ethambutol

Community-acquired pneumonia
- *Adult:* **PO/IV** 500 mg **IV** q24hr × 2 doses, then 500 mg **PO** q24hr × 7-10 days

Pelvic inflammatory disease
- *Adult:* **PO/IV** 500 mg **IV** q24hr × 2 doses, then 500 mg **PO** q24hr × 7-10 days

Cervicitis, chlamydia, chancroid, nongonococcal urethritis, syphilis
- *Adult:* **PO** 1 g single dose

Gonorrhea
- *Adult:* **PO** 2 g single dose

Endocarditis prophylaxis
- *Adult:* **PO** 500 mg 1 hr prior to procedure
- *Child:* **PO** 15 mg/kg 1 hr prior to procedure

Lower respiratory tract infections, acute skin/soft tissue infections, acute pharyngitis/tonsillitis
- *Child, 3-day regimen:* **PO** 5-10 mg/kg/day × 3 days

Acute otitis media
- *Child:* **PO** 30 mg/kg as a single dose or 10 mg/kg/day × 3 days or 10 mg/kg as a single dose on day 1 (max 500 mg/day), then 5 mg/kg on days 2-5 (max 250 mg/day)

Prevention of acute otitis media
- *Child:* **PO** 10 mg/kg q wk × 6 mo

Legionnaire's disease/early Lyme disease (unlabeled)
- *Adult:* **PO** 500 mg/day

Available forms: Tabs 250, 500, 600 mg; powder for inj 500 mg; powder for oral susp 1 g/packet; susp 100, 200 mg/5 ml

SIDE EFFECTS

CNS: Dizziness, headache, vertigo, somnolence, myasthenia gravis
CV: Palpitations, chest pain
EENT: Hearing loss, tinnitus, loss of smell (anosmia)
GI: Nausea, vomiting, diarrhea, **hepatotoxicity,** abdominal pain, stomatitis, heartburn, dyspepsia, flatulence, melena, **cholestatic jaundice, pseudomembranous colitis,** tongue discoloration
GU: Vaginitis, moniliasis, nephritis
HEMA: Anemia
INTEG: Rash, urticaria, pruritus, photosensitivity
SYST: **Angioedema, Stevens-Johnson syndrome, toxic epidermal necrolysis**

Contraindications: Hypersensitivity to azithromycin, erythromycin, or any macrolide

Precautions: Pregnancy (B), breastfeeding; geriatric patients; renal/hepatic/cardiac disease; <6 mo for otitis media; <2 yr for pharyngitis, tonsillitis

PHARMACOKINETICS

PO: Peak 2-4 hr, duration 24 hr
IV: Peak end of inf; duration 24 hr; half-life 11-57 hr; excreted in bile, feces; urine primarily as unchanged product; may be an inhibitor of P-glycoprotein

INTERACTIONS

- Toxicity: ergotamine

⚠ Dysrhythmias: pimozide; fatal reaction

Increase: effects of oral anticoagulants, digoxin, theophylline, methylPREDNISolone, cycloSPORINE, bromocriptine, disopyramide, triazolam, carbamazepine, phenytoin, tacrolimus, nelfinavir
Decrease: clearance of triazolam
Decrease: absorption of azithromycin—aluminum, magnesium antacids

Drug/Herb

- Do not use acidophilus with antiinfectives; separate by several hours

Drug/Lab Test

Increase: CPK, ALT, AST, bilirubin, BUN, creatinine, alk phos

NURSING CONSIDERATIONS

Assess:

- I&O ratio; report hematuria, oliguria in renal disease
- Hepatic studies: AST, ALT; CBC with differential
- Renal studies: urinalysis, protein, blood
- C&S before product therapy; product may be taken as soon as culture is taken; C&S may be repeated after treatment
- For superinfection: sore throat, mouth, tongue; fever, fatigue, diarrhea, anogenital pruritus
- Bowel pattern before, during treatment
- Respiratory status: rate, character, wheezing, tightness in chest; discontinue product if these occur

Administer:

PO route

- Susp 1 hr before meals or 2 hr after meals; reconstitute 1 g packet for susp with 60 ml water, mix, rinse glass with more water and have patient drink to consume all medication; packets not for pediatric use

IV route

- Reconstitute 500 mg of product/4.8 ml sterile water for inj (100 mg/ml); shake, dilute with ≥250 ml 0.9% NaCl, 0.45% NaCl, or LR to 1-2 mg/ml; diluted solution is stable for 24 hr or 7 days if refrigerated
- Give 500 mg or more/hr; never give IM or as a bolus

Perform/provide:

- Storage at room temperature

Evaluate:

- Therapeutic response: C&S negative for infection; decreased signs of infection

Teach patient/family:

⚠ To report sore throat, fever, fatigue, severe diarrhea, anal/genital itching (may indicate superinfection)

- Not to take aluminum/magnesium-containing antacids simultaneously with this product (PO)

B

▲ To notify nurse of diarrhea stools, dark urine, pale stools, yellow discoloration of eyes or skin, severe abdominal pain
- To complete dosage regimen

Treatment of hypersensitivity: Withdraw product, maintain airway, administer epinephrine, aminophylline, O_2, IV corticosteroids

azithromycin ophthalmic

See Appendix B

Rarely Used

aztreonam (℞)

(az-tree'oh-nam)

Azactam

Func. class.: Antibiotic—miscellaneous

Uses: Urinary tract infection; septicemia; skin, muscle, bone infection, lower respiratory tract, intraabdominal infections; and other infections caused by gram-negative organisms

DOSAGE AND ROUTES

Urinary tract infections
- *Adult:* **IM/IV** 500 mg-1 g q8-12hr

Systemic infections
- *Adult:* **IM/IV** 1-2 g q8-12hr
- *Child:* **IM/IV** 90-120 mg/kg/day divided q6-8hr; max 8 g/day **IV**

Severe systemic infections
- *Adult:* **IM/IV** 2 g q6-8hr; do not exceed 8 g/day

Continue treatment for 48 hr after negative culture or until patient is asymptomatic

Contraindications: Hypersensitivity to this product, penicillins, cephalosporins, severe renal disease

bacitracin topical

See Appendix B

baclofen (℞)

(bak'loe-fen)

Lioresal, Lioresal Intrathecal

Func. class.: Skeletal muscle relaxant, central acting

Chem. class.: GABA chlorophenyl derivative

Do not confuse:
Lioresal/Lotensin

Action: Inhibits synaptic responses in CNS by stimulating GABAb receptor subtype, which decreases neurotransmitter function; decreases frequency, severity of muscle spasms

Uses: Spasticity in spinal cord injury, multiple sclerosis

Unlabeled uses: Neuropathic pain, hiccups, trigeminal neuralgia/nystagmus, recurrent priapism

DOSAGE AND ROUTES

- *Adult:* **PO** 5 mg tid × 3 days, then 10 mg tid × 3 days, then 15 mg tid × 3 days, then 20 mg tid × 3 days, then titrated to response, not to exceed 80 mg/day; **INTRATHECAL** use implantable intrathecal inf pump, use screening trial of 3 separate bol doses if needed 24 hr apart (50 mcg/ml, 75 mcg/1.5 ml, 100 mcg/2 ml); patients who do not respond to 100 mcg should not be considered for chronic IT therapy; initial: double screening dose that produced result and give over 24 hr, increase by 10%-30% q24hr only; maintenance: 1200-1500 mcg/day
- *Child >2-7 yr:* **PO** 10-15 mg/day divided q8hr titrate every 3 days by 5-15 mg/day to max 40 mg/day
- *Child ≥8 yr:* As above, max 60 mg/day
- *Child:* **INTRATHECAL** Initial test dose same as adult; for small children, initial dose of 25 mcg/dose may be used; 25-1200 mcg/day inf, titrated to response in screening phase
- *Geriatric:* **PO** 5 mg bid-tid

Neuropathic pain including trigeminal neuralgia (unlabeled)

• *Adult:* **PO** 5 mg tid, may increase by 5 mg q3days; max 80 mg/day

Hiccups (unlabeled)

• *Adult:* **PO** 10 mg qid

Recurrent priapism (unlabeled)

• *Adult:* **PO** 40 mg at bedtime

Available forms: Tabs 10, 20 mg; intrathecal inj 10 mg/20 ml (500 mcg/ml), 10 mg/5 ml (2000 mcg/ml); pharmacy can prepare extemperaneous liquid preparations

SIDE EFFECTS

CNS: *Dizziness, weakness, fatigue, drowsiness,* headache, *disorientation,* insomnia, paresthesias, tremors; **seizures, life-threatening CNS depression, coma; CNS infection** (IT)

CV: Hypotension, chest pain, palpitations, edema; **cardiovascular collapse (IT)**

EENT: Nasal congestion, blurred vision, mydriasis, tinnitus

GI: *Nausea,* constipation, *vomiting,* increased AST, alk phos, abdominal pain, dry mouth, anorexia

GU: Urinary frequency, hematuria

INTEG: Rash, pruritus

RESP: Dyspnea; respiratory failure (IT)

Contraindications: Hypersensitivity

Precautions: Pregnancy (C), breastfeeding, geriatric patients, peptic ulcer disease, renal/hepatic disease, stroke, seizure disorder, diabetes mellitus

Black Box Warning: Abrupt discontinuation

PHARMACOKINETICS

PO: Onset 3-4 days, peak 2-3 hr, duration >8 hr, half-life 2½-4 hr, partially metabolized in liver, excreted in urine (unchanged)

INTRATHECAL: CSF levels with plasma levels 100 times oral route, peak 4 hr, duration 4-8 hr

BOLUS: Onset ½-1 hr

CONT INF: Onset 6-8 hr, peak 24-48 hr

INTERACTIONS

Increase: CNS depression—alcohol, tricyclics, opiates, barbiturates, sedatives, hypnotics, MAOIs

Increase: hypotension—antihypertensives

Drug/Herb

Increase: CNS depression—chamomile, hops, kava, skullcap, valerian

Drug/Lab Test

Increase: AST, alk phos, blood glucose

NURSING CONSIDERATIONS

Assess:

• B/P, weight, blood glucose, and hepatic function periodically

⚠ For increased seizure activity in seizure disorders; this product decreases seizure threshold

• I&O ratio; check for urinary frequency

• EEG in epileptic patients; poor seizure control has occurred in patients taking this product

• Allergic reactions: rash, fever, respiratory distress

• Severe weakness, numbness in extremities

• Tolerance: increased need for medication, more frequent requests for medication, increased pain

• For withdrawal symptoms: CNS depression, dizziness, drowsiness, psychiatric symptoms

Administer:

PO route

• With meals for GI symptoms

IT route

• For screening, dilute to a concentration of 50 mcg/ml with NaCl for inj (preservative-free), give test dose over 1 min; watch for decreasing muscle tone or frequency of spasm; if inadequate, use 2 more test doses q24hr; maintenance inf via implantable pump 500-2000 mcg/ml

• Dosage, as individual titration is required

• Do not use IT inj IV, IM, SUBCUT, epidural

Additive compatibilities: Morphine

Perform/provide:

- Storage in tight container at room temperature
- Assistance with ambulation if dizziness or drowsiness occurs

Evaluate:

- Therapeutic response: decreased pain, spasticity

Teach patient/family:

- Not to discontinue medication quickly; hallucinations, spasticity, tachycardia will occur; product should be tapered off over 1-2 wk
- Not to take with alcohol, other CNS depressants
- To avoid hazardous activities if drowsiness or dizziness occurs; rise slowly to prevent orthostatic hypotension
- To avoid using OTC medication: cough preparations, antihistamines, unless directed by prescriber
- To notify prescriber if nausea; headache; tinnitus; insomnia; confusion; constipation; inadequate, painful urination continues
- May require 1-2 months for full response

Treatment of overdose: Induce emesis of conscious patient, activated charcoal, dialysis, physostigmine to reduce life-threatening CNS side effects

balsalazide (℞)

(ball-sal′a-zide)

Colazal

Func. class.: GI antiinflammatory

Chem. class.: Salicylate derivative

Do not confuse:

Colazal/Clozaril

Action: Delivered intact to the colon, bioconverted to 5-ASA

Uses: Active, mild to moderate ulcerative colitis in adults and children

DOSAGE AND ROUTES

- *Adult:* **PO** 2250 mg (three 750 mg caps) tid × 8-12 wk, max 6.75 g/day
- *Adolescent and child 5-12 yr:* **PO** 2250 mg (three 750 mg caps) tid × 8 wk

Available forms: Caps 750 mg

SIDE EFFECTS

CNS: Headache, insomnia, fatigue, fever, dizziness

EENT: Dry eyes, rhinitis, sinusitis, blurred vision

GI: Nausea, vomiting, abdominal pain, diarrhea

MS: Arthralgia, back pain, myalgia

SYST: **Anaphylaxis**

Contraindications: Hypersensitivity to salicylates/5-aminosalicylates

Precautions: Pregnancy (B), breastfeeding, children <5 yr, pyloric stenosis, renal disease, colitis, hepatitis

PHARMACOKINETICS

Low and variably absorbed, peak 1½ hr, excreted in feces as metabolites, protein binding 99%, metabolized to mesalamine

INTERACTIONS

Increase: myelosuppression—mercaptopurine

Increase: effect—warfarin, azathioprine

Decrease: effect—thioguanine

- Avoid use of varicella virus vaccine live

Drug/Lab Test

Increase: AST, ALT, GGT, LDH, bilirubin, alk phos

False positive: urinary glucose test

NURSING CONSIDERATIONS

Assess:

- Renal studies: BUN, creatinine, urinalysis (long-term therapy)
- Allergic reaction: rash, dermatitis, urticaria, pruritus, dyspnea, bronchospasm
- Myelosuppression: CBC

Administer:

- Whole; do not crush or chew tabs; cap can be opened and contents sprinkled on applesauce
- With food in evenly divided doses
- With resuscitative equipment available; severe allergic reactions may occur

• Total daily dose evenly spaced to minimize GI intolerance

Perform/provide:

• Storage in tight, light-resistant container at room temperature

Evaluate:

• Therapeutic response: absence of fever, mucus in stools, resolution of symptoms of ulcerative colitis

Teach patient/family:

• To notify prescriber if symptoms do not improve, if colitis symptoms worsen, if rash, hives, or respiratory problems occur

⚠ High Alert

basiliximab (℞)

(bas-ih-liks′ih-mab)

Simulect

Func. class.: Immunosuppressant

Chem. class.: Murine/human monoclonal antibody (interleukin-2) receptor antagonist

Action: Binds to and blocks the IL-2 receptor, which is selectively expressed on the surface of activated T lymphocytes; impairs the immune system to antigenic challenges

Uses: Acute allograft rejection in renal transplant patients when used with cycloSPORINE and corticosteroids

Unlabeled uses: Liver transplant rejection prophylaxis, graft-versus-host disease

DOSAGE AND ROUTES

• *Adult/child <35 kg:* **IV** 20 mg × 2 doses; 1st dose within 2 hr before transplant surgery; 2nd dose given 4 days after transplantation

• *Child 2-15 yr:* **IV** 12 mg/m^2 × 2 doses; 1st dose within 2 hr before transplant surgery; 2nd dose given 4 days after transplantation

Available forms: Powder for inj 10, 20 mg

SIDE EFFECTS

CNS: Pyrexia, chills, tremors, headache, insomnia, weakness, dizziness

CV: Chest pain, angina, **cardiac failure,** hypotension, *hypertension, edema*

GI: Vomiting, nausea, diarrhea, constipation, abdominal pain, **GI bleeding,** *gingival hyperplasia, stomatitis*

INTEG: Acne, pruritus

META: Acidosis, hypercholesterolemia, hyperuricemia, hypo/hyperkalemia, hypocalcemia, hypophosphatemia

MISC: Infection, moniliasis, **anaphylaxis,** anemia, allergic reaction, dysuria, CMV infection, candidiasis

MS: Arthralgia, myalgia

RESP: Dyspnea, wheezing, **pulmonary edema,** *cough*

Contraindications: Breastfeeding, hypersensitivity, exposure to viral infections

Precautions: Pregnancy (B), children, geriatric patients

Black Box Warning: Infections

PHARMACOKINETICS

Peak ½ hr (adults); terminal half-life 7 days (adult), 9½ days (children)

INTERACTIONS

• Immunosuppression: other immunosuppressants

Drug/Herb

Increase: immunosuppression—astragalus, echinacea, melatonin, safflower

Decrease: immunosuppression—ginseng, maitake, mistletoe, schisandra, St. John's wort, turmeric

Drug/Lab Test

Increase: cholesterol, BUN, uric acid, creatinine, K, Ca, blood glucose, Hgb, Hct

Decrease: Hgb, Hct, platelets, magnesium, phosphate

NURSING CONSIDERATIONS

Assess:

• For infection: increased temp, WBC, sputum, urine

• Blood studies: Hgb, WBC, platelets during treatment q mo; if leukocytes are <3000/mm^3, product should be discontinued

• Hepatic studies: alk phos, AST, ALT, bilirubin

• Hepatotoxicity: dark urine, jaundice, itching, light-colored stools; product should be discontinued

⚠ Anaphylaxis, hypersensitivity: dyspnea, wheezing, rash, pruritus, hypotension, tachycardia; if severe hypersensitivity reactions occur, product should not be used again

Administer:

• All medications PO if possible; avoid IM inj, since infection may occur

IV route

• After adding 5 ml sterile water for inj, shake gently to dissolve, reconstitute to a vol of 50 ml with 0.9% NaCl or D_5, gently invert bag, do not shake, give over ½ hr, do not admix

Evaluate:

• Therapeutic response: absence of graft rejection

Teach patient/family:

• To report fever, chills, sore throat, fatigue, since serious infection may occur
• To avoid crowds, persons with known upper respiratory tract infections
• To use contraception during treatment

beclomethasone (℞)

(be-kloe-meth′a-sone)

Beclodisk ♣, QVAR

Func. class.: Corticosteroid, synthetic

Chem. class.: Glucocorticoid

Do not confuse:
beclomethasone/betamethasone

Action: Prevents inflammation by suppression of migration of polymorphonuclear leukocytes, fibroblasts, reversal of increased capillary permeability and lysosomal stabilization; does not suppress hypothalamus and pituitary function

Uses: Chronic asthma, allergic/vasomotor rhinitis, nasal polyps

DOSAGE AND ROUTES

• *Adult:* **INH** 40-80 mcg bid (alone) or 40-160 mcg bid (with inhaled corticosteroids); max 320 mcg bid
• *Child 5-12 yr:* **INH** 40 mcg bid; max 80 mcg bid

Available forms: Oral inh 40, 80, 250 ♣mcg/metered spray

SIDE EFFECTS

CNS: Headache

EENT: Hoarseness, candidal infections of oral cavity, sore throat

GI: Dry mouth, dyspepsia

MISC: **Angioedema, adrenal insufficiency,** facial edema, Churg-Strauss syndrome (rare)

RESP: **Bronchospasm,** wheezing, cough

Contraindications: Hypersensitivity, status asthmaticus (primary treatment), nonasthmatic bronchial disease; bacterial, fungal, viral infections of mouth, throat, lungs

Precautions: Pregnancy (C), breastfeeding, children <12 yr, nasal disease/surgery

PHARMACOKINETICS

INH: Onset 1-4 wk; excreted in feces, urine (metabolites); half-life 2.8 hr; crosses placenta; metabolized in lungs, liver (by CYP3A)

NURSING CONSIDERATIONS

Assess:

• For fungal infection in mucous membranes
• Adrenal function periodically for HPA axis suppression during prolonged therapy, monitor growth/development

Administer:

• Oral aerosol: shake well, use spacer
• Titrated dose, use lowest effective dose

Perform/provide:

• Gum, rinsing of mouth for dry mouth

Evaluate:

• Therapeutic response: decreased dyspnea, wheezing, dry crackles

Teach patient/family:

• To gargle/rinse mouth after each use to prevent oral fungal infections
• That in times of stress, systemic corticosteroids may be needed to prevent adrenal insufficiency; do not discontinue oral product abruptly, taper slowly

- To notify prescriber if therapeutic response decreases; dosage adjustment may be needed
- Proper administration technique
- Clean inhaler by wiping with dry cloth
- All aspects of product usage, including cushingoid symptoms
- The symptoms of adrenal insufficiency: nausea, anorexia, fatigue, dizziness, dyspnea, weakness, joint pain, depression

beclomethasone nasal agent

See Appendix B

benazepril (℞)

(ben-aze'uh-pril)

Lotensin

Func. class.: Antihypertensive

Chem. class.: Angiotensin-converting enzyme (ACE) inhibitor

Action: Selectively suppresses renin-angiotensin-aldosterone system; inhibits ACE, preventing conversion of angiotensin I to angiotensin II

Uses: Hypertension, alone or in combination with thiazide diuretics

Unlabeled uses: CHF, diabetic nephropathy, proteinuria, renal impairment

DOSAGE AND ROUTES

- *Adult:* **PO** 10 mg/day initially, then 20-40 mg/day divided bid or daily (without a diuretic); 5 mg **PO** daily (with a diuretic); max 80 mg/day
- *Geriatric:* **PO** 5-10 mg/day initially

Renal dose

- *Adult:* **PO** CCr <30 ml/min 5 mg **PO** daily, max 40 mg/day

Renal impairment due to diabetic nephropathy (unlabeled)

- *Adult:* **PO** 10 mg/day

Heart failure (unlabeled)

- *Adult:* **PO** 2-20 mg/day

Available forms: Tabs 5, 10, 20, 40 mg

SIDE EFFECTS

CNS: Anxiety, hypertonia, insomnia, paresthesia, headache, dizziness, fatigue
CV: Hypotension, postural hypotension, syncope, palpitations, angina
GI: Nausea, constipation, vomiting, gastritis, melena, diarrhea
GU: Increased BUN, creatinine, decreased libido, impotence, UTI
INTEG: Rash, flushing, sweating
META: Hyperkalemia, hyponatremia
MISC: **Angioedema**
MS: Arthralgia, arthritis, myalgia
RESP: Cough, asthma, bronchitis, dyspnea, sinusitis

Contraindications: Breastfeeding, children, hypersensitivity to ACE inhibitors

Black Box Warning: Pregnancy (D)

Precautions: Geriatric patients, impaired renal/hepatic function, dialysis patients, hypovolemia, blood dyscrasias, CHF, COPD, asthma, bilateral renal artery stenosis

PHARMACOKINETICS

Peak 1-2 hr fasting, 2-4 hr after food; protein binding 89%-95%; half-life 10-11 hr; metabolized by liver (metabolites); excreted in urine 33%

INTERACTIONS

Increase: hypotension—phenothiazines, nitrates, acute alcohol ingestion, diuretics, other antihypertensives
Increase: hyperkalemia—potassium-sparing diuretics, potassium supplements
Increase: myelosuppression—azathioprine
Increase: serum levels of lithium, digoxin
Decrease: hypotensive effects—NSAIDs

Drug/Herb

Increase: toxicity/death—aconite
Increase: antihypertensive effect—barberry, betony, black catechu, black cohosh, bloodroot, broom, burdock, cat's claw, dandelion, goldenseal, hawthorn, Irish moss, Jamaican dogwood, kelp, khella, mistletoe, parsley

Increase or decrease: antihypertensive effect—astragalus, cola tree
Decrease: antihypertensive effect—coltsfoot, guarana, khat, licorice, pineapple, yohimbe

Drug/Lab Test
Increase: AST, ALT, alk phos, bilirubin, uric acid, blood glucose
Positive: ANA titer
False positive: ANA titer

NURSING CONSIDERATIONS

Assess:

- Blood studies: neutrophils, decreased platelets; WBC with differential baseline and q3mo, if neutrophils <1000/mm^3 discontinue treatment, recommended in collagen-vascular disease
- B/P at peak/trough level of product, orthostatic hypotension, syncope when used with diuretic
- Renal studies: protein, BUN, creatinine; increased levels may indicate nephrotic syndrome; monitor urine for protein, increased LFTs, uric acid and glucose may be increased
- Potassium levels, although hyperkalemia rarely occurs
- Allergic reactions: rash, fever, pruritus, urticaria; product should be discontinued if antihistamines fail to help
- Renal symptoms: polyuria, oliguria, frequency, dysuria
- Edema in feet, legs daily, weight daily in CHF; monitor for cough

Administer:

- Do not discontinue product abruptly

Perform/provide:

- Storage in tight container at 86° F (30° C) or less

Evaluate:

- Therapeutic response: decrease in B/P

Teach patient/family:

- Not to use OTC products (cough, cold, allergy) unless directed by prescriber; do not use salt substitutes containing potassium without consulting prescriber
- The importance of complying with dosage schedule, even if feeling better
- To notify prescriber of pregnancy, product will need to be discontinued
- To rise slowly to sitting or standing position to minimize orthostatic hypotension
- To notify prescriber of mouth sores, sore throat, fever, swelling of hands or feet, irregular heartbeat, chest pain
- To report excessive perspiration, dehydration, vomiting, diarrhea; may lead to fall in B/P
- That product may cause dizziness, fainting, light-headedness; may occur during first few days of therapy
- That product may cause skin rash or impaired perspiration
- How to take B/P, and normal readings for age-group

Treatment of overdose: 0.9% NaCl IV INF, hemodialysis

⚠ High Alert

bendamustine (℞)

(ben-da-muss'teen)
Treanda
Func. class.: Antineoplastic alkylating agent
Chem. class.: Nitrogen mustard

Action: Cross-linking DNA that causes single strand and double strand breaks, inhibits several mitotic checkpoints, combines alkylating and antimetabolite properties

Uses: Chronic lymphocytic leukemia, non-Hodgkin's lymphoma

Unlabeled uses: Mantle cell lymphoma (MCL)

DOSAGE AND ROUTES

Chronic lymphocytic leukemia

- *Adult:* **IV INF** 100 mg/m^2 over 30 min on days 1, 2 q28days up to 6 cycles

Non-Hodgkin's lymphoma

- *Adult:* **IV INF** 120 mg/m^2 over 60 min on days 1, 2 q21days up to 8 cycles

Mantle cell lymphoma (unlabeled)
• *Adult:* **IV INF** 90 mg/m^2 on days 1, 2 with rituximab on day 1 q28 days for 6 cycles

Available forms: Powder for inj 100 mg

SIDE EFFECTS

CNS: Asthenia, fatigue, fever, headache
CV: Hypertension, **hypertensive crisis**
GI: Nausea, vomiting, diarrhea, hyperbilirubinemia, constipation, stomatitis, anorexia
GU: **Renal failure**
HEMA: **Thrombocytopenia, leukopenia, anemia, lymphocytopenia, neutropenia, secondary malignancy, toxic epidermal necrolysis, tumor lysis syndrome**
INTEG: Bulbous rash, pruritus
META: Hyperuricemia
SYST: **Anaphylaxis,** infection, dehydration, **severe skin toxicities**

Contraindications: Fetal harm may occur, breastfeeding, children, hepatic disease, renal impairment, hypersensitivity to this product or mannitol

Precautions: Hyperuricemia, infusion-related reactions, myelosuppression, infection, skin-reactions

PHARMACOKINETICS

95% protein binding, metabolized by hydrolysis via CYP450 1A2, two metabolites are produced, half-life 40 min, 90% excreted unchanged (feces)

INTERACTIONS

• Do not use with clozapine due to risk of agranulocytosis

Increase: bleeding risk—aspirin, anticoagulants, NSAIDs, platelet inhibitors, thrombolytics

Increase: myelosuppression—myelosuppressive agents

Increase: toxicity—other antineoplastics, radiation, cimetidine

Increase: adverse reactions, decreased antibody reaction—live vaccines

Increase: bendamustine—CYP1A2 inhibitors (atazanavir, cimetidine, ciprofloxacin, enoxacin, ethyl estradiol, fluvoxamine, mexiletine, norfloxacin, tacrine, thiabendazole, zileuton)

Decrease: bendamustine—CYP1A2 inducers (barbiturates, carbamazepine, rifampin)

Drug/Lab Test

Increase: LFTs

NURSING CONSIDERATIONS

Assess:

• CBC, differential, platelet count weekly; withhold product if WBC is <1000 or platelet count is <75,000; notify prescriber of results
• Hepatic studies: AST, ALT, bilirubin
• Renal studies: BUN, serum uric acid, urine CCr before, during therapy; I&O ratio; report fall in urine output of 30 ml/hr; electrolytes
• Monitor for cold, cough, fever (may indicate beginning infection)
• Bleeding: hematuria, guaiac, bruising, petechiae, mucosa, orifices q8hr
• For tumor lysis syndrome

Administer:

• Blood transfusions or RBC colony-stimulating factors to counter anemia
• Antiemetic 30-60 min before giving product to prevent vomiting
• All medications PO, if possible avoid IM inj if platelets are <100,000/mm^3

Intermittent IV INF route

• Prepare in biologic cabinet wearing gown, gloves, mask; avoid contact with skin; can cause burning and staining the skin brown; use cytotoxic handling procedures
• After diluting 100 mg product/20 ml sterile water for inj (5 mg/ml), sol should be clear, colorless to pale yellow, completely dissolve in 5 min; if particulate is present, do not use
• Within 30 min of reconstitution, withdraw the volume needed and further dilute in 500 ml NS or $D_{2.5}/_{0.45}$%NS to a final conc 0.2-0.6 mg/ml; doses ≤100 mg/m^2, give over 30 min; doses >100 mg/m^2, give over 60 min

Perform/provide:

- Storage of reconstituted sol in refrigerator for 24 hr, or room temperature for 3 hr; protect from light; store vials at room temperature

Evaluate:

- Therapeutic response: improvement in blood counts and morphology

Teach patient/family:

- To avoid use of aspirin, ibuprofen, razors, commercial mouthwash
- To report signs of anemia (fatigue, irritability, SOB, faintness)
- To report signs of infection

benzocaine topical

See Appendix B

Rarely Used

benzonatate (℞)

(ben-zoe′na-tate)

Tessalon Perles

Func. class.: Antitussive, nonopioid

Uses: Nonproductive cough

DOSAGE AND ROUTES

- *Adult and child:* **PO** 100 mg up to tid, max 600 mg/day

Contraindications: Hypersensitivity

benztropine (℞)

(benz′troe-peen)

Apo-Benztropine ✦, benztropine mesylate, Cogentin

Func. class.: Cholinergic blocker, antiparkinson's agent

Chem. class.: Tertiary amine

Action: Blockade of central acetylcholine receptors

Uses: Parkinson's symptoms, EPS associated with neuroleptic products, acute dystonic reactions, hypersalivation

DOSAGE AND ROUTES

Product-induced EPS

- *Adult:* **IM/IV** 1-4 mg daily-bid; give **PO** dose as soon as possible; **PO** 1-2 mg bid/tid, increase by 0.5 mg q5-6days
- *Child:* **IM/IV** 0.02-0.05 mg/kg/dose 1-2×/day
- *Geriatric:* **PO** 0.5 mg daily-bid, increase by 0.5 mg q5-6days; max 4 mg/day

Parkinson's symptoms

- *Adult:* **PO** 1-2 mg/day in 1-2 divided doses, increase 0.5 mg q5-6days titrated to patient response, max 6 mg/day

Acute dystonic reactions

- *Adult:* **IM/IV** 1-2 mg, may increase to 1-2 mg bid **(PO)**

Available forms: Tabs 0.5, 1, 2 mg; inj 1 mg/ml

SIDE EFFECTS

CNS: Anxiety, restlessness, irritability, delusions, hallucinations, headache, sedation, depression, incoherence, dizziness, memory loss; *confusion,* delirium (geriatric patients)

CV: Palpitations, tachycardia, hypotension, bradycardia

EENT: Blurred vision, photophobia, dilated pupils, difficulty swallowing, dry eyes, mydriasis, increased intraocular tension, closed-angle glaucoma

GI: Dryness of mouth, constipation, nausea, vomiting, abdominal distress, **paralytic ileus,** epigastric distress

GU: Hesitancy, retention, dysuria

INTEG: Rash, urticaria, dermatoses

MISC: Increased temperature, flushing, decreased sweating, **hyperthermia, heat stroke,** numbness of fingers

MS: Muscular weakness, cramping

Contraindications: Children <3 yr, hypersensitivity, closed-angle glaucoma, myasthenia gravis, GI/GU obstruction, peptic ulcer, megacolon, prostate hypertrophy

Precautions: Pregnancy (C), breastfeeding, children, geriatric patients, tachycardia, renal/hepatic disease, substance abuse history, dysrhythmias, hypotension, hypertension, psychiatric patients

PHARMACOKINETICS

PO: Onset 1 hr, duration 6-10 hr
IM/IV: Onset 15 min, duration 6-10 hr

INTERACTIONS

Increase: anticholinergic effect—antihistamines, phenothiazines, tricyclics, disopyramide, quinidine
Decrease: absorption—antidiarrheals
Drug/Herb
Increase: benztropine effect—butterbur, jimsonweed
Increase: constipation—black catechu
Decrease: benztropine effect—jaborandi, kava, pill-bearing spurge

NURSING CONSIDERATIONS

Assess:
- I&O ratio; commonly causes decreased urinary output; urinary hesitancy, retention; palpate bladder if retention occurs
- Parkinsonism, EPS: shuffling gait, muscle rigidity, involuntary movements, loss of balance
- Constipation; increase fluids, bulk, exercise if this occurs
- Mental status: affect, mood, CNS depression, worsening of mental symptoms during early therapy
- Use caution in hot weather; product may increase susceptibility to stroke by decreasing sweating
- For benztropine "buzz" or "high," patients may imitate EPS

Administer:
PO route
- With or after meals to prevent GI upset; may give with fluids other than water
- At bedtime to avoid daytime drowsiness in patient with parkinsonism

IM route
- Use for dystonic reactions only

IV, direct route
- Undiluted IV (1 mg = 1 ml) give 1 mg/1 min; keep in bed for at least 1 hr after dose

Syringe compatibilities: Metoclopramide
Y-site compatibilities: Fluconazole, tacrolimus

Perform/provide:
- Storage at room temperature
- Hard candy, gum, frequent drinks, to relieve dry mouth

Evaluate:
- Therapeutic response: absence of involuntary movements

Teach patient/family:
- That tabs may be crushed and mixed with food
- Not to discontinue this product abruptly; to taper off over 1 wk, or withdrawal symptoms may occur (EPS, tremors, insomnia, tachycardia, restlessness)
- To avoid driving, other hazardous activities; drowsiness may occur
- To avoid OTC medication: cough, cold preparations with alcohol, antihistamines unless directed by prescriber
- To change positions slowly to prevent orthostatic hypotension
- To use good oral hygiene, frequent sips of water, sugarless gum for dry mouth

Rarely Used

beractant (℞)
(ber-ak'tant)
Survanta
Func. class.: Natural lung surfactant

Uses: Prevention and treatment (rescue) of respiratory distress syndrome in premature infants

DOSAGE AND ROUTES

- *Newborn:* **INTRATRACHEAL INSTILL** 4 doses can be administered in the 1st 48 hr of life; give doses no more frequently than q6hr; each dose is 100 mg of phospholipids/kg birth weight (4 ml/kg)

betamethasone (℞)

(bay-ta-meth'a-sone)
Betnelan ✦, Betnesol ✦, Celestone, Cel-U-Jec, Selestoject ✦

Func. class.: Corticosteroid, synthetic, long-acting

Do not confuse:
betamethasone/beclomethasone

Action: Decreases inflammation by suppressing migration of polymorphonuclear leukocytes, fibroblasts, reversal of increased capillary permeability and lysosomal stabilization

Uses: Immunosuppression, severe inflammation, prevention of neonatal respiratory distress syndrome (by administration to mother)

Unlabeled uses: Churg-Strauss syndrome, multiple myeloma, polyarteritis nodosa, polychondritis, pulmonary edema, temporal arteritis, Wegener's granulomatosis, prevention of hyaline membrane disease

DOSAGE AND ROUTES

- *Adult:* **PO** 0.6-7.2 mg/day; **IM/IV** 0.6-7.2 mg/day in joint or soft tissue (sodium phosphate)
- *Child:* **PO** 17.5 mcg/kg/day in 3 divided doses; **IM** 17.5 mcg/kg/day in 3 divided doses every 3rd day or 5.8-8.75 mcg/kg/day as a single dose (adrenal insufficiency)

Other uses

- *Child:* **PO** 62.5-250 mcg/kg/day in 3 divided doses; **IM** 20.8-125 mcg/kg/day of the base q12-24hr

Maintenance in acute rheumatic carditis/polymyositis/SLE/temperol arteritis/Churg-Strauss syndrome/ mixed connective tissue disease/ polyarteritis nodosa/relapsing polychondritis/polymyalgia rheumatica/vasculitis/Wegener's granulomatosis (unlabeled)

- *Adult:* **PO** 0.6-7.2 mg/day as a single or divided dose
- *Child:* **PO** 62.5-250 mcg/kg/day

Available forms: Tabs 500, 600 mcg; effervescent tabs 500 mcg ✦; syr 600 mcg/5 ml; ext rel tab 1 mg; sol for inj (phosphate) 3 mg/ml; susp for inj (phosphate/acetate) 6 mg/ml

SIDE EFFECTS

CNS: Depression, flushing, sweating, headache, bruising, mood changes

CV: Hypertension, **circulatory collapse, thrombophlebitis, embolism,** tachycardia, **necrotizing angiitis, CHF**

EENT: Fungal infections, increased intraocular pressure, blurred vision

GI: Diarrhea, nausea, abdominal distention, **GI hemorrhage,** *increased appetite,* **pancreatitis**

HEMA: **Thrombocytopenia**

INTEG: Acne, poor wound healing, ecchymosis, bruising, petechiae

MS: Fractures, osteoporosis, weakness

Contraindications: Children <2 yr, psychosis, hypersensitivity, idiopathic thrombocytopenia, acute glomerulonephritis, amebiasis, fungal infections, nonasthmatic bronchial disease, AIDS, TB, threadworm, high doses in traumatic brain injury

Precautions: Pregnancy (C), breastfeeding, diabetes mellitus, glaucoma, osteoporosis, seizure disorders, ulcerative colitis, CHF, myasthenia gravis, renal disease, esophagitis, peptic ulcer

PHARMACOKINETICS

Metabolized in liver, excreted in urine as metabolites, crosses placenta

PO: Onset 1-2 hr, peak 1 hr, duration 3 days

IM/IV: Onset 10 min, peak 4-8 hr, duration 1-1½ days

INTERACTIONS

Increase: GI bleeding—NSAIDs, alcohol, salicylates, indomethacin

Increase: effects of betamethasone—CYP3A4 inhibitors (erythromycin, ketoconazole, itraconazole, ritonavir, saquinavir, indinavir)

Increase: hypokalemia—thiazides, loop diuretics, ticarcillin, amphotericin B, piperacillin
Increase: tendon rupture—fluoroquinolones
Decrease: action of betamethasone—barbiturates, rifampin, phenytoin
Decrease: effects of anticoagulants, antidiabetics, insulin, isoniazid, toxoids, vaccines, salicylates, oral contraceptives, somatrem, somatropin

Drug/Herb
Increase: hypokalemia—aloe, buckthorn, cascara sagrada, Chinese rhubarb, rhubarb, senna
Increase: corticosteroid effects—goldenseal, hawthorn, hops, lemon balm, licorice, lily of the valley, mistletoe, perilla, pheasant's eye, squill

Drug/Food
- Grapefruit juice should be avoided

Drug/Lab Test
Increase: cholesterol, sodium, blood glucose, uric acid, calcium, urine glucose
Decrease: calcium, potassium, T_4, T_3, thyroid ^{131}I uptake test, urine 17-OHCS, 17-KS, PBI
False negative: skin allergy tests

NURSING CONSIDERATIONS

Assess:
- Infection: increased temp, WBC even after withdrawal of medication; product masks infection symptoms
- Potassium depletion: paresthesias, fatigue, nausea, vomiting, depression, polyuria, dysrhythmias, weakness
- Edema, hypo/hypertension, cardiac symptoms
- Mental status: affect, mood, behavioral changes, aggression
- Potassium, blood glucose, urine glucose while on long-term therapy; hypokalemia and hyperglycemia
- Weight daily; notify prescriber of weekly gain >5 lb
- B/P q4hr, pulse; notify prescriber if chest pain occurs
- I&O ratio; be alert for decreasing urinary output and increasing edema
- Plasma cortisol levels during long-term therapy (normal level: 138-635 nmol/L SI units when drawn at 8 AM)

Administer:

PO route
- With food or milk to decrease GI symptoms

IM route
- Inj deeply in large muscle mass, rotate sites, avoid deltoid, use 21G needle
- In one dose in AM to prevent adrenal suppression, avoid SUBCUT administration; may damage tissue

IV route
- After shaking suspension (parenteral)
- Only sodium phosphate product; give >1 min; may be given by IV INF in compatible sol
- Titrated dose; use lowest effective dose

Y-site compatibilities: Heparin, hydrocortisone, potassium chloride, vit B/C

Perform/provide:
- Assistance with ambulation in patient with bone tissue disease to prevent fractures

Evaluate:
- Therapeutic response: ease of respirations, decreased inflammation

Teach patient/family:
- That ID as corticosteroid user should be carried
- To notify prescriber if therapeutic response decreases; dosage adjustment may be needed
- ⚠ Not to discontinue abruptly; adrenal crisis can result
- To avoid all OTC products unless directed by prescriber
- All aspects of product usage including cushingoid symptoms
- The symptoms of adrenal insufficiency: nausea, anorexia, fatigue, dizziness, dyspnea, weakness, joint pain

betamethasone topical
See Appendix B

betamethasone (augmented) topical

See Appendix B

betaxolol ophthalmic

See Appendix B

bethanechol (℞)

(be-than′e-kole)
bethanechol chloride,
Urabeth, Urecholine
Func. class.: Urinary tract stimulant, cholinergic
Chem. class.: Synthetic choline ester

Action: Stimulates muscarinic ACH receptors directly; mimics effects of parasympathetic nervous system stimulation; stimulates gastric motility, stimulates micturition; increases lower esophageal sphincter pressure

Uses: Urinary retention (postoperative, postpartum), neurogenic atony of bladder with retention

Unlabeled uses: Ileus

DOSAGE AND ROUTES

- *Adult:* **PO** 10-50 mg bid-qid; **SUBCUT** 5 mg tid-qid prn
- *Child:* **PO** 0.3-0.6 mg/kg/day divided in 3-4 doses/day

Test dose

- *Adult:* **SUBCUT** 2.5 mg repeated 15-30 min intervals × 4 doses to determine effective dose

Ileus (unlabeled)

- *Adult:* **PO/SUBCUT** 10-20 mg tid-qid; before meals (PO)

Available forms: Tabs 5, 10, 25, 50 mg; inj 5 mg/ml

SIDE EFFECTS

CNS: Dizziness, headache, malaise

CV: Hypotension, bradycardia, reflex tachycardia, **cardiac arrest, circulatory collapse**

EENT: Miosis, increased salivation, lacrimation, blurred vision

GI: Nausea, bloody diarrhea, belching, vomiting, cramps, fecal incontinence

GU: Urgency

INTEG: Rash, urticaria, flushing, increased sweating

RESP: **Acute asthma, dyspnea, bronchoconstriction**

Contraindications: Hypersensitivity, severe bradycardia, asthma, severe hypotension, hyperthyroidism, peptic ulcer, parkinsonism, seizure disorders, CAD, COPD, coronary occlusion, mechanical obstruction, peritonitis, recent urinary or GI surgery, GI/GU obstruction

Precautions: Pregnancy (C), breastfeeding, children <8 yr, hypertension

PHARMACOKINETICS

PO: Onset 30-90 min, duration 6 hr
SUBCUT: Onset 5-15 min, duration 2 hr

INTERACTIONS

Increase: severe hypotension—ganglionic blockers

Increase: action or toxicity—cholinergic agonists, anticholinesterase agents

Decrease: action of anticholinergics, procainamide, quinidine

Drug/Herb

Increase: cholinergic effect—jaborandi tree

Decrease: effects—jimsonweed, scopolia

Drug/Lab Test

Increase: AST, lipase/amylase, bilirubin, BSP

NURSING CONSIDERATIONS

Assess:

- B/P, pulse; observe after parenteral dose for 1 hr
- I&O ratio; check for urinary retention or urge incontinence
- Bradycardia, hypotension, bronchospasm, headache, dizziness, seizures, respiratory depression; product should be discontinued if toxicity occurs

Administer:
- To avoid nausea and vomiting, take on an empty stomach

SUBCUT route

▲ Parenteral dose by SUBCUT route; use of IM, IV may result in cardiac arrest

▲ Only with atropine sulfate available for cholinergic crisis

- Only after all other cholinergics have been discontinued
- Increased doses if tolerance occurs

Perform/provide:
- Storage at room temperature
- Bedpan/urinal if given for urinary retention

Evaluate:
- Therapeutic response: absence of urinary retention, abdominal distention

Teach patient/family:
- To take product exactly as prescribed; 1 hr before meals or 2 hr after meals
- To make position changes slowly; orthostatic hypotension may occur
- To avoid driving, hazardous activities until effects are known

Treatment of overdose: Administer atropine 0.6-1.2 mg IV or IM (adult)

▲ High Alert

bevacizumab (℞)

(beh-va-kiz′you-mab)

Avastin

Func. class.: Antineoplastic—miscellaneous

Chem. class.: Monoclonal antibody

Action: DNA-derived monoclonal antibody selectively binds to and inhibits activity of human vascular endothelial growth factor (VEGF) to reduce microvascular growth and inhibition of metastatic disease progression

Uses: Metastatic carcinoma of the colon or rectum in combination with 5-FU IV; metastatic breast cancer, renal cell carcinoma, glioblastoma

Unlabeled uses: Adjunctive in pancreatic/neovascular/renal/ovarian cancer; (wet) macular degeneration

DOSAGE AND ROUTES

Colorectal cancer
- *Adult:* **IV INF** 5 mg/kg q14days given over 90 min; if well tolerated, the next inf may be given over 60 min; if 60-min infs are well tolerated, subsequent infs may be given over 30 min

Metastatic breast cancer (previously received chemotherapy)
- *Adult:* **IV** 10 mg/kg on days 1, 15 with paclitaxel 90 mg/m^2 on days 1, 8, 15, given q28days

Metastatic breast cancer (have not received chemotherapy)
- *Adult:* **IV** 7.5 mg/kg or 15 mg/kg with docetaxel (100 mg/m^2 IV), repeat q3wk

Metastatic renal cell carcinoma
- *Adult:* **IV** 10 mg/kg q2wk with interferon alfa 9 million units SUBCUT 3×/wk up to 52 wk

Single agent (unlabeled)
- *Adult:* **IV** 10 mg/kg q2wk given over 60-90 min

Advanced pancreatic cancer (unlabeled)
- *Adult:* **IV** 10 mg/kg on days 1, 15 with gemcitabine 1000 mg/m^2 on days 1, 8, 15 in 28-day cycle

Metastatic renal cell cancer (unlabeled)
- *Adult (single agent):* **IV** 10 mg/kg over 60-90 min q2wk; may be given in combination with other products

Ovarian cancer (unlabeled)
- *Adult:* **IV** 15 mg/kg q21days until unacceptable toxicity or disease progression

Neovascular (wet) macular degeneration (unlabeled)
- *Adult:* **INTRAVITREOUS INJ** 1.25 mg q mo

Available forms: Inj 25 mg/ml

SIDE EFFECTS

CNS: Asthenia, dizziness, **intracranial hemorrhage** (malignant glioma)

CV: **Deep vein thrombosis,** hypertension, hypotension, **hypertensive crisis**

GI: Nausea, vomiting, anorexia, diarrhea, constipation, abdominal pain, colitis, stomatitis, **GI hemorrhage/perforation**

GU: Proteinuria, urinary frequency/urgency, **nephrotic syndrome**
HEMA: **Leukopenia, neutropenia, thrombocytopenia, microangiopathic hemolytic anemia**
META: Bilirubinemia, hypokalemia
MISC: **Exfoliative dermatitis, hemorrhage,** non-GI fistula formation, alopecia
RESP: Dyspnea, upper respiratory tract infection

Contraindications: Hypersensitivity
Precautions: Pregnancy (C), breastfeeding, children, geriatric patients, CHF, blood dyscrasias, CV disease, hypertension

Black Box Warning: GI perforation, wound dehiscence

PHARMACOKINETICS

Half-life 20 days, steady state 100 days

INTERACTIONS

- Avoid concurrent use with sunitab; microangiopathic hemolytic anemia may occur

NURSING CONSIDERATIONS

Assess:

- B/P q3-4wk, more frequently if hypertension develops
- For symptoms of infection; may be masked by product
- CNS reaction: dizziness, confusion
- For CHF: crackles, jugular vein distention, dyspnea during treatment

⚠ GU status: (proteinuria) nephrotic syndrome may occur; monitor urinalysis for increasing protein level; product should be held if protein ≥2 g/24 hr, resume when <2 g/24 hr

⚠ For GI perforation, serious bleeding, nephrotic syndrome, hypertensive crisis, product should be discontinued permanently; surgery, product should be discontinued temporarily

Administer:

- Do not give by IV bolus, or IV push
- Give as IV inf over 90 min for first dose and 60 min thereafter, if well tolerated

Evaluate:

- Therapeutic response: decrease in size of tumors

Teach patient/family:

- To avoid hazardous tasks, since confusion, dizziness may occur
- To report signs of infection: sore throat, fever, diarrhea, vomiting
- Not to become pregnant while taking this product or for several months after discontinuing treatment
- Notify prescriber if pregnant or planning a pregnancy
- Report bleeding, changes in urinary patterns, edema
- Avoid immunizations

bicalutamide (℞)

(bye-kal-u'ta-mide)
Casodex
Func. class.: Antineoplastic hormone
Chem. class.: Nonsteroidal antiandrogen

Action: Binds to cytosolic androgen in target tissue, which competitively inhibits the action to androgens
Uses: Stage D-2 metastatic prostate cancer in combination with luteinizing hormone–releasing hormone (LHRH) analog
Unlabeled uses: Recurrent priapism

DOSAGE AND ROUTES

- *Adult:* **PO** 50 mg/day with LHRH

Recurrent priapism (unlabeled)

- *Adult:* **PO** 50 mg every other day

Available forms: Tabs 50 mg

SIDE EFFECTS

CNS: Dizziness, paresthesia, insomnia, anxiety, neuropathy, headache
CV: **CHF**, edema, *hot flashes,* hypertension, chest pain,
GI: *Diarrhea, constipation, nausea,* vomiting, increased hepatic enzymes, anorexia, dry mouth, melena, abdominal pain

GU: Nocturia, hematuria, UTI, impotence, gynecomastia, urinary incontinence, frequency, dysuria, retention, urgency, breast tenderness, decreased libido
INTEG: Rash, sweating, dry skin, pruritus, alopecia
MISC: Infection, anemia, dyspnea, bone pain, headache, asthenia, *back pain,* flu-like symptoms
Contraindications: Pregnancy (X), women, hypersensitivity
Precautions: Breastfeeding, geriatric patients, renal/hepatic disease

PHARMACOKINETICS

Well absorbed; peak 31½ hr; metabolized by liver; excreted in urine, feces; half-life 5.8 days; 96% protein binding

INTERACTIONS

Increase: anticoagulation—anticoagulants
Increase: bicalutamide effects—CYP3A4 inhibitors (amiodarone, antiretrovirals, protease inhibitors, clarithromycin, dalfopristin, quinupristin, delavirdine, efavirenz, erythromycin, fluoxetine, fluvoxamine, imatinib, mifepristone, RU-486, nefazodone, some azole antifungals)
Decrease: bicalutamide effects—CYP3A4 inducers (barbiturates, bosentan, carbamazepine, dexamethasone, nevirapine, oxcarbazepine, phenytoins, rifabutin, rifampin, rifapentine)

Drug/Herb
- Do not use with St. John's wort

Drug/Food
- Do not use with grapefruit juice

Drug/Lab Test
Increase: AST, ALT, bilirubin, BUN, creatinine
Decrease: Hgb, WBC

NURSING CONSIDERATIONS

Assess:
- For diarrhea, constipation, nausea, vomiting
- For hot flashes, gynecomastia (assure patient that these are common side effects)
- Prostate specific antigen, LFTs

Administer:
- At same time each day, either AM or PM, with/without food
- With LHRH treatment; start at same time for both products

Evaluate:
- Therapeutic response: decreased tumor size, decreased spread of malignancy

Teach patient/family:
- To recognize, report signs of anemia, hepatoxicity, renal toxicity
- That hair may be lost, but this is reversible after therapy is completed
- Not to use other products, unless approved by prescriber
- To report severe diarrhea
- To use contraception while taking this product

bimatoprost ophthalmic

See Appendix B

bisacodyl (℞, OTC)

(bis-a-koe′dill)
Bisac-Evac, Bisaco-Lax, Bisacolax ✱, Carter's Little Pills, Dacodyl, Deficol, Dulcagen, Dulcolax, Feen-a-Mint, Fleet Laxative, Laxit ✱, Modane, Reliable Gentle Laxative, Therelax
Func. class.: Laxative, stimulant
Chem. class.: Diphenylmethane

Action: Acts directly on intestine by increasing motor activity; thought to irritate colonic intramural plexus
Uses: Short-term treatment of constipation, bowel or rectal preparation for surgery, examination

DOSAGE AND ROUTES

- *Adult and child ≥12 yr:* **PO** 10-15 mg in PM or AM; may use up to 30 mg for

bowel or rectal preparation; **RECT** 10 mg, single dose; 30 ml enema
• *Child 6-11 yr:* **PO** 5 mg as a single dose; **RECT** 5 mg as a single dose
Available forms: Tabs 5 mg; enteric-coated tabs 5 mg; supp 5, 10 mg; enema 10 mg/30 ml

SIDE EFFECTS

CNS: Muscle weakness
GI: Nausea, vomiting, anorexia, cramps, diarrhea, rectal burning (suppositories)
META: Protein-losing enteropathy, alkalosis, hypokalemia, **tetany,** electrolyte, fluid imbalances
Contraindications: Hypersensitivity, rectal fissures, abdominal pain, nausea, vomiting, appendicitis, acute surgical abdomen, ulcerated hemorrhoids, acute hepatitis, fecal impaction, intestinal/biliary tract obstruction
Precautions: Pregnancy (C), breastfeeding

PHARMACOKINETICS

Small amounts metabolized by liver; excreted in urine, bile, feces, breast milk
PO: Onset 6-10 hr
RECT: Onset 15-60 min

INTERACTIONS

Increase: gastric irritation—antacids, milk, H_2-blockers, gastric acid pump inhibitors
Drug/Herb
Increase: action—flax, lily of the valley, pheasant's eye, senna, squill

NURSING CONSIDERATIONS

Assess:
• Blood, urine electrolytes if product is used often by patient
• I&O ratio to identify fluid loss
• Cause of constipation; identify whether fluids, bulk, or exercise missing from lifestyle, constipating products
• Cramping, rectal bleeding, nausea, vomiting; if these symptoms occur, product should be discontinued

Administer:
PO route
• Swallow tabs whole; do not break, crush, or chew tabs
• Alone only with water for better absorption; do not take within 1 hr of other products or within 1 hr of antacids, milk, H_2 antagonists; do not take enteric product with proton pump inhibitors
• In AM or PM
Evaluate:
• Therapeutic response: decrease in constipation
Teach patient/family:
• Not to use laxatives for long-term therapy; bowel tone will be lost
• That normal bowel movements do not always occur daily
• Not to use in presence of abdominal pain, nausea, vomiting
• To notify prescriber if constipation is unrelieved or if symptoms of electrolyte imbalance occur: muscle cramps, pain, weakness, dizziness

bismuth subsalicylate (OTC)

(bis′muth sub-sal-iss′uh-late)
Bismatrol, Kaopectate, Kao-Tin, Kapectolin, K-Pek, Peptic Relief, Pepto-Bismol, Pink Bismuth ♣
Func. class.: Antidiarrheal, weak antacid
Chem. class.: Salicylate

Do not confuse:
Kaopectate/Kayoxalate
Action: Inhibits prostaglandin synthesis responsible for GI hypermotility, intestinal inflammation; stimulates absorption of fluid and electrolytes; binds toxins produced by *Escherichia coli*
Uses: Diarrhea (cause undetermined), prevention of diarrhea when traveling; may be included to treat *Helicobacter pylori,* heartburn, indigestion, nausea

DOSAGE AND ROUTES

Antidiarrheal

• *Adult:* **PO** 2 tabs or 30 ml (15 ml extra/max strength) q30min or 2 tabs q60min, max 4.2 g/24 hr

Antiulcer (unlabeled)

• *Adult/adolescent:* **PO** 524 mg q30-60min or 1048 mg q1hr, max 4.2 g/24 hr; given with metronidazole or tetracycline

Available forms: Tabs 262 mg; chewable tabs 262 mg; susp 87 mg/5 ml, 130 mg/15 ml, 262 mg/15 ml, 525 mg/15 ml

SIDE EFFECTS

CNS: Confusion, twitching, **neurotoxicity (high doses)**

EENT: Hearing loss, tinnitus, metallic taste, blue gums, black tongue

GI: Increased fecal impaction (high doses), dark stools, constipation, diarrhea, nausea

HEMA: Increased bleeding time

Contraindications: Children <3 yr, children with chickenpox, history of GI bleeding, renal disease, flulike symptoms, hypersensitivity to this product or salicylates

Precautions: Pregnancy (C), breastfeeding, geriatric patients, anticoagulant therapy, immobility, gout, diabetes mellitus, bleeding disorders, previous hypersensitivity to NSAIDs, *Clostridium difficile*–associated diarrhea when used with antiinfectives for *H. pylori*

PHARMACOKINETICS

PO: Onset 1 hr, peak 2 hr, duration 4 hr

INTERACTIONS

Increase: toxicity—salicylates, methotrexate

Increase: effects of oral anticoagulants, oral antidiabetics

Decrease: absorption of tetracycline, quinolones

Drug/Herb

Increase: absorption of bismuth—sarsaparilla

Increase: antidiarrheal effect—nutmeg

Drug/Lab Test

Interference: radiographic studies of GI system

NURSING CONSIDERATIONS

Assess:

• Electrolytes (K, Na, Cl) if diarrhea is severe or continues long term; assess skin turgor or other signs of dehydration

• Bowel pattern before product therapy, after treatment

Administer:

PO route

• Increased fluids to rehydrate the patient

• Shake liquid before using

Evaluate:

• Therapeutic response: decreased diarrhea or absence of diarrhea when traveling

Teach patient/family:

• To chew or dissolve in mouth; do not swallow whole; shake liquid before using

• To avoid other salicylates unless directed by prescriber; not to give to children, possibility of Reye's syndrome

• That stools may turn black; tongue may darken; impaction may occur in debilitated patients

• To stop use if symptoms do not improve within 2 days or become worse, or if diarrhea is accompanied by high fever

bisoprolol (℞)

(bis-oh'pro-lole)

Zebeta

Func. class.: Antihypertensive

Chem. class.: β_1-Blocker

Do not confuse:

Zebeta/DiaBeta/Zetia

Action: Preferentially and competitively blocks stimulation of β_1-adrenergic receptors within cardiac muscle (decreases rate of SA node discharge, increases recovery time), slows conduction of AV node, decreases heart rate, which decreases O_2 consumption in myocardium; decreases renin-aldosterone-angiotensin

system; inhibits β_2-receptors in bronchial and vascular smooth muscle at high doses
Uses: Mild to moderate hypertension
Unlabeled uses: Stable angina, stable CHF

DOSAGE AND ROUTES

Hypertension
• *Adult:* **PO** 5 mg/day; may increase if necessary to 20 mg/day; max 40 mg/day
Renal/hepatic dose
• *Adult:* **PO** 2.5 mg, titrate upward
Angina (unlabeled)
• *Adult:* **PO** 5-20 mg/day
Heart failure (unlabeled)
• *Adult:* **PO** 1.25 mg/day × 48 hr, then 2.5 mg/day for 1st mo, then 5 mg/day
Available forms: Tabs 5, 10 mg

SIDE EFFECTS

CNS: Vertigo, headache, insomnia, fatigue, dizziness, mental changes, memory loss, hallucinations, depression, lethargy, drowsiness, strange dreams, catatonia, peripheral neuropathy
CV: **Ventricular dysrhythmias, profound hypotension, bradycardia, CHF,** cold extremities, postural hypotension, **2nd- or 3rd-degree heart block**
EENT: Sore throat; dry, burning eyes
ENDO: Increased hypoglycemic response to insulin
GI: Nausea, diarrhea, vomiting, **mesenteric arterial thrombosis,** ischemic colitis, flatulence, gastritis, gastric pain
GU: Impotence, decreased libido
HEMA: **Agranulocytosis, thrombocytopenia,** purpura, eosinophilia
INTEG: Rash, flushing, alopecia, pruritus, sweating
MISC: Facial swelling, weight gain, decreased exercise tolerance
MS: Joint pain, arthralgia
RESP: **Bronchospasm,** dyspnea, wheezing, cough, nasal stuffiness
Contraindications: Hypersensitivity to β-blockers, cardiogenic shock, heart block (2nd, 3rd degree), sinus bradycardia, CHF, cardiac failure
Precautions: Pregnancy (C), breastfeeding, children, major surgery, diabetes mellitus, thyroid/renal/hepatic disease, COPD, asthma, well-compensated heart failure, aortic or mitral valve disease, peripheral vascular disease, myasthenia gravis

Black Box Warning: Abrupt discontinuation

PHARMACOKINETICS

Peak 2-4 hr, half-life 9-12 hr, 50% excreted unchanged in urine, protein binding 30%-36%, metabolized in liver to inactive metabolites

INTERACTIONS

Increase: hypotension—reserpine, guanethidine
Increase: myocardial depression—calcium channel blockers
Increase: antihypertensive effect—ACE inhibitors, α blockers, calcium channel blockers, diuretics
Increase: bradycardia—digoxin, amiodarone
Increase: peripheral ischemia—ergots
Increase: antidiabetic effect—antidiabetics
Decrease: antihypertensive effect—NSAIDs, salicylates
Drug/Herb
• Toxicity/death: aconite
Increase: β-blocking effect—betel palm, butterbur, cola tree, figwort, fumitory, guarana, hawthorn, lily of the valley, motherwort, plantain
Decrease: β-blocking effect—coenzyme Q10, St. John's wort, yohimbe
Drug/Lab Test
Increase: AST, ALT, ANA titer, blood glucose, BUN, uric acid, K, lipoprotein
Interference: glucose/insulin tolerance tests

NURSING CONSIDERATIONS

Assess:
• B/P during beginning treatment, periodically thereafter; pulse q4hr: note rate, rhythm, quality

- Apical/radial pulse before administration; notify prescriber of any significant changes (pulse <50 bpm)
- Baselines in renal, hepatic studies before therapy begins
- I&O, weight daily, watch for CHF: increased weight, jugular vein distention, dyspnea, crackles
- Edema in feet, legs daily
- Skin turgor, dryness of mucous membranes for hydration status, especially geriatric patients

Administer:

- Product before meals, bedtime; tab may be crushed or swallowed whole, may give without regard to meals
- Reduced dosage in renal/hepatic dysfunction

Perform/provide:

- Storage protected from light, moisture; place in cool environment

Evaluate:

- Therapeutic response: decreased B/P after 1-2 wk

Teach patient/family:

- Not to discontinue product abruptly; may cause precipitate angina, rebound hypertension; evaluate noncompliance
- Not to use OTC products containing α-adrenergic stimulants (such as nasal decongestants, OTC cold preparations) unless directed by prescriber
- To report bradycardia, dizziness, confusion, depression, fever, cold extremities
- To take pulse at home; advise when to notify prescriber
- To avoid alcohol, smoking, sodium intake
- To comply with weight control, dietary adjustments, modified exercise program
- To carry emergency ID to identify product taking, allergies
- To avoid hazardous activities if dizziness is present

⚠ To report symptoms of CHF: difficulty breathing, especially on exertion or when lying down, night cough, swelling of extremities

- That if diabetic, may mask signs of hypoglycemia, or alter blood glucose levels

Treatment of overdose: Lavage, IV atropine for bradycardia, IV theophylline for bronchospasm; digoxin, O_2, diuretic for cardiac failure; hemodialysis, IV glucose for hypoglycemia; IV diazepam (or phenytoin) for seizures

⚠ High Alert

bivalirudin (℞)

(bye-val-i-rue′din)

Angiomax

Func. class.: Anticoagulant

Chem. class.: Thrombin inhibitor

Action: Direct inhibitor of thrombin that is highly specific; able to inhibit free and clot-bound thrombin

Uses: Unstable angina in patients undergoing percutaneous transluminal coronary angioplasty (PTCA), used with aspirin; heparin-induced thrombocytopenia; heparin-induced thrombocytopenia with thrombosis syndrome

Unlabeled uses: Acute MI, DVT prophylaxis

DOSAGE AND ROUTES

PCI/PTCA

- *Adult:* **IV BOL** 0.75 mg/kg, then **IV INF** 1.75 mg/kg/hr for 4 hr; another **IV INF** may be used at 0.2 mg/kg/hr for ≤20 hr; this product is intended to be used with aspirin (325 mg/day) adjusted to body weight

HIT/HITTS

- *Adult:* **IV BOL** 0.75 mg/kg, then **CONT INF** 1.75 mg/kg/hr for duration of procedure

Renal dose

- *Adult:* **IV** GFR 30-59 ml/min give 1.75 mg/kg/hr; GFR 10-29 ml/min give 1 mg/kg/hr; dialysis-dependent patients give 0.25 mg/kg/hr

Acute MI (unlabeled)

- *Adult:* **IV BOL** 0.25 mg/kg, then **CONT IV INF** 0.5 mg/kg/hr × 12 hr, then 0.25 mg/kg/hr for subsequent 36 hr used with streptokinase

DVT prophylaxis (unlabeled)

• *Adult:* **SUBCUT** 1 mg/kg q8hr in those undergoing orthopedic surgery

Available forms: Inj, lyophilized 250 mg/vial

SIDE EFFECTS

CNS: Headache, insomnia, anxiety, nervousness

CV: Hypo/hypertension, bradycardia

GI: Nausea, vomiting, abdominal pain, dyspepsia

HEMA: **Hemorrhage, thrombocytopenia**

MISC: Pain at inj site, pelvic pain, urinary retention, fever

MS: Back pain

Contraindications: Hypersensitivity, active bleeding, cerebral aneurysm, intracranial hemorrhage, recent surgery, CVA

Precautions: Pregnancy (B), breastfeeding, children, geriatric patients, renal function impairment, hepatic disease, asthma, blood dyscrasias, thrombocytopenia, GI ulcers, hypertension

PHARMACOKINETICS

Excreted in urine, half-life 25 min, duration 1 hr, no protein binding

INTERACTIONS

Increase: bleeding risk—anticoagulants, aspirin, treprostinil, thrombolytics

Drug/Herb

Increase: bleeding risk—agrimony, alfalfa, angelica, anise, bilberry, black haw, bogbean, buchu, cat's claw, chamomile, chondroitin, devil's claw, dong quai, evening primrose, fenugreek, feverfew, fish oils, garlic, ginger, ginkgo, ginseng, horse chestnut, Irish moss, kava, kelp, kelpware, khella, licorice, lovage, lungwort, meadowsweet, motherwort, mugwort, nettle, papaya, parsley (large amts), pau d'arco, pineapple, poplar, prickly ash, red clover, safflower, saw palmetto, senega, skullcap, tonka bean, turmeric, wintergreen, yarrow

Decrease: anticoagulant effect—coenzyme Q10, flax, glucomannan, goldenseal, guar gum

NURSING CONSIDERATIONS

Assess:

• Baseline and periodic ACT, APTT, PT, INR, TT, platelets, Hgb, Hct

⚠ Bleeding: check arterial and venous sites, IM inj sites, catheters; all punctures should be minimized; fall in B/P or Hct that may indicate hemorrhage

• Fever, skin rash, urticaria

• CV status: BP, watch for hypo/hypertension, bradycardia

• Neurologic status: any focal or generalized deficits should be reported immediately

Administer:

• Prior to PTCA, give with aspirin, 325 mg

IV, direct route

• Dilute by adding 5 ml of sterile water for inj/250 mg bivalirudin, swirl until dissolved, further dilute in 50 ml of D_5W or 0.9% NaCl (5 mg/ml), give by bolus inj 0.75 mg/kg, then intermittent infusion

CONT IV INF route

• To each 250-mg vial add 5 ml of sterile water for inj, swirl until dissolved, further dilute in 500 ml D_5W or 0.9% NaCl (0.5 mg/ml); give inf after bolus dose at a rate of 1.75 mg/kg/hr; may give an additional inf at 0.2 mg/kg/hr

Perform/provide:

• Storage of reconstituted vials in refrigerator up to 24 hr; store diluted concentration at room temperature for 24 hr

Evaluate:

• Therapeutic response: anticoagulation in PTCA; resolution of heparin-induced thrombocytopenia and thrombosis syndrome

Teach patient/family:

• Reason for product and expected results

• To report black, tarry stools; blood in urine; difficulty breathing

⚠ High Alert

bleomycin (℞)

(blee-oh-mye′sin)

Blenoxane

Func. class.: Antineoplastic, antibiotic

Chem. class.: Glycopeptide

Action: Inhibits synthesis of DNA, RNA, protein; derived from *Streptomyces verticillus;* phase specific in the G_2 and M phases; a nonvesicant, sclerosing agent

Uses: Cancer of head, neck, penis, cervix, vulva of squamous cell origin, Hodgkin's/non-Hodgkin's disease, lymphosarcoma, reticulum cell sarcoma, testicular carcinoma, as a sclerosing agent for malignant pleural effusion

Unlabeled uses: Cutaneous T-cell lymphoma (CTCL) hemangioma, Kaposi's sarcoma, malignant ascites, verruca plantaris/vulgaris

DOSAGE AND ROUTES

- *Adult and child:* **SUBCUT/IV/IM** 0.25-0.5 units/kg 1-2 times/wk or 10-20 units/m^2, then 1 unit/day or 5 units/wk; may also be given by **CONT INF;** do not exceed total dose, 400 units in lifetime

Hodgkin's disease (test dose)

- *Adult and child (unlabeled):* **IM/IV/SUBCUT** ≤2 units for first 2 doses followed by 24 hr observation

Malignant pleural effusion

- *Adult:* 60 units diluted in 100 ml of 0.9% NaCl intrapleural inj given through a thoracostomy tube following drainage of excess pleural fluid and complete lung expansion, remove after 4 hr

Cutaneous T-cell lymphoma (CTCL) (unlabeled)

- *Adult:* **IV** 15 units twice weekly with vinBLAStine and predniSONE

Kaposi's sarcoma (unlabeled)

- *Adult:* **IV** 15 units q2wk with DOXOrubicin and vinCRIStine

Malignant ascites (unlabeled)

- *Adult:* **INTRACAVITARY** 60 units mixed in 50-100 ml 0.9% NaCl and injected into pleural space

Available forms: Powder for inj, 15, 30 units/vial

SIDE EFFECTS

CNS: Pain at tumor site, headache, confusion

GI: ***Nausea, vomiting, anorexia, stomatitis, weight loss,*** ulceration of mouth, lips

IDIOSYNCRATIC REACTION: Hypotension, confusion, fever, chills, wheezing

INTEG: ***Rash, hyperkeratosis, nail changes, alopecia,*** pruritus, acne, striae, peeling, hyperpigmentation

RESP: **Fibrosis, pneumonitis,** wheezing, **pulmonary toxicity**

SYST: **Anaphylaxis,** radiation recall, Raynaud's phenomenon

Contraindications: Pregnancy (D), breastfeeding, hypersensitivity, prior idiosyncratic reaction

Precautions: Patients >70 yr old, renal/hepatic, respiratory disease

Black Box Warning: Fever, pulmonary fibrosis

PHARMACOKINETICS

Half-life 2 hr; when CCr >35 ml/min, half-life is increased in lower clearance; metabolized in liver; 50% excreted in urine (unchanged)

INTERACTIONS

- Avoid live virus vaccines concurrently

Increase: toxicity—other antineoplastics, radiation therapy, general anesthesia

Decrease: serum phenytoin levels—phenytoin, fosphenytoin

Drug/Lab Test

Increase: uric acid

NURSING CONSIDERATIONS

Assess:

- IM test dose in lymphoma 1-2 units before 1st 2 doses

• Pulmonary function tests: chest x-ray before and during therapy; should be obtained q2wk during treatment, pulmonary diffusion capacity for carbon monoxide (DLCO) monthly, if <40% of pretreatment value, stop treatment; treat pulmonary infection prior to treatment
• Temp q4hr; fever may indicate beginning infection
• Serum creatinine
• Dyspnea, crackles, unproductive cough, chest pain, tachypnea, fatigue, increased pulse, pallor, lethargy
• Effects of alopecia and skin color on body image; discuss feelings about body changes
• Buccal cavity q8hr for dryness, sores, ulceration, white patches, oral pain, bleeding, dysphagia
• Local irritation, pain, burning, discoloration at inj site

⚠ Symptoms indicating anaphylaxis: rash, pruritus, urticaria, purpuric skin lesions, itching, flushing, wheezing, hypotension; have emergency equipment available

Administer:
• Antiemetic 30-60 min before giving product to prevent vomiting, continue antiemetics 6-10 hr after treatment
• Topical or systemic analgesics for pain of stomatitis as ordered; antihistamines and antipyretics for fever and chills

IM/SUBCUT route
• After reconstituting 15 units/1-5 ml sterile H_2O, D_5W, 0.9% NaCl, or bacteriostatic water for inj, rotate inj sites; do not use products containing benzyl alcohol when giving to neonates

Intrapleural route
• 60 units/50-100 ml of 0.9% NaCl, administered by MD through thoracotomy tube

IV route
• Using cytotoxic handling procedures
• After reconstituting 15 units or less/5 ml or more of D_5W or 0.9% NaCl; after further diluting with 50-100 ml D_5W or 0.9% NaCl, give 15 units or less/10 min through Y-tube or 3-way stopcock

In lymphoma, two test doses 2-5 units before initial dose; monitor for anaphylaxis

Additive compatibilities: Amikacin, cephapirin, dexamethasone, diphenhydrAMINE, fluorouracil, gentamicin, heparin, hydrocortisone, phenytoin, streptomycin, tobramycin, vinBLAStine, vinCRIStine

Solution compatibilities: 0.9% NaCl

Syringe compatibilities: Cisplatin, cyclophosphamide, DOXOrubicin, droperidol, fluorouracil, furosemide, heparin, leucovorin, methotrexate, metoclopramide, mitomycin, vinBLAStine, vinCRIStine

Y-site compatibilities: Allopurinol, amifostine, aztreonam, cefepime, cisplatin, cyclophosphamide, DOXOrubicin, DOXOrubicin liposome, droperidol, filgrastim, fludarabine, fluorouracil, granisetron, heparin, leucovorin, melphalan, methotrexate, metoclopramide, mitomycin, ondansetron, paclitaxel, piperacillin/tazobactam, sargramostim, teniposide, thiotepa, vinBLAStine, vinCRIStine, vinorelbine

Perform/provide:
• Storage for 2 wk after reconstituting if refrigerated or 24 hr at room temperature; discard unused portions
• Deep-breathing exercises with patient tid-qid; place in semi-Fowler's position
• Liquid diet: carbonated beverage; gelatin may be added if patient is not nauseated or vomiting
• Rinsing of mouth tid-qid with water, club soda; brushing of teeth with baking soda bid-tid with soft brush or cotton-tipped applicators for stomatitis; use unwaxed dental floss
• HOB raised to facilitate breathing

Evaluate:
• Therapeutic response: decrease in size of tumor

Teach patient/family:
• To report any complaints, side effects to nurse or prescriber
• To report any changes in breathing, coughing, fever

- That hair may be lost during treatment, and wig or hairpiece may make patient feel better; that new hair may be different in color, texture
- To avoid foods with citric acid, hot or rough texture
- To report any bleeding, white spots, ulcerations in mouth; to examine mouth daily and report symptoms
- To use contraception during treatment, avoid breastfeeding
- Not to receive vaccines during treatment

boric acid otic

See Appendix B

bortezomib (℞)

(bor-tez'oh-mib)

Velcade

Func. class.: Antineoplastic—miscellaneous

Chem. class.: Proteasome inhibitor

Action: A reversible inhibitor of chymotrypsin-like activity in mammalian cells. Causes a delay in tumor growth by disrupting normal homeostatic mechanisms

Uses: Multiple myeloma previously untreated or when at least two other treatments have failed; mantle cell lymphoma

Unlabeled uses: Non-Hodgkin's lymphoma (NHL)

DOSAGE AND ROUTES

Multiple myeloma (previously untreated)

- *Adult:* **IV BOL** Give for 9 6-wk cycles; cycle 1-4, 1.3 mg/m^2/dose given on days 1, 4, 8, 11, then a 10-day rest period (days 12-21) and again on days 22, 25, 29, 32, then a 10-day rest period (days 33-42) given with melphalan (9 mg/m^2/day on days 1-4) and predniSONE (60 mg/m^2/day on days 1-4); this 6-wk cycle is considered one course; in cycles 5-9, give bortezomib 1.3 mg/m^2/dose on days 1, 8, 22, 29 with melphalan (9 mg/m^2/day on days 1-4) and predniSONE (60 mg/m^2/day on days 1-4); this 6-wk cycle is considered one course; at least 72 hr should elapse between consecutive doses

Mantle cell lymphoma

- *Adult:* **IV BOL** 1.3 mg/m^2/dose days 1, 4, 8, 11 followed by 10-day rest period (days 12 to 21); max 8 cycles

Neuropathic pain

- Grade 1 with pain or grade 2: Reduce to 1 mg/m^2
- Grade 2 with pain or grade 3: Hold product until toxicity resolves, then start at 0.7 mg/m^2 q wk
- Grade 4 hematologic toxicities, withhold use

Other types of B-cell NHL (excluding MCL) (unlabeled)

- *Adult:* **IV BOL** 1.5 mg/m^2 on days 1, 4, 8, 11 followed by 10-day rest period days 12-21; max 8 cycles

Available forms: Lyophilized powder for inj 3.5 mg

SIDE EFFECTS

CNS: Anxiety, insomnia, dizziness, headache, *peripheral neuropathy,* rigors, paresthesia

CV: Hypotension, edema, CHF

GI: Abdominal pain, *constipation, diarrhea,* dyspepsia, nausea, *vomiting,* anorexia

HEMA: Anemia, **neutropenia, thrombocytopenia**

MISC: Dehydration, weight loss, herpes zoster, rash, pruritus, blurred vision

MS: Fatigue, malaise, weakness, arthralgia, bone pain, muscle cramps, myalgia, back pain, tumor lysis syndrome

RESP: Cough, pneumonia, dyspnea, URI

Contraindications: Pregnancy (D), breastfeeding, hypersensitivity to this product, boron, or mannitol

Precautions: Children, geriatric patients, peripheral neuropathy, renal/hepatic disease, hypotension

PHARMACOKINETICS

Half-life 9-15 hr, protein binding 83%, metabolized by CYP450 enzymes (3A4, 2D6, 2C19, 2C9, 1A2)

INTERACTIONS

• Do not use hematopoietic progenitor cells (sargramostim, GM-CSF, filgrastim, G-CSF) within 24 hr of chemotherapy
• Oral hypoglycemics: may result in hypo/hyperglycemia
Increase: risk for bleeding—anticoagulants, NSAIDs, platelet inhibitors, salicylates, thrombolytics
Increase: hypotension—antihypertensives
Increase: peripheral neuropathy—amiodarone, antivirals (amprenavir; atazanavir; didanosine, ddI; lamirudine, 3TC; ritonavir; stavudine, d4T; zidovudine, ZDV), chloramphenicol, cisplatin, colchicine, cycloSPORINE, dapsone, disulfiram, docetaxel, gold salts, HMG-CoA reductase inhibitors, iodoquinol, INH, metronidazole, nitrofurantoin, oxaliplatin, paclitaxel, penicillamine, phenytoin, sulfasalazine, thalidomide, vinBLAStine, vinCRIStine, zalcitabine ddc, isoniazid, statins, and others
Increase: toxicity or decrease efficacy when administered with products that induce or inhibit CYP3A4

Drug/Herb

Increase: toxicity or decrease efficacy—St. John's wort

NURSING CONSIDERATIONS

Assess:

• Hematologic status: platelets, CBC throughout treatment
• For extravasation at inj site
• B/P, fluid status, peripheral neuropathy symptoms

Administer:

• Reconstitute each vial with 3.5 ml 0.9% NaCl
• Use protective clothing during handling, preparation, avoid contact with skin

Evaluate:

• Therapeutic response: improvement of multiple myeloma symptoms

Teach patient/family:

• To use contraception while on this product, pregnancy (D), avoid breastfeeding
• To monitor blood glucose levels if diabetic
• To contact prescriber of new or worsening peripheral neuropathy, severe vomiting, diarrhea
• To avoid driving, operating machinery until effect is known
• To avoid using other medications unless approved by prescriber

bosentan (℞)

(boh'sen-tan)
Tracleer
Func. class.: Vasodilator
Chem. class.: Endothelin receptor antagonist

Action: Peripheral vasodilation occurs via antagonism of the effect of endothelin on endothelium and vascular smooth muscle

Uses: Pulmonary arterial hypertension with WHO class III, IV symptoms

Unlabeled uses: Septic shock to improve microcirculatory blood flow, functional class II pulmonary arterial hypertension

DOSAGE AND ROUTES

• *Adult >40 kg and child >12 yr:* **PO** 62.5 mg bid × 4 wk, then 125 mg bid
• *Adult <40 kg and child >12 yr:* **PO** 62.5 mg bid

Available forms: Tabs 62.5, 125 mg

SIDE EFFECTS

CNS: Headache, flushing, fatigue, fever
CV: Hypo/hypertension, **hypertensive crisis,** palpitations, edema of lower limbs
GI: Abnormal hepatic function, diarrhea, dyspepsia, **hepatotoxicity**

HEMA: **Anemia, leukopenia, neutropenia, lymphopenia, thrombocytopenia**
INTEG: Pruritus, **anaphylaxis,** rash, **Stevens-Johnson syndrome, toxic epidermal necrolysis**
MISC: Oligospermia, tumor lysis syndrome
SYST: **Secondary malignancy**
Contraindications: Pregnancy (X), hypersensitivity, CVA, CAD
Precautions: Breastfeeding, children, geriatric patients, mitral stenosis
Black Box Warning: Hepatic disease

PHARMACOKINETICS

Metabolized by CYP2C9, CYP3A4, and possibly CYP2C19; metabolized by the liver; terminal half-life 5 hr; steady state 3-5 days

INTERACTIONS

- Do not coadminister cycloSPORINE and bosentan; bosentan is increased, cycloSPORINE is decreased
- Do not coadminister glyBURIDE with bosentan; glyBURIDE is decreased significantly, bosentan also is decreased, hepatic enzymes may be increased

Increase: bosentan effects—CYP2C9, CYP3A4 inhibitors
Increase: bosentan level—ketoconazole
Decrease: effects of warfarin, hormonal contraceptives, statins
Decrease: effects of simvastatin, other statins, hormonal contraceptives, warfarin
Drug/Lab Test
Increase: ALT, AST
Decrease: Hgb, Hct

NURSING CONSIDERATIONS

Assess:
- B/P, pulse during treatment until stable
- Hepatic studies: AST, ALT, bilirubin; hepatic enzymes may increase; if ALT/AST >3 and ≤5 × ULN, decrease dose or interrupt treatment and monitor AST/ALT q2wk; if >2 × ULN and bilirubin >2 × upper limit of normal or signs of hepatitis, hepatic disease, stop treatment
- Blood studies: Hct, Hgb may be decreased
- Hepatic involvement: vomiting, jaundice; product should be discontinued

Administer:
- Do not stop product abruptly, taper

Perform/provide:
- Storage at room temperature

Evaluate:
- Therapeutic response: decrease in pulmonary hypertension

Teach patient/family:
- To report jaundice, dark urine, joint pain, fatigue, malaise, bruising, easy bleeding; may indicate blood dyscrasias
- To avoid pregnancy; to use nonhormonal form of contraception
- Lab work will be required periodically

brimonidine ophthalmic

See Appendix B

brinzolamide ophthalmic

See Appendix B

bromfenac ophthalmic

See Appendix B

bromocriptine (℞)

(broe-moe-krip'teen)
Apo-Bromocriptine ♣, Cycloset, Parlodel, Parlodel Snap Tabs, PMS-Bromocriptine
Func. class.: DOPamine receptor agonist, antiparkinson agent
Chem. class.: Ergot alkaloid derivative

Do not confuse:
Parlodel/pindolol/Provera
Action: Inhibits prolactin release by activating postsynaptic DOPamine receptors;

activation of striatal DOPamine receptors may be reason for improvement in Parkinson's disease

Uses: Parkinson's disease, amenorrhea/galactorrhea caused by hyperprolactinemia, infertility, acromegaly, pituitary adenomas, adjunct in type 2 diabetes

Unlabeled uses: Neuroleptic malignant syndrome, alcoholism, premenstrual syndrome, mastalgia, cocaine withdrawal, premenstrual breast symptoms

DOSAGE AND ROUTES

Hyperprolactinemia

- *Adult:* **PO** 1.25-2.5 mg with meals; may increase by 2.5 mg q3-7days, usual 2.5-15 mg/day

Acromegaly

- *Adult:* **PO** 1.25-2.5 mg × 3 days at bedtime; may increase by 1.25-2.5 mg q3-7 days; usual range 20-30 mg/day, max 100 mg/day

Parkinson's disease

- *Adult:* **PO** 1.25 mg bid with meals, may increase q2-4wk by 2.5 mg/day, max 100 mg/day; levodopa should be continued while bromocriptine is being instituted

Pituitary adenoma

- *Adult:* **PO** 1.25 mg bid-tid, may increase over several weeks to 10-20 mg/day

Type 2 diabetes (Cycloset only)

- *Adult:* **PO** (initially) 0.8 mg daily in AM within 2 hr of waking, titrate by 0.8 mg/day no more than q wk to max 1.6-4.8 mg/day

Neuroleptic malignant syndrome (unlabeled)

- *Adult:* **PO** 2.5-5 mg 2-6 ×/day

Cocaine withdrawal (unlabeled)

- *Adult:* **PO** 0.625 mg qid × 42 days

Alcoholism (unlabeled)

- *Adult:* **PO** 7.5 mg/day

Mastalgia (unlabeled)

- *Adult:* **PO** 2.5-7.5 bid, starting 10-14 days prior to menses; discontinue when menses begin

Available forms: Caps 5 mg; tabs 2.5 mg; cycloset tabs 0.8 mg

SIDE EFFECTS

CNS: Headache, depression, restlessness, anxiety, nervousness, confusion, **seizures,** *hallucinations,* dizziness, fatigue, drowsiness, abnormal involuntary movements, psychosis

CV: Orthostatic hypotension, decreased B/P, palpitation, extrasystole, **shock,** dysrhythmias, bradycardia, **MI**

EENT: Blurred vision, diplopia, burning eyes, nasal congestion

GI: Nausea, vomiting, anorexia, cramps, constipation, diarrhea, dry mouth, GI hemorrhage

GU: Frequency, retention, incontinence, diuresis

INTEG: Rash on face, arms; alopecia; coolness, pallor of fingers, toes; peripheral edema

Contraindications: Severe ischemic disease, uncontrolled hypertension, severe peripheral vascular disease, hypersensitivity to ergot, bromocriptine, migraine, preeclampsia

Precautions: Pregnancy (B), breastfeeding, children, renal/hepatic disease, pituitary tumors, peptic ulcer disease, sulfite hypersensitivity, pulmonary fibrosis, dementia, GI bleeding, bipolar disorder

PHARMACOKINETICS

Peak 1-3 hr, duration 4-8 hr, 90%-96% protein bound, half-life 3 hr, metabolized by liver (inactive metabolites), 85%-98% of dose excreted in feces, >90% of absorbed dose undergoes first-pass metabolism

INTERACTIONS

- Disulfiram-like reaction: alcohol

Increase: action of antihypertensives, levodopa

Decrease: action of bromocriptine—phenothiazines, oral contraceptives, progestins, estrogens, haloperidol, loxapine, methyldopa, metoclopramide, MAOIs, reserpine

Drug/Herb

Increase: serotonin effect—horehound

Decrease: bromocriptine effect—chaste tree fruit, kava

Drug/Lab Test

Increase: growth hormone, AST, ALT, CK, BUN, uric acid, alk phos

NURSING CONSIDERATIONS

Assess:

• B/P; establish baseline, compare with other reading; this product decreases B/P

• Parkinson's symptoms: pill-rolling, shuffling gait, restlessness, tremors, postural instability, before and during treatment

• For resolution of symptoms of neuroleptic malignant syndrome: decreased temp, seizures, sweating, pulse

• Change in size of soft tissue volume, in acromegaly

Administer:

• With meal to prevent GI symptoms

• At bedtime so dizziness, orthostatic hypotension do not occur

Perform/provide:

• Storage at room temperature in tight, light resistant container

Evaluate:

• Therapeutic response (Parkinson's disease): decreased dyskinesia, decreased slow movements, decreased drooling

Teach patient/family:

• That tabs may be crushed and mixed with food

• To change position slowly to prevent orthostatic hypotension

• To use contraceptives during treatment with this product; pregnancy may occur; to use methods other than oral contraceptives

• That therapeutic effect for Parkinson's disease may take 2 mo

• To avoid hazardous activity if dizziness occurs

• To report symptoms of MI immediately

brompheniramine (℞)

(brome-fen-ir′a-meen)

Bidhist, BPM, brompheniramine, BroveX, BroveX CT, J-Tan, J-Tan PD, Lo Hist 12, Lodrane 24, TanaCof-XR, VaZol

Func. class.: Antihistamine

Chem. class.: Alkylamine, H_1-receptor antagonist

Action: Acts on blood vessels, GI, respiratory system by competing with histamine for H_1-receptor site; decreases allergic response by blocking histamine

Uses: Allergy symptoms, rhinitis, urticaria

DOSAGE AND ROUTES

• *Adult and child >12 yr:* **PO** 4-8 mg q6-8hr, max 48 mg/day; **EXT-REL** 6-12 mg bid-tid, max 48 mg/day

• *Child 6-12 yr:* **PO** 2 mg q6-8hr, max 24 mg/day; **EXT REL** 6-12 mg/day

• *Child 2-6 yr:* 1 mg q6-8hr, max 12 mg/day

Available forms: Tabs 4 mg; elix 2 mg/5 ml; caps 4 mg; chew tabs 12 mg; ext rel tabs 6 mg; ext rel caps 12 mg; liquid 8 mg, 12 mg/5 ml

SIDE EFFECTS

CNS: ***Dizziness, drowsiness,*** poor coordination, fatigue, anxiety, euphoria, confusion, paresthesia, neuritis, paradoxical excitation (children, elderly)

CV: Hypotension, palpitations, tachycardia

EENT: Blurred vision, dilated pupils, tinnitus, nasal stuffiness, dry nose, throat, mouth

GI: Nausea, vomiting, anorexia, constipation, diarrhea

GU: Retention, dysuria, frequency, impotence

HEMA: **Thrombocytopenia, agranulocytosis, hemolytic anemia (rare)**

INTEG: Photosensitivity

RESP: Thick secretions, wheezing, chest tightness

Contraindications: Children <2 yr, hypersensitivity to H_1-receptor antagonists, acute asthma attack, lower respiratory tract disease

Precautions: Pregnancy (C), breastfeeding, increased intraocular pressure, renal/cardiac disease, hypertension, bronchial asthma, seizure disorder, stenosed peptic ulcers, hyperthyroidism, prostatic hypertrophy, bladder neck obstruction, closed-angle glaucoma

PHARMACOKINETICS

PO: Peak 2-5 hr, duration to 48 hr; metabolized in liver, excreted by kidneys, excreted in breast milk, half-life 12-34 hr

INTERACTIONS

• Incompatible with aminophylline, insulins, pentobarbital

Increase: CNS depression—barbiturates, opiates, hypnotics, tricyclics, alcohol

Increase: anticholinergic effect—MAOIs

Drug/Herb

Increase: effect—hops, Jamaican dogwood, kava, khat, senega

Increase: anticholinergic effect—corkwood, henbane leaf

Drug/Lab Test

Interference: skin allergy tests

NURSING CONSIDERATIONS

Assess:

• Be alert for urinary retention, frequency, dysuria; product should be discontinued if these occur

• CBC during long-term therapy

• Blood dyscrasias: thrombocytopenia, agranulocytosis (rare) during long-term therapy

• Respiratory status: rate, rhythm, increase in bronchial secretions, wheezing, chest tightness

Administer:

PO route

• Do not break, crush, or chew ext rel forms

• With meals if GI symptoms occur; absorption may slightly decrease

Perform/provide:

• Hard candy, gum, frequent rinsing of mouth for dryness

• Storage in tight container at room temperature

Evaluate:

• Therapeutic response: absence of running or congested nose or rashes

Teach patient/family:

• All aspects of product use; to notify prescriber if confusion/sedation/hypotension occurs

• To avoid driving, other hazardous activities if drowsiness occurs

• To avoid use of alcohol, other CNS depressants while taking product

budesonide (℞)

(byoo-des′oh-nide)

Entocort EC, Pulmicort, Pulmicort Flexhaler, Pulmicort Respules, Rhinocort, Rhinocort Aqua

Func. class.: Glucocorticoid

Chem. class.: Nonhalogenated

Action: Prevents inflammation by depression of migration of polymorphonuclear leukocytes, fibroblasts, reversal of increased capillary permeability and lysosomal stabilization; does not suppress hypothalamus and pituitary function

Uses: Rhinitis; prophylaxis for asthma; Crohn's disease

Unlabeled uses: Microscopic colitis

DOSAGE AND ROUTES

Rhinitis (Rhinocort Aqua)

• *Adult and child >6 yr:* **SPRAY/INH** 256 mcg/day (2 sprays in each nostril AM, PM or 4 sprays in each nostril, AM)

Asthma

• *Adult and child ≥6 yr:* **INH** 400-600 mcg/day

Crohn's disease/microscopic colitis (unlabeled)

• *Adult:* **PO** 9 mg/day AM × 8 wk

Available forms: Dry powder for INH 90, 180 mcg/actuation (Pulmicort Flexhaler); inh susp 0.25 mg/2 ml, 0.5 mg/2 ml (Pulmicort Respules); 32 mcg/actuation (Rhinocort Aqua)

SIDE EFFECTS

CNS: ***Headache,*** insomnia, hypertonia, syncope, dizziness, drowsiness

CV: Chest pain, hypertension, sinus tachycardia, palpitation

EENT: ***Sinusitis, pharyngitis,*** rhinitis, oral candidiasis

ENDO: Adrenal insufficiency, growth suppression in children

GI: Dry mouth, dyspepsia, nausea, vomiting, abdominal pain

MISC: Ecchymosis, fever, ***hypersensitivity,*** flulike symptoms, epistaxis, dysuria

MS: Back pain, myalgias, fractures

RESP: Nasal irritation, cough, nasal bleeding, ***respiratory infections,*** **bronchospasm**

Contraindications: Hypersensitivity, status asthmaticus

Precautions: Pregnancy (C), inhaled form (B); breastfeeding, children, TB, fungal, bacterial, systemic viral infections; ocular herpes simplex; nasal septal ulcers; hepatic disease (caps)

PHARMACOKINETICS

Peak: Respules 4-6 wk, Rhinocort Aqua 2 wk, half-life 2-3.6 hr

Onset: Respules 2-8 days, Rhinocort Aqua 10 hr

Enters breast milk

INTERACTIONS

• Avoid using with products metabolized by CYP3A4 inhibition

• Avoid concurrent use of varicella live vaccine in pediatric patients

Decrease: budesonide metabolism—ketoconazole, cimetidine

Drug/Herb

Increase: hypokalemia—aloe, buckthorn, Chinese rhubarb, licorice, senna, St. John's wort

NURSING CONSIDERATIONS

Assess:

• Respiratory status: rate, rhythm, increase in bronchial secretions, wheezing, chest tightness; provide fluids to 2 L/day to decrease thickness of secretions; check for oral candidiasis

• For bronchospasm, stop treatment and give bronchodilator

• With viral infections, corticosteroid use can mask infections

• For increased intraocular pressure, discontinue use if increase occurs

Administer:

PO route (Crohn's disease)

• Swallow caps whole; do not break, crush, or chew

• May repeat 8-wk course if needed; may taper to 6 mg/day for 2 wk before cessation

Inhalation route (asthma)

• Use scissors to open pouch

Perform/provide:

• Storage at 59°-86° F (15°-30° C); keep away from heat, open flame

Evaluate:

• Therapeutic response: absence of asthma, rhinitis

Teach patient/family:

• To notify prescriber of pharyngitis, nasal bleeding, oral candidiasis

• Not to exceed recommended dose; adrenal suppression may occur

• To carry emergency ID identifying steroid use

• To read and follow package directions

• To prevent exposure to infections, especially viral

• To avoid taking with grapefruit juice (capsule PO)

• To use good oral hygiene if using nebulizer or inhaler

• To avoid breastfeeding

• That burning or stinging may occur with first few doses of inhalation use

budesonide nasal agent

See Appendix B

bumetanide (℞)

(byoo-met′a-nide)

Bumex

Func. class.: Loop diuretic, antihypertensive

Chem. class.: Sulfonamide derivative

Do not confuse:

Bumex/Buprenex/Permax

Action: Acts on ascending loop of Henle by inhibiting reabsorption of chloride, sodium

Uses: Edema in CHF, renal/hepatic disease, ascites, heart failure

Unlabeled uses: Hypercalcemia, hypertension

DOSAGE AND ROUTES

• *Adult:* **PO** 0.5-2.0 mg/day; may give 2nd or 3rd dose at 4-5 hr intervals, max 10 mg/day; may be given on alternate days or intermittently; **IV/IM** 0.5-1.0 mg; may give 2nd or 3rd dose at 2-3 hr intervals, not to exceed 10 mg/day

• *Child:* **PO/IM/IV** 0.02-0.1 mg/kg q12hr, max 10 mg/day

Hypercalcemia (unlabeled)

• *Adult:* **IV** 1-2 mg q1-4hr to maintain urine output of 200-250 ml/hr; give saline before 1st dose of this product

Hypertension (unlabeled)

• *Adult and adolescent:* **PO** 0.5-2 mg/day, max 10 mg/day in 2 divided doses

Available forms: Tabs 0.5, 1, 2 mg; inj 0.25 mg/ml

SIDE EFFECTS

CNS: Headache, fatigue, weakness, dizziness

CV: **Chest pain,** hypotension, **circulatory collapse,** ECG changes, dehydration

EENT: Loss of hearing

ELECT: Hypokalemia, hypochloremic alkalosis, hypomagnesemia, hyperuricemia, hypocalcemia, hyponatremia

ENDO: Hyperglycemia

GI: Nausea, diarrhea, dry mouth, vomiting, anorexia, cramps, upset stomach, abdominal pain, **acute pancreatitis, jaundice**

GU: Polyuria, **renal failure,** glycosuria, premature ejaculation

HEMA: **Thrombocytopenia, leukopenia, granulocytopenia, hemoconcentration**

INTEG: Rash, pruritus, purpura, **Stevens-Johnson syndrome,** sweating, photosensitivity

MS: Muscular cramps, arthritis, stiffness

Contraindications: Hypersensitivity to sulfonamides, anuria, hepatic coma

Black Box Warning: Electrolyte imbalance

Precautions: Pregnancy (C), breastfeeding, neonates, ascites, severe renal disease, hepatic cirrhosis, blood dyscrasias, ototoxicity, hyperuricemia, hypokalemia

Black Box Warning: Dehydration

PHARMACOKINETICS

Excreted by kidneys (50% unchanged), feces (20%); crosses placenta; excreted in breast milk; protein binding >91%; half-life 1-1½ hr, 6-15 hr neonates

PO: Onset ½-1 hr, peak 1-2 hr, duration 3-6 hr

IM: Onset 40 min, peak 1-2 hr, duration 4-6 hr

IV: Onset 5 min, peak 15-30 min, duration 3-6 hr

INTERACTIONS

• Ototoxicity: aminoglycosides

• Hypokalemia: potassium-wasting products

Increase: toxicity—lithium, digoxin

Increase: diuresis, electrolyte loss—metolazone

Decrease: diuretic effect—indomethacin, NSAIDs, probenecid

Decrease: antidiabetic effects—antidiabetics

Drug/Herb

- Severe photosensitivity: St. John's wort

Increase: effect—aloe, cucumber, dandelion, horsetail, pumpkin, Queen Anne's lace

Increase: hypotension—khella

NURSING CONSIDERATIONS

Assess:

- For tinnitus, obtain audiometric testing for long-term IV treatment
- Weight, I&O daily to determine fluid loss; if urinary output decreases or azotemia occurs, product should be discontinued; the safest dosage schedule is on alternate days
- B/P lying, standing; postural hypotension may occur
- Electrolytes: K, Na, Cl; include BUN, blood glucose, CBC, serum creatinine, blood pH, ABGs, uric acid, Ca, Mg, severe electrolyte imbalances should be corrected before starting treatment
- Blood glucose if patient is diabetic; blood uric acid levels in those with gout
- Improvement in edema of feet, legs, sacral area daily if medication is being used in CHF
- Signs of metabolic alkalosis: drowsiness, restlessness
- Signs of hypokalemia: postural hypotension, malaise, fatigue, tachycardia, leg cramps, weakness
- Rashes, temp elevation daily
- Confusion, especially in geriatric patients; take safety precautions if needed
- For digoxin toxicity in patients taking digoxin products (anorexia, nausea, vomiting, confusion, paresthesia, muscle cramps); lithium toxicity in those taking lithium

Administer:

- In AM to avoid interference with sleep if using product as a diuretic
- Potassium replacement if potassium is <3.0

PO route

- With food if nausea occurs; absorption may be decreased slightly

IV, direct route

- Direct IV undiluted slowly over at least 2 min through Y-tube or 3-way stopcock or heplock

Intermittent IV INF route

- Dilute in LR, D_5W, 0.9% NaCl (rarely given by this method), give over 12 hr in renal disease

Additive compatibilities: Floxacillin, furosemide

Syringe compatibilities: Doxapram

Y-site compatibilities: Allopurinol, amifostine, aztreonam, cefepime, cisatracurium, cladribine, clarithromycin, diltiazem, docetaxel, etoposide, filgrastim, granisetron, lorazepam, melphalan, meperidine, morphine, piperacillin/tazobactam, propofol, remifentanil, teniposide, thiotepa, vinorelbine

Evaluate:

- Therapeutic response: decreased edema, B/P

Teach patient/family:

- To increase fluid intake to 2-3 L/day unless contraindicated, to take potassium supplement, to rise slowly from lying or sitting position
- To recognize adverse reactions: muscle cramps, weakness, nausea, dizziness
- To take with food or milk for GI symptoms
- To take early in day to prevent nocturia
- To use sunscreen to prevent photosensitivity

Treatment of overdose: Lavage if taken orally; monitor electrolytes; administer dextrose in saline; monitor hydration, CV, renal status

B

buprenorphine (℞)

(byoo-pre-nor′feen)
Buprenex, Subutex
Func. class.: Opioid analgesic, partial agonist
Chem. class.: Thebaine derivative

Controlled Substance Schedule V (Parenteral); Schedule III (Tablet)

Do not confuse:
Buprenex/Bumex

Action: Depresses pain impulse transmission at the spinal cord level by interacting with opioid receptors

Uses: Moderate to severe pain

Unlabeled uses: Cocaine withdrawal, opiate agonist withdrawal

DOSAGE AND ROUTES

• *Adult:* **IM/IV** 0.3 mg q6hr prn, reduce dosage in geriatric patients, may repeat after 30-60 min; **EPIDURAL** (unlabeled) 4 mcg/kg or 2 mcg/kg (epidural inj), remove over 48 hr
• *Child 2-12 yr:* **IM/IV** 2-6 mcg/kg q4-6hr

Opiate dependence (unlabeled)
• *Adult/adolescent ≥16 yr:* **SL** 8 mg day 1, 16 mg day 2, then maintenance titrate q2days; maintenance 16 mg daily

Available forms: Inj 0.3 mg/ml (1-ml vials); SL tab 2, 8 mg as base

SIDE EFFECTS

CNS: Drowsiness, dizziness, confusion, headache, sedation, euphoria, **increased intracranial pressure,** amnesia
CV: Palpitations, bradycardia, change in B/P, tachycardia
EENT: Tinnitus, blurred vision, *miosis,* diplopia
GI: Nausea, vomiting, anorexia, constipation, cramps, dry mouth
GU: Increased urinary output, dysuria, urinary retention
INTEG: Rash, urticaria, bruising, flushing, diaphoresis, pruritus
RESP: **Respiratory depression,** dyspnea, hypo/hyperventilation

Contraindications: Hypersensitivity

Precautions: Pregnancy (C), breastfeeding, substance abuse/alcoholism, increased intracranial pressure, MI (acute), severe heart disease, respiratory depression, renal/hepatic/pulmonary disease, hypothyroidism, Addison's disease

PHARMACOKINETICS

Metabolized by liver by CYP3A4, excreted by kidneys/feces, crosses placenta, excreted in breast milk, half-life 2½-3½ hr, 96% bound to plasma proteins
IM: Onset 10-30 min, peak ½ hr, duration 6 hr
SL: Onset, peak, duration unknown, half-life 37 hr
IV: Onset 1 min, peak 5 min, duration 6 hr, half-life 2.2 hr

INTERACTIONS

Increase: effect with other CNS depressants—alcohol, opioids, sedative/hypnotics, antipsychotics, skeletal muscle relaxants, MAOIs
Increase: buprenorphine effect—CYP3A4 inhibitors (erythromycin, indinavir, ketoconazole, ritonavir, saquinavir)
Decrease: buprenorphine effect—CYP3A4 inducers (carbamazepine, phenobarbital, phenytoin, rifampin)

Drug/Herb
Increase: CNS depression—gotu kola, Jamaican dogwood, kava, lavender, mistletoe, nettle, pokeweed, poppy, senega, St. John's wort, valerian
Increase: anticholinergic effect—corkwood

NURSING CONSIDERATIONS

Assess:
• I&O ratio; check for decreasing output; may indicate urinary retention
• Bowel pattern, severe constipation can occur
• CNS changes, dizziness, drowsiness, hallucinations, euphoria, LOC, pupil reac-

tion; withdrawal in opioid-dependent persons; if dependence occurs, within 2 wk of discontinuing product withdrawal symptoms will occur

- Allergic reactions: rash, urticaria
- Respiratory dysfunction: respiratory depression, character, rate, rhythm; notify prescriber if respirations are <12/min
- Need for pain medication, tolerance; location, intensity, severity

Administer:

- Long-term use is not recommended

IM route

- In deep muscle mass

IV, direct route

- Undiluted over 3-5 min (0.3 mg over 2 min), titrate to patient response
- With antiemetic if nausea, vomiting occur
- When pain is beginning to return; determine dosage interval by patient response

Additive compatibilities: Bupivacaine, diphenhydrAMINE, droperidol, glycopyrrolate, haloperidol, hydrOXYzine, promethazine, scopolamine

Syringe compatibilities: Glycopyrrolate, haloperidol, heparin, midazolam

Y-site compatibilities: Allopurinol, amifostine, aztreonam, cefepime, cisatracurium, cladribine, filgrastim, granisetron, melphalan, piperacillin/tazobactam, propofol, remifentanil, teniposide, thiotepa, vinorelbine

Evaluate:

- Therapeutic response: decrease in pain, absence of grimacing

Teach patient/family:

- To report any symptoms of CNS changes, allergic reactions
- That tolerance may result when used for extended periods, but long-term use is not recommended
- To avoid hazardous activities such as driving unless reaction is known

Treatment of overdose: Naloxone 0.4 mg ampule diluted in 10 ml 0.9% NaCl given by direct IV push 0.02 mg q2min (adult)

*buPROPion (℞)

(byoo-proe′pee-on)
Aplenzin, Budeprion SR, buPROPion, Wellbutrin, Wellbutrin SR, Wellbutrin XL, Zyban

Func. class.: Antidepressant—miscellaneous smoking deterrent
Chem. class.: Aminoketone

Do not confuse:
buPROPion/busPIRone
Zyban/Diovan/Zagam

Action: Inhibits reuptake of DOPamine

Uses: Depression (Wellbutrin), smoking cessation (Zyban); seasonal affective disorder

Unlabeled uses: Neuropathic pain, enhancement of weight loss, ADHD (attention deficit hyperactivity disorder)

DOSAGE AND ROUTES

Depression

- *Adult:* **PO** 100 mg bid initially, then increase after 3 days to 100 mg tid if needed; may increase after 1 mo to 150 mg tid; **ER/SR** initially 150 mg AM, increase to 300 mg/day if initial dose is tolerated; Aplenzin 174 mg q AM, may increase to 348 mg q AM on day 4, may increase to 522 mg after several weeks if needed
- *Geriatric:* **PO** 50-100 mg/day, may increase by 50-100 mg q3-4days

Smoking cessation

- *Adult:* **PO** 150 mg bid, begin with 150 mg/day × 3 days, then 300 mg/day; continue for 7-12 wk; max 300 mg/day

ADHD (unlabeled)

- *Adult:* **PO** 100 mg bid, after ≥3 days titrate to 100 mg tid; SR 300 mg/day, 200 mg 8 AM, 100 mg 4 PM

Diabetic neuropathy/postherpetic neuralgia (unlabeled)

- *Adult:* **PO** SR 150-300 mg/day

Available forms: Tabs 75, 100 mg; sus rel tabs (SR) 150; ext rel tab (XL) 100, 150, 200, 300 mg; (SR-12 hr, XL-24 hr); tab ext rel (Aplenzin) 174, 348, 522 mg

B

SIDE EFFECTS

CNS: Headache, agitation, dizziness, akinesia, bradykinesia, confusion, **seizures**, delusions, *insomnia, sedation, tremors,* **suicidal ideation**

CV: Dysrhythmias, hypertension, palpitations, *tachycardia,* hypotension, **complete AV block; QRS prolongation (overdose)**

EENT: Blurred vision, auditory disturbance

GI: Nausea, vomiting, anorexia, diarrhea, *dry mouth,* increased appetite, *constipation,* altered taste

GU: Impotence, urinary frequency, retention, *menstrual irregularities*

INTEG: Rash, pruritus, *sweating,* **Stevens-Johnson syndrome**

MISC: Weight loss or gain

Contraindications: Hypersensitivity, eating disorders, seizure disorders

Precautions: Pregnancy (C), breastfeeding, geriatric patients, renal/hepatic disease, recent MI, cranial trauma, seizure disorder

Black Box Warning: Children <18 yr, suicidal thinking/behavior (young adults)

PHARMACOKINETICS

Onset 2-4 wk, half-life 14 hr, extensively metabolized by liver, some conversion to active metabolites, steady state 1½-5 wk

INTERACTIONS

⚠ ***Increase:*** adverse reactions, seizures—levodopa, MAOIs, phenothiazines, antidepressants, benzodiazepines, alcohol, theophylline, systemic steroids

Increase: buPROPion toxicity—ritonavir

Increase: buPROPion level—cimetidine

Increase: buPROPion effect—CYP2D6/CYP2B6 inhibitors

Decrease: buPROPion effect—carbamazepine, cimetidine, phenobarbital, phenytoin or other products (CYP450, CYP2D6)

Decrease: buPROPion effect—CYP2D6, CYP2B6 inducers

Drug/Herb

Increase: CNS depression—hops, kava, lavender

Increase: anticholinergic effect—belladonna, corkwood, jimsonweed

NURSING CONSIDERATIONS

Assess:

- Hepatic/renal function in patients with hepatic or kidney impairment
- For increased risk of seizures; if patient has excessively used CNS depressants and OTC stimulants, dosage of buPROPion should not be exceeded
- For smoking cessation after 7-12 wk; if progress has not been made, product should be discontinued
- Mental status: mood, sensorium, affect, suicidal tendencies, increase in psychiatric symptoms

Administer:

PO route

- When switching to Aplenzin from Wellbutrin, Wellbutrin SR or XL, use these equivalents 174 mg buPROPion HBr = 150 mg buPROPion HCl; 348 mg buPROPion HBr = 300 mg buPROPion HCl; 522 mg buPROPion HBr = 450 mg buPROPion HCl
- Do not break, crush, or chew sus rel, ext rel tab
- In evenly spaced times to prevent seizures; seizure risk increases with high doses
- Increased fluids, bulk in diet if constipation occurs
- With food or milk for GI symptoms
- Sugarless gum, hard candy, or frequent sips of water for dry mouth
- Avoid giving at night to prevent insomnia

Perform/provide:

- Assistance with ambulation during beginning therapy, since sedation occurs
- Safety measures, primarily in geriatric patients

Evaluate:

- Therapeutic response: decreased depression, ability to function in daily activities, ability to sleep throughout the night, smoking cessation

Teach patient/family:

- That therapeutic effects may take 2-4 wk; not to increase dose without prescriber's approval; that treatment for smoking cessation lasts 7-12 wk
- To use caution in driving, other activities requiring alertness; sedation, blurred vision may occur
- To avoid alcohol ingestion, other CNS depressants, alcohol may increase risk of seizures
- Not to use with nicotine patches unless directed by prescriber, may increase B/P
- To notify prescriber immediately if urinary retention occurs
- That risk of seizures is increased when dose is exceeded, or if patient has seizure disorder

⚠ That suicidal ideas, behaviors, hostility, depression may occur in children or young adults

- To notify prescriber if pregnancy is suspected or planned

Treatment of overdose: ECG monitoring; lavage, activated charcoal; administer anticonvulsant

*busPIRone (℞)

(byoo-spye'rone)

BuSpar, BuSpar Dividose, VanSpar

Func. class.: Antianxiety, sedative

Chem. class.: Azaspirodecanedione

Do not confuse:
busPIRone/buPROPion

Action: Acts by inhibiting the action of serotonin (5-HT); has shown little potential for abuse, a good choice in substance abuse

Uses: Management and short-term relief of generalized anxiety disorders

Unlabeled uses: Autism

DOSAGE AND ROUTES

- *Adult:* **PO** 5 mg tid; may increase by 5 mg/day q2-3days, max 60 mg/day

Autism with anxiety (unlabeled)

- *Adult:* **PO** 5-15 mg tid after titration, max 60 mg/day
- *Child ≥5 yr:* **PO** 0.2-0.6 mg/kg/day, max 60 mg/day; use titration to higher dose

Available forms: Tabs 5, 7.5, 10, 15, 30 mg

SIDE EFFECTS

CNS: Dizziness, headache, depression, stimulation, insomnia, nervousness, light-headedness, numbness, paresthesia, incoordination, nightmares, *tremors,* excitement, involuntary movements, confusion, akathisia, hostility

CV: Tachycardia, palpitations, hypo/hypertension, **CVA, CHF, MI**

EENT: Sore throat, tinnitus, blurred vision, nasal congestion; red, itching eyes; change in taste, smell

GI: Nausea, dry mouth, diarrhea, constipation, flatulence, increased appetite, rectal bleeding

GU: Frequency, hesitancy, menstrual irregularity, change in libido

INTEG: Rash, edema, pruritus, alopecia, dry skin

MISC: Sweating, fatigue, weight gain, fever

MS: Pain, weakness, muscle cramps, spasms

RESP: Hyperventilation, chest congestion, shortness of breath

Contraindications: Children <18 yr, hypersensitivity

Precautions: Pregnancy (B), breastfeeding, geriatric patients, impaired hepatic/renal function

PHARMACOKINETICS

Peak 40-90 min, half-life 2-3 hr, rapidly absorbed, metabolized by liver (CYP3A4), excreted in feces, protein binding 86%

INTERACTIONS

Increase: busPIRone—product metabolized by CYP450, 3A4 (erythromycin, itra-

conazole, nefazodone, ketoconazole, ritonavir)
Increase: B/P—procarbazine, MAOIs; do not use together
Increase: CNS depression—psychotropic products, alcohol (avoid use)
Increase: serotonin syndrome—SSRIs
Decrease: busPIRone effects—rifampin
Decrease: busPIRone action—products induced by CYP3A4 (rifampin, phenytoin, phenobarbital, carbamazepine, dexamethasone)

Drug/Herb

Increase: CNS depression—cowslip, kava, Queen Anne's lace, valerian

Drug/Food

Increase: peak concentration of busPIRone—grapefruit juice

NURSING CONSIDERATIONS

Assess:

- B/P (lying, standing), pulse; if systolic B/P drops 20 mm Hg, hold product, notify prescriber
- CNS reactions, since some reactions may be unpredictable
- Mental status: mood, sensorium, affect, sleeping pattern, drowsiness, dizziness; withdrawal symptoms when dose is reduced or product discontinued

Administer:

- With food or milk for GI symptoms, avoid grapefruit juice
- Crushed if patient unable to swallow medication whole
- Sugarless gum, hard candy, frequent sips of water for dry mouth

Perform/provide:

- Assistance with ambulation during beginning therapy; drowsiness, dizziness occur
- Safety measures if drowsiness occurs
- Check to see PO medication swallowed

Evaluate:

- Therapeutic response: decreased anxiety, restlessness, sleeplessness

Teach patient/family:

- That product may be taken consistently with or without food
- To avoid OTC preparations unless approved by prescriber; avoid large amounts of grapefruit juice
- To avoid activities requiring alertness, since drowsiness may occur
- To avoid alcohol ingestion, other psychotropic medications, unless directed by prescriber
- Not to discontinue medication abruptly after long-term use; if dose is missed, do not double
- To rise slowly because fainting may occur, especially geriatric patients
- That drowsiness may worsen at beginning of treatment
- That 1-2 wk of therapy may be required before therapeutic effects occur

⚠ High Alert

busulfan (℞)

(byoo-sul′fan)

Busulfex, Myleran

Func. class.: Antineoplastic alkylating agent
Chem. class.: Bifunctional alkylating agent

Do not confuse:

Myleran/Leukeran

Action: Changes essential cellular ions to covalent bonding with resultant alkylation; this interferes with normal biologic function of DNA; activity is not phase specific; action is due to myelosuppression

Uses: Chronic myelocytic leukemia, bone marrow ablation, stem cell transplant preparation in CML

DOSAGE AND ROUTES

Chronic myelocytic (granulocytic) leukemia

- *Adult:* **PO** 4-8 mg/day initially, reduce dose if WBC reach 30,000-40,000/mm^3, stop if WBC ≤20,000/mm^3, maintenance 1-3 mg/day
- *Child:* **PO** 0.06-0.12 mg/kg/day or 1.8-4.6 mg/m^2/day; discontinue if WBC ≤20,000/mm^3

Allogenic hemopoietic stem cell transplantation in chronic myelogenous leukemia

• *Adult:* **IV** 0.8 mg/kg over 2 hr, q6hr × 4 days (total 16 doses); give cyclophosphamide **IV** 60 mg/kg over 1 hr daily for 2 days, starting after 16th dose of busulfan

Available forms: Tabs 2 mg; inj 6 mg/ml

SIDE EFFECTS

PO route

CV: Hypotension, **thrombosis,** *chest pain,* **tachycardia, atrial fibrillation, heart block, pericardial effusion, cardiac tamponade** (high dose with cyclophosphamide)

GI: Anorexia, constipation, diarrhea, dry mouth, nausea, vomiting

RESP: **Alveolar hemorrhage,** atelectasis, cough, hemoptysis, hypoxia, pleural effusion, pneumonia, sinusitis, **pulmonary fibrosis**

IV route

CNS: **Cerebral hemorrhage, coma, seizures,** *anxiety, depression, dizziness, headache,* encephalopathy, *weakness,* mental changes

EENT: Pharyngitis, epistaxis, cataracts

GI: Nausea, vomiting, *diarrhea, weight loss*

GU: Impotence, sterility, amenorrhea, gynecomastia, **renal toxicity,** hyperuremia, adrenal insufficiency–like syndrome

HEMA: **Thrombocytopenia, leukopenia, pancytopenia, severe bone marrow depression**

INTEG: Dermatitis, hyperpigmentation, alopecia

OTHER: **Chromosomal aberrations**

RESP: **Irreversible pulmonary fibrosis,** pneumonitis

Contraindications: Pregnancy (D) 3rd trimester, breastfeeding, radiation, chemotherapy, blastic phase of chronic myelocytic leukemia, hypersensitivity

Precautions: Childbearing-age women and men, leukopenia, anemia, hepatotoxicity, renal toxicity, seizures, tumor lysis syndrome, hyperkalemia, hyperphosphatemia, hypocalcemia, hyperuricemia

Black Box Warning: Thrombocytopenia, neutropenia, secondary malignancy

PHARMACOKINETICS

Well absorbed orally, excreted in urine, crosses placenta, excreted in breast milk, half-life 2.5 hr

INTERACTIONS

Increase: hepatotoxicity—thioguanine

Increase: cardiac tamponade—cyclophosphamide

Increase: toxicity—other antineoplastics, radiation

Increase: risk for bleeding—anticoagulants, salicylates

Increase: antibody response—live virus vaccines

Decrease: busulfan level—phenytoin

Decrease: busulfan clearance—acetaminophen, itraconazole

Drug/Lab Test

False positive: breast, bladder, cervix, lung cytology tests

NURSING CONSIDERATIONS

Assess:

• CBC, differential, platelet count weekly; withhold product if WBC is $<15,000/mm^3$ or platelet count is $<150,000/mm^3$; notify prescriber of results; institute thrombocytopenia precautions; levels to withhold product will be different in children

• Bone marrow status prior to chemotherapy; seizure history

• Pulmonary function tests, chest x-ray films before, during therapy; chest film should be obtained q2wk during treatment; pulmonary fibrosis may occur up to 10 yr after treatment with busulfan

• Renal studies: BUN, serum uric acid, urine CCr before, during therapy; monitor ALT, alk phos, bilirubin, uric acid before and during treatment

• I&O ratio; report fall in urine output <30 ml/hr

- Monitor for cold, fever, sore throat (may indicate beginning infection)
- Bleeding: hematuria, guaiac, bruising or petechiae, mucosa or orifices q8hr, no rectal temps
- Dyspnea, crackles, nonproductive cough, chest pain, tachypnea
- Inflammation of mucosa, breaks in skin; use viscous xylocaine for oral pain

Administer:

PO route

- Give at same time daily, on empty stomach

IV route

- Prepared in biologic cabinet, using gloves, gown, mask; dilute with 10 times volume of product with D_5W or 0.9% NaCl, (0.5 mg/ml). When withdrawing product, use needle with 5-micron filter provided, remove amount needed, remove filter and inject product into diluent; always add product to diluent, not vice versa; stable for 8 hr room temperature (using D_5W) or 12 hr refrigerated
- Give antiemetics before IV route, on schedule
- In those with history of seizures give phenytoin prior to IV route, to prevent seizures (using 0.9% NaCl) give by central venous catheter over 2 hr q6hr × 4 days, use infusion pump, do not admix

Perform/provide:

- Comprehensive oral hygiene
- Strict medical asepsis, protective isolation if WBC levels are low
- Increase fluid intake to 2-3 L/day to prevent urate deposits, calculi formation
- Store in tight container

Evaluate:

- Therapeutic response: decreased exacerbations of chronic myelocytic leukemia

Teach patient/family:

- About protective isolation precautions
- To avoid use of products containing aspirin or ibuprofen, razors, commercial mouthwash
- Use effective contraception during and at least 3 mo after treatment; avoid breastfeeding
- To report signs of anemia (fatigue, headache, irritability, faintness, shortness of breath); symptoms of infection; jaundice
- To report symptoms of bleeding (hematuria, tarry stools)
- Avoid vaccinations
- Avoid crowds, or persons with known infections
- That impotence or amenorrhea can occur, are reversible after discontinuing treatment
- To report any changes in breathing or coughing even several years after treatment

butoconazole vaginal antifungal

See Appendix B

butorphanol (℞)

(byoo-tor′fa-nole)

Stadol

Func. class.: Opioid analgesic

Chem. class.: Mixed opioid antagonist, partial agonist

Controlled Substance Schedule IV

Do not confuse:

Stadol/Haldol/sotalol

Action: Depresses pain impulse transmission at the spinal cord level by interacting with opioid receptors

Uses: Moderate to severe pain, general anesthesia induction/maintenance, headache, migraine, preanesthesia

Unlabeled uses: Pruritus

DOSAGE AND ROUTES

- *Adult:* **IM** 1-4 mg q3-4hr prn; **IV** 0.5-2 mg q3-4hr prn; **INTRANASAL,** 1 spray in one nostril q3-4hr; may give another dose 1-1½ hr later; repeat if needed q3-4hr
- *Geriatric:* **IV** ½ adult dose at 2× the interval; **INTRANASAL,** may repeat q1-2hr

Severe pain

- *Adult:* **INTRANASAL,** 1 spray in each nostril q3-4hr

Renal dose

• *Adult:* **INTRANASAL** max 1 mg, followed by 1 mg in 90-120 min; **IM/IV** give 50% of dose (0.5 mg **IV,** 1 mg **IM**) do not repeat within 6 hr

Opioid induced pruritus (unlabeled)

• *Adult:* **INTRANASAL** 1 mg (1 spray) in each nostril q4-6hr

Intractable pruritus with inflammatory skin or systemic disease (unlabeled)

• *Adult:* **INTRANASAL** 1-4 mg/day

Available forms: Inj 1, 2 mg/ml; nasal spray 10 mg/ml

SIDE EFFECTS

CNS: Drowsiness, dizziness, confusion, headache, sedation, euphoria, weakness, hallucinations

CV: Palpitations, bradycardia, hypotension

EENT: Tinnitus, blurred vision, miosis, diplopia, nasal congestion, unpleasant taste

GI: Nausea, vomiting, anorexia, constipation, cramps

GU: Increased urinary output, dysuria, urinary retention

INTEG: Rash, urticaria, bruising, flushing, diaphoresis, pruritus

RESP: **Respiratory depression,** pulmonary hypertension, URI, sinusitis

Contraindications: Hypersensitivity to this product or preservative, addiction (opioid), CHF, myocardial infarction

Precautions: Pregnancy (C), breastfeeding, children <18 yr, addictive personality, increased intracranial pressure, respiratory depression, renal/hepatic disease, bowel impaction

PHARMACOKINETICS

Metabolized by liver, excreted by kidneys, crosses placenta, excreted in breast milk, half-life 2-9 hr, protein binding 80%

IM: Onset 5-10 min, peak ½ hr, duration 3-4 hr

INTRANASAL: Onset within 15 min, peak 1-2 hr, duration 4-5 hr

IV: Onset 1 min, peak 5 min, duration 2-4 hr

INTERACTIONS

⚠ Severe, fatal reactions: MAOIs

Increase: CNS effects—alcohol, opioids, sedative/hypnotics, antipsychotics, skeletal muscle relaxants, other CNS depressants

Drug/Herb

Increase: anticholinergic effect—corkwood

Increase: CNS depression—chamomile, Jamaican dogwood, kava, lavender, mistletoe, nettle, pokewood, poppy, senega, skullcap, St. John's wort, valerian

NURSING CONSIDERATIONS

Assess:

• For decreasing output; may indicate urinary retention

⚠ For withdrawal symptoms in opioid-dependent patients: PE, vascular occlusion, abscesses, ulcerations

• CNS changes: dizziness, drowsiness, hallucinations, euphoria, LOC, pupil reaction

• Allergic reactions: rash, urticaria

• Respiratory dysfunction: respiratory depression, character, rate, rhythm; notify prescriber if respirations are <10/min

• Need for pain medication, physical dependence

Administer:

• With antiemetic if nausea, vomiting occur

• When pain is beginning to return; determine dosage interval by patient response

IM route

• Deeply in large muscle mass

IV route

• Undiluted at a rate of <2 mg/>3-5 min, titrate to patient response

Syringe compatibilities: Atropine, chlorproMAZINE, cimetidine, diphenhydrAMINE, droperidol, fentanyl, hydrOXYzine, meperidine, methotrimeprazine, metoclopramide, midazolam, morphine, pentazocine,perphenazine, prochlorperazine, promethazine, scopolamine, thiethylperazine

Y-site compatibilities: Allopurinol, amifostine, aztreonam, cefepime, cisatracurium, cladribine, DOXOrubicin liposome, enalaprilat, esmolol, filgrastim, fludarabine, granisetron, labetalol, melphalan, paclitaxel, piperacillin/tazobactam, propofol, remifentanil, sargramostim, tenoposide, thiotepa, vinorelbine

Perform/provide:

- Storage in light-resistant container at room temperature
- Assistance with ambulation
- Safety measures: night-light, call bell within easy reach, especially geriatric patients

Evaluate:

- Therapeutic response: decrease in pain

Teach patient/family:

- To report any symptoms of CNS changes, allergic reactions
- That physical dependency may result when used for extended periods
- That withdrawal symptoms may occur: nausea, vomiting, cramps, fever, faintness, anorexia
- To avoid hazardous activities; drowsiness may occur

Treatment of overdose: Naloxone HCl (Narcan) 0.2-0.8 mg IV, O_2, IV fluids, vasopressors

calcitonin (rDNA) (℞)

(kal-sih-toh′nin)

Fortical

calcitonin (salmon) (℞)

Calcimar, Miacalcin, Miacalcin Nasal Spray, Osteocalcin, Salmonine

Func. class.: Parathyroid agents (calcium regulator)

Chem. class.: Polypeptide hormone

Action: Decreases bone resorption, blood calcium levels; increases deposits of calcium in bones; opposes parathyroid hormone

Uses: Paget's disease, postmenopausal osteoporosis, hypercalcemia

Unlabeled uses: Bone/neuropathic pain, diabetic neuropathy, osteolytic metastases, osteoporosis prophylaxis, phantom limb pain

DOSAGE AND ROUTES

rDNA

Paget's disease

- *Adult:* **SUBCUT** 0.5 mg/day initially; may require 0.5 mg bid × 6 mo, then decrease until symptoms reappear

Salmon

Postmenopausal osteoporosis

- *Adult:* **SUBCUT/IM** 100 international units/day; **INTRANASAL** 200 international units (1 spray) daily alternating nostrils daily, activate pump before 1st dose

Paget's disease

- *Adult:* **SUBCUT/IM** 100 international units/day, maintenance 50-100 international units daily or every other day

Hypercalcemia

- *Adult:* **SUBCUT/IM** 4 international units/kg q12hr, increase to 8 international units/kg q12hr if response is unsatisfactory

Neuropathic pain/phantom limb pain/diabetic neuropathy (unlabeled)

- *Adult:* **IV/SUBCUT** 100-200 international units/day; in phantom limb pain **IV** 200 international units over 20 min, and a second inf was given

Bone pain due to osteoporosis, osteolytic metastases (unlabeled)

- *Adult:* **SUBCUT** 50-100 international units/day or **INTRANASAL** 200 international units in one nostril/day

Available forms: Inj 200 international units/ml; nasal spray 200 international units/actuation

SIDE EFFECTS

CNS: Headache, tetany, chills, weakness, dizziness, fever

CV: Chest pressure

EENT: Nasal congestion, eye pain

GI: Nausea, diarrhea, vomiting, anorexia, abdominal pain, salty taste, epigastric pain

GU: Diuresis, nocturia, urine sediment, frequency

INTEG: Rash, flushing, pruritus of earlobes, edema of feet, reaction at inj site
MS: Swelling, tingling of hands, backache
RESP: Dyspnea
SYST: **Anaphylaxis**

Contraindications: Hypersensitivity to this product or fish

Precautions: Pregnancy (C), breastfeeding, children, renal disease, osteogenic sarcoma, pernicious anemia

PHARMACOKINETICS

IM/SUBCUT: Onset 15 min, peak 4 hr, duration 8-24 hr, metabolized by kidneys, excreted as inactive metabolites via kidneys

INTERACTIONS

Decrease: lithium effect

NURSING CONSIDERATIONS

Assess:

- GI symptoms, polyuria, flushing, head swelling, tingling, headache; may indicate hypercalcemia
- Nutritional status; diet for sources of vit D (milk, some seafood), calcium (dairy products, dark green vegetables), phosphates
- BUN, creatinine, uric acid, chloride, electrolytes, urine pH, urinary calcium, magnesium, phosphate, urinalysis (calcium should be kept at 9-10 mg/dl, vit D 50-135 international units/dl), alk phos baseline, q3-6mo, monitor urine hydroproline in Paget's disease, biochemical markers of bone formation/absorption, radiologic evidence of fracture; bone density (osteoporosis)
- Increased product level, since toxic reactions occur rapidly; have parenteral calcium on hand if calcium level drops too low; check for tetany (irritability, paresthesia, nervousness, muscle twitching, seizures, tetanic spasms)
- Urine for sediment

Administer:

SUBCUT route (rDNA)

- By SUBCUT route only; rotate inj sites; use within 6 hr of reconstitution; give at bedtime to minimize nausea, vomiting

IM route (Salmon)

- After test dose of 10 international units/ml, 0.1 ml intradermally; watch 15 min; give only with epinephrine and emergency meds available
- IM inj slowly in deep muscle mass; rotate sites, preferred route if volume is >2 ml

Perform/provide:

- Storage at <77° F (25° C); protect from light

Evaluate:

- Therapeutic response: calcium levels 9-10 mg/dl, decreasing symptoms of Paget's disease

Teach patient/family:

- The method of inj if patient will be responsible for self-medication
- To report difficulty swallowing or any change in side effects to prescriber immediately

Nasal

- To use alternating nostrils for nasal spray; use after allowing to warm to room temperature, prime to get full spray

calcitriol (℞)

(kal-sih-try′ole)

Calcijex, Rocaltrol, vitamin D_3

Func. class.: Parathyroid agent (calcium regulator)

Chem. class.: Vit D hormone

Do not confuse:
calcitriol/Calciferol

Action: Increases intestinal absorption of calcium, provides calcium for bones, increases renal tubular resorption of phosphate

Uses: Hypocalcemia in chronic renal disease, hyperparathyroidism pseudohypoparathyroidism

Unlabeled uses: Osteopetrosis, osteoporosis, osteoporosis prophylaxis, rickets, familial hypophosphatemia

DOSAGE AND ROUTES

Hypocalcemia

• *Adult:* **IV** 0.5 mcg tid, initially; may increase by 0.25-0.5 mcg/dose q2-4wk; 0.5-3 mcg tid maintenance

Predialysis

• *Adult:* **PO** 0.25 mcg/day, max 0.5 mcg/day

Hypocalcemia during chronic dialysis

• *Adult:* **PO** 0.5-3 mcg/day
• *Child:* **PO** 0.25-2 mcg/day

Renal osteodystrophy

• *Adult:* **PO** 0.25 mcg every other day-3 mcg/day
• *Child:* **PO** 0.014-0.041 mcg/kg/day

Hypoparathyroidism

• *Adult:* **PO** 0.25-2.7 mcg/day
• *Child <1 yr:* **PO** 0.04-0.08 mcg/kg/day
• *Child 1-5 yr:* **PO** 0.25-0.75 mcg daily

Rickets (unlabeled)

• *Adult and child:* **PO** 1 mcg/day

Familial hypophosphatemia (unlabeled)

• *Adult:* **PO** 2 mcg/day
• *Child:* **PO** 0.015-0.02 mcg/kg/day, maintenance 0.03-0.06 mcg/kg/day; max 2 mcg/day

Postmenopausal osteoporosis (unlabeled)

• *Adult:* **PO** 0.25 mcg bid, adjust to serum calcium levels

Osteopetrosis (unlabeled)

• *Child:* **PO** High-dose calcitriol 1-2 mcg/kg/day, given in 4-6 divided doses

Osteoporosis prophylaxis in corticosteroid therapy (unlabeled)

• *Adult:* **PO** 0.5-1 mcg/day

Available forms: Caps 0.25, 0.5 mcg; inj 1 mcg; oral sol 1 mcg/ml

SIDE EFFECTS

CNS: Drowsiness, headache, vertigo, fever, lethargy, hallucinations
CV: Palpitations, hypertension
EENT: Blurred vision, photophobia
GI: Nausea, diarrhea, vomiting, jaundice, anorexia, dry mouth, constipation, cramps, metallic taste
GU: Polyuria, hypercalciuria, hyperphosphatemia, hematuria, thirst
MS: Myalgia, arthralgia, decreased bone development, weakness
SYST: **Anaphylaxis**

Contraindications: Hypersensitivity, hyperphosphatemia, hypercalcemia, vit D toxicity

Precautions: Pregnancy (C), breastfeeding, renal calculi, CV disease

PHARMACOKINETICS

PO: Absorbed readily from GI tract, peak 10-12 hr, duration 3-5 days, half-life 3-6 hr, undergoes hepatic recycling, excreted in bile

INTERACTIONS

• Hypercalcemia: thiazide diuretics, calcium supplements
• Cardiac dysrhythmias: cardiac glycosides, verapamil
• Hypermagnesemia: magnesium antacids
• Toxicity: other vit D products

Increase: metabolism of vit D—phenytoin

Decrease: absorption of calcitriol—cholestyramine, mineral oil, fat-soluble vitamins

Drug/Food

• Large amounts of high-calcium foods may cause hypercalcemia

Drug/Lab Test

False increase: cholesterol
Interference: alk phos, electrolytes

NURSING CONSIDERATIONS

Assess:

• BUN, urinary calcium, AST, ALT, cholesterol, creatinine, albumin, uric acid, chloride, magnesium, electrolytes, urine pH, phosphate; may increase calcium, should be kept at 9-10 mg/dl, vit D 50-135 international units/dl, phosphate 70 mg/dl
• Alk phos; may be decreased
• For increased product level, since toxic reactions may occur rapidly
• For dry mouth, metallic taste, polyuria, bone pain, muscle weakness, headache, fatigue, change in LOC, dysrhythmias, in-

creased respirations, anorexia, nausea, vomiting, cramps, diarrhea, constipation; may indicate hypercalcemia

- Renal status: decreased urinary output (oliguria, anuria), edema in extremities, weight gain 5-7 lb, periorbital edema
- Nutritional status, diet for sources of vit D (milk, some seafood); calcium (dairy products, dark green vegetables), phosphates (dairy products) must be avoided

Administer:

PO route

- Do not break, crush, or chew caps
- Give without regard to meals

IV route

- Give by direct IV over 1 min

Perform/provide:

- Storage protected from light, heat, moisture
- Restriction of sodium, potassium if required
- Restriction of fluids if required for chronic renal failure

Evaluate:

- Therapeutic response: calcium 9-10 mg/dl, decreasing symptoms of hypocalcemia, hypoparathyroidism

Teach patient/family:

- The symptoms of hypercalcemia (renal stones, nausea, vomiting, anorexia, lethargy, thirst, bone or flank pain)
- About foods rich in calcium
- To avoid products with sodium: cured meats, dairy products, cold cuts, olives, beets, pickles, soups, meat tenderizers in chronic renal failure
- To avoid products with potassium: oranges, bananas, dried fruit, peas, dark green leafy vegetables, milk, melons, beans in chronic renal failure
- To avoid OTC products containing calcium, potassium, or sodium in chronic renal failure
- To avoid all preparations containing vit D
- To monitor weight weekly, maintain fluid intake

calcium carbonate (PO-OTC, IV-℞)

Alka-Mints, Amitone, Apo-Cal ✤, Calcarb, Calci-Chew, Calci-Mix, Calcilac, Calcite ✤, Calglycine ✤, Cal-Plus, Calsan ✤, Caltrate, Chooz, Dicarbosil, Equilet, Liquid-Cal, Maalox Antacid Caplets, Mallamint, Mylanta Lozenges ✤, Nephro-Calci, Nu-Cal ✤, Os-Cal 500, Oysco, Oystercal, Oyst-Cal, Rolaids Calcium Rich, Surpass, Surpass Extra Strength, Titralac, Tums, Tums E-X

calcium acetate (OTC)

(kal'see-um ass'e-tate)

Calphron, PhosLo

Func. class.: Antacid, calcium supplement

Chem. class.: Calcium product

Do not confuse:

Os-Cal/Asacol

Action: Neutralizes gastric acidity

Uses: Antacid, calcium supplement; not suitable for chronic therapy, hyperphosphatemia, hypertension in pregnancy, osteoporosis, prevention, treatment of hypocalcemia, hypoparathyroidism

Unlabeled uses: Duodenal ulcer, PMS, stress gastritis

DOSAGE AND ROUTES

Antacid

- *Adult:* **PO** 0.5-1.5 g or 2 pieces of gum 1 hr after meals and at bedtime

Prevention of hypocalcemia, depletion, osteoporosis

- *Adult:* **PO** 1200 mg/day

Hyperphosphatemia

- *Adult:* **PO** 1 g or more in divided doses

Hypertension in pregnancy

- *Adult:* **PO** 500 mg tid during 3rd trimester

Duodenal ulcer/stress gastritis (unlabeled)
- *Adult:* **PO** 80-140 mEq q1-3hr

PMS (unlabeled)
- *Adult:* **PO** (Tums EX, Tums Calcium for Life PMS) Chew 2 tabs bid

Available forms: *calcium carbonate:* chewable tabs 350, 420, 450, 500, 750, 1000, 1250 mg; tabs 500, 600, 650, 667, 1000, 1250, 1500 mg; gum 300, 450, 500 mg; susp 1250 mg/5 ml; caps 1250 mg; powder 6.5 g/packet; *calcium acetate:* tabs 250 mg (65 mg Ca), 667 mg (169 mg Ca), 668 mg (169 mg Ca), 1 g (250 mg Ca); caps 500 mg (125 mg Ca)

SIDE EFFECTS

GI: Constipation, anorexia, nausea, vomiting, flatulence, diarrhea, rebound hyperacidity, eructation

GU: Calculi, hypercalciuria

Contraindications: Hypersensitivity, hypercalcemia, hyperparathyroidism, bone tumors

Precautions: Pregnancy (C), breastfeeding, geriatric patients, fluid restriction, decreased GI motility, GI obstruction, dehydration, renal disease

PHARMACOKINETICS

⅓ of dose absorbed by small intestine, onset 20 min, duration 20-180 min, excreted in feces and urine, crosses placenta, must have adequate vit D for absorption

INTERACTIONS

Increase: digoxin toxicity—hypercalcemia

Increase: plasma levels of quinidine, amphetamines

Increase: hypercalcemia—thiazide diuretics

Decrease: levels of salicylates, calcium channel blockers, ketoconazole, iron salts, tetracyclines, fluoroquinolones, phenytoin, etidronate, risedronate, atenolol

Drug/Herb

Increase: action/side effects—lily of the valley, pheasant's eye, shark cartilage, squill

Drug/Lab Test

False increase: chloride

False positive: benzodiazepines

False decrease: magnesium, oxylate, lipase

NURSING CONSIDERATIONS

Assess:
- Calcium (serum, urine), calcium should be 8.5-10.5 mg/dl, urine calcium should be 150 mg/day, monitor weekly
- ⚠ Milk-alkali syndrome: nausea, vomiting, disorientation, headache
- Constipation; increase bulk in the diet if needed
- Hypercalcemia: headache, nausea, vomiting, confusion; hypocalcemia: paresthesia, twitching colic, dysrhythmias, Chvostek's/Trousseau's signs
- Those taking digoxin for toxicity
- Antacid—for abdominal pain, heartburn indigestion before and after administration

Administer:

PO route
- As antacid 1 hr after meals and at bedtime
- As supplement 1½ hr after meals and at bedtime
- Only with regular tablets or capsules; do not give with enteric-coated tablets
- Laxatives or stool softeners if constipation occurs

Evaluate:
- Therapeutic response: absence of pain, decreased acidity; decreased hyperphosphatemia in renal failure (acetate)

Teach patient/family:
- To increase fluids to 2 L unless contraindicated, to add bulk to diet for constipation, notify prescriber of constipation
- Not to switch antacids unless directed by prescriber, not to use as antacid for >2 wk without approval by prescriber
- That therapeutic dose recommendations are figured as elemental calcium

• Avoid excessive use of alcohol, caffeine, tobacco
• Avoid spinach, cereals, dairy products in large amounts

CALCIUM SALTS

calcium chloride (℞)
calcium gluceptate (℞)
calcium gluconate (℞)
Kalcinate
calcium lactate (℞)
Cal-Lac

Func. class.: Electrolyte replacement—calcium product

Action: Cation needed for maintenance of nervous, muscular, skeletal function; enzyme reactions; normal cardiac contractility; coagulation of blood; affects secretory activity of endocrine, exocrine glands

Uses: Prevention and treatment of hypocalcemia, hypermagnesemia, hypoparathyroidism, neonatal tetany, cardiac toxicity caused by hyperkalemia, lead colic, hyperphosphatemia, vit D deficiency, osteoporosis prophylaxis, calcium antagonist toxicity (calcium channel blocker toxicity)

Unlabeled uses: Electrolyte abnormalities in cardiac arrest, CPR

DOSAGE AND ROUTES

Calcium chloride
• *Adult:* **IV** 500 mg-1 g q1-3days as indicated by serum calcium levels, give at <1 ml/min; **IV** 200-800 mg injected in ventricle of heart

Calcium gluceptate
• *Adult:* **IV** 5-20 ml; **IM** 2-5 ml

Calcium gluconate
• *Adult:* **PO** 0.5-2 g bid-qid; **IV** 0.5-2 g at 0.5 ml/min (10% solution); max **IV** dose 3 g
• *Child:* **PO/IV** 500 mg/kg/day in divided doses

Calcium lactate
• *Adult:* **PO** 325 mg-1.3 g tid with meals
• *Child:* **PO** 500 mg/kg/day in divided doses

Available forms: Many; check product listings

SIDE EFFECTS

CV: Shortened QT, heart block, hypotension, bradycardia, **dysrhythmias; cardiac arrest (IV)**
GI: Vomiting, nausea, constipation
HYPERCALCEMIA: Drowsiness, lethargy, muscle weakness, headache, constipation, **coma,** anorexia, nausea, vomiting, polyuria, thirst
INTEG: Pain, burning at IV site, severe venous thrombosis, necrosis, extravasation

Contraindications: Hypercalcemia, digoxin toxicity, ventricular fibrillation, renal calculi

Precautions: Pregnancy (C), breastfeeding, children, respiratory/renal disease, cor pulmonale, digitalized patient, respiratory failure, diarrhea, dehydration

PHARMACOKINETICS

Crosses placenta, enters breast milk, excreted via urine and feces, half-life unknown, protein binding 40%-50%
PO: Onset, peak, duration unknown, absorption from GI tract
IV: Onset immediate, duration ½-2 hr

INTERACTIONS

Increase: milk-alkali syndrome—antacids
Increase: dysrhythmias—digoxin glycosides
Increase: toxicity—verapamil
Increase: hypercalcemia—thiazide diuretics
Decrease: absorption of fluoroquinolones, tetracyclines, iron salts, phenytoin, thyroid hormones, when calcium is taken PO
Decrease: effects of atenolol, verapamil

Drug/Herb
Increase: action/side effects—lily of the valley, pheasant's eye, shark cartilage, squill
Drug/Lab Test
Increase: 11-OHCS
Decrease: 17-OHCS
False decrease: magnesium

NURSING CONSIDERATIONS

Assess:

- ECG for decreased QT and T wave inversion: hypercalcemia, product should be reduced or discontinued, consider cardiac monitoring
- Calcium levels during treatment (8.5-11.5 g/dl is normal level); urine calcium if hypercaluria occurs
- Cardiac status: rate, rhythm, CVP (PWP, PAWP if being monitored directly)
- Hypocalcemia: muscle twitching, paresthesia, dysrhythmias, laryngospasm
- Digitalized patients closely; an increase in calcium, increases digoxin toxicity risk

Administer:

PO route

- With or following meals to enhance absorption

IM route

- IM inj may cause severe burning, necrosis, tissue sloughing; warm sol to body temp before administering (only gluconate/gluceptate)

IV route

- Undiluted or diluted with equal amounts of NS to a 5% sol for inj, give 0.5-1 ml/min
- Through small-bore needle into large vein; if extravasation occurs, necrosis will result (IV)
- Remain recumbent ½ hr after IV dose

Calcium chloride

Additive compatibilities: Amikacin, amphotericin B, ampicillin, ascorbic acid, bretylium, ceftriaxone, cephapirin, chloramphenicol, DOPamine, hydrocortisone, isoproterenol, lidocaine, methicillin, norepinephrine, penicillin G potassium, penicillin G sodium, pentobarbital, phenobarbital, verapamil, vit B/C

Syringe compatibilities: Milrinone

Y-site compatibilities: Inamrinone, DOBUTamine, epinephrine, esmolol, morphine, paclitaxel

Calcium gluceptate

Additive compatibilities: Ascorbic acid inj, isoproterenol, lidocaine, norepinephrine, phytonadione, sodium bicarbonate

Calcium gluconate

Additive compatibilities: Amikacin, aminophylline, ascorbic acid inj, bretylium, cephapirin, chloramphenicol, cisatracurium, corticotropin, dimenhyDRINATE, DOXOrubicin liposome, erythromycin, furosemide, heparin, hydrocortisone, lidocaine, magnesium sulfate, methicillin, norepinephrine, penicillin G potassium, penicillin G sodium, phenobarbital, potassium chloride, remifentanil, tobramycin, vancomycin, verapamil, vit B/C

Syringe compatibilities: Aldesleukin, allopurinol, amifostine, aztreonam, cefazolin, cefepime, ciprofloxacin, cladribine, DOBUTamine, enalaprilat, epinephrine, famotidine, filgrastim, granisetron, heparin/hydrocortisone, labetalol, melphalan, midazolam, netilmicin, piperacillin/tazobactam, potassium chloride, prochlorperazine, propofol, sargramostim, tacrolimus, teniposide, thiotepa, tolazoline, vinorelbine, vit B/C

Perform/provide:

- Seizure precautions: padded side rails, decreased stimuli (noise, light); place airway suction equipment, padded mouth gag if Ca levels are low
- Store at room temperature

Evaluate:

- Therapeutic response: decreased twitching, paresthesias, muscle spasms, absence of tremors, seizures, dysrhythmias, dyspnea, laryngospasm, negative Chvostek's sign, negative Trousseau's sign

Teach patient/family:

- To add foods high in vit D
- To add calcium-rich foods to diet: dairy products, shellfish, dark green leafy vegetables; decrease oxalate-rich and zinc-rich foods: nuts, legumes, chocolate, spinach, soy

• To prevent injuries, avoid immobilization

Rarely Used

calfactant (℞)

(cal-fak'tant)

Infasurf

Func. class.: Natural lung surfactant extract

Uses: Prevention and treatment (rescue) of respiratory distress syndrome in premature infants

DOSAGE AND ROUTES

• *Newborn*: **INTRATRACHEAL INSTILL:** 3 ml/kg of birth weight, given as 2 doses of 1.5 ml/kg, repeat doses of 3 ml/kg of birth wt until up to 3 doses 12 hr apart have been given

Rarely Used

canakinumab

(kan-a-kin-ue-mab)

Ilaris

Func.class.: Monoclonal antibody

Uses: Cryopyrin-associated periodic syndromes (CAPS)

DOSAGE AND ROUTES

• *Adult:* **SUBCUT:** 150 mg q8wk, slowly inject a vial with 1 ml preservative-free, sterile water for injection

Contraindications: Hypersensitivity

candesartan (℞)

(can-deh-sar'tan)

Atacand

Func. class.: Antihypertensive

Chem. class.: Angiotensin II receptor (type AT_1) antagonist

Action: Blocks the vasoconstrictor and aldosterone-secreting effects of angiotensin II; selectively blocks the binding of angiotensin II to the AT_1 receptor found in tissues

Uses: Hypertension, alone or in combination; CHF NYHA Class II-IV and ejection fraction ≤40%

DOSAGE AND ROUTES

• *Adult:* **PO** Single agent 16 mg/day initially in patients who are not volume depleted, range 8-32 mg/day; with diuretic, or volume depletion 2-32 mg/day as single dose or divided bid

Renal disease

• *Adult*: **PO** Give lowest possible dose

Available forms: Tabs 4, 8, 16, 32 mg

SIDE EFFECTS

CNS: Dizziness, fatigue, headache

CV: Chest pain, peripheral edema, hypotension

EENT: Sinusitis, rhinitis, pharyngitis

GI: Diarrhea, nausea, abdominal pain, vomiting

GU: **Renal failure**

MS: Arthralgia, pain

RESP: Cough, upper respiratory infection

SYST: **Angioedema**

Contraindications: Hypersensitivity

Black Box Warning: Pregnancy (D) 2nd/3rd trimesters

Precautions: Pregnancy (C) 1st trimester, breastfeeding, children, geriatric patients, hypersensitivity to ACE inhibitors, volume-depletion, renal/hepatic impairment

PHARMACOKINETICS

Peak 3-4 hr, protein binding 99%, half-life 9-12 hr, extensively metabolized, excreted in urine (33%) and feces (67%)

INTERACTIONS

Increase: lithium level—lithium

Increase: hypokalemia—potassium, potassium-sparing diuretics

Increase: hypotension—ACE inhibitors, β-blockers, calcium channel blockers, α-blockers

Decrease: effect—salicylates, NSAIDs

Drug/Herb

Increase: effect—barberry, betony, black catechu, black cohosh, bloodroot, broom, burdock, cat's claw, dandelion, goldenseal, Irish moss, Jamaican dogwood, kelp, khella, mistletoe, parsley, Queen Anne's lace, rue

Increase: toxicity/death—aconite

Increase or decrease: effect—astragalus, cola tree

Decrease: effect—coltsfoot, guarana, khat, licorice, yohimbine

NURSING CONSIDERATIONS

Assess:

- For angioedema: facial swelling, difficulty breathing (rare)
- For pregnancy, this product can cause fetal death when given in pregnancy
- Response and adverse reactions especially in renal disease
- B/P, pulse q4hr; note rate, rhythm, quality; electrolytes: K, Na, Cl; baselines in renal/hepatic studies before therapy begins

Administer:

- Without regard to meals

Evaluate:

- Therapeutic response: decreased B/P

Teach patient/family:

- To comply with dosage schedule, even if feeling better
- To notify prescriber of mouth sores, fever, swelling of hands or feet, irregular heartbeat, chest pain
- That excessive perspiration, dehydration, vomiting, diarrhea may lead to fall in B/P; to consult prescriber if these occur
- That product may cause dizziness, fainting; light-headedness may occur
- To rise slowly to sitting or standing position to minimize orthostatic hypotension
- To notify prescriber immediately if pregnant; not to use during breastfeeding
- To avoid all OTC medications, unless approved by prescriber; to inform all health care providers of medication use
- To use proper technique for obtaining B/P and acceptable parameters

capecitabine (℞)

(cap-eh-sit'ah-bean)

Xeloda

Func. class.: Antineoplastic, antimetabolite

Chem. class.: Fluoropyrimidine carbamate

Do not confuse:

Xeloda/Xenical

Action: Competes with physiologic substrate of DNA synthesis, thus interfering with cell replication in the S phase of cell cycle (before mitosis), also interferes with RNA and protein synthesis; product is converted to 5-FU

Uses: Monotherapy for paclitaxel, anthracycline resistant, metastatic breast, colorectal cancer when 5-FU monotherapy is preferred; treatment of colorectal cancer patients who have undergone complete resection of their primary tumor

Unlabeled uses: Pancreatic cancer, metastatic colorectal cancer

DOSAGE AND ROUTES

- *Adult:* **PO** 2500 mg/m^2/day in 2 divided doses q12hr at end of meal × 2 wk, then 1 wk rest period; given in 3 wk cycles; may be combined with docetaxel, when capecitabine dose is lowered; follow the NCIC (National Cancer Institute of Canada) common toxicity criteria

Renal dose

- *Adult:* **PO** CCr 30-50 ml/min, decrease initial dose to 75% of usual dose

Available forms: Tabs 150, 500 mg

SIDE EFFECTS

CNS: Dizziness, *headache, paresthesia, fatigue,* insomnia

GI: Nausea, vomiting, anorexia, diarrhea, stomatitis, abdominal pain, constipation, dyspepsia, **intestinal obstruction, necrotizing enterocolitis**

HEMA: **Neutropenia, lymphopenia, thrombocytopenia,** anemia

INTEG: Hand and foot syndrome, dermatitis, nail disorder

OTHER: Hyperbilirubinemia, *eye irritation, edema, myalgia,* limb pain, *pyrexia*, dehydration
RESP: Cough, dyspnea
Contraindications: Pregnancy (D), hypersensitivity to 5-FU, infants, severe renal impairment (CCr <30 ml/min), DPD deficiency
Precautions: Breastfeeding, children, geriatric patients, renal/hepatic disease

PHARMACOKINETICS

Readily absorbed, peak 1½ hr, food decreases absorption, extensively metabolized in the liver, elimination half-life 45 min

INTERACTIONS

Increase: toxicity—leucovorin
Increase: capecitabine levels—antacids (aluminum, magnesium)
Increase: phenytoin level—phenytoin
Black Box Warning: *Increase:* bleeding risk—anticoagulants
Drug/Food
Increase: absorption, give within 30 min of a meal

NURSING CONSIDERATIONS

Assess:
- CBC (RBC, Hct, Hgb), differential, platelet count weekly; withhold product if WBC is <4000/mm^3, platelet count is <75,000/mm^3, or RBC, Hct, Hgb low; notify prescriber of these results; frequently monitor INR in those receiving warfarin concurrently
- Renal studies: BUN, serum uric acid, urine CCr, electrolytes before and during therapy
- Monitor temp q4hr; fever may indicate beginning infection; no rectal temps
- Hepatic studies before and during therapy: bilirubin, ALT, AST, alk phos, as needed or monthly
- Bleeding: hematuria, heme-positive stools, bruising or petechiae, mucosa or orifices q8hr
- Dyspnea, crackles, unproductive cough, chest pain, tachypnea, fatigue, increased pulse, pallor, lethargy; personality changes, with high doses
- For hand and foot syndrome: paresthesia, tingling, painful/painless swelling, blistering, erythema with severe pain of hands or feet
- For toxicity: severe diarrhea, nausea, vomiting, stomatitis, fever
- Buccal cavity q8hr for dryness, sores or ulceration, white patches, oral pain, bleeding, dysphagia
- GI symptoms: frequency of stools, cramping; if severe diarrhea occurs, fluid and electrolytes may need to be given

Administer:
- With water within ½ hr of breakfast and dinner

Perform/provide:
- Rinsing of mouth tid-qid with water, club soda; brushing of teeth bid-tid with soft brush or cotton-tipped applicators for stomatitis; use unwaxed dental floss

Evaluate:
- Therapeutic response: decreased tumor size, spread of malignancy

Teach patient/family:
- To avoid foods with citric acid, hot or rough texture if stomatitis is present; take with water within 30 min of end of meal
- To avoid pregnancy while on this product; to avoid breastfeeding
- Not to double dose, if dose is missed
- ⚠ To immediately report severe diarrhea, vomiting, stomatitis, fever over 100° F (37.8° C), hand and foot syndrome, anorexia
- To report signs of infection: increased temp, sore throat, flulike symptoms
- To report signs of anemia: fatigue, headache, faintness, shortness of breath, irritability
- To report bleeding; to avoid use of razors, commercial mouthwash

captopril (℞)

(kap'toe-pril)

Capoten, Novo-Captopril ✦

Func. class.: Antihypertensive

Chem. class.: Angiotensin-converting enzyme (ACE) inhibitor

Do not confuse:
captopril/Capitrol/carvedilol

Action: Selectively suppresses renin-angiotensin-aldosterone system; inhibits ACE; preventing conversion of angiotensin I to angiotensin II

Uses: Hypertension, CHF, left ventricular dysfunction after MI, diabetic nephropathy

Unlabeled uses: Acute MI, hypertensive emergency/urgency, scleroderma renal crisis (SRC)

DOSAGE AND ROUTES

Malignant hypertension

- *Adult:* **PO** 25 mg increasing q2hr until desired response, not to exceed 450 mg/day

Hypertension

- *Adult:* **PO** initial dose: 12.5-25 mg bid-tid; may increase to 50 mg bid-tid at 1-2 wk intervals; usual range: 25-150 mg bid-tid; max 450 mg
- *Child:* **PO** 0.3-0.5 mg/kg/dose, titrate up to 6 mg/kg/day in 2-4 divided doses
- *Neonate:* **PO** 0.05-0.1 mg/kg bid-tid, may increase as needed

CHF

- *Adult:* **PO** 25 mg bid-tid; may increase to 50 mg bid-tid; after 14 days, may increase to 150 mg tid if needed

LVD after MI

- *Adult:* **PO** 50 mg tid, may begin treatment 3 days after MI; give 6.25 mg as a single dose, then 12.5 mg tid, increase to 25 mg tid for several days, then to 50 mg tid

Diabetic nephropathy

- *Adult:* **PO** 25 mg tid

Renal dose

- *Adult:* **PO** CCr >50 ml/min, no change; CCr 10-50 ml/min, decrease dose by 25%; CCr <10 ml/min, decrease dose by 50%

Acute MI (unlabeled)

- *Adult:* **PO** 6.25-12.5 mg tid, increased to 25 mg tid gradually

Hypertensive emergency/urgency (unlabeled)

- *Adult:* **PO** 25 mg, may repeat q30min

Available forms: Tabs 12.5, 25, 50, 100 mg

SIDE EFFECTS

CNS: Fever, chills

CV: *Hypotension,* postural hypotension, *tachycardia,* angina

GI: Loss of taste, increased LFTs

GU: Impotence, dysuria, nocturia, proteinuria, **nephrotic syndrome, acute reversible renal failure**, polyuria, oliguria, urinary frequency

HEMA: **Neutropenia, agranulocytosis, pancytopenia, thrombocytopenia,** anemia

INTEG: Rash, pruritus

MISC: **Angioedema,** hyperkalemia

RESP: **Bronchospasm,** *dyspnea, cough*

Contraindications: Breastfeeding, children, hypersensitivity, heart block, potassium-sparing diuretics, bilateral renal artery stenosis, angioedema

Black Box Warning: Pregnancy (D)

Precautions: Dialysis patients, hypovolemia, leukemia, scleroderma, SLE, blood dyscrasias, CHF, diabetes mellitus, thyroid/renal/hepatic disease, COPD, asthma

PHARMACOKINETICS

Peak 1 hr; duration 2-6 hr; half-life <2 hr, increased in renal disease; metabolized by liver (metabolites); excreted in urine; crosses placenta; excreted in breast milk, small amounts; protein binding 25%-30%

INTERACTIONS

- Do not use with potassium-sparing diuretics, sympathomimetics, potassium supplements

Increase: possible toxicity—lithium, digoxin
Increase: hypoglycemia—insulin, oral antidiabetics
Increase: hypotension—diuretics, other antihypertensives, phenothiazines, nitrates, acute alcohol ingestion
Decrease: captopril effect—antacids, NSAIDs, salicylates

Drug/Herb
Increase: toxicity/death—aconite
Increase: antihypertensive effect—barberry, betony, black catechu, black cohosh, bloodroot, broom, burdock, cat's claw, dandelion, goldenseal, Irish moss, Jamaican dogwood, kelp, khella, mistletoe, parsley
Increase or decrease: antihypertensive effect—astragalus, cola tree
Decrease: antihypertensive effect—coltsfoot, guarana, khat, licorice, yohimbe

Drug/Lab Test
Increase: AST, ALT, alk phos, bilirubin, uric acid, glucose
False positive: urine acetone, ANA titer

NURSING CONSIDERATIONS

Assess:

- Blood studies: decreased platelets; WBC with differential baseline and periodically q3mo, if neutrophils <1000/mm^3, discontinue treatment (recommended with collagen-vascular or renal disease)
- B/P, pulse rates baseline, frequently
- Renal studies: protein, BUN, creatinine; watch for raised levels that may indicate nephrotic syndrome
- Baselines in renal, hepatic studies before therapy begins and periodically, increased LFTs, uric acid and glucose may be increased
- Edema in feet, legs daily, weight daily in CHF
- Allergic reaction: rash, fever, pruritus, urticaria; discontinue product if antihistamines fail to help
- Symptoms of CHF: edema, dyspnea, wet crackles, B/P

Administer:

- 1 hr before or 2 hr after meals
- May crush tab and dissolve in water; give within ½ hr; make sure tab is completely dissolved

Perform/provide:

- Storage in tight container at 86° F (30° C) or less

Evaluate:

- Therapeutic response: decrease in B/P in hypertension, edema, moist crackles (CHF)

Teach patient/family:

- That tabs may be crushed and mixed with food; to take 1 hr before or 2 hr after meals; not to discontinue product abruptly; if dose is missed, take as soon as remembered, but not if almost time for next dose; do not double doses
- Not to use OTC products (cough, cold, or allergy) unless directed by prescriber; avoid salt substitutes, high-potassium or high-sodium foods
- To avoid sunlight or wear sunscreen if in sunlight; photosensitivity may occur
- To comply with dosage schedule, even if feeling better
- To rise slowly to sitting or standing position to minimize orthostatic hypotension
- To notify prescriber of mouth sores, sore throat, fever, swelling of hands or feet, irregular heartbeat, chest pain, signs of angioedema
- That excessive perspiration, dehydration, vomiting; diarrhea may lead to fall in B/P; consult prescriber if these occur
- That dizziness, fainting, lightheadedness may occur during first few days of therapy
- That skin rash or impaired perspiration may occur
- How to take B/P and when to notify prescriber
- To report if pregnancy is suspected or planned

Treatment of overdose: 0.9% NaCl IV/INF; hemodialysis

carbachol ophthalmic

See Appendix B

carbamazepine (℞)

(kar-ba-maz′e-peen)

Apo-Carbamazepine ✦, Carbatrol, Epitol, Equetro, Novo-Carbamaz ✦, Tegretol, Tegretol CR ✦, Tegretol-XR, Teril

Func. class.: Anticonvulsant

Chem. class.: Iminostilbene derivative

Do not confuse:
Tegretol/Toradol

Action: Exact mechanism unknown; appears to decrease polysynaptic responses and block posttetanic potentiation

Uses: Tonic-clonic, complex-partial, mixed seizures; trigeminal neuralgia, bipolar disorder

Unlabeled uses: Neurogenic pain, psychotic behavior with dementia, diabetic neuropathy, agitation, hiccups

DOSAGE AND ROUTES

Seizures

- *Adult and child >12 yr:* **PO** 200 mg bid, may be increased by 200 mg/day in weekly intervals, give in divided doses q6-8hr; maintenance 800-1200 mg/day, max 1600 mg/day (adult); max child 12-15 yr 1000 mg/day; max child >15 yr 1200 mg/day; adjustment is needed to minimum dose to control seizures; **EXT REL** give bid; rectal administration of **ORAL SUSP** 200 mg/10 ml or 6 mg/kg as a single dose
- *Child 6-12 yr:* **PO** tabs 100 mg bid or susp 50 mg qid; may increase by <100 mg q wk; max 1000 mg/day **EXT REL** tabs daily-bid
- *Child <6 yr:* **PO** 10-20 mg/kg/day in 2-3 divided doses, may increase q wk

Trigeminal neuralgia

- *Adult:* **PO** 100 mg bid with meals; may increase 100 mg q12hr until pain subsides, not to exceed 1200 mg/day; maintenance is 200-400 mg bid

Bipolar disorder

- *Adult:* **PO** (Equetro only) 200 mg bid, may adjust dose by 200 mg/day to desired response, max 1600 mg/day

Agitation due to dementia (unlabeled)

- *Adult:* **PO** 100 mg bid, may increase to 250-300 mg/day

Hiccups (unlabeled)

- *Adult:* **PO** 200 mg tid

Available forms: Chewable tabs 100, 200 mg; tabs 200 mg; ext rel tabs (XR) 100, 200, 400 mg; oral susp 100 mg/5 ml; ext rel caps 100, 200, 300 mg

SIDE EFFECTS

CNS: Drowsiness, dizziness, unsteadiness, confusion, fatigue, **paralysis,** headache, hallucinations, **worsening of seizures,** speech disturbance, **suicidal thoughts/behaviors**

CV: **Hypertension, CHF, dysrhythmias, AV block,** hypotension, aggravation of cardiac artery disease

EENT: Tinnitus, dry mouth, blurred vision, diplopia, nystagmus, conjunctivitis

ENDO: SIADH (geriatric patients)

GI: Nausea, constipation, diarrhea, anorexia, vomiting, abdominal pain, stomatitis, glossitis, increased hepatic enzymes, **hepatitis, hepatic porphyria**

GU: Frequency, retention, albuminuria, glycosuria, impotence, increased BUN, **renal failure**

HEMA: **Thrombocytopenia, leukopenia, agranulocytosis, leukocytosis, aplastic anemia, eosinophilia,** increased PT

INTEG: Rash, **Stevens-Johnson syndrome,** urticaria, photosensitivity, **toxic epidermal necrolysis**

RESP: Pulmonary hypersensitivity (fever, dyspnea, pneumonitis)

Contraindications: Pregnancy (D), hypersensitivity to carbamazepine or tricyclics, AV or bundle branch block

Black Box Warning: Bone marrow depression

Precautions: Breastfeeding, children <6 yr, glaucoma, cardiac/renal/hepatic disease, psychosis, alcoholism, hepatic porphyria

Black Box Warning: Hematologic disease, Asian patients, agranulocytosis, leukopenia, neutropenia, thrombocytopenia

PHARMACOKINETICS

Onset slow; peak 4-5 hr; metabolized by liver; excreted in urine, feces; crosses placenta, blood-brain barrier; excreted in breast milk; half-life 18-65 hr then 8-29 hr after 1st month; protein binding 76%; metabolized by CYP3A4

INTERACTIONS

• CNS toxicity: lithium

⚠ Fatal reaction: MAOIs

Increase: carbamazepine levels—CYP3A inhibitors (cimetidine, clarithromycin, danazol, diltiazem, erythromycin, fluoxetine, fluvoxamine, isoniazid, propoxyphene, valproic acid, verapamil, voriconazole)

Increase: effects of desmopressin, lithium, lypressin, vasopressin

Decrease: carbamazepine effect—CYP1A2, CYP2C9 substrates

Decrease: effect of CYP3A inducers

Decrease: effects of benzodiazepines, doxycycline, felbamate, haloperidol, oral contraceptives, phenobarbital, phenytoin, primidone, theophylline, thyroid hormones, warfarin

Decrease: carbamazepine levels—CYP3A4 inducers (cisplatin, darunavir, delavirdine, DOXOrubicin, felbamate, nefazodone, oxcarbazepine, phenobarbital, phenytoin, primidone, rifampin, theophylline)

Drug/Herb

Decrease: carbamazepine metabolism, increased levels—quinine, ginkgo

Decrease: anticonvulsant effect—ginseng, santonica

Drug/Food

Increase: peak concentration of carbamazepine—grapefruit juice

NURSING CONSIDERATIONS

Assess:

• Asian patients for serious skin reaction; genetic test prior to administration

• For seizures: character, location, duration, intensity, frequency, presence of aura

• For trigeminal neuralgia: facial pain including location, duration, intensity, character, activity that stimulates pain

• Renal studies: urinalysis, BUN, urine creatinine q3mo

⚠ Blood studies: RBC, Hct, Hgb, reticulocyte counts q wk for 4 wk then q3-6mo, if on long-term therapy; if myelosuppression occurs, product should be discontinued

• Hepatic studies: ALT, AST, bilirubin

• Product levels during initial treatment or when changing dose; should remain at 4-12 mcg/ml; anorexia may indicate increased blood levels

⚠ Mental status: mood, sensorium, affect, behavioral changes, suicidal thoughts/behaviors; if mental status changes, notify prescriber

• Eye problems: need for ophthalmic examinations before, during, after treatment (slit lamp, funduscopy, tonometry)

• Allergic reaction: purpura, red, raised rash; if these occur, product should be discontinued

⚠ Blood dyscrasias: fever, sore throat, bruising, rash, jaundice

⚠ Toxicity: bone marrow depression, nausea, vomiting, ataxia, diplopia, CV collapse, Stevens-Johnson syndrome

Administer:

PO route

• Do not crush or chew ext rel tab; ext rel cap may be opened and the beads sprinkled over food; patient should chew chewable tab, not swallow it whole

• With food, milk to decrease GI symptoms

• Shake oral susp before use

• Mix an equal amount of water, D_5W, 0.9% NaCl when giving by NG tube, flush tube with 100 ml of above sol

Perform/provide:
- Storage at room temperature
- Hard candy, gum, frequent rinsing for dry mouth

Evaluate:
- Therapeutic response: decreased seizure activity, document on patient's chart

Teach patient/family:
- To carry emergency ID stating patient's name, products taken, condition, prescriber's name, phone number
- To avoid driving, other activities that require alertness usually the first 3 days of treatment
- Not to discontinue medication quickly after long-term use
- To report immediately chills, rash, light-colored stools, dark urine, yellowing of skin and eyes, abdominal pain, sore throat, mouth ulcers, bruising, blurred vision, dizziness
- That urine may turn pink to brown

Treatment of overdose: Lavage, VS

carbidopa-levodopa (℞)

(kar-bi-doe′pa) (lee-voe-doe′pa)

Atamet, carbidopa/levodopa, Parcopa, Sinemet, Sinemet CR

Func. class.: Antiparkinson agent
Chem. class.: Catecholamine

Action: Decarboxylation of levodopa in periphery is inhibited by carbidopa; more levodopa is made available for transport to brain and conversion to DOPamine in the brain

Uses: Parkinson's disease, parkinsonism resulting from carbon monoxide, chronic manganese intoxication, cerebral arteriosclerosis

Unlabeled uses: Restless leg syndrome

DOSAGE AND ROUTES

Beginning therapy for those not taking levodopa

- *Adult:* **PO** 25 mg carbidopa/100 mg levodopa tid, may increase daily or every other day by 1 tab to desired response (8 tabs/day); **EXT REL** tabs 50 mg carbidopa/200 mg levodopa bid

For those not taking levodopa ER

- 50 mg carbidopa/200 mg levodopa bid

For those taking levodopa ER

- Begin treatment with 10% more levodopa/day given q4-8hr, may increase or decrease dose q3days

For those taking levodopa <1.5 g/day

- *Adult:* **PO** 25 mg carbidopa/100 mg levodopa tid-qid, may increase daily to desired response

For those taking levodopa >1.5 g/day

- *Adult:* **PO** 25 mg carbidopa/250 mg levodopa tid-qid, may increase daily to desired response

Restless leg syndrome (RLS) (unlabeled)

- *Adult:* **PO** 25 mg carbidopa/100 mg levodopa, 1 tab at bedtime, may repeat if awakening within 2 hr or 50 mg carbidopa/200 mg levodopa sus rel tab 1-2 tabs 1 hr before bedtime

Available forms: Tabs 10 mg carbidopa/100 mg levodopa, 25 mg carbidopa/100 mg levodopa, 25 mg carbidopa/250 mg levodopa; ext rel tab 25 mg/100 mg, 50 mg carbidopa/200 mg levodopa (Sinemet CR); oral disintegrating tab (Parcopa) 10 mg carbidopa/100 mg levodopa, 25 mg carbidopa/100 mg levodopa; 25 mg carbidopa/250 mg levodopa

SIDE EFFECTS

CNS: Involuntary choreiform movements, hand tremors, fatigue, headache, anxiety, twitching, numbness, weakness, confusion, agitation, insomnia, nightmares, psychosis, hallucination, hypomania, severe depression, dizziness

CV: Orthostatic hypotension, tachycardia, hypertension, palpitation

EENT: Blurred vision, diplopia, dilated pupils

GI: Nausea, vomiting, anorexia, abdominal distress, dry mouth, flatulence, dysphagia, bitter taste, diarrhea, constipation

HEMA: **Hemolytic anemia, leukopenia, agranulocytosis**

INTEG: Rash, sweating, alopecia

MISC: Urinary retention, incontinence, weight change, dark urine

Contraindications: Hypersensitivity, closed-angle glaucoma, malignant melanoma, history of malignant melanoma or undiagnosed skin lesions resembling melanoma

Precautions: Pregnancy (C), breastfeeding, diabetes, closed-angle glaucoma, respiratory/cardiac/renal/hepatic disease, MI with dysrhythmias, seizures, peptic ulcer, depression

PHARMACOKINETICS

PO: Onset 30 min, peak 1-3 hr, excreted in urine (metabolites)

EXT REL: Onset 4-6 hr

INTERACTIONS

- Hypertensive crisis: nonselective MAOIs

Increase: effects of levodopa—antacids, metoclopramide

Decrease: effects of levodopa—anticholinergics, hydantoins, papaverine, pyridoxine, benzodiazepines

Decrease: absorption of levodopa—protein

Drug/Herb

Increase: Parkinson symptoms—kava, octacosanol

Decrease: action, increased EPS—Indian snakeroot

Drug/Lab Test

Increase: BUN, AST, ALT, bilirubin, alk phos, LDH

Decrease: VMA, BUN, creatinine

False positive: urine ketones (dipstick), Coombs' test

False negative: urine glucose

False increase: uric acid, urine protein

NURSING CONSIDERATIONS

Assess:

- For Parkinson's symptoms: tremors, pill rolling, drooling, akinesia, rigidity before and during treatment
- B/P, respiration; orthostatic B/P
- Mental status: affect, mood, behavioral changes, depression, complete suicide assessment
- Muscle twitching, blepharospasm that may indicate toxicity
- Renal, hepatic, hematopoietic tests, also for diabetes, acromegaly if on long-term therapy

Administer:

- Pyridoxine (B_6) is not effective in reversing Sinemet or Sinemet CR

PO route

- Do not crush or chew ext rel tabs; they may be broken in half
- Oral disintegrating tab by gently removing from bottle, placing on tongue and swallowing with saliva; after it dissolves, liquid is not necessary
- Product until NPO before surgery
- Adjust dosage to response
- With meals if GI symptoms occur; limit protein taken with product
- Only after nonselective MAOIs have been discontinued for 2 wk; if previously on levodopa, discontinue for at least 12 hr before change to carbidopa-levodopa

Evaluate:

- Therapeutic response: decrease in akathisia/bradykinesis, tremor, rigidity, improved mood

Teach patient/family:

- To change positions slowly to prevent orthostatic hypotension
- To report side effects: twitching, eye spasms; indicate overdose
- To use product as prescribed; if discontinued abruptly, parkinsonian crisis, neuroleptic malignant syndrome (NMS) may occur; gradually taper
- That urine, sweat may darken
- To use physical activities to maintain mobility, lessen spasms
- That improvement may not occur for 2-4 mo

⚠ High Alert

carboplatin (℞)
(kar-boe-pla'-tin)
Paraplatin, Paraplatin-AQ ♣
Func. class.: Antineoplastic alkylating agent
Chem. class.: Platinum coordination compound

Do not confuse:
carboplatin/cisplatin
Paraplatin/Platinol

Action: Produces interstrand DNA cross-links and, to a lesser extent, DNA-protein cross-links; activity is not cell cycle phase specific

Uses: Initial treatment of advanced ovarian cancer in combination with other agents; palliative treatment of ovarian carcinoma recurrent after treatment with other antineoplastic agents

Unlabeled uses: Acute lymphocytic leukemia (ALL), acute myelogenous leukemia (AML), bladder/breast/head/neck/lung/testicular cancer, bone marrow ablation, malignant glioma, neuroblastoma, non-Hodgkin's lymphoma, osteogenic sarcoma, soft-tissue sarcoma, stem-cell transplant preparation, Wilm's tumor, stage I seminoma

DOSAGE AND ROUTES

- *Adult (single agent):* **IV INF** initially 300 mg/m^2 given with cyclophosphamide, q4-6wk; refractory tumors 360 mg/m^2 single dose, may repeat q4wk, as needed, do not repeat until neutrophils >2000/mm^3 and platelets >100,000/mm^3

Renal dose

- *Adult (single agent):* **IV INF** CCr 41-59 ml/min 250 mg/m^2, CCr 16-40 ml/min 200 mg/m^2, do not use in CCr <15 ml/min

AML/ALL (unlabeled)

- *Adult:* **CONT IV INF** 315 mg/m^2/day × 5 days

Wilms' tumor (unlabeled)

- *Child:* **IV** 160 mg/m^2 × 5 days with etoposide

Osteogenic sarcoma (unlabeled)

- *Child:* **IV** 200-300 mg/m^2 with ifosfamide and etoposide (ICE)

Neuroblastoma/soft-tissue sarcoma (unlabeled)

- *Child:* **IV** 300-600 mg/m^2 q4wk or 400 mg/m^2/day for 2 days q4wk or 160 mg/m^2/day × 5 days q4wk

Available forms: Lyophilized powder for inj 50-, 150-, 450-mg vials; aqueous sol for inj 50 mg/5-ml vial, 150 mg/15-ml vial, 450 mg/45-ml vial, 600 mg/60-ml vial

SIDE EFFECTS

CNS: **Seizures, central neurotoxicity,** *peripheral neuropathy,* dizziness, confusion

CV: Cardiac abnormalities

EENT: Tinnitus, hearing loss, *vestibular toxicity,* visual changes

GI: *Severe nausea, vomiting,* diarrhea, weight loss, mucositis, anorexia, constipation, taste change

HEMA: **Thrombocytopenia, leukopenia, pancytopenia, neutropenia, anemia,** bleeding

INTEG: *Alopecia,* dermatitis, rash, erythema, pruritus, urticaria

META: Hypomagnesemia, hypocalcemia, hypokalemia, hyponatremia, hyperuremia

SYST: **Anaphylaxis**

Contraindications: Pregnancy (D), breastfeeding, hypersensitivity to this product, platinum products, mannitol; significant bleeding, aluminum products used to prepare or administer carboplatin

Black Box Warning: Severe bone marrow depression

Precautions: Geriatric patients, radiation therapy within 1 mo, other cancer chemotherapy within 1 mo, renal/hepatic disease

Black Box Warning: Anemia, infection

PHARMACOKINETICS

Initial half-life 1-2 hr, postdistribution half-life 2½-6 hr, not bound to plasma proteins, excreted by the kidneys

INTERACTIONS

Increase: nephrotoxicity or ototoxicity—aminoglycosides, amphotericin B
Increase: bleeding risk—aspirin, NSAIDs, thrombolytic agents
Increase: toxicity—radiation, bone marrow suppressants
Increase: myelosuppression—myelosuppressives
Decrease: phenytoin levels
Drug/Lab Test
Increase: AST, BUN, alk phos, bilirubin, creatinine

NURSING CONSIDERATIONS

Assess:
- CBC, differential, platelet count weekly; withhold product if neutrophil count is <2000/mm³ or platelet count is <100,000/mm³; notify prescriber of results
- Renal studies: BUN, creatinine, serum uric acid, urine CCr before and during therapy; I&O ratio; report fall in urine output to <30 ml/hr
- Monitor temp q4hr (may indicate beginning of infection)
- Hepatic studies tests before and during therapy (bilirubin, AST, ALT, LDH) as needed or monthly; jaundice of skin, sclera, dark urine, clay-colored stools, itchy skin, abdominal pain, fever, diarrhea

⚠ For anaphylaxis: hypotension, rash, pruritus, wheezing, tachycardia; notify prescriber after discontinuing product, resuscitation equipment should be available
- Bleeding; hematuria, stool guaiac, bruising or petechiae, mucosa or orifices q8hr
- Dyspnea, crackles, unproductive cough, chest pain, tachypnea
- Effects of alopecia on body image; discuss feelings about body changes

Administer:
- Antiemetic 30-60 min before giving product and prn for vomiting

IV route
- Using cytotoxic handling procedures
- After diluting 10 mg/ml of sterile water for inj, D_5W, NS (10 mg/ml); then further dilute with the same sol 1-4 mg/ml; give over 15 min or more (intermittent INF)
- IV INF over 5-6 hr; do not use needles or IV administration sets containing aluminum; may cause precipitate or loss of potency

Additive compatibilities: Cisplatin, etoposide, floxuridine, ifosfamide, ifosfamide/etoposide, paclitaxel

Solution compatibilities: D_5/0.2% NaCl, D_5/0.45% NaCl, D_5/0.9% NaCl, 0.9% NaCl, D_5W, sterile water for inj

Y-site compatibilities: Allopurinol, amifostine, aztreonam, cefepime, cladribine, DOXOrubicin liposome, filgrastim, fludarabine, granisetron, melphalan, ondansetron, paclitaxel, piperacillin/tazobactam, propofol, sargramostim, teniposide, thiotepa, vinorelbine

Perform/provide:
- Storage protected from light at room temperature; reconstituted sol stable for 8 hr at room temperature

Evaluate:
- Therapeutic response: decreasing size of tumor, spread of malignancy

Teach patient/family:
- To report ringing/roaring in the ears, numbness, tingling in face, extremities, weight gain
- That impotence or amenorrhea can occur; reversible after treatment is discontinued, to notify prescriber if pregnancy is suspected or planned; contraception should be used if patient is fertile
- Not to breastfeed during treatment
- To avoid OTC products with aspirin, NSAIDs, alcohol or receiving vaccinations during treatment

⚠ To notify prescriber immediately of fever, fatigue, sore throat, bleeding, bruis-

ing, chills, back pain, blood in stools, dyspnea
• That hair may be lost during treatment; a wig or hairpiece may make patient feel better; new hair may be different in color, texture
• To avoid crowds, persons with known infections; avoid use of razors, stiff-bristle toothbrush

carboprost (℞)

(kar'boe-prost)
Hemabate, Prostin/15M ♣
Func. class.: Oxytocic, abortifacient
Chem. class.: Prostaglandin

Action: Stimulates uterine contractions, causing complete abortion in approximately 16 hr
Uses: Abortion at 13-20 wk gestation, postpartum hemorrhage caused by uterine atony not controlled by other methods
Unlabeled uses: Hemorrhagic cystitis

DOSAGE AND ROUTES

To induce abortion
• *Adult:* **IM** 250 mcg, then 250 mcg q1½-3½hr, may increase to 500 mcg if no response, not to exceed 12 mg total dose
Postpartum hemorrhage
• *Adult:* **IM** 250 mcg, repeat at 15-90 min intervals; max total dosage 2 mg
Hemorrhagic cystitis (unlabeled)
• *Adult:* **INTRAVESICULAR** 0.8 mg/dl in 50 ml of saline instilled into the bladder for 60 min, q6hr × 4 doses
Available forms: Inj 250 mcg/ml

SIDE EFFECTS

CNS: *Fever, chills,* headache
GI: *Nausea, vomiting, diarrhea*
Contraindications: Hypersensitivity, severe CV/respiratory/renal/hepatic disease, PID
Precautions: Pregnancy (C), asthma, anemia, jaundice, diabetes mellitus, seizure disorders, past uterine surgery

PHARMACOKINETICS

Peak 15-60 min, excreted in urine (major metabolites)

INTERACTIONS

Increase: action—other oxytocics

NURSING CONSIDERATIONS

Assess:
• B/P, pulse; watch for change that may indicate hemorrhage
• Respiratory rate, rhythm, depth; notify prescriber of abnormalities
• For length, duration of contraction; notify prescriber of contractions lasting over 1 min or absence of contractions; watch for signs of uterine rupture
• For incomplete abortion, pregnancy must be terminated by another method; product is teratogenic
Administer:
• In deep muscle mass; rotate inj sites if additional doses are given
Perform/provide:
• Storage in refrigerator
Evaluate:
• Therapeutic response: expulsion of fetus, control of bleeding
Teach patient/family:
• To report increased blood loss, abdominal cramps, increased temp, foul-smelling lochia

carisoprodol (℞)

(kar-eye-soe-proe'dole)
carisoprodol, Soma, Soprodol 350, Vanadom
Func. class.: Skeletal muscle relaxant, central acting
Chem. class.: Meprobamate congener

Do not confuse:
Soma/Soma Compound
Action: Depresses CNS by blocking interneuronal activity in descending reticular formation, spinal cord, producing sedation

Uses: Relieving pain, stiffness in musculoskeletal disorders

DOSAGE AND ROUTES

• *Adult and child >12 yr:* **PO** 350 mg tid and at bedtime, max 3 wk

Available forms: Tabs 350 mg

SIDE EFFECTS

CNS: Dizziness, weakness, drowsiness, headache, tremor, depression, insomnia, ataxia, irritability, **seizures**

CV: Postural hypotension, tachycardia

EENT: Diplopia, temporary loss of vision

GI: Nausea, vomiting, hiccups, epigastric discomfort

HEMA: Eosinophilia

INTEG: Rash, pruritus, fever, facial flushing, **erythema multiforme**

RESP: Asthmatic attacks

SYST: **Angioedema, anaphylaxis**

Contraindications: Hypersensitivity, intermittent porphyria

Precautions: Pregnancy (C), breastfeeding, geriatric patients, Asian patients, renal/hepatic disease, addictive personality

PHARMACOKINETICS

PO: Onset ½ hr; peak 4 hr; duration 4-6 hr; extensively metabolized by liver, substrate of CYP2C19; excreted in urine; crosses placenta; excreted in breast milk (large amounts); half-life 8 hr

INTERACTIONS

• Do not use together with meprobamate

Increase: CNS depression—alcohol, tricyclics, opioids, barbiturates, sedatives, hypnotics

Drug/Herb

Increase: CNS depression—chamomile, kava, skullcap, valerian

Drug/Lab Test

Increase: AST, alk phos, blood glucose

NURSING CONSIDERATIONS

Assess:

• Pain, stiffness, mobility, activities of daily living baseline and throughout treatment

• ECG in seizure patients; poor seizure control has occurred with patients taking this product

• Idiosyncratic reaction (weakness, dizziness, blurred vision, confusion, euphoria), anaphylaxis within a few minutes or hours of 1st to 4th dose

• Allergic reactions: rash, fever, respiratory distress

• CNS depression: dizziness, drowsiness, psychiatric symptoms

Administer:

• With meals for GI symptoms

• For short term 2-3 wk, potential for habituation

Perform/provide:

• Storage in tight container at room temperature

• Assistance with ambulation if dizziness, drowsiness occurs, especially geriatric patients

Evaluate:

• Therapeutic response: decreased pain, spasticity

Teach patient/family:

• Not to take with alcohol, other CNS depressants

• To avoid hazardous activities if drowsiness, dizziness occur

• To avoid using OTC medication: cough preparations, antihistamines, unless directed by prescriber

• To report allergic reaction immediately: rash, swelling of tongue/lips, hives, dyspnea

Treatment of overdose: Activated charcoal, dialysis, lavage

⚠ High Alert

carmustine (℞)

(kar-mus′teen)

BiCNU, Gliadel

Func. class.: Antineoplastic alkylating agent

Chem. class.: Nitrosourea

Action: Alkylates DNA, RNA; is able to inhibit enzymes that allow synthesis of amino acids in proteins; activity is not cell cycle phase specific

Uses: Brain tumors such as glioblastoma, medulloblastoma, brain stem glioma, astrocytoma, ependymoma, metastatic brain tumors; multiple myeloma (with predniSONE), non-Hodgkin's, Hodgkin's disease, other lymphomas; GI, breast, bronchogenic, renal carcinomas, other lymphomas; wafer, as adjunct to surgery/radiation in newly diagnosed high-grade malignant glioma patients; in recurrent glioblastoma multiforme patients as an adjunct to surgery

Unlabeled uses: Malignant melanoma, bone marrow ablation, mycosis fungoides, stem cell transplant preparation

DOSAGE AND ROUTES

• *Adult:* **IV** 75-100 mg/m^2 over 1-2 hr × 2 days or 150-200 mg/m^2 × 1 dose q6-8wk or 40 mg/m^2/day × 5 days q6wk; if WBC is 3000-3999/mm^3 give 50% of dose; if WBC is 2000-2999/mm^3 and platelets are 25,000-75,000/mm^3 give 25% of dose; withhold dose if WBC is <2000/mm^3 and platelets are <25,000/mm^3

• *Adult:* **INTRACAVITARY** Up to 8 wafers inserted into resection cavity

Malignant melanoma (unlabeled)

• *Adult:* **IV** 75-100 mg/m^2/day for 2 days q6wk or 200 mg/m^2 as a slow inf q6-8wk

Stem cell transplant/bone marrow ablation (unlabeled)

• *Adult:* **IV** 450-600 mg/m^2 as a single dose or two divided doses q12hr at a rate of no more than 3 mg/m^2/min

Available forms: Powder for inj 100 mg; wafer 7.7 mg (intracavitary)

SIDE EFFECTS

GI: Nausea, vomiting, anorexia, stomatitis, **hepatotoxicity**

GU: Azotemia, **renal failure**

HEMA: **Thrombocytopenia, leukopenia, myelosuppression, anemia**

INTEG: Pain, burning, hyperpigmentation at inj site

RESP: **Fibrosis, pulmonary infiltrate**

SYST: **Secondary malignant neoplastic disease**

Contraindications: Pregnancy (D), breastfeeding, hypersensitivity, leukopenia, thrombocytopenia

Precautions: Dental disease, extravasation, females, infection, leukopenia, neutropenia, secondary malignancy, thrombocytopenia

Black Box Warning: Bone marrow suppression, pulmonary fibrosis

PHARMACOKINETICS

Degraded within 15 min; crosses blood-brain barrier; 70% excreted in urine within 96 hr; 10% excreted as CO_2, fate of 20% is unknown

INTERACTIONS

Increase: bleeding risk—aspirin, anticoagulants

Increase: myelosuppression—myelosuppressive agents

Increase: toxicity: other antineoplastics, radiation, cimetidine

Increase: adverse reactions, decreased antibody reaction—live vaccines

Decrease: effects of digoxin, phenytoins

NURSING CONSIDERATIONS

Assess:

• CBC, differential, platelet count weekly; withhold product if WBC is <4000 or platelet count is <100,000; notify prescriber of results

• Hepatic studies: AST, ALT, bilirubin

• Pulmonary function tests, chest x-ray films before, during therapy; chest film

should be obtained q2wk during treatment; monitor for dyspnea, cough, pulmonary fibrosis; infiltrate occurs after high doses or several low-dose courses
- Renal studies: BUN, serum uric acid, urine CCr before, during therapy; I&O ratio; report fall in urine output of 30 ml/hr
- Monitor for cold, cough, fever (may indicate beginning infection)
- Bleeding: hematuria, guaiac, bruising, petechiae, mucosa, orifices q8hr

Administer:
- Blood transfusions or RBC colony-stimulating factors to counter anemia
- Antiemetic 30-60 min before giving product to prevent vomiting
- All medications PO, if possible, avoid IM inj if platelets are <100,000/mm^3

Wafer route
- If wafers are broken in several pieces, they should not be used
- Foil pouches may be kept at room temperature for 6 hr if unopened

IV route
- Prepare in biologic cabinet wearing gown, gloves, mask; avoid contact with skin; can cause burning and staining the skin brown; use cytotoxic handling procedures
- After diluting 100 mg product/3 ml ethyl alcohol (provided); then further dilute 27 ml sterile H_2O for inj; then dilute with 100-500 ml 0.9% NaCl or D_5W, give over 1 hr or more, reduce rate if discomfort is felt; use only glass containers, protect from light
- Flush IV line after carmustine with 10 ml 0.9% NaCl to prevent irritation at site

Y-site compatibilities: Amifostine, aztreonam, cefepime, filgrastim, fludarabine, granisetron, melphalan, ondansetron, piperacillin/tazobactam, sargramostim, teniposide, thiotepa, vinorelbine

Perform/provide:
- Storage of reconstituted sol in refrigerator for 24 hr, or room temperature for 8 hr, protect from light
- Rinsing of mouth tid-qid with water or club soda; use of sponge brush for stomatitis
- Warm compresses at inj site for inflammation; reduce flow rate if patient complains of burning at inf site

Evaluate:
- Therapeutic response: decreasing size of tumor, spread of malignancy

Teach patient/family:
- To report any changes in breathing or coughing, avoid smoking
- To avoid foods with citric acid, hot or rough texture if stomatitis is present; to report any bleeding, white spots, ulceration in mouth to prescriber; tell patient to examine mouth daily
- To avoid use of aspirin, ibuprofen, razors, commercial mouthwash
- To report signs of anemia (fatigue, irritability, shortness of breath, faintness); to report signs of infection (sore throat, fever); pulmonary toxicity can occur up to 15 yr after treatment
- To use contraception during treatment; avoid breastfeeding
- Not to receive live vaccines during treatment

carteolol ophthalmic

See Appendix B

carvedilol (℞)

(kar-ved′i-lole)

Coreg, Coreg CR

Func. class.: Antihypertensive, α/β-adrenergic blocker

Do not confuse:
carvedilol/captopril/carteolol

Action: A mixture of nonselective α/β-adrenergic blocking activity; decreases cardiac output, exercise-induced tachycardia, reflex orthostatic tachycardia; causes vasodilation, reduction in peripheral vascular resistance

Uses: Essential hypertension alone or in combination with other antihypertensives, CHF, LV dysfunction following MI, cardiomyopathy

Unlabeled uses: Angina, pediatric patients

DOSAGE AND ROUTES

Essential hypertension

• *Adult:* **PO** 6.25 mg bid × 7-14 days; if tolerated well, then increase to 12.5 mg bid × 7-14 days; if tolerated well, may be increased (if needed) to 25 mg bid; not to exceed 50 mg/day; **EXT REL** cap 20 mg/day, may increase after 7-14 days to 40 mg/day

Congestive heart failure

• *Adult:* **PO** 3.125 mg bid × 2 wk; if tolerated well, give 6.25 mg bid × 2 wk, then double q2wk to max dose, 25 mg-bid <85 kg or 50 mg bid >85 kg; **EXT REL** caps (Coreg CR) 10 mg/day × 2 wk

Cardiomyopathy

• *Adult:* **PO** 6.25-25 mg bid

Angina (unlabeled)

• *Adult:* **PO** 25-50 mg bid

Available forms: Tabs 3.125, 6.25, 12.5, 25 mg; ext rel cap 10, 20, 40, 80 mg

SIDE EFFECTS

CNS: Dizziness, fatigue, weakness, somnolence, insomnia, ataxia, hyperesthesia, paresthesia, vertigo, depression, headache

CV: **Bradycardia,** *postural hypotension,* dependent edema, peripheral edema, **AV block,** extrasystoles, hypo/hypertension, palpitations, peripheral ischemia, **CHF, pulmonary edema**

GI: Diarrhea, abdominal pain, increased alk phos, ALT, AST

GU: Decreased libido, *impotence,* UTI

INTEG: Rash

MISC: Injury, back pain, viral infection, hypertriglyceridemia, **thrombocytopenia,** *hyperglycemia*

RESP: Rhinitis, pharyngitis, dyspnea, **bronchospasm**

Contraindications: Hypersensitivity, asthma, class IV decompensated cardiac failure, 2nd- or 3rd-degree heart block, cardiogenic shock, severe bradycardia, pulmonary edema

Precautions: Pregnancy (C), breastfeeding, children, geriatric patients, cardiac failure, hepatic injury, peripheral vascular disease, anesthesia, major surgery, diabetes mellitus, thyrotoxicosis, emphysema, chronic bronchitis, renal disease

Black Box Warning: Abrupt discontinuation

PHARMACOKINETICS

Peak 1-2 hr; readily and extensively absorbed PO; >98% protein binding; extensively metabolized by liver; excreted through bile into feces; terminal half-life 7-10 hr with increases in geriatric patients, hepatic disease

INTERACTIONS

Increase: conduction disturbances—calcium channel blockers

Increase: bradycardia, hypotension—levodopa, MAOIs, reserpine

Increase: hypoglycemia—antidiabetic agents

Increase: concentrations of digoxin

Increase: toxicity of carvedilol—cimetidine, other antihypertensives, nitrates, acute alcohol ingestion

Decrease: heart rate, B/P—clonidine

Decrease: carvedilol levels—rifampin, NSAIDs, thyroid medications

Drug/Herb

Increase: toxicity/death—aconite

Increase: antihypertensive effect—barberry, betony, black catechu, black cohosh, bloodroot, broom, burdock, cat's claw, dandelion, goldenseal, hawthorn, Irish moss, Jamaican dogwood, kelp, khella, mistletoe, parsley

Increase or decrease: antihypertensive effect—astragalus, cola tree

Decrease: antihypertensive effect—coltsfoot, guarana, khat, licorice

Drug/Lab Test

Increase: ANA titer, blood glucose, BUN, potassium, triglycerides, uric acid

NURSING CONSIDERATIONS

Assess:

⚠ Renal studies, including protein, BUN, creatinine; watch for increased levels that may indicate nephrotic syndrome; obtain baselines in renal, hepatic studies before beginning treatment; I&O, weight daily

- Hepatic studies, jaundice; if LFTs are elevated, product should be discontinued
- B/P during beginning treatment, periodically thereafter; pulse q4hr, note rate, rhythm, quality; apical/radial pulse before administration; notify prescriber of significant changes
- Edema in feet, legs daily, fluid overload: dyspnea, weight gain, jugular vein distention, fatigue, crackles

Administer:

- Pulse: if <50 bpm, hold product, call prescriber
- Product before meals, bedtime; tabs may be crushed or swallowed whole; do not break, crush, or chew ext rel cap
- Reduced dosage in renal dysfunction; may give with food

Evaluate:

- Therapeutic response: decreased B/P in hypertension

Teach patient/family:

- To comply with dosage schedule, even if feeling better, that improvement may take several weeks
- To rise slowly to sitting or standing position to minimize orthostatic hypotension
- To report bradycardia, dizziness, confusion, depression, fever, weight gain, SOB, cold extremities, rash, sore throat, bleeding, or bruising
- To weigh, take pulse, B/P at home; advise if weight gain >2 lb/day or 5 lb/wk and when to notify prescriber

⚠ Not to discontinue product abruptly, taper over 1-2 wk; life-threatening dysrhythmias may occur

- To avoid hazardous activities until stabilized on medication; dizziness may occur
- To avoid all OTC medications unless approved by prescriber
- To carry emergency ID with product name, prescriber at all times
- To inform all health care providers of products, supplements taken

caspofungin (℞)

(cas-po-fun′gin)

Cancidas

Func. class.: Antifungal, systemic

Chem. class.: Echinocandin

Action: Inhibits an essential component in fungal cell walls; causes direct damage to fungal cell wall

Uses: Treatment of invasive aspergillosis, and candidemia that has responded to other treatment including peritonitis, intraabdominal abscesses; susceptible species: *Aspergillus flavus, A. fumigatus, A. terreus, Candida albicans, C. glabrata, C. krusei, C. lusitaniae, C. parapsilosis, C. tropicalis,* esophageal candidiasis; empirical therapy for presumed fungal infection in febrile, neutropenic patients

Unlabeled uses: *Aspergillus niger,* fungal infections in premature neonates, neonates, infants, children <2 yr

DOSAGE AND ROUTES

- *Adult:* **IV** Loading dose 50-70 mg on day 1, then 50 mg/day maintenance dose depending on condition; max 70 mg/day
- *Adolescent/child/infant ≥3 mo:* **IV INF** 70 mg/m^2 as a loading dose, then 50 mg/m^2/day; (max 70 mg/day)
- *Neonate and infant <3 mo (unlabeled):* **IV** 25 mg/m^2/day

Available forms: Powder for inj 50, 70 mg

SIDE EFFECTS

CNS: Dizziness, *headache*

CV: Sinus tachycardia

GI: Abdominal pain, *nausea, anorexia, vomiting, diarrhea, increased AST, ALT, alk phos*

HEMA: Thrombophlebitis, vasculitis, anemia

INTEG: Rash, pruritus, inj site pain
META: Hypokalemia
MS: Myalgia
RESP: **Acute respiratory distress syndrome (ARDS)**
SYST: **Anaphylaxis**

Contraindications: Hypersensitivity to this product or other echinocandins including mannitol

Precautions: Pregnancy (C), breastfeeding, children, geriatric patients, severe hepatic disease

PHARMACOKINETICS

Metabolized in liver to inactive metabolites; excretion in feces, urine; phase II terminal half-life 9-11 hr; phase III terminal half-life 40-50 hr; protein binding 97%

INTERACTIONS

Increase: plasma concentrations—cycloSPORINE; may need dosage reduction

Decrease: caspofungin levels—carbamazepine, dexamethasone, efavirenz, nelfinavir, nevirapine, phenytoin, rifampin

Decrease: tacrolimus levels

Drug/Lab Test

Increase: AST, ALT

NURSING CONSIDERATIONS

Assess:

- For signs and symptoms of infection; clearing of cultures during treatment; obtain culture baseline and throughout; product may be started as soon as culture is taken (esophageal candidiasis); monitor cultures during HSCT, for prevention of *Candida* infections
- Hepatic studies before and during treatment: bilirubin, AST, ALT, alk phos, as needed; obtain baseline in renal studies
- For hypersensitivity: rash, pruritus, facial swelling; also for phlebitis
- GI symptoms: frequency of stools, cramping; if severe diarrhea occurs, electrolytes may need to be given

Administer:

IV route

- Allow to warm to room temperature
- May administer a loading dose on day 1 of treatment
- Do not admix; do not use with dextrose
- Reconstitute 50-mg vial or 70-mg vial with 10.5 ml 0.9% NaCl, sterile water for inj, or bacteriostatic water for inj (5 mg/ml; or 7 mg/ml); swirl to dissolve, withdraw 10 ml reconstituted solution and further dilute with 250 ml 0.9% NaCl, 0.45% NaCl, 0.225% NaCl, RL; run over 1 hr or more

Perform/provide:

- Storage at room temperature for up to 24 hr, or refrigerated 48 hr; store reconstituted solution at room temperature for 1 hr prior to preparation of solution for administration

Evaluate:

- Therapeutic response: decreased symptoms of *Candida* infections or *Aspergillus* infections

Teach patient/family:

- To notify prescriber if pregnancy is suspected or planned; use nonhormonal form of contraception while taking this product
- To avoid breastfeeding while taking this product
- To inform prescriber of renal/hepatic disease
- To report bleeding, facial swelling, wheezing, difficulty breathing, itching, rash, hives, increasing warmth, flushing; anaphylaxis can occur

cefaclor

See cephalosporins—2nd generation

cefadroxil

cefazolin

See cephalosporins—1st generation

cefdinir

cefditoren pivoxil

cefepime

cefixime

cefotaxime

See cephalosporins—3rd generation

cefotetan

cefoxitin

See cephalosporins—2nd generation

cefpodoxime

See cephalosporins—3rd generation

cefprozil

See cephalosporins—2nd generation

ceftazidime

ceftibuten

ceftizoxime

ceftriaxone

See cephalosporins—3rd generation

cefuroxime

See cephalosporins—2nd generation

⚠ High Alert

celecoxib (℞)

(sel-eh-cox′ib)

Celebrex

Func. class.: Nonsteroidal antiinflammatory, antirheumatic

Chem. class.: COX-2 inhibitor

Do not confuse:

Celebrex/Celexa/Cerebra/Cerebyx

Action: Inhibits prostaglandin synthesis by selectively inhibiting cyclooxygenase 2 (COX-2), an enzyme needed for biosynthesis

Uses: Acute, chronic rheumatoid arthritis, osteoarthritis, familial adenomatous polyposis (FAP), acute pain, primary dysmenorrhea, ankylosing spondylitis, juvenile rheumatoid arthritis (JRA)

Unlabeled uses: Colorectal adenoma prophylaxis

DOSAGE AND ROUTES

Do not exceed recommended dose, deaths have occurred

Acute pain/primary dysmenorrhea

• *Adult:* **PO** 400 mg initially, then 200 mg if needed on first day, then 200 mg bid prn on subsequent days; start with ½ dose in poor CYP2C9 metabolizers

Osteoarthritis

• *Adult:* **PO** 200 mg/day as a single dose or 100 mg bid; start with ½ dose in poor CYP2C9 metabolizers

Rheumatoid arthritis

• *Adult:* **PO** 100-200 mg bid; start with ½ dose in poor CYP2C9 metabolizers

Ankylosing spondylitis

• *Adult:* **PO** 200 mg/day or in divided dose (bid); start with ½ dose in poor CYP2C9 metabolizers

Familial adenomatous polyposis (FAP)

• *Adult:* **PO** 400 mg bid; start with ½ dose in poor CYP2C9 metabolizers

Juvenile rheumatoid arthritis (JRA)

• *Adolescent and child ≥2 yr (>25 kg):* **PO** 100 mg bid; start with ½ dose in poor CYP2C9 metabolizers

• *Child ≥2 yr (10-25 kg):* **PO** 50 mg bid; start with ½ dose in poor CYP2C9 metabolizers

Hepatic disease

• *Adult:* **PO** (Child-Pugh B) Reduce dose by 50%

Colorectal adenoma prophylaxis (unlabeled)

• *Adult:* **PO** 400 mg bid × 6 mo

Available forms: Caps 50, 100, 200, 400 mg

SIDE EFFECTS

CNS: Fatigue, anxiety, depression, nervousness, paresthesia, dizziness, insomnia

CV: **Stroke, MI, tachycardia, CHF,** angina, palpitations, dysrhythmias, hypertension, fluid retention

EENT: Tinnitus, hearing loss, blurred vision, glaucoma, cataract, conjunctivitis, eye pain
GI: Nausea, anorexia, vomiting, constipation, dry mouth, diverticulitis, gastritis, gastroenteritis, hemorrhoids, hiatal hernia, stomatitis, **GI bleeding/ulceration**
GU: **Nephrotoxicity:** ***dysuria,*** **hematuria, oliguria, azotemia,** cystitis, UTI
HEMA: **Blood dyscrasias,** epistaxis, bruising, anemia, **platelet aggregation**
INTEG: **Serious, sometimes fatal Stevens-Johnson syndrome, toxic epidermal necrolysis,** purpura, rash, pruritus, sweating, erythema, petechiae, photosensitivity, alopecia
RESP: Pharyngitis, shortness of breath, pneumonia, coughing
Contraindications: Pregnancy (D) 3rd trimester, hypersensitivity to salicylates, iodides, other NSAIDs, sulfonamides

Black Box Warning: CABG

Precautions: Pregnancy (C) 1st/2nd trimesters, breastfeeding, children <18 yr, geriatric patients, bleeding, GI/renal/hepatic/cardiac disorders, PVD, hypertension, severe dehydration, asthma

Black Box Warning: GI bleeding/perforation, peptic ulcer disease, MI, stroke

PHARMACOKINETICS

Well absorbed, crosses placenta, bound to plasma proteins, metabolized by 2C9 in liver, very little excreted by kidneys/feces, peak 3 hr, half-life 11 hr, protein binding 87%

INTERACTIONS

Increase: bleeding risk—anticoagulants, SSRIs, antiplatelets, thrombolytics, salicylates, alcohol
Increase: adverse reactions—glucocorticoids, NSAIDs, aspirin
Increase: toxicity—lithium, antineoplastics, biphosphonates
Increase: celecoxib blood level—fluconazole
Decrease: effect of aspirin, ACE inhibitors, thiazide diuretics, furosemide

Drug/Herb

- Severe photosensitivity: St. John's wort

Increase: celecoxib effect—bearberry, bilberry
Increase: gastric irritation—arginine, gossypol
Increase: bleeding risk—bogbean, saw palmetto, turmeric, garlic, ginger, gingko

Drug/Lab Test

Increase: ALT, AST, BUN

NURSING CONSIDERATIONS

Assess:

- For pain of rheumatoid arthritis, osteoarthritis; check ROM, inflammation of joints, characteristics of pain
- For cardiac disease that may be worse after taking this product
- FAP clients for decreasing number of polyps
- Blood counts during therapy; watch for decreasing platelets; if low, therapy may need to be discontinued, restarted after hematologic recovery

⚠ For blood dyscrasias (thrombocytopenia): bruising, fatigue, bleeding, poor healing

- GI toxicity: black, tarry stools; abdominal pain

Administer:

- Do not break, crush, chew, or dissolve caps; caps may be opened into applesauce or soft food, ingest immediately with water
- With a full glass of water to enhance absorption
- With food or milk to decrease gastric symptoms, do not increase dose

Evaluate:

- Therapeutic response: decreased pain, inflammation in arthritic conditions; decreased number of polyps

Teach patient/family:

⚠ **Do not exceed recommended dose; notify prescriber immediately of chest pain, skin eruptions; stop product**

- To check with prescriber to determine when product should be discontinued prior to surgery

• That product must be continued for prescribed time to be effective; to avoid other NSAIDs, aspirin, sulfonamides
• To notify prescriber if pregnancy is planned or suspected
⚠ To notify prescriber of GI symptoms: black, tarry stools; cramping or rash; edema of extremities, weight gain
⚠ To report bleeding, bruising, fatigue, malaise since blood abnormalities do occur
• To report possible respiratory infection: fever, shortness of breath, coughing, painful swallowing

cephalexin

See cephalosporins—1st generation

CEPHALOSPORINS—1ST GENERATION

cefadroxil (℞)
(sef-a-drox′ill)
cefadroxil, Duricef

cefazolin (℞)
(sef-a′zoe-lin)
Ancef, cefazolin

cephalexin (℞)
(sef-a-lex′in)
Apo-Cephalex ♣, cephalexin, Keflex, Novo-Lexin ♣, Nu-Cephalex ♣, Panixine

cephradine (℞)
(sef′ra-deen)
cephradine, Velosef

Func. class.: Antiinfective
Chem. class.: Cephalosporin (1st generation)

Do not confuse:
cephalexin/cefaclor

Action: Inhibits bacterial cell wall synthesis, rendering cell wall osmotically unstable, leading to cell death; lysis mediated by cell wall autolytic enzymes

Uses:
cefadroxil: Gram-negative bacilli: *Escherichia coli, Proteus mirabilis, Klebsiella* (UTI only); gram-positive organisms: *Streptococcus pneumoniae, Streptococcus pyogenes, Staphylococcus aureus;* upper, lower respiratory tract, urinary tract, skin infections, otitis media; tonsillitis; and UTIs
cefazolin: Gram-negative bacilli: *Haemophilus influenzae, Escherichia coli, Proteus mirabilis, Klebsiella;* gram-positive organisms: *Staphylococcus aureus;* upper, lower respiratory tract, urinary tract, skin infections, bone, joint, biliary, genital infections, endocarditis, surgical prophylaxis, septicemia
cephalexin: Gram-negative bacilli: *Haemophilus influenzae, Escherichia coli, Proteus mirabilis, Klebsiella;* gram-positive organisms: *Streptococcus pneumoniae, Streptococcus pyogenes, Staphylococcus aureus;* upper, lower respiratory tract, urinary tract, skin, bone infections, otitis media
cephradine: Gram-negative bacilli: *Haemophilus influenzae, Escherichia coli, Proteus mirabilis, Klebsiella;* gram-positive organisms: *Streptococcus pneumoniae, Streptococcus pyogenes, Staphylococcus aureus;* serious respiratory tract, skin infections, UTIs, otitis media

DOSAGE AND ROUTES

cefadroxil
• *Adult:* **PO** 1-2 g/day or q12hr in divided doses, give a loading dose of 1 g initially
• *Child:* **PO** 30 mg/kg/day in divided doses bid

Renal dose
• *Adult:* **PO** CCr 25-50 ml/min 500 mg q12hr; CCr 10-24 ml/min 500 mg q24hr; CCr <10 ml/min 500 mg q36hr

Available forms: Caps 500 mg; tabs 1 g; oral susp 250, 500 mg/5 ml

cefazolin
Life-threatening infections
• *Adult:* **IM/IV** 1-2 g q6hr; max 12 g/day
• *Child >1 mo:* **IM/IV** 100 mg/kg in 3-4 divided doses; max 6 g/day

Mild/moderate infections

• *Adult:* **IM/IV** 250 mg-1 g q8hr

• *Child >1 mo:* **IM/IV** 25-50 mg/kg in 3-4 equal doses

Renal dose

• *Adult:* **IM/IV** Following loading dose CCr 35-54 ml/min, dose q8hr; CCr 10-34 ml/min, 50% of dose q12hr; CCr <10 ml/min, 50% of dose q18-24hr

• *Child:* **IM/IV** CCr >70 ml/min, no dosage adjustment; CCr 40-70 ml/min following loading dose, reduce dose to 7.5-30 mg/kg q12hr; CCr 20-39 ml/min, give 3.125-12.5 mg/kg after loading dose q12hr; CCr 5-19 ml/min, 2.5-10 mg/kg after loading dose q24hr

Available forms: Inj 250, 500 mg, 1, 5, 10, 20 g; inf 500 mg, 1 g/50-ml vial

cephalexin

Moderate infections

• *Adult:* **PO** 250-500 mg q6hr, max 4 g/day

• *Child:* **PO** 25-50 mg/kg/day in 4 equal doses, max 4 g/day

Moderate skin infections

• *Adult:* **PO** 500 mg q12hr

Endocarditis prophylaxis

• 2 g 1 hr before procedure

Severe infections

• *Adult:* **PO** 500 mg-1 g q6hr

• *Child:* **PO** 50-100 mg/kg/day in 4 equal doses, max 4 g/day

Renal dose

• *Adult:* **PO** CCr 10-40 ml/min 250-500 mg, then 250-500 mg q8-12hr; CCr <10 ml/min 250-500 mg, then 250-500 mg q12-24hr

Available forms: Caps 250, 500 mg; tabs 250, 500 mg, 1 g; oral susp 125 mg, 250 mg/5ml

cephradine

• *Adult:* **PO** 250 mg-1 g q6-12hr

• *Child >1 yr:* **PO** 6-12 mg/kg q6hr

Renal dose

• *Adult:* **PO** CCr >20 ml/min 500 mg q6hr; CCr 5-20 ml/min 250 mg q6hr

Available forms: Caps 250, 500 mg; oral susp 125 mg, 250 mg/5 ml

SIDE EFFECTS

CNS: Headache, dizziness, weakness, paresthesia, fever, chills, **seizures** (high doses)

GI: Nausea, vomiting, ***diarrhea, anorexia,*** pain, glossitis, bleeding; increased AST, ALT, bilirubin, LDH, alk phos; abdominal pain, **pseudomembranous colitis**

GU: Proteinuria, vaginitis, pruritus, candidiasis, increased BUN, **nephrotoxicity, renal failure**

HEMA: **Leukopenia, thrombocytopenia, agranulocytosis,** anemia, **neutropenia, lymphocytosis, eosinophilia, pancytopenia, hemolytic anemia**

INTEG: Rash, urticaria, dermatitis

RESP: Dyspnea

SYST: **Anaphylaxis, serum sickness,** superinfection, **Stevens-Johnson syndrome**

Contraindications: Hypersensitivity to cephalosporins, infants <1 mo

Precautions: Pregnancy (B), breastfeeding, hypersensitivity to penicillins, renal disease

PHARMACOKINETICS

cefadroxil: Peak 1-1½ hr, duration 12-24 hr, half-life 1-2 hr, 20% bound by plasma proteins, crosses placenta, excreted in breast milk

cefazolin

IM: Peak ½-2 hr, duration 6-12 hr, half-life 1½-2¼ hr

IV: Peak 10 min, duration 6-12 hr, eliminated unchanged in urine, 70%-86% protein bound

cephalexin: Peak 1 hr, duration 6-12 hr, half-life 30-72 min, 5%-15% bound by plasma proteins, 90%-100% eliminated unchanged in urine, crosses placenta, excreted in breast milk

cephradine: Peak 1-2 hr, duration 6-12 hr, half-life 0.75-1.5 hr, 20% bound by plasma proteins, 80%-90% eliminated unchanged in urine, crosses placenta, excreted in breast milk

INTERACTIONS

Increase: protime—anticoagulants; use cautiously

Increase: toxicity—aminoglycosides, loop diuretics, probenecid

Drug/Herb

- Do not use acidophilus with antiinfectives; separate by several hours

Drug/Lab Test

Increase: AST, ALT, alk phos, LDH, BUN, creatinine, bilirubin

False positive: urinary protein, direct Coombs' test, urine glucose

Interference: cross-matching

NURSING CONSIDERATIONS

Assess:

- Sensitivity to penicillin and other cephalosporins

⚠ Nephrotoxicity: increased BUN, creatinine

- I&O daily
- Blood studies: AST, ALT, CBC, Hct, bilirubin, LDH, alk phos, Coombs' test monthly if patient is on long-term therapy
- Electrolytes: K, Na, Cl monthly if patient is on long-term therapy
- Bowel pattern daily; if severe diarrhea occurs, product should be discontinued; may indicate pseudomembranous colitis
- Urine output: if decreasing, notify prescriber; may indicate nephrotoxicity

⚠ Anaphylaxis: rash, urticaria, pruritus, chills, fever, joint pain; angioedema; may occur few days after therapy begins; discontinue product, notify prescriber immediately, keep emergency equipment nearby

- Bleeding: ecchymosis, bleeding gums, hematuria, stool guaiac daily

⚠ Overgrowth of infection: perineal itching, fever, malaise, redness, pain, swelling, drainage, rash, diarrhea, change in cough, sputum

Administer:

cefadroxil

- For 10-14 days to ensure organism death, prevent superinfection
- With food if needed for GI symptoms
- Shake susp, refrigerate, discard after 2 wk
- After C&S completed

cefazolin

- IV; check for irritation, extravasation often; dilute in 10 ml sterile H_2O for inj and run over 3-5 min; may be further diluted with 50-100 ml of NS, D_5W sol and run over ½-1 hr by Y-tube or 3-way stopcock
- For 10-14 days to ensure organism death, prevent superinfection
- After C&S completed

Additive compatibilities: Aztreonam, clindamycin, famotidine, fluconazole, metronidazole, verapamil

Syringe compatibilities: Heparin, vit B

Y-site compatibilities: Acyclovir, allopurinol, amifostine, atracurium, aztreonam, calcium gluconate, cyclophosphamide, diltiazem, DOXOrubicin liposome, enalaprilat, esmolol, famotidine, filgrastim, fluconazole, fludarabine, foscarnet, heparin, hydromorphone, insulin (regular), labetalol, lidocaine, magnesium sulfate, melphalan, meperidine, midazolam, morphine, multivitamins, ondansetron, perphenazine, pancuronium, remifentanil, sargramostim, tacrolimus, teniposide, theophylline, thiotepa, vecuronium, vit B/C, warfarin

cephalexin

- Shake susp, refrigerate, discard after 2 wk
- For 10-14 days to ensure organism death, prevent superinfection
- With food if needed for GI symptoms
- After C&S

cephradine

- Shake suspension well before each dose
- For 10-14 days to ensure organism death, prevent superinfection
- With food if needed for GI symptoms
- After C&S

Evaluate:

- Therapeutic response: decreased symptoms of infection, negative C&S

Teach patient/family:

- To use yogurt or buttermilk to maintain intestinal flora, decrease diarrhea
- To take all medication prescribed for length of time ordered

⚠ To report sore throat, bruising, bleeding, joint pain (may indicate blood dyscrasias [rare]); diarrhea with mucus, blood, may indicate pseudomembranous colitis

Treatment of anaphylaxis: Epinephrine, antihistamines; resuscitate if needed

CEPHALOSPORINS—2ND GENERATION

cefaclor (℞)
(sef′a-klor)
Ceclor, Raniclor

cefotetan (℞)
(sef′oh-tee-tan)
Cefotan

cefoxitin (℞)
(se-fox′i-tin)
Mefoxin

cefprozil (℞)
(sef-proe′zill)
Cefzil

cefuroxime (℞)
(sef-yoor-ox′eem)
Ceftin, cefuroxime, Zinacef

loracarbef (℞)
(lor-a-kar′beff)
Lorabid

Func. class.: Antiinfective
Chem. class.: Cephalosporin (2nd generation)

Do not confuse:
cefaclor/cephalexin
Cefotan/Ceftin
cefprozil/cefazolin/cefuroxime
Cefzil/Ceftin

Action: Inhibits bacterial cell wall synthesis, rendering cell wall osmotically unstable, leading to cell death by binding to cell wall membrane

Uses:
cefaclor: Gram-negative bacilli: *Haemophilus influenzae, Escherichia coli, Proteus mirabilis, Klebsiella;* gram-positive organisms: *Streptococcus pneumoniae, Streptococcus pyogenes, Staphylococcus aureus;* respiratory tract, urinary tract, skin, bone, joint infections, otitis media

cefotetan: Gram-negative organisms: *Haemophilus influenzae, Escherichia coli, Enterobacter aerogenes, Proteus mirabilis, Klebsiella, Citrobacter, Salmonella, Shigella, Acinetobacter, Bacteroides fragilis, Neisseria, Serratia;* gram-positive organisms: *Streptococcus pneumoniae, Streptococcus pyogenes, Staphylococcus aureus;* upper and lower, serious respiratory tract, urinary tract, skin, bone, joint, gynecologic, gonococcal, intraabdominal infections

cefoxitin: Gram-negative bacilli: *Haemophilus influenzae, Escherichia coli, Proteus, Klebsiella, Bacteroides fragilis, Neisseria gonorrhoeae;* gram-positive organisms: *Streptococcus pneumoniae, Streptococcus pyogenes, Staphylococcus aureus;* anaerobes including *Clostridium,* lower respiratory tract, urinary tract, skin, bone, gynecologic, gonococcal infections, septicemia, peritonitis

cefprozil: Pharyngitis/tonsillitis, otitis media, secondary bacterial infection of acute bronchitis, and acute bacterial exacerbation of chronic bronchitis and uncomplicated skin and skin structure infections; acute sinusitis

cefuroxime: Gram-negative bacilli: *Haemophilus influenzae, Escherichia coli, Neisseria, Proteus mirabilis, Klebsiella;* gram-positive organisms: *Streptococcus pneumoniae, Streptococcus pyogenes, Staphylococcus aureus;* serious lower respiratory tract, urinary tract, skin, bone, joint, gonococcal infections, septicemia, meningitis

loracarbef: Gram-negative bacilli: *Haemophilus influenzae, Escherichia coli, Proteus mirabilis, Klebsiella;* gram-positive organisms: *Streptococcus pneumoniae, Streptococcus pyogenes, Staph-*

ylococcus aureus; upper and lower respiratory tract, urinary tract, skin infections, otitis media, pharyngitis, tonsillitis

DOSAGE AND ROUTES

cefaclor

• *Adult:* **PO** 250-500 mg q8hr, not to exceed 4 g/day

• *Child >1 mo:* **PO** 20-40 mg/kg/day in divided doses q8hr, or total daily dose may be divided and given q12hr, not to exceed 1 g/day

Available forms: Caps 250, 500 mg; oral susp 125, 187, 250, 375 mg/5 ml; chew tabs (Raniclor) 250, 375 mg

cefotetan

• *Adult:* **IM/IV** 1-2 g q12hr × 5-10 days

Renal dose

• *Adult:* **IM/IV** CCr 10-30 ml/min, give dose q24hr or ½ dose q12hr; CCr <10 ml/min, give dose q48hr or ½ dose q24hr

Perioperative prophylaxis

• *Adult:* **IV** 1-2 g ½-1 hr before surgery

Available forms: Inj 1, 2, 10 g

cefoxitin

• *Adult:* **IM/IV** 1-2 g q6-8hr

Renal dose

• *Adult:* **IM/IV** After loading dose CCr 30-50 ml/min 1-2 g q8-12hr; CCr 10-29 ml/min 1-2 g q12-24hr; CCr <10 ml/min 0.5-1 g q12-24hr

Uncomplicated gonorrhea (outpatient)

• *Adult/adolescent/child ≥45 kg:* **IM** 2 g as single dose with 1 g **PO** probenecid at same time

Severe infections

• *Adult:* **IM/IV** 2 g q4hr

• *Child ≥3 mo:* **IM/IV** 80-160 mg/kg/day divided q4-6hr; max 12 g/day

Available forms: Powder for inj 1, 2, 10 g

cefprozil

Renal dose

• CCr <30 ml/min 50% of dose

Upper respiratory infections

• *Adult:* **PO** 500 mg q24hr × 10 days

Otitis media

• *Child 6 mo-12 yr:* **PO** 15 mg/kg q12hr × 10 days

Lower respiratory infections

• *Adult:* **PO** 500 mg q12hr × 10 days

Skin/skin structure infections

• *Adult:* **PO** 250-500 mg q12hr × 10 days

Available forms: Tabs 250, 500 mg; susp 125, 250 mg/5 ml

cefuroxime

• *Adult and child:* **PO** 250 mg q12hr; may increase to 500 mg q12hr in serious infections

• *Adult:* **IM/IV** 750 mg-1.5 g q8hr for 5-10 days

Urinary tract infections

• *Adult:* **PO** 125 mg q12hr; may increase to 250 mg q12hr if needed

Otitis media

• *Child <2 yr:* **PO** 125 mg bid

• *Child >2 yr:* **PO** 250 mg bid

Surgical prophylaxis

• *Adult:* **IV** 1.5 g ½-1 hr preoperative

Severe infections

• *Adult:* **IM/IV** 1.5 g q6hr; may give up to 3 g q8hr for bacterial meningitis

• *Child >3 mo:* **IM/IV** 50-100 mg/kg/day; may give up to 200-240 mg/kg/day **IV** in divided doses for bacterial meningitis (not recommended)

• Dosage reduction indicated in severe renal impairment (CCr <20 ml/min)

Uncomplicated gonorrhea

• *Adult:* 1.5 g **IM** as single dose with oral probenecid in 2 separate sites

Available forms: Tabs 125, 250, 500 mg; inj 150, 750 mg, 1.5, 7.5 g; inj 750 mg; 1.5 g powder; susp 125, 250 mg/5 ml

loracarbef

• *Adult and child >13 yr:* **PO** 200-400 mg q12hr

• *Child <12 yr:* **PO** 15-30 mg/kg/day in 2 divided doses q12hr

Renal dose

• CCr 10-49 ml/min 50% of dose; CCr <10 ml/min q3-5days

Available forms: Caps 200, 400 mg; oral susp 100 mg, 200 mg/5 ml

SIDE EFFECTS

CNS: Dizziness, headache, fatigue, paresthesia, fever, chills, confusion

C

GI: Diarrhea, nausea, vomiting, anorexia, dysgeusia, glossitis, bleeding; increased AST, ALT, bilirubin, LDH, alk phos; abdominal pain, loose stools, flatulence, heartburn, stomach cramps, colitis, jaundice, **pseudomembranous colitis**

GU: Vaginitis, pruritus, candidiasis, increased BUN, **nephrotoxicity, renal failure,** pyuria, dysuria, reversible interstitial nephritis

HEMA: **Leukopenia, thrombocytopenia, agranulocytosis,** anemia, **neutropenia, lymphocytosis, eosinophilia, pancytopenia, hemolytic anemia, leukocytosis, granulocytopenia**

INTEG: Rash, urticaria, dermatitis, **Stevens-Johnson syndrome**

RESP: Dyspnea

SYST: Anaphylaxis, **serum sickness,** superinfection

Contraindications: Hypersensitivity to cephalosporins or related antibiotics, seizures

Precautions: Pregnancy (B), breastfeeding, children, GI/renal disease

PHARMACOKINETICS

cefaclor

PO: Peak ½-1 hr, half-life 36-54 min, 25% bound by plasma proteins, 60%-85% eliminated unchanged in urine in 8 hr, crosses placenta, excreted in breast milk (low concentrations)

cefotetan

IM/IV: Peak 1½-3 hr, half-life 3-5 hr, 70%-90% bound by plasma proteins, 50%-80% eliminated unchanged in urine, crosses placenta, excreted in breast milk

cefoxitin

Half-life 1 hr; 65%-80% bound by plasma proteins; 90%-100% eliminated unchanged in urine; crosses placenta, blood-brain barrier; eliminated in breast milk; not metabolized

IM: Peak 15-60 min

IV: Peak 3 min

cefprozil

PO: Peak 1.5 hr, plasma protein binding 35%-45%, elimination half-life 25 hr, extensively metabolized to an active metabolite

cefuroxime

65% excreted unchanged in urine, half-life 1-2 hr in normal renal function

loracarbef

PO: Peak 1 hr, half-life 1 hr, excreted in urine as unchanged product

INTERACTIONS

Increase: effect/toxicity—aminoglycosides, furosemide, probenecid

Increase: bleeding risk (cefotetan)—anticoagulants, thrombolytics, NSAIDs, antiplatelets, plicamycin, valproic acid

Decrease: absorption of cephalosporin—antacids

Decrease: effect of cephalosporin—H_2-blockers

Drug/Herb

• Do not use acidophilus with antiinfectives; separate by several hours

Increase: bleeding risk (cefotetan)—angelica, anise, arnica, bogbean, boldo, celery, chamomile, clove, fenugreek, feverfew, garlic, ginger, ginkgo, ginseng *(Panax)*, horse chestnut, horseradish, licorice, meadowsweet, prickly ash, onion, papain, passion flower, poplar, red clover, turmeric, willow

Drug/Lab Test

False increase: creatinine (serum urine), urinary 17-KS

False positive: urinary protein, direct Coombs' test, urine glucose testing (Clinitest)

Interference: cross-matching

NURSING CONSIDERATIONS

Assess:

⚠ Nephrotoxicity: increased BUN, creatinine

• I&O ratio

• Blood studies: AST, ALT, CBC, Hct, bilirubin, LDH, alk phos, Coombs' test q mo if patient is on long-term therapy

• Electrolytes: K, Na, Cl q mo if patient is on long-term therapy

• Bowel pattern daily; if severe diarrhea occurs, product should be discontinued; may indicate pseudomembranous colitis

• Urine output; if decreasing, notify prescriber (may indicate nephrotoxicity)

⚠ Anaphylaxis: rash, flushing, urticaria, pruritus, dyspnea, discontinue product, notify prescriber, have emergency equipment available

• Bleeding: ecchymosis, bleeding gums, hematuria, stool guaiac daily

⚠ Overgrowth of infection: perineal itching, fever, malaise, redness, pain, swelling, drainage, rash, diarrhea, change in cough, sputum

Administer:

• Do not break, crush, or chew ext rel tabs or caps

• On an empty stomach 1 hr before or 2 hr after a meal

cefaclor

• Shake susp, refrigerate, discard after 2 wk

• For 10-14 days to ensure organism death, prevent superinfection

• With food if needed for GI symptoms

• After C&S completed

cefotetan

• IV direct after diluting 1 g/10 ml sterile H_2O for inj and give over 3-5 min; may be diluted further with 50-100 ml of NS or D_5W, shake; run over ½-1 hr by Y-tube or 3-way stopcock; discontinue primary inf during administration

• May be stored 96 hr refrigerated or 24 hr room temperature

Y-site compatibilities: Allopurinol, amifostine, aztreonam, diltiazem, famotidine, filgrastim, fluconazole, fludarabine, heparin, insulin (regular), melphalan, meperidine, morphine, paclitaxel, remifentanil, sargramostim, tacrolimus, teniposide, theophylline, thiotepa

cefoxitin

• IV after diluting 1 g or less/10 ml or more D_5W, NS and give over 3-5 min; may be diluted further with 50-100 ml of normal saline or D_5W; run over ½-1 hr by Y-tube or 3-way stopcock; discontinue primary inf during administration; by cont inf at prescribed rate; may store 96 hr refrigerated or 24 hr room temperature

• For 10-14 days to ensure organism death, prevent superinfection

• After C&S completed

Additive compatibilities: Amikacin, cimetidine, clindamycin, gentamicin, kanamycin, multivitamins, sodium bicarbonate, tobramycin, verapamil, vit B/C

Syringe compatibilities: Heparin, insulin

Y-site compatibilities: Acyclovir, amifostine, amphotericin B cholesteryl sulfate complex, aztreonam, cyclophosphamide, diltiazem, DOXOrubicin liposome, famotidine, fluconazole, foscarnet, hydromorphone, magnesium sulfate, meperidine, morphine, ondansetron, perphenazine, remifentanil, teniposide, thiotepa

cefprozil

• For 10-14 days to ensure organism death, prevent superinfection

• After C&S

• Refrigerate/shake susp prior to use

cefuroxime

• For 10-14 days to ensure organism death, prevent superinfection

• With food if needed for GI symptoms

• After C&S

Additive compatibilities: Clindamycin, floxacillin, furosemide, metronidazole, netilmicin

Y-site compatibilities: Acyclovir, allopurinol, amifostine, atracurium, aztreonam, cyclophosphamide, diltiazem, famotidine, fludarabine, foscarnet, hydromorphone, melphalan, meperidine, morphine, ondansetron, pancuronium, perphenazine, remifentanil, sargramostim, tacrolimus, teniposide, thiotepa, vecuronium

loracarbef

• Oral susp should be shaken before giving; store for 2 wk at room temperature, discard after 2 wk

• 1 hr before or 2 hr after a meal

• After C&S is completed

• For 7 days to ensure organism death, prevent superinfection

Evaluate:

• Therapeutic response: negative C&S

Teach patient/family:

• If diabetic, to use blood glucose testing

- To complete full course of product therapy, to report persistent diarrhea
- To use yogurt or buttermilk to maintain intestinal flora, decrease diarrhea
- To notify prescriber if breastfeeding or of any side effects

⚠ To report sore throat, bruising, bleeding, joint pain (may indicate blood dyscrasias [rare]); diarrhea with mucus, blood, may indicate pseudomembranous colitis

Treatment of anaphylaxis: Epinephrine, antihistamines; resuscitate if needed

CEPHALOSPORINS—3RD GENERATION

cefdinir (℞)
(sef′dih-ner)
Omnicef

cefditoren pivoxil (℞)
(sef-dit′oh-ren pih-vox′il)
Spectracef

cefepime (℞)
(sef′e-peem)
Maxipime

cefixime (℞)
(sef-icks′ime)
Cefixime, Suprax

cefotaxime (℞)
(sef-oh-taks′eem)
Claforan

cefpodoxime (℞)
(sef-poe-docks′eem)
Vantin

ceftazidime (℞)
(sef′tay-zi-deem)
Ceptaz, Fortaz, Tazicef, Tazidime

ceftibuten (℞)
(sef-ti-byoo′tin)
Cedax

ceftizoxime (℞)
(sef-ti-zox′eem)
Cefizox

ceftriaxone (℞)
(sef-try-ax′one)
Rocephin

Func. class.: Broad-spectrum antibiotic
Chem. class.: Cephalosporin (3rd generation)

Do not confuse:
ceftazidime/ceftizoxime
Vantin/Ventolin

Action: Inhibits bacterial cell wall synthesis, rendering cell wall osmotically unstable, leading to cell death

Uses:

cefdinir: Community-acquired pneumonia, otitis media, sinusitis, pharyngitis, skin and skin structure infections, acute exacerbations of chronic bronchitis, gram-negative bacilli: *Haemophilus influenzae, Haemophilus parainfluenzae, Moraxella catarrhalis;* gram-positive organisms: *Streptococcus pneumoniae, Streptococcus pyogenes, Staphylococcus aureus (MSSA)*

cefditoren pivoxil: Acute bacterial exacerbation of chronic bronchitis caused by *Haemophilus influenzae, Haemophilus parainfluenzae, Streptococcus pneumoniae, Moraxella catarrhalis*; pharyngitis/tonsillitis caused by *Streptococcus pyogenes*; uncomplicated skin and skin structure infections caused by *Staphylococcus aureus, Streptococcus pyogenes;* community-acquired pneumonia

cefepime: Gram-negative bacilli: *Escherichia coli, Proteus, Klebsiella;* gram-positive organisms: *Streptococcus pneumoniae, Streptococcus pyogenes, Staphylococcus aureus;* lower respiratory tract, urinary tract, skin, bone infections, febrile neutropenia intraabdominal infection

cefixime: Uncomplicated UTI *(Escherichia coli, Proteus mirabilis)*, pharyngitis and tonsillitis *(Streptococcus pyogenes)*, otitis media *(Haemophilus influenzae), Moraxella catarrhalis,* acute bronchitis and acute exacerbations of chronic bronchitis *(Streptococcus pneumoniae, H. influenzae)*, uncomplicated gonorrhea

cefotaxime: Gram-negative organisms: *Haemophilus influenzae, Haemophilus parainfluenzae, Escherichia coli, Enterococcus faecalis, Neisseria gonorrhoeae, Neisseria meningitidis, Proteus mirabilis, Klebsiella, Citrobacter, Serratia, Salmonella, Shigella Pseudomonas;* gram-positive organisms: *Streptococcus pneumoniae, Streptococcus pyogenes, Staphylococcus aureus;* serious lower respiratory tract, urinary tract, skin, bone, gonococcal infections; bacteremia, septicemia, meningitis, skin, skin structure infections, CNS infections; perioperative prophylaxis

cefpodoxime: Gram-negative bacilli: *Neisseria gonorrhoeae, Haemophilus influenzae, Escherichia coli, Proteus mirabilis, Klebsiella;* gram-positive organisms: *Streptococcus pneumoniae, Streptococcus pyogenes, Staphylococcus aureus;* upper and lower respiratory tract, urinary tract, skin infections; otitis media, sexually transmitted diseases

ceftazidime: Gram-negative organisms: *Haemophilus influenzae, Escherichia coli, Enterobacter aerogenes, Pseudomonas aeruginosa, Proteus mirabilis, Klebsiella, Citrobacter, Enterobacter, Salmonella, Shigella, Acinetobacter, Bacteroides fragilis, Neisseria, Serratia;* gram-positive organisms: *Streptococcus pneumoniae, Streptococcus pyogenes, Staphylococcus aureus;* serious upper/lower respiratory tract, urinary tract, skin, gynecologic, bone, joint, intraabdominal infections; septicemia, meningitis, febrile neutropenia

ceftibuten: Pharyngitis/tonsillitis, otitis media, secondary bacterial infection of acute bronchitis

ceftizoxime: Gram-negative bacilli: *Haemophilus influenzae, Escherichia coli, Enterobacter aerogenes, Proteus mirabilis, Klebsiella, Enterobacter;* gram-positive organisms: *Streptococcus pneumoniae, Streptococcus pyogenes, Staphylococcus aureus;* serious lower respiratory tract, urinary tract, skin, intraabdominal infections, septicemia, meningitis, bone and joint infections, PID caused by *Neisseria gonorrhoeae*

ceftriaxone: Gram-negative bacilli: *Haemophilus influenzae, Escherichia coli, Enterobacter aerogenes, Proteus mirabilis, Klebsiella, Citrobacter, Enterobacter, Salmonella, Shigella, Acinetobacter, Bacteroides fragilis, Neisseria, Serratia;* gram-positive organisms: *Streptococcus pneumoniae, Streptococcus pyogenes, Staphylococcus aureus;* serious lower respiratory tract, urinary tract, skin, gonococcal, intraabdominal infections, septicemia, meningitis, bone, joint infections, otitis media, PID

DOSAGE AND ROUTES

cefdinir

Uncomplicated skin and skin structure infections/community-acquired pneumonia

• *Adult and child ≥13 yr:* **PO** 300 mg q12hr × 10 days

• *Child 6 mo-12 yr:* **PO** 7 mg/kg q12hr or 14 mg/kg q24hr × 10 days

Acute exacerbations of chronic bronchitis/acute maxillary sinusitis

• *Adult and child ≥13 yr:* **PO** 300 mg q12hr or 600 mg q24hr × 10 days or 300 mg bid × 5 days in some infections

Pharyngitis/tonsillitis

• *Adult and child ≥13 yr:* **PO** 300 mg q12hr or 600 mg q24hr × 10 days

• *Child 6 mo-12 yr:* **PO** 7 mg/kg q12hr × 5-10 days or 14 mg/kg q24hr × 10 days

Renal dose

• CCr <30 ml/min 300 mg/day (adult); 7 mg/kg/day (child)

Available forms: Caps 300 mg; susp 125 mg, 250 mg/5 ml

cefditoren pivoxil

• *Adult:* **PO** 200-400 mg bid

Renal dose

• *Adult:* **PO** CCr 30-50 ml/min, max 200 mg bid; CCr <30 ml/min, max 200 mg daily

Available forms: Tabs 200 mg

cefepime

Febrile neutropenia

• *Adult:* **IV** 2 g q8hr × 7 days or until neutropenia resolves

Urinary tract infections (mild to moderate)

• *Adult:* **IV/IM** 0.5-1 g q12hr × 7-10 days

Urinary tract infections (severe)

• *Adult:* **IV** 2 g q12hr × 10 days

Pneumonia (moderate to severe)

• *Adult:* **IV** 1-2 g q12hr × 10 days

• Dosage reduction indicated in renal impairment (CCr <50 ml/min)

Uncomplicated gonorrhea

• **IM** 2 g as a single dose with 1 g **PO** probenecid at the same time

Available forms: Powder for inj 500 mg, 1, 2 g

cefixime

• *Adult:* **PO** 400 mg/day as a single dose or 200 mg q12hr

• *Child >50 kg or >12 yr:* **PO** Use adult dosage

• *Child <50 kg or <12 yr:* **PO** 8 mg/kg/day as a single dose or 4 mg/kg q12hr

Renal dose

• CCr 21-60 ml/min give 75% of dose; CCr <20 ml/min give 50% of dose

Available forms: Tabs 400 mg; powder for oral susp 100 mg/5 ml

cefotaxime

• *Adult:* **IM/IV** 1-2 g q12hr

• *Child 1 mo-12 yr:* **IM/IV** 50-180 mg/kg/day divided q6hr

Severe infections

• *Adult:* **IM/IV** 2 g q4hr, not to exceed 12 g/day

• *Child 1 mo-12 yr:* **IM/IV** 50-180 mg/kg/day in 4-6 divided doses

Uncomplicated gonorrhea

• *Adult:* **IM** 1 g

• Dosage reduction indicated for severe renal impairment (CCr <30 ml/min)

Available forms: Powder for inj 500 mg, 1, 2, 10 g; inj 1, 2 g premixed frozen

cefpodoxime

Pneumonia

• *Adult >13 yr:* **PO** 200 mg q12hr for 14 days

Uncomplicated gonorrhea

• *Adult >13 yr:* **PO** 200 mg, single dose

Skin and skin structure

• *Adult >13 yr:* **PO** 400 mg q12hr for 7-14 days

Pharyngitis and tonsillitis

• *Adult >13 yr:* **PO** 100 mg q12hr for 10 days

• *Child 5 mo-12 yr:* **PO** 5 mg/kg q12hr (max 100 mg/dose or 200 mg/day) × 5-10 days

Uncomplicated UTI

• *Adult >13 yr:* **PO** 100 mg q12hr for 7 days; dosing interval increased in presence of severe renal impairment

Acute otitis media

• *Child 5 mo-12 yr:* **PO** 5 mg/kg q12hr for 10 days

Available forms: Tabs 100, 200 mg; granules for susp 50 mg, 100 mg/5 ml

ceftazidime

- *Adult:* **IV/IM** 1-2 g q8-12hr × 5-10 days
- *Child:* **IV** 30-50 mg/kg q8hr not to exceed 6 g/day
- *Neonate:* **IV** 30-50 mg/kg q12hr

Renal dose

- CCr <50 ml/min give q12hr; CCr 10-30 ml/min give q24hr; CCr <10 ml/min give q48-72hr

Available forms: Inj 250, 500 mg, 1, 2, 6 g

ceftibuten

- *Adult:* **PO** 400 mg/day × 10 days
- *Child 6 mo-12 yr:* **PO** 9 mg/kg/day × 10 days

Renal dose

- CCr 30-49 ml/min give 200 mg q24hr; CCr 5-29 ml/min give 100 mg q24hr

Available forms: Caps 400 mg; susp 90 mg, 180 mg/5 ml

ceftizoxime

- *Adult:* **IM/IV** 1-2 g q8-12hr, may give up to 4 g q8hr in life-threatening infections
- *Child >6 mo:* **IM/IV** 50 mg/kg q6-8hr

Renal dose

- CCr <50-80 ml/min give 500-1500 mg q8hr; CCr 5-49 ml/min give 250-1000 mg q12hr

PID

- *Adult:* **IV** 2 g q8hr, may increase to 4 g q8hr in severe infections

Available forms: Powder for inj 500 mg, 1, 2, 10 g; premixed 1 g, 2 g/50 ml

ceftriaxone

- *Adult:* **IM/IV** 1-2 g/day, max 2 g q12-24hr
- *Child:* **IM/IV** 50-75 mg/kg/day in equal doses q12hr

Uncomplicated gonorrhea

- *Adult:* 250 mg **IM** as single dose
- Reduce dosage in severe renal impairment (CCr <10 ml/min)

Meningitis

- *Adult and child:* **IM/IV** 100 mg/kg/day in equal doses q12hr, max 4 g/day

Surgical prophylaxis

- *Adult:* **IV** 1 g ½-2 hr preop

Available forms: Inj 250, 500 mg, 1, 2, 10 g

SIDE EFFECTS

CNS: Headache, dizziness, weakness, paresthesia, fever, chills, **seizures,** dyskinesia (cefdinir)

CV: **Heart failure,** syncope (cefdinir)

GI: Nausea, vomiting, diarrhea, anorexia, pain, glossitis, **bleeding;** increased AST, ALT, bilirubin, LDH, alk phos; abdominal pain, **pseudomembranous colitis;** cholestasis (cefotaxime)

GU: **Proteinuria,** vaginitis, pruritus, candidiasis, increased BUN, **nephrotoxicity, renal failure**

HEMA: **Leukopenia, thrombocytopenia, agranulocytosis,** anemia, **neutropenia, lymphocytosis, eosinophilia, pancytopenia, hemolytic anemia**

INTEG: Rash, urticaria, dermatitis

RESP: Dyspnea

SYST: **Anaphylaxis, serum sickness, Stevens-Johnson syndrome, toxic epidermal necrolysis**

Contraindications: Hypersensitivity to cephalosporins, infants <1 mo

Precautions: Pregnancy (B), breastfeeding, children, hypersensitivity to penicillins, GI/renal disease

PHARMACOKINETICS

cefdinir

Unchanged in urine; crosses placenta, blood-brain barrier; eliminated in breast milk, not metabolized; 60%-70% protein binding

cefditoren pivoxil

Well absorbed after it is broken down (prodrug), distribution widely, half-life 100 min, onset rapid, peak 0.5-3 hr, duration 12 hr, 88% protein binding

cefepime

Peak 79 min; half-life 2 hr; 20% bound by plasma proteins; 90% excreted unchanged in urine; crosses placenta, blood-brain barrier; excreted in breast milk, not metabolized

cefixime

PO: Peak 1-2 hr, half-life 3-4 hr, 65% bound by plasma proteins, 50% eliminated unchanged in urine, crosses placenta, excreted in breast milk

cefotaxime

Half-life 1 hr, 35%-65% is bound by plasma proteins, 40%-65% is eliminated unchanged in urine in 24 hr, 25% metabolized to active metabolites, excreted in breast milk (small amounts)

IM: Onset 30 min

IV: Onset 5 min

cefpodoxime

Half-life 1 hr, 25% bound by plasma proteins, 30% eliminated unchanged in urine in 8 hr, crosses placenta, excreted in breast milk

ceftazidime

IM/IV: Peak 1 hr, half-life 1-2 hr, 90% bound by plasma proteins, 80% eliminated unchanged in urine, crosses placenta, excreted in breast milk

ceftibuten

PO: Peak 2-3 hr; plasma protein binding 65%, elimination half-life 2 hr, extensively metabolized to an active metabolite

ceftizoxime

Half-life 1.6 hr, 90% bound by plasma proteins, 36%-60% eliminated unchanged in urine, crosses placenta, excreted in breast milk

IM: Peak 1 hr

IV: Onset 5 min

ceftriaxone

Half-life 5-8 hr, 90% bound by plasma proteins, 35%-60% eliminated unchanged in urine, crosses placenta, excreted in breast milk

IM: Peak 2-3 hr

IV: Onset 5 min

INTERACTIONS

Increase: bleeding—anticoagulants, thrombolytics, plicamycin, valproic acid, NSAIDs

Increase: toxicity—aminoglycosides, furosemide, probenecid

Decrease: absorption of cefdinir—iron

Drug/Herb

• Do not use acidophilus with antiinfectives; separate by several hours

Increase: bleeding risk (cefoperazone)—angelica, anise, arnica, bogbean, boldo, celery, chamomile, clove, fenugreek, feverfew, garlic, ginger, ginkgo, ginseng *(Panax)*, horse chestnut, horseradish, licorice, meadowsweet, prickly ash, onion, papain, passion flower, poplar, red clover, turmeric, willow

Drug/Food

Decrease: absorption—iron-rich cereal, infants formula

Drug/Lab Test

Increase: ALT, AST, alk phos, LDH, bilirubin, BUN, creatinine

False increase: creatinine (serum urine), urinary 17-KS

False positive: urinary protein, direct Coombs' test, urine glucose

Interference: cross-matching

NURSING CONSIDERATIONS

Assess:

• Sensitivity to penicillin, other cephalosporins

⚠ Nephrotoxicity: increased BUN, creatinine; urine output: if decreasing, notify prescriber; may indicate nephrotoxicity

• Blood studies: AST, ALT, CBC, Hct, bilirubin, LDH, alk phos, Coombs' test monthly if patient is on long-term therapy

• Electrolytes: K, Na, Cl monthly if patient is on long-term therapy

• Bowel pattern daily; if severe diarrhea occurs, product should be discontinued; may indicate pseudomembranous colitis

• IV site for extravasation, phlebitis

⚠ Anaphylaxis: rash, urticaria, pruritus, chills, fever, joint pain, angioedema; may occur few days after therapy begins

• Bleeding: ecchymosis, bleeding gums, hematuria, stool guaiac

⚠ Overgrowth of infection: perineal itching, fever, malaise, redness, pain, swelling, drainage, rash, diarrhea, change in cough, sputum

Administer:

• Change IV site q72hr

cefdinir

• Oral susp after adding 39 ml water to the 60-ml bottle; 65 ml water to the

120-ml bottle; discard unused portion after 10 days; give without regard to food
• After C&S completed

cefditoren pivoxil
• For 10 days to ensure organism death, prevent superinfection
• With food for GI symptoms
• After C&S completed

cefepime
• IV after diluting in 50-100 ml or more D_5, NS and give over 30 min
• For 7-10 days to ensure organism death, prevent superinfection

Solution compatibilities: 0.9% NaCl, D_5, D_5W, 0.5%, 10% lidocaine, bacteriostatic water for inj with parabens/benzyl alcohol

Y-site compatibilities: Doxorubicin liposome

cefixime
• For 10-14 days to ensure organism death, prevent superinfection
• Do not break, crush, or chew tab
• Without regard to food

cefotaxime
• IV after diluting 1 g/10 ml D_5W, NS, sterile H_2O for inj and give over 3-5 min by Y-tube or 3-way stopcock; may be diluted further with 50-100 ml of normal saline or D_5W; run over ½-1 hr; discontinue primary inf during administration; or may be diluted in larger vol of sol and given as a cont inf over 6-24 hr
• For 10-14 days to ensure organism death, prevent superinfection
• Thaw frozen container at room temperature or refrigeration; do not force thaw by immersion or microwave; visually inspect container for leaks

Additive compatibilities: Clindamycin, metronidazole, verapamil

Syringe compatibilities: Heparin, ofloxacin

Y-site compatibilities: Acyclovir, amifostine, aztreonam, cyclophosphamide, diltiazem, famotidine, fludarabine, hydromorphone, lorazepam, magnesium sulfate, melphalan, meperidine, midazolam, morphine, ondansetron, perphenazine, sargramostim, teniposide, thiotepa, tolazoline, vinorelbine

cefpodoxime
• Do not break, crush, or chew tabs
• For 10-14 days to ensure organism death, prevent superinfection
• Without regard to food

Y-site compatibilities: Famotidine, fluconazole, fludarabine, insulin (regular), meperidine, morphine, sargramostim

ceftazidime
• IV after diluting 1 g/10 ml sterile H_2O for inj, shake, invert needle, push plunger, insert needle through stopper and keep in sol, expel bubbles and give over 3-5 min; may be diluted further with 50-100 ml of normal saline or D_5W; run over ½-1 hr, give through Y-tube or 3-way stopcock, discontinue primary inf during administration; store for 96 hr refrigerated, 24 hr room temperature
• For 5-10 days to ensure organism death, prevent superinfection

Syringe compatibilities: Hydromorphone

Additive compatibilities: Ciprofloxacin, clindamycin, fluconazole, metronidazole, ofloxacin

Y-site compatibilities: Acyclovir, allopurinol, amifostine, aztreonam, ciprofloxacin, diltiazem, enalaprilat, esmolol, famotidine, filgrastim, fludarabine, foscarnet, granisetron, heparin, hydromorphone, labetalol, meperidine, melphalan, morphine, ondansetron, paclitaxel, ranitidine, remifentanil, tacrolimus, teniposide, theophylline, thiotepa, vinorelbine, zidovudine

ceftibuten
• For 10 days to ensure organism death, prevent superinfection
• Without regard to food

ceftizoxime
• IV after diluting 1 g/10 ml sterile water, shake and give over 3-5 min; may be diluted further with 50-100 ml NS or D_5W give through Y-tube or 3-way stopcock; run over ½-1 hr
• For 10-14 days to ensure organism death, prevent superinfection

Additive compatibilities: Clindamycin

Y-site compatibilities: Acyclovir, allopurinol, amphotericin B cholesteryl sulfate complex, aztreonam, DOXOrubicin liposome, enalaprilat, esmolol, famotidine, fludarabine, foscarnet, hydromorphone, labetalol, melphalan, meperidine, morphine, ondansetron, remifentanil, sargramostim, teniposide, vinorelbine

ceftriaxone

- For 10-14 days to ensure organism death, prevent superinfection
- IM inj deeply in large muscle mass
- IV after diluting 250 mg/2.4 ml D_5W, H_2O for inj, 0.9% NaCl; may be further diluted with 50-100 ml NS, D_5W, $D_{10}W$, shake; run over ½-1 hr
- Do not mix with calcium salts

Additive compatibilities: Amino acids or sodium bicarbonate, metronidazole

Y-site compatibilities: Acyclovir, allopurinol, aztreonam, cisatracurium, diltiazem, DOXOrubicin liposome, fludarabine, foscarnet, heparin, melphalan, meperidine, methotrexate, morphine, paclitaxel, remifentanil, sargramostim, tacrolimus, teniposide, theophylline, vinorelbine, warfarin, zidovudine

Evaluate:

- Therapeutic response: decreased symptoms of infection; negative C&S

Teach patient/family:

- If diabetic, to check blood glucose

⚠ To report sore throat, bruising, bleeding, joint pain; may indicate blood dyscrasias (rare); diarrhea with mucus, blood, may indicate pseudomembranous colitis

- To report persistent diarrhea
- Cefditoren can be taken with oral contraceptives

Treatment of anaphylaxis: Epinephrine, antihistamines; resuscitate if needed

cephradine

See cephalosporins—
1st generation

certolizumab (℞)

(ser'tue-liz'oo-mab)

Cimzia

Func. class.: Biologic response modifier

Chem. class: Anti-tissue necrosis factor (anti-TNF) agent

Action: Monoclonal antibody that neutralizes the activity of tumor necrosis factor alpha (TNF-α) found in Crohn's disease; decreased infiltration of inflammatory cells

Uses: Crohn's disease (moderate-severe), rheumatoid arthritis (moderate-severe)

Unlabeled uses: Moderate-severe chronic plaque psoriasis, fistulizing Crohn's disease

DOSAGE AND ROUTES

Crohn's disease (moderate-severe)

- *Adult:* **SUBCUT** 400 mg given as 2 inj at wk 0, 2, 4; if clinical response occurs, give 400 mg q4wk

Rheumatoid arthritis (moderate to severe)

- *Adult:* **SUBCUT** 400 mg q2wk × 3 doses, then 200 mg q2wk; given with methotrexate

Crohn's disease (fistulizing)/ intolerant to infliximab (unlabeled)

- *Adult:* **SUBCUT** 400 mg wk 0, 2, 4, then 400 mg q4wk

Available forms: Powder for inj 400 mg kit

SIDE EFFECTS

CNS: Dizziness, syncope, peripheral neuropathy, fever, **seizures, demyelinating disease of CNS**

CV: Hypotension, **heart failure, MI, cardiac dysrhythmia**

EENT: Optic neuritis, retinal hemorrhage, uveitis

GI: Increased LFTs, **hepatitis, bowel obstruction**

GU: UTI, renal disease

HEMA: **Anemia, aplastic anemia, pancytopenia, thrombocytopenia**

INTEG: *Rash, urticaria,* **angioedema**
MISC: **Anaphylaxis,** antibody formation, arthralgia, bleeding, infection, lupuslike symptoms, lymphadenopathy, **malignancies, serum sickness, suicidal ideation**
RESP: Dyspnea, upper respiratory tract infection

Contraindications: Influenza, IV administration, sepsis, hypersensitivity

Black Box Warning: Infection

Precautions: Pregnancy (B), breastfeeding, children, geriatric patients, AIDS, coagulopathy, diabetes, fungal infection, heart failure, hepatitis, human antichimeric antibody, immunosuppression, leukopenia, MS, cancer, neurologic/renal disease, surgery, thrombocytopenia, TB, vaccinations

PHARMACOKINETICS

Peak 54-171 hr, terminal half-life 14 days

INTERACTIONS

- Do not administer live vaccines, toxoids concurrently

Increase: possible infections—abatacept, adalimumab, anakinra, etanercept, immunosuppressive agents, infliximab, rilonacept

Increase: possible malignancies—adalimumab, etanercept, infliximab

NURSING CONSIDERATIONS

Assess:

- Antinuclear antibody test (ANA), hepatitis B serology, CBC
- For rheumatoid arthritis, ROM, pain
- GI symptoms: nausea, vomiting, abdominal pain, hepatitis, increased LFTs
- Periodic blood counts (CBC)
- CV status: B/P, pulse, chest pain

⚠ Allergic reaction, anaphylaxis: rash, dermatitis, urticaria, dyspnea, hypotension, fever, chills; discontinue if severe, administer epinephrine, corticosteroids, antihistamines; assess for allergies to murine proteins before starting therapy

- Infections: discontinue if infection occurs; do not administer to patients with active infections
- Identify TB, risk for HBV before beginning treatment; a TB test should be obtained, if present; TB should be treated prior to receiving infliximab

Administer:

SUBCUT route

- Give by SUBCUT only
- Reconstitution: allow to warm to room temperature; add 1 ml sterile water for inj to each vial; two vials will be needed for Crohn's disease
- Gently swirl; do not shake; full reconstitution may take up to 30 min; reconstituted product may remain at room temperature for up to 2 hr or refrigerated up to 24 hr
- If the reconstituted product has been refrigerated, allow to warm to room temperature
- Use two syringes and 2 20G needles
- Withdraw reconstituted sol from each vial into separate syringes; each will contain 200 mg; switch 20G to 23G needle; inject into 2 separate sites in abdomen or thigh

Perform/provide:

- Storage in refrigerator; do not freeze

Evaluate:

- Therapeutic response: absence of fever, mucus in stools

Teach patient/family:

- Not to breastfeed while taking this product
- To notify prescriber of GI symptoms, hypersensitivity reactions
- Not to operate machinery, drive if dizziness, vertigo occur

cetirizine (℞, OTC)

(se-teer′i-zeen)

Zyrtec

Func. class.: Antihistamine (2nd generation, peripherally selective)

Chem. class.: Piperazine, H_1-histamine antagonist

Do not confuse:

Zyrtec/Xanax/Zantac

Action: Acts on blood vessels, GI, respiratory system by competing with histamine for H_1-receptor site; decreases allergic response by blocking pharmacologic effects of histamine; minimal anticholinergic, sedative action

Uses: Rhinitis, allergy symptoms, chronic idiopathic urticaria

Unlabeled uses: Asthma, atopic dermatitis

DOSAGE AND ROUTES

- *Adult and child ≥6 yr:* **PO** 5-10 mg/day
- *Child 2-5 yr:* **PO** 2.5 mg/day, may increase to 5 mg/day or 2.5 mg bid
- *Child 1-2 yr:* **PO** 2.5 mg/day, may increase to 2.5 mg q12hr
- *Child 6-11 mo:* **PO** 2.5 mg/day
- *Geriatric:* **PO** 5 mg/day, may increase to 10 mg/day

Self-treatment of hay fever/other respiratory allergies

- *Adult/adolescent/child ≥6 yr:* **PO** 10 mg/day; **ORAL SOL** 5-10 mg/day

Renal dose

- *Adult:* **PO** CCr 11-31 ml/min 5 mg/day

Hemodialysis

- *Adult:* **PO** 5 mg/day

Hepatic dose

- *Adult:* **PO** 5 mg/day

Atopic dermatitis (unlabeled)

- *Child 6-12 yr:* **PO** 5-10 mg/day
- *Child 1-2 yr:* **PO** 0.25 mg/kg bid

Available forms: Tabs 5, 10 mg; syr 5 mg/5 ml

SIDE EFFECTS

CNS: Headache, stimulation, *drowsiness,* sedation, *fatigue,* confusion, blurred vision, tinnitus, restlessness, tremors, paradoxical excitation in children or geriatric patients

GI: Dry mouth, increase LFTs, constipation

INTEG: Rash, eczema, photosensitivity, urticaria

RESP: Thickening of bronchial secretions, dry nose, throat

Contraindications: Breastfeeding, newborn or premature infants, hypersensitivity to this product or hydrOXYzine, severe hepatic disease

Precautions: Pregnancy (B), children, geriatric patients, respiratory disease, angle-closure glaucoma, prostatic hypertrophy, bladder neck obstruction, asthma

PHARMACOKINETICS

Absorption rapid; onset ½ hr; peak 1-2 hr; duration 24 hr; protein binding 93%; half-life decreased in children, increased in renal/hepatic disease

INTERACTIONS

Increase: CNS depression—alcohol, opiates, sedative/hypnotics, other CNS depressants

Increase: anticholinergic/sedative effect—MAOIs

Drug/Herb

Increase: effect—hops, Jamaican dogwood, kava, senega, valerian

Increase: anticholinergic effect—corkwood

Drug/Food

- Food prolongs absorption by 1.7 hr

Drug/Lab Test

False negative: skin allergy tests

NURSING CONSIDERATIONS

Assess:

- Allergy symptoms: pruritus, urticaria, watering eyes, baseline and during treatment

• Respiratory status: rate, rhythm, increase in bronchial secretions, wheezing, chest tightness

Administer:

• Without regard to meals

Perform/provide:

• Hard candy, gum, frequent rinsing of mouth for dryness
• Storage in tight, light-resistant container

Evaluate:

• Therapeutic response: absence of running or congested nose or rashes

Teach patient/family:

• All aspects of product use; to notify prescriber if confusion, sedation, hypotension occur
• To avoid driving, other hazardous activity if drowsiness occurs
• To avoid alcohol, other CNS depressants, OTC antihistamines
• To avoid exposure to sunlight; burns may occur
• To use sugarless gum, candy, frequent sips of water to minimize dry mouth
• Not to breastfeed

Treatment of overdose: Administer diazepam, vasopressors, phenytoin IV

cetrorelix (℞)

(set-roe-ree'lix)
Cetrotide
Func. class.: Gonadotropin-releasing hormone antagonist
Chem. class.: Synthetic decapeptide

Action: Inhibitor of pituitary gonadotropin secretion; initially increases LH and FSH, induces a rapid suppression of gonadotropin secretion

Uses: For inhibition of premature LH surges in women undergoing controlled ovarian hyperstimulation

Unlabeled uses: Benign prostatic hyperplasia (BPH), endometriosis

DOSAGE AND ROUTES

Single-dose regimen

• *Adult:* **SUBCUT** 3 mg when serum estradiol level is at appropriate stimulation response, usually on stimulation day 7; if hCG has not been given within 4 days after inj of 3 mg cetrorelix, give 0.25 mg daily until day of hCG administration

Multiple-dose regimen

• *Adult:* **SUBCUT** 0.25 mg is given on stimulation day 5 (either morning or evening) or 6 (morning) and continued daily until day hCG is given

BPH (unlabeled)

• *Adult (male):* **SUBCUT** 5 mg bid ×2 days, then 1 mg/day

Endometriosis (unlabeled)

• *Adult (female):* **SUBCUT** 3 mg q wk

Available forms: Inj 0.25, 3 mg

SIDE EFFECTS

CNS: Headache
CV: Edema
ENDO: Ovarian hyperstimulation syndrome, abdominal pain (gyn)
GI: Nausea, vomiting, diarrhea
INTEG: Pain on inj; local site reactions, bruising, pruritus
OTHER: Rapid weight gain
RESP: Shortness of breath
SYST: **Fetal death, anaphylaxis**

Contraindications: Pregnancy (X), breastfeeding, hypersensitivity, latex allergy, renal disease

Precautions: Geriatric patients

PHARMACOKINETICS

Excreted in feces/urine, half-life depends on dosage, metabolized to metabolites, protein binding 86%

NURSING CONSIDERATIONS

Assess:

• Serum progesterone, LH; ovarian ultrasound day 7-14
• For suspected pregnancy, product should not be used
• For latex allergy, product should not be used
• For ALT, AST, GGT, alk phos
⚠ For anaphylaxis during first infusion

Administer:

• SUBCUT using abdomen, 1 inch away from navel or upper thigh; swab inj area with disinfectant; clean a 2-inch circle and

allow to dry; pinch up area between thumb and finger; insert needle 45-90 degrees to surface; if positioned correctly, no blood will be drawn back into syringe; reposition needle without removing it; rotate inj sites
• Do not administer if patient is pregnant

Perform/provide:
• Protection from light

Evaluate:
• Therapeutic response: pregnancy

Teach patient/family:
• To report abdominal pain, vaginal bleeding, nausea, vomiting, diarrhea, shortness of breath, peripheral edema
• To teach self-administration technique if needed

cetuximab (℞)

(se-tux′i-mab)
Erbitux
Func. class.: Antineoplastic—miscellaneous, monoclonal antibody
Chem. class.: Epidermal growth factor receptor inhibitor

Action: Not fully understood; binds to epidermal growth factor receptors (EGFRs); inhibits phosphorylation and activation of receptor-associated kinase, resulting in inhibition of cell growth

Uses: Alone or in combination with irinotecan for EGFRs expressing metastatic colorectal carcinoma, head/neck cancer

Unlabeled uses: Front-line use in non–small cell lung cancer in combination with cisplatin and vinorelbine

DOSAGE AND ROUTES

• *Adult*: **IV INF** 400 mg/m^2 loading dose given over 120 min, max inf rate 5 ml/min; weekly maintenance dose (all other inf) is 250 mg/m^2 given over 60 min, max inf rate 5 ml/min; premedicate with an H_1 antagonist (diphenhydrAMINE 50 mg IV); dosage adjustments are made for inf reactions or dermatologic toxicity; other protocols are used

Non–small cell lung cancer (NSCLC) (unlabeled)
• *Adult:* **IV** 400 mg/m^2 over 120 min (max 5 ml/min) the 1st week with weekly inf of 250 mg/m^2 over 60 min (max 5 ml/min) with cisplatin 80 mg/m^2 on day 1, and vinorelbine 25 mg/m^2 on days 1, 8

Available forms: Inj 50-ml, single-use vial with 100 mg of cetuximab (2 mg/ml)

SIDE EFFECTS

CNS: Headache, insomnia, depression
GI: Nausea, diarrhea, vomiting, anorexia, mouth ulceration, dehydration, constipation, abdominal pain
HEMA: **Leukopenia, anemia**
INTEG: Rash, pruritus, acne, dry skin, **toxic epidermal necrolysis, angioedema,** *blepharitis, cheilitis, cellulitis, cysts, alopecia, skin/nail disorder,* **acute infusion reactions, other skin toxicities**
MISC: Conjunctivitis, asthma, malaise, fever, **renal failure,** hypomagnesemia
MS: Back pain
RESP: **Interstitial lung disease,** *cough, dyspnea,* **pulmonary embolus,** *peripheral edema*
SYST: **Anaphylaxis, sepsis, infection**

Contraindications: Hypersensitivity to this product or murine proteins

Precautions: Pregnancy (C), breastfeeding, children, geriatric patients, CV/renal/hepatic disease, ocular, pulmonary disorders

Black Box Warning: Arrhythmias, CAD, infusion-related reactions, radiation

PHARMACOKINETICS

Half-life 114 hr, steady state by 3rd wkly inf, peak 168-235 g/ml, trough 41-85 g/ml

INTERACTIONS

Drug/Lab
Increase: LFTs

NURSING CONSIDERATIONS

Assess:

⚠ Pulmonary changes: lung sounds, cough, dyspnea; interstitial lung disease may occur, may be fatal; discontinue therapy if confirmed

⚠ Toxic epidermal necrosis, angioedema, anaphylaxis

- GI symptoms: frequency of stools, dehydration, abdominal pain, stomatitis
- For K-RAS mutations in metastatic colorectal carcinoma; if K-RAS mutation on codon 12 or 13 is detected, then patient should not receive anti-EGFR antibody therapy

Administer:

Intermittent IV INF route

- Using cytoxic handling procedures
- By IV inf only, do not give by IV push or bolus
- Do not shake or dilute
- Inf pump: draw up volume of a vial using appropriate syringe/needle (a vented spike or other appropriate transfer device); fill Erbitux into sterile evacuated container/bag, repeat until calculated volume has been put into the container; use a new needle for each vial; give through in-line filter (low protein binding 0.22-micrometer); affix inf line and prime before starting inf, max rate 5 ml/min; flush line at end of inf with 0.9% NaCl
- Syringe pump: Draw up volume of a vial using appropriate syringe/needle (a vented spike); place syringe into syringe driver of a syringe pump and set rate; use an in-line filter 0.22-micrometer (low protein binding); connect inf line and start inf after priming; repeat until calculated volume has been given
- Use a new needle and filter for each vial, max 5 ml/min rate; use 0.9% NaCl to flush line after inf
- Do not piggyback to patient inf line
- Observe patient for adverse reactions for 1 hr after inf
- Inf reactions: if mild (grade 1 or 2) reduce all doses by 50%; if severe (grade 3 or 4) permanently discontinue

Perform/provide:

- Storage refrigerated 36° F-46° F, discard unused portions

Evaluate:

- Therapeutic response: Decrease growth, spread of EGFR expressing metastatic colorectal, head/neck carcinoma

Teach patient/family:

- To report adverse reactions immediately: shortness of breath, severe abdominal pain, skin eruptions
- Reason for treatment, expected results
- Use contraception during treatment, pregnancy (C), avoid breastfeeding
- To wear sunscreen and hats to limit sun exposure; sun exposure can exacerbate any skin reactions
- To avoid crowds, persons with known infections

charcoal, activated (OTC)

Actidose-Aqua, Actidose with Sorbitol, CharcoAid, Charcoal Plus, Charcocaps, Liqui-Char

Func. class.: Antiflatulent; antidote

Action: Binds poisons, toxins, irritants; increases adsorption in GI tract; inactivates toxins and binds until excreted

Uses: Poisoning, overdose

Unlabeled uses: Diarrhea, flatulence

DOSAGE AND ROUTES

Children should not get more than 1 dose of products with sorbitol

Poisoning

- Tabs/caps should not be used in poisonings
- *Adult and child:* **PO** 30-100 g or 1 g/kg, minimum dose 30 g/250 ml of water, may give 20-40 g q6hr for 1-2 days in severe poisoning, take with plenty of water

Diarrhea/flatulance (unlabeled)

- *Adult:* **PO** (CharcoCaps) 520 mg (2 caps) after meals or prn, max 4.16 g (16 cap)/day

Available forms: Powder 15, 25 ♣, 30, 40, 120, 240 g/container; oral susp 12.5 g/60 ml, 15 g/72 ml, 15 g/120 ml, 25 g/120 ml, 30 g/120 ml, 50 g/240 ml; Canada 15 g/120 ml, 25 g/125 ml, 50 g/225 ml, 50 g/250 ml

• Tabs/caps should not be used in poisonings

SIDE EFFECTS

GI: Nausea, black stools, vomiting, constipation, diarrhea, abdominal pain
OTHER: **Pulmonary aspiration**
Contraindications: Hypersensitivity to this product, unconsciousness, semiconsciousness, poisoning of cyanide, mineral acids, alkalis, gag reflex depression, ethanol intoxication, intestinal obstruction, absent bowel sounds
Precautions: Pregnancy (C), hypersensitivity to quinidine, quinine

PHARMACOKINETICS

PO: Excreted in feces, not absorbed, excreted unchanged in feces

INTERACTIONS

• Inactivation of acetylcysteine
Decrease: effects of acarbose, carbamazepine, digoxin, ipecac, phenytoin

NURSING CONSIDERATIONS

Assess:
• Respiration, pulse, B/P to determine charcoal effectiveness if taken for barbiturate/opiate poisoning, intact gag reflex, serum electrolytes
Administer:
PO route
• After inducing vomiting unless vomiting contraindicated (i.e., cyanide or alkalis)
• After mixing with water or fruit juice to form thick syrup; do not use dairy products, chocolate syrup to mix charcoal
• Repeat dose if vomiting occurs soon after dose; give with a laxative to promote elimination
• After spacing at least 1 hr before or after other products, or absorption will be decreased
NG route
• Through a nasogastric tube if patient unable to swallow
Perform/provide:
• Container closed tightly to prevent absorption of gases
Evaluate:
• Therapeutic response: LOC alert (poisoning)
Teach patient/family:
• That stools will be black
• How to prevent further poisonings

chloral hydrate (℞)

(klor-al hye′drate)
Aquachloral, chloral hydrate, Novo-Chlorhydrate ♣, PMS-chloral hydrate ♣, Somnote
Func. class.: Sedative/hypnotic, nonbarbiturate
Chem. class.: Chloral derivative

Controlled Substance Schedule IV (USA), Schedule F (Canada)
Action: Reduction product trichloroethanol produces mild cerebral depression, which causes sleep
Uses: Sedation, short-term treatment of insomnia, anxiety, alcohol withdrawal

DOSAGE AND ROUTES

Sedation
• *Adult:* **PO/RECT** 250 mg tid after meals; max 2 g/day
• *Child:* **PO** 25-50 mg/kg tid; max 500 mg tid
Insomnia
• *Adult:* **PO/RECT** 500 mg-1 g ½ hr before bedtime; max 2 g/day
• *Child:* **PO/RECT** 50-75 mg/kg (one dose)
Alcohol withdrawal
• *Adult:* **PO/RECT** 500 mg-1 g q6hr; max 2 g/day
Postoperative pain/adjunct
• *Adult:* **PO** 250 mg tid after meals; max 2 g/day
Procedure sedation
• *Child:* **PO/RECT** 25-50 mg/kg; max 100 mg/kg or 2 g

Renal disease

• *Adult:* **PO/RECT** CCr <50 ml/min, avoid use

Available forms: Caps 500 mg; syr 250 mg, 500 mg/5 ml; supp 325, 650 mg

SIDE EFFECTS

CNS: *Drowsiness,* dizziness, stimulation, nightmares, ataxia, hangover (rare), lightheadedness, headache, paranoia, hallucinations

CV: Hypotension, **dysrhythmias**

GI: *Nausea, vomiting, flatulence, diarrhea,* unpleasant taste, **gastric necrosis,** abdominal pain

HEMA: **Eosinophilia, leukopenia**

INTEG: *Rash,* urticaria, **angioedema,** fever, purpura, eczema

RESP: **Depression**

Contraindications: Hypersensitivity to this product or triclofos, severe renal/hepatic disease, GI disorders (oral forms), gastritis

Precautions: Pregnancy (C), breastfeeding, geriatric patients, severe cardiac disease, depression, suicidal individuals, asthma, intermittent porphyria, esophagitis, gastric/duodenal ulcers, gastritis

PHARMACOKINETICS

PO: Onset 30 min-1 hr, duration 4-8 hr

RECT: Onset slow, duration 4-8 hr, metabolized by liver, excreted by kidneys (inactive metabolite) and feces, crosses placenta, excreted in breast milk, metabolite is highly protein bound

INTERACTIONS

Increase: action—oral anticoagulants, furosemide

Increase: action of both products—alcohol, CNS depressants

Decrease: effects of phenytoin

Drug/Herb

Increase: sedative effect—catnip, chamomile, clary, cowslip, hops, kava, lavender, mistletoe, nettle, pokeweed, poppy, Queen Anne's lace, senega, skullcap, valerian

Increase: hypotension—black cohosh

Drug/Lab Test

Interference: urine catecholamines, urinary 17-OHCS

NURSING CONSIDERATIONS

Assess:

• Mental status: mood, sensorium, affect, memory (long and short term)

• Physical dependency: more frequent requests for medication, tremors, anxiety, pinpoint pupils

• Respiratory dysfunction: respiratory depression, character, rate, rhythm; hold product if respirations <10/min or if pupils dilated (rare)

• History of substance abuse, cardiac disease, gastritis

Administer:

• Do not break, crush, or chew caps

• On empty stomach with full glass of water or juice for best absorption and to decrease corrosion

• After meals to decrease GI symptoms if using for sedation

• ½-1 hr before bedtime for sleeplessness

Perform/provide:

• Assistance with ambulation after receiving dose, especially geriatric patients

• Safety measure: night-light, call bell within easy reach

• Check to see PO medication swallowed

• Check dose of syrup carefully; fatal overdoses have occurred

• Storage in dark container, suppositories in refrigerator

Evaluate:

• Therapeutic response: ability to sleep at night, decreased amount of early morning awakening if taking product for insomnia

Teach patient/family:

• To avoid driving, other activities requiring alertness

• To avoid alcohol ingestion, CNS depressants; serious CNS depression may result

- Not to discontinue medication quickly after long-term use; product should be tapered over 1-2 wk, delirium may occur
- That effects may take 2 nights for benefits to be noticed
- Alternative measures to improve sleep (reading, exercise several hours before bedtime, warm bath, warm milk, TV, self-hypnosis, deep breathing)
- Avoid breastfeeding

Treatment of overdose: Lavage, activated charcoal; monitor electrolytes, vital signs

chlorambucil (℞)

(klor-am′byoo-sil)

Leukeran

Func. class.: Antineoplastic alkylating agent

Chem. class.: Nitrogen mustard

Do not confuse:
Leukeran/leucovorin/Leukine

Action: Alkylates DNA, RNA; inhibits enzymes that allow synthesis of amino acids in proteins; activity is not cell cycle phase specific

Uses: Chronic lymphocytic leukemia, non-Hodgkin's/Hodgkin's disease, other lymphomas

Unlabeled uses: Macroglobulinemia ovarian, testicular carcinoma, Behçet's syndrome, Churg-Strauss syndrome, dermatomyositis, hydatidiform mole, thrombocytopenic purpura (ITP), lupus nephritis, nephrotic syndrome, pneumonitis, polyarteritis nodosa, polymyositis, rheumatoid arthritis, SLE, Wegener's granulomatosis, choriocarcinoma

DOSAGE AND ROUTES

- *Adult:* **PO** 0.1-0.2 mg/kg/day for 3-6 wk initially, then 4-10 mg/day maintenance
- *Geriatric:* **PO** initially ≤2-4 mg/day
- *Child:* **PO** 0.1-0.2 mg/kg/day (4.5 mg/m²/day) in divided doses or 4.5 mg/m²/day as 1 dose or in divided doses × 3-6 wk

Nephrotic syndrome

- *Child:* **PO** 0.1-0.2 mg/kg/day with predniSONE × 8-12 wk

Macroglobulinemia (unlabeled)

- *Adult:* **PO** 2-10 mg/day × 9 days, or 8 mg/m²/day with predniSONE × 10 days, repeat q6-8wk as needed

Intractable idiopathic uveitis/Behçet's syndrome/Churg-Strauss syndrome/polyarteritis nodosa/Wegener's granulomatosis (unlabeled)

- *Adult:* **PO** 0.2 mg/kg/day

Dermatomyositis/pneumonitis/lupus nephritis/polymyositis related to SLE/rheumatoid arthritis (unlabeled)

- *Adult:* **PO** 0.1-0.2 mg/kg/day

Available forms: Tabs 2 mg

SIDE EFFECTS

CNS: **Seizures,** tremors, confusion, agitation, ataxia, hallucinations

GI: Nausea, vomiting, diarrhea, weight loss, **hepatoxicity,** *jaundice*

GU: Hyperuremia

HEMA: **Thrombocytopenia, leukopenia, pancytopenia** (prolonged use), **permanent bone marrow depression**

INTEG: Alopecia (rare), dermatitis, rash, **Stevens-Johnson syndrome**

RESP: **Fibrosis, pneumonitis**

Contraindications: Breastfeeding, radiation therapy within 1 mo, chemotherapy within 1 mo, thrombocytopenia, recent smallpox vaccination

Black Box Warning: Pregnancy (D)

Precautions: Children, *Pneumococcus* vaccination, tumor lysis syndrome

Black Box Warning: Bone marrow suppression, infertility, secondary malignancy

PHARMACOKINETICS

Well absorbed orally, metabolized in liver, excreted in urine, half-life 2 hr

INTERACTIONS

• Filgrastim, sargramostim contraindicated 24 hr prior to or after chemotherapy
• Not to be used in combination with nalidixic acid
Increase: toxicity—other antineoplastics, radiation
Increase: bleeding risk—anticoagulants, salicylates

NURSING CONSIDERATIONS

Assess:
• Bleeding: hematuria, guaiac, bruising or petechiae, mucosa or orifices q8hr
• Jaundice of skin, sclera, dark urine, clay-colored stools, itchy skin, abdominal pain, fever, diarrhea
• Dyspnea, crackles, unproductive cough, chest pain, tachypnea
• Effects of alopecia on body image; discuss feelings about body changes (rare)
• CBC, differential, platelet count weekly; withhold product if WBC is <2000 or granulocyte count is <1000/mm^3; notify prescriber of results
• Pulmonary function tests, chest x-ray films before, during therapy; chest film should be obtained q2wk during treatment
• Renal studies: BUN, serum uric acid, urine CCr before, during therapy; I&O ratio; report urine output of <30 ml/hr
• Monitor temp q4hr (may indicate beginning infection)
• Hepatic studies before, during therapy (bilirubin, AST, ALT, LDH) as needed or monthly
Administer:
• All products PO if possible, avoid IM inj when platelets <100,000/mm^3
• Allopurinol to maintain uric acid levels, alkalinization of urine; increase fluid intake to 2-3 L/day to prevent urate deposits, calculi formation
Perform/provide:
• Storage in tight container, amber glass, store in refrigerator
Evaluate:
• Therapeutic response: decreased size of tumor, spread of malignancy
Teach patient/family:
• To report signs of infection: increased temp, sore throat, persistent cough, flu-like symptoms
• To report signs of anemia: fatigue, headache, faintness, shortness of breath, irritability, seizures, jaundice, bruising
• To report bleeding; avoid use of razors, commercial mouthwash
• To avoid use of aspirin products, ibuprofen
• To avoid vaccinations during treatment
• To use contraception during and several months after completion of therapy; may cause irreversible gonadal suppression; avoid breastfeeding
• To report any changes in breathing or coughing
• To drink 2-3 L of fluid daily unless contraindicated; report drop in urine output

chloramphenicol (℞)

(klor-am-fen′i-kole)
chloramphenicol,
Chloromycetin,
Pentamycetin ✦
Func. class.: Antiinfective—miscellaneous
Chem. class.: Dichloroacetic acid derivative

Action: Binds to 50S ribosomal subunit, which interferes with or inhibits protein synthesis
Uses: Infections caused by *Haemophilus influenzae, Salmonella typhi, Rickettsia, Neisseria, Staphylococcus, Streptococcus, Escherichia coli* mycoplasma, meningitis, bacteremia, abdominal skin, soft tissue infections; not to be used if less toxic products can be used
Unlabeled uses: *Bacillus anthracis,* glanders, melioidosis, plague, plague prophylaxis, psittacosis, *Stenotrophomonas maltophilia,* tularemia

DOSAGE AND ROUTES

• *Adult and child:* **PO/IV** 50-75 mg/kg/day in divided doses q6hr, 100 mg/kg/day (for meningitis only) max 4 g/day
• *Premature infant and neonate:* **IV** 25 mg/kg/day in divided doses q12-24hr
Available forms: Inj 1 g, caps 250 mg

SIDE EFFECTS

CNS: Headache, *depression,* confusion, peripheral neuritis
CV: **Gray syndrome in newborns: failure to feed, pallor, cyanosis, abdominal distention, irregular respiration, vasomotor collapse**
EENT: Optic neuritis, blindness
GI: *Nausea, vomiting, diarrhea,* abdominal pain, xerostomia, glossitis, colitis, pruritus ani
HEMA: **Anemia, thrombocytopenia, aplastic anemia, granulocytopenia, leukopenia, acute generalized exanthematous pustulosis (AGEP) (rare)**
INTEG: Itching, urticaria, contact dermatitis, rash
Contraindications: Hypersensitivity, severe renal/hepatic disease, minor infections, labor, influenza, tympanic membrane perforation
Precautions: Pregnancy (C), breastfeeding, infants, children, renal/hepatic disease, ulcerative colitis, pseudomembranous colitis

Black Box Warning: Bone marrow suppression

PHARMACOKINETICS

Absorbed well (PO), completely (IV); distributed widely, metabolized in liver; excreted in kidneys, unchanged; half-life 1½-4 hr
PO: Peak 1-2 hr, onset 15 min
IV: Peak inf end, onset rapid

INTERACTIONS

Increase: action of barbiturates, anticoagulants, hydantoins, iron products, antidiabetics
Decrease: action of vit B_{12}, folic acid, penicillins, rifampin

Drug/Herb
• Do not use acidophilus with antiinfectives; separate by several hours

NURSING CONSIDERATIONS

Assess:
• Signs of infection, anemia
⚠ Any patient with compromised renal system; product is excreted slowly in poor renal system function; toxicity may occur rapidly
• Hepatic studies: AST, ALT
• Blood studies: WBC, RBC, Hct, Hgb, platelets, serum iron, reticulocytes; product should be discontinued if bone marrow is depressed
• Renal studies: urinalysis, protein, blood, BUN, creatinine
• C&S before product therapy; may be given as soon as culture is taken
• Product level in impaired renal, hepatic systems; peak 15-20 mg/ml 3 hr after dose, trough 5-10 mg/ml prior to next dose
• Bowel pattern before, during treatment
• Skin eruptions, itching, dermatitis after administration
• Allergies before treatment, reaction of each medication
⚠ Neonates for beginning Gray syndrome: cyanosis, abdominal distention, irregular respiration, failure to feed; product should be discontinued immediately

Administer:
• Product must be taken in equal intervals around clock to maintain blood levels
• IM route not recommended

PO route
⚠ Do not break, crush, or chew caps
• Give oral form on empty stomach with full glass of water
• Store cap in airtight container at room temperature

IV route
• After diluting 1 g/10 ml of sterile H_2O for inj or D_5W (10% sol); give >1 min; may be further diluted in 50-100 ml of D_5W; give through Y-tube, 3-way stopcock, or additive inf set; run over ½-1 hr

Additive compatibilities: Amikacin, aminophylline, ascorbic acid, calcium chloride or gluconate, cephalothin, cephapirin, colistimethate, corticotropin, cyanocobalamin, dimenhyDRINATE, DOPamine, ephedrine, heparin, hydrocortisone, kanamycin, lidocaine, magnesium sulfate, metaraminol, methicillin, methyldopate, methylPREDNISolone, metronidazole, nafcillin, oxacillin, oxytocin, penicillin G potassium, penicillin G sodium, pentobarbital, phenylephrine, phytonadione, plasma protein fraction, potassium chloride, promazine, ranitidine, sodium bicarbonate, thiopental, verapamil, vit B/C

Syringe compatibilities: Ampicillin, cloxacillin, heparin, methicillin, penicillin G sodium

Y-site compatibilities: Acyclovir, cyclophosphamide, enalaprilat, esmolol, foscarnet, hydromorphone, labetalol, magnesium sulfate, meperidine, morphine, perphenazine, tacrolimus

Perform/provide:

- Reconstituted sol at room temperature 30 days

Evaluate:

- Therapeutic response: decreased symptoms of infection

Teach patient/family:

- All aspects of product therapy: culture may be taken after complete course of medication
- To report sore throat, fever, fatigue, unusual bleeding, bruising; could indicate bone marrow depression (may occur weeks or months after termination of product)

Treatment of hypersensitivity:

- Withdraw product, maintain airway, administer epinephrine, aminophylline, O_2, IV corticosteroids

chloramphenicol ophthalmic

See Appendix B

chloramphenicol otic

See Appendix B

chlordiazepoxide (℞)

(klor-dye-az-e-pox′ide)
Apo-Chlordiazepoxide ♣, Librium, Novo-Poxide ♣

Func. class.: Antianxiety
Chem. class.: Benzodiazepine, long-acting

Controlled Substance Schedule IV

Do not confuse:
Librium/Librax

Action: Potentiates the actions of GABA, especially in the limbic system, reticular formation

Uses: Short-term management of anxiety, acute alcohol withdrawal, preoperatively for relaxation

DOSAGE AND ROUTES

Mild anxiety

- *Adult:* **PO** 5-10 mg tid-qid
- *Geriatric:* **PO** 5 mg bid initially, increase as needed
- *Child >6 yr:* **PO** 5 mg bid-qid, max 10 mg bid-tid

Severe anxiety

- *Adult:* **PO** 20-25 mg tid-qid; **IM/IV** 50-100 mg initially, then 25-50 mg tid or 25-50 mg initially in geriatric patients

Preoperatively

- *Adult:* **PO** 5-10 mg tid-qid on day before surgery

Alcohol withdrawal

- *Adult:* **PO** 50-100 mg q4-6hr prn, max 300 mg/day

Renal disease

- *Adult:* **PO** CCr <10 ml/min give 50% dose

Liver disease

- *Adult:* **PO** 5 mg bid-qid

Available forms: Caps 5, 25 mg

SIDE EFFECTS

CNS: Dizziness, drowsiness, confusion, headache, anxiety, tremors, stimulation, fatigue, depression, insomnia, hallucinations

CV: Orthostatic hypotension, edema, **ECG changes, tachycardia,** hypotension

EENT: Blurred vision, tinnitus, mydriasis

GI: Constipation, dry mouth, nausea, vomiting, anorexia, diarrhea

GU: Irregular periods, decreased libido

HEMA: **Agranulocytosis**

INTEG: Rash, dermatitis, itching

Contraindications: Pregnancy (D), breastfeeding, children <6 yr, hypersensitivity to benzodiazepines, closed-angle glaucoma, psychosis

Precautions: Geriatric patients, debilitated, renal/hepatic disease, suicidal ideation, abrupt discontinuation

PHARMACOKINETICS

PO: Onset 30 min, peak within 2 hr, duration 4-6 hr, metabolized by liver, excreted by kidneys, crosses placenta, excreted in breast milk, half-life 5-30 hr (increased in geriatric patients)

INTERACTIONS

Increase: CNS depression—CNS depressants, alcohol

Increase: chlordiazepoxide—cimetidine, disulfiram, fluoxetine, isoniazid, ketoconazole, metoprolol, oral contraceptives, propranolol, valproic acid

Decrease: action of levodopa

Decrease: action of chlordiazepoxide—CYP3A4 inhibitors (protease inhibitors, barbiturates, rifamycins)

Drug/Herb

Decrease: effect—cowslip, kava, Queen Anne's lace, St. John's wort, valerian

Drug/Lab Test

False increase: 17-OHCS

False positive: pregnancy test (some methods)

NURSING CONSIDERATIONS

Assess:

- B/P (lying, standing), pulse; if systolic B/P drops 20 mm Hg, hold product, notify prescriber
- Blood studies: CBC during long-term therapy; blood dyscrasias have occurred rarely
- Hepatic studies: AST, ALT, bilirubin, creatinine, LDH, alk phos during long-term therapy
- I&O; may indicate renal dysfunction
- For ataxia, oversedation in geriatric patients, debilitated patients
- Mental status: mood, sensorium, affect, sleeping pattern, drowsiness, dizziness
- Physical dependency, withdrawal symptoms: headache, nausea, vomiting, muscle pain, weakness after long-term use
- Suicidal tendencies, paradoxic reactions such as excitement, stimulation, acute rage
- For pregnancy; product should be avoided during pregnancy

Administer:

PO route

- With food or milk for GI symptoms
- Crushed if patient is unable to swallow medication whole

Perform/provide:

- Assistance with ambulation during beginning therapy, since drowsiness/dizziness occurs
- Check to see PO medication has been swallowed if patient is depressed, suicidal
- Sugarless gum, hard candy, frequent sips of water for dry mouth

Evaluate:

- Therapeutic response: decreased anxiety, restlessness, sleeplessness

Teach patient/family:

- That product may be taken with food
- Not to use product for everyday stress or use longer than 4 mo, unless directed by prescriber
- Not to take more than prescribed amount; may be habit forming
- To avoid OTC preparations unless approved by prescriber
- To avoid driving, activities that require alertness; drowsiness may occur

- To avoid alcohol ingestion, other psychotropic medications, unless directed by prescriber
- Not to discontinue medication abruptly after long-term use; may precipitate seizures
- To rise slowly or fainting may occur, especially geriatric patients
- That drowsiness may be worse at beginning of treatment
- To notify prescriber if pregnancy is suspected or planned

Treatment of overdose: Lavage, VS, supportive care, give flumazenil

chloroquine (℞)

(klor'oh-kwin)

Aralen Phosphate, chloroquine phosphate

Func. class.: Antimalarial

Chem. class.: Synthetic 4-aminoquinoline derivative

Action: Inhibits parasite replications, transcription of DNA to RNA by forming complexes with DNA of parasite

Uses: Malaria of *Plasmodium vivax, P. malariae, P. ovale, P. falciparum* (some strains), amebiasis

Unlabeled uses: Discoid lupus erythematosus, polymorphous light eruption, rheumatoid arthritis, ulcerative colitis

DOSAGE AND ROUTES

Malaria suppression

- *Adult and child:* **PO** 5 mg base/kg/wk (child) or 500 mg (300 mg base)/wk (adult) on same day of week, max 300 mg base; treatment should begin 1-2 wk before exposure and for 8 wk after leaving endemic area; if treatment begins after exposure, 600 mg base for adult and 10 mg base/kg for children in 2 divided doses 6 hr apart

Extraintestinal amebiasis

- *Adult:* **PO** 250 mg (150 mg base) qid × 2 days, then 250 mg (150 mg base) bid × 2-3 wk
- *Child:* **PO** 10 mg/kg/day × 2-3 wk, max 300 mg/day

Rheumatoid arthritis/discoid lupus erythematosus (unlabeled)

- *Adult and adolescent:* **PO** 250 mg/day

Available forms: Tabs 250 mg (150 mg base), 500 mg (300 mg base) phosphate

SIDE EFFECTS

CNS: Headache, stimulation, fatigue, **seizures,** psychosis

CV: Hypotension, **heart block, asystole with syncope,** ECG changes

EENT: Blurred vision, corneal changes, retinal changes, difficulty focusing, tinnitus, vertigo, deafness, photophobia, corneal edema

GI: Nausea, vomiting, anorexia, diarrhea, cramps

HEMA: **Thrombocytopenia, agranulocytosis, hemolytic anemia, leukopenia**

INTEG: Pruritus, pigmentary changes, skin eruptions, lichen planus–like eruptions, eczema, **exfoliative dermatitis**

Contraindications: Hypersensitivity, retinal field changes

Precautions: Pregnancy (C), breastfeeding, children, blood dyscrasias, severe GI disease, neurologic disease, alcoholism, hepatic disease, G6PD deficiency, psoriasis, eczema, seizures, preexisting auditory damage

Black Box Warning: Infection

PHARMACOKINETICS

Metabolized in liver; excreted in urine, feces, breast milk; crosses placenta

PO: Peak 1-3 hr, half-life 3-5 days

IM: Peak 30 min

INTERACTIONS

• Reduced oral clearance and metabolism of chloroquine: cimetidine

Increase: effects—2D6 inhibitors (amiodarone, chlorpheniramine, fluoxetine, haloperidol, ritonavir, paroxetine, terbinafine, ticlopidine); CYP3A4 inhibitors (diltiazem, verapamil, itraconazole, ketoconazole, erythromycin, doxycycline, clarithromycin)

Decrease: action of chloroquine—magnesium, aluminum compounds, kaolin; do not use concurrently

NURSING CONSIDERATIONS

Assess:

• Ophthalmic test if long-term treatment or dosage >150 mg/day

• Hepatic studies q wk: AST, ALT, bilirubin

• Blood studies: CBC, since blood dyscrasias occur

• ECG during therapy; watch for depression of T waves, widening of QRS complex

• Allergic reactions: pruritus, rash, urticaria

• Blood dyscrasias: malaise, fever, bruising, bleeding (rare)

• For ototoxicity (tinnitus, vertigo, change in hearing); audiometric testing should be done before, after treatment

⚠ For toxicity: blurring vision; difficulty focusing; headache; dizziness; decreased knee, ankle reflexes, seizures, CV collapse; product should be discontinued immediately and IV fluids given

Administer:

• Product in mg or base; they are different

PO route

• Before or after meals at same time each day to maintain product level

Additive compatibilities: Promethazine

Perform/provide:

• Storage in tight, light-resistant container at room temperature; keep inj in cool environment

Evaluate:

• Therapeutic response: decreased symptoms of infection

Teach patient/family:

• To take with meals or immediately after meals

• To use sunglasses in bright sunlight to decrease photophobia

• That urine may turn rust or brown color

• To report hearing, visual problems, fever, fatigue, bruising, bleeding, which may indicate blood dyscrasias

Treatment of overdose: Induce vomiting, gastric lavage, administer barbiturate (ultrashort-acting), vasopressor; tracheostomy may be necessary

chlorothiazide (℞)

(klor-oh-thye′a-zide)

Diuril

Func. class.: Diuretic

Chem. class.: Thiazide; sulfonamide derivative

Do not confuse:

chlorothiazide/chlorproMAZINE/chlorthalidone/chlorproPAMIDE

Action: Acts on distal tubule and thick ascending limb of the loop of Henle by increasing excretion of water, sodium, chloride, potassium, magnesium

Uses: Hypertension, diuresis, CHF, edema

DOSAGE AND ROUTES

Hypertension

• *Adult:* **PO/IV** 500 mg-2 g/day may divide bid

Edema

• *Adult:* **IV** 250 mg q6-12hr

• *Child >6 mo:* **PO** 10-20 mg/kg/day may divide bid

• *Child <6 mo:* **PO** up to 40 mg/kg/day in 2 doses

Available forms: Tabs 250, 500 mg; powder for inj 500 mg; oral susp 250 mg/5 ml

SIDE EFFECTS

CNS: Paresthesia, headache, *dizziness, fatigue*
CV: Irregular pulse, orthostatic hypotension, volume depletion
EENT: Blurred vision
ELECT: *Hypokalemia,* hypercalcemia, hyponatremia, hypomagnesemia
GI: *Nausea, vomiting, anorexia,* constipation, diarrhea, pancreatitis, GI irritation, **hepatitis**
GU: *Urinary frequency,* polyuria, incontinence
HEMA: **Aplastic anemia, hemolytic anemia, leukopenia, agranulocytosis, thrombocytopenia, neutropenia**
INTEG: *Rash,* urticaria, purpura, photosensitivity, fever, alopecia
META: Hyperglycemia, *hyperuricemia,* increased creatinine, BUN
SYST: **Anaphylaxis**

Contraindications: Breastfeeding, hypersensitivity to thiazides or sulfonamides, hepatic coma, anuria, renal decompensation

Precautions: Pregnancy (B), geriatric patient, hypokalemia, renal/hepatic disease, gout, COPD, SLE, diabetes mellitus, hyperlipidemia

PHARMACOKINETICS

PO: Onset 2 hr, peak 4 hr, duration 6-12 hr, crosses placenta, excreted in breast milk, excreted unchanged by kidneys, half-life 2 hr; not well absorbed

INTERACTIONS

• Hypokalemia: ticarcillin, glucocorticoids, amphotericin, mezlocillin, piperacillin

Increase: toxicity—lithium, nondepolarizing skeletal muscle relaxants, digoxin, allopurinol

Increase: hypotension—other antihypertensives, alcohol, nitrates

Decrease: absorption of thiazides—cholestyramine, colestipol

Decrease: diuretic action—NSAIDs

Drug/Herb

• Hypokalemia: chronic use aloe, buckthorn, cascara sagrada, Chinese rhubarb, gossypol, licorice, nettle, senna
• Severe photosensitivity: St. John's wort

Increase: diuretic effect—aloe, cucumber, dandelion, horsetail, pumpkin, Queen Anne's lace

Drug/Lab Test

Increase: Ca, amylase, parathyroid test, CPK

Decrease: PBI

False negative: phentolamine and tyramine tests

Interference: urine steroid tests

NURSING CONSIDERATIONS

Assess:

• Weight, I&O daily to determine fluid loss; effect of product may be decreased if used daily
• Rate, depth, rhythm of respirations; effect of exertion
• B/P lying, standing; postural hypotension may occur, especially in geriatric patients
• Electrolytes: K, Na, Cl; include BUN, blood glucose, CBC, serum creatinine, blood pH, ABGs, uric acid, Ca, Mg
• Glucose in urine if patient is diabetic
• Signs of metabolic alkalosis: drowsiness, restlessness
• Rashes, temp elevation daily
• Confusion, especially in geriatric patients; take safety precautions if needed

Administer:

• In AM to avoid interference with sleep if using product as a diuretic
• Potassium replacement if potassium < 3 mg/dl
• With food if nausea occurs; absorption may be decreased slightly; dehydration may occur; tablets may be crushed
• After shaking suspension

IV route

• After diluting 0.5 g/18 ml or more of sterile water for inj; may be diluted further with 0.9% NaCl, D_5W, check for extravasation; give over 5 min (0.5 g/5 min)

Additive compatibilities: Cimetidine, lidocaine, nafcillin, ranitidine, sodium bicarbonate

Evaluate:

- Therapeutic response: improvement in edema of feet, legs, sacral area daily if medication is being used for CHF; decreased B/P; increased urinary output

Teach patient/family:

- To rise slowly from lying or sitting position; orthostatic hypotension may occur
- To notify prescriber of muscle weakness, cramps, nausea, dizziness
- That product may be taken with food or milk; to take at same time each day; not to double dose
- That blood glucose may be increased in diabetics
- To take early in day to avoid nocturia
- To use sunscreen; use protective clothing to prevent photosensitivity
- To weigh weekly and notify prescriber of change of >3 lb
- To eat diet high in potassium if recommended by prescriber; teach high-potassium foods
- Not to take OTC medications without consulting prescriber

Treatment of overdose: Lavage if taken orally; monitor electrolytes; administer dextrose in saline; monitor hydration, CV, renal status

C

chlorpheniramine

(OTC, ℞)

(klor-fen-ir′a-meen)

Aller-Chlor, Allergy, Chlo-Amine, Chlorate, chlorpheniramine maleate, Chlor-Trimeton, Chlor-Tripolon ✦, Novo-Pheniram ✦, PediaCare Allergy Formula, Phenetron, Telachlor, Teldrin

Func. class.: Antihistamine (1st generation, nonselective)

Chem. class.: Alkylamine, H_1-receptor antagonist

Do not confuse:

Teldrin/Tedral

Action: Acts on blood vessels, GI system, respiratory system, by competing with histamine for H_1-receptor site; decreases allergic response by blocking histamine

Uses: Allergy symptoms, rhinitis, conjunctivitis (allergic)

DOSAGE AND ROUTES

- *Adult and child ≥12 yr:* **PO** 2-4 mg tid-qid, not to exceed 24 mg/day; **TIME-REL** 8-12 mg bid-tid, not to exceed 24 mg/day; **IM/IV/SUBCUT** 5-40 mg/day, max 40 mg/day
- *Child 6-12 yr:* **PO** 2 mg q4-6hr, not to exceed 12 mg/day; **SUS REL** 8 mg bedtime or daily, **SUS REL** not recommended for child <6 yr; **SUBCUT** 87.5 mcg/kg or 2.5 mg/m^2 q6hr
- *Child 2-5 yr:* **PO** 1 mg q4-6hr, not to exceed 4 mg/day

For self-treatment of hay fever or other upper respiratory allergies

- *Adult/adolescent/child ≥12 yr:* **PO** 4 mg q4-6hr, max 24 mg/24 hr
- *Child 6-11 yr:* **PO** 2 mg q4-6hr, max 12 mg/24 hr

Available forms: Chewable tabs 2 mg; tabs 4, 8, 12 mg; ext rel tabs 8, 12 mg; ext rel caps 8, 12 mg; syr 1 mg/5 ml, 2 mg/5 ml, 2.5 mg/5 ml; inj 10, 100 mg/ml

SIDE EFFECTS

CNS: ***Dizziness, drowsiness,*** poor coordination, fatigue, anxiety, euphoria, confusion, paresthesia, neuritis
EENT: Blurred vision; dilated pupils; tinnitus; nasal stuffiness; dry nose, throat, mouth
GI: Nausea, anorexia, diarrhea
GU: ***Retention,*** dysuria, urinary frequency
HEMA: **Thrombocytopenia, agranulocytosis, hemolytic anemia**
INTEG: Photosensitivity
RESP: Increased thick secretions, wheezing, chest tightness

Contraindications: Newborns/neonates

Precautions: Pregnancy (B), breastfeeding, geriatric patients, increased intraocular pressure, cardiac/renal disease, hypertension, asthma, seizure disorder, hyperthyroidism, prostatic hypertrophy, GI obstruction, peptic ulcer disease, emphysema, hypersensitivity to H_1-receptor antagonists, lower respiratory tract disease, stenosed peptic ulcers, bladder neck obstruction, closed-angle glaucoma

PHARMACOKINETICS

PO: Onset ½ hr, duration 4-12 hr
PO-ER: Duration 8-24 hr
IM/IV/SUBCUT: Duration 4-12 hr, detoxified in liver, excreted by kidneys (metabolites/free drug), half-life 12-15 hr

INTERACTIONS

Increase: CNS depression—barbiturates, opiates, hypnotics, tricyclics, alcohol
Increase: effect of chlorpheniramine—MAOIs
Increase: anticholinergic action—atropine, phenothiazines, quinidine, haloperidol

Drug/Herb
Increase: effect—hops, Jamaican dogwood, kava, khat, senega
Increase: anticholinergic effect—corkwood, henbane leaf

Drug/Lab Test
False negative: skin allergy tests

NURSING CONSIDERATIONS

Assess:
- Be alert for urinary retention, frequency, dysuria; product should be discontinued
- Respiratory status: rate, rhythm, increase in bronchial secretions, wheezing, chest tightness

Administer:
- Avoid concurrent use with other CNS depressants

PO route
- Do not break, crush, or chew ext rel forms
- With meals for GI symptoms; absorption may slightly decrease

IV route
- Undiluted at ≥10 mg/1 min
- Use only 10 mg/ml form for IV use

Perform/provide:
- Hard candy, gum, frequent rinsing of mouth for dryness
- Storage in tight container at room temperature

Evaluate:
- Therapeutic response: absence of running, congested nose, rashes, conjunctivitis

Teach patient/family:
- All aspects of product use; to notify prescriber of confusion/sedation/hypotension, difficulty voiding
- To avoid driving, other hazardous activity if drowsiness occurs, especially geriatric patients
- To avoid concurrent use of alcohol

Treatment of overdose: Administer diazepam, vasopressors, phenytoin IV

*chlorproMAZINE (℞)

(klor-proe′ma-zeen)
Chlorpromanyl ♣, chlorproMAZINE HCl, Largactil ♣, Novo-ChlorproMAZINE ♣, Thorazine, Thor-Prom

Func. class.: Antipsychotic/ antiemetic
Chem. class.: Phenothiazine-aliphatic

Do not confuse:
chlorproMAZINE/chlorproPAMIDE/ prochlorperazine

Action: Depresses cerebral cortex, hypothalamus, limbic system, which control activity aggression; blocks neurotransmission produced by DOPamine at synapse; exhibits a strong α-adrenergic, anticholinergic blocking action; mechanism for antipsychotic effects is unclear

Uses: Psychotic disorders, mania, schizophrenia, anxiety, intractable hiccups in adults, nausea, vomiting; preoperatively for relaxation; acute intermittent porphyria, behavioral problems in children, nonpsychotic, demented patients, Tourette's syndrome

Unlabeled uses: Vascular headache, agitation, dementia, neonatal abstinence syndrome

DOSAGE AND ROUTES

Psychosis

• *Adult:* **PO** 10-50 mg q1-4hr initially, then increase up to 2 g/day if necessary; **IM** 10-50 mg q1-4hr, usual dose 300-800 mg/day

• *Geriatric:* 10-25 mg daily-bid, increase by 10-25 mg/day q4-7days, max 800 mg/ day

• *Child >6 mo:* **PO** 0.5 mg/kg q4-6hr; **IM** 0.5 mg/kg q6-8hr; **RECT** 1 mg/kg q6-8hr

Nausea and vomiting

• *Adult:* **PO** 10-25 mg q4-6hr prn; **IM** 25-50 mg q3hr prn; **RECT** 50-100 mg q6-8hr prn, not to exceed 400 mg/day; **IV** 25-50 mg daily-qid

• *Child ≥6 mo:* **PO** 0.55 mg/kg q4-6hr; **IM** q6-8hr; **RECT** 1.1 mg/kg q6-8hr; max **IM** ≤5 yr or ≤22.7 kg, 40 mg; max **IM** 5-10 yr or 22.7-45.5 kg, 75 mg

Intractable hiccups

• *Adult:* **PO** 25-50 mg tid-qid; **IM** 25-50 mg (only if PO dose does not work); **IV** 25-50 mg in 500-1000 ml **NS** (only for severe hiccups)

Available forms: Tabs 10, 25, 50, 100, 200 mg; sus rel caps 30, 75, 150, 200, 300 mg; syr 10, 25, 100 mg/5 ml; conc 30, 40, 100 mg/ml; supp 25, 100 mg; inj 25 mg/ml

SIDE EFFECTS

CNS: EPS: pseudoparkinsonism, akathisia, dystonia, tardive dyskinesia, **seizures,** *headache,* **neuroleptic malignant syndrome,** dizziness

CV: Orthostatic hypotension, hypertension, **cardiac arrest,** ECG changes, **tachycardia**

EENT: Blurred vision, glaucoma, dry eyes

ENDO: SIADH

GI: Dry mouth, nausea, vomiting, anorexia, constipation, diarrhea, cholestatic jaundice, weight gain

GU: Urinary retention, enuresis, impotence, amenorrhea, gynecomastia, breast engorgement

HEMA: Anemia, **leukopenia, leukocytosis, agranulocytosis**

INTEG: Rash, photosensitivity, dermatitis

RESP: **Laryngospasm,** dyspnea, **respiratory depression**

SYST: **Death in geriatric patients with dementia**

Contraindications: Children <6 mo, hypersensitivity, circulatory collapse, liver damage, cerebral arteriosclerosis, coronary disease, severe hypo/hypertension, blood dyscrasias, coma, brain damage, bone marrow depression, alcohol/ barbiturate withdrawal, closed-angle glaucoma

Precautions: Pregnancy (C), breastfeeding, geriatric patients, seizure disorders, hypertension, hepatic/cardiac disease, prostatic enlargement, Parkinson's disease, pulmonary disease

Black Box Warning: Dementia

PHARMACOKINETICS

Metabolized by liver, excreted in urine (metabolites), crosses placenta, enters breast milk, 95% bound to plasma proteins, elimination half-life 10-30 hr

PO: Absorption variable, widely distributed, onset erratic 30-60 min, duration 4-6 hr

PO-ER: Onset 30-60 min, peak unknown, duration 10-12 hr

IM: Well absorbed, peak 15-20 min, duration 4-8 hr

RECT: Onset erratic, duration 3 hr

IV: Onset 5 min, peak 10 min, duration unknown

INTERACTIONS

Increase: other CNS depressants, alcohol, barbiturate anesthetics, antihistamines, sedatives/hypnotics, antidepressants

Increase: toxicity—epinephrine

Increase: agranulocystosis—antithyroid agents

Increase: effects of both products—β-adrenergic blockers, alcohol

Increase: anticholinergic effects—anticholinergics, antidepressants, antiparkinsonian agents

Increase: valproic acid level

Decrease: lowered seizure threshold—anticonvulsants

Decrease: absorption—aluminum hydroxide, magnesium hydroxide antacids

Decrease: antiparkinson activity—levodopa, bromocriptine

Decrease: serum chlorproMAZINE—lithium, barbiturates

Decrease: anticoagulant effect—warfarin

Drug/Herb

Increase: action—cola tree, hops, nettle, nutmeg

Increase: anticholinergic effect—henbane leaf

Increase: EPS—betel palm, kava

Drug/Lab Test

Increase: hepatic studies, cardiac enzymes, cholesterol, blood glucose, prolactin, bilirubin, PBI, cholinesterase, ^{131}I, alk phos, leukocytes, granulocytes, platelets

Decrease: hormones (blood and urine)

False positive: pregnancy tests, PKU

False negative: urinary steroids, 17-OHCS

NURSING CONSIDERATIONS

Assess:

- Mental status: orientation, mood, behavior, presence and type of hallucinations before initial administration and monthly
- Any potentially reversible causes of behavior problems in the geriatric patients before and during therapy
- Swallowing of PO medication; check for hoarding or giving of medication to other patients
- I&O ratio; palpate bladder if low urinary output occurs, especially in geriatric patients
- Bilirubin, CBC, LFTs, ocular exam; agranulocytosis may occur, monthly
- Urinalysis recommended before, during prolonged therapy
- Affect, orientation, LOC, reflexes, gait, coordination, sleep pattern disturbances
- B/P sitting, standing, lying; take pulse and respirations q4hr during initial treatment; establish baseline before starting treatment; report drops of 30 mm Hg; obtain baseline ECG, Q-wave and T-wave changes
- Dizziness, faintness, palpitations, tachycardia on rising

⚠ For neuroleptic malignant syndrome: hyperpyrexia, muscle rigidity, increased CPK, altered mental status, for acute dystonia (check chewing, swallowing, eyes, pill rolling)

- EPS including akathisia (inability to sit still, no pattern to movements), tardive dyskinesia (bizarre movements of the jaw, mouth, tongue, extremities), pseudoparkinsonism (rigidity, tremors, pill rolling, shuffling gait)
- Skin turgor daily

• Constipation, urinary retention daily; increase bulk, H_2O in diet

Administer:

• IM, inject in deep muscle mass, do not give SUBCUT

• Rectal after placing in refrigerator for ½ hr if too soft to insert

• Anticholinergic agent for EPS if ordered

PO route

• Do not break, crush, or chew ext rel caps

• With full glass of water, milk; or with food to decrease GI upset

• Product in liquid form mixed in glass of juice or cola if hoarding is suspected

• Periodically attempt dosage reduction in behavioral problems

• Avoid use with CNS depressants

IV route

• After diluting 1 mg/1 ml with NS, give 1 mg or less/2 min or more; may be further diluted in 500-1000 ml of NS

Additive compatibilities: Ascorbic acid, ethacrynate, netilmicin, theophylline, vit B/C

Syringe compatibilities: Atropine, benztropine, butorphanol, diphenhydrAMINE, doxapram, droperidol, fentanyl, glycopyrrolate, hydromorphone, hydrOXYzine, meperidine, metoclopramide, midazolam, morphine, pentazocine, perphenazine, prochlorperazine, promazine, promethazine, scopolamine

Y-site compatibilities: Amsacrine, cisatracurium, cisplatin, cladribine, cyclophosphamide, cytarabine, DOXOrubicin, DOXOrubicin liposome, famotidine, filgrastim, fluconazole, granisetron, heparin, hydrocortisone, ondansetron, potassium chloride, propofol, teniposide, thiotepa, vinorelbine, vit B/C

Perform/provide:

• Supervised ambulation until stabilized on medication; do not involve in strenuous exercise program because fainting is possible; patient should not stand still for long periods

• Increased fluids and roughage to prevent constipation

• Candy, gum, sips of water for dry mouth

• Storage in tight, light-resistant container, oral sol in amber bottle

Evaluate:

• Therapeutic response: decrease in emotional excitement, hallucinations, delusions, paranoia, reorganization of patterns of thought, speech, increase in target behaviors

Teach patient/family:

• To use good oral hygiene; frequent rinsing of mouth, sugarless gum, candy, ice chips for dry mouth

• To avoid hazardous activities until product response is determined

• That orthostatic hypotension occurs often and to rise gradually from sitting or lying position

• To remain lying down for at least 30 min after IM inj

• To avoid hot tubs, hot showers, tub baths, since hypotension may occur; that in hot weather, heat stroke may occur; take extra precautions to stay cool

• To avoid abrupt withdrawal of this product or EPS may result; product should be withdrawn slowly

• To avoid OTC preparations (cough, hay fever, cold) unless approved by prescriber, since serious product interactions may occur; avoid use with alcohol, increased drowsiness may occur

• To use a sunscreen and sunglasses to prevent burns

• To take antacids 2 hr before or after this product

• To report sore throat, malaise, fever, bleeding, mouth sores; CBC should be drawn and product discontinued

• Contraceptive measures

• That urine may turn pink or reddish-brown

Treatment of overdose: Lavage if orally ingested; provide airway; *do not induce vomiting or use epinephrine*

chlorthalidone (℞)

(klor-thal′i-done)
Apo-Chlorthalidone ✦, chlorthalidone, Hygroton, Thalitone, Uridon ✦
Func. class.: Diuretic
Chem. class.: Thiazide-like phthalimidine derivative

Do not confuse:
Uridon/Vicodin
Hygroton/Regroton

Action: Acts on distal tubule and by blocking the reabsorption of sodium and chloride resulting in increasing excretion of water, sodium, chloride, potassium, magnesium, bicarbonate, possible arteriolar dilation

Uses: Edema, hypertension, edema in CHF

DOSAGE AND ROUTES

Hypertension
- *Adult:* **PO** 25-100 mg/day or 100 mg 3×/wk

Edema
- *Adult:* **PO** 50-100 mg/day or 100 mg on alternate day, max 200 mg/day
- *Geriatric:* **PO** 12.5-25 mg/day or every other day

Available forms: Tabs 25, 50, 100 mg

SIDE EFFECTS

CNS: Paresthesia, headache, *dizziness, weakness,* fever
CV: Hypertension, orthostatic hypotension, palpitations, volume depletion
EENT: Blurred vision
ELECT: *Hypokalemia,* hypomagnesemia, hypercalcemia, hyponatremia, hypochloremia
GI: *Nausea, vomiting, anorexia,* constipation, diarrhea, pancreatitis, GI irritation, jaundice
GU: *Urinary frequency,* polyuria, **uremia,** glucosuria, impotence
HEMA: **Aplastic anemia, hemolytic anemia, leukopenia, agranulocytosis, thrombocytopenia, neutropenia**
INTEG: Rash, urticaria, purpura, photosensitivity
META: *Hyperglycemia, hyperuremia,* increased creatinine, BUN, gout

Contraindications: Hypersensitivity to thiazides or sulfonamides, anuria, renal decompensation, breastfeeding

Precautions: Pregnancy (B), geriatric patients, hypokalemia, renal/hepatic disease, gout, diabetes mellitus, hyperlipidemia, SLE, hypotension, CCr <25 ml/min

PHARMACOKINETICS

Onset 2 hr, peak 6 hr, duration 24-72 hr, excreted unchanged by kidneys, crosses placenta, enters breast milk, half-life 40 hr

INTERACTIONS

Increase: hyperglycemia, hypotension—diazoxide
Increase: hypokalemia—glucocorticoids, amphotericin B
Increase: toxicity of lithium, nondepolarizing skeletal muscle relaxants, allopurinol
Increase: hypotensive effect—alcohol
Decrease: absorption of thiazides—cholestyramine, colestipol

Drug/Herb
- Potassium deficiency: chronic use of buckthorn, cascara sagrada, Chinese rhubarb, gossypol, licorice, nettle, senna

Increase: severe photosensitivity—St. John's wort
Increase: hypotension—cucumber, dandelion, khella, horsetail, pumpkin, Queen Anne's lace

Drug/Lab Test
Increase: Amylase, bilirubin, calcium, cholesterol, creatinine, low-density lipoproteins, serum/urine glucose (diabetics), triglycerides, uric acid
Decrease: PBI, parathyroid test, magnesium, potassium, sodium, urinary calcium

NURSING CONSIDERATIONS

Assess:

- Weight, I&O daily to determine fluid loss; effect of product may be decreased if used daily
- Rate, depth, rhythm of respiration, effect of exertion, B/P lying, standing; postural hypotension may occur
- Electrolytes: K, Mg, Na, Cl; include BUN, blood glucose, CBC, serum creatinine, blood pH, ABGs, uric acid, Ca
- Blood glucose levels if patient is diabetic
- Signs of metabolic alkalosis: drowsiness, restlessness
- Signs of hypokalemia: postural hypotension, malaise, fatigue, tachycardia, leg cramps, weakness
- Rashes, temp elevation daily
- Confusion, especially in geriatric patients; take safety precautions if needed

Administer:

- In AM to avoid interference with sleep if using product as a diuretic
- Potassium replacement if potassium less than 3 mg/dl
- With food if nausea occurs; absorption may be decreased slightly

Evaluate:

- Therapeutic response: improvement in edema of feet, legs, sacral area daily if medication used in CHF

Teach patient/family:

- To rise slowly from lying or sitting position
- To notify prescriber of muscle weakness, cramps, nausea, dizziness
- That product may be taken with food or milk
- To maintain adequate potassium intake
- That blood glucose may be increased in diabetics
- To use sunscreen to protect against photosensitivity
- To take early in day to avoid nocturia

Treatment of overdose: Lavage if taken orally, monitor electrolytes, administer dextrose in NS, monitor hydration, CV, renal status

cholestyramine (℞)

(koe-less-tir′a-meen)
LoCHOLEST, LoCHOLEST Light, Prevalite, Questran, Questran Light
Func. class.: Antilipemic
Chem. class.: Bile acid sequestrant

Action: Absorbs, combines with bile acids to form insoluble complex that is excreted through feces; loss of bile acids lowers cholesterol levels

Uses: Primary hypercholesterolemia, pruritus associated with biliary obstruction

Unlabeled uses: Diarrhea caused by excess bile acid

DOSAGE AND ROUTES

- *Adult:* **PO** 4 g/day or bid, max 24 g/day
- *Child:* **PO** 240 mg/kg/day in 3 divided doses with food or drink, max 8 g/day titrated up over several weeks to decrease GI effects

Available forms: Powder for susp 4 g cholestyramine/packet or scoop; tab 1 g

SIDE EFFECTS

CNS: Headache, dizziness, drowsiness, vertigo, tinnitus, anxiety

GI: Constipation, abdominal pain, nausea, fecal impaction, hemorrhoids, flatulence, vomiting, steatorrhea, peptic ulcer

HEMA: **Bleeding,** increased PT

INTEG: Rash, irritation of perianal area, tongue, skin

META: Decreased vit A, D, K, red cell folate content; **hyperchloremic acidosis**

MS: Muscle, joint pain

Contraindications: Hypersensitivity; biliary obstruction; hyperlipidemia III, IV, V

Precautions: Pregnancy (C), breastfeeding, children

PHARMACOKINETICS

PO: Excreted in feces, LDL lowered in 4-7 days, serum cholesterol lowered in 1 mo

INTERACTIONS

Decrease: absorption of warfarin; thiazides; cardiac glycosides; propranolol; corticosteroids; iron; thyroid hormones; fat-soluble vitamins; clindamycin; acetaminophen; amiodarone; penicillin G; tetracyclines; clofibrate; gemfibrozil; glipiZIDE; phenytoin; vit A, D, E, K

Drug/Herb

Increase: effect—glucomannan

Decrease: gotu kola

Drug/Lab Test

Increase: AST, ALT, alk phos

Decrease: sodium, potassium

Interfere: cholecystography

NURSING CONSIDERATIONS

Assess:

- Cardiac glycoside level, if both products are being administered
- For signs of vit A, D, K deficiency
- Fasting LDL, HDL, total cholesterol, triglyceride levels, electrolytes if on extended therapy
- Bowel pattern daily; increase bulk, H_2O in diet for constipation

Administer:

- Product daily or bid; give all other medications 1 hr before cholestyramine or 4-6 hr after cholestyramine to avoid poor absorption
- Product mixed with applesauce or stirred into beverage (2-6 oz), let stand for 2 min; do not take dry, avoid inhaling powder
- Supplemental doses of vit A, D, K, if levels are low

Evaluate:

- Therapeutic response: decreased cholesterol level (hyperlipidemia); diarrhea, pruritus (excess bile acids)

Teach patient/family:

⚠ The symptoms of hypoprothrombinemia: bleeding mucous membranes, dark tarry stools, hematuria, petechiae; report immediately

- That PKU patients should avoid Questran Light (contains aspartame and phenylalanine)
- The importance of compliance
- That risk factors should be decreased: high-fat diet, smoking, alcohol consumption, absence of exercise
- That GI side effects will resolve with continued use

choline salicylate (℞)

(koe'leen sa-liss'ih-late)

Arthropan

choline/magnesium salicylates (℞)

CMT, Tricosal, Trilisate

Func. class.: Nonopioid analgesic

Chem. class.: Salicylate

Action: Blocks pain impulses in CNS that occur in response to inhibition of prostaglandin synthesis; antipyretic action results from inhibition of hypothalamic heat-regulating center to produce vasodilation to allow heat dissipation

Uses: Mild to moderate pain or fever including arthritis, juvenile rheumatoid arthritis

DOSAGE AND ROUTES

435 mg of choline salicylate = 325 mg of aspirin

Choline salicylate

- *Adult and child >12 yr:* **PO** 870-1740 mg qid; max 6×/day

Pain/fever

- *Adult:* **PO** 435-870 mg q3-4hr prn

Choline/magnesium salicylates

- *Adult:* **PO** 1500 mg bid
- *Child >37 kg:* **PO** 2.2 g of salicylate/day divided bid
- *Child <37 kg:* **PO** 50 mg of salicylate/kg/day divided bid

Available forms: *Choline salicylate:* liq 870 mg/5 ml; *choline/magnesium salicylate:* tabs 500, 750, 1000 mg; liquid 500 mg/5 ml

SIDE EFFECTS

CNS: Stimulation, drowsiness, dizziness, confusion, **seizures,** headache, flushing, hallucinations, **coma**

CV: Rapid pulse, pulmonary edema

EENT: Tinnitus, hearing loss
ENDO: Hypoglycemia, hyponatremia, hypokalemia
GI: Nausea, vomiting, GI bleeding, diarrhea, heartburn, anorexia, **hepatitis, hepatotoxicity**
HEMA: **Thrombocytopenia, agranulocytosis, leukopenia, neutropenia, hemolytic anemia,** increased PT
INTEG: Rash, urticaria, bruising, sweating
RESP: Wheezing, hyperpnea, hyperventilation

Contraindications: Children <3 yr, vit K deficiency, children with flulike symptoms, hypersensitivity to salicylates, GI bleeding, bleeding disorders, Reye's syndrome

Precautions: Pregnancy (C), breastfeeding, anemia, renal/hepatic disease, Hodgkin's disease

PHARMACOKINETICS

Absorbed via GI tract; onset 15-30 min; metabolized by liver; crosses placenta; excreted in breast milk, by kidneys; half-life 2-3 hr; large doses 9-17 hr

INTERACTIONS

Increase: gastric ulcer—steroids, antiinflammatories, NSAIDs
Increase: bleeding—alcohol, aspirin, heparin, plicamycin
Increase: effects of anticoagulants, insulin, methotrexate, thrombolytic agents, penicillins, phenytoin, valproic acid, oral hypoglycemics, sulfonamides
Increase: salicylate levels—urinary acidifiers, ammonium chloride, nizatidine
Decrease: effects of choline salicylate: antacids (high doses), urinary alkalizers, corticosteroids
Decrease: effects of probenecid, spironolactone, sulfinpyrazone, sulfonylamides, NSAIDs, β-blockers

Drug/Herb

Increase: bleeding risk—bilberry, bogbean, chondroitin, horse chestnut, Irish moss, kelpware, pansy

Drug/Lab Test

Increase: coagulation studies, LFTs, serum uric acid, amylase, CO_2, urinary protein
Decrease: serum K, cholesterol
Interference: VMA, TSH, 5-HIAA

NURSING CONSIDERATIONS

Assess:

- Pain: location, intensity, character baseline and 1-2 hr after dose
- Hepatic studies: AST, ALT, bilirubin, creatinine (long-term therapy)
- Renal studies: BUN, urine creatinine (long-term therapy); decreased urine output
- Blood studies: CBC, Hct, Hgb, PT (long-term therapy)
- I&O ratio; decreasing output may indicate renal failure (long-term therapy)

⚠ Hepatotoxicity: dark urine; clay-colored stools; yellowing of skin, sclera; itching; abdominal pain; fever; diarrhea (long-term therapy)

- Allergic reactions: rash, urticaria; product may have to be discontinued
- Ototoxicity: tinnitus, ringing, roaring in ears; audiometric testing needed before, after long-term therapy
- Edema in feet, ankles, legs
- Product history; many interactions

Administer:

- Mixed with fruit juice, carbonated beverage, water

Evaluate:

- Therapeutic response: decreased pain, fever, stiffness of joints

Teach patient/family:

- To report any symptoms of hepatotoxicity, renal toxicity, visual changes, ototoxicity, allergic reactions, bleeding (long-term therapy)
- Not to exceed recommended dosage; acute poisoning may result
- To read label on other OTC products; many contain aspirin
- That therapeutic response takes 2 wk (arthritis)
- To avoid alcohol ingestion; GI bleeding may occur

• That if anticoagulants are given with this product, this product should be decreased 2 wk before surgery

Treatment of overdose: Lavage, activated charcoal, monitor electrolytes, VS

cidofovir (℞)

(si-doh-foh'veer)

Vistide

Func. class.: Antiviral

Chem. class.: Nucleotide analog

Action: Suppresses cytomegalovirus (CMV) replication by selective inhibition of viral DNA synthesis

Uses: CMV retinitis in patients with HIV, used with probenecid

Unlabeled uses: Adenovirus, condylomata acuminata, eczema vaccination, Epstein-Barr, generalized vaccinia, herpes genitalis/simplex, HPV, molluscum contagiosum, vaccinia necrosum, vaccinia, varicella-zoster, variola

DOSAGE AND ROUTES

• *Adult:* **IV** 5 mg/kg q wk × 2 wk, then 3 mg/kg q2wk, give with probenecid

Renal dose

• *Adult:* **IV** CCr <55 ml/min, do not use; SCr increase of 0.3-0.4 mg/dl above baseline, decrease dose to 3 mg/kg; SCr increase of ≥0.5 mg/dl above baseline or ≥2+ proteinuria, discontinue

Available forms: Inj 75 mg/ml

SIDE EFFECTS

CNS: Fever, chills, **coma,** confusion, abnormal thought, *dizziness,* bizarre dreams, *headache,* psychosis, tremors, somnolence, paresthesia, *amnesia, anxiety, insomnia,* **seizures**

CV: Dysrhythmias, hypo/hypertension

EENT: Retinal detachment in CMV retinitis

GI: Abnormal LFTs, *nausea, vomiting, anorexia, diarrhea,* abdominal pain, **hemorrhage**

GU: **Hematuria,** increased creatinine, BUN, **nephrotoxicity**

HEMA: **Granulocytopenia, thrombocytopenia, irreversible neutropenia, anemia, eosinophilia**

INTEG: Rash, alopecia, pruritus, acne, urticaria, pain at inj site, phlebitis

RESP: Dyspnea

Contraindications: Hypersensitivity to this product or probenecid, sulfa products

Black Box Warning: Proteinuria, renal disease/failure

Precautions: Pregnancy (C), breastfeeding, children <6 mo, geriatric patients, preexisting cytopenias, renal function impairment, platelet count <25,000/mm^3

Black Box Warning: Neutropenia, infertility, secondary malignancy

PHARMACOKINETICS

Terminal half-life 2.6 hr

INTERACTIONS

• Nephrotoxicity: amphotericin B, foscarnet, aminoglycosides, pentamidine IV, NSAIDs, salicylates; wait 7 days after use to begin cidofovir

NURSING CONSIDERATIONS

Assess:

• Culture before treatment is initiated; cultures of blood, urine, and throat may all be taken; CMV is not confirmed by this method; the diagnosis is made by an ophthalmic exam

• Renal, hepatic, increased hemopoietic studies and BUN; serum creatinine, AST, ALT, creatinine, CCr, A-G ratio, baseline and drip treatment, blood counts should be done q2wk; watch for decreasing granulocytes, Hgb; if low, therapy may have to be discontinued and restarted after hematologic recovery; blood transfusions may be required

• For GI symptoms: severe nausea, vomiting, diarrhea; severe symptoms may necessitate discontinuing product

• Electrolytes and minerals: calcium, phosphorus, magnesium, sodium, potassium; watch closely for tetany during first administration

- For symptoms of blood dyscrasias (anemia, granulocytopenia); bruising, fatigue, bleeding, poor healing
- Allergic reactions: flushing, rash, urticaria, pruritus
- For leukopenia, neutropenia, thrombocytopenia: WBCs, platelets q2 days during 2×/day dosing and q wk thereafter; check for leukopenias, with daily WBC count in patients with prior leukopenia, with other nucleoside analogs, or for whom leukopenia counts are <1000 cells/mm^3 at start of treatment
- Monitor serum creatinine or CCr at least q2wk; give only to those with creatinine levels ≤1.5 mg/dl, CCr >55 ml/min, urine protein <100 mg/dl

Administer:

Intermittent IV INF route

- Dilute in 100 ml 0.9% saline sol before administration; probenecid must be given PO 2 g 3 hr prior to the cidofovir inf and 1 g at 2 and 8 hr after ending the cidofovir inf; give 1 L of 0.9% saline sol IV with each INF of cidofovir, give saline INF over 1-2 hr period immediately prior to cidofovir; patient should be given a 2nd L if the patient can tolerate the fluid load (2nd L given at time of cidofovir or immediately afterward and should be given over a 1-3 hr period)
- Mix under strict aseptic conditions using gloves, gown, and mask, and using precautions for antineoplastic
- Slowly; do not give by bolus IV, SUBCUT inj
- Use diluted sol within 12 hr, do not refrigerate or freeze; do not use sol with particulate matter or discoloration
- Refrigerate up to 24 hr, allow to warm to room temperature before using

Evaluate:

- Therapeutic response: decreased symptoms of CMV

Teach patient/family:

- To notify prescriber if sore throat, swollen lymph nodes, malaise, fever occur; may indicate other infections
- To report perioral tingling, numbness in extremities, paresthesias; report rash immediately
- That serious product interactions may occur if OTC products are ingested; check first with prescriber
- That product is not a cure, but will control symptoms
- That regular ophthalmic exams must be continued
- That major toxicities may necessitate discontinuing product
- To use contraception during treatment and that infertility may occur; men should use barrier contraception for 90 days after treatment

Treatment of overdose: Discontinue product; use hemodialysis, and increase hydration

cilostazol (℞)

(sih-los'tah-zol)

Pletal

Func. class.: Platelet aggregation inhibitor

Chem. class.: Quinolinone derivative

Do not confuse:

Pletal/Plendil

Action: Reversibly inhibits cellular phosphodiesterase; inhibits platelet aggregation induced by thrombin, ADP, collagen, arachidonic acid, epINEPHrine, stress

Uses: Intermittent claudication

Unlabeled uses: Buerger's disease, percutaneous coronary intervention (PCI)

DOSAGE AND ROUTES

- *Adult:* **PO** 100 mg bid taken ≥30 min before or 2 hr after breakfast and dinner or 50 mg bid if using products that inhibit CYP3A4 and CYP2C19; 12 wk of treatment may be needed for beneficial effect

PCI to prevent acute coronary thrombosis/Buerger's disease (unlabeled)

- *Adult:* **PO** 100 mg bid

Available forms: Tabs 50, 100 mg

SIDE EFFECTS

CNS: Dizziness, headache

CV: Palpitations, tachycardia, nodal dysrhythmia, postural hypotension

EENT: Blindness, diplopia, ear pain, tinnitus, retinal hemorrhage

GI: Nausea, vomiting, *diarrhea,* GI discomfort, colitis, cholelithiasis, ulcer, esophagitis, gastritis, anorexia, *flatulence, dyspepsia*

GU: Cystitis, frequency, vaginitis, **vaginal hemorrhage,** hematuria

HEMA: **Bleeding (epistaxis, hematuria, retinal hemorrhage, GI bleeding), thrombocytopenia,** anemia, **polycythemia, aplastic anemia**

INTEG: Rash, urticaria, dry skin, **Stevens-Johnson syndrome**

MISC: Back pain, headache, infection, myalgia, peripheral edema, chills, fever, malaise, diabetes mellitus

RESP: Cough, pharyngitis, rhinitis, asthma, pneumonia

Contraindications: Hypersensitivity, acute MI, active bleeding conditions, hemostatic conditions

Black Box Warning: CHF

Precautions: Pregnancy (C), breastfeeding, children, geriatric patients, past hepatic disease, cardiac/renal disease, increased bleeding risk, low platelet count, platelet dysfunction

PHARMACOKINETICS

95%-98% protein binding; metabolism-hepatic extensively by CYP3A4, 2C19 enzymes; excreted urine (74%), feces (20%); half-life 11-13 hr

INTERACTIONS

Increase: bleeding tendencies—anticoagulants, NSAIDs, thrombolytics, abciximab, eptifibatide, tirofiban, ticlopidine

Increase: cilostazol levels—CYP3A4 inhibitors, CYP2C19 inhibitors; diltiazem, erythromycin, clarithromycin, verapamil, protease inhibitors, omeprazole; exercise caution when coadministering with fluvoxamine, fluoxetine, ketoconazole, isoniazid, gemfibrozil, omeprazole, itraconazole, voriconazole, fluconazole and reduce dose to 50 mg bid

Decrease: cilostazol levels—CYP3A4 inducers

Drug/Herb

Increase: bleeding risk—agrimony, alfalfa, angelica, anise, bilberry, black haw, bogbean, buchu, chondroitin, dong quai, fenugreek, feverfew, garlic, ginger, ginkgo, ginseng, green tea, horse chestnut, Irish moss, kelp, kelpware, khella, lovage, lungwort, meadowsweet, motherwort, mugwort, nettle, papaya, parsley (large amt), pau d'arco, pineapple, poplar, prickly ash, safflower, saw palmetto, senega, tonka bean, turmeric, wintergreen, white willow, yarrow

Decrease: action—chamomile, coenzyme Q10, flax, glucomannan, goldenseal, St. John's wort

Drug/Food

- Do not use with grapefruit juice, toxicity may occur

NURSING CONSIDERATIONS

Assess:

- For underlying CV disease since CV risk is great; for CV lesions with repeated oral administration; do not administer to patients with CHF of any severity; for severe headache, signs of toxicity
- Blood studies: CBC q2wk, Hct, Hgb, PT

Administer:

- Give bid 1 hr before or 2 hr after meals; do not give with grapefruit juice

Evaluate:

- Therapeutic response: improved walking distance and duration, decreased pain

Teach patient/family:

- To report any unusual bleeding
- To report side effects such as diarrhea, skin rashes, subcutaneous bleeding
- That effects may take 2-4 wk, treatment of up to 12 wk may be required for necessary effect
- That reading the patient package insert is necessary
- That it is best to discontinue tobacco use

• That there are many drug and herb interactions, obtain approval by prescriber before use

cimetidine (OTC, ℞)

(sye-met'i-deen)

Apo-Cimetidine ♣, cimetidine, Major Acid Reducer, Novo-Cimetidine ♣, Peptol ♣, Tagamet, Tagamet HB

Func. class.: H_2-histamine receptor antagonist

Chem. class.: Imidazole derivative

Action: Inhibits histamine at H_2-receptor site in the gastric parietal cells, which inhibits gastric acid secretion

Uses: Short-term treatment of duodenal and gastric ulcers and maintenance; management of GERD (PO) and Zollinger-Ellison syndrome; prevention of upper GI bleeding; prevent, relieve heartburn, acid indigestion, upper GI bleeding

Unlabeled uses: Prevention of aspiration pneumonitis, stress ulcers, angioedema, molluscum contagiosum, NSAID-induced ulcer prophylaxis, verruca vulgaris

DOSAGE AND ROUTES

Short-term treatment of active ulcers

• *Adult:* **PO** 300 mg qid with meals, at bedtime × 8 wk or 400 mg bid, 800 mg at bedtime; after 8 wk give bedtime dose only; **IV BOL** 300 mg/20 ml 0.9% NaCl over 1-2 min q6hr; **IV INF** 300 mg/50 ml D_5W over 15-20 min; **IM** 300 mg q6hr, not to exceed 2400 mg/day

• *Child:* **PO** 20-40 mg/kg/day; **IM/IV** 5-10 mg/kg q6-8hr

Prophylaxis of duodenal ulcer

• *Adult and child >16 yr:* 400 mg at bedtime or 300 mg bid

GERD

• *Adult:* **PO** 800-1600 mg/day in divided doses

Hypersecretory conditions (Zollinger-Ellison syndrome)

• *Adult:* **PO/IM/IV** 300-600 mg q6hr; may increase to 12 g/day if needed; OTC use up to 200 mg daily or bid, max 2×/wk

Upper GI bleeding prophylaxis

• *Adult:* **IV** 50 mg/hr; lowered in renal disease

Renal disease

• *Adult:* **PO/IV** CCr <30 ml/min 300 mg q12hr

Aspiration pneumonitis prophylaxis (unlabeled)

• *Adult:* **IM/IV** 300 mg **IM** 1 hr before anesthesia, then 300 mg **IV** q4hr until patient is alert, max 2400 mg/day

Severe urticaria/angioedema (unlabeled)

• *Adult:* **IV** 300 mg, diluted appropriately, in combination with an H_1-blocker

Molluscum contagiosum (unlabeled)

• *Child:* **PO** 40 mg/kg/day × 2 mo

Verruca vulgaris (unlabeled)

• *Child:* **PO** 30-40 mg/kg/day × 2 mo

Available forms: Tabs 100, 200, 300, 400, 800 mg; liq 200, 300 mg/5 ml; inj 300 mg/2 ml, 300 mg/50 ml 0.9% NaCl

SIDE EFFECTS

CNS: Confusion, headache, depression, dizziness, anxiety, weakness, psychosis, tremors, **seizures**

CV: Bradycardia, tachycardia, **dysrhythmias**

GI: Diarrhea, abdominal cramps, **paralytic ileus, jaundice**

GU: Gynecomastia, galactorrhea, impotence, increase in BUN, creatinine

HEMA: **Agranulocytosis, thrombocytopenia, neutropenia, aplastic anemia, increase in PT**

INTEG: Urticaria, rash, alopecia, sweating, flushing, **exfoliative dermatitis**

RESP: **Pneumonia**

Contraindications: Hypersensitivity

Precautions: Pregnancy (B), breastfeeding, children <16 yr, geriatric patients, organic brain syndrome, renal/hepatic disease

PHARMACOKINETICS

Half-life 1½-2 hr; 30%-40% metabolized by liver, excreted in urine (unchanged), crosses placenta, enters breast milk

PO: Onset 30 min, peak 45-90 min; duration 4-5 hr, well absorbed

IM/IV: Onset 10 min, peak ½ hr, duration 4-5 hr, well absorbed (IM)

INTERACTIONS

Increase: toxicity due to CYP450 pathway—benzodiazepines, β-blockers, calcium channel blockers, carbamazepine, chloroquine, lidocaine, metronidazole, moricizine, phenytoin, quinidine, quinine, sulfonylureas, theophylline, tricyclics, valproic acid, warfarin

Decrease: absorption of cimetidine—antacids, sucralfate

Decrease: absorption—ketoconazole, itraconazole

Drug/Lab Test

Increase: alk phos, AST, creatinine, prolactin

False positive: Gastroccult, Hemoccult tests

False negative: TB skin tests

NURSING CONSIDERATIONS

Assess:

- Gastric pH (5 or more should be maintained), also epigastric pain and duration, intensity; aggravating, ameliorating factors
- I&O ratio, BUN, creatinine, CBC with differential periodically

Administer:

- With meals for prolonged product effect; antacids 1 hr before or 1 hr after cimetidine

IV route

- After diluting 300 mg/20 ml of 0.9% NaCl for inj; give ≥5 min; may be diluted 300 mg/50 ml of D_5W; run over 15-20 min; or total daily dose (900 mg) diluted in 100-1000 ml D_5W given over 24 hr

Additive compatibilities: AcetaZOLAMIDE, amikacin, aminophylline, atracurium, cefoperazone, cefoxitin, chlorothiazide, clindamycin, colistimethate, dexamethasone, digoxin, epinephrine, erythromycin, ethacrynate, floxacillin, flumazenil, furosemide, gentamicin, insulin (regular), isoproterenol, lidocaine, lincomycin, meropenem, metaraminol, methylPREDNISolone, norepinephrine, nitroprusside, penicillin G potassium, phytonadione, polymyxin B, potassium chloride, protamine, quinidine, tacrolimus, vancomycin, verapamil, vit B/C

Syringe compatibilities: Atropine, butorphanol, cephalothin, diazepam, diphenhydrAMINE, doxapram, droperidol, fentanyl, glycopyrrolate, heparin, hydromorphone, hydrOXYzine, lorazepam, meperidine, midazolam, morphine, nafcillin, nalbuphine, penicillin G sodium, pentazocine, perphenazine, prochlorperazine, promazine, promethazine, scopolamine

Y-site compatibilities: Acyclovir, amifostine, aminophylline, amrinone, atracurium, aztreonam, cisatracurium, cisplatin, cladribine, cyclophosphamide, cytarabine, diltiazem, DOXOrubicin, DOXOrubicin liposome, enalaprilat, esmolol, filgrastim, fluconazole, fludarabine, foscarnet, gallium, granisetron, haloperidol, heparin, hetastarch, idarubicin, labetalol, melphalan, meropenem, methotrexate, midazolam, ondansetron, paclitaxel, pancuronium, piperacillin/tazobactam, propofol, remifentanil, sargramostim, tacrolimus, teniposide, theophylline, thiotepa, tolazoline, vecuronium, vinorelbine, zidovudine

Perform/provide:

- Storage of diluted sol at room temperature up to 48 hr

Evaluate:

- Therapeutic response: decreased pain in abdomen; healing of ulcers, absence of gastroesophageal reflux, gastric pH 5

Teach patient/family:

- That gynecomastia, impotence may occur, are reversible
- To avoid driving, other hazardous activities until patient is stabilized on this medication; drowsiness or dizziness may occur

• To avoid black pepper, caffeine, alcohol, harsh spices, extremes in temperature of food
• To avoid OTC preparations: aspirin, cough, cold preparations; condition may worsen
• That smoking decreases the effectiveness of the product
• That product must be taken exactly as prescribed and continued for prescribed time to be effective; doses not to be doubled
• To report bruising, fatigue, malaise; blood dyscrasias may occur
• To report to prescriber diarrhea, black tarry stools, sore throat, rash

cinacalcet (℞)

(sin-a-kal'set)
Sensipar
Func. class.: Calcium receptor agonist
Chem. class.: Polypeptide hormone

Action: Directly lowers PTH levels by increasing sensitivity of calcium sensing receptors to extracellular calcium
Uses: Hypercalcemia in parathyroid carcinoma, secondary hyperparathyroidism in chronic kidney disease on dialysis, primary hyperparathyroidism

DOSAGE AND ROUTES

Parathyroid carcinoma
• *Adult:* **PO** 30 mg bid, titrate q2-4wk, with sequential doses of 30 mg bid, 60 mg bid, 90 mg bid, 90 mg tid-qid to normalize calcium levels
Secondary hyperparathyroidism
• *Adult:* **PO** 30 mg/day, titrate no more frequently than 2-4 wk with sequential doses of 30, 60, 90, 120, 180 mg/day
Available forms: Tabs 30, 60, 90 mg

SIDE EFFECTS

CNS: Dizziness, asthenia, **seizures,** tetany, hallucinations, depression
CV: Hypertension, dysrhythmia exacerbation
GI: Nausea, diarrhea, vomiting, anorexia
MISC: Access infection, noncardiac chest pain, hypocalcemia
MS: Myalgia
Contraindications: Hypersensitivity
Precautions: Pregnancy (C), breastfeeding, children, seizure disorders, hepatic disease, hypocalcemia

PHARMACOKINETICS

93%-97% bound to plasma; proteins metabolized by CYP3A4, 2D6, 1A2; half-life 30-40 hr; renal excretion of metabolites (80% renal, 15% feces)

INTERACTIONS

• Drugs metabolized by CYP3A4 (ketoconazole, erythromycin, itraconazole), CYP2D6 (flecainide, vinBLAStine, thioridazine, tricyclics): adjustments may be necessary
Drug/Food
Increase: action by high-fat meal

NURSING CONSIDERATIONS

Assess:
• Hypocalcemia: cramping, seizures, tetany, myalgia, paresthesia
• Calcium, phosphorous within 1 wk and iPTH 1-4 wk after initiation or dosage adjustment when maintenance is established; measure calcium, phosphorus monthly; iPTH q1-3mo, target range 150-300 pg/ml for iPTH level; biochemical markers of bone formation/resorption, radiologic evidence of fracture
• If calcium <8.4 mg/dl, do not start therapy
Administer:
• Swallow tabs whole; do not break, crush, or chew
• Can be used alone or in combination with vit D sterols and/or phosphate binders
Secondary hyperthyroidism
• Titrate q2-4wk to target iPTH consistent with National Kidney Foundation–Kidney Disease Outcomes Quality Initiative (NKF-K/DOQI) for chronic kidney disease patient on dialysis of 150-300 pg/ml; if iPTH drops below 150-300 pg/

ml, reduce dose of cinacalcet and/or vit D sterols or discontinue treatment

Perform/provide:

• Storage at <77° F (25° C)

Evaluate:

• Therapeutic response: calcium levels 9-10 mg/dl, decreasing symptoms of hypercalcemia

Teach patient/family:

• Take with food or shortly after a meal

• Report immediately: cramping, seizures, muscle pain, tingling, tetany

ciprofloxacin (℞)

(sip-ro-floks'a-sin)

Cipro, Cipro XR, ProQuin XR

Func. class.: Antiinfective—broad-spectrum

Chem. class.: Fluoroquinolone

Do not confuse:

ciprofloxacin/cephalexin

Action: Interferes with conversion of intermediate DNA fragments into high-molecular-weight DNA in bacteria; DNA gyrase inhibitor

Uses: Infection caused by susceptible *Escherichia coli, Enterobacter cloacae, Proteus mirabilis, Klebsiella pneumoniae, Proteus vulgaris, Citrobacter freundii, Serratia marcescens, Pseudomonas aeruginosa, Staphylococcus aureus, Staphylococcus epidermidis, Enterobacter, Campylobacter jejuni, Salmonella;* chronic bacterial prostatitis, acute sinusitis, postexposure inhalation anthrax, infectious diarrhea, typhoid fever, complicated intraabdominal infections, nosocomial pneumonia, urinary tract infections

Unlabeled uses: *Acinetobacter/woffii, Aeromonas hydrophila,* brucellosis, *Burkholderia, pseudomallei,* chancroid, cholera, dental infection, *Edwardsiella tarda,* endocarditis, *Enterobacter aerogenes,* granuloma inguinale, *Klebsiella oxytoca,* Legionnaire's disease, melioidosis, meningococcal infection prophylaxis, *Pasteurella multocida,* PID, periodontitis, pharyngitis, *Salmonella sp., Stenotrophomonas maltophilia,* tularemia, *Vibrio cholerae/parahaemolyticus/vulnificus, Yersinia enterocolitica*

DOSAGE AND ROUTES

Uncomplicated urinary tract infections

• *Adult:* **PO** 100-250 mg q12hr × 3 days or 500 mg × q24hr × 3 days

Complicated/severe urinary tract infections

• *Adult:* **PO** 500 mg q12hr or 1000 mg q24hr × 7-14 days; **IV** 400 mg q12hr

Pyelonephritis, acute uncomplicated

• *Adult:* **PO** 1000 mg q24hr × 7-14 days

Respiratory, bone, skin, joint infections

• *Adult:* **PO** 500-750 mg q12hr × 7-14 days; **IV** 400 mg q12hr

Nosocomial pneumonia

• *Adult:* **IV** 400 mg q8hr × 10-14 days

Intraabdominal infections, complicated

• *Adult:* **PO** 500 mg q12hr × 7-14 days; **IV** 400 mg q12hr × 7-14 days, usually given with metronidazole

Acute sinusitis, mild/moderate

• *Adult:* **PO** 500 mg q12hr × 10 days; **IV** 400 mg q12hr × 10 days

Inhalational anthrax (postexposure)

• *Adult:* **PO** 500 mg q12hr × 60 days; **IV** 400 mg q12hr × 60 days

• *Child:* **PO** 15 mg/kg/dose, max 500 mg/dose; **IV** max 400 mg/dose × 60 days

Infectious diarrhea

• *Adult:* **PO** 500 mg q12hr × 5-7 days

Chronic bacterial prostatis

• *Adult:* **PO** 500 mg q12hr × 28 days; **IV** 400 mg q12hr × 28 days

Renal disease

• CCr 30-50 ml/min; **PO** 250-500 mg q12hr; CCr 5-29 ml/min; **PO** 250-500 mg q18hr; **IV** 200-400 mg q18-24hr

Available forms: Tabs 100, 250, 500, 750 mg; ext rel tabs (XR) 500, 1000 mg; inj 200 mg/20 ml, 400 mg/40 ml, 200 mg/100 ml D_5, 400 mg/200 ml D_5; oral susp 250 mg, 500 mg/5 ml

SIDE EFFECTS

CNS: Headache, dizziness, fatigue, insomnia, depression, *restlessness*, **seizures,** confusion

GI: Nausea, diarrhea, increased ALT, AST, dry mouth, flatulence, heartburn, *vomiting*, oral candidiasis, dysphagia, **pseudomembranous colitis**

HEMA: **Bone marrow depression**

INTEG: Rash, pruritus, urticaria, photosensitivity, flushing, fever, chills, **toxic epidermal necrolysis**

MISC: **Anaphylaxis, Stevens-Johnson syndrome,** visual impairment, QT prolongation

MS: Tremor, arthralgia, tendinitis, **tendon rupture**

Contraindications: Hypersensitivity to quinolones

Precautions: Pregnancy (C), breastfeeding, children, geriatric patients, renal disease, epilepsy, QT prolongation, hypokalemia

Black Box Warning: Tendon pain/rupture, tendinitis

PHARMACOKINETICS

PO: Peak 1 hr; half-life 3-4 hr; excreted in urine as active product, metabolites

INTERACTIONS

Increase: nephrotoxicity—cycloSPORINE

Increase: ciprofloxacin levels—probenecid; monitor for toxicity

Increase: levels of theophylline, warfarin, monitor blood levels

Increase: QT prolongation—astemizole, droperidol, probucol, class IA/III antidysrhythmics, tricyclics, tetracyclines, local anesthetics, phenothiazines, haloperidol, risperidone, sertindole, ziprasidone, alfuzosin, arsenic trioxide, bepridil, β-agonists, chloroquine, clozapine, cyclobenzapine, dasatinib, dolasetron, droperidol, flecainide, halofantrine, halogenated anesthetics, lapatinib, levomethadyl, macrolides, methadone, octreotide, ondansetron, paliperidone, palonosetron, pentamidine, probucol, propafenone, ranolazine, sunitinib, tacrolimus, terfenadine, vardenafil, vorinostat

Decrease: ciproflaxin absorption—antacids containing magnesium, aluminum; zinc, iron, sucralfate, enteral feedings, calcium

Drug/Herb

- Do not use acidophilus with antiinfectives; separate by several hours
- Possible toxicity: yerba maté

Decrease: effect—fennel

Drug/Food

Increase: effect of caffeine

Decrease: absorption—dairy products, food

Drug/Lab Test

Increase: AST, ALT, BUN, creatinine, LDH, bilirubin, alk phos, glucose, proteinuria, albuminuria

Decrease: WBC, glucose

NURSING CONSIDERATIONS

Assess:

- Infection: WBC, temperature prior to and periodically
- CNS symptoms: headache, dizziness, fatigue, insomnia, depression
- Renal, hepatic studies: BUN, creatinine, AST, ALT
- I&O ratio, urine pH <5.5 is ideal

⚠ Anaphylaxis: fever, flushing, rash, urticaria, pruritus, dyspnea

- For tendon pain, especially in children

Administer:

- Not to use theophylline with this product, will cause toxicity
- Use caution when giving with antidysrhythmics IA and III

PO route

- Do not break, crush, or chew XR (ext rel) product
- 2 hr before or 2 hr after antacids, zinc, iron, calcium

IV route

- Over 1 hr as an INF, comes in premixed plastic INF container or diluted 20- or 40-ml vial to a final conc of 0.5-2 mg/ml of NS or D_5W; give through Y-tube or 3-way stopcock
- After clean-catch urine for C&S

Additive compatibilities: Amikacin, aztreonam, ceftazidime, cycloSPORINE, gentamicin, metronidazole, netilmicin, piperacillin, potassium acetate, potassium chloride, potassium phosphates, prednisoLONE, promethazine, propofol, ranitidine, Ringer's, sodium chloride, tobramycin, vit B/C

Y-site compatibilities: Amifostine, amino acids, aztreonam, calcium gluconate, ceftazidime, cisatracurium, digoxin, diltiazem, diphenhydrAMINE, DOBUTamine, DOPamine, DOXOrubicin liposome, gallium, gentamicin, granisetron, hydrOXYzine, lidocaine, lorazepam, metoclopramide, midazolam, midodrine, piperacillin, potassium acetate, potassium chloride, potassium phosphates, prednisoLONE, promethazine, propofol, ranitidine, remifentanil, Ringer's, sodium chloride, tacrolimus, teniposide, thiotepa, tobramycin, verapamil

Perform/provide:
- Limited intake of alkaline foods, products: milk, dairy products, alkaline antacids, sodium bicarbonate
- Increase in fluids to 3 L/day to avoid crystallization in kidneys

Evaluate:
- Therapeutic response: decreased pain, frequency, urgency, C&S; absence of infection

Teach patient/family:
- Not to take any products containing magnesium or calcium (such as antacids), iron, or aluminum with this product or within 2 hr of product
- To report tendon pain, chest pain, palpitations
- If dizziness occurs, to ambulate, perform activities with assistance
- To complete full course of product therapy, not to double or miss doses
- To contact prescriber if adverse reaction occurs or if inflammation or pain in tendon occurs
- To use frequent rinsing of mouth, sugarless candy or gum for dry mouth
- To contact prescriber if taking theophylline

ciprofloxacin ophthalmic

See Appendix B

⚠ High Alert

cisplatin (℞)

(sis′pla-tin)

Platinol ✤, Platinol-AQ

Func. class.: Antineoplastic alkylating agent

Chem. class.: Platinum complex

Do not confuse:
cisplatin/carboplatin
Platinol/Paraplatin

Action: Alkylates DNA, RNA; inhibits enzymes that allow synthesis of amino acids in proteins; activity is not cell cycle phase specific

Uses: Advanced bladder cancer, adjunctive in metastatic testicular cancer, osteosarcoma, soft tissue sarcomas, adjunctive in metastatic ovarian cancer, head, neck cancer, esophagus, prostate, lung and cervical cancer, lymphoma

Unlabeled uses: Astrocytoma, breast/gastric/head/neck/hepatocellular/lung/penile cancer, carcinoid, desmoid tumor, Hodgkin's disease, malignant glioma, malignant melanoma, neuroblastoma, non-Hodgkin's lymphoma (NHL), osteogenic sarcoma

DOSAGE AND ROUTES

Dosage protocols may vary

Metastatic testicular cancer
- *Adult:* **IV** 20 mg/m^2/day × 5 days, repeat q3wk for 2 cycles or more, depending on response

Advanced bladder cancer
- *Adult:* **IV** 50-70 mg/m^2 q3-4wk

Metastatic ovarian cancer
- *Adult:* **IV** 100 mg/m^2 q4wk or 75-100 mg/m^2 q3wk with cyclophosphamide; mix with 2 L NaCl and 37.5 g mannitol over 6 hr

Breast cancer (unlabeled)

• *Adult:* **IV** 60 mg as a single dose on days 23, 30 of a 60-day cycle with other antineoplastics

Hodgkin's/non-Hodgkin's lymphoma (unlabeled)

• *Adult and child:* **IV INF** 100 mg/m^2 24 hr continuous inf day 1 of a 4-day regimen with cytarabine/dexamethasone q3-4wk

Gastric cancer (unlabeled)

• *Adult:* **IV** 75 mg/m^2 on day 1 with docetaxel 75 mg/m^2 and fluorouracil 750 mg/m^2 on days 1-5, q21days

Available forms: Inj 0.5 ✱, 1 mg/ml

SIDE EFFECTS

CNS: **Seizures,** peripheral neuropathy

CV: Cardiac abnormalities

EENT: *Tinnitus, hearing loss, vestibular toxicity,* blurred vision, altered color perception

GI: *Severe nausea, vomiting, diarrhea, weight loss*

GU: **Renal tubular damage,** renal insufficiency, impotence, sterility, amenorrhea, gynecomastia, hyperuremia

HEMA: **Thrombocytopenia, leukopenia, pancytopenia**

INTEG: *Alopecia,* dermatitis

META: Hypomagnesemia, hypocalcemia, hypokalemia, hypophosphatemia

RESP: **Fibrosis**

SYST: **Anaphylaxis**

Contraindications: Pregnancy (D), breastfeeding, radiation therapy or chemotherapy within 1 mo, thrombocytopenia, recent smallpox vaccination, aluminum products used to prepare or administer cisplatin

Black Box Warning: Preexisting hearing impairment, bone marrow suppression, platinum compound hypersensitivity, renal disease/failure

Precautions: Geriatric patients, pneumococcus vaccination

PHARMACOKINETICS

Absorption complete, metabolized in liver, excreted in urine, half-life 30-100 hr, accumulates in body tissues for several months, enters breast milk

INTERACTIONS

Increase: bleeding risk—aspirin, NSAIDs, alcohol

Increase: ototoxicity—bumetanide, ethacrynic acid, furosemide

Increase: myelosuppression—myelosuppressive agents, radiation

Increase: nephrotoxicity—aminoglycosides, loop diuretics, salicylates

Decrease: effects of phenytoin

Decrease: antibody response—live virus vaccines

Drug/Lab Test

Increase: uric acid, BUN, creatinine

Decrease: CCr, calcium, phosphate, potassium, magnesium

Positive: Coombs' test

NURSING CONSIDERATIONS

Assess:

For bone marrow depression

• CBC, differential, platelet count weekly; withhold product if WBC is <4000 or platelet count is <100,000; notify prescriber of results

• Renal studies: BUN, creatinine, serum uric acid, urine CCr before, electrolytes during therapy; dose should not be given if BUN <25 mg/dl; creatinine <1.5 mg/dl; I&O ratio; report fall in urine output of <30 ml/hr

⚠ For anaphylaxis: wheezing, tachycardia, facial swelling, fainting; discontinue product and report to prescriber; resuscitation equipment should be nearby

• Monitor temp q4hr (may indicate beginning infection)

• Hepatic studies before, during therapy (bilirubin, AST, ALT, LDH) as needed or monthly

⚠ Bleeding: hematuria, guaiac, bruising or petechiae, mucosa or orifices q8hr; obtain prescription for viscous lidocaine (Xylocaine)

• Effects of alopecia on body image; discuss feelings about body changes
• Jaundice of skin, sclera; dark urine; clay-colored stools; itchy skin; abdominal pain; fever; diarrhea
• Edema in feet, joint pain, stomach pain, shaking, peripheral neuropathy

Administer:

IV route

• Do not use aluminum equipment during any preparation or administration, will form precipitate; do not refrigerate unopened powder or solution, protect from sunlight
• Prepare in biologic cabinet using gown, gloves, mask; do not allow product to come in contact with skin; use soap and water if contact occurs; use cytoxic handling procedures
• Hydrate patient with 0.9% NaCl over 8-12 hr before treatment
• Epinephrine, antihistamines, corticosteroids for hypersensitivity reaction
• Antiemetic 30-60 min before giving product and prn
• Allopurinol to maintain uric acid levels, alkalinization of urine
• Diuretic (furosemide 40 mg IV) or mannitol after infusion

Intermittent IV INF route

• Dilute 10 mg/10 ml or 50 mg/50 ml sterile H_2O for inj; withdraw prescribed dose, dilute ½ dose with 1000 ml D_5 0.2 NaCl or D_5 0.45 NaCl with 37.5 g mannitol; IV INF is given over 3-4 hr; use a 0.45-µm filter; total dose 2 L over 6-8 hr; check site for irritation, phlebitis

CONT IV INF route

• Give over 24 hr × 5 days

Additive compatibilities: Carboplatin, cyclophosphamide with etoposide, etoposide, etoposide with floxuridine, floxuridine, floxuridine with leucovorin, hydrOXYzine, ifosfamide, ifosfamide with etoposide, leucovorin, magnesium sulfate, mannitol, ondansetron

Solution compatibilities: D_5/0.225% NaCl, D_5/0.45% NaCl, D_5/0.9% NaCl, D_5/0.45% NaCl with mannitol 1.875%, D_5/0.33% NaCl with KCl 20 mEq and mannitol 1.875%, 0.9% NaCl, 0.45% NaCl, 0.3% NaCl, 0.225% NaCl

Syringe compatibilities: Bleomycin, cyclophosphamide, doxapram, DOXOrubicin, droperidol, fluorouracil, furosemide, heparin, leucovorin, methotrexate, metoclopramide, mitomycin, vinBLAStine, vinCRIStine

Y-site compatibilities: Allopurinol, aztreonam, bleomycin, chlorproMAZINE, cimetidine, cladribine, cyclophosphamide, dexamethasone, diphenhydrAMINE, DOXOrubicin, DOXOrubicin liposome, droperidol, famotidine, filgrastim, fludarabine, fluorouracil, furosemide, ganciclovir, granisetron, heparin, hydromorphone, leucovorin, lorazepam, melphalan, methotrexate, methylPREDNISolone, metoclopramide, mitomycin, morphine, ondansetron, paclitaxel, prochlorperazine, promethazine, propofol, ranitidine, sargramostim, teniposide, vinBLAStine, vinCRIStine, vinorelbine

Perform/provide:

• Comprehensive oral hygiene
• All medications PO, if possible, avoid IM inj when platelets <100,000/mm^3
• Increase fluid intake to 2-3 L/day to prevent urate deposits, calculi formation; promote elimination of product

Evaluate:

• Therapeutic response: decreased tumor size, spread of malignancy

Teach patient/family:

• To report signs of infection: increased temp, sore throat, flulike symptoms
• To report signs of anemia: fatigue, headache, faintness, shortness of breath, irritability
• To report bleeding, bruising, petechiae: avoid use of razors, commercial mouthwash
• To avoid aspirin, ibuprofen, NSAIDs, alcohol; may cause GI bleeding
• To report any complaints or side effects to nurse or prescriber
• That impotence or amenorrhea can occur; reversible after discontinuing treatment
• To report any changes in breathing, coughing

• To maintain adequate fluids; report decreased urine output, flank pain
• That hair may be lost during treatment; a wig or hairpiece may make patient feel better; new hair may be different in color, texture
• To report numbness, tingling in face or extremities, poor hearing or joint pain, swelling
• Not to receive vaccinations during treatment
• To use contraception during treatment and 4 mo after; this product may cause infertility; avoid breastfeeding

citalopram (℞)

(sigh-tal′oh-pram)
Celexa
Func. class.: Antidepressant
Chem. class.: Selective serotonin reuptake inhibitor (SSRI)

Do not confuse:
Celexa/Celebrex/Cerebyx/Cerebra
Action: Inhibits CNS neuron uptake of serotonin but not of norepinephrine; weak inhibitor of CYP450 enzyme system, making it more appealing than other products
Uses: Major depressive disorder
Unlabeled uses: Premenstrual disorders, panic disorder, social phobia, impulsive aggression in children, obsessive-compulsive disorder in adolescents, treatment of psychotic symptoms in nondepressed demented patients, anxiety, hot flashes, menopause, adjunct in schizophrenia, PTSD

DOSAGE AND ROUTES

Depression
• *Adult:* **PO** 20 mg/day AM or PM, may increase if needed to 40 mg/day after 1 wk; maintenance: after 6-8 wk of initial treatment, continue for 24 wk (32 wk total), reevaluate long-term usefulness (max 60 mg/day)
Hepatic dose/geriatric
• *Adult:* **PO** 20 mg/day, may increase to 40 mg/day if no response
Panic disorder (unlabeled)
• *Adult:* **PO** 20-60 mg/day
Premenstrual dysphoria/social phobia (unlabeled)
• *Adult:* **PO** 20-40 mg/day, used intermittently in premenstrual dysphoria
Available forms: Tabs 10, 20, 40 mg; oral sol 10 mg/5 ml

SIDE EFFECTS

CNS: Headache, nervousness, insomnia, drowsiness, anxiety, tremor, dizziness, fatigue, sedation, poor concentration, abnormal dreams, agitation, **convulsions,** apathy, euphoria, hallucinations, delusions, psychosis, **suicidal attempts, malignant neuroleptic-like syndrome reactions**
CV: Hot flashes, palpitations, angina pectoris, **hemorrhage,** hypertension, tachycardia, 1st-degree AV block, bradycardia, *MI,* thrombophlebitis
EENT: Visual changes, ear/eye pain, photophobia, tinnitus
GI: Nausea, diarrhea, dry mouth, anorexia, dyspepsia, constipation, cramps, vomiting, taste changes, flatulence, decreased appetite
GU: Dysmenorrhea, decreased libido, urinary frequency, UTI, amenorrhea, cystitis, impotence, urine retention
INTEG: Sweating, rash, pruritus, acne, alopecia, urticaria
MS: Pain, arthritis, twitching
RESP: Infection, pharyngitis, nasal congestion, sinus headache, sinusitis, cough, dyspnea, bronchitis, asthma, hyperventilation, pneumonia
SYST: Asthenia, viral infection, fever, allergy, chills; hyponatremia (geriatric patients)
Contraindications: Hypersensitivity
Precautions: Pregnancy (C), breastfeeding, geriatric patients, renal/hepatic disease, seizure disorder
Black Box Warning: Children, suicidal ideation

PHARMACOKINETICS

Metabolized in liver by CYP1A2, CYP2D6; excreted in urine; steady state 28-35 days; peak 2-4 hr; half-life 35 hr

INTERACTIONS

⚠ Fatal reactions: do not use with MAOIs
⚠ ***Increase:*** QTc interval—pimoside, quinolones, ziprasidone; do not use together
Increase: effect of tricyclics, use cautiously
Increase: serotonin syndrome—serotonin receptor agonists, SSRIs
Increase: bleeding risk—NSAIDs, salicylates, thrombolytics, anticoagulants
Increase: CNS effects—barbiturates, sedative/hypnotics, other CNS depressants
Increase: citalopram levels—macrolides, azole antifungals
Increase: plasma levels of β-blockers
Increase: serotonergic effects—lithium, MAOIs, trazodone, SNRIs (venlafaxine, duloxetine)
Decrease: citalopram levels—carbamazepine, clonidine

Drug/Herb

⚠ ***Increase:*** serotonin syndrome—St. John's wort, SAM-e; fatal reaction may occur; do not use concurrently
Increase: CNS stimulation—yohimbe

Drug/Lab Test

Increase: serum bilirubin, blood glucose, alk phos
Decrease: VMA, 5-HIAA
False increase: urinary catecholamines

NURSING CONSIDERATIONS

Assess:

- Mental status: mood, sensorium, affect, suicidal tendencies, increase in psychiatric symptoms, depression, panic
- B/P (lying/standing), pulse q4hr; if systolic B/P drops 20 mm Hg, hold product, notify prescriber; take vital signs q4hr in patients with CV disease
- Weight q wk; appetite may decrease or increase with product
- ECG for flattening of T wave, bundle branch, AV block, dysrhythmias in cardiac patients
- Alcohol consumption; if alcohol is consumed, hold dose until AM

Administer:

- With food or milk for GI symptoms
- Crushed if patient is unable to swallow medication whole
- Dosages at bedtime if oversedation occurs during the day; may take entire dose at bedtime

Perform/provide:

- Storage at room temperature; do not freeze
- Assistance with ambulation during therapy, since drowsiness, dizziness occur
- Safety measures primarily in geriatric patients
- Check to see if PO medication swallowed
- Sugarless gum, hard candy, frequent sips of water for dry mouth

Evaluate:

- Therapeutic response: decreased depression

Teach patient/family:

- That therapeutic effect may take 4-6 wk, may have increased anxiety first 5-7 days of therapy
- To use caution in driving, other activities requiring alertness because of drowsiness, dizziness, blurred vision
- To avoid alcohol ingestion, other CNS depressants
- That suicidal ideas, behavior may occur in children or young adults
- To notify prescriber if pregnant or plan to become pregnant or breastfeed
- The effects of serotonin syndrome: nausea/vomiting, tremors; if symptoms occur discontinue immediately and notify prescriber

clarithromycin (℞)

(klare-ith'row-my-sin)
Biaxin, Biaxin XL
Func. class.: Antiinfective
Chem. class.: Macrolide

Action: Binds to 50S ribosomal subunits of susceptible bacteria and suppresses protein synthesis

Uses: Mild to moderate infections of the upper and lower respiratory tract, uncomplicated skin and skin structure infections caused by *Streptococcus pneumoniae, Mycoplasma pneumoniae, Legionella pneumophila, Moraxella catarrhalis, Neisseria gonorrhoeae, Corynebacterium diphtheriae, Listeria monocytogenes, Haemophilus influenzae, Streptococcus pyogenes, Staphylococcus aureus, Mycobacterium avium* complex (MAC), complex infection in AIDS patients, *Mycobacterium avium intracellulare, Helicobacter pylori* in combination with omeprazole

Unlabeled uses: Endocarditis prophylaxis, dyspepsia, gastric ulcer, Legionnaire's disease, pertussis, SARS

DOSAGE AND ROUTES

Acute exacerbation of chronic bronchitis

- *Adult:* **PO** 250-500 mg q12hr × 7-14 days or 1000 mg/day × 7 days (XL)

Pharyngitis/tonsillitis

- *Adult:* **PO** 250 mg q12hr × 10 days

Community-acquired pneumonia

- *Adult:* **PO** 250 mg q12hr × 7-14 days or 1000 mg/day × 7 days (XL)

Endocarditis prophylaxis

- *Adult:* **PO** 500 mg 1 hr before procedure

MAC prophylaxis/treatment

- *Adult:* **PO** 500 mg bid, will require an additional antiinfective for active infection

H. pylori *infection*

- *Adult:* **PO** 500 mg bid plus omeprazole 2 × 20 mg q AM (days 1-14), then omeprazole 20 mg q AM (days 15-28)

Acute maxillary sinusitis

- *Adult:* **PO** 500 mg q12hr × 14 days

Most infections

- *Child:* **PO** 7.5 mg/kg q12hr × 10 days, max 500 mg/dose for MAC

Renal dose

- *Adult/child:* **PO** CCr <30 ml/min reduce dose by 50%

Legionnaire's disease/SARS/ whooping cough/gastric ulcer/ dyspepsia* (H. pylori) *(unlabeled)

- *Adult:* **PO** 500 mg q12hr, may be used in combination for some of these conditions

Available forms: Tabs 250, 500 mg; oral susp 125 mg/5 ml, 250 mg/5 ml; ext rel tab (XL) 500 mg

SIDE EFFECTS

CV: **Ventricular dysrhythmias, QT prolongation**

GI: Nausea, vomiting, diarrhea, **hepatotoxicity,** *abdominal pain,* stomatitis, heartburn, anorexia, *abnormal taste,* **pseudomembranous colitis**

GU: Vaginitis, moniliasis

HEMA: Leukopenia, thrombocytopenia, increased INR

INTEG: Rash, urticaria, pruritus, **Stevens-Johnson syndrome, toxic epidermal necrolysis**

MISC: Headache, hearing loss

Contraindications: Hypersensitivity to this product or macrolide antibiotics

Precautions: Pregnancy (C), breastfeeding, geriatric patients, renal/hepatic disease, QT prolongation

PHARMACOKINETICS

Peak 2 hr; duration 12 hr; half-life 4-6 hr; metabolized by liver; excreted in bile, feces; possible inhibition of P-glycoprotein

INTERACTIONS

Increase: dysrhythmias—cisapride, pimozide

Increase: levels, increase toxicity—alprazolam, busPIRone, carbamazepine, cycloSPORINE, digoxin, disopyramide, ergots, felodipine, fluconazole, omeprazole, tacrolimus, theophylline
Increase: oral anticoagulants effect—digoxin, theophylline, carbamazepine
Increase: levels of HMG-CoA reductase inhibitors
Increase: action, risk of toxicity—all products metabolized by CYP3A enzyme system
Increase: effect of calcium channel blockers, midazolam, benzodiazepines, tacrolimus
Increase: QT prolongation—class IA, III antidysrhythmics
Increase or decrease action: zidovudine
Decrease: levels—rifampin, rifabutin
Drug/Herb
• Do not use acidophilus with antiinfectives; separate by several hours
Drug/Lab Test
Increase: 17-OHCS/17-KS, AST, ALT, BUN, creatinine, LDH, total bilirubin
Decrease: folate assay, WBC

NURSING CONSIDERATIONS

Assess:
• For infection: wound characteristics, urine, stool, sputum, WBC, temp
• Cardiac function due to QT effects
• For ulcers: abdominal pain, bleeding in stools, emesis
• Renal, hepatic studies; report hematuria, oliguria
• C&S before product therapy; product may be given as soon as culture is taken; C&S may be repeated after treatment
• Bowel pattern before, during treatment
• Skin eruptions, itching
• Respiratory status: rate, character, wheezing, tightness in chest; discontinue product
• Allergies before treatment, reaction of each medication
Administer:
• Do not break, crush, or chew tabs
• Adequate intake of fluids (2 L) during diarrhea episodes
• q12hr to maintain serum level
Perform/provide:
• Storage at room temperature
Evaluate:
• Therapeutic response: C&S negative for infection
Teach patient/family:
• To take with full glass H_2O; may give with food to decrease GI symptoms
⚠ To report sore throat, fever, fatigue; may indicate superinfection
⚠ To notify nurse of diarrhea, dark urine, pale stools, yellow discoloration of eyes or skin, severe abdominal pain
• To take at evenly spaced intervals; complete dosage regimen
• To notify prescriber if pregnancy is suspected or planned
Treatment of hypersensitivity: Withdraw product, maintain airway, administer epinephrine, aminophylline, O_2, IV corticosteroids

clevidipine (℞)

(klev-id'i-peen)
Cleviprex
Func. class.: Calcium channel blocker (L-type)
Chem. class.: Dihydropyridine

Action: L-type calcium channels mediate the influx of calcium during depolarization in arterial smooth muscle, reduces mean arterial B/P by decreasing systemic vascular resistance
Uses: Reduction of B/P when oral therapy is not feasible

DOSAGE AND ROUTES

• *Adult:* **CONT IV** 1-2 mg/hr; dose may be doubled q90sec initially; as B/P reaches goal, adjust dose less frequently (5-10 min), with smaller increases in dose; most patients require 4-6 mg/hr, max 32 mg/hr; no more than 1000 ml should be infused per 24 hr period due to lipid load restrictions
Available forms: Single dose vial 50, 100 ml (0.5 mg/ml), intravenous emulsion

SIDE EFFECTS

CNS: Headache
CV: Hypotension, **MI, sinus tachycardia,** syncope, **reflex tachycardia, atrial fibrillation**
GI: Nausea, vomiting
GU: Renal failure

Contraindications: Hypersensitivity to this product, eggs or soya lecithin; defective lipid metabolism; severe aortic stenosis, pancreatitis

Precautions: Pregnancy (C), labor, breastfeeding, children <18 yr, heart failure, hyperlipidemia, chronic hypertension, pheochromocytoma

PHARMACOKINETICS

Onset 2-4 min; half-life initially 1 min, terminal 15 min; metabolized via esterases in blood, extravascular tissues; excreted in urine 63%-74%, feces 7%-22%; protein binding >99%

NURSING CONSIDERATIONS

Assess:

- Cardiac status: B/P, pulse, respiration, ECG; some patients have developed severe angina, acute MI after calcium channel blockers if obstructive CAD is severe; if not transitioned to other antihypertensive therapies following clevidipine infusion, patients should be monitored ≥8 hr for rebound hypertension; monitor for rebound hypertension following product stoppage
- I&O ratio, weight daily; peripheral edema, dyspnea, jugular vein distention, crackles

Administer:

- Do not give through same line as other medications
- Gently invert several times before use; do not use if discolored or particulate matter is present
- Give through central or peripheral line
- Use infusion device

Perform/provide:

- Storage of vials in refrigerator, do not freeze; leave vials in carton until use; product is photosensitive, but protection from light during administration is not required

Evaluate:

- Therapeutic response: decreased B/P

Teach patient/family:

- To notify prescriber immediately if neurological symptoms, visual changes, or symptoms of CHF occur
- To continue follow up for hypertension

C

clindamycin HCl (℞)
(klin-da-my′sin)
Cleocin HCl

clindamycin palmitate (℞)
Cleocin Pediatric, Dalacin C Palmitate

clindamycin phosphate (℞)
Cleocin Phosphate, Dalacin C, Dalacin C Phosphate

Func. class.: Antiinfective—miscellaneous
Chem. class.: Lincomycin derivative

Action: Binds to 50S subunit of bacterial ribosomes, suppresses protein synthesis

Uses: Infections caused by staphylococci, streptococci, *Rickettsia, Fusobacterium, Actinomyces, Peptococcus, Bacteroides, Pneumocystis jiroveci*

Unlabeled uses: Acne rosacea, *Bacillus anthracis,* dental infections, folliculitis, malaria, pemphigus, periodontitis, *Pneumocystis jiroveci* pneumonia (PCP), toxoplasmosis

DOSAGE AND ROUTES

- *Adult:* **PO** 150-450 mg q6-8hr, max 1.8 g/day; **IM/IV** 1.2-1.8 g/day in 2-4 divided doses, max 4800 mg/day
- *Child >1 mo:* **PO** 8-25 mg/kg/day in divided doses q6-8hr; **IM/IV** 20-40 mg/kg/day in divided doses q6-8hr (3-4 equal doses)

• *Child <1 mo:* **IM/IV** 15-20 mg/kg/day divided q6-8hr

PID

• *Adult:* **IV** 900 mg q8hr plus gentamicin

Bacterial endocarditis prophylaxis

• *Adult:* 600 mg 1 hr prior to procedure

P. jiroveci *pneumonia (unlabeled)*

• *Adult:* **PO** 1200-1800 mg/day in divided doses with 15-30 mg primaquine/day

Available forms: *HCl:* caps 75, 150, 300 mg; *palmitate:* oral sol 75 mg/5 ml; *phosphate:* inj 150, 300, 600 mg base/4 ml; 900 mg base/ml; inj inf in D_5 300 mg, 600 mg, 900 mg

SIDE EFFECTS

GI: Nausea, vomiting, abdominal pain, diarrhea, **pseudomembranous colitis,** anorexia, weight loss, increased AST, ALT, bilirubin, alk phos; jaundice

GU: Vaginitis, urinary frequency

HEMA: **Leukopenia, eosinophilia, agranulocytosis, thrombocytopenia, polyarthritis**

INTEG: Rash, urticaria, pruritus, erythema, pain, abscess at inj site

SYST: **Stevens-Johnson syndrome, exfoliative dermatitis**

Contraindications: Hypersensitivity to this product or lincomycin, tartrazine dye; ulcerative colitis/enteritis

Black Box Warning: Pseudomembranous colitis

Precautions: Pregnancy (B), breastfeeding, geriatric patients, GI/renal/hepatic disease, asthma, allergy

Black Box Warning: Diarrhea

PHARMACOKINETICS

PO: Peak 45 min, duration 6 hr

IM: Peak 3 hr; duration 8-12 hr; half-life 2½ hr; metabolized in liver; excreted in urine, bile, feces as inactive metabolites; crosses placenta; excreted in breast milk

INTERACTIONS

• May block clindamycin effect: erythromycin, chloramphenicol

Increase: neuromuscular blockade—neuromuscular blockers

Decrease: absorption—kaolin

Drug/Herb

• Do not use acidophilus with antiinfectives; separate by several hours

Drug/Lab Test

Increase: alk phos, bilirubin, CPK, AST, ALT

NURSING CONSIDERATIONS

Assess:

• Hepatic studies: AST, ALT if on long-term therapy

• Blood studies: WBC, RBC, Hct, Hgb, platelets, serum iron, reticulocytes; product should be discontinued if bone marrow depression occurs

• C&S before product therapy; product may be given as soon as culture is taken

• B/P, pulse in patient receiving product parenterally

• Bowel pattern before, during treatment; if severe diarrhea occurs, product should be discontinued; may indicate pseudomembranous colitis

• Skin eruptions, itching, dermatitis after administration

• Respiratory status: rate, character, wheezing, tightness in chest

• Allergies before treatment, reaction of each medication

Administer:

• That product must be taken in equal intervals around clock to maintain blood levels

PO route

• Do not break, crush, or chew caps

• Orally with at least 8 oz H_2O

IM route

• IM deep inj; rotate sites; do not give >600 mg in single IM inj

IV route

• By inf only; do not administer bolus dose; dilute 300 mg or less/50 ml or more of D_5W, NS; may be further diluted in greater amounts of D_5W, NS and given as a cont inf in acute PID; give first dose 10 mg/min over ½ hr, then 0.75 mg/min; increased rates may be used to keep serum blood levels higher; run >10 min; no more than 1200 mg in a single 1-hr inf

Additive compatibilities: Amikacin, ampicillin, aztreonam, cefazolin, cefepime, cefonicid, cefotaxime, cefoxitin, ceftazidime, ceftizoxime, cefuroxime, cephalothin, cimetidine, fluconazole, heparin, hydrocortisone, kanamycin, methylPREDNISolone, metoclopramide, metronidazole, netilmicin, ofloxacin, penicillin G, piperacillin, potassium chloride, sodium bicarbonate, tobramycin, verapamil, vit B/C

Syringe compatibilities: Amikacin, aztreonam, gentamicin, heparin

Y-site compatibilities: Amifostine, amiodarone, amphotericin B cholesteryl, amsacrine, aztreonam, cefpirome, cisatracurium, cyclophosphamide, diltiazem, DOXOrubicin liposome, enalaprilat, esmolol, fludarabine, foscarnet, granisetron, heparin, hydromorphone, labetalol, magnesium sulfate, melphalan, meperidine, midazolam, morphine, multivitamins, ondansetron, perphenazine, piperacillin/tazobactam, propofol, remifentanil, sargramostim, tacrolimus, teniposide, theophylline, thiotepa, vinorelbine, vit B/C, zidovudine

Perform/provide:

- Storage at room temperature (caps) up to 2 wk (reconstituted)
- Epinephrine, suction, tracheostomy set, endotracheal intubation equipment on unit
- Adequate intake of fluids (2 L) during diarrhea episodes

Evaluate:

- Therapeutic response: decreased temp, negative C&S

Teach patient/family:

- To take oral product with full glass of water; antiperistaltic products may worsen diarrhea
- All aspects of product therapy: need to complete entire course of medication to ensure organism death (10-14 days); culture may be taken after medication course completed
- ⚠ To report sore throat, fever, fatigue; may indicate superinfection
- To take with food to reduce GI symptoms
- To notify nurse or prescriber of diarrhea

Treatment of hypersensitivity:

- Withdraw product; maintain airway; administer epinephrine, aminophylline, O_2, IV corticosteroids

clindamycin topical

See Appendix B

clobetasol topical

See Appendix B

*clomiPHENE (℞)

(kloe′mi-feen)

Clomid, clomiphene citrate, Serophene

Func. class.: Ovulation stimulant

Chem. class.: Nonsteroidal antiestrogenic

Do not confuse:

clomiPHENE/clomiPRAMINE

Action: Increases LH, FSH release from the pituitary, which increases maturation of ovarian follicle, ovulation, development of corpus luteum

Uses: Female infertility (ovulatory failure)

Unlabeled uses: Oligospermia

DOSAGE AND ROUTES

- *Adult:* **PO** 50-100 mg/day × 5 days or 50-100 mg/day beginning on day 5 of cycle; may be repeated until conception occurs or 3 cycles of therapy have been completed

Oligospermia (unlabeled)
- *Adult (men):* **PO** 25 mg/day × 25 days, then 5 days off cycle each mo

Available forms: Tabs 50 mg

SIDE EFFECTS

CNS: Headache, depression, restlessness, anxiety, nervousness, fatigue, insomnia, dizziness, flushing

CV: Vasomotor flushing, phlebitis, **deep-vein thrombosis**

EENT: Blurred vision, diplopia, photophobia

GI: Nausea, vomiting, constipation, abdominal pain, bloating

GU: Polyuria, urinary frequency, **birth defects, spontaneous abortions,** multiple ovulation, breast pain, oliguria, abnormal uterine bleeding, ovarian cyst, hypertrophy of ovary

INTEG: Rash, dermatitis, urticaria, alopecia

Contraindications: Pregnancy (X), hypersensitivity, hepatic disease, undiagnosed uterine bleeding, uncontrolled thyroid or adrenal dysfunction, intracranial lesion, ovarian cysts, endometrial carcinoma

Precautions: Hypertension, depression, seizures, diabetes mellitus, abnormal ovarian enlargement, ovarian hyperstimulation

PHARMACOKINETICS

Metabolized in liver, excreted in feces

INTERACTIONS

Drug/Lab Test

Increase: FSH/LH, BSP, thyroxine, TBG

NURSING CONSIDERATIONS

Assess:
- For LFTs before therapy: AST, ALT, alk phos
- Serum progesterone, urinary excretion of pregnanediol to identify occurrence of ovulation
- Ovarian size, cervical condition by pelvic examination
- For endometrial carcinoma in women over 35 by endometrial biopsy

Administer:
- After discontinuing estrogen therapy
- At same time daily to maintain product level

Evaluate:
- Therapeutic response: fertility

Teach patient/family:
- That multiple births are common
- To notify prescriber immediately if low abdominal pain occurs; may indicate ovarian cyst, cyst rupture
- To notify prescriber of photophobia, blurred vision, diplopia, abnormal bleeding, hot flashes, nausea, vomiting, headache
- That if dose is missed, to double it next time; if more than one dose is missed, to call prescriber
- That response usually occurs 4-10 days after last day of treatment
- The method for taking, recording basal body temp to determine whether ovulation has occurred
- If ovulation can be determined (there is a slight decrease in temp, then a sharp increase for ovulation), to attempt coitus 3 days before and every other day until after ovulation
- If pregnancy is suspected, to notify prescriber immediately

*clomiPRAMINE (℞)

(kloe-mip′ra-meen)

Anafranil

Func. class.: Antidepressant, tricyclic

Chem. class.: Tertiary amine

Do not confuse:
clomiPRAMINE/clomiPHENE/desipramine/Norpramin

Action: Potentiates serotonin and norepinephrine; also increases DOPamine metabolism; moderate anticholinergic effect

Uses: Obsessive-compulsive disorder

Unlabeled uses: Panic disorder, autism, depression, premature ejaculation, dysphoria, phobias, anxiety, agoraphobia

DOSAGE AND ROUTES

Obsessive-compulsive disorder

• *Adult:* **PO** 25 mg at bedtime and increase gradually over 4 wk to 75-250 mg/day in divided doses

• *Child 10-18 yr:* **PO** 25 mg/day gradually increased; max 3 mg/kg/day or 200 mg/day, whichever is smaller

Autism (unlabeled)

• *Adult:* **PO** 25 mg/day, may increase to 75-100 mg/day, max 250 mg/day

• *Child:* **PO** 25 mg/day, may increase if needed

Premature ejaculation (unlabeled)

• *Adult:* **PO** 25-50 mg/day

Depression (unlabeled)

• *Adult:* **PO** 25 mg at bedtime and increase gradually over 4 wk to 75-250 mg/day in divided doses

• *Child 10-18 yr:* **PO** 25-50 mg/day gradually increased; max 3 mg/kg/day, whichever is smaller

Available forms: Caps 25, 50, 75 mg

SIDE EFFECTS

CNS: Dizziness, tremors, mania, **seizures,** aggressiveness, EPS, drowsiness, headache, **neuroleptic malignant syndrome**

CV: Hypotension, tachycardia, **cardiac arrest**

EENT: Blurred vision

ENDO: Galactorrhea, hyperprolactinemia

GI: Constipation, dry mouth, nausea, dyspepsia, weight gain, **hepatic toxicity**

GU: Delayed ejaculation, anorgasmia, urinary retention, decreased libido

HEMA: **Agranulocytosis, neutropenia, pancytopenia**

INTEG: Diaphoresis, photosensitivity

META: Hyponatremia

SYST: **Suicide in children/adolescents**

Contraindications: Hypersensitivity, immediate post-MI

Precautions: Pregnancy (C), breastfeeding, geriatric patients, seizures, cardiac disease, glaucoma

Black Box Warning: Children, suicidal ideation

PHARMACOKINETICS

Onset ≥2 wk (depression), 4-10 wk (OCD); peak 2-6 hr; extensively bound to tissue and plasma proteins; demethylated in liver; active metabolites excreted in urine (50%-60%), feces (24%-32%); half-life 20-30 hr; steady state 1-2 wk; metabolized by CYP1A2, CYP2D6

INTERACTIONS

Increase: hypertensive crisis, seizures, hypertensive episode—MAOIs

Increase: clomiPRAMINE levels—cimetidine, fluoxetine, fluvoxamine, sertraline; do not use together

Increase: hypertensive effect—clonidine, epinephrine, norepinephrine

Increase: clomiPRAMINE level—CYP1A2, CYP2D6

Increase: CNS depression—alcohol, CNS depressants, general anesthetics

Increase: QT prolongation—other tricyclics, phenothiazines, quinolones

Decrease: effect of clonidine, levodopa, skeletal muscle relaxants, haloperidol, opiates

Decrease: clomiPRAMINE levels—barbiturates, carbamazepine, phenytoin

Drug/Herb

• Serotonin syndrome: SAM-e, St. John's wort; do not use concurrently

Increase: CNS depression—hops, kava, lavender, valerian

Increase: anticholinergic effect—belladonna, corkwood, henbane, jimsonweed

Increase: clomiPRAMINE action—scopolia root

Drug/Lab Test

Increase: prolactin, TBG, AST, ALT

Decrease: serum thyroid hormone (T_3, T_4)

NURSING CONSIDERATIONS

Assess:

- B/P (lying, standing), pulse q4hr; if systolic B/P drops 20 mm Hg, withhold product, notify prescriber; take VS q4hr in patients with CV disease
- For neuroleptic malignant syndrome: hyperpyrexia, rigidity, irregular pulse, diaphoresis
- ECG for flattening of T wave, QTc prolongation, bundle branch block, AV block, dysrhythmias in cardiac patients
- Blood studies: CBC, leukocytes, differential, cardiac enzymes if patient is receiving long-term therapy
- Hepatic studies: AST, ALT, bilirubin
- Mental status: mood, sensorium, affect, suicidal tendencies; increase in psychiatric symptoms: depression, panic, frequency of obsessive-compulsive behaviors; watch closely for evidence of suicidal thoughts in children/adolescents, seizure disorders
- Urinary retention, constipation; constipation more likely in children
- Withdrawal symptoms: headache, nausea, vomiting, muscle pain, weakness; not usual unless product discontinued abruptly
- Alcohol consumption; if alcohol consumed, withhold dose until AM

Administer:

- Do not break, crush, or chew caps
- Increased fluids, bulk in diet for constipation, especially geriatric patients
- With food or milk for GI symptoms
- After titration, may be given as a single dose at bedtime, to reduce daytime sedation

Perform/provide:

- Storage in tight container at room temperature; do not freeze
- Assistance with ambulation during beginning therapy, since drowsiness/dizziness occurs
- Safety measures, primarily in geriatric patients
- Checking to see PO medication swallowed
- Gum, hard candy, or frequent sips of water for dry mouth

Evaluate:

- Therapeutic response: decreased anxiety, depression

Teach patient/family:

- That the effects may take 4-6 wk
- About risk of seizures
- To use caution in driving, other activities requiring alertness because of drowsiness, dizziness, blurred vision
- To avoid alcohol ingestion, other CNS depressants
- Not to discontinue medication quickly after long-term use; may cause nausea, headache, malaise
- That suicidal ideas/behavior may occur in children/young adults
- To wear sunscreen, protective clothing to prevent photosensitivity
- To notify prescriber if pregnancy is planned or suspected
- That men may experience a high incidence of sexual dysfunction

Treatment of overdose: ECG monitoring; induce emesis; lavage, activated charcoal; anticonvulsant; diazepam IV

clonazepam (℞)

(kloe-na′zi-pam)

Apo-Clonazepam ♣, Gen-Clonazepam ♣, Klonopin, Klonopin wafers, Novo-Clonazepam ♣, Nu-Clonazepam ♣, PMS-Clonazepam ♣, Rivotril ♣

Func. class.: Anticonvulsant

Chem. class.: Benzodiazepine derivative

Controlled Substance Schedule IV

Do not confuse:

clonazepam/lorazepam/clorazepate

Klonopin/clonidine

Action: Inhibits spike, wave formation in absence seizures (petit mal), decreases amplitude, frequency, duration, spread of discharge in minor motor seizures

Uses: Absence, atypical absence, akinetic, myoclonic seizures, Lennox-Gastaut syndrome, panic disorder

Unlabeled uses: Anxiety, insomnia, nystagmus, restless leg syndrome

DOSAGE AND ROUTES

• *Adult:* **PO** Not to exceed 1.5 mg/day in 3 divided doses; may be increased 0.5-1 mg q3days until desired response, max 20 mg/day; **RECT** 0.02 mg/kg

• *Geriatric:* **PO** 0.25 daily-bid initially, increase by 0.25/day q7-14days as needed

• *Child <10 yr or <30 kg:* **PO** 0.01-0.03 mg/kg/day in divided doses q8hr, not to exceed 0.05 mg/kg/day; may be increased 0.25-0.5 mg q3days until desired response, not to exceed 0.1-0.2 mg/kg/day; **RECT** 0.05-0.1 mg/kg

Restless leg syndrome (RLS) (unlabeled)

• *Adult:* **PO** 0.5 mg tid

Insomnia/anxiety (unlabeled)

• *Adult:* **PO** 0.125-0.25 mg at bedtime, titrate up q3-4days as needed

Available forms: Tabs 0.5, 1, 2 mg; orally disintegrating tabs 0.125, 0.25, 0.5, 1, 2 mg; wafer 0.125, 0.25, 0.5, 1, 2 mg

SIDE EFFECTS

CNS: Drowsiness, dizziness, confusion, behavioral changes, tremors, insomnia, headache, **suicidal tendencies,** slurred speech, anterograde amnesia

CV: Palpitations, bradycardia, tachycardia

EENT: Increased salivation, nystagmus, diplopia, abnormal eye movements

GI: Nausea, constipation, polyphagia, anorexia, xerostomia, diarrhea, gastritis, sore gums

GU: Dysuria, enuresis, nocturia, retention, libido changes

HEMA: **Thrombocytopenia, leukocytosis, eosinophilia**

INTEG: Rash, alopecia, hirsutism

RESP: **Respiratory depression,** dyspnea, congestion

Contraindications: Pregnancy (D), hypersensitivity to benzodiazepines, acute closed-angle glaucoma, psychosis, severe hepatic disease

Precautions: Breastfeeding, geriatric patients, open-angle glaucoma, chronic respiratory disease, renal/hepatic disease

PHARMACOKINETICS

PO: Peak 1-2 hr, metabolized by liver, excreted in urine, half-life 18-50 hr, duration 6-12 hr, protein binding 85%

INTERACTIONS

Increase: clonazepam effects—CYP3A4 inhibitors (azoles, cimetidine, clarithromycin, diltiazem, erythromycin, fluoxetine), oral contraceptives

Increase: CNS depression—alcohol, barbiturates, opiates, antidepressants, other anticonvulsants, general anesthetics, hypnotics, sedatives

Decrease: clonazepam effect—CYP3A4 inducers (carbamazepine, phenobarbital, phenytoin)

Drug/Herb

Increase: CNS depression—kava

Increase: clonazepam effect—ginkgo, melatonin

Decrease: clonazepam effect—ginseng, santonica, St. John's wort

Drug/Lab Test

Increase: AST, alk phos

NURSING CONSIDERATIONS

Assess:

• Renal studies: urinalysis, BUN, urine creatinine

• Blood studies: RBC, Hct, Hgb, reticulocyte counts q wk for 4 wk, then q mo

• Hepatic studies: ALT, AST, bilirubin, creatinine

• Product levels during initial treatment (therapeutic 20-80 ng/ml)

• Signs of physical withdrawal if medication suddenly discontinued

⚠ Mental status: mood, sensorium, affect, oversedation, behavioral changes, suicidal thoughts/behaviors; if mental status changes, notify prescriber

- Eye problems: need for ophthalmic exam before, during, after treatment (slit lamp, funduscopy, tonometry)
- Allergic reaction: red, raised rash; product should be discontinued

⚠ Blood dyscrasias: fever, sore throat, bruising, rash, jaundice

- Toxicity: bone marrow depression, nausea, vomiting, ataxia, diplopia, CV collapse

Administer:

PO route

- With food, milk for GI symptoms
- Avoid use with CNS depressants

Perform/provide:

- Storage at room temperature
- Assistance with ambulation during early part of treatment; dizziness occurs, especially geriatric patients

Evaluate:

- Therapeutic response: decreased seizure activity, document on patient's chart

Teach patient/family:

- To carry emergency ID bracelet stating name, products taken, condition, prescriber's name, phone number
- To avoid driving, other activities that require alertness
- To avoid alcohol ingestion; increased sedation may occur
- Not to discontinue medication quickly after long-term use; taper off over several wk

Treatment of overdose: Lavage, activated charcoal, flumazenil, monitor electrolytes, VS, administer vasopressors

clonidine (℞)

(klon′i-deen)

Apo-Clonidine ♣, Catapres, Catapres-TTS, clonidine HCl, Dixarit ♣, Duraclon, Novo-Clonidine ♣, Nu-Clonidine ♣

Func. class.: Antihypertensive

Chem. class.: Central α-adrenergic agonist

Do not confuse:

clonidine/Klonopin/clonazepam

Catapres/Cataflam/Catarase

Action: Inhibits sympathetic vasomotor center in CNS, which reduces impulses in sympathetic nervous system; blood pressure, pulse rate, cardiac output decrease, prevents pain signal transmission in CNS by α-adrenergic receptor stimulation of the spinal cord

Uses: Mild to moderate hypertension, used alone or in combination; severe pain in cancer patients (epidural)

Unlabeled uses: Opioid withdrawal, prevention of vascular headaches, treatment of menopausal symptoms, dysmenorrhea, attention deficit hyperactivity disorder (ADHD), autism, cycloSPORINE nephrotoxicity prophylaxis, diabetic neuropathy, ethanol withdrawal, Tourette's syndrome, hypertensive emergency

DOSAGE AND ROUTES

Hypertension

- *Adult:* **PO/TRANSDERMAL** 0.1 mg bid, then increase by 0.1-0.2 mg/day at weekly intervals, until desired response; range 0.2-0.6 mg/day in divided doses
- *Geriatric:* **PO** 0.1 mg at bedtime, may increase gradually
- *Child:* **PO** 5-10 mcg/kg/day in divided doses q8-12hr, max 0.9 mg/day

Severe pain

- *Adult:* **CONT EPIDURAL INF** 30 mcg/hr
- *Child:* **CONT EPIDURAL INF** 0.5 mcg/kg/hr, then titrate to response

Opioid withdrawal (unlabeled)

• *Adult:* **PO** 0.3-1.2 mg/day; may decrease by 50% × 3 days then decrease by 0.1-0.2 mg/day or discontinue

ADHD/tic disorders in children/ autism (unlabeled)

• *Child:* **PO** 0.05 mg/kg/day in 3-4 divided doses × 8 wk, max 0.3 mg/day

Menopausal symptoms (unlabeled)

• *Adult:* **TRANSDERMAL** 0.1 mg patch q1wk; **PO** 0.05-0.4 mg/day

Tourette's syndrome (unlabeled)

• *Adult:* **PO** 0.15-0.2 mg/day

Hypertensive emergency (unlabeled)

• *Adult:* **PO** 0.1-0.2 mg q1hr to a total of 0.6 mg

Available forms: Tabs 0.025 ♣, 0.1, 0.2, 0.3 mg; transdermal 2.5, 5, 7.5 mg delivering 0.1, 0.2, 0.3 mg/24 hr, respectively; inj 100, 500 mcg/ml

SIDE EFFECTS

CNS: Drowsiness, sedation, headache, fatigue, nightmares, insomnia, mental changes, anxiety, depression, hallucinations, delirium

CV: Orthostatic hypotension, palpitations, **CHF,** ECG abnormalities

EENT: Taste change, parotid pain

ENDO: Hyperglycemia

GI: Nausea, vomiting, malaise, constipation, *dry mouth*

GU: Impotence, dysuria, nocturia, gynecomastia

INTEG: Rash, alopecia, facial pallor, pruritus, hives, edema, burning papules, excoriation (transdermal patches)

MISC: Withdrawal symptoms

MS: Muscle, joint pain; leg cramps

Contraindications: Hypersensitivity; (epidural) bleeding disorders, anticoagulants

Precautions: Pregnancy (C), breastfeeding, children <12 yr (transdermal), geriatric patients, noncompliant patients, MI (recent), diabetes mellitus, chronic renal failure, Raynaud's disease, thyroid disease, depression, COPD, asthma

Black Box Warning: Labor

PHARMACOKINETICS

Absorbed well

PO: Onset ½ to 1 hr, peak 2-4 hr, duration 8-12 hr, half-life 6-12 hr

TRANSDERMAL: Onset 3 days; duration 1 wk; metabolized by liver (metabolites); excreted in urine (30% unchanged, inactive metabolites), feces; crosses blood-brain barrier; excreted in breast milk

INTERACTIONS

• AV block: verapamil

⚠ Life-threatening elevations of B/P: tricyclics, β-blockers

Increase: CNS depression—opiates, sedatives, hypnotics, anesthetics, alcohol

Increase: hypotensive effects—diuretics, other antihypertensive nitrates

Decrease: hypotensive effects—tricyclics, MAOIs, appetite suppressants, amphetamines, prazosin

Decrease: effect of levodopa

Drug/Herb

• Toxicity/death: aconite

Increase: antihypertensive effect—barberry, betony, black catechu, black cohosh, bloodroot, broom, burdock, cat's claw, dandelion, goldenseal, hawthorn, Irish moss, Jamaican dogwood, kelp, khella, mistletoe, parsley, Queen Anne's lace, rue

Decrease: antihypertensive effect—astragalus, capsicum peppers, cola tree, coltsfoot, guarana, khat, licorice, yohimbine

Drug/Lab Test

Increase: blood glucose

Decrease: VMA, urinary catecholamines, aldosterone

NURSING CONSIDERATIONS

Assess:

• Blood studies: neutrophils, decreased platelets

• Renal studies: protein, BUN, creatinine; increased levels may indicate nephrotic syndrome

• Baselines in renal, hepatic studies before therapy begins; potassium levels, although hyperkalemia rare
• B/P, pulse if used for hypertension, report significant changes
• For opiate withdrawal including fever, diarrhea, nausea, vomiting, cramps, insomnia, shivering, dilated pupils
• Pain: location, intensity, character; alleviating, aggravating factors, baseline and frequently
• Edema in feet, legs daily; monitor I&O; check for falling output
• Allergic reaction: rash, fever, pruritus, urticaria; product should be discontinued if antihistamines fail to help
• Allergic reaction from patches: rash, urticaria, angioedema; should not continue to use
• Symptoms of CHF: edema, dyspnea, wet crackles, B/P
• Renal symptoms: polyuria, oliguria, frequency

Administer:

PO route

• Give last dose at bedtime

Transdermal route

• Q wk; apply to site without hair; best absorption over chest or upper arm; rotate sites with each application; clean site before application; apply firmly, especially around edges

Epidural route

• Used for severe cancer pain
• May be used with opiates
• Use only if familiar with epidural infusion devices

Perform/provide:

• Storage of patches in cool environment, tablets in tight container

Evaluate:

• Therapeutic response: decrease in B/P in hypertension, decrease in withdrawal symptoms (opioid), decrease in pain

Teach patient/family:

• To avoid hazardous activities, since product may cause drowsiness
• To notify all health care providers of medication use
• Not to discontinue product abruptly or withdrawal symptoms may occur: anxiety, increased B/P, headache, insomnia, increased pulse, tremors, nausea, sweating
• Not to use OTC (cough, cold, or allergy) products unless directed by prescriber
• To comply with dosage schedule even if feeling better
• To rise slowly to sitting or standing position to minimize orthostatic hypotension, especially geriatric patients
• To notify prescriber of mouth sores, sore throat, fever, swelling of hands or feet, irregular heartbeat, chest pain, signs of angioedema
• About excessive perspiration, dehydration, vomiting; diarrhea may lead to fall in blood pressure; consult prescriber if these occur
• That product may cause dizziness, fainting; light-headedness may occur during first few days of therapy
• That product may cause dry mouth; use hard candy, saliva product, or frequent rinsing of mouth
• That compliance is necessary; not to skip or stop product unless directed by prescriber; tolerance may develop with long-term use
• That product may cause skin rash or impaired perspiration
• To use patch; patch comes in two parts: product patch and overlay to keep patch in place, do not trim or cut patch
• That response may take 2-3 days if product is given transdermally; instruct on administration of patch, if switching from tabs to patch, taper tabs to avoid withdrawal

Treatment of overdose: Supportive treatment; administer tolazoline, atropine, DOPamine prn

clopidogrel (℞)

(klo-pid'oh-grel)

Plavix

Func. class.: Platelet aggregation inhibitor

Chem. class.: Thienopyridine derivative

Do not confuse:
Plavix/Paxil/Elavil

Action: Inhibits ADP-induced platelet aggregation

Uses: Reducing the risk of stroke, MI, vascular death, peripheral arterial disease in high-risk patients, acute coronary syndrome, transient ischemic attack (TIA), unstable angina

Unlabeled uses: Cardiac surgery (infant and child), Kawasaki disease

DOSAGE AND ROUTES

Recent MI, stroke, peripheral arterial disease

• *Adult:* **PO** 75 mg/day with or without aspirin

Acute coronary syndrome

• *Adult:* **PO** loading dose 300 mg then 75 mg/day with aspirin

Cardiac surgery/other cardiac conditions (unlabeled)

• *Neonate/infant/child ≤2 yr:* **PO** 0.2 mg/kg/day for platelet inhibition

Available forms: Tabs 75 mg

SIDE EFFECTS

CNS: Headache, dizziness, depression, syncope, hypesthesia, neuralgia

CV: Edema, hypertension, chest pain

GI: Nausea, vomiting, diarrhea, constipation, GI discomfort, **GI bleeding, pancreatitis**

GU: **Glomerulonephritis**

HEMA: Epistaxis, purpura, **bleeding, neutropenia, aplastic anemia**

INTEG: Rash, pruritus

MISC: UTI, hypercholesterolemia, chest pain, fatigue, **intracranial hemorrhage, toxic epidermal necrolysis, Stevens-Johnson syndrome,** flulike syndrome

MS: Arthralgia, back pain

RESP: Upper respiratory tract infection, dyspnea, rhinitis, bronchitis, cough, **bronchospasm**

Contraindications: Hypersensitivity, active bleeding

Precautions: Pregnancy (B), breastfeeding, children, past hepatic disease, increased bleeding risk, neutropenia, agranulocytosis, renal disease, Asian/Black/Caucasian patients

PHARMACOKINETICS

Rapidly absorbed; peak 1-3 hr; metabolized by liver (CYP3A4); excreted in urine, feces; half-life 8 hr; plasma protein binding 95%; effect on platelets after 3-7 days

INTERACTIONS

• Avoids use with CYP2C19 inhibitors

Increase: bleeding risk—anticoagulants, aspirin, NSAIDs, abciximab, eptifibatide, tirofiban, thrombolytics, ticlopidine, SSRIs, treprostinil, rifampin

Increase: action of some NSAIDs, phenytoin, TOLBUTamide, tamoxifen, torsemide, fluvastatin, warfarin

Decrease: CYP3A4 inhibitors/substrates—atorvastatin, simvastatin, cerivastatin

Drug/Herb

Increase: clopidogrel effect—bogbean, dong quai, feverfew, garlic, ginger, ginkgo biloba, green tea, horse chestnut

Increase: gastric irritation—arginine

Decrease: clopidogrel effect—bilberry, saw palmetto

Drug/Lab Test

Increase: AST, ALT, bilirubin, uric acid, total cholesterol, nonprotein nitrogen (NPN)

NURSING CONSIDERATIONS

Assess:

⚠ Thrombotic/thrombocytic purpura: fever, thrombocytopenia, neurolytic anemia

• For symptoms of stroke, MI during treatment

• Hepatic studies: AST, ALT, bilirubin, creatinine (long-term therapy)
• Blood studies: CBC, differential, Hct, Hgb, PT, cholesterol (long-term therapy)

Administer:
• With food to decrease gastric symptoms

Evaluate:
• Therapeutic response: absence of stroke, MI

Teach patient/family:
• That blood work will be necessary during treatment
• To report any unusual bruising, bleeding to prescriber, that it may take longer to stop bleeding
• To take with food or just after eating to minimize GI discomfort
• To report diarrhea, skin rashes, subcutaneous bleeding, chills, fever, sore throat
• To tell all health care providers that clopidogrel is used; may be held 3-7 days before surgery

clorazepate (℞)

(klor-az′e-pate)

Apo-Clorazepate ♣, clorazepate, Gen-XENE, Novo-Clopate ♣, Tranxene, Tranxene-SD, Tranxene-SD Half Strength, Tranxene T-tab

Func. class.: Antianxiety, anticonvulsant, sedative/hypnotic

Chem. class.: Benzodiazepine, long-acting

Controlled Substance Schedule IV

Do not confuse:
clorazepate/clonazepam

Action: Potentiates the actions of GABA, especially in limbic system, reticular formation

Uses: Anxiety, acute alcohol withdrawal, adjunct in seizure disorders

Unlabeled uses: Insomnia

DOSAGE AND ROUTES

Anxiety
• *Adult:* **PO** 15-60 mg/day in divided doses or 7.5 mg tid; **EXT REL** 11.25-22.5 mg at bedtime, do not use **EXT REL** to initiate therapy
• *Geriatric:* **PO** 7.5 mg daily-bid

Alcohol withdrawal
• *Adult:* **PO** 30 mg then 30-60 mg in divided doses; day 2, 45-90 mg in divided doses; day 3, 22.5-45 mg in divided doses; day 4, 15-30 mg in divided doses; then gradually reduce daily dose to 7.5-15 mg

Seizure disorders
• *Adult and child >12 yr:* **PO** 7.5 mg tid; may increase by 7.5 mg/wk or less, max 90 mg/day
• *Child 9-12 yr:* **PO** 3.75-7.5 mg bid; may increase by 3.75 mg/wk or less, max 60 mg/day

Insomnia (unlabeled)
• *Adult:* **PO** 7.5-15 mg at bedtime
• *Geriatric:* **PO** 3.75-7.5 mg at bedtime; max 15 mg at bedtime

Available forms: Tabs 3.75, 7.5, 15 mg; ext rel tab (Tranxene-SD Half Strength) 11.25 mg; (Tranxene-SD) 22.5 mg

SIDE EFFECTS

CNS: Dizziness, drowsiness, confusion, headache, anxiety, tremors, stimulation, fatigue, depression, insomnia, hallucinations, lethargy

CV: Orthostatic hypotension, **ECG changes, tachycardia,** hypotension, chest pain

EENT: Blurred vision, tinnitus, mydriasis

GI: Constipation, dry mouth, nausea, vomiting, anorexia, diarrhea

INTEG: Rash, dermatitis, itching

Contraindications: Pregnancy (D), breastfeeding, children <9 yr, hypersensitivity to benzodiazepines, closed-angle glaucoma, psychosis

Precautions: Geriatric patients, debilitated, renal/hepatic disease, suicidal ideation, dependency problems

PHARMACOKINETICS

PO: Onset 1 hr; peak 1-2 hr; duration up to 24 hr; metabolized by liver; excreted by kidneys; crosses placenta, breast milk; half-life 30-200 hr; 97% protein binding

INTERACTIONS

Increase: clorazepate effects—CNS depressants, alcohol, valproic acid, antidepressants, MAOIs, cimetidine, oral contraceptives, disulfiram, fluoxetine, isoniazid, ketoconazole, propoxyphene, some β-blockers; CYP3A4 inhibitors

Decrease: clorazepate action—rifampin, barbiturates

Drug/Herb

Increase: CNS depression—catnip, chamomile, clary, cowslip, kava, mistletoe, nettle, pokeweed, poppy, Queen Anne's lace, senega, St. John's wort, valerian

Increase: hypotension—black cohosh

Drug/Lab Test

Increase: AST, ALT

Decrease: Hct

NURSING CONSIDERATIONS

Assess:

- B/P (lying, standing), pulse; if systolic B/P drops 20 mm Hg, hold product, notify prescriber
- Blood studies: CBC during long-term therapy; blood dyscrasias have occurred rarely
- Hepatic studies: AST, ALT, bilirubin, creatinine, LDH, alk phos
- I&O; may indicate renal dysfunction
- Mental status: mood, sensorium, affect, sleeping pattern, drowsiness, dizziness; for delirium, tremors, hallucination in alcohol withdrawal
- Physical dependency, withdrawal symptoms: headache, nausea, vomiting, muscle pain, weakness after long-term use
- Suicidal tendencies, anxiety level
- Seizures: location, duration, intensity

Administer:

- Do not break, crush, or chew ext rel product
- With food, milk for GI symptoms
- Crushed if patient cannot swallow whole (tab only)
- Do not use Tranxene-SD to start treatment

Perform/provide:

- Assistance with ambulation during beginning therapy because of drowsiness/dizziness, especially geriatric patients
- Check to see PO medication has been swallowed
- Sugarless gum, hard candy, frequent sips of water for dry mouth

Evaluate:

- Therapeutic response: decreased anxiety, restlessness, insomnia

Teach patient/family:

- That product may be taken with food
- That product is not to be used for everyday stress or used longer than 4 mo unless directed by prescriber; not to take more than prescribed amount; may be habit forming
- To avoid OTC preparations unless approved by prescriber
- To avoid driving, activities that require alertness; drowsiness may occur, especially in geriatric patients
- To avoid alcohol ingestion, other psychotropic medications, unless directed by prescriber
- Not to discontinue medication abruptly after long-term use; restlessness, insomnia, irritability may occur
- To rise slowly because fainting may occur
- That drowsiness may worsen at beginning of treatment

Treatment of overdose: Lavage, VS, supportive care, flumazenil

clotrimazole topical

See Appendix B

clotrimazole vaginal antifungal

See Appendix B

clozapine (℞)

(kloz'a-peen)

clozapine, Clozaril, Fazaclo

Func. class.: Antipsychotic

Chem. class.: Tricyclic dibenzodiazepine derivative

Do not confuse:
Clozaril/Clinoril/Colazal

Action: Interferes with DOPamine receptor binding with lack of EPS; also acts as an adrenergic, cholinergic, histaminergic, serotonergic antagonist

Uses: Management of psychotic symptoms in schizophrenic patients for whom other antipsychotics have failed, recurrent suicidal behavior; orally disintegrating tabs are not used for recurrent suicidal behavior

Unlabeled uses: Agitation, bipolar disorder, psychosis in dementia, tremor in Parkinson's disease

DOSAGE AND ROUTES

• *Adult:* **PO** 12.5 mg daily or bid; may increase by 25-50 mg/day; normal range 300-450 mg/day after 2 wk; do not increase dose more than 2 × per wk; max 900 mg/day; use lowest dose to control symptoms

Tremor in Parkinson's disease (unlabeled)

• *Adult:* **PO** 40 mg at bedtime

Dementia with multiple behavioral disturbances (unlabeled)

• *Geriatric:* **PO** 12.5 mg daily at bedtime, may increase by 12.5 mg every other day, max 50 mg/day

Available forms: Tabs 12.5, 25, 50, 100, 200 mg; orally disintegrating tabs 25, 100 mg

SIDE EFFECTS

CNS: **Neuroleptic malignant syndrome,** *sedation, salivation, dizziness, headache, tremors, sleep problems, akinesia, fever,* **seizures,** *sweating, akathisia, confusion, fatigue, insomnia,* depression, slurred speech, anxiety, *agitation,* dystonia

CV: Tachycardia, hypo/hypertension, chest pain, ECG changes, orthostatic hypotension

EENT: Blurred vision

GI: Drooling or excessive salivation, constipation, nausea, abdominal discomfort, vomiting, diarrhea, anorexia, *weight gain, dry mouth,* heartburn, *dyspepsia, gastroesophageal reflux*

GU: Urinary abnormalities, incontinence, ejaculation dysfunction, frequency, urgency, retention, dysuria

HEMA: **Leukopenia, agranulocytosis, eosinophilia**

MS: Weakness; pain in back, neck, legs; spasm, *rigidity*

OTHER: Diaphoresis

RESP: Dyspnea, nasal congestion

SYST: **Death in geriatric patients with dementia**

Contraindications: Hypersensitivity, severe granulocytopenia (WBC <3500 before therapy), coma

Black Box Warning: Myeloproliferative disorders, severe CNS depression, uncontrolled epilepsy

Precautions: Pregnancy (B), breastfeeding, children <16, geriatric patients, CV/pulmonary/cardiac/renal/hepatic disease, seizures, prostatic enlargement, closed-angle glaucoma

PHARMACOKINETICS

Bioavailability 27%-47%; 97% protein bound; completely metabolized by liver enzymes involved in metabolism CYP1A2, 2D6, 3A4; excreted in urine (50%) and feces (30%) (metabolites); half-life 8-12 hr

INTERACTIONS

Increase: CNS depression—CNS depressants, psychoactives, alcohol

Increase: clozapine level—caffeine, citalopram, fluoxetine, sertraline, ritonavir, risperidone, CYP1A2 inhibitors (fluvoxamine), CYP3A4 inhibitors (ketoconazole, erythromycin)

Increase: plasma concentration—warfarin, digoxin, other highly protein-bound products
Increase: hypotension, respiratory, cardiac arrest, collapse—benzodiazepines
Decrease: clozapine level—CYP1A2 inducers (carbamazepine, omeprazole, rifampin); phenobarbital

Drug/Herb

Increase: CNS depression—kava, St. John's wort
Increase: EPS—betel palm, kava
Increase: clozapine action—cola tree, hops, nettle, nutmeg

Drug/Lab Test

Increase: LFTs, cardiac enzymes, cholesterol, blood glucose, bilirubin, PBI, cholinesterase, ^{131}I
False positive: pregnancy tests, PKU
False negative: urinary steroids, 17-OHCS

NURSING CONSIDERATIONS

Assess:

- For myocarditis, if suspected, discontinue use; myocarditis usually occurs during first month of treatment
- For seizures, usually occurs with higher doses
- I&O ratio; obtain baseline before treatment begins; palpate bladder if low urinary output occurs
- Bilirubin, CBC, LFTs monthly; discontinue treatment if WBC <3000/mm^3 or ANC <1500/mm^3 test q wk; may resume when normal; if WBC <2000/mm^3 or ANC <1000/mm^3 discontinue
- Urinalysis is recommended before, during prolonged therapy
- Affect, orientation, LOC, reflexes, gait, coordination, sleep pattern disturbances
- B/P standing and lying; take pulse and respirations q4hr during initial treatment; establish baseline before starting treatment; report drops of 30 mm Hg
- Dizziness, faintness, palpitations, tachycardia on rising
- EPS including akathisia (inability to sit still, no pattern to movements), tardive dyskinesia (bizarre movements of the jaw, mouth, tongue, extremities), pseudoparkinsonism (rigidity, tremors, pill rolling, shuffling gait)

⚠ For neuroleptic malignant syndrome: tachycardia, seizures, fever, dyspnea, diaphoresis, increased or decreased B/P, notify prescriber immediately

- Constipation, urinary retention daily; if these occur, increase bulk, water in diet, especially geriatric patients, stool softeners, laxatives may be needed
- If diabetic, check blood glucose levels

Administer:

- Patient-specific registration required before administration; if WBC <3500 cells/mm^3 or ANC <2000 cells/mm^3, therapy should not be started
- Check for swallowing of PO medication; monitor for hoarding or giving of medication to other patients, if hospitalized; avoid giving patient over 7 days medication if outpatient
- Orally disintegrating tab: do not push through foil, leave in foil blister until ready to take, peel back foil, place tab in mouth, allow to dissolve, swallow; water is not needed

Perform/provide:

- Supervised ambulation until stabilized on medication; do not involve in strenuous exercise program because fainting is possible; patient should not stand still for long periods
- Storage in tight, light-resistant container

Evaluate:

- Therapeutic response: decrease in emotional excitement, hallucinations, delusions, paranoia, reorganization of patterns of thought, speech

Teach patient/family:

- About symptoms of agranulocytosis and need for blood tests q wk for 6 mo, then q2wk; report flulike symptoms
- That orthostatic hypotension often occurs, and to rise gradually from sitting or lying position; to avoid hot tubs, hot showers, tub baths; hypotension may occur
- To avoid abrupt withdrawal of this product because EPS may result; product should be withdrawn over 1-2 wk

- To avoid OTC preparations (cough, hay fever, cold) unless approved by prescriber, since serious product interactions may occur; avoid use with alcohol or CNS depressants, increased drowsiness may occur
- About compliance with product regimen
- About EPS and necessity for meticulous oral hygiene, since oral candidiasis may occur
- To report sore throat, malaise, fever, bleeding, mouth sores; if these occur, CBC should be drawn and product discontinued
- That heat stroke may occur in hot weather; take extra precautions to stay cool
- To avoid driving, other hazardous activities; seizures may occur
- To notify prescriber if pregnant or if pregnancy is intended, not to breastfeed

Treatment of overdose: Lavage, activated charcoal; provide an airway; do not induce vomiting

codeine (℞)

(koe′deen)

Paveral ♣

Func. class.: Opiate analgesic, antitussive

Chem. class.: Opiate, phenathrene derivative

Controlled Substance Schedule II, III, IV, V (depends on content)

Do not confuse:

codeine/Lodine/iodine/Cardene

Action: Depresses pain impulse transmission at the spinal cord level by interacting with opioid receptors, decreases cough reflex, GI motility

Uses: Moderate to severe pain

Unlabeled uses: Diarrhea, arthralgia, bone/dental pain, headache, migraine, myalgia, nonproductive cough

DOSAGE AND ROUTES

Pain

- *Adult:* **PO/IM/SUBCUT** 15-60 mg q4hr prn
- *Child 6-17 yr:* **PO** 3 mg/kg/day in divided doses q4hr prn

Cough

- *Adult:* **PO** 10-20 mg q4-6hr, not to exceed 120 mg/day

Renal disease

- *Adult:* **PO** CCr 10-50 ml/min 75% of dose; CCr <10 ml/min 50% of dose

Diarrhea (unlabeled)

- *Adult:* **PO** 30 mg; may repeat qid prn

Arthralgia/bone pain/back pain/ dental pain/headache/migraine/ myalgia (unlabeled)

- *Adult:* **PO/IM/SUBCUT** 15-60 mg q4-6hr
- *Child ≥3 yr:* **IM/SUBCUT** 0.5-1 mg/kg or 15 mg/m^2 (max 60 mg/dose) q4-6hr

Available forms: Inj tab 30, 60 mg; tabs 15, 30, 60 mg; inj 15, 30 mg/ml

SIDE EFFECTS

CNS: Drowsiness, sedation, dizziness, agitation, dependency, lethargy, restlessness, euphoria, **seizures,** hallucinations, headache, confusion

CV: Bradycardia, palpitations, orthostatic hypotension, tachycardia, **circulatory collapse**

GI: Nausea, vomiting, anorexia, constipation, dry mouth

GU: Urinary retention

INTEG: Flushing, rash, urticaria, pruritus

RESP: **Respiratory depression, respiratory paralysis,** dyspnea

SYST: **Anaphylaxis**

Contraindications: Breastfeeding, hypersensitivity to opiates, respiratory depression, increased intracranial pressure, seizure disorders, severe respiratory disorders

Precautions: Pregnancy (C), geriatric patients, cardiac dysrhythmias, prostatic hypertrophy, bowel impaction

PHARMACOKINETICS

Bioavailability 60%-90%; peak ½-1 hr; duration 4-6 hr; metabolized by liver (CYP3A4); excreted by kidneys, in breast milk; crosses placenta; half-life 3 hr; protein binding 7%; altered codeine metabolism occurs in different ethnic groups
PO: Onset 30-60 min
IM: Onset 10-30 min

INTERACTIONS

Increase: CNS depression—CYP2D6, alcohol, opiates, sedative/hypnotics, antipsychotics, skeletal muscle relaxants
⚠ ***Increase:*** toxicity—MAOIs, use cautiously
Drug/Herb
Increase: CNS depression—Jamaican dogwood, gotu kola, kava, lavender, mistletoe, nettle, pokeweed, poppy, senega, valerian
Increase: anticholinergic effect—corkwood
Decrease: codeine levels—St. John's wort
Drug/Lab Test
Increase: lipase, amylase

NURSING CONSIDERATIONS

Assess:
- I&O ratio; check for decreasing output; may indicate urinary retention, especially geriatric patients
- GI function: nausea, vomiting, constipation
- By using pain-scoring method
- Cough: type, duration, ability to raise secretion, for productive cough; do not use to suppress a productive cough
- CNS changes, dizziness, drowsiness, hallucinations, euphoria, LOC, pupil reaction
- Allergic reactions: rash, urticaria

⚠ Respiratory dysfunction: respiratory depression, character, rate, rhythm; notify prescriber if respirations are <10/min, shallow
- Need for pain medication, tolerance

Administer:
IM/SUBCUT route
- Do not use if precipitate is present
- Usually given IM/SUBCUT

IV route
- Give slowly by direct inj
- With antiemetic for nausea, vomiting
- When pain is beginning to return; determine dosage interval by patient response

Syringe compatibilities: Dimenhydrinate, glycopyrrolate, hydrOXYzine
Perform/provide:
- Storage in light-resistant container at room temperature
- Assistance with ambulation if needed
- Safety measures: top side rails, nightlight, call bell

Evaluate:
- Therapeutic response: decrease in pain, absence of grimacing, decreased cough; decreased diarrhea

Teach patient/family:
- Not to breastfeed
- To report any symptoms of CNS changes, allergic reactions
- That physical dependency may result after extended periods
- To change position slowly; orthostatic hypotension may occur
- To avoid hazardous activities if drowsiness, dizziness occurs
- To avoid alcohol, other CNS depressants unless directed by prescriber

Treatment of overdose: Naloxone 0.4 mg ampule diluted in 10 ml 0.9% NaCl and given by direct IV push 0.02 mg q2min (adult)

colchicine (℞)

(kol'chi-seen)
Colcrys, Colsalide
Func. class.: Antigout agent
Chem. class.: Colchicum autumnale alkaloid

Action: Inhibits microtubule formation of lactic acid in leukocytes, which decreases phagocytosis and inflammation in joints

Uses: Gout, gouty arthritis (prevention, treatment); to arrest progression of neurologic disability in MS

Unlabeled uses: Hepatic cirrhosis, Mediterranean fever, pericarditis, amyloidosis, Behçet's syndrome, biliary cirrhosis, dermatitis herpetiformis, idiopathic thrombocytopenic purpura, Paget's disease, pseudogout, pulmonary fibrosis

DOSAGE AND ROUTES

Gout prevention

• *Adult:* **PO** 0.6-1.8 mg/day depending on severity

Gout treatment

• *Adult:* **PO** 1.2 mg initially, then 0.6 mg 1 hr later (1.8 mg); those on strong CYP3A4 inhibitor (past 14 days) 0.6 mg initially, then 0.3 mg 1 hr later

Renal dose

• *Adult:* **PO** CCr <30 ml/min for acute gout, do not repeat course for 2 wk, familial mediterranean fever 0.3 mg daily increase cautiously

Mediterranean fever (unlabeled)

• *Adult:* **PO** 0.6 mg qhr × 4 doses, then q2hr × 2 doses, then 1.2 mg q12hr × 2 days

Amyloidosis/biliary cirrhosis/dermatitis herpetiformis/Paget's disease/Behçet's syndrome/chronic idiopathic thrombocytopenic purpura/pulmonary fibrosis (unlabeled)

• *Adult:* **PO** 0.5-0.6 mg bid-tid

Available forms: Tabs 0.5, 0.6, 1 ✱mg

SIDE EFFECTS

GI: Nausea, vomiting, anorexia, malaise, metallic taste, cramps, peptic ulcer, diarrhea

GU: Hematuria, **oliguria, renal damage**

HEMA: **Agranulocytosis, thrombocytopenia, aplastic anemia, pancytopenia**

INTEG: Chills, dermatitis, pruritus, purpura, erythema

MISC: Myopathy, alopecia, reversible azospermia, peripheral neuritis

Contraindications: Pregnancy (D) (injectable), serious GI, severe cardiac/renal/hepatic disorders, hypersensitivity

Precautions: Pregnancy (C) (PO), breastfeeding, children, geriatric patients, blood dyscrasias, hepatic disease

PHARMACOKINETICS

PO: Peak ½-2 hr, half-life 4.4 hr, deacetylates in liver, excreted in feces (metabolites/active product)

INTERACTIONS

Increase: toxicity—cycloSPORINE, clarithromycin, erythromycin

Increase: GI effects—NSAIDs, ethanol

Increase: bone marrow depression—radiation, bone marrow depressants, cycloSPORINE

Decrease: action of vit B_{12}, may cause reversible malabsorption

Drug/Lab Test

Increase: alk phos, AST

False positive: urine, RBC, Hgb

Interference: urinary 17-hydroxycorticosteroids

NURSING CONSIDERATIONS

Assess:

• For relief of pain, uric acid levels returning to normal

• I&O ratio; observe for decrease in urinary output

⚠ CBC, platelets, reticulocytes before, during therapy (q3mo), may cause aplastic anemia, agranulocytosis, decreased platelets

• For toxicity: weakness, abdominal pain, nausea, vomiting, diarrhea; product should be discontinued

Administer:

PO route

• With food for GI symptoms

Evaluate:

• Therapeutic response: decreased stone formation on x-ray, decreased pain in kidney region, absence of hematuria, decreased pain in joints

Teach patient/family:
- To avoid alcohol, OTC preparations that contain alcohol
- To report any pain, redness, or hard area, usually in legs; rash, sore throat, fever, bleeding, bruising, weakness, numbness, tingling
- The importance of complying with medical regimen (diet, weight loss, product therapy); the possibility of bone marrow depression occurring

Treatment of overdose: D/C medication, may need opioids to treat diarrhea

colesevelam (℞)
(coal-see-vel'am)
Welchol
Func. class.: Antilipemic
Chem. class.: Bile acid sequestrant

Action: Absorbs, combines with bile acids to form insoluble complex that is excreted through feces; loss of bile acids lowers cholesterol levels

Uses: Elevated LDL cholesterol, alone or in combination with HMG-CoA reductase inhibitor; type 2 diabetes (adjunct)

DOSAGE AND ROUTES

Monotherapy
- *Adult:* **PO** 3 625-mg tabs bid with meals or 6 tabs daily with a meal; may increase to 7 tabs if needed

Combination therapy
- *Adult:* **PO** 3 tabs bid with meals or 6 tabs daily with a meal given with an HMG-CoA reductase inhibitor

Type 2 diabetes, adjunct (to improve glycemic control)
- *Adult and geriatric:* **PO** Approx 3.8 g (6 tabs)/day or approx 1.9 g (3 tabs) bid

Available forms: Tabs 625 mg

SIDE EFFECTS

CNS: Headache, dizziness, drowsiness, vertigo, tinnitus

GI: Constipation, abdominal pain, nausea, fecal impaction, hemorrhoids, flatulence, vomiting, steatorrhea, peptic ulcer, GI obstruction

HEMA: Decreased red cell folate content; **bleeding**, increased PT

INTEG: Rash, irritation of perianal area, tongue, skin

META: Decreased vit A, D, K; **hyperchloremic acidosis**

MS: Muscle, joint pain

Contraindications: Hypersensitivity, biliary obstruction, dysphagia, bowel disease, primary biliary cirrhosis, triglycerides > 300 mg/dl, fat-soluble vitamin deficiency

Precautions: Pregnancy (C), breastfeeding, children

PHARMACOKINETICS

Excreted in feces, peak response 2 wk

INTERACTIONS

Decrease: absorption of diltiazem, gemfibrozil, glipiZIDE, mycophenolate, phenytoin, propranolol, warfarin, thiazides, digoxin, penicillin G, tetracyclines, corticosteroids, iron, thyroid, clindamycin, fat-soluble vitamins

Drug/Herb

Increase: effect—glucomannan

Decrease: antilipidemic effect—gotu kola

Drug/Lab Test

Increase: LFTs

NURSING CONSIDERATIONS

Assess:
- Cardiac glycoside level, if both products are being administered
- For signs of vit A, D, K deficiency
- Fasting LDL, HDL, total cholesterol, triglyceride levels, electrolytes if on extended therapy
- Bowel pattern daily; increase bulk, H_2O in diet for constipation

Administer:
- Swallow tabs whole; do not break, crush, or chew
- Drug daily or bid with meals; give all other medications 1 hr before colesevelam or 4 hr after colesevelam; to avoid poor absorption take with liquid
- Supplemental doses of vit A, D, K, if levels are low

Evaluate:

• Therapeutic response: decreased total cholesterol level, LDL cholesterol, apolipoproteins (hyperlipidemia); diarrhea, pruritus (excess bile acids)

Teach patient/family:

⚠ The symptoms of hypoprothrombinemia: bleeding mucous membranes, dark tarry stools, hematuria, petechiae; report immediately

• The importance of compliance; toxicity may result if doses missed

• That risk factors should be decreased: high-fat diet, smoking, alcohol consumption, absence of exercise

• Not to discontinue suddenly

colestipol (℞)

(koe-les′ti-pole)

Colestid

Func. class.: Antilipemic

Chem. class.: Bile acid sequestrant

Action: Absorbs, combines with bile acids to form insoluble complex excreted through feces; loss of bile acids lowers cholesterol levels

Uses: Primary hypercholesterolemia, xanthomas

Unlabeled uses: Digotoxin toxicity/overdose, pruritus, diarrhea due to increased bile acids after surgery

DOSAGE AND ROUTES

• *Adult:* **PO** Tabs 2 g daily-bid, may increase q1mo, max 16 g/day; powder 5-30 g mixed with liquid daily or in divided doses

Digotoxin toxicity/overdose, digoxin overdose (unlabeled)

• *Adult:* **PO** 10 g, then 5 g q6-8hr

Diarrhea/pruritus (unlabeled)

• *Adult:* **PO** Granules 5 g daily-bid, may increase by 5 g/day at 1-2 month intervals, max 30 g/day in 1-2 divided doses

Available forms: Powder/packet/scoop (granules) 5 g; tabs 1 g

SIDE EFFECTS

GI: Constipation, abdominal pain, nausea, fecal impaction, hemorrhoids, flatulence, vomiting, steatorrhea, peptic ulcer

HEMA: **Bleeding, increased PT**

INTEG: Rash, irritation of perianal area, tongue, skin

META: Decreased vit A, D, K, red folate content; **hyperchloremic acidosis**

Contraindications: Hypersensitivity, biliary obstruction

Precautions: Pregnancy (B), breastfeeding, children, bleeding disorders

PHARMACOKINETICS

PO: Onset 24-48 hr, peak/duration 30 days, excreted in feces

INTERACTIONS

Decrease: action of thiazides, digoxin, warfarin, penicillin G, gemfibrozil, glipiZIDE, propranolol, phenytoin, TOLBUTamide, tetracycline, corticosteroids, iron, thyroid agents, clindamycin, fat-soluble vitamins

Drug/Herb

Increase: lipidemic effect—glucomannan

Decrease: lipidemic effect—gotu kola

Drug/Lab Test

Increase: AST, ALT, alk phos, chloride, PO_4

Decrease: Na, K, Ca

NURSING CONSIDERATIONS

Assess:

• Fat consumption in diet

• Cardiac glycoside levels, if both products are being administered

• For signs of vit A, D, K deficiency

• Serum cholesterol, triglyceride levels, electrolytes (extended therapy)

• Bowel pattern daily; increase bulk, water in diet if constipation develops

Administer:

• Swallow tabs whole; do not break, crush, or chew; take tabs one at a time

• Product daily or bid; give all other medications 1 hr before colestipol or 4

hr after colestipol to avoid poor absorption
- Drug mixed in applesauce or stirred into beverage (2-6 oz); do not take dry; let stand for 2 min
- Supplemental doses of vit A, D, K if levels are low

Evaluate:
- Therapeutic response: decreased LDL cholesterol; decreased pruritus, diarrhea

Teach patient/family:

⚠ The symptoms of hypoprothrombinemia: bleeding mucous membranes; dark, tarry stools; hematuria, petechiae; report immediately
- That compliance is needed; not to miss or double doses
- That risk factors should be decreased: high-fat diet, smoking, alcohol consumption, absence of exercise

conivaptan (℞)

(kon-ih-vap'-tan)

Vaprisol

Func. class.: Vasopressin receptor antagonist

Action: Dual arginine vasopressin (AVP) antagonist with affinity for V_{1A}, V_2 receptors; level of circulating AVP in circulating blood is critical for regulation of water, electrolyte balance and is usually elevated in euvolemic/hypervolemic hyponatremia

Uses: Euvolemia hyponatremia in those hospitalized, not indicated for CHF, hypervolemic hyponatremia

DOSAGE AND ROUTES

- *Adult:* **IV INF** Loading dose 20 mg given over 30 min, then **CONT IV** over 24 hr; after 1 day, give for an additional 1-3 days as a **CONT INF** of 20 mg/day total, can be titrated up to 40 mg/day if serum sodium is not rising at the desired rate; max time 4 days

Available forms: 5 mg/ml (20 mg/4 ml) in single use ampule; 20 mg/100 ml in D_5 for injection

SIDE EFFECTS

CNS: Headache, confusion, insomnia

CV: **Atrial fibrillation,** hypo/hypertension, orthostatic hypotension, phlebitis

GI: Nausea, vomiting, constipation, dry mouth

GU: Hematuria, polyuria, UTI, pollakiuria

HEMA: Anemia

INTEG: Erythemia, inj site reaction

META: Dehydration, hypo/hyperglycemia, hypokalemia, hypomagnesia, hyponatremia

MISC: Oral candidiasis, pain, peripheral edema, pneumonia

Contraindications: Hypersensitivity, hypovolemia

Precautions: Pregnancy (C), breastfeeding, orthostatic disease, renal disease

PHARMACOKINETICS

Protein binding 99%, metabolized by CYP3A4, terminal half-life 5 hr

INTERACTIONS

Increase: plasma concentrations of conivaptan—CYP3A4 inhibitors

Decrease: plasma concentration of conivaptan—digoxin

NURSING CONSIDERATIONS

Assess:
- Renal, hepatic function
- Frequent sodium volume status; overly rapid correction of sodium concentration (>12 mEq/L per 24 hr) may result in osmotic demyelination syndrome
- Neurologic status: confusion, headache
- CV status: atrial fibrillation, hypo/hypertension, orthostatic hypotension; monitor B/P, pulse
- Monitor other electrolytes (magnesium and potassium)

Administer:

IV route
- Withdraw 4 ml (20 mg) of conivaptan, add to 100 ml D_5W, gently invert several times to mix, give over 30 min

CONT IV INF route

• Withdraw 4 ml (20 mg) of conivaptan, add to 250 ml D_5W, gently invert several times to mix, give over 24 hr; or 40 mg in 250 ml D_5W, gently invert several times to mix, give over 24 hr

Evaluate:

• Therapeutic response: correction of serum sodium levels

Teach patient/family:

• To avoid pregnancy, breastfeeding while taking this product

• To report neurologic changes: headache, insomnia, confusion

• Administrations procedure and expected result

• To report inj site pain, redness, swelling

CONTRACEPTIVES, HORMONAL

Monophasic, Oral

ethinyl estradiol/ desogestrel (℞)

Apri, Cesia, Desogen, Kariva, Mircette, Ortho-Cept, Reclipsen, Solia, Velivet

ethinyl estradiol/ drospirenone (℞)

Yasmin, Yaz 28

ethinyl estradiol/ ethynodiol (℞)

Kelnor 1/35, Zovia

ethinyl estradiol/ levonorgestrel (℞)

Alesse, Aviane-28, Enpresse, Jolessa, Lessina, Levlen, Levlite, Levora, Lutera, Nordette, Portia, Quasense, Seasonique, Sronyx

ethinyl estradiol/ norethindrone (℞)

Brevicon, Genora 0.5/35, Genora 1/35, Junel 21 1/20, Junel 21 1.5/20, Loestrin 21 1.5/30, Loestrin 21 1/20, Microgestin, Modicon, N.E.E 1/35, Nelova 0.5/35E, Nelova 1/35E, Norcept-E 1/35, Norethin 1/35E, Norinyl 1+35, Norlestrin 1/50, Norlestrin 2.5/50, Nortrel

ethinyl estradiol/ norgestimate (℞)

MonoNessa, Ortho-Cyclen, Previfem, Sprintec

ethinyl estradiol/ norgestrel (℞)

Cryselle, Lo/Ovral, Low-Ogestrel, Ogestrel, Ovral

mestranol/ norethindrone (℞)

Genora 1/50, Nelova 1/50m, Norethin 1/50m, Norinyl 1+50, Ortho-Novum 1/50

Biphasic, Oral
ethinyl estradiol/ norethindrone (℞)
Nelova 10/11, Ortho-Novum 10/11

Triphasic, Oral
ethinyl estradiol/ desogestrel (℞)
Cyclessa
ethinyl estradiol/ norethindrone (℞)
Necor 7/7/7, Nortrel 7/7/7, Ortho-Novum 7/7/7, Tri-Norinyl
ethinyl estradiol/ norgestimate (℞)
Ortho Tri-Cyclen, Ortho Tri-Cyclen Lo
ethinyl estradiol/ levonorgestrel (℞)
Enpresse, Tri-Levlen, Triphasil

Extended Cycle, Oral
ethinyl estradiol/ levonorgestrel (℞)
Seasonale

Progestin, Oral
norethindrone (℞)
Errin, Ortho Micronor, Camila, Jolivette, Nor-Q D

Progressive Estrogen, Oral
ethinyl estradiol/ norethindrone acetate (℞)
Estrostep, Estrostep Fe
Emergency
levonorgestrel/ethinyl estradiol (℞)
Preven
levonorgestrel (℞)
Plan B

medroxyprogesterone (℞)
Depo-Provera

Intrauterine
levonorgestrel (℞)
Mirena

Implant
etonogestrel (℞)
Implanon

Vaginal Ring
ethinyl estradiol/ etonogestrel (℞)
Nuva Ring

Transdermal
ethinyl estradiol/ norelgestromin (℞)
Ortho Evra

Action: Prevents ovulation by suppressing FSH, LH; *monophasic:* estrogen/ progestin (fixed dose) used during a 21-day cycle; ovulation is inhibited by suppression of FSH and LH; thickness of cervical mucus and endometrial lining prevents pregnancy; *biphasic:* ovulation is inhibited by suppression of FSH and LH; alteration of cervical mucus, endometrial lining prevents pregnancy; *triphasic:* ovulation is inhibited by suppression of FSH and LH; change of cervical mucus, endometrial lining prevents pregnancy; variable doses of estrogen/progestin combinations may be similar to natural hormonal fluctuations; *extended cycle:* estrogen/progestin continuous for 84 days, off for 7 days, result 4 menstrual periods/yr; *progressive estrogen:* constant progestin with 3 progressive doses of estrogen; *progestin-only pill, implant, intrauterine:* change of cervical mucus and endometrial lining prevents pregnancy; ovulation may be suppressed
Uses: To prevent pregnancy, regulation of menstrual cycle, treatment of acne in

women over 14 yr that other treatment has failed, emergency contraception; *injection:* inhibits gonadotropin secretion, ovulation, follicular maturation; *emergency:* inhibits ovulation and fertilization, decreases transport of sperm and egg from fallopian tube to uterus; *vaginal ring, transdermal:* inhibits ovulation, prevents sperm entry into uterus; *antiacne:* may decrease sex hormone binding globulin, results in decreased testosterone

DOSAGE AND ROUTES

Monophasic

• *Adult:* **PO** Take first tab on Sunday after start of menses × 21 days; skip 7 days, then repeat cycle; start on 1st day of menses × 21 days; skip 7 days, then repeat cycle; may contain 7 placebo tabs, where 1 tab is taken daily

Biphasic

• *Adult:* **PO** Take 10 days of small progestin, then large progestin; estrogen is the same during cycle; skip 7 days, then repeat cycle; may contain 7 placebo tabs, where 1 tab is taken daily

Triphasic

• *Adult:* **PO** Estrogen dose remains constant, progestin changes throughout 21 day cycle, some products contain 28 tabs per month

Extended cycle

• *Adult:* **PO** Start taking on first day of menses; continue for 84 days of active tab, then 7 days of placebo; repeat cycle

Progestin

• *Adult:* **PO** Start on 1st day of menses, then daily and continuously

Progressive estrogen

• *Adult:* **PO** Progestin dose remains constant, estrogen increases q7days throughout 21-day cycle, may include 7 placebo tabs for 28-day cycle

Emergency

• *Adult and adolescent:* Give within 72 hr of intercourse, repeat 12 hr later; **Plan B** 1 tab, then 1 tab 12 hr later; **Preven** 2 tab, then 2 tab 12 hr later; **Ovral (unlabeled)** 2 white tabs; **Lo/Ovral (unlabeled)** 4 white tabs; **Levlen (unlabeled), Nordette (unlabeled)** 4 orange tabs; **Triphasil (unlabeled), Tri-Levlen (unlabeled)** 4 yellow tabs

Injectable

• *Adult:* **IM (Depo-Provera)** 150 mg within 5 days of start of menses, or within 5 days postpartum (must not be breastfeeding); if breastfeeding, give 6 wk postpartum, repeat q3mo

Intrauterine

• *Adult:* To be inserted using the levonorgestrel releasing intrauterine system (LRIS) by those trained in procedure; inserted into uterine cavity within 7 days of the onset of menstruation; use should not exceed 5 years per implant

Vaginal ring

• *Adult:* **VAG** Insert 1 ring on or prior to day 5 of cycle, leave in place 3 wk; remove for 1 wk, then repeat

Transdermal

• *Adult:* **TD** Apply patch within 7 days of menses, change weekly × 3 wk; no patch wk 4, repeat cycle

Implant

• *Adult:* **SUBDERMAL** In inner side of upper arm on days 1-5 of menses, replace q3yr

Acne

• *Adult:* **PO (Ortho Tri-Cyclen)** Take daily × 21 days, off 7 days

SIDE EFFECTS

CNS: Depression, fatigue, dizziness, nervousness, anxiety, headache

CV: Increased B/P, **cerebral hemorrhage, thrombosis, pulmonary embolism,** fluid retention, edema

EENT: Optic neuritis, retinal thrombosis, cataracts

ENDO: Decreased glucose tolerance, increased TBG, PBI, T_4, T_3

GI: Nausea, vomiting, cramps, diarrhea, bloating, constipation, change in appetite, **cholestatic jaundice**

GU: Breakthrough bleeding, amenorrhea, spotting, dysmenorrhea, galactorrhea, endocervical hyperplasia, vaginitis, cystitis-like syndrome, breast change

HEMA: Increased fibrinogen, clotting factor

INTEG: Chloasma, melasma, acne, rash, urticaria, erythema, pruritus, hirsutism, alopecia, photosensitivity

Contraindications: Pregnancy (X), breastfeeding, women 40 and over, reproductive cancer, thrombophlebitis, MI, hepatic tumors, hepatic disease, CAD, CVA

Precautions: Depression, hypertension, renal disease, seizure disorders, lupus erythematosus, rheumatic disease, migraine headache, amenorrhea, irregular menses, breast cancer (fibrocystic), gallbladder disease, diabetes mellitus, heavy smoking, acute mononucleosis, sickle cell disease

PHARMACOKINETICS

Excreted in breast milk

INTERACTIONS

Decrease: oral contraceptives effectiveness—anticonvulsants, rifampin, analgesics, antibiotics, antihistamines, griseofulvin

Decrease: oral anticoagulants action

Drug/Herb

- Altered action: alfalfa, black cohosh, chaste tree

Decrease: oral contraceptives effect—saw palmetto, St. John's wort

Drug/Food

Increase: peak level—grapefruit juice

Drug/Lab Test

Increase: PT; clotting factors VII, VIII, IX, X; TBG, PBI, T_4, platelet aggregability, BSP, triglycerides, bilirubin, AST, ALT

Decrease: T_3, antithrombin III, folate, metyrapone test, GTT, 17-OHCS

NURSING CONSIDERATIONS

Assess:

- Glucose, thyroid function, LFTs
- Reproductive changes: change in breasts, tumors, positive Pap smear; product should be discontinued

Administer:

- PO with food for GI symptoms; give at same time each day
- Subdermal implant of 6 caps effective for 5 yr; then should be removed
- IM inj deep in large muscle mass after shaking suspension; ensure patient not pregnant if inj are 2 wk or more apart

Evaluate:

- Therapeutic response: absence of pregnancy, endometriosis, hypermenorrhea

Teach patient/family:

- About detection of clots using Homan's sign
- To use sunscreen or avoid sunlight; photosensitivity can occur
- To take at same time each day to ensure equal product level
- To report GI symptoms that occur after 4 mo
- To use another birth control method during 1st week of oral contraceptive use
- To take another tablet as soon as possible if one is missed
- That after product is discontinued, pregnancy may not occur for several months
- To report abdominal pain, change in vision, shortness of breath, change in menstrual flow, spotting, breakthrough bleeding, breast lumps, swelling, headache, severe leg pain
- That continuing medical care is needed: Pap smear and gynecologic examinations q6mo
- To notify health care providers and dentists of oral contraceptive

Rarely Used

corticotropin (ACTH) (℞)

(kor-ti-koe-troe′pin)

H.P. Acthar Gel

Func. class.: Pituitary hormone

Uses: Testing adrenocortical function, treatment of adrenal insufficiency caused by administration of corticosteroids (long term), MS, myasthenia gravis

DOSAGE AND ROUTES

Acute exacerbations of multiple sclerosis

• *Adult:* **IM** 80-120 units/day × 14-21 days

Infantile spasms

• *Infant:* **IM GEL** 20 units/day × 2 wk, increase if needed

Contraindications: Hypersensitivity, scleroderma, osteoporosis, CHF, peptic ulcer disease, hypertension, systemic fungal infections, smallpox vaccination, recent surgery, ocular herpes simplex, primary adrenocortical insufficiency/hyperfunction

cortisone (℞)

(kor′ti-sone)

Cortone ♣, Cortone Acetate

Func. class.: Corticosteroid, synthetic

Chem. class.: Glucocorticoid, short-acting

Action: Decreases inflammation by suppression of migration of polymorphonuclear leukocytes, fibroblasts, reversal of increased capillary permeability and lysosomal stabilization

Uses: Inflammation, severe allergy, adrenal insufficiency, collagen disorders; respiratory, dermatologic, rheumatic disorders

Unlabeled uses: Temporal arteritis, Churg-Strauss syndrome, mixed connective tissue disease, polyarteritis nodosa, relapsing polychondritis, polymyalgia rheumatica, vasculitis, Wegener's granulomatosis, multiple myeloma

DOSAGE AND ROUTES

• *Adult:* **PO** 25-300 mg/day or q2days, titrated to response

• *Child:* **PO** 0.7-10 mg/kg/day

Multiple myeloma/temporal arteritis/Churg-Strauss syndrome/mixed connective tissue disease/polyarteritis nodosa/relapsing polychondritis/polymyalgia rheumatica/vasculitis/Wegener's granulomatosis (unlabeled)

• *Adult:* **PO** 25-300 mg/day or alternate days

Available forms: Tabs 25 mg

SIDE EFFECTS

CNS: Depression, flushing, sweating, headache, mood changes

CV: Hypertension, **circulatory collapse, thrombophlebitis, embolism,** tachycardia, **necrotizing angiitis, CHF,** edema

EENT: Fungal infections, increased intraocular pressure, blurred vision, cataracts, glaucoma

GI: Diarrhea, nausea, abdominal distention, **GI hemorrhage,** increased appetite, **pancreatitis,** ulcerative esophagitis

HEMA: **Thrombocytopenia**

INTEG: Acne, poor wound healing, ecchymosis, bruising, petechiae, hirsutism

META: Sodium, fluid retention, potassium loss, diabetes

MS: Fractures, osteoporosis, weakness, loss of muscle mass

Contraindications: Pregnancy (D), children <2 yr, psychosis, hypersensitivity, idiopathic thrombocytopenia, acute glomerulonephritis, amebiasis, fungal infections, nonasthmatic bronchial disease, AIDS, TB, measles, varicella

Precautions: Breastfeeding, diabetes mellitus, glaucoma, osteoporosis, seizure disorders, ulcerative colitis, CHF, myasthenia gravis, renal/hepatic disease, esophagitis, peptic ulcer

PHARMACOKINETICS

Peak 2 hr, duration 1½ days, half-life 8-12 hr

INTERACTIONS

Increase: action of cortisone—salicylates, estrogens, indomethacin, oral

contraceptives, ketoconazole, macrolide antiinfectives
Increase: side effects—alcohol, salicylates, indomethacin, potassium-wasting diuretics
Increase: GI symptoms—salicylates, indomethacin, NSAIDs
Decrease: effects of anticoagulants, antidiabetics, toxoids, vaccines, salicylates
Decrease: cortisone action—barbiturates, rifampin, phenytoin, theophylline, acetylcholinesterases

Drug/Herb
Increase: potassium deficiency—aloe, buckthorn, cascara sagrada, Chinese rhubarb, rhubarb, senna
Increase: steroid effect—aloe, licorice, perilla

Drug/Lab Test
Increase: cholesterol, Na, blood glucose, uric acid, Ca, urine glucose
Decrease: Ca, K, T_4, T_3, thyroid ^{131}I uptake test, urine 17-OHCS, 17-KS
False negative: Skin allergy tests

NURSING CONSIDERATIONS

Assess:

- Potassium; blood glucose while on long-term therapy; hypokalemia and hyperglycemia may occur
- Weight daily; notify prescriber of weekly gain >5 lb
- B/P q4hr, pulse; notify prescriber if chest pain occurs
- I&O ratio; be alert for decreasing urinary output and increasing edema
- Plasma cortisol levels during long-term therapy (normal level: 138-635 nmol/L SI units if drawn at 8 AM)
- Infection: fever, WBC even after withdrawal of medication; product masks infection
- Potassium depletion: paresthesias, fatigue, nausea, vomiting, depression, polyuria, dysrhythmias, weakness
- Edema, hypertension, cardiac symptoms
- Mental status: affect, mood, behavioral changes, aggression

Administer:

- Titrated dose; use lowest effective dose
- In one dose in AM to prevent adrenal suppression
- With food or milk to decrease GI symptoms

Perform/provide:

- Assistance with ambulation in patient with bone tissue disease to prevent fractures

Evaluate:

- Therapeutic response: decreased inflammation

Teach patient/family:

- That medical ID as corticosteroid user should be carried at all times
- To notify prescriber if therapeutic response decreases; dosage adjustment may be needed

⚠ Not to discontinue abruptly or adrenal crisis can result

- To avoid all OTC products: salicylates, alcohol in cough products, cold preparations unless directed by prescriber; avoid high-sodium foods
- All aspects of product usage, including cushingoid symptoms
- The symptoms of adrenal insufficiency: nausea, anorexia, fatigue, dizziness, dyspnea, weakness, joint pain
- Avoid exposure to chickenpox and measles
- To take PO dose in AM with food or fluid (milk)

cromolyn (OTC, ℞)

(kroe′moe-lin)
Gastrocrom Intal, Nasalcrom, Rynacrom ✤
Func. class.: Antiasthmatic
Chem. class.: Mast cell stabilizer

Do not confuse:
Nasalcrom/Nasalide

Action: Stabilizes the membrane of the sensitized mast cell, preventing release of chemical mediators after an antigen-IgE interaction

Uses: Severe perennial bronchial asthma, prevention of exercise-induced broncho-

spasm, acute bronchospasm induced by environmental pollutants, mastocytosis, allergic rhinitis
Unlabeled uses: Food allergy, ulcerative colitis

DOSAGE AND ROUTES

Allergic rhinitis
• *Adult and child >2 yr:* **NASAL SOL** 1 spray in each nostril tid-qid, max 6 doses/day
To prevent exercise-induced bronchospasm
• *Adult and child >5 yr:* **INH** 2 metered sprays inhaled ≤1 hr prior to exercise
Bronchial asthma
• *Adult and child >5 yr:* **INH** 2 metered sprays using inhaler qid; **NEB** 20 mg qid by nebulization
Systemic mastocytosis
• *Adult and child >12 yr:* **PO** 200 mg qid ½ hr before meals and at bedtime
• *Child 2-12 yr:* **PO** 100 mg qid ½ before meals and at bedtime
Ulcerative colitis (unlabeled)
• *Adult:* **PO** (Gastrocrom) 200 mg qid 20 min before meals and at bedtime, may double dose after 2 wk
• *Child 2-14 yr:* **PO** (Gastrocrom) 100 mg qid 20 min before meals and at bedtime, may double dose after 2-3 wk
Available forms: Nasal sol 5.2 mg/metered spray (40 mg/ml); neb sol 20 mg/2 ml; aerosol 800 mcg/actuation; oral conc 100 mg/5 ml

SIDE EFFECTS

CNS: Headache, dizziness, neuritis, confusion, drowsiness
EENT: Throat irritation, cough, nasal congestion, burning eyes, nasal stinging, sneezing
GI: Nausea, vomiting, anorexia, dry mouth, bitter taste
GU: Urinary frequency, dysuria
INTEG: Rash, urticaria, angioedema
MS: Joint pain/swelling

Oral conc
CNS: Dizziness, headache, paresthesia, migraine, seizures, psychosis, anxiety, depression, hallucinations, insomnia
CV: Tachycardia, PVCs, palpitations
GI: Diarrhea, nausea, abdominal pain, constipation, dyspepsia, stomatitis, vomiting
HEMA: Polycythemia, neutropenia, pancytopenia
INTEG: Pruritus, rash, flushing, photosensitivity
Contraindications: Hypersensitivity to this product or lactose, status asthmaticus, acute asthma
Precautions: Pregnancy (B), breastfeeding, children <5 yr (aerosol); <2 yr (nebulizer); <2 yr (nasal sol); oral <2 yr; renal/hepatic disease, safety not established; cardiac dysrhythmias, CAD

PHARMACOKINETICS

Excreted unchanged in feces, half-life 80 min, 63%-76% protein binding

NURSING CONSIDERATIONS

Assess:
• Eosinophil count during treatment
• Respiratory status: rate, rhythm, characteristics, cough, wheezing, dyspnea
Administer:
• For oral conc: break open ampule, squeeze contents in glass of water, stir, drink
Perform/provide:
• Gargle, sip of water to decrease irritation in throat (INH/Neb)
Evaluate:
• Therapeutic response: decrease in asthmatic symptoms; congested, runny nose
Teach patient/family:
Nasal sol
• Blow nose, hold pump between fingers; if first use, spray in air until fine mist occurs, insert nozzle in nostril, spray and breathe in through nose, repeat in other nostril
Aerosol (not for Acute Asthma)
• Take cover off mouthpiece, shake gently, breathe out slowly, place mouthpiece

in mouth, close mouth around it, tilt head back, breathe in as the inhaler is depressed, remove, hold breath, then breathe out slowly

Inhalation

- Do not swallow sol
- Empty ampule into power driven nebulizer as directed; do not combine different meds

Oral

- To take ½ hr before meals and at bedtime

Rarely Used

crotamiton (℞)

(kroe-tam′i-ton)

Eurax

Func. class.: Scabicide

Uses: Scabies, pruritus

DOSAGE AND ROUTES

Scabies

- *Adult and child:* **CREAM** Wash area with soap, water; remove visible crusts; apply cream; apply another coat in 24 hr; remove with soap, water in 48 hr

Pruritus

- *Adult and child:* **CREAM** Massage into affected area, repeat as necessary

Contraindications: Hypersensitivity, skin inflammation, abrasions, breaks in skin, mucous membranes

cyanocobalamin (vit B_{12}) (OTC, ℞)

(sye-an-oh-koe-bal′a-min)

Alphamin, Anacobin ♣, Bedoz ♣, Cobex, Cobolin-M, Crystamine, Crysti-1000, Cyanabin ♣, Cyanoject, Cyomin, Ener-B, Hydrobexan, Hydro-Crysti-12

hydroxocobalamin (OTC, ℞)

Hydro Cobex, Hydroxycobal, LA-12, Nascobal, Neuroforte-R, Rubesol-1000, Rubramin PC, Shovite, Vibral LA, Vibral, Vitamin B_{12}

Func. class.: Vit B_{12}, water-soluble vitamin

Action: Needed for adequate nerve functioning, protein and carbohydrate metabolism, normal growth, RBC development, cell reproduction

Uses: Vit B_{12} deficiency, pernicious anemia, vit B_{12} malabsorption syndrome, Schilling test, increased requirements with pregnancy, thyrotoxicosis, hemolytic anemia, hemorrhage, renal/hepatic disease, nutritional supplementation

DOSAGE AND ROUTES

Cyanocobalamin

- *Adult:* **PO** Up to 1000 mcg/day **SUBCUT/IM** 30-100 mcg/day × 1 wk, then 100-200 mcg/mo

Schilling test

- *Adult and child:* **IM** 1000 mcg in 1 dose
- *Child:* **PO** Up to 1000 mcg/day **SUBCUT/IM** 30-50 mcg/day × 2 wk, then 100 mcg/mo; **NASAL** 500 mcg q wk

Hydroxocobalamin

- *Adult:* **SUBCUT/IM** 30-50 mcg/day × 5-10 days, then 100-200 mcg/mo
- *Child:* **SUBCUT/IM** 30-50 mcg/day × 5-10 days, then 30-50 mcg/mo

Available forms: *Cyanocobalamin:* tabs 25, 50, 100, 250, 500, 1000, 5000 mcg; ext rel tabs 100, 200, 500, 1000 mcg; lozenges 100, 250, 500 mcg; nasal jel 500 mcg/spray; inj 100, 1000 mcg/ml; *hydroxocobalamin:* inj 1000 mcg/ml

SIDE EFFECTS

CNS: Flushing, optic nerve atrophy
CV: **CHF**, peripheral vascular thrombosis, **pulmonary edema**
GI: Diarrhea
INTEG: Itching, rash, pain at inj site
META: Hypokalemia
SYST: **Anaphylactic shock**

Contraindications: Hypersensitivity, optic nerve atrophy

Precautions: Pregnancy (A), breastfeeding, children

PHARMACOKINETICS

Gastric intrinsic factor must be present for absorption to occur; stored in liver, kidneys, stomach; 50%-90% excreted in urine; crosses placenta; excreted in breast milk

INTERACTIONS

Increase: absorption—predniSONE

Decrease: absorption—aminoglycosides, anticonvulsants, colchicine, chloramphenicol, aminosalicylic acid, potassium preparations, cimetidine

Drug/Herb

Decrease: vit B_{12} absorption—goldenseal

Drug/Lab Test

False positive: intrinsic factor

NURSING CONSIDERATIONS

Assess:

- For vit B_{12} deficiency: red, beefy tongue; psychosis; pallor; neuropathy
- GI function: diarrhea, constipation
- Potassium levels during beginning treatment in megaloblastic anemia; q6mo in pernicious anemia; folic acid, plasma vit B_{12} (after 1 wk), reticulocyte counts
- Nutritional status: egg yolks, fish, organ meats, dairy products, clams, oysters: good sources of vit B_{12}
- For pulmonary edema, worsening of CHF in cardiac patients

Administer:

PO route

- With fruit juice to disguise taste; immediately after mixing
- With meals if possible for better absorption; large doses should not be used since most is excreted

IM route

- By IM inj for pernicious anemia for life unless contraindicated

Intranasal route

- Avoid use within 1 hr of hot fluids/food

IV route

- IV route not recommended but may be admixed in TPN solution

Additive compatibilities: Ascorbic acid, chloramphenicol, metaraminol, vit B/C

Solution compatibilities: Dextrose/Ringer's or lactated Ringer's combinations, dextrose/saline combinations, D_5W, $D_{10}W$, 0.45% NaCl, Ringer's or lactated Ringer's sol

Y-site compatibilities: Heparin, hydrocortisone, potassium chloride, vit B/C

Perform/provide:

- Protection from light and heat

Evaluate:

- Therapeutic response: decreased anorexia, dyspnea on exertion, palpitations, paresthesias, psychosis, visual disturbances

Teach patient/family:

- That treatment must continue for life for pernicious anemia
- To eat well-balanced diet
- To avoid contact with persons with infection; infections common

Treatment of overdose: Discontinue product

cyclobenzaprine (℞)

(sye-kloe-ben′za-preen)
Amrix, cyclobenzaprine HCl, Fexmid, Flexeril
Func. class.: Skeletal muscle relaxant, central acting
Chem. class.: Tricyclic amine salt

Do not confuse:
cyclobenzaprine/cyproheptadine
Action: Reduction of tonic muscle activity at the brain stem; may be related to antidepressant effects
Uses: Adjunct for relief of muscle spasm and pain in musculoskeletal conditions
Unlabeled uses: Fibromyalgia

DOSAGE AND ROUTES

Muscloskeletal disorders

- *Adult:* **PO** 5 mg tid × 1 wk, max 30 mg/day × 3 wk
- *Geriatric:* **PO** 5 mg tid

Fibromyalgia (unlabeled)

- *Adult:* **PO** 10 mg at bedtime, titrated up

Available forms: Tabs 5, 10 mg; ext rel tab 15, 30 mg

SIDE EFFECTS

CNS: Dizziness, weakness, drowsiness, headache, tremor, depression, insomnia, confusion, paresthesia, nervousness
CV: Postural hypotension, tachycardia, **dysrhythmias**
EENT: Diplopia, temporary loss of vision
GI: Nausea, vomiting, hiccups, dry mouth, constipation, hepatitis
GU: Urinary retention, frequency, change in libido
INTEG: Rash, pruritus, fever, facial flushing, sweating
Contraindications: Children <12 yr, acute recovery phase of myocardial infarction, dysrhythmias, heart block, CHF, hypersensitivity, intermittent porphyria, thyroid disease
Precautions: Pregnancy (B), breastfeeding, geriatric patients, renal/hepatic disease, addictive personality

PHARMACOKINETICS

PO: Onset 1 hr, peak 3-8 hr, duration 12-24 hr, half-life 1-3 days, metabolized by liver, excreted in urine, crosses placenta, excreted in breast milk

INTERACTIONS

- Do not use within 14 days of MAOIs, tramadol

Increase: QT interval—erythromycin, levaquin
Increase: CNS depression—alcohol, tricyclics, opiates, barbiturates, sedatives, hypnotics
Drug/Herb
Increase: CNS depression—kava

NURSING CONSIDERATIONS

Assess:

- For pain: location, duration, mobility, stiffness, baseline and periodically
- Allergic reactions: rash, fever, respiratory distress
- Severe weakness, numbness in extremities

Administer:

- Without regard to meals

Perform/provide:

- Storage in tight container at room temperature
- Assistance with ambulation if dizziness, drowsiness occur, especially geriatric patients

Evaluate:

- Therapeutic response: decreased pain, spasticity; muscle spasms of acute, painful musculoskeletal conditions generally short term; long-term therapy seldom warranted

Teach patient/family:

- Not to discontinue medication abruptly; insomnia, nausea, headache, spasticity, tachycardia will occur; product should be tapered off over 1-2 wk
- Not to take with alcohol, other CNS depressants
- To avoid hazardous activities if drowsiness/dizziness occurs

• To avoid using OTC medication: cough preparations, antihistamines, unless directed by prescriber
• To use gum, frequent sips of water for dry mouth

Treatment of overdose: Administer activated charcoal; use anticonvulsants if indicated; monitor cardiac function

cyclopentolate ophthalmic

See Appendix B

⚠ High Alert

cyclophosphamide (℞)

(sye-kloe-foss′fa-mide)

Cytoxan, Procytox ✤

Func. class.: Antineoplastic alkylating agent

Chem. class.: Nitrogen mustard

Do not confuse:
cyclophosphamide/cycloSPORINE
Cytoxan/Cytosar/Cytotec/cytarabine

Action: Alkylates DNA is responsible for cross-linking DNA strands; activity is not cell cycle phase specific

Uses: Hodgkin's disease; lymphomas; leukemia; cancer of female reproductive tract, breast, lung, prostate; multiple myeloma; neuroblastoma; retinoblastoma; Ewing's sarcoma; disseminated neuroblastoma

Unlabeled uses: Aplastic anemia, chronic idiopathic thrombocytopenic purpura, dermatomyositis, pneumonitis, polymyositis, SLE, scleroderma, RA, Behçet's syndrome, Churg-Strauss syndrome, polyarteritis nodosa, Wegener's granulomatosis, idiopathic pulmonary fibrosis, localized neuroblastoma, CLL

DOSAGE AND ROUTES

• *Adult:* **PO** Initially 1-5 mg/kg over 2-5 days, maintenance is 1-5 mg/kg; **IV** initially 40-50 mg/kg in divided doses over 2-5 days, maintenance 10-15 mg/kg q7-10 days, or 3-5 mg/kg q3days
• *Child:* **PO/IV** 2-8 mg/kg or 60-250 mg/m^2 in divided doses for 6 or more days; maintenance 10-15 mg/kg q7-10 days or 30 mg/kg q3-4wk; dose should be reduced by half when bone marrow depression occurs

Neuroblastoma

• *Child and infant:* **PO** 150 mg/m^2/day, days 1-7 with DOXOrubicin (**IV** 35 mg/m^2 on day 8) q21days × 5 cycles
• *Child:* **IV** 70 mg/kg/day with hydration on days 1 and 2 with DOXOrubicin and vinCRIStine q21days for courses 1, 2, 4, 6, alternating with cisplatin and etoposide q21days for courses 3, 5, 7

Breast cancer

• *Adult:* **PO** 100-200 mg/m^2/day or 2 mg/kg/day × 4-14 days; **IV** 500-1000 mg/m^2 on day 1 in combination with fluorouracil and methotrexate or DOXOrubicin or DOXOrubicin alone, also cyclophosphamide 600 mg/m^2, may be given dose-dense on day 1 of q14days with DOXOrubicin (60 mg/m^2) with growth factor support

Operable node-positive breast cancer IV (TAC regimen)

• *Adult:* **IV** 500 mg/m^2 with DOXOrubicin (50 mg/m^2 **IV**), then docetaxel (75 mg/m^2) **IV** given 1 hr later q3wk × 6 cycles

Aplastic anemia (unlabeled)

• *Adult:* **IV** 45-50 mg/kg divided over 5 days

Behçet's syndrome/Churg-Strauss syndrome/polyarteritis nodosa/uveitis/Wegener's granulomatosis (unlabeled)

• *Adult:* **PO** 1-2 mg/kg/day, **IV** 0.5-1 g/m^2

Rheumatoid arthritis (unlabeled)

• *Adult and child:* **PO** 1.5-2.5 mg/kg/day

CLL (unlabeled)

• *Adult:* **IV** 250 mg/m^2/day on days 1-3 with fludarabine 30 mg/m^2/day on days 1-3

Available forms: Inj 100, 200, 500 mg, 1, 2 g; tabs 25, 50 mg

SIDE EFFECTS

CNS: Headache, dizziness
CV: **Cardiotoxicity (high doses), myocardial fibrosis**
ENDO: SIADH, gonadal suppression
GI: Nausea, vomiting, diarrhea, weight loss, colitis, **hepatotoxicity**
GU: **Hemorrhagic cystitis,** *hematuria, neoplasms, amenorrhea, azoospermia, sterility, ovarian fibrosis*
HEMA: **Thrombocytopenia, leukopenia, pancytopenia; myelosuppression**
INTEG: Alopecia, dermatitis
META: Hyperuricemia
MISC: Secondary neoplasms, **anaphylaxis**
RESP: **Pulmonary fibrosis, interstitial pneumonia**

Contraindications: Pregnancy (D), breastfeeding, severely depressed bone marrow function, hypersensitivity, prostatic hypertrophy, bladder neck obstruction

Precautions: Radiation therapy, cardiac disease

PHARMACOKINETICS

Metabolized by liver, excreted in urine, half-life 4-6½ hr, 50% bound to plasma proteins

INTERACTIONS

Increase: neuromuscular blockade—succinylcholine
Increase: cyclophosphamide toxicity—barbiturates
Increase: action of warfarin
Increase: bone marrow depression—allopurinol, thiazides
Increase: hypoglycemia—insulin
Decrease: digoxin levels—digoxin
Decrease: cyclophosphamide effect—chloramphenicol, corticosteroids
Decrease: antibody response—live virus vaccines

Drug/Herb
Toxicity: St. John's wort

Drug/Lab Test
Increase: uric acid
Decrease: pseudocholinesterase
False positive: Pap smear
False negative: PPD, mumps, trichophytin, *Candida, Trichophyton,* Pap smear

NURSING CONSIDERATIONS

Assess:

- For hemorrhagic cystitis; renal studies: BUN, serum uric acid, urine CCr before, during therapy; I&O ratio; report fall in urine output <30 ml/hr
- CBC, differential, platelet count baseline, weekly; withhold product if WBC is <2500 or platelet count is <75,000; notify prescriber of results
- Pulmonary function tests, chest x-ray films before, during therapy; chest film should be obtained q2wk during treatment
- Monitor temp q4hr (elevated temp may indicate beginning infection)
- Hepatic studies before, during therapy (bilirubin, AST, ALT, LDH) as needed or monthly
- Bleeding: hematuria, guaiac, bruising or petechiae, mucosa or orifices q8hr
- Dyspnea, crackles, unproductive cough, chest pain, tachypnea
- Effects of alopecia on body image, discuss feelings about body changes
- Jaundice of skin, sclera; dark urine; clay-colored stools; itchy skin; abdominal pain; fever; diarrhea
- Buccal cavity q8hr for dryness, sores or ulceration, white patches, oral pain, bleeding, dysphagia; obtain prescription for viscous lidocaine (Xylocaine)

⚠ Symptoms indicating severe allergic reaction: rash, pruritus, urticaria, purpuric skin lesions, itching, flushing

Administer:

- In AM so product can be eliminated before bedtime
- Fluids IV or PO before chemotherapy to hydrate patient
- Antacid before oral agent, give after evening meal, before bedtime
- Antiemetic 30-60 min before giving product and prn
- Allopurinol or sodium bicarbonate to maintain uric acid levels, alkalinization of urine

IV route

- Using cytoxic handling procedures
- IV after diluting 100 mg/5 ml of sterile H_2O or bacteriostatic H_2O; shake; let stand until clear; may be further diluted in up to 250 ml D_5 or NS; give 100 mg or less/min through 3-way stopcock of glucose or saline inf
- Using 21, 23, 25G needle; check site for irritation, phlebitis

Additive compatibilities: Cisplatin with etoposide, fluorouracil, hydrOXYzine, methotrexate, methotrexate/fluorouracil, mitoxantrone, ondansetron

Solution compatibilities: Amino acids 4.25%/D_{25}, D_5/0.9% NaCl, D_5W, 0.9% NaCl

Syringe compatibilities: Bleomycin, cisplatin, doxapram, DOXOrubicin, droperidol, fluorouracil, furosemide, heparin, leucovorin, methotrexate, metoclopramide, mitomycin, vinBLAStine, vinCRIStine

Y-site compatibilities: Allopurinol, amifostine, amikacin, ampicillin, azlocillin, aztreonam, bleomycin, cefamandole, cefazolin, cefepime, cefoperazone, cefotaxime, cefoxitin, cefuroxime, cephalothin, cephapirin, chloramphenicol, chlorproMAZINE, cimetidine, cisplatin, cladribine, clindamycin, dexamethasone, diphenhydrAMINE, DOXOrubicin, DOXOrubicin liposome, doxycycline, droperidol, erythromycin, famotidine, filgrastim, fludarabine, fluorouracil, furosemide, gallium, ganciclovir, gentamicin, granisetron, heparin, hydromorphone, idarubicin, kanamycin, leucovorin, lorazepam, melphalan, methotrexate, methylPREDNISolone, metoclopramide, metronidazole, mezlocillin, minocycline, mitomycin, morphine, moxalactam, nafcillin, ondansetron, oxacillin, paclitaxel, penicillin G potassium, piperacillin, piperacillin/tazobactam, prochlorperazine, promethazine, propofol, ranitidine, sargramostim, sodium bicarbonate, teniposide, thiotepa, ticarcillin, ticarcillin-clavulanate, tobramycin, trimethoprim-sulfamethoxazole, vancomycin, vinBLAStine, vinCRIStine, vinorelbine

Perform/provide:

- Storage in tight container at room temperature
- Strict medical asepsis, protective isolation if WBC levels are low
- Increase fluid intake to 2-3 L/day to prevent urate deposits, calculi formation, reduce incidence of hemorrhagic cystitis
- Diet low in purines: organ meats (kidney, liver), dried beans, peas to maintain alkaline urine
- Rinsing of mouth tid-qid with water, club soda; brushing of teeth bid-tid with soft brush or cotton-tipped applicators for stomatitis; use unwaxed dental floss
- Warm compresses at inj site for inflammation

Evaluate:

- Therapeutic response: decreased tumor size, spread of malignancy

Teach patient/family:

- About protective isolation
- That amenorrhea can occur and may last up to 1 yr after therapy; reversible after stopping treatment
- To report any changes in breathing or coughing
- That hair may be lost during treatment; a wig or hairpiece may make patient feel better; new hair may be different in color, texture
- To avoid foods with citric acid, hot or rough texture
- To report any bleeding, white spots, ulcerations in mouth to prescriber; tell patient to examine mouth daily
- To report signs of infection: increased temperature, sore throat, flulike symptoms
- To report signs of anemia: fatigue, headache, faintness, shortness of breath, irritability
- To report bleeding (bruising, hematuria, petechiae): avoid use of razors, commercial mouthwash
- To use reliable contraception during and for 4 mo after treatment; do not breastfeed
- To avoid use of aspirin products, ibuprofen
- To avoid vaccinations during therapy

*cycloSPORINE (℞)

(sye'kloe-spor-een)

Gengraf, Neoral, Sandimmune, Pulminiq

Func. class.: Immunosuppressant

Chem. class.: Fungus-derived peptide

Do not confuse:
cycloSPORINE/cycloSERINE/cyclophosphamide

Action: Produces immunosuppression by inhibiting lymphocytes (T)

Uses: Organ transplants (liver, kidney, heart) to prevent rejection, rheumatoid arthritis, psoriasis

Unlabeled uses: Recalcitrant ulcerative colitis, aplastic anemia, Crohn's disease, GVHD, thrombocytopenia purpura, lupus, nephritis, myasthenia gravis, psoriatic arthritis, atopic dermatitis

DOSAGE AND ROUTES

Prevention of transplant rejection

• *Adult and child:* **PO** 15 mg/kg several hr before surgery, daily for 2 wk, reduce dosage by 2.5 mg/kg/wk to 5-10 mg/kg/day; **IV** 5-6 mg/kg several hr before surgery, daily, switch to PO form as soon as possible

Rheumatoid arthritis (Neoral/Gengraf)

• *Adult:* **PO** 2.5 mg/kg/day divided bid, may increase 0.5-0.75 mg/kg/day after 8-12 wk, max 4 mg/kg/day

Psoriasis (Neoral/Gengraf)

• *Adult:* **PO** 2.5 mg/kg/day divided bid, × 4 wk, then increase by 0.5 mg/kg/day q2wk, max 4 mg/kg/day

Idiopathic thrombocytopenia purpura (unlabeled)

• *Adult:* **PO** 1.25-2.5 mg/kg bid

Severe aplastic anemia (unlabeled)

• *Adult and child:* **PO** 12 mg/kg/day or 15 mg/kg/day (child) with antithymocyte globulin (ATG)

Atopic dermatitis (unlabeled)

• *Adult/adolescent/child ≥2 yr:* **PO** 5 mg/kg/day

Available forms: Oral sol 100 mg/ml; soft gel cap 25, 50, 100 mg; inj 50 mg/ml; sol for inh 300 mg/4.8 ml

SIDE EFFECTS

CNS: Tremors, headache, **seizures, confusion**

GI: Nausea, vomiting, diarrhea, *oral candida, gum hyperplasia,* **hepatotoxicity,** pancreatitis

GU: **Albuminuria, hematuria, proteinuria, renal failure**

INTEG: Rash, acne, ***hirsutism,*** pruritus

META: Hyperkalemia, hypomagnesemia, hyperlipidemia, hyperuricemia

MISC: Infection

Contraindications: Breastfeeding, hypersensitivity to polyxyethylated castor oil (inj only); psoriasis or RA in renal disease (Neoral/Gengraf); Gengraf/Neoral used with PUVA/UVB, methotrexate, coal tar; ocular infections

Black Box Warning: Uncontrolled, malignant hypertension, radiation in psoriasis, neoplastic disease, sunlight (UV) exposure, renal disease/failure

Precautions: Pregnancy (C), geriatric patients, severe hepatic disease

PHARMACOKINETICS

Peak 4 hr; highly protein bound; half-life (biphasic) 1.2 hr, 25 hr; metabolized in liver; excreted in feces, 6% in urine; crosses placenta; excreted in breast milk

INTERACTIONS

Increase: action, toxicity of cycloSPORINE—allopurinol, amiodarone, amphotericin B, androgens, azole antifungals, β-blockers, bromocriptine, calcium channel blockers, carvedilol, cimetidine, colchicine, corticosteroids, fluoroquinolones, foscarnet, imipenem-cilastatin, macrolides, metoclopramide, oral contraceptives, NSAIDs, melphalan, SSRIs

Increase: effects of digoxin, etoposide, HMG-CoA reductase inhibitors, methotrexate, potassium-sparing diuretics, sirolimus, tacrolimus

Decrease: cycloSPORINE action—anticonvulsants, nafcillin, orlistat, phenobarbital, phenytoin, probucol, rifamycins, sulfamethoxazole-trimethoprim, terbinafine, ticlopidine
Decrease: antibody reaction—live virus vaccines

Drug/Herb

Increase: immunosuppressant effect—safflower
Decrease: immunosuppressant effect—ginseng, maitake, mistletoe, schisandra, St. John's wort, turmeric

Drug/Food

- Slowed metabolism of product: grapefruit juice, food

NURSING CONSIDERATIONS

Assess:

- Renal studies: BUN, creatinine at least monthly during treatment, 3 mo after treatment
- Product blood level during treatment
- Hepatic studies: alk phos, AST, ALT, bilirubin; hepatotoxicity: dark urine, jaundice, itching, light-colored stools; product should be discontinued
- Serum lipids, magnesium, potassium, cycloSPORINE blood concentrations

⚠ For nephrotoxicity: 6 wk postop, acute tubular necrosis, CyA trough level >200 ng/ml, gradual rise in creatinine (0.15 mg/dl/day), creatinine plateau <25% above baseline, intracapsular pressure <40 mm Hg

⚠ For signs/symptoms of encephalopathy, lymphoma

Administer:

PO route

- Do not break, crush, or chew caps
- Use pipette provided to draw up oral sol; may mix with milk or juice, wipe pipette, do not wash
- For several days before transplant surgery; give at same time of day
- With corticosteroids
- With meals for GI upset or in chocolate milk, milk, or orange juice
- With oral antifungal for candida infections

Rheumatoid arthritis

- Give Neoral or Gengraf 2.5 mg/kg/day divided bid, may use with salicylates, NSAIDs, PO corticosteroids
- Always give the daily dose of Neoral/Gengraf in 2 divided doses on consistent schedule
- Give initial Sandimmune PO dose 4-12 hr prior to transplantation as a single dose of 15 mg/kg, continue the single daily dose for 1-2 wk, then taper 5%/wk to a maintenance dose 5-10 mg/kg/day

IV route

- After diluting each 50 mg/20-100 ml of 0.9% NaCl or D_5W; run over 2-6 hr, may give as a continuous inf over 24 hr; use an inf pump, glass inf bottles only
- For Sandimmune parenteral, give ⅓ of PO dose, initial dose 4-12 hr prior to transplantation as a single IV dose 5-6 mg/kg/day, continue the single daily dose until PO can be used

Additive compatibilities: Ciprofloxacin

Solution compatibilities: D_5W, NaCl 0.9%

Y-site compatibilities: Cefmetazole, propofol, sargramostim

Evaluate:

- Therapeutic response: absence of rejection

Teach patient/family:

- To report fever, chills, sore throat, fatigue, since serious infections may occur; tremors, bleeding gums, increased B/P
- To use contraceptive measures during treatment, for 12 wk after ending therapy
- To take at same time of day, every day; do not skip doses or double a missed dose; not to use with grapefruit juice or receive vaccines
- To limit UV exposure

cyproheptadine (℞)

(si-proe-hep'ta-deen)
cyproheptadine HCl,
PMS-Cyproheptadine ✱
Func. class.: Antihistamine, H_1-receptor antagonist
Chem. class.: Piperidine

Do not confuse:
cyproheptadine/cyclobenzaprine

Action: Acts on blood vessels, GI, respiratory system by competing with histamine for H_1-receptor site; decreases allergic response by blocking histamine

Uses: Allergy symptoms, rhinitis, pruritus, common cold, urticaria

Unlabeled uses: Appetite stimulant, management of vascular headache, nightmares, posttraumatic stress disorder

DOSAGE AND ROUTES

- *Adult:* **PO** 4 mg tid-qid, not to exceed 0.5 mg/kg/day
- *Geriatric:* **PO** 4 mg bid, may increase if needed
- *Child 6-14 yr:* **PO** 4 mg bid-tid, not to exceed 16 mg/day
- *Child 2-5 yr:* **PO** 2 mg bid-tid, not to exceed 12 mg/day

Nightmares, posttraumatic stress disorder (unlabeled)

- *Adult:* **PO** 4-12 mg nightly, max 32 mg

Available forms: Tabs 4 mg; syr 2 mg/5 ml

SIDE EFFECTS

CNS: Dizziness, drowsiness, poor coordination, fatigue, anxiety, euphoria, confusion, paresthesia, neuritis

CV: Hypotension, palpitations, tachycardia

EENT: Blurred vision, dilated pupils; tinnitus; nasal stuffiness; dry nose, throat, mouth

GI: Constipation, dry mouth, nausea, vomiting, anorexia, diarrhea, weight gain, increased appetite

GU: Retention, dysuria, urinary frequency

HEMA: **Hemolytic anemia, leukopenia, thrombocytosis, agranulocytosis**

INTEG: Rash, urticaria, photosensitivity

RESP: Increased thick secretions, wheezing, chest tightness

SYST: **Anaphylactic shock**

Contraindications: Hypersensitivity to H_1-receptor antagonist, breastfeeding, closed-angle glaucoma, neonates/infants, peptic ulcers, bladder-neck obstruction, prostatic hypertrophy

Precautions: Pregnancy (B), geriatric patients, cardiac disease, asthma, ileus, urinary retention, COPD

PHARMACOKINETICS

PO: Duration 4-6 hr; metabolized in liver; excreted by kidneys (65%-75%), feces (25%-35%); excreted in breast milk

INTERACTIONS

Increase: CNS depression—barbiturates, opiates, hypnotics, tricyclics, alcohol, and other CNS depressants

Increase: anticholinergic effect—MAOIs

Drug/Herb

Increase: CNS depression—hops, Jamaican dogwood, kava, khat, senega

Increase: anticholinergic effect—corkwood, henbane

Drug/Lab Test

False negative: skin allergy tests

NURSING CONSIDERATIONS

Assess:

- I&O ratio; be alert for urinary retention, frequency, dysuria; product should be discontinued
- CBC during long-term therapy
- Respiratory status: rate, rhythm, increase in bronchial secretions, wheezing, chest tightness
- Cardiac status: palpitations, increased pulse, hypotension

Administer:

- With meals for GI symptoms; absorption may slightly decrease

Perform/provide:

- Hard candy, gum, frequent rinsing of mouth for dryness
- Storage in airtight container at room temperature

Evaluate:

- Therapeutic response: absence of running or congested nose, rashes

Teach patient/family:

- All aspects of product use; to notify prescriber of confusion, sedation, hypotension
- To avoid driving, other hazardous activity if drowsiness occurs, especially geriatric patients
- To avoid concurrent use of alcohol, other CNS depressants
- To avoid breastfeeding

Treatment of overdose: Ipecac syrup or lavage, diazepam, vasopressors, phenytoin IV

⚠ High Alert

cytarabine (℞)

(sye-tare'a-been)

Ara-C, Cytosar ✦, cytosine arabinoside

cytarabine liposomal (℞)

DepoCyt

Func. class.: Antineoplastic, antimetabolite

Chem. class.: Pyrimidine nucleoside analog

Do not confuse:

Cytosar/Cytoxan/Cytovene

Action: Competes with physiologic substrate of DNA synthesis, thus interfering with cell replication in the S phase of the cell cycle (before mitosis)

Uses: Acute myelocytic leukemia, acute nonlymphocytic leukemia, chronic myelocytic leukemia, lymphomatous meningitis (IT)

Unlabeled uses: Hodgkin's/non-Hodgkin's lymphoma, malignant meningitis, mantle cell lymphoma

DOSAGE AND ROUTES

Acute nonlymphocytic/lymphocytic

- *Adult:* **IV INF** 200 mg/m^2/day × 5 days q2wk as single agent or 2-6 mg/kg/day (100-200 mg/m^2/day) as a single dose or 2-3 divided doses for 5-10 days until remission, used in combination; maintenance 70-200 mg/m^2/day for 2-5 days q mo; **SUBCUT/IM** maintenance 1 mg/kg q1-2×/wk

Meningeal leukemia

- *Adult and child:* **INTRATHECAL** 5-75 mg/m^2 variable daily × 4 days to q2-7days

Refractory acute Hodgkin's/refractory non-Hodgkin's lymphoma (unlabeled)

- *Adult:* **IV** 2 g/m^2/day; on day 5 q21days, with etoposide, methylPREDNISolone, and cisplatin

Available forms: Powder for inj 100, 500 mg, 1, 2 g; sus rel, (DepoCyt) liposomal for intrathecal use 10 mg/ml

SIDE EFFECTS

CNS: Neuritis, dizziness, headache, cerebellar syndrome, personality changes, ataxia, mechanical dysphasia, **coma; chemical arachnoiditis** (IT)

CV: Chest pain, **cardiopathy**

CYTARABINE SYNDROME: *Fever,* myalgia, bone pain, chest pain, *rash,* conjunctivitis, malaise (6-12 hr after administration)

EENT: Sore throat, conjunctivitis

GI: *Nausea, vomiting, anorexia, diarrhea, stomatitis,* **hepatotoxicity,** abdominal pain, hematemesis, **GI hemorrhage**

GU: Urinary retention, **renal failure, hyperuricemia**

HEMA: **Thrombophlebitis, bleeding, thrombocytopenia, leukopenia, myelosuppression, anemia**

INTEG: *Rash, fever,* freckling, cellulitis

META: Hyperuricemia

RESP: **Pneumonia,** dyspnea, **pulmonary edema** (high doses)

SYST: **Anaphylaxis**

Contraindications: Pregnancy (D), hypersensitivity

Precautions: Breastfeeding, children, renal/hepatic disease, tumor lysis syndrome, infection, hyperkalemia, hyperphosphatemia, hyperuricemia, hypocalcemia

Black Box Warning: Bone marrow suppression

PHARMACOKINETICS

INTRATHECAL: Half-life 100-236 hr; metabolized in liver; excreted in urine (primarily inactive metabolite); crosses blood-brain barrier, placenta
IV/SUBCUT: Distribution half-life 10 min, elimination half-life 1-3 hr

INTERACTIONS

- Do not use with live virus vaccines
- Do not use within 24 hr of chemotherapy—sargramostim, GM-CSF, filgrastim, G-CSF

Increase: toxicity—immunosuppressants, methotrexate, flucytosine, radiation, or other antineoplastics
Increase: bleeding risk—anticoagulants, platelet inhibitors, salicylates, thrombolytics, NSAIDs
Decrease: effects of oral digoxin, gentamicin

NURSING CONSIDERATIONS

Assess:

- CBC (RBC, Hct, Hgb), differential, platelet count weekly; withhold product if WBC is <1000/mm^3, platelet count is <50,000/mm^3, or RBC, Hct, Hgb low; notify prescriber of these results
- Renal studies: BUN, serum uric acid, urine CCr, electrolytes before and during therapy
- I&O ratio; report fall in urine output to <30 ml/hr
- Monitor temp q4hr; fever may indicate beginning infection; no rectal temps
- Hepatic studies before and during therapy: bilirubin, ALT, AST, alk phos, as needed or monthly; check for jaundice of skin, sclera; dark urine; clay-colored stools; pruritus; abdominal pain; fever; diarrhea
- Blood uric acid during therapy

⚠ For anaphylaxis: rash, pruritus, facial swelling, dyspnea; resuscitation equipment should be nearby

⚠ Chemical arachnoiditis (IT): headache, nausea, vomiting, fever; neck rigidity pain, meningism, CSF pleocytosis; may be decreased by dexamethasone

- Cytarabine syndrome 6-12 hr after inf: fever, myalgia, bone pain, chest pain, rash, conjunctivitis, malaise; corticosteroids may be ordered
- Bleeding: hematuria, heme-positive stools, bruising or petechiae, mucosa or orifices q8hr

⚠ Dyspnea, crackles, unproductive cough, chest pain, tachypnea, fatigue, increased pulse, pallor, lethargy; personality changes, with high doses; pulmonary edema may be fatal (rare)

- Buccal cavity q8hr for dryness, sores or ulceration, white patches, oral pain, bleeding, dysphagia
- Local irritation, pain, burning, discoloration at inj site
- GI symptoms: frequency of stools, cramping, antispasmodic may be used
- Acidosis, signs of dehydration: rapid respirations, poor skin turgor, decreased urine output, dry skin, restlessness, weakness

Administer:

- Antiemetic 30-60 min before giving product and prn
- Allopurinol to maintain uric acid levels and alkalinization of the urine
- Topical or systemic analgesics for pain

IT route

- Use preservative-free NS, add 5 ml/100-mg vial or 10 ml/500-mg vial; use immediately, discard unused product
- Use dexamethasone with IT administration

IV route

- After diluting 100 mg/5 ml of sterile H_2O for inj; given by direct IV over 1-3 min through free-flowing tubing (IV); may be further diluted in 50-100 ml NS or D_5W, given over 30 min to 24 hr depending on dose; also may be given by continuous inf

Additive compatibilities: Corticotropin, DAUNOrubicin with etoposide, etoposide, hydrOXYzine, lincomycin, mitoxantrone, ondansetron, potassium chloride, prednisoLONE, sodium bicarbonate, vinCRIStine

Solution compatibilities: Amino acids, D_5/LR, D_5/0.2% NaCl, D_5/0.9% NaCl, D_{10}/0.9% NaCl, D_5W, invert sugar 10% in electrolyte #1, Ringer's LR, 0.9% NaCl, sodium lactate ⅙ mol/L, TPN #57

Syringe compatibilities: Metoclopramide

Y-site compatibilities: Amifostine, amsacrine, aztreonam, cefepime, chlorproMAZINE, cimetidine, cladribine, dexamethasone, diphenhydrAMINE, DOXOrubicin liposome, droperidol, famitodine, filgrastim, fludarabine, gentamicin, granisetron, heparin, hydrocortisone, hydromorphone, idarubicin, lorazepam, melphalan, methotrexate, methylPREDNISolone, metoclopramide, morphine, ondansetron, paclitaxel, piperacillin/tazobactam, prochlorperazine, promethazine, propofol, ranitidine, sargramostim, sodium bicarbonate, teniposide, thiotepa, vinorelbine

Perform/provide:

- Strict medical asepsis and protective isolation if WBC levels are low
- Increase fluid intake to 2-3 L/day to prevent urate deposits and calculi formation, unless contraindicated
- Diet low in purines: absence of organ meats (kidney, liver), dried beans, peas to prevent increased urate deposits
- Rinsing of mouth tid-qid with water, club soda; brushing of teeth bid-tid with soft brush or cotton-tipped applicators for stomatitis; use unwaxed dental floss

Evaluate:

- Therapeutic response: decreased tumor size, spread of malignancy

Teach patient/family:

- To report any coughing, chest pain, changes in breathing; may indicate beginning pneumonia, pulmonary edema
- To avoid foods with citric acid, spicy or rough texture if stomatitis is present, use sponge brush and rinse with water after each meal; to report stomatitis: any bleeding, white spots, ulcerations in mouth; tell patient to examine mouth daily, report any symptoms
- To report signs of infection: increased temp, sore throat, flulike symptoms; avoid crowds, persons with infections
- To report signs of anemia: fatigue, headache, faintness, SOB, irritability
- To report bleeding; avoid use of razors, commercial mouthwash, salicylates, NSAIDs, anticoagulants
- To use thrombocytopenia precautions
- To take fluids to 3 L/day to prevent renal damage
- To use reliable contraception during treatment and 4 mo thereafter, do not breastfeed
- To avoid receiving vaccines during treatment
- That fever, headache, nausea, vomiting are likely to occur

⚠ High Alert

dacarbazine (℞)

(da-kar′ba-zeen)

dacarbazine, DTIC ♣, DTIC-Dome

Func. class.: Antineoplastic alkylating agent

Chem. class.: Cytotoxic triazine

Action: Alkylates DNA, RNA; inhibits DNA, RNA synthesis; also responsible for breakage, cross-linking DNA strands; activity is not cell cycle phase specific

Uses: Hodgkin's disease, malignant melanoma

Unlabeled uses: Malignant pheochromocytoma in combination with cyclophosphamide and vinCRIStine, metastatic soft tissue sarcoma in combination with other agents, carcinoma meningitis, neuroblastoma

DOSAGE AND ROUTES

Metastatic malignant melanoma

- *Adult:* **IV** 2-4.5 mg/kg/day × 10 days or 150-250 mg/m²/day × 5 days; repeat q3-4wk depending on response

Hodgkin's disease

- *Adult:* **IV** 150 mg/m^2/day × 5 days with other agents, repeat q4wk; or 375 mg/m^2 on days 1 and 15 when given in combination, repeat q28 days

Osteogenic sarcoma (unlabeled)

- *Adult and child:* **IV** 250 mg/m^2/day as a continuous inf × 4 days q28days

Soft tissue sarcoma (unlabeled)

- *Adult and child:* **IV** 250-300 mg/m^2/day as a continuous inf × 3 days q21-28 days

Carcinoma meningitis (unlabeled)

- *Adult:* **INTRATHECAL** 5-30 mg in a fixed dose 2-3 ×/wk until disease controlled

Available forms: Powder for inj 10, 100, 200 mg

SIDE EFFECTS

CNS: Facial paresthesia, flushing, fever, malaise; confusion, headache, **seizures, cerebral hemorrhage,** blurred vision (high doses)

GI: Nausea, anorexia, vomiting, **hepatotoxicity** (rare)

HEMA: **Thrombocytopenia, leukopenia,** anemia

INTEG: Alopecia, dermatitis, pain at inj site, photosensitivity; severe sun reactions (high doses)

MISC: Flulike symptoms, malaise, fever, myalgia, hypotension

SYST: **Anaphylaxis**

Contraindications: Breastfeeding, hypersensitivity

Precautions: Renal disease

Black Box Warning: Pregnancy (C) 1st trimester, radiation therapy, hepatic disease, bone marrow suppression, secondary malignancy

PHARMACOKINETICS

Metabolized by liver; excreted in urine; half-life 35 min, terminal 5 hr, 5% protein bound

INTERACTIONS

- Toxicity, bone marrow suppression: bone marrow suppressants, radiation, other antineoplastics
- Bleeding: salicylates, anticoagulants

Increase: adverse reaction; decrease antibody reaction—live virus vaccines

Increase: nephrotoxicity—aminoglycosides

Increase: ototoxicity—loop diuretics

Decrease: dacarbazine effect—phenytoin, phenobarbital

NURSING CONSIDERATIONS

Assess:

⚠ CBC, differential, platelet count weekly; withhold product if WBC <4000 or platelet count <75,000; notify prescriber of results

- Monitor temp q4hr (may indicate beginning infection)
- Hepatic studies before, during therapy (bilirubin, AST, ALT, LDH) as needed or monthly
- Bleeding: hematuria, guaiac, bruising or petechiae, mucosa or orifices q8hr
- Effects of alopecia on body image, discuss feelings about body changes
- Jaundice of skin, sclera; dark urine; clay-colored stools; itchy skin; abdominal pain; fever; diarrhea
- Inflammation of mucosa, breaks in skin

⚠ Hypersensitivity reactions, anaphylaxis, discontinue product, administer meds for anaphylaxis

Administer:

- Antiemetic 30-60 min before giving product to prevent vomiting, nausea; vomiting may subside after several doses
- Antibiotics for prophylaxis of infection

IV route

- After diluting 100 mg/9.9 ml of sterile H_2O for inj (10 mg/ml), give by direct IV over 1 min through Y-tube or 3-way stopcock; may be further diluted in 50-250 ml D_5W or NS for inj, given as an inf over ½ hr
- Watch for extravasation; give Na thiosulfate 10% 4 ml plus sterile H_2O 5 ml, 3-5 ml SUBCUT if needed

Additive compatibilities: Bleomycin, carmustine, cyclophosphamide, cytarabine, dactinomycin, DOXOrubicin, fluorouracil, mercaptopurine, methotrexate, ondansetron, vinBLAStine

Additive incompatibilities: Hydrocortisone sodium succinate, cysteine

Y-site compatibilities: Amifostine, aztreonam, filgrastim, fludarabine, granisetron, melphalan, ondansetron, paclitaxel, sargramostim, teniposide, thiotepa, vinorelbine

Perform/provide:

- Storage in light-resistant container, dry area
- Strict medical asepsis, protective isolation if WBC levels are low
- Increase fluid intake to 2-3 L/day to prevent urate deposits, calculi formation
- Warm compresses at infusion site for inflammation

Evaluate:

- Therapeutic response: decreased tumor size, spread of malignancy

Teach patient/family:

- That patient should avoid prolonged exposure to sun, wear sunscreen
- That hair may be lost during treatment; a wig or hairpiece may make the patient feel better; new hair may be different in color, texture
- To report signs of infection: fever, sore throat, flulike symptoms
- To report signs of anemia: fatigue, headache, faintness, SOB, irritability
- To report bleeding; avoid use of razors, commercial mouthwash
- To avoid use of aspirin products or ibuprofen
- To use reliable contraceptives during and for several months after therapy; do not breastfeed

⚠ High Alert

daclizumab (℞)

(dah-kliz′uh-mab)

Zenapax

Func. class.: Immunosuppressant

Chem. class.: Humanized IgG1 monoclonal antibody

Action: Binds to the IL-2 (interleukin-2) receptor antagonist

Uses: Acute allograft rejection in renal transplant patients

DOSAGE AND ROUTES

- *Adult:* **IV** Begin 24 hr prior to transplant, then 1 mg/kg as part of a regimen that includes cycloSPORINE and corticosteroids; mix calculated vol with 50 ml of 0.9% NaCl and give via peripheral/central vein over 15 min; do not admix; give q14 days for a total of 5 doses

Available forms: Inj 5 mg/ml

SIDE EFFECTS

CNS: Chills, tremors, dizziness, insomnia, headache, prickly sensation, fatigue

CV: Hypo/hypertension, **tachycardia, thrombosis,** bleeding, chest pain

GI: Vomiting, nausea, diarrhea, constipation, abdominal pain, pyrosis

GU: Oliguria, dysuria, **renal tubular necrosis,** renal damage, **hydronephrosis**

INTEG: Acne, impaired wound healing

MISC: Edema, peripheral edema, allergic reaction, **anaphylaxis, bleeding, thrombosis**

RESP: Dyspnea, wheezing, **pulmonary edema,** coughing, atelectasis, congestion, hypoxia

Contraindications: Hypersensitivity to this product or murine protein

Precautions: Pregnancy (C), breastfeeding, children <11 mo, geriatric patients, severe liver disease

Black Box Warning: Infection

INTERACTIONS

Drug/Herb

Increase: immunosuppressant effect—safflower

Decrease: immunosuppressant effect—ginseng, maitake, mistletoe, schisandra, St. John's wort, turmeric

NURSING CONSIDERATIONS

Assess:

- Blood studies: Hgb, WBC, platelets during treatment q mo; if leukocytes are <3000/mm^3, product should be discontinued
- Hepatic studies: alk phos, AST, ALT, bilirubin

⚠ Hepatotoxicity: dark urine, jaundice, itching, light-colored stools; product should be discontinued

⚠ For anaphylaxis, have corticosteroids, epinephrine available

- For fluid overload: weight gain, renal function studies; check lung sounds, VS

Administer:

- All other medications PO if possible
- Avoid IM inj, since infection may occur
- Protect undiluted sol from direct light; should be used with products for immunosuppression
- Do not give by direct bolus injection

Solution compatibilities: 0.9% NaCl

Perform/provide:

- Increased fluid intake during treatment
- Storage of unopened vials in refrigerator; do not shake or freeze; protect from light

Evaluate:

- Therapeutic response: absence of graft rejection

Teach patient/family:

- To report fever, chills, sore throat, fatigue, since serious infection may occur; rash, hives, difficulty breathing, since allergic reactions may occur; nausea, constipation, diarrhea, stomach pain, headache, fast heartbeat, swelling, tremors, chest pain, urinary tract bleeding, fever, cough, pain, redness at site
- To use contraception (women) before, during, and for 4 mo after treatment
- To avoid vaccinations during treatment
- To avoid hazardous activities, dizziness, blurred vision may occur
- To avoid crowds, persons with known upper respiratory infections

D

⚠ High Alert

dactinomycin (℞)

(dak-ti-noe-mye'sin)

Cosmegen

Func. class.: Antineoplastic, antibiotic

Do not confuse:
dactinomycin/daptomycin

Action: Inhibits DNA, RNA, protein synthesis; derived from *Streptomyces parvullus;* replication is decreased by binding to DNA, which causes strand splitting; cell cycle nonspecific; a vesicant

Uses: Sarcomas, trophoblastic tumors in women, testicular cancer, Wilms' tumor, rhabdomyosarcoma

Unlabeled uses: Kaposi's sarcoma, malignant melanoma, osteogenic sarcoma, ovarian cancer, soft tissue sarcoma

DOSAGE AND ROUTES

- *Adult:* **IV** 500 mcg/m^2/day × 5 days; stop product for 2-4 wk; then repeat cycle
- *Child:* **IV** 15 mcg/kg/day × 5 days, not to exceed 500 mcg/day; stop product until bone marrow recovery, then repeat cycle

Choriocarcinoma/hydatidiform mole

- *Adult:* **IV** 1250 mcg/m^2 q14days × 4 cycles

Wilms' tumor/childhood rhabdomyosarcoma/Ewing's sarcoma

- *Adult and child:* **IV** 15 mcg/kg/day × 5 days

Germ cell testicular cancer

- *Adult and child:* **IV** 1000 mcg/m^2 as a single dose on day 1

Malignant melanoma (unlabeled)

- *Adult:* **IV** 1-1.5 mg/m^2

Soft tissue sarcoma/Kaposi's sarcoma (unlabeled)
- *Adult:* **CONT IV INF** 15 mcg/kg/day × 5 days q3mo

Germ testicular/ovarian cancer (unlabeled)
- *Adult and child:* **IV** 1000 mcg/m^2 as a single dose on day 1, used with VAB-6 regimen

Available forms: Inj 0.5 mg/vial

SIDE EFFECTS

CNS: Malaise, fatigue, lethargy, fever
EENT: Chelitis, dysphagia, esophagitis
GI: *Nausea, vomiting, anorexia, stomatitis,* **hepatotoxicity**, abdominal pain, diarrhea
HEMA: **Thrombocytopenia, leukopenia, aplastic anemia**
INTEG: *Rash,* alopecia, pain at inj site, folliculitis, acne, desquamation, **extravasation**
MS: Myalgia

Contraindications: Children <6 mo, hypersensitivity, herpes infection

Black Box Warning: Pregnancy (D)

Precautions: Breastfeeding, renal/hepatic disease, bone marrow depression, tumor lysis syndrome, infection

Black Box Warning: Accidental exposure, extravasation, secondary malignancy

PHARMACOKINETICS

Half-life 36 hr; IV onset 2-5 min; concentrates in kidneys, liver, spleen; does not cross blood-brain barrier; excreted in feces and urine

INTERACTIONS

Increase: toxicity—other antineoplastics, radiation

Drug/Lab Test

Increase: uric acid

NURSING CONSIDERATIONS

Assess:
- CBC, differential, platelet count weekly; withhold product if WBC is <4000/mm^3 or platelet count is <75,000/mm^3; notify prescriber
- Renal studies: BUN, serum uric acid, urine CCr, electrolytes before, during therapy
- I&O ratio; report fall in urine output to <30 ml/hr
- Monitor temp q4hr; fever may indicate beginning infection
- Hepatic studies before, during therapy: bilirubin, AST, ALT, alk phos, as needed or monthly; check for jaundice of skin, sclera; dark urine; clay-colored stools; itchy skin; abdominal pain; fever; diarrhea
- Bleeding: hematuria, guaiac stools, bruising, petechiae, mucosa or orifices q8hr
- Food preferences; list likes, dislikes
- Effects of alopecia on body image; discuss feelings about body changes
- Inflammation of mucosa, breaks in skin
- Buccal cavity q8hr for dryness, sores, ulceration, white patches, oral pain, bleeding, dysphagia
- ⚠ Symptoms indicating severe allergic reaction: rash, pruritus, urticaria, purpuric skin lesions, itching, flushing
- GI symptoms: frequency of stools, cramping, nausea, vomiting, anorexia
- Acidosis, signs of dehydration: rapid respirations, poor skin turgor, decreased urine output, dry skin, restlessness, weakness, sunken eyeball in children

Administer:
- Antiemetic 30-60 min before giving product to prevent vomiting
- Increase fluids to 3 L/day

IV route
- After diluting 0.5 mg/1.1 ml of sterile H_2O for inj without preservative; use 2.2 ml (0.25 mg/ml), give by direct IV at 0.5 mg or less/min through Y-tube or 3-way stopcock if inf in progress; may be further diluted if required in 50 ml D_5W or NS for inf; run over 10-15 min; change needles between reconstitution and direct IV administration
- Hydrocortisone, sodium thiosulfate to infiltration area, and ice compress after stopping infusion

Y-site compatibilities: Allopurinol, amifostine, aztreonam, cefepime, fludarabine, granisetron, melphalan, ondansetron, sargramostim, teniposide, thiotepa, vinorelbine

Perform/provide:

- Strict hand-washing technique, gloves and protective covering
- Liquid diet: carbonated beverages; gelatin may be added if patient is not nauseated or vomiting
- Rinsing of mouth tid-qid with water, club soda; brushing of teeth bid-qid with soft brush or cotton-tipped applicators for stomatitis; use unwaxed dental floss to prevent injury
- Storage in cool, dark environment; do not expose to bright light or freeze
- Fluid increase to 3 L/day

Evaluate:

- Therapeutic response: decreased tumor size, spread of malignancy

Teach patient/family:

- That reliable contraception is needed during treatment and for 4-6 mo after discontinuing therapy; do not breastfeed
- To avoid vaccinations without order by prescriber
- That hair may be lost during treatment after 1-2 wk and that wig or hairpiece may make patient feel better; that new hair may be different in color, texture
- To avoid foods with citric acid, hot or rough texture when stomatitis is present
- To report any bleeding, white spots, ulcerations in mouth to prescriber; tell patient to examine mouth daily
- To avoid crowds, persons with known infection when granulocyte count is low

⚠ High Alert

dalteparin (℞)

(dahl'ta-pear-in)

Fragmin

Func. class.: Anticoagulant

Chem. class.: Low molecular weight heparin

Action: Inhibits factor Xa/IIa (thrombin) resulting in anticoagulation

Uses: Unstable angina/non–Q-wave MI; prevention of deep vein thrombosis in abdominal surgery, hip replacement or those with restricted mobility during acute illness, PE

Unlabeled uses: Antiphospholipid antibody, arterial thromboembolism (after heart valve surgery), cerebral thromboembolism

DOSAGE AND ROUTES

Hip replacement surgery/DVT prophylaxis

- *Adult:* **SUBCUT** 2500 international units 2 hr prior to surgery and 2nd dose in the evening the day of surgery (4-8 hr postop), then 5000 international units **SUBCUT** 1st postop day and daily 5-10 days

Unstable angina/non–Q-wave MI

- *Adult:* **SUBCUT** 120 international units/kg q12hr × 5-8 days, max 10,000 international units q12hr × 5-8 days, with concurrent aspirin, continue until stable

DVT, prophylaxis for abdominal surgery

- *Adult:* **SUBCUT** 2500 international units 1-2 hr prior to surgery and repeat daily × 5-10 days; in high-risk patients 5000 international units should be used

APLA (unlabeled)

- *Adult (female):* **SUBCUT** Antepartum 5000 international units/day with aspirin, maintain anti-factor Xa of 0.2-0.6 international units/ml

Cerebral thromboembolism (unlabeled)

- *Adult:* **SUBCUT** 120 international units/kg (max 10,000 international units) q12hr × 5-8 days, usually with aspirin therapy

Arterial thromboembolism prophylaxis (unlabeled)

• *Adult:* **SUBCUT** LMWH in combination with oral anticoagulants until INR is in therapeutic range × 2 consecutive days

Available forms: Prefilled syringes, 2500, 5000 international units/0.2 ml; 7500 international units/0.3 ml, 10,000, 25,000 international units/ml

SIDE EFFECTS

CNS: **Intracranial bleeding**

HEMA: **Thrombocytopenia**

INTEG: Pruritus, superficial wound infection

SYST: Hypersensitivity, **hemorrhage, anaphylaxis** possible

Contraindications: Hypersensitivity to this product, heparin, or pork products, benzyl alcohol; active major bleeding, hemophilia, leukemia with bleeding, thrombocytopenic purpura, cerebrovascular hemorrhage, cerebral aneurysm, those undergoing regional anesthesia for unstable angina, non–Q-wave MI, dalteparin-induced thrombocytopenia

Precautions: Pregnancy (B), breastfeeding, children, recent childbirth, geriatric patients; hepatic disease; severe renal disease; blood dyscrasias; bacterial endocarditis; acute nephritis; uncontrolled hypertension; recent brain, spine, eye surgery; congenital or acquired disorders; severe cardiac disease; peptic ulcer disease; hemorrhagic stroke; history of HIT; pericarditis; pericardial effusion; recent lumbar puncture; vasculitis; other diseases in which bleeding is possible

Black Box Warning: Epidural anesthesia

PHARMACOKINETICS

87% absorbed, excreted by kidneys, elimination half-life 3-5 hr, peak 4 hr, onset 1-2 hr, duration >12 hr

INTERACTIONS

Increase: bleeding risk—aspirin, oral anticoagulants, platelet inhibitors, NSAIDs, salicylates, thrombolytics

Drug/Herb

Increase: bleeding risk—agrimony, alfalfa, angelica, anise, bilberry, black haw, bogbean, bromelain, buchu, chondroitin, cinchona bark, dong quai, fenugreek, feverfew, garlic, ginger, ginkgo, ginseng, horse chestnut, Irish moss, kelp, kelpware, khella, lovage, lungwort, meadowsweet, motherwort, mugwort, nettle, papaya, parsley (large amts), pau d'arco, pineapple, poplar, prickly ash, safflower, saw palmetto, senega, tonka bean, turmeric, wintergreen, yarrow

Decrease: anticoagulant action—chamomile, coenzyme Q10, flax, glucomannan, goldenseal, guar gum

Drug/Lab Test

Increase: AST, ALT

NURSING CONSIDERATIONS

Assess:

• For blood studies (Hct, CBC, platelets, occult blood in stools) during treatment since bleeding can occur

⚠ For bleeding gums, petechiae, ecchymosis, black tarry stools, hematuria, epistaxis, decrease in Hct, B/P; may indicate bleeding, possible hemorrhage; notify prescriber immediately, product should be discontinued

⚠ For neurologic impairment frequently in those when neuraxial anesthesia has been used, spinal/epidural hematomas can occur, with paralysis

• For hypersensitivity: fever, skin rash, urticaria; notify prescriber immediately

• For needed dosage change q1-2wk; dose may need to be decreased if bleeding occurs

Administer:

• Cannot be used interchangeably (unit for unit) with unfractionated heparin or LMWHs

• Do not give IM or IV product route; approved is SUBCUT only; do not mix with other inj or sol
• Have patient sit or lie down; SUBCUT inj may be 2 inches from umbilicus in a U-shape, upper outer side of thigh, around navel, or upper outer quadrangle of the buttocks; rotate inj sites
• Changing needles is not recommended; change inj site daily; use at same time of day

Evaluate:
• Therapeutic response: absence of DVT

Teach patient/family:
• To avoid OTC preparations that contain aspirin; other anticoagulants, serious product interaction may occur unless approved by prescriber
• To use soft-bristle toothbrush to avoid bleeding gums, avoid contact sports, use electric razor, avoid IM inj
• To report any signs of bleeding: gums, under skin, urine, stools; unusual bruising

Treatment of overdose: Protamine sulfate 1% given IV; 1 mg protamine/100 anti-Xa international units of dalteparin given

dantrolene (℞)

(dan'troe-leen)
Dantrium
Func. class.: Skeletal muscle relaxant, direct acting
Chem. class.: Hydantoin

Do not confuse:
Dantrium/danazol

Action: Interferes with intracellular release of calcium from the sarcoplasmic reticulum necessary to initiate contraction; slows catabolism in malignant hyperthermia

Uses: Spasticity in multiple sclerosis, stroke, spinal cord injury, cerebral palsy, malignant hyperthermia

Unlabeled uses: Neuroleptic malignant syndrome

DOSAGE AND ROUTES

Spasticity
• *Adult:* **PO** 25 mg/day; may increase to 25-100 mg bid-qid, max 400 mg/day
• *Child:* **PO** 0.5 mg/kg/day given in divided doses bid; dosage may increase gradually, not to exceed 400 mg/day

Prevention of malignant hyperthermia
• *Adult and child:* **PO** 4-8 mg/kg/day in 3-4 divided doses × 1-2 days prior to procedures, give last dose 4 hr preop; **IV** 2.5 mg/kg prior to anesthesia

Malignant hyperthermia
• *Adult and child:* **IV** 1 mg/kg, may repeat to total dose of 10 mg/kg; **PO** 4-8 mg/kg/day in 4 divided doses × 3 days to prevent further hyperthermia; post-crisis follow-up 4-8 mg/kg/day for 1-3 days

Neuroleptic malignant syndrome (unlabeled)
• *Adult:* **PO** 100-300 mg/day in divided doses; **IV** 1.25-1.5 mg/kg

Available forms: Caps 25, 50, 100 mg; powder for inj 20 mg/vial

SIDE EFFECTS

CNS: *Dizziness, weakness, fatigue, drowsiness,* headache, disorientation, insomnia, paresthesias, tremors, **seizures**
CV: Hypotension, chest pain, palpitations
EENT: Nasal congestion, blurred vision, mydriasis
GI: **Hepatic injury,** *nausea,* constipation, vomiting, increased AST, alk phos, abdominal pain, dry mouth, anorexia, hepatitis, dyspepsia
GU: Urinary frequency, nocturia, impotence, crystalluria
HEMA: **Eosinophilia, aplastic anemia, leukopenia**
INTEG: Rash, pruritus, photosensitivity, extravasation (tissue necrosis)
RESP: Pleural effusion

Contraindications: Hypersensitivity, compromised pulmonary function, impaired myocardial function

Black Box Warning: Active hepatic disease

Precautions: Pregnancy (C), breastfeeding, geriatric patients, peptic ulcer disease, cardiac/renal/hepatic disease, stroke, seizure disorder, diabetes mellitus, ALS, COPD, MS, mannitol/gelatin hypersensitivity, labor, lactase deficiency, extravasation

Black Box Warning: Females

PHARMACOKINETICS

PO: Peak 5 hr, highly protein bound, half-life 8 hr, metabolized in liver, excreted in urine (metabolites), absorption poor (35%)

INTERACTIONS

• Considered incompatible in sol or syringe; compatibility unknown

Increase: dysrhythmias—verapamil

Increase: hepatotoxicity—estrogens, other hepatotoxics

Increase: CNS depression—alcohol, tricyclics, opiates, barbiturates, sedatives, hypnotics, antihistamines

NURSING CONSIDERATIONS

Assess:

• For increased seizure activity, ECG in epilepsy patient; poor seizure control has occurred

• I&O ratio; check for urinary retention, frequency, hesitancy, especially geriatric patients

• Hepatic function by frequent determination of AST, ALT, bilirubin, alk phos, GGTP; renal function studies, BUN, creatinine, CBC

• Allergic reactions: rash, fever, respiratory distress

• Severe weakness, numbness in extremities; prescriber should be notified and product discontinued

• Tolerance: increased need for medication, more frequent requests for medication, increased pain

• CNS depression: dizziness, drowsiness, insomnia, psychiatric symptoms

⚠ Signs of hepatotoxicity: jaundice, yellow sclera, pain in abdomen, nausea, fever; prescriber should be notified, product should be discontinued

Administer:

• Avoid use with other CNS depressants

PO route

• Do not crush or chew caps

• Caps may be opened, mixed with juice and swallowed

• With meals for GI symptoms

IV route

• IV after diluting 20 mg/60 ml sterile H_2O for inj without bacteriostatic agent (333 mcg/ml); shake until clear; give by rapid IV push through Y-tube or 3-way stopcock; follow by prescribed doses immediately; may also give by intermittent inf over 1 hr prior to anesthesia

Perform/provide:

• Storage in tight container at room temperature; protect diluted sol from light, use reconstituted solution within 6 hr

• Gum, frequent sips of water for dry mouth

• Assistance with ambulation if dizziness/drowsiness occurs

Evaluate:

• Therapeutic response: decreased pain, spasticity

Teach patient/family:

• Not to discontinue medication quickly; hallucinations, spasticity, tachycardia will occur; product should be tapered off over 1-2 wk; notify prescriber of abdominal pain, jaundiced sclera, clay-colored stools, change in color of urine

• That if improvement does not occur within 6 wk, prescriber may discontinue

• To avoid hazardous activities if drowsiness, dizziness occurs

• To avoid using OTC medication: cough preparations, antihistamines, other CNS depressants, alcohol, unless directed by prescriber

• To use sunscreen or stay out of the sun to prevent burns

Treatment of overdose: Activated charcoal, supportive care

dapiprazole ophthalmic

See Appendix B

daptomycin (℞)

(dap'toe-mye-sin)

Cubicin

Func. class.: Antiinfective—miscellaneous

Chem. class.: Lipopeptides

Action: A new class of antiinfective; it binds to the bacterial membrane and results in a rapid depolarization of the membrane potential, thus leading to inhibition of DNA, RNA, and protein synthesis

Uses: Complicated skin, skin structure infections caused by *Staphylococcus aureus* including methicillin-resistant strains, *Streptococcus pyogenes, Streptococcus agalactiae, Streptococcus dysgalactiae, Enterococcus faecalis* (vancomycin-susceptible strains)

Unlabeled uses: Bacteremia endocarditis, UTI, vancomycin-resistant enterococci (VRE), *Corynebacterium jeikeium, Staphylococcus haemolyticus, Enterococcus facium*

DOSAGE AND ROUTES

- *Adult:* **IV INF** 4 mg/kg over ½ hr diluted in 0.9% NaCl, give q24hr × 7-14 days
- *Adolescent/child/infant* ≥*5 mo (unlabeled):* **IV** 4-6 mg/kg/day

Renal dose

- *Adult:* **IV INF** CCr <30 ml/min, hemodialysis, CAPD 4 mg/kg q48hr

Bacteremia, endocarditis, UTI (unlabeled)

- *Adult:* **IV** 6 mg/kg/day

VRE (unlabeled)

- *Adult:* **IV** 4 mg/kg/day

Available forms: Lyophilized powder for inj 500 mg

SIDE EFFECTS

CNS: Headache, insomnia, dizziness, confusion, anxiety, fatigue, fever

CV: Hypo/hypertension, **heart failure,** chest pain

GI: Nausea, constipation, diarrhea, vomiting, dyspepsia, **pseudomembranous colitis,** abdominal pain

GU: **Nephrotoxicity**

HEMA: **Leukocytosis, anemia, thrombocytopenia**

INTEG: Rash, pruritus

MISC: Fungal infections, UTI, anemia

MS: Muscle pain or weakness, arthralgia, pain, **rhabdomyolysis**

RESP: Cough

SYST: **Anaphylaxis**

Contraindications: Hypersensitivity

Precautions: Pregnancy (B), breastfeeding, children, geriatric patients, GI/renal disease, myopathy, ulcerative/pseudomembranous colitis, rhabdomyolysis

PHARMACOKINETICS

Site of metabolism unknown, protein binding 92%, terminal half-life 8-9 hr, 78% excreted unchanged (urine)

INTERACTIONS

Increase: myopathy—HMG-CoA reductase inhibitors

Drug/Lab Test

Increase: CPK, AST, ALT, BUN, creatinine, albumin

NURSING CONSIDERATIONS

Assess:

- I&O ratio: report hematuria, oliguria, serum creatinine, BUN; nephrotoxicity may occur

⚠ Any patient with compromised renal system, toxicity may occur; BUN, creatinine

- Blood studies: CBC, CPK
- C&S, product may be given as soon as culture is taken
- B/P during administration; hypo/hypertension may occur
- Signs of infection
- Respiratory status: rate, character, wheezing
- Allergies before treatment, reaction of each medication

Administer:

IV route

- After reconstitution with 5 ml 0.9% NaCl (250 mg/5 ml) or 10 ml 0.9% NaCl (500 mg/10 ml), further dilution is needed with 0.9 NaCl, infuse over ½ hr

Solution compatibilities: 0.9% NaCl, LR

Evaluate:

- Therapeutic response: Negative culture

Teach patient/family:

- Allergies before treatment, reaction of each medication
- To report sore throat, fever, fatigue, could indicate superinfection

darbepoetin (℞)

(dar'bee-poh'eh-tin)

Aranesp

Func. class.: Hematopoietic agent

Chem. class.: Recombinant human erythropoietin

Action: Stimulates erythropoiesis by the same mechanism as endogenous erythropoietin; in response to hypoxia, erythropoietin is produced in the kidney and released into the bloodstream, where it interacts with progenitor stem cells to increase red cell production

Uses: Anemia associated with chronic renal failure, in patients on and not on dialysis, and anemia in nonmyeloid malignancies receiving coadministered chemotherapy

DOSAGE AND ROUTES

Correction of anemia in chronic renal failure

- *Adult:* **SUBCUT/IV** 0.45 mcg/kg as a single inj; every week titrate not to exceed a target Hgb of 12 g/dl

Chemotherapy treatment

- *Adult:* **SUBCUT** 2.25 mcg/kg/wk or 500 mcg q3wk

Epoetin alfa to darbepoetin conversion

- *Adult:* **SUBCUT/IV** (epoetin alfa <2500 units/wk) 6.25 mcg/wk; (epoetin alfa 2500-4999 units/wk) 12.5 mcg/wk; (epoetin alfa 5000-10,999 units/wk) 25 mcg/wk; (epoetin alfa 11,000-17,999 units/wk) 40 mcg/wk; (epoetin alfa 18,000-33,999 units/wk) 60 mcg/wk; (epoetin alfa 34,000-89,999 units/wk) 100 mcg/wk; (epoetin alfa >90,000 units/wk) 200 mcg/wk

Available forms: Sol for inj 25, 40, 60, 100, 150, 200, 300, 500 mcg/ml

SIDE EFFECTS

CNS: **Seizures**, sweating, headache, dizziness, **stroke**

CV: Hypo/hypertension, **cardiac arrest,** *angina pectoris,* **thrombosis, CHF, acute MI, dysrhythmias,** chest pain, transient ischemic attacks, edema

GI: Diarrhea, vomiting, nausea, abdominal pain, constipation

HEMA: **Red cell aplasia**

MISC: Infection, fatigue, fever, **death,** *fluid overload,* **vascular access hemorrhage,** dehydration, **sepsis**

MS: Bone pain, myalgia, limb pain, back pain

RESP: URI, dyspnea, cough, bronchitis, **PE**

SYST: Allergic reactions, **anaphylaxis**

Contraindications: Hypersensitivity to mammalian cell–derived products or human albumin, uncontrolled hypertension, red cell aplasia

Precautions: Pregnancy (C), breastfeeding, children, seizure disorder, porphyria, hypertension, sickle cell disease; vit B_{12}, folate deficiency, chronic renal failure, dialysis, latex hypersensitivity, CABG, angina, anemia

Black Box Warning: Hgb >12 g/dl, surgery

PHARMACOKINETICS

IV: Onset of increased reticulocyte count 2-6 wk; distributed to vascular space; absorption slow and rate-limiting; terminal half-life 49 hr (SUBCUT), 21 hr (IV); peak concentration at 34 hr; increased Hgb levels not generally observed until 2-6 wk after treatment initiated

INTERACTIONS

⚠ Do not use epoetin alfa with this product

Increase: darbepoetin alfa effect—androgens

Drug/Lab Test

Increase: WBC, platelets

Decrease: bleeding time

NURSING CONSIDERATIONS

Assess:

- For symptoms of anemia: fatigue, dyspnea, pallor

⚠ Serious allergic reactions: rash, urticaria; if anaphylaxis occurs, stop product, administer emergency treatment (rare)

- Renal studies: urinalysis, protein, blood, BUN, creatinine; monitor dialysis shunts; during dialysis, heparin may need to be increased
- Blood studies: ferritin, transferrin q mo; transferrin sat ≥20%, ferritin ≥100 ng/ml; Hgb 2×/wk until stabilized in target range (30%-33%), then at regular intervals; those with endogenous erythropoietin levels of <500 units/L respond to this agent; iron stores should be corrected before beginning therapy
- B/P; check for rising B/P as Hgb rises, antihypertensives may be needed

⚠ CV status: hypertension may occur rapidly leading to hypertensive encephalopathy; Hgb >12 g/dl may lead to death

- I&O; report drop in output to <50 ml/hr
- For seizures if Hgb is increased within 2 wk by 4 pts institute seizure precautions
- CNS symptoms: sweating, pain in long bones
- Dialysis patients: thrill, bruit of shunts, monitor for circulation impairment

Administer:

SUBCUT/IV route

- Without shaking; check for discoloration, particulate matter, do not use if present; do not dilute, do not mix with other products or solutions, discard unused portion, do not pool unused portions
- Subcut is typically used with those not requiring dialysis
- IV is given undiluted as direct, or bolus into IV tubing or venous line after completion of dialysis
- Adjust dosage every month or more

Evaluate:

- Therapeutic response: increase in reticulocyte count, Hgb/Hct; increased appetite, enhanced sense of well-being

Teach patient/family:

- To avoid driving or hazardous activity during beginning of treatment
- To monitor B/P, Hgb
- To take iron supplements, vit B_{12}, folic acid as directed
- To report side effects to prescriber, to comply with treatment regimen
- That menses and fertility may return; use contraception if want to
- Home administration procedures, if appropriate

darunavir (℞)

(dar-ue′na-vir)

Prezista

Func. class.: Antiretroviral

Chem. class.: Protease inhibitor

Action: Inhibits human immunodeficiency virus (HIV-1) protease; this prevents maturation of virus

Uses: HIV-1 in combination with ritonavir and other antiretrovirals

DOSAGE AND ROUTES

Treatment-Naive Patients

- *Adult:* **PO** 800 mg with ritonavir 100 mg daily

Treatment-Experienced Patients

- *Adult/child ≥6 yr/adolescent >40 kg:* **PO** 600 mg bid; with ritonavir 100 mg bid with food
- *Adolescent ≥30 kg, <40 kg and child ≥6:* **PO** 450 mg bid with ritonavir 60 mg bid

• *Adolescent ≥20 kg, <30 kg and child ≥6 yr:* **PO** 375 mg bid with ritonavir 50 mg bid

Available forms: Tabs 75, 150, 300, 400, 600 mg

SIDE EFFECTS

CNS: Headache, insomnia, dizziness, somnolence

GI: Diarrhea, abdominal pain, nausea, vomiting, anorexia, dry mouth

GU: Nephrolithiasis

INTEG: Rash

MS: Pain

OTHER: Asthenia, **insulin-resistant hyperglycemia,** hyperlipidemia, **ketoacidosis,** lipodystrophy

Contraindications: Hypersensitivity

Precautions: Pregnancy (B), breastfeeding, children, renal/hepatic disease, history of renal stones, diabetes, hypercholesterolemia, sulfonamide hypersensitivity, antimicrobial resistance, bleeding, elderly, immune reconstitution syndrome, pancreatitis

PHARMACOKINETICS

95% protein binding; metabolized by CYP3A; peak 2.5-4 hr; terminal half-life 15 hr; excreted in feces 79.5%, urine 13.9%

INTERACTIONS

⚠ Life-threatening dysrhythmias: ergots, midazolam, rifampin, pimozide, triazolam; do not use concurrently

Increase: myopathy—HMG-CoA reductase inhibitors (atorvastatin, lovastatin, simvastatin)

Increase: darunavir levels—CYP3A4 inhibitors: (ketoconazole, itraconazole)

Increase: levels of both products—clarithromycin, zidovudine

Decrease: darunavir levels—CYP3A4 inducers: (carbamazepine, phenytoin, fosphenytoin, phenobarbital), rifamycins, fluconazole, nevirapine, efavirenz

Decrease: levels of oral contraceptives

Drug/Herb

Decrease: darunavir levels—St. John's wort; avoid concurrent use

Drug/Food

Increase: darunavir absorption

NURSING CONSIDERATIONS

Assess:

• For complaints of lower back, flank pain; indicates kidney stones

• Signs of infection, anemia, the presence of other sexually transmitted diseases

• Hepatic studies: ALT, AST, bilirubin, amylase; all may be elevated

• Viral load, CD4 during treatment

• Bowel pattern before, during treatment; if severe abdominal pain with bleeding occurs, product should be discontinued; monitor hydration

• Skin eruptions: rash, urticaria, itching

• Allergies before treatment, reaction of each medication; place allergies on chart

Administer:

• With food and ritonavir

• Water to 1.5 L/day minimum to prevent nephrolithiasis

Evaluate:

• Therapeutic response: decreased viral load and increased CD4 count

Teach patient/family:

• To use nonhormonal birth control

• To take as prescribed; if dose is missed, take as soon as remembered up to 1 hr before next dose; do not double dose

• That product must be taken in equal intervals around the clock to maintain blood levels for duration of therapy

⚠ That hyperglycemia may occur; watch for increased thirst, weight loss, hunger, dry, itchy skin; notify prescriber

• To increase fluids to prevent kidney stones; if stone formation occurs, treatment may need to be interrupted

• That product does not cure AIDS, only controls symptoms; do not donate blood

dasatinib (℞)

(da-si'ti-nib)

Sprycel

Func. class.: Antineoplastic—miscellaneous

Chem. class.: Protein-tyrosine kinase inhibitor

Action: Inhibits BCR-ABL, SRC, LCK, YES, FYN, C-KIT, $EPHA_2$, and PDGFR-β tyrosine kinase created in chronic myeloid leukemia (CML)

Uses: Treatment of accelerated, chronic blast phase CML or acute lymphoblastic leukemia (ALL); chronic phase CML with resistance or intolerance to prior therapy

DOSAGE AND ROUTES

Accelerated or myeloid/lymphoid blast phase CML with resistance/intolerance to prior therapy

- *Adult:* **PO** 140 mg daily, titrated up to 180 mg bid in those resistant to therapy

Chronic phase CML with resistance/intolerance to prior therapy

- *Adult:* **PO** 100 mg daily either AM or PM

Dosage reduction for those taking a strong CYP3A4 inhibitor

- *Adult:* **PO** 20 mg daily

Available forms: Tabs 20, 50, 70, 100 mg

SIDE EFFECTS

CNS: **CNS hemorrhage,** headache, dizziness, insomnia, neuropathy, asthenia

CV: Dsyrhythmias, chest pain, CHF, pericardial effusion

GI: Nausea, **vomiting,** *anorexia, abdominal pain,* constipation, diarrhea, GI bleeding, muscositis, stomatitis

HEMA: **Neutropenia, thrombocytopenia, bleeding**

INTEG: Rash, pruritus

META: Fluid retention, edema, hypocalcemia, hypophosphatemia

MISC: Increased/decreased weight

MS: Pain, arthralgia, myalgia

RESP: Cough, dyspnea, pulmonary edema/hypertension, pneumonia, upper respiratory tract infection, **pleural effusion**

Contraindications: Pregnancy (D), hypersensitivity

Precautions: Breastfeeding, children, geriatric patients, QT prolongation, infection, thrombocytopenia, accidental exposure, edema, infertility, lactase deficiency, neutropenia

PHARMACOKINETICS

Metabolized by CYP3A4; 96% protein bound; peak 0.5-6 hr; excreted in feces (85%), small amount in urine (4%); terminal half-life 1.3-5 hr

INTERACTIONS

- Altered action of CYP3A4 substrates: alfentanil, cycloSPORINE, ergots, fentanyl, pimozide, quinidine, sirolimus, tacrolimus

Increase: dasatinib concentrations—ketoconazole, itraconazole, erythromycin, clarithromycin, nefazodone, protease inhibitors, telithromycin

Increase: plasma concentrations of simvastatin

Increase: QT prolongation—class IA/III antidysrhythmics and other drugs that increase QT prolongation

Decrease: dasatinib concentrations—CYP3A4 inducers (dexamethasone, phenytoin, carbamazepine, rifampin, phenobarbital), H_2 blockers (famotidine), proton pump inhibitors (omeprazole)

Drug/Herb

Decrease: dasatinib concentration—St. John's wort

NURSING CONSIDERATIONS

Assess:

- ANC and platelets; in chronic phase if ANC $<1 \times 10^9$/L and/or platelets $<50 \times 10^9$/L, stop until ANC $>1.5 \times 10^9$/L and platelets $>75 \times 10^9$/L; in accelerated phase/blast crisis if ANC $<0.5 \times 10^9$/L and/or platelets $<10 \times 10^9$/L, determine whether cytopenia is related to biopsy/aspirate, if not, reduce dose by 200 mg, if cytopenia continues, reduce dose by another 100 mg; if cytopenia continues for 4 wk, stop product until ANC ≥1 × 10^9/L

• For renal toxicity: if bilirubin >3 × IULN, withhold until bilirubin levels return to <1.5 × IULN

• For hepatotoxicity: monitor LFTs, before treatment and q mo; if liver transaminases >5 × IULN, withhold until transaminase levels return to <2.5 × IULN

• CBC, differential, platelet count weekly; withhold product if WBC is <3500/mm^3, or platelet count <100,000/mm^3; notify prescriber of these results; product should be discontinued

• Signs of fluid retention, edema: weigh, monitor lung sounds, assess for edema, some fluid retention is dose dependent

Administer:

• Do not break, crush, or chew tab

• After meal and with large glass of water

Perform/provide:

• Nutritious diet with iron, vitamin supplement

• Storage at 25° C (77° F)

Evaluate:

• Therapeutic response: decrease in leukemic cells or size of tumor

Teach patient/family:

• To report adverse reactions immediately: SOB, swelling of extremities, bleeding

• Reason for treatment, expected result

• To use contraception; pregnancy category (D)

High Alert

*DAUNOrubicin (℞)

(daw-noe-roo′bi-sin)

Cerubidine

*DAUNOrubicin citrate liposomal (℞)

DaunoXome

Func. class.: Antineoplastic, antibiotic

Chem. class.: Anthracycline glycoside

Do not confuse:

DAUNOrubicin/DOXOrubicin

Action: Inhibits DNA synthesis, primarily; derived from *Streptomyces coerulorubidus;* replication is decreased by binding to DNA, which causes strand splitting; cell cycle specific (S phase); a vesicant

Uses: Acute lymphocytic leukemia (ALL), acute myelogenous leukemia (AML); *liposomal:* Karposi's sarcoma

Unlabeled uses: *Liposomal:* Multiple myeloma, AML, breast cancer, non-Hodgkin's lymphoma

DOSAGE AND ROUTES

Use decreased dose for those >60 yr of age

DAUNOrubicin

• *Adult:* **IV** 45-60 mg/m^2/day × 3 days, then 2 days of subsequent courses in combination

• *Child:* **IV** 25-60 mg/m^2 depending on cycle

DAUNOrubicin citrate liposomal

• *Adult:* **IV** 40 mg/m^2 q2wk

Renal dose

• *Adult:* **IV** Serum CCr >3 mg/dl reduce dose by 50%

Hepatic dose

• *Adult:* **IV** Serum bilirubin 1.2-3 mg/dl reduce dose by 25%; bilirubin >3 mg/dl reduce dose by 50%

Available forms: Inj 20 mg powder/vial, sol for inj 5 mg/ml (DaunoXome); *liposomal:* dispersion for inj 2 mg/ml

SIDE EFFECTS

DAUNOrubicin

CNS: Fever, chills
CV: **Dysrhythmias, CHF, pericarditis, myocarditis,** peripheral edema
GI: Nausea, vomiting, anorexia, mucositis, **hepatotoxicity**
GU: Impotence, sterility, amenorrhea, gynecomastia, hyperuricemia
HEMA: **Thrombocytopenia, leukopenia, anemia**
INTEG: Rash, **extravasation,** dermatitis, reversible alopecia, cellulitis, thrombophlebitis at inj site
SYST: **Anaphylaxis**

DAUNOrubicin citrate liposomal

CNS: Fatigue, headache, depression, insomnia, dizziness, *malaise, neuropathy*
CV: Chest pain, edema
GI: Abdominal pain, stomatitis, *nausea, vomiting, diarrhea,* constipation
INTEG: Alopecia, pruritus, sweating
MISC: Allergic reactions, chest pain, fever, edema, flulike symptoms
MS: Rigors, arthralgia, back pain
RESP: Cough, dyspnea, rhinitis, sinusitis

Contraindications: Pregnancy (D), breastfeeding, hypersensitivity, systemic infections, cardiac disease, bone marrow depression

Precautions: Tumor lysis syndrome, MI, infection, thrombocytopenia, renal/hepatic disease; gout

Black Box Warning: Bone marrow suppression, cardiac disease, extravasation, renal failure

PHARMACOKINETICS

Half-life 18½ hr, liposome 55½ hr; metabolized by liver; crosses placenta; excreted in breast milk, urine, bile

INTERACTIONS

Increase: bleeding risk—NSAIDs, salicylates
Increase: toxicity—other antineoplastics, radiation, cyclophosphamide
Decrease: antibody reaction—live virus vaccines

Drug/Lab Test

Increase: uric acid

NURSING CONSIDERATIONS

Assess:

⚠ CBC, differential, platelet count weekly, leukocyte nadir within 2 wk after administration, recovery within 3 wk; do not administer if absolute granulocyte count is <750/mm^3 (liposome)

- Blood, urine uric acid levels baseline and during therapy
- Renal studies: BUN, urine CCr, electrolytes baseline, before each dose
- I&O ratio; report fall in urine output to <30 ml/hr
- Monitor temp q4hr; fever may indicate beginning infection
- Hepatic studies baseline, before each dose: bilirubin, AST, ALT, alk phos; check for jaundice of skin, sclera; dark urine; clay-colored stools; itchy skin; abdominal pain; fever; diarrhea
- Chest x-ray, echocardiography, radionuclide angiography, ECG; watch for ST-T wave changes, low QRS and T, possible dysrhythmias (sinus tachycardia, heart block, PVCs); watch for CHF (jugular vein distention, weight gain, edema, crackles), may occur after 2-6 mo of treatment
- Bleeding: hematuria, guaiac stools, bruising or petechiae, mucosa or orifices q8hr
- Effects of alopecia on body image; discuss feelings about body changes
- Buccal cavity q8hr for dryness, sores or ulceration, white patches, oral pain, bleeding, dysphagia
- Local irritation, pain, burning at inj site
- GI symptoms: frequency of stools, cramping
- Acidosis, signs of dehydration: rapid respirations, poor skin turgor, decreased urine output, dry skin, restlessness, weakness

Administer:

- Antiemetic 30-60 min before giving product and 6-10 hr after treatment to prevent vomiting

• Allopurinol or sodium bicarbonate to reduce uric acid levels, alkalinization of urine

IV route (Cerubidine)

• After diluting 20 mg/4 ml sterile H_2O for inj (5 mg/ml), rotate, further dilute in 10-15 ml 0.9% NaCl; give over 3-5 min by direct IV through Y-tube or 3-way stopcock of inf of D_5 or 0.9% NaCl; or dilute in 50 ml 0.9% NaCl and give over 10-15 min; or dilute in 100 ml and give over 30 min

• Hydrocortisone for extravasation; apply ice compress after stopping inf

Additive compatibilities: Cytarabine/etoposide, hydrocortisone; not recommended for admixing

Solution compatibilities: $D_{3.3}$/0.3% NaCl, D_5W, Normosol R, Ringer's, 0.9% NaCl

Y-site compatibilities: Amifostine, filgrastim, granisetron, melphalan, methotrexate, ondansetron, sodium bicarbonate, teniposide, thiotepa, vinorelbine

IV route (DaunoXome)

• Dilute with D_5W to (1 mg/ml) give over 60 min, do not use in-line filter, reconstituted sol may be stored ≤6 hr refrigerated; do not admix

Perform/provide:

• Increased fluid intake to 2-3 L/day to prevent urate and calculi formation

• Rinsing of mouth tid-qid with water, club soda; brushing of teeth bid-qid with soft brush or cotton-tipped applicators for stomatitis; use unwaxed dental floss

Evaluate:

• Therapeutic response: decreased tumor size, spread of malignancy

Teach patient/family:

• To report signs of infection, bleeding, bruising, SOB, swelling, change in heart rate

• That hair may be lost during treatment and wig or hairpiece may make patient feel better; tell patient that new hair may be different in color, texture

• To avoid pregnancy while on this product, and 4 mo thereafter; do not breastfeed

• To avoid foods with citric acid, hot or rough texture

• To report any bleeding, white spots, ulcerations in mouth; tell patient to examine mouth daily

• That urine and other body fluids may be red-orange for 48 hr

• To avoid vaccines while taking this product

• To avoid crowds, those with known infections

• To avoid alcohol, aspirin, NSAIDs

decitabine (℞)

(de-sit'-a-been)

Dacogen

Func. class.: DNA demethylation agent

Chem. class.: Cytosine analog

Action: Incorporated into DNA and inhibits DNA methylation, halting growth of rapid proliferation of blasts

Uses: Treatment of naïve and experienced myelodysplasic syndrome

Unlabeled uses: Chronic myelogenous leukemia (CML)

DOSAGE AND ROUTES

• *Adult:* **CONT IV** First treatment cycle: 15 mg/m^2 over 3 hr, q8hr × 3 days; subsequent treatment cycles: repeat above cycle q6wk for at least 4 cycles; a partial or complete response may take more than 4 cycles

Available forms: Powder for injection, lyophilized 50 mg, in single-dose vial

SIDE EFFECTS

CNS: Headache, anxiety, dizziness, hypoesthesia, insomnia, confusion

CV: Edema, murmur, hypotension

GI: Nausea, anorexia, vomiting, diarrhea, constipation, stomatitis, abdominal pain, dyspepsia

HEMA: **Neutropenia, thrombocytopenia, leukopenia, anemia**

INTEG: Alopecia, ecchymosis, erythema, pallor, petechiae, pruritus, rash, swelling face, urticaria, hematoma, cellulitis
META: Decreased potassium, sodium, magnesium, albumin; increased bilirubin, increased/decreased glucose
MS: Myalgia, arthralgia, back pain, chest wall pain, pain in limbs
RESP: Cough, crackles, hypoxia, pharyngitis, pneumonia, pulmonary edema
Contraindications: Pregnancy (D), breastfeeding, children, hypersensitivity to this product, severe neurotoxicity, severe blood dyscrasias
Precautions: Men (men should not father a child while receiving treatments or for 2 mo after treatment ends), severe renal/hepatic disease, dental work, infections, thrombocytopenia

PHARMACOKINETICS

Protein binding <1%; may be metabolized by the liver, granulocytes, intestinal epithelium, whole blood; terminal half-life 0.2-0.8 hr; data is limited

INTERACTIONS

- Do not use with live virus vaccines

NURSING CONSIDERATIONS

Assess:

- CBC (RBC, Hct, Hgb), differential, platelet count weekly; withhold product if WBC <4000/mm^3, platelets <75,000/mm^3, or RBC, Hct, Hgb is low; notify prescriber of results
- Renal studies: BUN, serum uric acid, urine CCr, electrolytes before and during therapy
- Monitor temp q4hr; fever may indicate beginning infection; no rectal temps
- Hepatic studies before and during treatment: bilirubin, AST, ALT, alk phos, as needed or monthly
- Bleeding: hematuria, heme-positive stools, bruising or petechiae, mucosa or orifices daily; blood dyscrasias can occur
- Dyspnea, crackles, unproductive cough, chest pain, tachypnea, fatigue, increased pulse, pallor, lethargy, personality changes
- Buccal cavity daily for dryness, ulceration, white patches, oral pain, bleeding, dysphagia
- GI symptoms: frequency of stools, cramping; if severe diarrhea occurs, electrolytes may need to be given

Administer:

- Use procedures for handling and disposal of products

Perform/provide:

- Rinsing of mouth tid-qid with water or club soda, brushing teeth tid with soft toothbrush or cotton tipped applicator for stomatitis; use unwaxed dental floss
- Storage at room temperature, away from light

Evaluate:

- Therapeutic response: decreased blast count

Teach patient/family:

- To report bleeding; not to use commercial mouthwashes, razors
- To report signs of infection: increased temp, sore throat, flulike symptoms
- To report signs of anemia: fatigue, headache, faintness, SOB, irritability
- To avoid citric acid, rough-textured foods, if stomatitis is present
- To notify prescriber if pregnancy is suspected or planned; use contraception while taking this product
- To avoid breastfeeding while taking this product
- Not to operate machinery or perform other hazardous activities while taking this product
- That men should not father a child while taking this product, pregnancy category (D)
- To inform prescriber of renal/hepatic disease
- Not to receive vaccinations while taking this product
- To drink 2-3 L of fluids per day unless contraindicated

Rarely Used

deferasirox (℞)

(def-a'sir-ox)

Exjade

Func. class.: Heavy metal chelating agent

Uses: Chronic iron overload, transfusion hemosiderosis

DOSAGE AND ROUTES

• *Adult and child >2 yr:* **PO** 20-30 mg/kg/day; oral dispersion tablet is dissolved in water <1 g in 3.5 oz; >1 g in 7 oz or more; give on empty stomach at least 30 min before meals

Contraindications: Breastfeeding, children, hypersensitivity, severe renal/hepatic disease

Rarely Used

deferoxamine (℞)

(de-fer-ox'a-meen)

Desferal

Func. class.: Heavy metal chelator

Do not confuse:
deferoxamine/cefuroxime

Uses: Acute, chronic iron intoxication, hemochromatosis, hemosiderosis

DOSAGE AND ROUTES

Acute iron toxicity

• *Adult and child:* **IM/IV** 1 g, then 500 mg q4hr × 2 doses, then 500 mg q4-12hr as needed, max 15 mg/kg/hr or 6 g/24 hr

Chronic iron toxicity

• *Adult and child:* **IM** 500 mg-1 g/day plus **IV INF** 2 g given by separate line with each unit of blood, max 15 mg/kg/hr or 6 g/24 hr; **SUBCUT** 1-2 g over 8-24 hr by SUBCUT inf pump

Iron overload due to transfusion-dependent anemias

• *Adult:* **IM** 0.5-1 g/day plus **IV** 2 g per unit of blood, max 1 g/day with no blood; 6 g/day with 3 or more units of blood or packed RBC

Contraindications: Children <3 yr, hypersensitivity, anuria, severe renal disease

delavirdine (℞)

(de-la-veer'deen)

Rescriptor

Func. class.: Antiretroviral

Chem. class.: Nonnucleoside reverse transcriptase inhibitor (NNRTI)

Action: Binds directly to reverse transcriptase and blocks RNA, DNA, polymerase, causing a disruption of the enzyme's site

Uses: HIV-1 in combination with other antiretrovirals

DOSAGE AND ROUTES

• *Adult and child ≥16 yr:* **PO** 400 mg tid, max 1200 mg/day

Available forms: Tabs 100, 200 mg

SIDE EFFECTS

CNS: Headache, fatigue, anxiety, insomnia, fever

GI: Diarrhea, abdominal pain, nausea, anorexia, vomiting, dyspepsia, **hepatotoxicity**

GU: **Nephrotoxicity**

HEMA: **Neutropenia, leukopenia, thrombocytopenia, anemia, granulocytopenia**

INTEG: Rash, pruritus

MISC: Cough

MS: Pain, myalgia

SYST: **Stevens-Johnson syndrome**

Contraindications: Hypersensitivity

Precautions: Pregnancy (C), breastfeeding, children, hepatic disease, achlorhydria, antimicrobial resistance, exfoliative dermatitis, hepatitis, immune reconstitution syndrome

PHARMOCOKINETICS:

98% protein bound, half-life 5.8 hr, peak 1 hr, duration 8 hr, extensively metabolized by CYP3A4, excreted in urine/feces

INTERACTIONS

⚠ Serious life-threatening adverse reaction: amphetamines, ergots, benzodiazepines, calcium channel blockers, sedative/hypnotics, antidysrhythmics, sildenafil, pimozide, cisapride, alprazolam, astemizole, midazolam, terfenadine, opiates, triazolam

Increase: levels of alprazolam, clarithromycin, dapsone, ergots, felodipine, midazolam, nifedipine, indinavir, saquinavir, lovastatin, simvastatin, atorvastatin, other CYP3A4, 2D6 inhibitors

Increase: delavirdine levels—fluoxetine, ketoconazole

Increase: levels of both products—quinidine, warfarin, clarithromycin

Decrease: delavirdine levels—antacids, anticonvulsants, rifamycins, protease inhibitors, didanosine

Decrease: action of oral contraceptives, didanosine

Drug/Herb

Decrease: delavirdine level—St. John's wort

NURSING CONSIDERATIONS

Assess:

- For signs of infection, anemia
- Hepatic studies: ALT, AST; renal studies
- C&S before product therapy; product may be taken as soon as culture is taken; repeat C&S after treatment; determine the presence of other sexually transmitted disease
- Bowel pattern before, during treatment; if severe abdominal pain with bleeding occurs, product should be discontinued; monitor hydration
- For skin eruptions; rash, urticaria, itching
- For allergies before treatment, reaction to each medication; place allergies on chart
- Plasma delavirdine concentrations (trough 10 micromolar)
- CBC, blood chemistry, plasma HIV RNA, absolute CD4+/CD8+/cell counts/%, serum β-2 microglobulin, serum ICD+24 antigen levels
- For signs of delavirdine toxicity: severe nausea/vomiting, maculopapular rash

Administer:

- Dispersion by adding 4 tab/3-4 oz water, let stand, stir, swallow, rinse glass, swallow; use only 100 mg tabs for dispersion
- Do not give within 1 hr of antacids or didanosine

Evaluate:

- Therapeutic response: increased CD4 cell count, decreased viral load, improvement in symptoms of HIV

Teach patient/family:

- To take as prescribed; if dose is missed, take as soon as remembered up to 1 hr before next dose; do not double dose
- That tabs may be dissolved in ½ cup of water, stir, when dissolved, drink right away, rinse cup with water, and drink that to get all medication
- To make sure health care provider knows of all the medications being taken
- That if severe rash, mouth sores, swelling, aching muscles/joints, or eye redness occur, stop taking and notify health care provider
- Not to breastfeed if taking this product
- That this product is not a cure, only controls symptoms

demecarium ophthalmic

See Appendix B

denileukin diftitox (℞)

(den-ih-loo'kin dif'tih-tox)
Ontak
Func. class.: Antineoplastic—miscellaneous
Chem. class.: Fusion protein

Action: A recombinant DNA-derived cytotoxic protein that interacts with high-affinity IL-2 receptors on the cell surface and inhibits cellular protein synthesis

Uses: Cutaneous T-cell lymphoma that expresses CD25 component of the IL-2 receptor

Unlabeled uses: Non-Hodgkin's lymphoma, psoriasis

DOSAGE AND ROUTES

- *Adult:* **IV** 9-18 mcg/kg/day given for 5 days q21days, infused over ≥15 min

Available forms: Sol for inj, frozen 150 mcg/ml

SIDE EFFECTS

CNS: Dizziness, paresthesia, nervousness, confusion, insomnia

CV: Hypotension, vasodilation, tachycardia, thrombosis, hypertension, dysrhythmias, capillary leak syndrome

EENT: Persistent visual impairment

GI: Nausea, anorexia, vomiting, diarrhea, constipation, dyspepsia, dysphagia

GU: Hematuria, albuminuria, pyuria, creatinine increase

HEMA: **Thrombocytopenia, leukopenia,** anemia

INTEG: Rash, pruritus, sweating

META: Hypoalbuminemia, edema, hypocalcemia, weight decrease, dehydration, hypokalemia

MISC: Fever, chills, asthenia, infection, pain, headache, chest pain, flulike symptoms, **serious infection, capillary leak syndrome**

MS: Myalgia, arthralgia

RESP: Dyspnea, cough, pharyngitis, rhinitis

Contraindications: Hypersensitivity to denileukin, diphtheria toxin, IL-2

Precautions: Pregnancy (C), breastfeeding, children, geriatric patients, CAD, *Escherichia coli,* protein hypersensitivity, immunosuppression, peripheral vascular disease

Black Box Warning: Capillary leak syndrome, infusion-related reactions, visual disturbances

PHARMACOKINETICS

Concentrates in liver/kidneys, metabolized by proteolytic degradation

INTERACTIONS

Increase: bone marrow depression—radiation, other antineoplastics

Decrease: antibody reaction—live vaccines

NURSING CONSIDERATIONS

Assess:

- CBC, differential, platelet count weekly; withhold product if WBC <4000/mm^3 or platelet count <75,000/mm^3; notify prescriber of results
- Monitor temp q4hr (may indicate beginning infection)
- Hepatic studies before, during therapy (bilirubin, AST, ALT, LDH) as needed or monthly
- Bleeding: hematuria, guaiac, bruising or petechiae, mucosa or orifices q8hr
- Jaundice of skin, sclera; dark urine; clay-colored stools; itchy skin; abdominal pain; fever; diarrhea
- For vascular leak syndrome after 2 wk of treatment (hypotension, edema, hypoalbuminemia); monitor weight, B/P, serum albumin, edema
- Obtain CD25 expression on skin biopsy samples

Administer:

- Antiemetic 30-60 min before giving product to prevent vomiting
- Antibiotics for prophylaxis of infection

IV route

- Do not shake vigorously
- Prepare and hold sol in plastic syringes or soft plastic IV bags only, no glass containers
- Draw calculated dose from vial, inject into empty IV inf bag, for each 1 ml of product removed from vial, no more than 9 ml of sterile saline without preservative should be added to IV bag; infuse over ≥15 min; do not give by bolus; do not admix with other products; do not use a filter
- Use within 6 hr, discard unused portions

Perform/provide:

- Storage in light-resistant container, dry area
- Warm compresses at inf site for inflammation

Evaluate:

- Therapeutic response: decreased tumor size, spread of malignancy

Teach patient/family:

- To report signs of infection: fever, sore throat, flulike symptoms
- To report signs of anemia: fatigue, headache, faintness, SOB, irritability
- To report bleeding; avoid use of razors, commercial mouthwash
- To avoid use of aspirin products, NSAIDs, or ibuprofen
- To use reliable contraception; avoid breastfeeding

desipramine (℞)

(dess-ip'ra-meen)

Apo-Desipramine ♣, desipramine HCl, Norpramin, Pertofrane ♣

Func. class.: Antidepressant, tricyclic

Chem. class.: Dibenzazepine, secondary amine

Action: Blocks reuptake of norepinephrine, serotonin into nerve endings, increasing action of norepinephrine, serotonin in nerve cells

Uses: Depression

Unlabeled uses: Chronic pain, postherpetic neuralgia, ADHD, bulimia, diabetic neuropathy, panic disorder, social phobia

DOSAGE AND ROUTES

Major depression

- *Adult:* **PO** 50-75 mg/day in 1-4 divided doses, titrate by 25-50 mg q wk up to 300 mg/day in single or divided doses
- *Geriatric:* **PO** 25 mg/day at bedtime, titrate q wk, may increase to 150 mg/day
- *Adolescent:* **PO** 25-50 mg/day in divided doses, max 150 mg/day
- *Child 6-12 yr:* **PO** 1-3 mg/kg/day in divided doses; give >3 mg/kg/day with close medical monitoring; max 5 mg/kg/day

ADHD/bulimia nervosa (unlabeled)

- *Adult:* **PO** 25 mg tid, may titrate to 200 mg/day by 25-50 mg/day at weekly intervals

Neuropathic pain/postherpetic neuralgia (unlabeled)

- *Adult:* **PO** 10-25 mg at bedtime

Diabetic neuropathy (unlabeled)

- *Adult:* **PO** 75-150 mg

Available forms: Tabs 10, 25, 50, 75, 100, 150 mg

SIDE EFFECTS

CNS: Dizziness, drowsiness, confusion, headache, anxiety, tremors, stimulation, weakness, insomnia, nightmares, EPS (geriatric patients), increased psychiatric symptoms, paresthenia, suicidal ideation

CV: Orthostatic hypotension, ECG changes, tachycardia, hypertension, palpitations

EENT: Blurred vision, tinnitus, mydriasis, ophthalmoplegia

GI: Diarrhea, dry mouth, nausea, vomiting, **paralytic ileus,** increased appetite, cramps, epigastric distress, jaundice, **hepatitis,** stomatitis, constipation, weight gain

GU: Retention, **acute renal failure**

HEMA: **Agranulocytosis, thrombocytopenia, eosinophilia, leukopenia**

INTEG: Rash, urticaria, sweating, pruritus, photosensitivity

Contraindications: Hypersensitivity to tricyclics, closed-angle glaucoma, acute MI

Precautions: Pregnancy (C), breastfeeding, geriatric patients, severe depression, increased intraocular pressure, seizure disorder, CV disease, prostatic hypertrophy, thyroid disease

Black Box Warning: Children <18 yr, suicidal patients

PHARMACOKINETICS

Well absorbed, widely distributed, protein binding 92%, extensively metabolized in the liver, half-life 12-24 hr

INTERACTIONS

Increase: CNS depression—alcohol, barbiturates, opioids, CNS depressants

Increase: desipramine level—cimetidine, diltiazem, fluvoxamine, fluoxetine, paroxetine, sertraline, verapamil

Increase: life-threatening B/P elevations, do not use concurrently—clonidine

Increase: hypertension—epinephrine, norepinephrine

Increase: hyperpyrexia, seizures, excitation, do not use with 14 days of MAOIs

Increase: QT interval—tricyclics

Drug/Herb

Increase: serotonin syndrome, avoid concurrent use—St. John's Wort, SAM-e

Increase: CNS depression—chamomile, hops, kava, valerian

Decrease: seizure threshold, do not use concurrently—evening primrose oil

Drug/Lab Test

Increase: serum bilirubin, blood glucose, alk phos

NURSING CONSIDERATIONS

Assess:

- B/P (lying, standing), pulse q4hr; if systolic B/P drops 20 mm Hg, hold product, notify prescriber; take VS q4hr in patients with cardiovascular disease
- Blood studies: CBC, leukocytes, differential, cardiac enzymes if patient is receiving long-term therapy
- Hepatic studies: AST, ALT, bilirubin
- Weight q wk; appetite may increase with this product
- ECG for flattening T wave, bundle branch block, AV block, dysrhythmias in cardiac patients
- EPS primarily in geriatric patients: rigidity, dystonia, akathisia
- Seizure activity in those with a history of seizures
- Mental status: mood, sensorium, affect, suicidal tendencies, increase in psychiatric symptoms: depression, panic
- Urinary retention, constipation; constipation most likely in children
- Withdrawal symptoms: headache, nausea, vomiting, muscle pain, weakness; not usual unless product discontinued abruptly
- Alcohol consumption; if consumed, hold dose until morning

Administer:

- Increased fluids, bulk in diet for constipation, especially in geriatric patients
- With food or milk for GI symptoms
- Crushed if patient is unable to swallow medication whole
- Dosage at bedtime if oversedation occurs during day; may take entire dose at bedtime; geriatric patients may not tolerate once-daily dosing
- Gum, hard candy, frequent sips of water for dry mouth

Perform/provide:

- Storage at room temperature
- Assistance with ambulation during beginning of therapy for drowsiness/dizziness
- Safety measures, primarily in the geriatric patient
- Check to see that PO medication is swallowed

Evaluate:

- Therapeutic response: decreased depression

Teach patient/family

- That therapeutic effects may take 2-3 wk

• That suicidal thoughts and behavior may occur
• To use caution in driving, other activities requiring alertness because of drowsiness, dizziness, blurred vision
• To avoid alcohol ingestion, other CNS depressants
• Not to discontinue medication quickly after long-term use; may cause nausea, headache, malaise
• To wear sunscreen or large hat, since photosensitivity occurs

Treatment of overdose: ECG monitoring; lavage, activated charcoal; administer anticonvulsant

desloratadine (℞)

(des'lor-at'ah-deen)
Clarinex, Clarinex RediTabs
Func. class.: Antihistamine, 2nd generation
Chem. class.: Selective histamine (H_1)-receptor antagonist

Action: Binds to peripheral histamine receptors, providing antihistamine action without sedation
Uses: Seasonal/perennial allergic rhinitis, chronic idiopathic urticaria

DOSAGE AND ROUTES

• *Adult and child ≥12 yr:* **PO** 5 mg/day
• *Child 6-11 yr:* **PO** 2.5 mg/day
• *Child 1-5 yr:* **PO** 1.25 mg/day
• *Child 6-11 mo:* **PO** 1 mg/day

Hepatic/renal dose
• *Adult:* **PO** 5 mg every other day

Available form: Tabs 5 mg; orally disintegrating tabs 2.5, 5 mg (Reditabs); syr 0.5 mg/ml

SIDE EFFECTS

CNS: Sedation (more common with increased doses), headache, psychomotor hyperactivity, **seizures,** fatigue
GI: **Hepatitis,** nausea, dry mouth
MISC: Flulike symptoms

Contraindications: Hypersensitivity, infants/neonates
Precautions: Pregnancy (C), breastfeeding, child, asthma, renal/hepatic impairment

PHARMACOKINETICS

Onset antihistamine effect 1 hr, relief as early as 1 day, duration up to 24 hr, peak 1½ hr, elimination half-life 8½-28 hr, metabolized in liver to active metabolites, excreted in urine

INTERACTIONS

Drug/Food
• Food may prolong time to peak with orally disintegrating tabs

NURSING CONSIDERATIONS

Assess:
• Allergy: hives, rash, rhinitis; monitor respiratory status; test interaction, antigen skin test

Administer:
• Without regard to meals
• Do not remove RediTabs from blister until ready to use
• RediTabs directly on tongue; may take with or without water

Perform/provide:
• Storage in tight container at room temperature

Evaluate:
• Therapeutic response: absence of running or congested nose, other allergy symptoms

Teach patient/family:
• To avoid driving, other hazardous activities if drowsiness occurs; observe caution until product's effects on the patient are known
• That product may cause photosensitivity; use sunscreen or stay out of the sun to prevent burns

desmopressin (℞)

(des-moe-press'in)

DDAVP, Minirin, Octostim ✱, Stimate

Func. class.: Pituitary hormone

Chem. class.: Synthetic antidiuretic hormone

Action: Promotes reabsorption of water by action on renal tubular epithelium; causes smooth muscle constriction, increase in plasma factor VIII levels, which increases platelet aggregation resulting in vasopressor effect, similar to vasopressin

Uses: Hemophilia A, von Willebrand's disease type 1, nonnephrogenic diabetes insipidus, symptoms of polyuria/polydipsia caused by pituitary dysfunction, nocturnal enuresis

Unlabeled uses: Cardiopulmonary bypass, sickle cell disease, uremic bleeding

DOSAGE AND ROUTES

Primary nocturnal enuresis

• *Adult and child ≥6 yr:* **PO** 0.2 mg at bedtime, may be increased to max 0.6 mg at bedtime

Diabetes insipidus

• *Adult:* **INTRANASAL** 0.1-0.4 ml/day in divided doses (1-4 sprays with pump); **IV/SUBCUT** 0.5-1 ml/day in divided doses

• *Child 3 mo to 12 yr:* **INTRANASAL** 0.05-0.3 ml/day in divided doses

Hemophilia/von Willebrand's disease

• *Adult and child >3 mo:* **IV** 0.3 mcg/kg in NaCl over 15-30 min; may repeat if needed

Antihemorrhagic

• *Adult and child >3 mo:* **IV** 0.3 mcg/kg

• *Adult and child <50 kg:* **INTRANASAL** 1 spray in one nostril

• *Adult and child >50 kg:* 1 spray each nostril

Cardiopulmonary bypass (unlabeled)

• *Adult:* **IV** 0.3 mcg/kg with aminocaproic acid given as a single postop dose

Sickle cell disease (unlabeled)

• *Adult:* **SUBCUT/IV** 0.3 mcg/kg with a high fluid intake

Uremic bleeding (unlabeled)

• *Adult:* **SUBCUT/IV** 0.2-0.4 mcg/kg/dose

Available forms: Inj 4, 15 mcg/ml, Rhihal Tube del 2.5 mg/vial (0.1 mg/ml); tabs 0.1, 0.2 mg; nasal spray pump 10 mcg/spray (0.1 mg/ml); nasal sol 1.5 mg/ml (150 mcg/dose)

SIDE EFFECTS

CNS: Drowsiness, headache, lethargy, flushing

CV: Increased B/P, palpitations, tachycardia

EENT: Nasal irritation, congestion, rhinitis

GI: Nausea, heartburn, cramps

GU: Vulval pain

META: Hyponatremia, hyponatremia-induced seizures

SYST: **Anaphylaxis (IV)**

Contraindications: Hypersensitivity, nephrogenic diabetes insipidus, severe renal disease

Precautions: Pregnancy (B), breastfeeding, coronary artery disease, hypertension, cystic fibrosis, thrombus

PHARMACOKINETICS

PO: Onset 1 hr, peak 4-7 hr

INTRANASAL: Onset 1 hr; peak 1-4 hr; duration 8-20 hr; half-life 8 min, 76 min (terminal)

IV: Onset 1 min, peak ½ hr, duration >3 hr

INTERACTIONS

Increase: antidiuretic action—carbamazepine, chlorpropamide, clofibrate

Decrease: antidiuretic action—lithium, alcohol, demeclocycline, heparin, large doses of epinephrine

NURSING CONSIDERATIONS

Assess:

• Pulse, B/P when giving IV or SUBCUT

• I&O ratio, weight daily; check for

edema in extremities; if water retention is severe, diuretic may be prescribed

- Water intoxication: lethargy, behavioral changes, disorientation, neuromuscular excitability
- Intranasal use: nausea, congestion, cramps, headache; usually decreased with decreased dose; for nasal mucosa changes: congestion, edema, discharge, scarring (nasal route)

⚠ For severe allergic reaction including anaphylaxis (IV route)

- Urine vol/osmolality and plasma osmolality (diabetes insipidus)
- Factor VIII coagulant activity before using for hemostasis
- Nocturnal enuresis: frequency of enuresis before and during treatment

Administer:

- Undiluted over 1 min in diabetes insipidus
- Diluted, one single dose/50 ml of 0.9% NaCl (adult and child >10 kg), a single dose/10 ml as an IV inf over 15-30 min in von Willebrand's disease or hemophilia A

Perform/provide:

- Storage in refrigerator or cool environment

Evaluate:

- Therapeutic response: absence of severe thirst, decreased urine output, decreased osmolality

Teach patient/family:

- The proper technique for nasal instillation: to insert tube into nostril to instill product
- To avoid OTC products: cough, hay fever products, since these preparations may contain epinephrine, decrease product response; do not use with alcohol, adverse reactions may occur
- To wear emergency ID specifying therapy
- That if dose is missed, take when remembered up to 1 hr before next dose; do not double dose; avoid fluids from 1 hr to up to 8 hr after PO dose
- To report to prescriber upper respiratory infection, nasal congestion

desonide topical

See Appendix B

desoximetasone topical

See Appendix B

desoxyephedrine nasal agent

See Appendix B

dexamethasone (℞)

(dex-ah-meth'a-sone)

Decadron, Deronil ✦ Dexasone ✦, Dexon, Hexadrol, Mymethasone

dexamethasone acetate (℞)

Dalalone DP, Dalalone LA, Decadron-LA, Decaject-LA, Dexacen LA-8, Dexasone-LA, Dexone LA, Solurex-LA

dexamethasone sodium phosphate (℞)

Dalalone, Decadron Phosphate, Decaject, Dexacen-4, Dexone, Hexadrol Phosphate, Solurex

Func. class.: Corticosteroid, synthetic

Chem. class.: Glucocorticoid, long acting

Do not confuse:

Decadron/Percodan

Action: Decreases inflammation by suppression of migration of polymorphonuclear leukocytes, fibroblasts, reversal of increased capillary permeability and lysosomal stabilization

Uses: Inflammation, allergies, neoplasms, cerebral edema, septic shock, collagen disorders

Unlabeled uses: ARDS, bone pain, bronchopulmonary dysplasia (BPD), Churg-Strauss syndrome, endophthalmitis, hyaline membrane disease prophylaxis, infertility with clomiPHENE, laryngeal edema prophylaxis, mixed connective tissue disease, polychondritis, polyarteritis nodosa, pulmonary edema, temporal arteritis, Wegener's granulomatosis, pediatric bacterial meningitis, cancer chemotherapy (nausea/vomiting), croup

DOSAGE AND ROUTES

Inflammation

• *Adult:* **PO** 0.75-9 mg/day in divided doses q6-12hr or phosphate **IM** 0.5-9 mg/day divided q6-12hr, or acetate **IM** 4-16 mg q1-3wk

• *Child:* **PO** 0.024-0.34 mg/kg/day in divided doses q6-12hr

Anaphylactic shock

• *Adult:* **IV** (Phosphate) single dose 1-6 mg/kg or **IV** 40 mg q2-6hr as needed up to 72 hr

Cerebral edema

• *Adult:* **IV** (Phosphate) 10 mg, then 4-6 mg **IM** q6hr × 2-4 days, then taper over 1 wk

• *Child:* Loading dose 1-2 mg/kg **(PO/IM/IV)** then 1-1.5 mg/kg/day, max 16 mg/day divided q4-6hr for 2-4 days, then taper down q wk

Adrenocortical insufficiency

• *Adult:* **PO** 0.5-9 mg/day in divided doses

• *Child:* **PO** 0.03-0.3 mg/kg/day divided in 2-4 doses

Suppression test

• *Adult:* **PO** 1 mg at 11 PM or 0.5 mg q6hr × 48 hr

ARDS (unlabeled)

• *Adult:* **IM/IV** (dexamethasone sodium phosphate) 0.5-9 mg/day in 2-4 divided doses

• *Child:* **IM/IV** (dexamethasone sodium phosphate) 0.06-0.3 mg/kg/day or 1.2-10 mg/m^2 in divided doses q6-12hr

Bone pain (unlabeled)

• *Adult:* **PO/IV** 12-20 mg/day in divided doses

Pediatric bacterial meningitis (unlabeled)

• *Child and infant >2 mo:* **IV** 0.15 mg/kg qid × first 2 days of antibiotics

Croup (unlabeled)

• *Child:* **PO** 0.024-0.34 mg/kg/day or 0.66-10 mg/m^2/day in 2-4 divided doses; a single dose of 0.6 mg/kg has been used for mild to moderate croup; **IM/IV** 0.06-0.3 mg/kg/day or 1.2-10 mg/m^2/day in divided doses q6-12hr, a single dose of 0.6 mg/kg IM has been used for severe croup

Available forms: *Dexamethasone:* tabs 0.25, 0.5, 0.75, 1, 1.5, 2, 4, 6 mg; elix 0.5 mg/5 ml; oral sol 0.5 mg/5 ml, 1 mg/1 ml; *inj acetate:* 8, 16 mg/ml; *inj phosphate:* 4, 10, 20, 24 mg/ml

SIDE EFFECTS

CNS: Depression, flushing, sweating, headache, mood changes, euphoria, psychosis, **seizures,** insomnia

CV: Hypertension, **circulatory collapse, thrombophlebitis, embolism,** tachycardia, edema, cardiomyopathy

EENT: Fungal infections, increased intraocular pressure, blurred vision, cataracts, glaucoma

ENDO: HPA suppression, hyperglycemia, sodium, fluid retention

GI: Diarrhea, nausea, abdominal distention, **GI hemorrhage,** *increased appetite,* **pancreatitis**

HEMA: **Thrombocytopenia,** transient leukocytosis

INTEG: Acne, poor wound healing, ecchymosis, petechiae, hirsutism

META: Hypokalemia

MS: Fractures, osteoporosis, weakness, arthralgia, myopathy

Contraindications: Children <2 yr, psychosis, hypersensitivity to corticosteroids or benyl alcohol; idiopathic thrombocytopenia, acute glomerulonephritis, amebiasis, fungal infections, nonasthmatic bronchial disease, AIDS, TB, ocular infection, glaucoma

Precautions: Pregnancy (C), breastfeeding, diabetes mellitus, osteoporosis, seizure disorders, ulcerative colitis, CHF, myasthenia gravis, renal disease, peptic ulcer, esophagitis

PHARMACOKINETICS

Half-life 36-54 hr
PO: Onset 1 hr, peak 1-2 hr, duration 2½ days
IM: (Acetate) Peak 8 hr, duration 6 days-3 wk

INTERACTIONS

Increase: side effects—alcohol, salicylates, indomethacin, amphotericin B, digoxin, cycloSPORINE, diuretics
Increase: dexamethasone action—salicylates, estrogens, indomethacin, oral contraceptives, ketoconazole, macrolide antiinfectives
Decrease: dexamethasone action—cholestyramine, colestipol, barbiturates, rifampin, ephedrine, phenytoin, theophylline, antacids
Decrease: effect of anticoagulants, anticonvulsants, antidiabetics, ambenonium, neostigmine, isoniazid, toxoids, vaccines, anticholinesterases, salicylates, somatrem

Drug/Herb

- Potassium deficiency: aloe, buckthorn, cascara sagrada, Chinese rhubarb, senna

Increase: corticosteroid effect—aloe, licorice, perilla

Drug/Lab Test

Increase: cholesterol, sodium, blood glucose, uric acid, calcium, urine glucose
Decrease: calcium, K, T_4, T_3, thyroid ^{131}I uptake test, urine 17-OHCS, 17-KS, PBI
False negative: skin allergy tests

NURSING CONSIDERATIONS

Assess:

- Potassium, blood, urine glucose while on long-term therapy; hypokalemia and hyperglycemia
- Weight daily; notify prescriber of weekly gain >5 lb
- B/P q4hr, pulse; notify prescriber of chest pain
- I&O ratio; be alert for decreasing urinary output, increasing edema
- Plasma cortisol levels during long-term therapy (normal: 138-635 nmol/L SI units when drawn at 8 AM); prolonged use can cause cushingoid symptoms
- Infection: fever, WBC even after withdrawal of medication; product masks infection
- Potassium depletion: paresthesias, fatigue, nausea, vomiting, depression, polyuria, dysrhythmias, weakness
- Edema, hypertension, cardiac symptoms
- Mental status: affect, mood, behavioral changes, aggression

Administer:

- Titrated dose; use lowest effective dose
- IM inj deeply in large muscle mass; rotate sites; avoid deltoid; use 21G needle
- In one dose in AM to prevent adrenal suppression; avoid SUBCUT administration, may damage tissue
- With food or milk to decrease GI symptoms

IV route

- Undiluted direct over 1 min or less or diluted with 0.9% NaCl or D_5W and give as an IV inf at prescribed rate
- After shaking suspension (parenteral); do not give suspension IV

Dexamethasone sodium phosphate
Additive compatibilities: Aminophylline, bleomycin, cimetidine, floxacillin, furosemide, granisetron, lidocaine, meropenem, mitomycin, nafcillin, netilmicin, ondansetron, prochlorperazine, ranitidine, verapamil
Syringe compatibilities: Granisetron, metoclopramide, ranitidine, sufentanil
Y-site compatibilities: Acyclovir, allopurinol, amifostine, amikacin, amphotericin B cholesteryl, amsacrine, aztreonam, cefepime, cefpirome, cisatracurium, cisplatin, cladribine, cyclophosphamide, cytarabine, DOXOrubicin, DOXOrubicin liposome, famotidine, filgrastim, fluconazole, fludarabine, foscarnet, granisetron, heparin, lorazepam, melphalan, meperidine, meropenem, morphine, ondansetron, paclitaxel, piperacillin/tazobactam, potassium chloride, propofol, remifentanil, sargramostim, sodium bicarbonate, sufentanil, tacrolimus, teniposide, theophylline, thiotepa, vinorelbine, vit B/C, zidovudine

Perform/provide:

- Assistance with ambulation in patient with bone tissue disease to prevent fractures

Evaluate:

- Therapeutic response: decreased inflammation

Teach patient/family:

- That ID as corticosteroid user should be carried
- To contact prescriber if surgery, trauma, stress occurs; dose may need to be adjusted
- To notify prescriber if therapeutic response decreases; dosage adjustment may be needed

⚠ Not to discontinue abruptly or adrenal crisis can result

- Symptoms of adrenal insufficiency: nausea, anorexia, fatigue, dizziness, dyspnea, weakness, joint pain
- To avoid OTC products: salicylates, alcohol in cough products, cold preparations unless directed by prescriber
- To teach patient all aspects of product usage, including cushingoid symptoms; to notify health care provider of infection
- Avoid exposure to chickenpox or measles, persons with infection

dexamethasone ophthalmic

See Appendix B

dexamethasone topical

See Appendix B

dexlansoprazole (℞)

(dex-lan-so-prey′zole)

Kapidex

Func. class.: Antiulcer, proton pump inhibitor

Chem. class.: Benzimidazole

Action: Suppresses gastric secretion by inhibiting hydrogen/potassium ATPase enzyme system in gastric parietal cell; characterized as gastric acid pump inhibitor, since it blocks final step of acid production

Uses: Gastroesophageal reflux disease (GERD), severe erosive esophagitis, heartburn

DOSAGE AND ROUTES

Erosive esophagitis

- *Adult:* **PO** 60 mg daily for up to 8 wk; maintenance: **PO** 30 mg daily for up to 6 months

GERD

- *Adult:* **PO** 30 mg daily × 4 wk

Available forms: Del rel caps 30, 60 mg

SIDE EFFECTS

CNS: Headache, dizziness, confusion, agitation, amnesia, depression, **anxiety, seizures,** insomnia, migraine

CV: Chest pain, angina, bradycardia, palpitations, **CVA**, hypertension, **MI**

EENT: Tinnitus

GI: Diarrhea, abdominal pain, vomiting, nausea, constipation, flatulence, colitis, dysgeusia

HEMA: Anemia, **neutropenia, thrombocytopenia, pernicious anemia, thrombosis**

INTEG: Rash, urticaria, pruritus

META: Gout

MS: Arthralgia, mylagia

RESP: Upper respiratory infections, cough, epistaxis, dyspnea, **pneumonia**

SYST: Anaphylaxis

Contraindications: Hypersensitivity

Precautions: Pregnancy (B), breastfeeding, children, proton pump hypersensitivity, gastric cancer, hepatic disease, vit B_{12} deficiency

PHARMACOKINETICS

Absorption 57%-64%; plasma half-life 1-2 hr; protein binding 96.1%-98.8%; extensively metabolized in liver; excreted in urine, feces; clearance decreased in the geriatric patient, renal/hepatic impairment, peak dual 1-2 hr, 4-5 hr

INTERACTIONS

Increase: dexlansoprazole effect—CYP2C19, 3A4 inhibitors (fluvoxamine, voriconazole)

- Dexlansoprazole absorption: sucralfate

Decrease: absorption of ketoconazole, itraconazole, iron, delavirdine, ampicillin, calcium carbonate

NURSING CONSIDERATIONS

Assess:

- GI system: bowel sounds q8hr, abdomen for pain, swelling, anorexia
- Hepatic studies: AST, ALT, alk phos during treatment

Administer:

- Swallow caps whole; do not crush or chew caps; caps may be opened and contents sprinkled on food, use immediately; do not chew contents of capsule

Evaluate:

- Therapeutic response: absence of epigastric pain, swelling, fullness

Teach patient/family:

- To report severe diarrhea; product may have to be discontinued
- That diabetic patient should know that hypoglycemia may occur
- To avoid hazardous activities; dizziness may occur
- To avoid alcohol, salicylates, ibuprofen; may cause GI irritation

dexmedetomidine (℞)

(dex-med-eh-tom′o-deen)

Precedex

Func. class.: Sedative, α_2 adrenoceptor agonist

Action: Produces α_2 agonist activity seen at low and moderate doses, also α_1 at high doses

Uses: Sedation in mechanically ventilated, intubated patients in ICU

DOSAGE AND ROUTES

- *Adult:* **IV** Loading dose of 1 mcg/kg over 10 min then 0.2-0.7 mcg/kg/hr; do not use for more than 24 hr
- *Child and infant (unlabeled):* **IV** 0.28 mcg/kg/hr for 24 hr to mechanically ventilated patients

Available forms: Inj 100 mcg/ml

SIDE EFFECTS

CV: Bradycardia, hypotension, hypertension, **atrial fibrillation, infarction, cardiac arrest**

GI: Nausea, thirst

GU: Oliguria

HEMA: Leukocytosis, anemia

MISC: Hyperkalemia

RESP: **Pulmonary edema, pleural effusion, hypoxia,** respiratory acidosis

Contraindications: Hypersensitivity, chronic hypertension

Precautions: Pregnancy (C), breastfeeding, children, geriatric patients, respiratory depression, severe respiratory disorders, cardiac dysrhythmias, hypovolemia, diabetes, CV/renal/hepatic disease

PHARMACOKINETICS

Rapid distribution, excreted in urine, metabolized in liver, protein binding 94%, elimination half-life 2 hr

INTERACTIONS

Increase: CNS depression—alcohol, opioids, sedative/hypnotics, antipsychotics, skeletal muscle relaxants, inhalational anesthetics

Increase: hypotension—antihypertensives

NURSING CONSIDERATIONS

Assess:

- Inj site: phlebitis, burning, stinging
- Cardiac status: B/P, heart rate, ECG for changes: atrial fibrillation, monitor geriatric patients more closely
- CNS changes: movement, jerking, tremors, dizziness, LOC, pupil reaction
- Respiratory dysfunction: respiratory depression, character, rate, rhythm; notify prescriber if respirations are <10/min

Administer:

IV route

- After diluting with D_5W 0.9% NaCl, withdraw 2 ml of product and add to 48 ml of 0.9% NaCl to a total of 50 ml, shake to mix well, use controlled inf device
- Only with resuscitative equipment available
- Only by qualified persons trained in ICU sedation

Solution compatibilities: LR, D_5W, 0.9% NaCl, 20% mannitol

Additive compatibilities: Atracurium, atropine, etomidate, fentanyl, glycopyrrolate, midazolam, mivacurium, morphine, pancuronium, phenylephrine, succinylcholine, thiopental, vecuronium

Perform/provide:

- Safety measures: side rails, nightlight, call bell within easy reach

Evaluate:

- Therapeutic response: induction of anesthesia

dexmethylphenidate (℞)

(dex'meth-ul-fen'ih-dayt)

Focalin, Focalin XR

Func. class.: Central nervous system (CNS) stimulant, psychostimulant

Controlled Substance Schedule II

Action: Increases release of norepinephrine and DOPamine into the extraneuronal space, also blocks reuptake of norepinephrine and DOPamine into the presynaptic neuron; mode of action in treating attention deficit hyperactivity disorder (ADHD) is unknown

Uses: ADHD

DOSAGE AND ROUTES

- *Child >6 yr:* **PO** 2.5 mg bid with doses at least 4 hr apart, gradually increase to a maximum of 20 mg/day (10 mg bid); for those taking methylphenidate, use ½ of methylphenidate dose initially, then increase as needed to a max of 20 mg/day; **EXT REL** 5 mg/day, may adjust to 20 mg/day in 5 mg increments
- *Adult:* **PO EXT REL** 10 mg/day, may adjust to 20 mg/day in 10-mg increments

Available forms: Tabs 2.5, 5, 10 mg; ext rel caps 5, 10, 20 mg (Focalin XR)

SIDE EFFECTS

CNS: Dizziness, headache, drowsiness, nervousness, insomnia, **toxic psychosis, neuroleptic malignant syndrome (rare),** Gilles de la Tourette's syndrome

CV: Palpitations, B/P changes, angina, **dysrhythmias, tachycardia**

GI: Nausea, anorexia, abnormal hepatic function, **hepatic coma,** *abdominal pain*

HEMA: **Leukopenia, anemia, thrombocytopenic purpura**

INTEG: **Exfoliative dermatitis,** urticaria, rash, erythema multiforme

MISC: Fever, arthralgia, scalp hair loss

Contraindications: Breastfeeding, children <6 yr, hypersensitivity to methylphenidate, anxiety, history of Gilles de la Tourette's syndrome, tics, psychosis, glaucoma, concurrent treatment with MAOIs or within 14 days of discontinuing treatment with MAOIs

Precautions: Pregnancy (C), hypertension, depression, seizures, CV disorders, alcoholism

Black Box Warning: Substance abuse

PHARMACOKINETICS

Readily absorbed, elimination half-life 2.2 hr, metabolized by liver, excreted by kidneys

PO: Peak 1½ hr, onset ½-1 hr, duration 4 hr

PO-ER: Onset unknown, peak 4 hr, duration 8 hr

INTERACTIONS

⚠ ***Increase:*** hypertensive crisis—MAOIs or within 14 days of MAOIs, vasopressors

Increase: sympathomimetic effect—decongestants, vasoconstrictors

Increase: effects of anticonvulsants, tricyclics, SSRIs, coumarin anticoagulants (warfarin)
Decrease: effects of antihypertensives
Drug/Herb
• Synergistic effect: melatonin
Increase: stimulant effect—horsetail, yohimbe

NURSING CONSIDERATIONS

Assess:
• VS, B/P; may reverse antihypertensives; check patients with cardiac disease more often for increased B/P
• CBC, differential platelet counts during long-term therapy, urinalysis; in diabetes: blood glucose, urine glucose; insulin changes may have to be made, because eating will decrease
• Height, growth rate q3mo in children; growth rate may be decreased
• Mental status: mood, sensorium, affect, stimulation, insomnia, aggressiveness
⚠ Withdrawal symptoms: headache, nausea, vomiting, muscle pain, weakness
• Appetite, sleep, speech patterns
• For attention span, decreased hyperactivity in persons with ADHD
Administer:
• Twice daily at least 4 hr apart; ext rel once a day
• Without regard to meals
Evaluate:
• Therapeutic response: decreased hyperactivity or ability to stay awake
Teach patient/family:
• To decrease caffeine consumption (coffee, tea, cola, chocolate); may increase irritability, stimulation
• To take early in day to prevent insomnia
• To avoid OTC preparations unless approved by prescriber
• To taper off product over several weeks to avoid depression, increased sleeping, lethargy
• To avoid alcohol ingestion
• To avoid hazardous activities until stabilized on medication
• To get needed rest; patients will feel more tired at end of day
• Notify all health care workers, including school nurse, of medication and schedule
• Discuss information instructions provided in patient information section

Treatment of overdose: Administer fluids; hemodialysis or peritoneal dialysis; antihypertensive for increased B/P; administer short-acting barbiturate before lavage

D

dextran 40 (℞)

(deks′tran)
Dextran 40, Gentran 40, LMD 10%, Rheomacrodex
Func. class.: Plasma volume expander
Chem. class.: Low-molecular-weight polysaccharide

Action: Similar to human albumin, which expands plasma volume by drawing fluid from interstitial space to intravascular space

Uses: Expand plasma volume, prophylaxis of embolism, thrombosis

DOSAGE AND ROUTES

Shock
• *Adult:* **IV INF** 500 ml over 15-30 min, total dose in 24 hr not to exceed 20 ml/kg; subsequent doses given slowly; if given >24 hr, not to exceed 10 ml/kg/day; not to exceed therapy >5 days
• *Child:* **IV** Total dose ≤20 ml/kg during first 24 hr, then ≤10 ml/kg/day if needed

Thrombosis/embolism
• *Adult:* **IV INF** 500-1000 ml, then 500 ml/day × 3 days, then 500 ml q2-3 days × 2 wk if needed

Available forms: 10% dextran 40/D_5W, 10% dextran 40/0.9% NaCl

SIDE EFFECTS

CV: Hypotension, **cardiac arrest, CHF**
GI: Nausea, vomiting, increased AST, ALT

GU: **Osmotic nephrosis, renal failure, stasis,** hyponatremia
HEMA: Decreased hematocrit, platelet function; **increased bleeding/coagulation times, thrombocytopenia**
INTEG: Rash, urticaria, pruritus, **angioedema,** chills, fever, flushing
RESP: Wheezing, dyspnea, **bronchospasm, pulmonary edema**
SYST: **Anaphylaxis**

Contraindications: Hypersensitivity

Precautions: Pregnancy (C), active hemorrhage, sodium restriction, bowel surgery, thrombocytopenia, renal failure, CHF (severe), extreme dehydration, pulmonary edema, bleeding disorders

PHARMACOKINETICS

IV: Expands blood vol 1-2 × amount infused, excreted in urine and feces

INTERACTIONS

- Incompatible with chlortetracycline, phytonadione, promethazine

Drug/Lab Test

False increase: blood glucose, urinary protein, bilirubin, total protein

Interference: Rh test, blood typing/crossmatching

NURSING CONSIDERATIONS

Assess:

- VS q5min × 30 min; Hgb/Hct, if falling by 30%, notify prescriber
- CVP during infusion (5-10 cm H_2O—normal range)
- Urine output q1hr; watch for increase in urinary output (common); if output does not increase, decrease or discontinue infusion
- I&O ratio and specific gravity, urine osmolarity; if specific gravity is very low, renal clearance is low, product should be discontinued
- Allergy: rash, urticaria, pruritus, wheezing, dyspnea, bronchospasm, product should be discontinued immediately

⚠ Circulatory overload: increased pulse, respirations, SOB, wheezing, chest tightness, chest pain

- Dehydration after infusion: decreased output, decreased specific gravity of urine, increased temp, poor skin turgor, increased specific gravity, dry skin

Administer:

IV route

- After prescribed dilution; may give initial 500 mg at 15-30 min; distribute remainder of daily dose over 8-24 hr
- After crossmatch is drawn, if blood is to be given also
- D_5W sol in heart failure patients as ordered

Additive compatibilities: Cloxacillin

Y-site compatibilities: Enalaprilat, famotidine

Perform/provide:

- Storage at constant temperature (15° C-30° C [59° F-86° F]); discard unused portions, protect from freezing

Evaluate:

- Therapeutic response: increased plasma volume

Teach patient/family:

- Signs of bleeding: bruising, blood in urine or black tarry stools

dextran 70/75 (℞)

(deks'tran)

Dextran 75, Gentran 70, Gentran 75, Macrodex

Func. class.: Plasma volume expander

Chem. class.: High-molecular-weight polysaccharide

Action: Similar to human albumin, which expands plasma volume by drawing fluid from interstitial spaces to intravascular space

Uses: Expand plasma volume in hypovolemic shock or impending shock

DOSAGE AND ROUTES

- *Adult:* **IV INF** 500-1000 ml not to exceed 20-40 ml/min, max 10 ml/kg/24 hr if therapy >24 hr

Available forms: 70/75 dextran in 0.9% NaCl, D_5%

SIDE EFFECTS

CV: Hypotension, **cardiac arrest, acute CHF**

GI: Nausea, vomiting, increased AST, ALT

GU: **Osmotic nephrosis, renal failure, stasis,** hypernatremia

HEMA: Decreased hematocrit, platelet function; **increased bleeding/coagulation times**

INTEG: Rash, urticaria, pruritus, **angioedema,** chills, fever, flushing

RESP: Wheezing, dyspnea, **bronchospasm, pulmonary edema**

SYST: **Anaphylaxis**

Contraindications: Hypersensitivity, renal failure, CHF (severe), extreme dehydration

Precautions: Pregnancy (C), active hemorrhage

PHARMACOKINETICS

IV: Onset within mins, duration 12 hr, expands blood vol 1-2 × amount infused; excreted in urine and feces

INTERACTIONS

Drug/Lab Test

False increase: blood glucose, urinary protein, bilirubin, total protein

Interference: Rh test, blood typing/crossmatching

NURSING CONSIDERATIONS

Assess:

- VS q5min × 30 min; Hgb/Hct, if falling by 30%, notify prescriber
- CVP during infusion (5-10 cm H_2O—normal range)
- Urine output q1hr; watch for increase in urinary output (common); if output does not increase, decrease or discontinue infusion
- I&O ratio and specific gravity, urine osmolarity; if specific gravity is very low, renal clearance is low, product should be discontinued
- Allergy: rash, urticaria, pruritus, wheezing, dyspnea, bronchospasm; product should be discontinued immediately
- ⚠ Circulatory overload: increased pulse, respirations, SOB, wheezing, chest tightness, chest pain
- Dehydration after infusion: decreased output, increased temp, poor skin turgor, increased specific gravity, dry skin

Administer:

- After prescribed dilution, may give initial 500 mg at 20-40 ml/min, reduce flow to lowest rate
- After crossmatch is drawn, if blood is also to be given
- D_5W sol in heart failure patients as ordered

Perform/provide:

- Storage at constant temperature (<25° C [77° F]); discard unused portions; do not use unless clear

Evaluate:

- Therapeutic response: increased plasma volume

Teach patient/family:

- Signs of bleeding: bruising, blood in urine, black tarry stools

dextroamphetamine (℞)

(dex-troe-am-fet′a-meen)

Dexedrine, dextroamphetamine, Liquadd

Func. class.: Cerebral stimulant

Chem. class.: Amphetamine

Controlled Substance Schedule II

Action: Increases release of norepinephrine, DOPamine in cerebral cortex to reticular activating system

Uses: Narcolepsy, attention deficit disorder with hyperactivity (ADHD)

Unlabeled uses: Obesity

DOSAGE AND ROUTES

Narcolepsy

- *Adult:* **PO** 5 mg bid, titrate daily dose by no more than 10 mg/wk, max 60 mg/day
- *Child 6-12 yr:* **PO** 5 mg/day, titrate daily dose by no more than 5 mg/day at weekly intervals

ADHD

• *Adult:* **PO** 5-60 mg/day in divided doses

• *Child 3-5 yr:* **PO** 2.5 mg/day increasing by 2.5 mg/day at weekly intervals, max 40 mg/day

• *Child >6-12 yr:* **PO** 5 mg daily-bid increasing by 5 mg/day at weekly intervals

Obesity, exogenous (unlabeled)

• *Adult and adolescent:* **PO** 5-30 mg/dose given 30-60 min before meals, use for 3-6 wk only

Available forms: Tabs 5, 10 mg; oral sol 5 mg/5 ml

SIDE EFFECTS

*CNS: **Hyperactivity, insomnia, restlessness, talkativeness,*** dizziness, headache, chills, stimulation, dysphoria, irritability, aggressiveness, tremor, dependence, addiction

*CV: **Palpitations, tachycardia,*** hypertension, decrease in heart rate, **dysrhythmias**

*GI: **Anorexia,*** dry mouth, diarrhea, constipation, weight loss, metallic taste

GU: Impotence, change in libido

INTEG: Urticaria

Contraindications: Hypersensitivity to sympathomimetic amines, hyperthyroidism, hypertension, glaucoma, severe arteriosclerosis, substance abuse, anxiety, anorexia nervosa, tartrazine dye hypersensitivity

Black Box Warning: CV disease, substance abuse

Precautions: Pregnancy (C), breastfeeding, children <3 yr, depression, Gilles de la Tourette's disorder

PHARMACOKINETICS

Onset 1 hr; peak 2 hr; duration 4-20 hr; metabolized by liver; urine excretion pH dependent; crosses placenta, breast milk; half-life 6-8 hr (child), 10-12 hr (adult)

INTERACTIONS

⚠ Hypertensive crisis: MAOIs or within 14 days of MAOIs

Increase: dextroamphetamine effect—acetaZOLAMIDE, antacids, sodium bicarbonate

Increase: CNS effect—haloperidol, tricyclics, phenothiazines

Decrease: absorption of barbiturates, phenytoin

Decrease: dextroamphetamine effect—ascorbic acid, ammonium chloride

Decrease: effect of adrenergic blockers, antidiabetics

Drug/Herb

• Serotonin syndrome: St. John's wort

Increase: stimulant effect—khat

Decrease: stimulant effect—eucalyptus

Drug/Food

Increase: amine effect—caffeine

NURSING CONSIDERATIONS

Assess:

• VS, B/P; this product may reverse antihypertensives; check patients with cardiac disease often

• CBC, urinalysis; in diabetes: blood glucose, urine glucose; insulin changes may be required, since eating will decrease

• Height, growth rate in children; growth rate may be decreased

• Mental status: mood, sensorium, affect, stimulation, insomnia, irritability

• Tolerance or dependency: an increased amount may be used to get same effect; will develop after long-term use

• Overdose: pain, fever, dehydration, insomnia, hyperactivity

Administer:

• At least 6 hr before bedtime to avoid sleeplessness

• Use calibrated measuring device for oral sol

Perform/provide:

• Gum, hard candy, frequent sips of water for dry mouth

• Storage of tabs and caps at room temperature; store oral sol at room temperature, protect from light

Evaluate:

• Therapeutic response: increased CNS stimulation, decreased drowsiness

Teach patient/family:

- To take before meals (obesity)
- To decrease caffeine consumption (coffee, tea, cola, chocolate); may increase irritability, stimulation
- To avoid OTC preparations unless approved by prescriber
- To taper product over several weeks; depression, increased sleeping, lethargy
- To avoid alcohol ingestion
- To avoid hazardous activities until stabilized on medication
- To get needed rest; patient will feel more tired at end of day

Treatment of overdose: Administer fluids, hemodialysis, or peritoneal dialysis; antihypertensive for increased B/P, ammonium Cl for increased excretion

dextromethorphan

(OTC)

(dex-troe-meth-or′fan)

Buckley's DM, Cap Honey, Creo-Terpin, Delsym, dextromethorphan, ElixSure Cough, Hold DM, PediaCare Long Acting Cough, Robafan, Robitussin Cough with honey, Robitussin Maximum Strength, Scot-Tussin DM Cough Chasers, Sucrets Cough Control, Triaminic Long Acting Cough, Tylenol Childrens Simply Cough, Vicks Formula 44 Cough Relief, Wal-Tussin, Zicam Cough Max Mist

Func. class.: Antitussive, nonopioid
Chem. class.: Levorphanol derivative

Action: Depresses cough center in medulla by direct effect

Uses: Nonproductive cough caused by colds or inhaled irritants

DOSAGE AND ROUTES

- *Adult and child ≥12 yr:* **PO** 10-20 mg q4hr, or 30 mg q6-8hr, not to exceed 120 mg/day; **SUS-REL LIQ** 60 mg q12hr, not to exceed 120 mg/day
- *Child 6-12 yr:* **PO** 5-10 mg q4hr; **SUS-REL LIQ** 30 mg bid, **LOZ** 5-10 mg q1-4hr; max 60 mg/day
- *Child 4-6 yr:* **PO** 2.5-7.5 mg q4-8hr, max 30 mg/day; **SUS REL** 15 mg bid
- *Child <4 yr:* Not recommended

Available forms: Loz 5 mg; liq 7.5, 15 mg/5 ml; syr 10 mg/5 ml, 15 mg/5 ml, 15 mg/15 ml, 30 mg/15 ml; gel caps 15 mg; caps 15 mg; spray mist 6 mg/accuation

SIDE EFFECTS

CNS: Dizziness, sedation, confusion, ataxia, fatigue

GI: Nausea

Contraindications: Hypersensitivity

Precautions: Pregnancy (C), fever, hepatic disease, asthma/emphysema, chronic cough

PHARMACOKINETICS

PO: Onset 15-30 min, duration 3-6 hr

SUS: Duration 12 hr, terminal half-life 11 hr, metabolized by the liver, excreted via kidneys

INTERACTIONS

- Do not give with MAOIs or within 2 wk of MAOIs; avoid furazolidone, linezolid, procarbazine (MAOI activity)

Increase: CNS depression—alcohol, antidepressants, antihistamines, opioids, sedative/hypnotics

Increase: adverse reactions—amiodarone, quinidine, serotonin receptor agonist, sibutramine, SSRI

NURSING CONSIDERATIONS

Assess:

- Cough: type, frequency, character, including sputum

Administer:

- Decreased dose to geriatric patients; metabolism may be slowed

Perform/provide:

- Increased fluids to liquefy secretions
- Humidification of patient's room

Evaluate:

• Therapeutic response: absence of cough

Teach patient/family:

• To avoid driving, other hazardous activities until patient is stabilized on this medication

• To avoid smoking, smoke-filled rooms, perfumes, dust, environmental pollutants, cleaners that increase cough

• To avoid alcohol, CNS depressants

• To notify prescriber if cough persists over a few days

dextrose (D-glucose) (℞)

Glucose, Glutose, Insta-Glucose

Func. class.: Caloric, parenteral solution

Action: Needed for adequate utilization of amino acids; decreases protein, nitrogen loss; prevents ketosis

Uses: Increases intake of calories; increases fluids in patients unable to take adequate fluids, calories orally; acute hypoglycemia

DOSAGE AND ROUTES

• *Adult and child:* **IV** Depends on individual requirements

Hypoglycemia

• *Adult:* **PO/IV** 10-25 mg

Available forms: Inj 2.5%, 5%, 10%, 20%, 25%, 30%, 38.5%, 40%, 50%, 60%, 70%; oral gel 40%; chew tab 5 g

SIDE EFFECTS

CNS: Confusion, **loss of consciousness,** dizziness

CV: Hypertension, **CHF, pulmonary edema, intracranial hemorrhage**

ENDO: Hyperglycemia, rebound hypoglycemia, hyperosmolar syndrome, hyperglycemic nonketotic syndrome, aluminum toxicity, hypokalemia, hypomagnesium

GI: Nausea

GU: Glycosuria, osmotic diuresis

INTEG: Chills, flushing, warm feeling, rash, urticaria, extravasation necrosis

RESP: Pulmonary edema

Contraindications: Hyperglycemia, delirium tremens, hemorrhage (cranial/spinal), CHF, anuria, allergy to corn products

Precautions: Cardiac/renal/hepatic disease, diabetes mellitus, carbohydrate intolerance

INTERACTIONS

Increase: fluid retention/electrolyte excretion—corticosteroids

NURSING CONSIDERATIONS

Assess:

• Electrolytes (K, Na, Ca, Cl, Mg), blood glucose, ammonia, phosphate

• Inj site for extravasation: redness along vein, edema at site, necrosis, pain; hard, tender area; site should be changed immediately

• Monitor temp q4hr for increased fever, indicating infection; if infection suspected, infusion is discontinued, tubing, bottle, catheter tip cultured

• Serum glucose in patients receiving hypotonic glucose 50% and over

• Nutritional status: calorie count by dietitian

Administer:

• Only (4%) protein and dextrose (up to 12.5%) via peripheral vein; stronger sol: central IV administration

• May be given undiluted via prepared sol; give 10% sol, 5 ml/15 sec; 10% sol, 1000 ml/3 hr or more; 20% sol, 500 ml/½-1 hr; 50% sol, 10 ml/min; control rate, rapid inf may cause fluid shifts

• Oral glucose preparations (gel, chew tabs) are to be used in conscious patients only; check serum blood glucose 10 min after first dose

• After changing IV catheter, dressing q24hr with aseptic technique

Evaluate:

• Therapeutic response: increased weight

Teach patient/family:
- The reason for dextrose inf
- To review hypoglycemia/hyperglycemia symptoms
- To review blood glucose monitoring procedure

diazepam (℞)

(dye-az′-e-pam)
Apo-Diazepam ✽, Diastat, Diazemuls ✽, diazepam, Diazepam Intensol, Novodiapam ✽, PMS-Diazepam ✽, Valium, Vivol ✽

Func. class.: Antianxiety, anticonvulsant, skeletal muscle relaxant, central acting
Chem. class.: Benzodiazepine, long-acting

Controlled Substance Schedule IV
Do not confuse:
diazepam/Ditropan/lorazepam

Action: Potentiates the actions of GABA, especially in limbic system, reticular formation; enhances presympathetic inhibition, inhibits spinal polysynaptic afferent paths

Uses: Anxiety, acute alcohol withdrawal, adjunct in seizure disorders; preoperatively as a relaxant, skeletal muscle relaxation; rectally for acute repetitive seizures

Unlabeled uses: Agitation, benzodiazepine withdrawal, chloroquine overdose, insomnia, seizure prophylaxis

DOSAGE AND ROUTES

Anxiety/convulsive disorders
- *Adult:* **PO** 2-10 mg bid-qid; **IM/IV** 2-10 mg q3-4hr
- *Geriatric:* **PO** 1-2 mg daily-bid, increase slowly as needed
- *Child >6 mo:* **IM/IV** 0.04-0.3 mg/kg/dose q2-4hr, max 0.6 mg/kg in an 8 hr period

Precardioversion
- *Adult:* **IV** 5-15 mg 5-10 min precardioversion

Preendoscopy
- *Adult:* **IV** 2.5-20 mg; **IM** 5-10 mg ½ hr preendoscopy

Muscle relaxation
- *Adult:* **PO** 2-10 mg tid-qid or **EXT REL** 15-30 mg/day; **IV/IM** 5-10 mg repeat in 2-4 hr
- *Geriatric:* **PO** 2-5 mg bid-qid; **IV/IM** 2-5 mg, may repeat in 2-4 hr

Tetanic muscle spasms
- *Child >5 yr:* **IM/IV** 5-10 mg q3-4hr prn
- *Infant >30 days:* **IM/IV** 1-2 mg q3-4hr prn

Status epilepticus
- *Adult:* **IV/IM** 5-10 mg, 2 mg/min, may repeat q10-15min, not to exceed 30 mg; may repeat in 2-4 hr if seizures reappear
- *Child >5 yr:* **IM** 1 mg q2-5min; **IV** 1 mg slowly
- *Child 1 mo-5 yr:* **IV** 0.2-0.5 mg slowly; **IM** 0.2-0.5 mg slowly q2-5min up to 5 mg, may repeat in 2-4 hr prn

Seizures other than status epilepticus
- *Adult:* **RECT** 0.2 mg/kg, may repeat 4-12 hr later
- *Child 6-11 yr:* **RECT** 0.3 mg/kg, may repeat 4-12 hr later
- *Child 2-5 yr:* **RECT** 0.5 mg/kg, may repeat 4-12 hr later

Alcohol withdrawal
- *Adult:* **IV** 10 mg initially, then 5-10 mg q3-4hr prn

Benzodiazepine withdrawal (unlabeled)
- *Adult:* **PO** Taper 0.5-2 mg over 4-16 wk

Febrile seizure prophylaxis (unlabeled)
- *Child 6 mo-5 yr:* **PO** 0.33 mg/kg q8hr until afebrile for ≥24 hr

Available forms: Tabs 2, 5, 10 mg; inj 5 mg/ml; oral sol 5 mg/5 ml, 5 mg/ml; gel, rectal delivery system 10 mg, twin packs; ext rel cap 15 mg

SIDE EFFECTS

CNS: Dizziness, drowsiness, confusion, headache, anxiety, tremors, stimulation, fatigue, depression, insomnia, hallucinations, ataxia, fatigue

CV: Orthostatic hypotension, **ECG changes, tachycardia,** hypotension

EENT: Blurred vision, tinnitus, mydriasis, nystagmus

GI: Constipation, dry mouth, nausea, vomiting, anorexia, diarrhea

HEMA: **Neutropenia**

INTEG: Rash, dermatitis, itching

RESP: **Respiratory depression**

Contraindications: Pregnancy (D), hypersensitivity to benzodiazepines, closed-angle glaucoma, coma, myasthenia gravis, ethanol intoxication, hepatic disease, sleep apnea

Precautions: Breastfeeding, children <6 mo, geriatric patients, debilitated, renal disease, asthma, bipolar disorder, COPD, CNS depression, labor, Parkinson's disease, neutropenia, psychosis, seizures, substance abuse, smoking

PHARMACOKINETICS

Metabolized by liver via CYP2C19, CYP3A4; excreted by kidneys; crosses placenta; excreted in breast milk; crosses the blood-brain barrier; half-life 20-50 hr; more reliable by mouth; 99% protein binding

PO: Rapidly absorbed, onset ½ hr, duration 2-3 hr

IM: Onset 15-30 min, duration 1-1½ hr, absorption slow and erratic

RECT: Peak 1.5 hr

IV: Onset immediate, duration 15 min-1 hr

INTERACTIONS

Increase: toxicity—barbiturates, SSRIs, cimetidine, CNS depressants, valproic acid, CYP3A4 inhibitors

Increase: CNS depression—CNS depressants, alcohol

Decrease: diazepam metabolism—oral contraceptives, valproic acid, disulfiram, isoniazid, propranolol

Decrease: diazepam effect—CYP3A4 inducers (rifampin, barbiturates, carbamazepine, ethotoin, phenytoin, fosphenytoin)

Drug/Herb

Increase: diazepam action—cowslip, goldenseal, kava, melatonin, mistletoe, pokeweed, poppy, Queen Anne's lace, valerian

Decrease: diazepam effect—cola tree, St. John's wort

Drug/Lab Test

Increase: AST/ALT, serum bilirubin

Decrease: RAIU

False increase: 17-OHCS

NURSING CONSIDERATIONS

Assess:

- B/P (lying, standing), pulse; respiratory rate; if systolic B/P drops 20 mm Hg, hold product, notify prescriber; respirations q5-15min if given IV
- Blood studies: CBC during long-term therapy; blood dyscrasias (rare); hepatic studies: ALT, AST
- Degree of anxiety; what precipitates anxiety and whether product controls symptoms
- For alcohol withdrawal symptoms, including hallucinations (visual, auditory), delirium, irritability, agitation, fine to coarse tremors
- For seizure control and type, duration, intensity of seizures
- For muscle spasms; pain relief
- Hepatic studies: AST, ALT, bilirubin, creatinine, LDH, alk phos
- IV site for thrombosis or phlebitis, which may occur rapidly
- Mental status: mood, sensorium, affect, sleeping pattern, drowsiness, dizziness, suicidal tendencies
- Physical dependency, withdrawal symptoms: headache, nausea, vomiting, muscle pain, weakness after long-term use

Administer:

- With food or milk for GI symptoms; crushed if patient is unable to swallow medication whole
- Sugarless gum, hard candy, frequent sips of water for dry mouth

• Reduced opioid dose by ⅓ if given concomitantly with diazepam
• Concentrate: use calibrated dropper only; mix with water, juice, pudding, applesauce; to be consumed immediately

Rectal route

• Do not use more than 5 ×/mo or for an episode q5days

IV route

• Into large vein; give IV 5 mg or less/1 min or total dose over 3 min or more (children, infants); continuous inf is not recommended; inject as close to vein insertion as possible; do not dilute or mix with other products

Additive compatibilities: Netilmicin, verapamil

Syringe compatibilities: Cimetidine

Y-site compatibilities: Cefmetazole, DOBUTamine, nafcillin, quinidine, sufentanil

Perform/provide:

• Assistance with ambulation during beginning therapy, for drowsiness, dizziness, safety measures
• Check to see PO medication has been swallowed

Evaluate:

• Therapeutic response: decreased anxiety, restlessness, insomnia

Teach patient/family:

• That product may be taken with food
• That product is not to be used for everyday stress or used longer than 4 mo unless directed by prescriber; no more than prescribed amount; may be habit forming
• To avoid OTC preparations unless approved by prescriber
• To avoid driving, activities that require alertness; drowsiness may occur
• To avoid alcohol, other psychotropic medications unless directed by prescriber; that smoking may decrease diazepam effect by increasing diazepam metabolism
• Not to discontinue medication abruptly after long-term use, gradually taper
• To rise slowly or fainting may occur, especially in geriatric patients
• That drowsiness may worsen at beginning of treatment
• To avoid use during pregnancy

Treatment of overdose: Lavage, VS, supportive care, flumazenil

diazoxide (℞)

(dye-az-ox'ide)
diazoxide parenteral,
Proglycem
Func. class.: Antihypertensive
Chem. class.: Vasodilator

Action: Vasodilates arteriolar smooth muscle by direct relaxation; a reduction in B/P with concomitant increases in heart rate, cardiac output; reduces release of insulin from the pancreas

Uses: Hypertensive crisis when urgent decrease of diastolic pressure required (IV); increase blood glucose levels in hyperinsulinism

DOSAGE AND ROUTES

Hypoglycemia

• *Adult and child:* **PO** 3-8 mg/kg/day in 2-3 divided doses q8-12hr
• *Infants and neonates:* **PO** 8-15 mg/kg/day in 2-3 divided doses 8-12 hr

Hypertension

• *Adult:* **IV BOL** 1-3 mg/kg rapidly up to a max of 150 mg in a single inj; dose may be repeated at 5-15 min intervals until desired response is achieved; give IV in 30 sec or less
• *Child:* **IV BOL** 1-2 mg/kg rapidly; administration same as adult, not to exceed 150 mg

Available forms: Caps 50 mg; oral susp 50 mg/ml; inj 15 mg/ml, 300 mg/20 ml

SIDE EFFECTS

CNS: *Headache,* sleepiness, euphoria, anxiety, EPS, confusion, tinnitus, blurred vision, dizziness, weakness, **seizures, cerebral ischemia, paralysis**

CV: **Hypotension,** T-wave changes, angina pectoris, palpitations, **supraventricular tachycardia, edema,** rebound hypertension, **shock, MI**

ENDO: Hyperglycemia in diabetics, transient hyperglycemia in nondiabetics, increased uric acid
GI: Nausea, vomiting, dry mouth
GU: Breast tenderness; increased BUN, fluid, electrolyte imbalances; Na, water retention
HEMA: Decreased Hgb, Hct, **thrombocytopenia**
INTEG: Rash

Contraindications: Hypersensitivity to thiazides, sulfonamides, hypertension of aortic coarctation or AV shunt, pheochromocytoma, dissecting aortic aneurysm, hypoglycemia

Precautions: Pregnancy (C), breastfeeding, children, tachycardia, fluid, electrolyte imbalances, impaired cerebral or cardiac circulation

PHARMACOKINETICS

Half-life 20-36 hr; excreted slowly in urine; crosses blood-brain barrier, placenta; highly protein bound (>90%)
PO: Onset 1 hr; peak 8-12 hr; duration 4-20 hr
IV: Onset 1-2 min, peak 5 min, duration 3-12 hr

INTERACTIONS

Increase: hyperglycemia—sulfonylureas
Increase: severe hypotension—antihypertensives
Increase: hyperuricemic, antihypertensive effects of diazoxide—thiazide diuretics
Decrease: anticonvulsant effect—hydantoins
Decrease: antihypertensive effect—NSAIDs, salicylates

Drug/Herb
- Toxicity/death: aconite

NURSING CONSIDERATIONS

Assess:
- B/P q5min until stabilized, then q1hr × 2 hr, then q4hr
- Pulse, jugular venous distention q4hr
- Electrolytes, blood studies: K, Na, Cl, CO_2, CBC, serum glucose
- Weight daily, I&O
- Edema in feet, legs daily
- Skin turgor, mucous membranes for hydration status
- Crackles, dyspnea, orthopnea
- IV site for extravasation
- Signs of CHF: dyspnea, edema, wet crackles
- Postural hypotension, take B/P sitting, standing

Administer:
- Undiluted; give over ½ min or less
- To patient in recumbent position; keep in that position for 1 hr after administration

Syringe compatibilities: Heparin

Perform/provide:
- Store protected from light

Evaluate:
- Therapeutic response: decreased B/P, primarily diastolic pressure

Treatment of overdose: DOPamine, or norepinephrine for hypotension, Trendelenburg maneuver

dibucaine topical

See Appendix B

diclofenac epolamine (℞)

(dye-kloe'fen-ak)

Flector

diclofenac potassium (℞)

Cataflam, Voltaren Rapide ✦, Zipsor

diclofenac sodium (℞)

Apo-Dilo ✦, Cambia, Novo-Difenac ✦, Solaraze Topical Gel, Voltaren, Voltaren Topical Gel, Voltaren XR

Func. class.: Nonsteroidal antiinflammatory products (NSAIDs), nonopioid analgesic

Chem. class.: Phenylacetic acid

Do not confuse:
Cataflam/Catapres

Action: Inhibits prostaglandin synthesis by decreasing enzyme needed for biosynthesis; analgesic, antiinflammatory, antipyretic

Uses: Acute, chronic RA; osteoarthritis; ankylosing spondylitis; analgesia; primary dysmenorrhea; patch: mild-moderate pain

Unlabeled uses: Arthralgia, headache, migraine, bone pain, myalgia

DOSAGE AND ROUTES

Osteoarthritis

- *Adult:* **PO** (Cataflam) 50 mg bid-tid, max 150 mg/day; **DEL REL** (Voltaren) 50 mg bid-tid, or 75 mg bid, max 150 mg/day; **EXT REL** (Voltaren-XR) 100 mg daily, max 150 mg/day; **TOP GEL** 1% (Voltaren gel) 4 g for each of lower extremities qid, max 16 g/day; 2 g for each of upper extremities qid, max 8 g/day

Rheumatoid arthritis

- *Adult:* **PO** (Cataflam) 50 mg tid-qid, max 225 mg/day; **DEL REL** (Voltaren) 50 mg tid-qid or 75 mg bid, max 225 mg/day; **EXT REL** (Voltaren-XR) 100 mg daily, may increase to 200 mg/day, max 225 mg/day

Ankylosing spondylitis

- *Adult:* **PO DEL REL** (Voltaren) 25 mg qid and 25 mg at bedtime, max 125 mg/day

Acute migraine with/without aura

- *Adult:* **PO** (powder for oral sol) (Cambia) 50 mg as a single dose, mix contents of packet in 1-2 oz water

Mild to moderate pain

- *Adult:* **PO** (Zipsor) 25 mg qid

Dysmenorrhea or nonrheumatic inflammatory conditions

- *Adult:* **PO** (Cataflam) 50 mg tid or 100 mg initially, then 50 mg tid, max 200 mg 1st day, then 150 mg/day

Pain of strains/sprains

- *Adult:* **TOP PATCH** (Flector) apply patch to area bid

Actinic keratosis

- *Adult:* **TOP GEL** (Solaraze) apply to area bid

Prevention of heterotropic ossification (unlabeled)

- *Adult:* **PO** 50 mg tid × 3 wk

Renal dose

- *Avoid:* Use of Voltaren gel in advanced renal disease

Available forms: *Epolamine:* topical patch 1.3%; *potassium:* tabs 50 mg; tabs liquid filled 25 mg; *sodium:* delayed rel tabs (enteric-coated) 25, 50, 75, 100 mg; oral sol

SIDE EFFECTS

CNS: Dizziness, headache, drowsiness, fatigue, tremors, confusion, insomnia, anxiety, depression, nervousness, paresthesia, muscle weakness

CV: **CHF,** tachycardia, peripheral edema, palpitations, **dysrhythmias,** hypo/hypertension, fluid retention, **MI, stroke**

EENT: Tinnitus, hearing loss, blurred vision, **laryngeal edema**

GI: Nausea, anorexia, vomiting, diarrhea, **jaundice, cholestatic hepatitis,** constipation, flatulence, cramps, dry mouth, peptic ulcer, GI bleeding, **hepatotoxicity**

GU: **Nephrotoxicity: dysuria, hematuria, oliguria, azotemia, cystitis, UTI**
HEMA: **Blood dyscrasias,** epistaxis, bruising
INTEG: Purpura, rash, pruritus, sweating, erythema, petechiae, photosensitivity, alopecia
RESP: Dyspnea, hemoptysis, pharyngitis, **bronchospasm,** rhinitis, SOB
SYST: **Anaphylaxis**

Contraindications: Hypersensitivity to aspirin, iodides, other NSAIDs, asthma, serious CV disease

Black Box Warning: Treatment of perioperative pain (CABG) surgery

Precautions: Pregnancy (C) 1st trimester, breastfeeding, children, not recommended in 2nd half of pregnancy, bleeding disorders, GI disorders, cardiac disorders, hypersensitivity to other antiinflammatory agents, CCr <30 ml/min

Black Box Warning: GI bleeding, MI, stroke

PHARMACOKINETICS

PO: Peak 2-3 hr, TOP Patch, peak 12 hr; elimination half-life 2.5 hr, 99% bound to plasma proteins, metabolized in liver to metabolite, excreted in urine

INTERACTIONS

• Hyperkalemia: potassium-sparing diuretics
• Need for dosage adjustment: antidiabetics

Increase: anticoagulant effect—anticoagulants, NSAIDs, platelet inhibitors, salicylates, thrombolytics, SSRIs
Increase: toxicity—phenytoin, lithium, cycloSPORINE, methotrexate
Increase: GI side effects—aspirin, other NSAIDs, biphosphonates, corticosteroids
Decrease: antihypertensive effect—β-blockers, diuretics, ACE inhibitors

Drug/Herb

• Severe photosensitivity: St. John's wort

Increase: bleeding risk—bogbean, chondroitin, garlic, ginger, ginkgo, saw palmetto, turmeric
Increase: gastric irritation—arginine, gossypol
Increase: NSAIDs effect—bearberry, bilberry

NURSING CONSIDERATIONS

Assess:

• For pain: location, character, aggravating, alleviating factors, ROM, before and 1 hr after dose
• Blood counts during therapy; watch for decreasing platelets; if low, therapy may need to be discontinued, restarted after hematologic recovery
• For clients with asthma, aspirin hypersensitivity, nasal polyps; may develop hypersensitivity
• LFTs (may be elevated) and uric acid (may be decreased—serum; increased—urine) periodically; also BUN, creatinine, electrolytes (may be elevated)

⚠ Blood dyscrasias (thrombocytopenia): bruising, fatigue, bleeding, poor healing

Administer:

PO route

• Do not break, crush, or chew enteric products
• Take with a full glass of water to enhance absorption, remain upright for ½ hr; if dose is missed, take as soon as remembered within 2 hr if taking 1-2 ×/day; do not double doses

Topical route (patch) (Flector)

• Wash hands before handling patch
• Remove and release liner before administration
• Use only on normal, intact skin
• Remove before bath, shower, swimming
• Discard removed patch in trash away from children, pets

Topical route (gel)

• Apply to intact skin
• Use only for osteoarthritis, mild-moderate pain

Perform/provide

• Storage of patches at room temperature in resealable envelope provided

Evaluate:

• Therapeutic response: decreased inflammation in joints, decreased inflammation after cataract surgery

Teach patient/family:
- That product must be continued for prescribed time to be effective; to contact prescriber prior to surgery as when to discontinue this product
- To report bleeding, bruising, fatigue, malaise; blood dyscrasias do occur
- To avoid aspirin, alcoholic beverages, NSAIDs, or other OTC medications unless approved by prescriber
- To take with food, milk, or antacids to avoid GI upset, to swallow whole
- To use caution when driving; drowsiness, dizziness may occur
- To report hepatotoxicity: flulike symptoms, nausea, vomiting, jaundice, pruritus, lethargy
- To use sunscreen to prevent photosensitivity
- To report respiratory difficulty, trouble swallowing
- To notify all providers that product is being used

diclofenac ophthalmic

See Appendix B

Rarely Used

dicyclomine (℞)

(dye-sye'kloe-meen)

Bentyl, Bentylol ♣, dicyclomine HCL, Formulex ♣, Lomine ♣

Func. class.: Gastrointestinal anticholinergic

Uses: Treatment of peptic ulcer disease in combination with other products; infant colic, urinary incontinence, IBS

DOSAGE AND ROUTES

- *Adult:* **PO** 10-20 mg tid-qid; **IM** 20 mg q4-6hr; max 160 mg/day
- *Child >2 yr:* **PO** 10 mg tid-qid
- *Child 6 mo-2 yr:* **PO** 5 mg tid-qid

Contraindications: Hypersensitivity to anticholinergics, closed-angle glaucoma, GI obstruction, myasthenia gravis, paralytic ileus, GI atony, toxic megacolon

didanosine (℞)

(dye-dan'oh-seen)

ddI, dideoxyinosine, Videx Pediatric, Videx EC

Func. class.: Antiretroviral

Chem. class.: Nucleoside reverse transcriptase inhibitor (NRTI)

Action: Nucleoside analog incorporating into cellular DNA by viral reverse transcriptase, thereby terminating the cellular DNA chain

Uses: HIV-1 infection in combination with other antiretrovirals

Unlabeled uses: Hepatitis B, HIV prophylaxis

DOSAGE AND ROUTES

- *Adult >60 kg:* **PO DEL REL** caps 400 mg/day
- *Adult <60 kg:* **PO DEL REL** caps 250 mg/day
- *Child:* **PO** (child BSA 1.1-1.4 m^2); recon pedi powder 125 mg q8-12hr; **PO** (child BSA 0.8-1 m^2); recon pedi powder 94 mg q8-12hr; **PO** (child BSA 0.5-0.7 m^2); recon pedi powder 62 mg q8-12hr; **PO** (child BSA <0.4 m^2); recon pedi powder 31 mg q8-12hr

Renal dose
- *Adult >60 kg:* **PO** (Videx EC cap) CCr 30-59 ml/min 200 mg/day; CCr 10-29 ml/min 125 mg/day; CCr <10 ml/min 125 mg/day
- *Adult <60 kg:* **PO** (Videx EC cap) CCr 30-59 ml/min 125 mg/day; CCr 10-29 ml/min 125 mg/day; CCr <10 ml/min avoid use

Available forms: Powder for oral sol 10 mg/ml; del rel caps 125, 200, 250, 400

SIDE EFFECTS

CNS: **Peripheral neuropathy, seizures,** confusion, *anxiety*, hypertonia, abnormal thinking, asthenia, *insomnia*, **CNS depression,** pain, dizziness, chills, fever

CV: Hypertension, vasodilation, dysrhythmia, syncope, **CHF**, palpitation
EENT: Ear pain, otitis, photophobia, visual impairment, retinal depigmentation
GI: **Pancreatitis,** ***diarrhea, nausea***, vomiting, ***abdominal pain***, constipation, stomatitis, dyspepsia, liver abnormalities, flatulence, taste perversion, dry mouth, oral thrush, melena, increased ALT, AST, alk phos, amylase, **hepatic failure**
GU: Increased bilirubin, uric acid
HEMA: **Leukopenia, granulocytopenia, thrombocytopenia, anemia**
INTEG: ***Rash, pruritus,*** alopecia, ecchymosis, hemorrhage, petechiae, sweating
MS: Myalgia, arthritis, myopathy, muscular atrophy
RESP: Cough, pneumonia, dyspnea, asthma, epistaxis, hypoventilation, sinusitis
SYST: **Lactic acidosis, anaphylaxis**
Contraindications: Hypersensitivity, lactic acidosis, pancreatitis, phenylketonuria
Precautions: Pregnancy (B), breastfeeding, children, renal disease, sodium-restricted diets, elevated amylase, preexisting peripheral neuropathy, hyperuricemia, gout, CHF

Black Box Warning: Hepatic disease, lactic acidosis, pancreatitis

PHARMACOKINETICS

PO: Peak 0.67 hr, del rel 2 hr; elimination half-life 1.62 hr; extensive metabolism is thought to occur; administration within 5 min of food will decrease absorption (50%); excreted urine/feces

INTERACTIONS

Increase: didanosine level—allopurinol, tenofovir, adjust dose as needed
Increase: side effects from magnesium, aluminum antacids
Decrease: absorption—ketoconazole, dapsone
Decrease: concentrations of fluoroquinolones, other antiretrovirals, itraconazole, tetracyclines
Decrease: didanosine level—methadone

Drug/Food

- Any food decreases rate of absorption 50%
- Do not use with acidic juices

NURSING CONSIDERATIONS

Assess:

- Peripheral neuropathy: tingling or pain in hands and feet, distal numbness; onset usually occurs 2-6 mo after beginning treatment, may persist if product is not discontinued

⚠ Pancreatitis: abdominal pain, nausea, vomiting, elevated hepatic enzymes; product should be discontinued, since condition can be fatal

- For anaphylaxis, lactic acidosis
- Children by dilated retinal exam q6mo to rule out retinal depigmentation
- CBC, differential, platelet count q mo; withhold product if WBC is <4000 or platelet count is <75,000; notify prescriber of results; alk phos, monitor amylase; viral load, CD4 count
- Renal studies: BUN, serum uric acid, urine CCr before, during therapy
- Temp q4hr, may indicate beginning infection
- Hepatic studies before, during therapy (bilirubin, AST, ALT) as needed or q mo

Administer:

- Pediatric powder for oral sol after preparation by pharmacist; dilution is required using purified USP water, then antacid (10 mg/ml), refrigerate, shake before use
- On an empty stomach ≥30 min before or 2 hr after meals
- Adjust dose in renal impairment

Perform/provide:

- Cleanup of powdered products; use wet mop or damp sponge
- Storage of tabs, caps in tightly closed bottle at room temperature; store oral sol after dissolving at room temperature ≤4 hr

Evaluate:

- Therapeutic response: absence of infection; symptoms of HIV

Teach patient/family:
- To avoid use with alcohol
- To report numbness/tingling in extremities
- To take on an empty stomach; not to take dapsone at same time as ddI; do not mix powder with fruit juice, chew tab or crush and dissolve in water; drink powder immediately after mixing
- To report signs of infection: increased temp, sore throat, flulike symptoms
- To report signs of anemia: fatigue, headache, faintness, SOB, irritability
- To report bleeding; avoid use of razors, commercial mouthwash
- That hair may be lost during therapy (rare); a wig or hairpiece may make patient feel better
- That product does not cure, only controls symptoms

Rarely Used

diflunisal (℞)

(dye-floo′ni-sal)

diflunisal, Dolobid

Func. class.: Nonsteroidal anti-inflammatory/analgesic (nonopioid)

Uses: Mild to moderate pain or fever including arthritis; 3-4 times more potent than aspirin

DOSAGE AND ROUTES

- *Adult:* **PO** Loading dose 1 g; then 250-1000 mg/day in 2 divided doses, q12hr, not to exceed 1500 mg/day
- *Geriatric:* **PO** ½ adult dose

Contraindications: Pregnancy (3rd trimester), children <12 yr, hypersensitivity to salicylates, bleeding disorders, vit K deficiency, Reye's syndrome, anemia, dehydration

Black Box Warning: GI bleeding, perioperative pain of CABG, MI, stroke

difluprednate ophthalmic

See Appendix B

⚠ High Alert

digoxin (℞)

(di-jox′in)

digoxin, Lanoxicaps, Lanoxin

Func. class.: Cardiac glycoside, inotropic, antidysrhythmic

Chem. class.: Digoxin preparation

Do not confuse:

Lanoxin/Lasix/Lonox/Lomotil/Xanax/Levoxine

Action: Inhibits the sodium-potassium ATPase, which makes more calcium available for contractile proteins, resulting in increased cardiac output (positive inotropic effect); increases force of contraction; decreases heart rate (negative chronotropic effect); decreases AV conduction speed

Uses: Heart failure, atrial fibrillation, atrial flutter, atrial tachycardia, cardiogenic shock, paroxysmal atrial tachycardia, rapid digitalization in these disorders

Unlabeled uses: Atrial flutter, paroxysmal supraventricular tachycardia (PSVT) treatment/prophylaxis

DOSAGE AND ROUTES

- *Adult:* **IV digitalizing dose** 0.6-1 mg given as 50% of the dose initially, additional fractions given at 4-8 hr intervals; **PO digitalizing dose** 0.75-1.25 mg given as 50% of the dose initially, additional fractions given at 4-8 hr intervals; **maintenance** 0.125-0.5 mg/day (tabs), or 0.350-0.5 mg/day (gelatin cap)
- *Child >10 yr:* **IV digitalizing dose** 8-12 mcg/kg given as 50% of the dose initially, additional fractions given at 4-8 hr intervals; **PO digitalizing dose** 0.01-0.015 mg/kg given as 50% of the dose initially, additional fractions given at 6-8 hr intervals; **maintenance** 25%-35% of the loading dose daily as a single dose
- *Child 5-10 yr:* **IV digitalizing dose** 0.015-0.03 mg/kg given as 50% of the dose initially, additional fractions given at 4-8 hr intervals; **PO digitalizing dose**

0.02-0.035 mg/kg given as 50% of the dose initially, additional fractions given at 6-8 hr intervals; **maintenance** 25%-35% of the loading dose daily in 2 divided doses

• *Child 2-5 yr:* **IV digitalizing dose** 0.025-0.035 mg/kg given as 50% of the dose initially, additional fractions given at 4-8 hr intervals; **PO digitalizing dose** 0.03-0.04 mg/kg given as 50% of the dose initially, additional fractions given at 6-8 hr intervals; **maintenance** 25%-35% of the loading dose daily in 2 divided doses

• *Child 1-2 yr:* **IV digitalizing dose** 0.03-0.05 mg/kg given as 50% of the dose initially, additional fractions given at 4-8 hr intervals; **PO digitalizing dose** 0.035-0.06 mg/kg given as 50% of the dose initially, additional fractions given at 4-8 hr intervals; **maintenance** 25%-35% of the loading dose daily in 2 divided doses

• *Infant:* **IV digitalizing dose** 0.02-0.03 mg/kg given as 50% of the dose initially, additional fractions given at 4-8 hr intervals; **PO digitalizing dose** 0.025-0.035 mg/kg given as 50% of the dose initially, additional fractions given at 6-8 hr intervals; **maintenance** 25%-35% of the loading dose daily in 2 divided doses

• *Infant, premature:* **IV digitalizing dose** 0.015-0.025 mg/kg given as 50% of the dose initially, additional fractions given at 4-8 hr intervals; **PO digitalizing dose** 0.02-0.03 mg/kg given as 50% of the dose initially, additional fractions given at 6-8 hr intervals; **maintenance** 20%-30% of the loading dose daily in 2 divided doses

Available forms: Caps 0.05, 0.1, 0.2 mg; elix 0.05 mg/ml; tabs 0.125, 0.25, 0.5 mg; inj 0.5 ♣, 0.25 mg/ml; pediatric inj 0.1 mg/ml

SIDE EFFECTS

CNS: Headache, drowsiness, apathy, confusion, disorientation, fatigue, depression, hallucinations

CV: **Dysrhythmias,** *hypotension,* bradycardia, **AV block**

EENT: Blurred vision, yellow-green halos, photophobia, diplopia

GI: Nausea, vomiting, anorexia, abdominal pain, diarrhea

Contraindications: Hypersensitivity to digoxin, ventricular fibrillation, ventricular tachycardia, carotid sinus syndrome, 2nd- or 3rd-degree heart block

Precautions: Pregnancy (C), breastfeeding, geriatric patients, renal disease, acute MI, AV block, severe respiratory disease, hypothyroidism, sinus nodal disease, hypokalemia

PHARMACOKINETICS

Half-life 1.5 days, excreted in urine

PO: Onset ½-2 hr, peak 6-8 hr, duration 3-4 days

IV: Onset 5-30 min, peak 1-5 hr, duration variable

INTERACTIONS

• Hypercalcemia, hypomagnesemia, digoxin toxicity: thiazides, parenteral calcium

• Hypokalemia, digoxin toxicity: diuretics, amphotericin B, carbenicillin, ticarcillin, corticosteroids

Increase: digoxin levels—propantheline, quinidine, verapamil, amiodarone, anticholinergics, diltiazem, NIFEdipine

Increase: bradycardia—β-adrenergic blockers, antidysrythmics

Increase: cardiac dysrhythmia risk—sympathomimetics

Decrease: digoxin absorption—antacids, kaolin/pectin

Decrease: digoxin level—thyroid agents, cholestyramine, colestipol, metoclopramide

Drug/Herb

• Forms insoluble complex: blackroot

• Bradycardia: Indian snakeroot

• Cardiac toxicity: aconite, hawthorn, horsetail

Increase: digoxin action—aloe, betel palm, broom, buckthorn, cascara sagrada, castor, Chinese rhubarb, figwort, fumitory, hawthorn, khat, kudzu, licorice, lily of the valley, Mayapple, mistletoe,

motherwort, night-blooming cereus, oleander, pheasant's eye, purple foxglove, Queen Anne's lace, rhubarb, rue, senna, Siberian ginseng, squill, yellow dock
Increase: hypokalemia—cocoa, coffee, cola, guarana, horsetail, licorice, yerba maté
Decrease: digoxin absorption—psyllium
Decrease: digoxin effect—beth root, goldenseal, St. John's wort
Drug/Lab Test
Increase: CPK

NURSING CONSIDERATIONS

Assess:
- Apical pulse for 1 min before giving product; if pulse <60 in adult or <90 in an infant, take again in 1 hr; if <60 in adult, call prescriber; note rate, rhythm, character; monitor ECG continuously during parenteral loading dose
- Electrolytes: K, Na, Cl, Mg, Ca; renal function studies: BUN, creatinine; blood studies: ALT, AST, bilirubin, Hct, Hgb before initiating treatment and periodically thereafter
- I&O ratio, daily weights; monitor turgor, lung sounds, edema
- Monitor product levels (therapeutic level 0.5-2 ng/ml)
- Cardiac status: apical pulse, character, rate, rhythm

Administer:
PO route
- Do not break, crush, or chew caps
- PO with or without food; may crush tabs, only mix with food/fluids
- Potassium supplements if ordered for potassium levels <3, or foods high in potassium: bananas, orange juice

IV route
- Undiluted or 1 ml of product/4 ml sterile H_2O, D_5, or NS; give >5 min through Y-tube or 3-way stopcock; during digitalization close monitoring is necessary

Additive compatibilities: Bretylium, cimetidine, floxacillin, furosemide, lidocaine, ranitidine, verapamil
Syringe compatibilities: Heparin, milrinone
Y-site compatibilities: Amrinone, cefmetazole, ciprofloxacin, cisatracurium, diltiazem, famotidine, meperidine, meropenem, midazolam, milrinone, morphine, potassium chloride, propofol, remifentanil, tacrolimus, vit B/C

Perform/provide:
- Storage protected from light

Evaluate:
- Therapeutic response: decreased weight, edema, pulse, respiration, crackles; increased urine output; serum digoxin level (0.5-2 ng/ml)

Teach patient/family:
- Not to stop product abruptly; teach all aspects of product, to take exactly as ordered; how to monitor heart rate
- To avoid OTC medications, herbal remedies since many adverse product interactions may occur; do not take antacid at same time
- To notify prescriber of loss of appetite, lower stomach pain, diarrhea, weakness, drowsiness, headache, blurred or yellow vision, rash, depression, toxicity
- The toxic symptoms of this product and when to notify prescriber
- To maintain a sodium-restricted diet as ordered
- To report shortness of breath, difficulty breathing, weight gain, edema, persistent cough

Treatment of overdose: Discontinue product; give potassium; monitor ECG; give adrenergic-blocking agent, digoxin immune FAB

digoxin immune FAB (ovine) (℞)

(di-jox'in im-myoon' FAB)
Digibind, DigiFab
Func. class.: Antidote—digoxin specific

Action: Antibody fragments bind to free digoxin or digitoxin to reverse toxicity by not allowing digoxin or digitoxin to bind to sites of action
Uses: Life-threatening digoxin toxicity

DOSAGE AND ROUTES

1 (38-mg) vial binds 0.5 mg digoxin

Digoxin toxicity (known amount) (tabs, oral sol, IM)

• *Adult and child:* **IV** dose (mg) = dose ingested (mg) × 0.8/1000 × 38 or 40 mg vial

Toxicity (known amount) (cap, IV)

• *Adult and child:* **IV** dose = dose ingested (mg)/0.5 × 38 or 40 mg vial

Toxicity (known amount) by serum digoxin concentrations (SDCs)

• *Adult and child:* **IV** SDC (ng/ml) × kg of weight/100 × 38 or 40 mg vial

Digoxin toxicity (unknown amount)

• *Adult and child >20 kg:* **IV** 228 mg (6 vials)

• *Infant and child <20 kg:* **IV** 38 mg (1 vial)

Acute ingestion

• *Adult:* **IV** 380 mg (10 vials)

Life-threatening ingestion

• *Adult:* **IV** 760 mg (20 vials)

Skin test

• *Adult:* **ID** 9.5 mcg

Available forms: Inj 38 mg/vial (binds 0.5 mg digoxin), 40 mg/vial (binds 0.5 mg digoxin)

SIDE EFFECTS

CV: **CHF,** ventricular rate increase, **atrial fibrillation,** low cardiac output, hypotension

INTEG: Hypersensitivity, allergic reactions, facial swelling, redness, phlebitis

META: **Hypokalemia**

MISC: **Anaphylaxis** (rare)

RESP: **Impaired respiratory function, rapid respiratory rate**

Contraindications: Mild digoxin toxicity, hypersensitivity to this product, papain or ovine protein

Precautions: Pregnancy (C), breastfeeding, children, geriatric patients, renal/cardiac disease, allergy to ovine proteins, hypocalcemia, heart failure

PHARMACOKINETICS

IV: Peaks after completion of inf; onset 30 min (variable); not known if crosses placenta, breast milk; half-life biphasic—14-20 hr, prolonged in renal disease; excreted by kidneys

INTERACTIONS

• Considered incompatible with all products in syringe or sol

Drug/Lab Test

Interference: immunoassay digoxin

NURSING CONSIDERATIONS

Assess:

• Hypokalemia: ST depression, flat T waves, presence of U wave, ventricular dysrhythmia; potassium levels may decrease rapidly

• CHF: Dyspnea, crackles, peripheral edema, B/P, volume overload

Administer:

• Test doses have proven to be ineffective in the general population; only use test dose in those with known allergies or those previously treated with digoxin immune FAB

• For test dose dilute 0.1 ml or reconstituted product (9.5 mg/ml) in 9.9 ml sterile isotonic saline, inj 0.1 ml (1 : 100 dilution) ID and observe for wheal with erythema; read in 20 min

• For scratch test place 1 gtt of sol on skin and make a scratch through the drop with a sterile needle; read in 20 min

• After diluting 38 mg/4 ml of sterile H_2O for inj 10 mg/ml mix; may be further diluted with normal saline, sol should be clear, colorless

• By bolus if cardiac arrest is imminent or IV over 30 min using a 0.22-μm filter

Perform/provide:

• Storage of reconstituted sol for up to 4 hr in refrigerator

• Do not freeze DigiFab

Evaluate:

• Therapeutic response: correction of digoxin toxicity; check digoxin levels 0.5-2 ng/ml; digitoxin level 9-25 ng/ml

Teach patient/family:
- The purpose of medication; to report delayed hypersensitivity; fever, chills, itching, swelling, dyspnea

dihydrotachysterol (℞)
(dye-hye-droh-tak-iss'ter-ole)
DHT Intensol ✤, Hytakerol
Func. class.: Parathyroid agent (calcium regulator)
Chem. class.: Vit D analog

Action: Increases intestinal absorption of calcium for bones, increases renal tubular absorption of phosphate; regulates calcium levels by regulating calcitonin, parathyroid hormone
Uses: Hypoparathyroidism, pseudohypoparathyroidism, postoperative tetany
Unlabeled uses: Renal osteodystrophy, familial hypophosphatemia

DOSAGE AND ROUTES

Hypoparathyroidism/pseudohypoparathyroidism
- *Adult:* **PO** 0.75-2.5 mg/day × 4 days, maintenance 0.2-1 mg/day regulated by serum calcium levels
- *Neonate:* **PO** 0.05-0.1 mg/day
- *Infant and child:* **PO** 1-5 mg daily × 4 days then 0.5-1.5 mg daily

Rickets (vit D–resistant)
- *Child:* **PO** 0.25-1 mg/day

Renal osteodystrophy (unlabeled)
- *Adult:* **PO** 0.1-0.6 mg/day
- *Child:* **PO** 0.1-0.5 mg/day

Hypophosphatemia (unlabeled)
- *Adult and child:* **PO** 0.5-2 mg/day, maintenance 0.2-1.5 mg/day

Available forms: Tabs 0.125, 0.2, 0.4 mg; caps 0.125 mg; oral sol 0.2, 0.25 mg/5 ml, 0.2 mg/ml ✤ (Intensol)

SIDE EFFECTS

CNS: Drowsiness, headache, vertigo, fever, lethargy, depression
CV: **Dysrhythmias**, hypertension
EENT: Tinnitus
GI: Nausea, diarrhea, vomiting, jaundice, anorexia, dry mouth, constipation, cramps, metallic taste, thirst
GU: Polyuria, hypercalciuria, hyperphosphatemia, hematuria, nocturia, renal calculi
MS: Myalgia, arthralgia, decreased bone development, weakness, ataxia
Contraindications: Hypersensitivity, renal disease, hyperphosphatemia, hypercalcemia, hypervitaminosis D
Precautions: Pregnancy (C), breastfeeding, renal calculi, CV disease

PHARMACOKINETICS

PO: Onset 2 wk, duration 2-9 wk, readily absorbed from small intestine, metabolized by liver, excreted in feces (active/inactive)

INTERACTIONS

- Hypercalcemia: thiazide diuretics, calcium supplements
- Cardiac dysrhythmias: cardiac glycosides, verapamil

Decrease: dihydrotachysterol absorption—cholestyramine, colestipol mineral oil
Decrease: dihydrotachysterol effect—corticosteroids, phenytoin, barbiturates
Drug/Lab Test
False increase: cholesterol

NURSING CONSIDERATIONS

Assess:
- BUN, urinary Ca, AST, ALT, cholesterol, creatinine, alk phos, uric acid, chlorine, magnesium, electrolytes, urine pH, phosphate; may increase calcium, should be kept at 9-10 mg/dl, vit D 50-135 international units/dl, phosphate 70 mg/dl
- Alk phos: may be decreased
- For increased blood level, since toxic reactions may occur rapidly
- For dry mouth, metallic taste, polyuria, bone pain, muscle weakness, headache, fatigue, tinnitus, change in LOC, irregular pulse, dysrhythmias, increased respirations, anorexia, nausea, vomiting, cramps, diarrhea, constipation; may indicate hypercalcemia

• Renal status: decreased urinary output (oliguria, anuria), edema in extremities, weight gain >5 lb, periorbital edema
• Nutritional status, diet for sources of vit D (milk, some seafood), calcium (dairy products, dark green vegetables), phosphates (dairy products) must be avoided

Administer:
• Do not break, crush, or chew caps
• PO, may be increased q4wk depending on blood level

Perform/provide:
• Storage in tight, light-resistant containers at room temperature
• Restriction of sodium, potassium if required
• Restriction of fluids if required for chronic renal failure

Evaluate:
• Therapeutic response: prevention of bone deficiencies

Teach patient/family:
• The symptoms of hypercalcemia
• About foods rich in calcium, vit D

⚠ High Alert

diltiazem (℞)

(dil-tye′a-zem)

Apo-Diltiaz ♣, Cardizem, Cardizem CD, Cardizem LA, Cartia XT, Dilacor-XR, Diltia XR, diltiazem, Novo-Diltiazem ♣, Nu-Diltiaz, Ratio-Diltiazem CD, Syn-Diltiazem ♣, Taztia XT, Tiamate, Tiazac, Tiazem

Func. class.: Calcium channel blocker, antiarrhythmic class IV, antihypertensive
Chem. class.: Benzothiazepine

Do not confuse:
Cardizem/Cardene

Action: Inhibits calcium ion influx across cell membrane during cardiac depolarization; produces relaxation of coronary vascular smooth muscle, dilates coronary arteries, slows SA/AV node conduction times, dilates peripheral arteries

Uses: **PO** Angina pectoris due to coronary artery spasm, hypertension, **IV** atrial fibrillation, flutter, paroxysmal supraventricular tachycardia

Unlabeled uses: Unstable angina, proteinuria, cardiomyopathy, diabetic neuropathy

DOSAGE AND ROUTES

Prinzmetal's or variant angina, chronic stable angina
• *Adult:* **PO** 30 mg qid, increasing dose gradually to 180-360 mg/day in divided doses or (SR) 60-120 mg bid; may increase to 240-360 mg/day or 120 or 180 mg **EXT REL** (LA, CD, XT, XR products) **PO** daily

Atrial fibrillation/flutter, paroxysmal supraventricular tachycardia
• *Adult:* **IV BOL** 0.25 mg/kg over 2 min initially, then 0.35 mg/kg may be given after 15 min; if no response, may give **CONT INF** 5-15 mg/hr for up to 24 hr

Hypertension
• *Adult:* **PO** or 180-240 mg **(EXT REL)** daily

Rapid ventricular rate secondary to dysrhythmias (unlabeled)
• *Adolescent/child/infant >7 months:* **IV BOL** 0.25 mg/kg over 5 min, then **CONT IV INF** 0.11 mg/kg/hr

Available forms: Tabs 30, 60, 90, 120 mg; ext rel tabs 120, 180, 240, 300, 360, 420 mg; ext rel caps 60, 90, 120, 180, 240, 300, 360, 420 mg; inj 5 mg/ml (5, 10 ml)

SIDE EFFECTS

CNS: Headache, fatigue, drowsiness, dizziness, depression, weakness, insomnia, tremor, paresthesia

CV: **Dysrhythmia,** *edema,* **CHF,** bradycardia, hypotension, palpitations, **heart block**

GI: Nausea, vomiting, diarrhea, gastric upset, *constipation,* increased LFTs

GU: Nocturia, polyuria, **acute renal failure**

INTEG: Rash, flushing, photosensitivity, burning, pruritus at inj site
RESP: Rhinitis, dyspnea, pharyngitis
Contraindications: Sick sinus syndrome, AV heart block, hypotension <90 mm Hg systolic, acute MI, pulmonary congestion, cardiogenic shock
Precautions: Pregnancy (C), breastfeeding, children, CHF, aortic stenosis, bradycardia, GERD, hepatic disease, hiatal hernia, ventricular dysfunction, elderly

PHARMACOKINETICS

Onset 30-60 min; peak 2-3 hr immediate rel, 10-14 hr ext rel, 6-11 hr sus rel; half-life 3½-9 hr; metabolized by liver; excreted in urine (96% as metabolites)

INTERACTIONS

Increase: effect, toxicity—theophylline
Increase: effects of β-blockers, digoxin, lithium, carbamazepine, cycloSPORINE, anesthetics, HMG-CoA reductase inhibitors, benzodiazepines, lovastatin, methylPREDNISolone
Increase: effects of diltiazem—cimetidine

Drug/Herb

Increase: diltiazem effect—barberry, betel palm, burdock, goldenseal, khat, khella, lily of the valley, plantain
Decrease: diltiazem effect—yohimbe

Drug/Food

Increase: hypotensive effects—grapefruit juice

NURSING CONSIDERATIONS

Assess:

- Cardiac status: B/P, pulse, respiration, ECG and intervals PR, QRS, QT; if systolic B/P <90 mm Hg or HR <50 bpm, hold dose, notify prescriber

Administer:

PO route

- Cardiazem LA ext rel tab 24 hr: Give daily, either AM or PM, without regard to meals
- Dilacor XR/Diltia XT ext rel cap 24 hr: Give daily, take on empty stomach, swallow whole, do not cut, crush, chew, open
- Tiazac, Tiztia XT: Give daily without regard to meals
- Conventional regular-rel tab: Give before meals and at bedtime
- Cardizem CD or equivalent (Cartia XT): Generic ext rel cap 24 hr: Give daily, without regard to meals
- May sprinkle (reg tab) on applesauce for administration after crushing

Oral suspension (unlabeled)

- Grind 16, 90 mg diltiazem reg rel tab into fine powder
- In separate container, mix 60 ml Ora-Sweet and 60 ml Ora-Plus
- Add small amount of sol to powder to form paste, add geometric amounts of base to achieve desired vol, place in amber container

IV route

- IV undiluted over 2 min or diluted 125 mg/100 ml, 250 mg/250 ml of D_5W, 0.9% NaCl, D_5/0.45% NaCl, give 10 mg/hr, may increase by 5 mg/hr to 15 mg/hr, continue inf up to 24 hr

Y-site compatibilities: Albumin, amikacin, amphotericin B, aztreonam, bretylium, bumetanide, cefazolin, cefotaxime, cefotetan, cefoxitin, ceftazidime, ceftriaxone, cefuroxime, cimetidine, ciprofloxacin, clindamycin, digoxin, DOBUTamine, DOPamine, doxycycline, epinephrine, erythromycin, esmolol, fentanyl, fluconazole, gentamicin, hetastarch, hydromorphone, imipenem-cilastatin, labetalol, lidocaine, lorazepam, meperidine, metoclopramide, metronidazole, midazolam, milrinone, morphine, multivitamins, niCARdipine, nitroglycerin, norepinephrine, oxacillin, penicillin G potassium, pentamidine, piperacillin, potassium chloride, potassium phosphates, ranitidine, sodium nitroprusside, theophylline, ticarcillin, ticarcillin/clavulanate, tobramycin, trimethoprim-sulfamethoxazole, vancomycin, vecuronium

Perform/provide:

- Storage in tight container at room temperature

Evaluate:

• Therapeutic response: decreased anginal pain, decreased B/P

Teach patient/family:

• How to take pulse, B/P before taking product; record or graph should be kept
• To avoid hazardous activities until stabilized on product, dizziness is no longer a problem
• To limit caffeine consumption, avoid grapefruit juice
• To avoid OTC products unless directed by prescriber
• The importance of complying with all areas of medical regimen: diet, exercise, stress reduction, product therapy
• To change position slowly
⚠ To report dizziness, SOB, palpitations
• Not to discontinue abruptly

Treatment of overdose: Atropine for AV block, vasopressor for hypotension

*dimenhyDRINATE (OTC, ℞)

(dye-men-hye′dri-nate)

Apo-Dimenhydrinate ✤, Calm-X, Children's Dramamine, dimenhyDRINATE, Dimetabs, Dramamine, Dramanate, Dymenate, Gravol ✤, Gravol L/A ✤, Nauseatol ✤, Novo-Dimenate ✤, PMS-Dimenhydrinate ✤, Travamine ✤,

Func. class.: Antiemetic, antihistamine, anticholinergic

Chem. class.: H_1-receptor antagonist, ethanolamine derivative

Do not confuse:
dimenhyDRINATE/diphenhydrAMINE

Action: Competes with histamine for H_1 receptors in GI tract, blood vessels, respiratory tract; central anticholinergic activity, which results in decreased vestibular stimulation and blockade of chemoreceptor trigger zone

Uses: Motion sickness, nausea, vomiting, vertigo

Unlabeled uses: Hyperemesis gravidarum, Ménière's syndrome

DOSAGE AND ROUTES

• *Adult:* **PO** 50-100 mg q4hr; **IM/IV** 50 mg q4hr as needed (Canada only)
• *Child 6-12 yr:* **PO** 25-50 mg q6-8hr prn, max 150 mg/day
• *Child 2-5 yr:* **PO** 12.5-25 mg q6-8hr, max 75 mg/day

Available forms: Tabs 50 mg; inj 50 mg/ml ✤; elixir 15 mg/5 ml ✤; chew tabs 50 mg

SIDE EFFECTS

CNS: ***Drowsiness,*** restlessness, headache, dizziness, insomnia, confusion, nervousness, tingling, vertigo

CV: Hypertension, ***hypotension***, palpitation

EENT: ***Dry mouth,*** blurred vision, diplopia, nasal congestion, photosensitivity

GI: Nausea, anorexia, vomiting, ***constipation***

INTEG: Rash, urticaria, fever, chills, flushing

MISC: **Anaphylaxis**

Contraindications: Hypersensitivity

Precautions: Pregnancy (B), breastfeeding, children, geriatric patients, cardiac dysrhythmias, asthma, prostatic hypertrophy, bladder-neck obstruction, closed-angle glaucoma, stenosing peptic ulcer, pyloroduodenal obstruction

PHARMACOKINETICS

PO/IM: Onset 15-30 min, duration 4-6 hr

INTERACTIONS

Increase: effect—alcohol, anticholinergic, tricyclics, MAOIs, opiates, sedative/hypnotics, other CNS depressants

Drug/Herb

Increase: anticholinergic effect—corkwood, henbane, jimsonweed, scopolia

Increase: effect—hops, Jamaican dogwood, khat, senega

Drug/Lab Test

False negative: allergy skin testing

NURSING CONSIDERATIONS

Assess:

- VS, B/P; check patients with cardiac disease more often
- Signs of toxicity of other products or masking of symptoms of disease: brain tumor, intestinal obstruction
- Observe for drowsiness, dizziness

Administer:

- IM inj in large muscle mass; aspirate to avoid IV administration (Canada only)
- Tablets may be swallowed whole, chewed, or allowed to dissolve

IV route (Canada only)

- After diluting 50 mg/10 ml of NaCl inj; give 50 mg or less over 2 min

Additive compatibilities: Amikacin, calcium gluconate, chloramphenicol, corticotropin, erythromycin, heparin, hydrOXYzine, methicillin, norepinephrine, penicillin G potassium, pentobarbital, phenobarbital, potassium chloride, prochlorperazine, vancomycin, vit B/C

Syringe compatibilities: Atropine, diphenhydrAMINE, droperidol, fentanyl, heparin, hydromorphone, meperidine, metoclopramide, morphine, pentazocine, perphenazine, ranitidine, scopolamine

Y-site compatibilities: Acyclovir

- Therapeutic response: absence of nausea, vomiting

Teach patient/family:

- To avoid hazardous activities, activities requiring alertness; dizziness may occur; instruct patient to request assistance with ambulation
- To avoid alcohol, other depressants

dinoprostone (℞)

(dye-noe-prost'one)

Cervidil Vaginal Insert,

Prepidil, Endocervical Gel,

Prostin E Vaginal Suppository

Func. class.: Oxytocic, abortifacient

Chem. class.: Prostaglandin E_2

D

Do not confuse:

Prepidil/bepridil

Action: Stimulates uterine contractions, causing abortion; acts within 30 hr for complete abortion

Uses: Abortion during 2nd trimester, benign hydatidiform mole, expulsion of uterine contents in fetal deaths to 28 wk, missed abortion, to efface and dilate the cervix in pregnancy at term

DOSAGE AND ROUTES

Abortifacient/2nd trimester/missed abortion/benign hydatidiform mole/intrauterine fetal death

- *Adult:* **VAG SUPP** 20 mg, repeat q3-5hr until abortion occurs, max dose is 240 mg

Cervical ripening

- *Adult:* **GEL** warm to room temperature, choose correct length shielded catheter (10 or 20 mm), fill catheter by pushing plunger; patient should remain recumbent for 15-30 min; insert one 10 mg insert

Available forms: Vag supp 20 mg; gel 0.5 mg/3 g (prefilled syringe); vag insert 10 mg

SIDE EFFECTS

CNS: Headache, dizziness, chills, fever

CV: Hypotension, **dysrhythmias**

EENT: Blurred vision

FETAL: Bradycardia (i.e., deceleration)

GI: Nausea, vomiting, diarrhea

GU: Vaginitis, vaginal pain, vulvitis, vaginismus

INTEG: Rash, skin color changes

MS: Leg cramps, joint swelling, weakness

GEL: Uterine contractile abnormality, GI side effects, back pain, fever

INSERT: Uterine hyperstimulation, fever, nausea, vomiting, diarrhea, abdominal pain

SUPPOSITORY: **Uterine rupture, anaphylaxis**

Contraindications: Hypersensitivity, C-section, surgery

Precautions: Pregnancy (C), cardiac/renal/hepatic disease, asthma, anemia, jaundice, diabetes mellitus, seizure disorders, hypertension, glaucoma, uterine fibrosis, cervical stenosis, pelvic surgery, pelvic inflammatory disease, respiratory disease

Black Box Warning: Hypotension, diarrhea, fever, vomiting

INTERACTIONS

Increase: effect—other oxytocics

Decrease: oxytocic effect—alcohol

PHARMACOKINETICS

Metabolized in spleen, kidney, lungs; excreted in urine

GEL: Onset 10 min, peak 30-45 min

SUPP: Onset 10 min, duration 2-3 hr

NURSING CONSIDERATIONS

Assess:

- Cervical ripening: dilation, effacement of cervix and uterine contraction, fetal heart tones, check for contractions over 1 min
- For fever that occurs ½ hr after suppository insertion (abortion)
- Respiratory rate, rhythm, depth; notify prescriber of abnormalities, pulse, B/P, temp
- Vaginal discharge: check for itching, irritation; indicates vaginal infection

Administer:

- By gel: after warming to room temperature, remove seal from end of syringe, and remove the protective end cap and insert into plunger stopper assembly; make sure patient is in dorsal position
- Antiemetic/antidiarrheal before administration of this product

Evaluate:

- Therapeutic response: expulsion of fetus

Teach patient/family:

- To remain supine for 10-15 min after insertion of supp 2 hr after insert, 15-30 min after gel
- To report excessive cramping, bleeding, chills, fever
- Some methods of pain, comfort control
- Avoid intercourse, tub baths, douches, tampon use for at least 2 wk

*diphenhydrAMINE (OTC, Rx)

(dye-fen-hye'dra-meen)

Allerdryl ✦, AllerMax ✦, Allermed, Banophen, Benadryl, Benadryl 25, Benadryl Kapseals, Benahist 10, Benahist 50, Ben-Allergin-50, Benoject-10, Benoject-50, Benylin Cough, Bydramine, Compoz, Diphenadryl, Diphen Cough, Diphenhist, diphenhydrAMINE HCl, Dormin, Genahist, Hydramine, Hydramyn, Hydril, Hyrexin-50, Insomnal ✦, Nidryl, Nighttime Sleep Aid, Nordryl, Nordryl Cough, Nytol, Phendry, Siladryl, Sleep-Eze 3, Sominex 2, Tusstat, Twilite, Uni-Bent Cough, Wehydryl

Func. class.: Antihistamine (1st generation, nonselective)

Chem. class.: Ethanolamine derivative, H_1-receptor antagonist

Do not confuse:

diphenhydrAMINE/dicyclomine

diphenhydrAMINE/dimenhyDRINATE

Action: Acts on blood vessels, GI, respiratory system by competing with histamine for H_1-receptor site; decreases allergic response by blocking histamine

Uses: Allergy symptoms, rhinitis, motion sickness, antiparkinsonism, nighttime sedation, infant colic, nonproductive cough, insomnia in children

Unlabeled uses: Nystagmus

DOSAGE AND ROUTES

• *Adult and child >12 yr:* **PO** 25-50 mg q4-6hr, max 300 mg/day; **IM/IV** 10-50 mg, max 300 mg/day

• *Child 6-12 yr:* **PO/IM/IV** 5 mg/kg/day in 4 divided doses, max 150 mg/day

Nighttime sleep aid

• *Adult and child ≥12 yr:* **PO** 25-50 mg at bedtime

Antitussive (syrup only)

• *Adult and child ≥12 yr:* **PO** 25 mg q4hr, max 150 mg/24 hr

• *Child 6-12 yr:* **PO** 12.5 mg q4hr, max 75 mg/24 hr

Renal disease

• CCr >50 ml/min give dose q6hr; CCr 10-50 ml/min dose q6-12hr; CCr <10 ml/min dose q12-18hr

Peripheral vestibular nystagmus (unlabeled)

• *Adult:* **PO** 25-50 mg q4-6hr up to 48 hr

Available forms: Caps 25, 50 mg; tabs 25, 50 mg; chew tabs 12.5 mg; elix 12.5 mg/5 ml; syr 12.5 mg/5 ml; inj 10, 50 mg/ml; orally disintegrating tabs 12.5, 25 mg

SIDE EFFECTS

CNS: Dizziness, drowsiness, poor coordination, fatigue, anxiety, euphoria, confusion, paresthesia, neuritis, **seizures**

CV: Hypotension, palpitations

EENT: Blurred vision, dilated pupils, tinnitus, nasal stuffiness, dry nose, throat, mouth

GI: Nausea, anorexia, diarrhea

GU: Retention, dysuria, frequency

HEMA: **Thrombocytopenia, agranulocytosis, hemolytic anemia**

INTEG: Photosensitivity

MISC: **Anaphylaxis**

RESP: Increased thick secretions, wheezing, chest tightness

Contraindications: Hypersensitivity to H_1-receptor antagonist, acute asthma attack, lower respiratory tract disease, neonates

Precautions: Pregnancy (B), breastfeeding, children <2 yr, increased intraocular pressure, cardiac/renal disease, hypertension, bronchial asthma, seizure disorder, stenosed peptic ulcers, hyperthyroidism, prostatic hypertrophy, bladder neck obstruction

PHARMACOKINETICS

Metabolized in liver, excreted by kidneys, crosses placenta, excreted in breast milk, half-life 2-7 hr

PO: Peak 1-3 hr, duration 4-7 hr

IM: Onset ½ hr, peak 1-4 hr, duration 4-7 hr

IV: Onset immediate, duration 4-7 hr

INTERACTIONS

Increase: CNS depression—barbiturates, opiates, hypnotics, tricyclics, alcohol

Increase: diphenhydrAMINE effect—MAOIs

Drug/Herb

Increase: anticholinergic effect—corkwood, henbane

Increase: effect—hops, Jamaican dogwood, khat, senega

Drug/Lab Test

False negative: skin allergy tests

NURSING CONSIDERATIONS

Assess:

• Be alert for urinary retention, frequency, dysuria; product should be discontinued

• CBC during long-term therapy; blood dyscrasias may occur

• Respiratory status: rate, rhythm, increase in bronchial secretions, wheezing, chest tightness

Administer:

⚠ Avoid use in children <2 yr; death has occurred

• With meals for GI symptoms; absorption rate may slightly decrease

- Deep IM in large muscle; rotate site
- At bedtime only if using for sleep aid

IV route

- Undiluted; give 25 mg/1 min or may be diluted with 0.9% NaCl, 0.45% NaCl, D_5W, 0.9% NaCl, $D_{10}W$, LR, Ringer's

Additive compatibilities: Amikacin, aminophylline, ascorbic acid, bleomycin, cephapirin, erythromycin, hydrocortisone, lidocaine, methyldopate, nafcillin, netilmicin, penicillin G potassium, penicillin G sodium, polymyxin B, vit B/C

Syringe compatibilities: Atropine, butorphanol, chlorproMAZINE, cimetidine, dimenhyDRINATE, droperidol, fentanyl, fluphenazine, glycopyrrolate, hydromorphone, hydrOXYzine, meperidine, metoclopramide, midazolam, morphine, nalbuphine, pentazocine, perphenazine, prochlorperazine, promazine, promethazine, ranitidine, scopolamine, sufentanil

Y-site compatibilities: Abciximab, aldesleukin, amifostine, amsacrine, ciprofloxacin, cisatracurium, cisplatin, cladribine, cyclophosphamide, cytarabine, DOXOrubicin, DOXOrubicin liposome, famotidine, filgrastim, fluconazole, fludarabine, gallium, granisetron, heparin, hydrocortisone, idarubicin, melphalan, meperidine, meropenem, methotrexate, ondansetron, paclitaxel, piperacillin/tazobactam, potassium chloride, propofol, remifentanil, sargramostim, sufentanil, tacrolimus teniposide, thiotepa, vinorelbine, vit B/C

Perform/provide:

- Hard candy, gum, frequent rinsing of mouth for dryness
- Storage in tight container at room temperature

Evaluate:

- Therapeutic response: absence of running or congested nose or rashes, improved sleep

Teach patient/family:

- All aspects of product use; to notify prescriber of confusion, sedation, hypotension
- To avoid driving, other hazardous activity if drowsiness occurs
- That photosensitivity may occur
- To avoid concurrent use of alcohol, other CNS depressants
- To avoid breastfeeding

Treatment of overdose: Administer diazepam, vasopressors, phenytoin IV

diphenoxylate/atropine (℞)

(dye-fen-ox'ee-late/a'troe-peen)

Lomotil, Lonox

difenoxin/atropine (℞)

(dye-fen-ox'in/a'troe-peen)

Motofen

Func. class.: Antidiarrheal

Chem. class.: Phenylpiperidine derivative opiate agonist

Controlled Substance Schedule V

diphenoxylate/atropine

Controlled Substance Schedule IV

difenoxin/atropine (US)

Do not confuse:

Lomotil/Lamictal/Lamasil/Lanoxin/Lasix/Ludomil

Action: Inhibits gastric motility by acting on mucosal receptors responsible for peristalsis

Uses: Acute nonspecific and acute exacerbations of chronic functional diarrhea

DOSAGE AND ROUTES

Diphenoxylate/atropine

- *Adult:* **PO** 5 mg qid titrated to patient response needed, not to exceed 8 tabs/24 hr
- *Child 2-12 yr:* **PO** (liquid only) 0.3-0.4 mg/kg/day in 4 divided doses

Difenoxin/atropine

- *Adult*: **PO** 2 tabs, then 1 tab after each loose stool or q3-4hr prn, max 8 tabs/day

Available forms: *diphenoxylate/atropine:* tabs 2.5 mg with atropine 0.025 mg; liquid 2.5 mg with atropine 0.025 mg/5 ml; *difenoxin/atropine:* tabs 1 mg difenoxin/0.025 atropine

SIDE EFFECTS

CNS: *Dizziness, drowsiness, lightheadedness, headache,* fatigue, nervousness, insomnia, confusion
EENT: Burning eyes, blurred vision
GI: *Nausea, vomiting, dry mouth, epigastric distress,* constipation, **paralytic ileus, toxic megacolon**
MISC: **Anaphylaxis, angioedema**
RESP: **Respiratory depression**

Contraindications: Children <2 yr, hypersensitivity, pseudomembranous colitis, severe electrolyte imbalances, diarrhea associated with organisms that penetrate intestinal mucosa

Precautions: Pregnancy (C), breastfeeding, hepatic disease, ulcerative colitis, severe hepatic disease, substance abuse, dehydration

PHARMACOKINETICS

PO: Onset 40-60 min, peak 2 hr, duration 3-4 hr, terminal half-life 12-14 hr, metabolized in liver to active metabolite; excreted in urine and feces

INTERACTIONS

- Do not use with MAOIs; hypertensive crisis may occur

Increase: action of alcohol, opioids, barbiturates, other CNS depressants, anticholinergics

Decrease: GI motility, possible toxic megacolon—amantadine, antimuscarinics, amoxapine, diphenhydrAMINE, clozapine, clemastine, cyclobenzaprine, loperamide, maprotiline, phenothiazines, tricyclics, disopyramide, olanzapine

Drug/Herb

Increase: antidiarrheal action—nutmeg

NURSING CONSIDERATIONS

Assess:

- Electrolytes (K, Na, Cl) if on long-term therapy
- Bowel pattern before; for rebound constipation after termination of medication; bowel sounds
- Response after 48 hr; if none, product should be discontinued
- Abdominal distention, toxic megacolon, which may occur in ulcerative colitis
- Hepatic studies if on long-term therapy

Administer:

- For 48 hr only; if no response, product should be discontinued

Evaluate:

- Therapeutic response: decreased diarrhea

Teach patient/family:

- To avoid OTC products unless directed by prescriber (may contain alcohol); do not use alcohol or CNS depressants
- Not to exceed recommended dose
- That product may be habit forming
- Not to engage in hazardous activities; drowsiness may occur, not to use for longer than 48 hr for acute diarrhea

dipivefrin ophthalmic

See Appendix B

dipyridamole (℞)

(dye-peer-id'a-mole)

Apo-Dipyridamole ✤, dipyridamole ✤, Novo-Dipiradol ✤, Persantine, Persantine IV

Func. class.: Coronary vasodilator, antiplatelet agent

Chem. class.: Nonnitrate

Action: Inhibits adenosine uptake, which produces coronary vasodilation; increases oxygen saturation in coronary tissues, coronary blood flow; acts on small resistance vessels with little effect on vascular resistance; may increase development of collateral circulation; decreases platelet aggregation by the inhibition of phosphodiesterase (an enzyme)

Uses: Prevention of transient ischemic attacks, inhibition of platelet adhesion to prevent myocardial reinfarction, thromboembolism, with warfarin in prosthetic heart valves, prevention of coronary bypass graft occlusion with aspirin; IV form used to evaluate CAD; used as alternative

to exercise in thallium myocardial perfusion imaging to evaluate CAD
Unlabeled uses: Cardiomyopathy, MI prophylaxis, proteinuria, TIA, valvular heart disease

DOSAGE AND ROUTES

TIA
• *Adult:* **PO** 50 mg tid, 1 hr before meals, not to exceed 400 mg/day
Inhibition of platelet adhesion
• *Adult:* **PO** 75-100 mg qid in combination with aspirin or warfarin
Thallium myocardial perfusion imaging
• *Adult:* **IV** 570 mcg/kg
Available forms: Tabs 25, 50, 75 mg; inj 10 mg/2 ml

SIDE EFFECTS

CNS: Headache, dizziness, weakness, fainting, syncope; IV: transient cerebral ischemia, weakness
CV: Postural hypotension; IV: **MI**
GI: Nausea, vomiting, anorexia, diarrhea
INTEG: Rash, flushing
RESP: IV: **Bronchospasm**
Contraindications: Hypersensitivity
Precautions: Pregnancy (B), breastfeeding, hypotension

PHARMACOKINETICS

PO: Peak 1.25 hr, duration 6 hr, therapeutic response may take several months, metabolized in liver, excreted in bile, undergoes enterohepatic recirculation

INTERACTIONS

• Prevention of coronary vasodilation: theophylline
Increase: digoxin effect—digoxin
Increase: bleeding risk—NSAIDs, cefamandole, cefotetan, cefoperazone, plicamycin, valproic acid, salicylates, sulfinpyrazole, anticoagulants, thrombolytics
Drug/Herb
• Gastric irritation: arginine
Increase: antiplatelet effect—bogbean, dong quai, feverfew, garlic, ginger, ginkgo, grapeseed, primrose
Decrease: antiplatelet effect—bilberry, saw palmetto

NURSING CONSIDERATIONS

Assess:
• B/P, pulse during treatment until stable; take B/P lying, standing; orthostatic hypotension is common
• Cardiac status: chest pain, what aggravates or ameliorates condition
Administer:
PO route
• On an empty stomach: 1 hr before meals or 2 hr after; give with 8 oz water for better absorption
IV route
• IV after diluting to at least 1:2 ratio using D_5W, 0.45% NaCl, or 0.9% NaCl to a total vol of 20-50 ml; give over 4 min; do not give undiluted
Perform/provide:
• Storage at room temperature
Evaluate:
• Therapeutic response: decreased platelet adhesion
Teach patient/family:
• That medication is not a cure; may have to be taken continuously in evenly spaced doses only as directed
• To avoid hazardous activities until stabilized on medication; dizziness may occur
• To rise slowly from sitting or lying to prevent orthostatic hypotension
• Not to use alcohol or OTC medications unless approved by prescriber

disopyramide (℞)

(dye-soe-peer'a-mide)
disopyramide, Norpace, Norpace CR, Rythmodan ✤, Rythmodan-LA ✤
Func. class.: Antidysrhythmic (Class IA)
Chem. class.: Nonnitrate

Action: Prolongs duration of action potential and effective refractory period; reduces disparity in refractory period between normal and infarcted myocardium; prevents increased myocardial excitability and conduction contractility

Uses: PVCs, ventricular tachycardia, supraventricular tachycardia

Unlabeled uses: Atrial flutter, fibrillation

DOSAGE AND ROUTES

- *Adult:* **PO** 100-200 mg q6hr; **CONT REL CAPS** 200-400 mg q12hr
- *Child 12-18 yr:* **PO** 6-15 mg/kg/day, in divided doses q6hr
- *Child 5-12 yr:* **PO** 10-15 mg/kg/day, in divided doses q6hr
- *Child 1-4 yr:* **PO** 10-20 mg/kg/day, in divided doses q6hr
- *Child <1 yr:* **PO** 10-30 mg/kg/day, in divided doses q6hr

Renal dose

- *Adult:* **PO** CCr >40 ml/min 100 mg q6hr; CCr 30-40 ml/min dose q8hr; CCr 15-30 ml/min dose q12hr; CCr <15 ml/min dose q24hr

Available forms: Caps 100, 150 mg; ext rel caps (CR) 100, 150 mg; ext rel tabs 150 mg ♣

SIDE EFFECTS

CNS: Headache, dizziness, psychosis, fatigue, depression, paresthesias, insomnia

CV: Hypotension, bradycardia, angina, PVCs, tachycardia, increased QRS, QT segments, **cardiac arrest**, edema, weight gain, AV block, **CHF**, syncope, chest pain

EENT: Blurred vision; dry nose, throat, eyes; angle-closure glaucoma

GI: Dry mouth, constipation, nausea, anorexia, flatulence, diarrhea, vomiting

GU: Urinary retention, hesitancy, impotence

HEMA: **Thrombocytopenia, agranulocytosis,** anemia (rare), decreased Hgb, Hct

INTEG: Rash, pruritus, urticaria

META: Hypoglycemia, hypokalemia

MS: Weakness, pain in extremities

Contraindications: Hypersensitivity, 2nd- or 3rd-degree block, cardiogenic shock, CHF (uncompensated), sick sinus syndrome

Black Box Warning: QT prolongation

Precautions: Pregnancy (C), breastfeeding, children, geriatric patients, diabetes mellitus, renal/hepatic disease, myasthenia gravis, closed-angle glaucoma, cardiomyopathy, conduction abnormalities, potassium imbalance

Black Box Warning: Arrhythmias, MI, torsade de pointes

PHARMACOKINETICS

PO: Peak 30 min-3 hr; duration 6-12 hr; half-life 4-10 hr; metabolized in liver; excreted in feces, urine, breast milk; crosses placenta

INTERACTIONS

Increase: disopyramide effect—quinidine, procainamide, propranolol, lidocaine, atenolol, other antidysrhythmics, erythromycin

Increase: side effects, urinary retention—anticholinergics

Decrease: disopyramide effect—phenytoin, rifampin, phenobarbital

Drug/Herb

- Toxicity/death: aconite

Increase: action—aloe, broom, buckthorn, cascara sagrada, Chinese rhubarb, figwort, fumitory, goldenseal, kudzu, licorice, senna

Increase: serotonin effect—horehound

Decrease: antiarrhythmic action—coltsfoot

Drug/Lab Test

Increase: hepatic enzymes, lipids, BUN, creatinine

Decrease: Hgb/Hct, blood glucose

NURSING CONSIDERATIONS

Assess:

- B/P, apical pulse for 1 min; if <60, check again in 1 hr; if still <60, notify prescriber; for rebound hypertension after 1-2 hr
- ECG; check for increased QT, widening QRS; product should be discontinued

⚠ CHF: crackles, jugular vein distention, weight gain, peripheral edema, dyspnea
- For dehydration or hypovolemia, I&O ratio, electrolytes (Na, K, Cl)
- Renal, hepatic studies (AST, ALT, bilirubin, BUN, creatinine) during treatment
- Diabetics for signs of hypoglycemia (rare)
- Constipation: increased bulk in diet, water, stool softeners, or laxatives needed
- Cardiac rate, respiration: rate, rhythm, character
- Urinary hesitancy, frequency, or a change in I&O ratio; check for edema daily; check for toxicity

Administer:
- Do not break, crush, or chew sus rel cap; give 1 hr before or 2 hr after meals
- Sugar-free gum, frequent sips of water for dry mouth

Evaluate:
- Therapeutic response: decreased dysrhythmias

Teach patient/family:
- To take product exactly as prescribed; if dose is missed, take within 3-4 hr of next dose; do not double dose
- To avoid alcohol, or severe hypotension may occur; to avoid OTC products, or serious product interactions may occur
- To make position change slowly during early therapy to prevent orthostatic hypotension
- To avoid hazardous activities if dizziness or blurred vision occurs
- The importance of complying with product regimen; tell patient that this product does not cure condition

Treatment of overdose: O_2, artificial ventilation, ECG, DOPamine for circulatory depression, diazepam or thiopental for seizures

Rarely Used

disulfiram (℞)

(dye-sul'fi-ram)

Antabuse

Func. class.: Alcohol deterrent

Uses: Chronic alcoholism (as adjunct)

DOSAGE AND ROUTES
- *Adult:* **PO** 250-500 mg/day × 1-2 wk, then 125-500 mg/day until fully socially recovered

Contraindications: Pregnancy (X), breastfeeding, ADD, hypersensitivity, psychoses, CV disease

Black Box Warning: Alcohol intoxication

*DOBUTamine (℞)

(doe-byoo'ta-meen)

DOBUTamine

Func. class.: Adrenergic direct-acting β_1-agonist, cardiac stimulant

Chem. class.: Catecholamine

Do not confuse:
DOBUTamine/DOPamine

Action: Causes increased contractility, increased cardiac output without marked increase in heart rate by acting on β_1-receptors in heart; minor α and β_2 effects

Uses: Cardiac decompensation due to organic heart disease or cardiac surgery

Unlabeled uses: Cardiogenic shock in children; congenital heart disease in children undergoing cardiac cath

DOSAGE AND ROUTES
- *Adult and child:* **IV INF** 2-20 mcg/kg/min; may increase to 40 mcg/kg/min if needed

Available forms: Inj 12.5 mg/ml

SIDE EFFECTS
CNS: Anxiety, headache, dizziness, fatigue

CV: Palpitations, tachycardia, hyper/hypotension, PVCs, angina

ENDO: Hypokalemia
GI: Heartburn, nausea, vomiting
MS: Muscle cramps (leg)
RESP: Dyspnea

Contraindications: Hypersensitivity, idiopathic hypertrophic subaortic stenosis

Precautions: Pregnancy (B), breastfeeding, children, hypertension, CAD, MI, hypovolemia, dysrhythmias

PHARMACOKINETICS

IV: Onset 1-2 min, peak 10 min, half-life 2 min, metabolized in liver (inactive metabolites), excreted in urine

INTERACTIONS

Increase: severe hypertension—guanethidine

Increase: dysrhythmias—general anesthetics, bretylium

Increase: pressor effect, dysrhythmias—atomoxetine, COMT inhibitors, tricyclics, MAOIs, oxytocics

Decrease: DOBUTamine action—other β-blockers

NURSING CONSIDERATIONS

Assess:

- Hypovolemia; if present, correct first; administer cardiac glycoside before DOBUTamine
- Oxygenation/perfusion deficit (check B/P, chest pain, dizziness, loss of consciousness)
- Heart failure: S_3 gallop, dyspnea, neck vein distention, bibasilar crackles in patients with CHF, cardiomyopathy, palpate peripheral pulses; report if extremities become cold or mottled or if peripheral pulses decrease
- ECG during administration continuously; if B/P increases, product is decreased; CVP or PCWP, cardiac output during inf; report changes
- Serum electrolytes, urine output

⚠ Sulfite sensitivity, which may be life-threatening

Administer:

IV route

- Diluting each 250 mg/10 ml of sterile H_2O or D_5W for inj; may be further diluted in 50 ml or more given at prescribed rate; should be gradually increased to desired rate; use a CVP catheter or large peripheral vein, use inf pump, titrate to patient response
- Standard concentrations are 250 mcg/ml-1000 mcg/ml, max 5 mg of DOBUTamine/ml

Additive compatibilities: Amiodarone, atracurium, atropine, DOPamine, enalaprilat, epinephrine, flumazenil, hydrALAZINE, isoproterenol, lidocaine, meperidine, meropenem, metaraminol, morphine, nitroglycerin, norepinephrine, phentolamine, phenylephrine, procainamide, propranolol, ranitidine

Syringe compatibilities: Heparin, ranitidine

Y-site compatibilities: Amifostine, amiodarone, amrinone, atracurium, aztreonam, bretylium, calcium chloride, calcium gluconate, ciprofloxacin, cisatracurium, cladribine, diazepam, diltiazem, DOPamine, DOXOrubicin liposome, enalaprilat, epinephrine, famotidine, fentanyl, fluconazole, granisetron, haloperidol, hydromorphone, insulin (regular), labetalol, lidocaine, lorazepam, magnesium sulfate, meperidine, milrinone, morphine, niCARdipine, nitroglycerin, norepinephrine, pancuronium, potassium chloride, propofol, ranitidine, remifentanil, sodium nitroprusside, streptokinase, tacrolimus, theophylline, thiotepa, tolazoline, vecuronium, verapamil, zidovudine

Perform/provide:

- Storage of reconstituted solution for 24 hr if refrigerated

Evaluate:

- Therapeutic response: increased B/P with stabilization, increased urine output

Teach patient/family:

- The reason for product administration; to report dyspnea, chest pain, numbness of extremities, headache, IV site discomfort

Treatment of overdose: Administer a β_1-adrenergic blocker; reduce IV or discontinue, ensure oxygenation/ventilation; for severe tachydysrhythmias (ventricular) give lidocaine or propranolol

docetaxel (℞)

(doe-se-tax'el)
Taxotere
Func. class.: Antineoplastic—miscellaneous
Chem. class.: Taxane

Do not confuse:
Taxotere/Taxol

Action: Inhibits reorganization of microtubule network needed for interphase and mitotic cellular functions; also causes abnormal bundles of microtubules during cell cycle and multiple esters of microtubules during mitosis

Uses: Locally advanced or metastatic breast cancer, non–small cell lung cancer, androgen independent metastatic prostate cancer, post-surgery operable node-positive breast cancer, induction treatment of locally advanced squamous cell of the head/neck, adjuvant treatment of breast cancer with carboplatin and trastuzumab

Unlabeled uses: Malignant melanoma, ovarian cancer, front-line use with bevacizumab for metastatic breast cancer

DOSAGE AND ROUTES:

• Other regimens are used

Locally advanced or metastatic breast cancer after failure of other chemotherapy

• *Adult:* **IV** 60-100 mg/m^2 given over 1 hr q3wk; if neutrophil count is <500 cells/mm^3 for >1 wk, reduce dose by 25%

Operable node-positive breast cancer

• *Adult:* **IV** (TAC regimen) 75 mg/m^2 1 hr after doxorubicin 50 mg/m^2 and cyclophosphamide 500 mg/m^2 q3wk × 6 cycles

Adjuvant treatment of operable stage I-III invasive breast cancer in combination with cyclophosphamide

• *Adult:* **IV** (TAC regimen) docetaxel 75 mg/m^2 with cyclophosphamide 600 mg/m^2 q21days × 4 cycles

Locally advanced or metastatic non–small-cell lung cancer after failure of cisplatin chemotherapy

• *Adult:* **IV** 75 mg/m^2 over 1 hr q3wk; if neutrophil count is <500 cells/mm^3 for >1 wk, reduce dose to 55 mg/m^2; if patient develops grade 3 peripheral neuropathy, stop product

Unreactable, locally advanced or metastatic non–small cell lung cancer previously treated with chemotherapy

• *Adult:* **IV** 75 mg/m^2 over 1 hr, then cisplatin 75 mg/m^2 **IV** given over 30-60 min q3wk; reduce dose to 65 mg/m^2 in those with hematologic or nonhematologic toxicities

Androgen-independent metastatic prostate cancer

• *Adult:* **IV** 75 mg/m^2 given over 1 hr q3wk, with 5 mg predniSONE **PO** bid continuously; give dexamethasone 8 mg **PO** at 12 hr, 3 hr, and 1 hr prior to docetaxel; if neutrophil count is <500 cells/mm^3 for more than 1 wk or other toxicities occur, reduce dose to 60 mg/m^2

Adjuvant post-surgery treatment of operable node-positive breast cancer

• *Adult:* **IV** 75 mg/m^2 over 1 hr, given 1 hr after DOXOrubicin 50 mg/m^2, cyclophosphamide 500 mg/m^2 q3wk × 6 cycles

Squamous cell of head/neck

• *Adult:* **IV** 75 mg/m^2 over 1 hr, then cisplatin 75 mg/m^2 over 1 hr on day 1, then 5FU 750 mg/m^2/day **CONT INF** × 5 days, repeat cycle q3wk

Advanced ovarian cancer/ metastatic melanoma (unlabeled)

• *Adult:* **IV** 100 mg/m^2 over 1 hr q3wk

Available forms: Inj 20, 80 mg in single-dose vials

SIDE EFFECTS

CNS: **Seizures**

CV: *Hypotension,* fluid retention, peripheral edema, flushing, **MI, sinus tachycardia**

GI: *Nausea, vomiting, diarrhea,* **hepatotoxicity,** stomatitis, colitis

HEMA: **Neutropenia, leukopenia, thrombocytopenia, anemia,** bleeding, infections, **myelosuppression**

INTEG: *Alopecia,* nail pain, rash, skin eruptions

MISC: Amenorrhea, fever of unknown origin, **secondary malignancy, Stevens-Johnson syndrome**

MS: *Arthralgia, myalgia,* back pain

NEURO: *Peripheral neuropathy*

RESP: Dyspnea, **pulmonary edema, fibrosis, embolism**

SYST: *Hypersensitivity reactions,* **AML, death**

Contraindications: Pregnancy (D), breastfeeding, hypersensitivity to this product or severe hepatic disease, bilirubin exceeding upper normal limit, or severely elevated ALT, AST, alk phos

Black Box Warning: Other products with polysorbate 80, neutropenia of $<1500/mm^3$

Precautions: Children, cardiovascular disease, pulmonary disorders, bone marrow depression, herpes zoster, pleural effusion

Black Box Warning: Edema, hepatic disease, lung cancer, taxane hypersensitivity

PHARMACOKINETICS

Metabolized in liver, excreted in feces, terminal half-life 11.1 hr

INTERACTIONS

- Altered docetaxel levels: cycloSPORINE, erythromycin, ketoconazole, troleadomycin

Increase: myelosuppression—other antineoplastics, radiation

Decrease: immune response—live virus vaccines

NURSING CONSIDERATIONS

Assess:

- CBC, differential, platelet count prior to and q wk; withhold product if WBC is $<1500/mm^3$ or platelet count is $<100,000/mm^3$, notify prescriber
- Monitor temp q4hr (may indicate beginning of infection)
- CV status: B/P, edema, flushing
- Hepatic studies before, during therapy (bilirubin, AST, ALT, LDH) prn or q mo; check for jaundiced skin and sclera, dark urine, clay-colored stools, itchy skin, abdominal pain, fever, diarrhea
- CNS changes: confusion, paresthesias, dysethenia, pain, weakness; if severe, product should be discontinued
- VS during 1st hr of inf, check IV site for signs of infiltration

⚠ Hypersensitive reactions, anaphylaxis including hypotension, dyspnea, angioedema, generalized urticaria; discontinue infusion immediately

- Bone marrow depression: bleeding, hematuria, guaiac, bruising or petechiae, mucosa or orifices q8hr; obtain prescription for viscous lidocaine (Xylocaine); avoid invasive procedures
- Effects of alopecia on body image; discuss feelings about body changes

Administer:

- Antiemetic 30-60 min before giving product and prn

IV route

- Using cytotoxic handling procedures
- Allow vials to warm to room temperature; withdraw all diluent and inject in vial of docetaxel; rotate gently to mix; allow to stand to decrease foaming, then withdraw the required amount (10 mg/ml) and inject in 250 ml of 0.9% wall or D_5W; mix gently; give over 1 hr

Y-site compatibilities: Acyclovir, amikacin, aminophylline, ampicillin/sulbactam, butorphanol, calcium gluconate, cefepime, cefotetan, ceftazidime, ceftriaxone, cimetidine, diphenhydrAMINE, droperidol, famotidine, fluconazole, furosemide, ganciclovir, gentamicin, granisetron, haloperidol, heparin, hydrocortisone, hydromorphone, lorazepam, magnesium sulfate, mannitol, meperidine, mesna, metoclopramide, morphine, ondansetron, potassium chloride, prochlorperazine, ranitidine, sodium bicarbonate, vancomycin, zidovudine

Perform/provide:

• Confirmation that dexamethasone was given 12 hr and 6 hr before infusion begins

• Storage of prepared sol up to 27 hr in refrigerator

Evaluate:

• Therapeutic response: decreased tumor size, spread of malignancy

Teach patient/family:

• To report signs of infection: fever, sore throat, flulike symptoms

• To report signs of anemia: fatigue, headache, faintness, SOB, irritability

• To report bleeding; avoid use of razors, commercial mouthwash

• To avoid use of aspirin, ibuprofen

• To report any complaints or side effects to nurse or prescriber

• That hair may be lost during treatment; a wig or hairpiece may make patient feel better; new hair may be different in color and texture

• That pain in muscles and joints 2-5 days after inf is common

• To use barrier contraception; avoid breastfeeding

• To avoid receiving vaccinations while on this product

docosanol topical

See Appendix B

docusate calcium (OTC)

(dok'yoo-sate cal'see-um)

DC Softgels, Dioctocal, Pro-Cal-Sof, Sulfolax, Surfak

docusate sodium (OTC)

Colace, Correctol Extra Gentle, Diocto, Docu DOK, DOS, DSS, Dulcolax Stool Softener Ex-Lax, Fleet Sof-Lax Modane, Regulex ♣, Silace, Therevac SB

Func. class.: Laxative, emollient; stool softener

Chem. class.: Anionic surfactant

Action: Increases water, fat penetration in intestine; allows for easier passage of stool

Uses: Prevention of dry, hard stools

DOSAGE AND ROUTES

• *Adult:* **PO** 50-300 mg/day (sodium) or 240 mg (calcium or potassium) prn; **ENEMA** 4 ml

• *Child >12 yr:* **ENEMA** 2 ml

• *Child 6-12 yr:* **PO** 40-150 mg/day (sodium) in divided doses

• *Child 3-6 yr:* **PO** 20-60 mg/day (sodium) in divided doses

• *Child <3 yr:* **PO** 10-40 mg/day (sodium) in divided doses

Available forms: *Calcium:* 240 mg; *sodium:* caps 50, 100, 250 mg; tabs 100 mg; syr 20 mg/5 ml, 50 mg/15 ml, 100 mg/30 ml, 150 mg/15 ml; oral sol 10, 50 mg/ml; enema 283 mg/3.9 cap

SIDE EFFECTS

EENT: Bitter taste, throat irritation

GI: Nausea, anorexia, cramps, diarrhea

INTEG: Rash

Contraindications: Hypersensitivity, obstruction, fecal impaction, nausea/vomiting

Precautions: Pregnancy (C), breastfeeding

PHARMACOKINETICS

Onset 12-72 hr

INTERACTIONS

- Toxicity: mineral oil

Drug/Herb

Increase: laxative action—flax, senna

NURSING CONSIDERATIONS

Assess:

- Cause of constipation; identify whether fluids, bulk, or exercise are missing from lifestyle, constipating products
- Cramping, rectal bleeding, nausea, vomiting; if these symptoms occur, product should be discontinued

Administer:

- Swallow tabs whole; do not break, crush, or chew
- Oral sol: diluted in milk, fruit juice to decrease bitter taste
- In morning or evening (oral dose)

Perform/provide:

- Storage in cool environment; do not freeze

Evaluate:

- Therapeutic response: decrease in constipation

Teach patient/family:

- That normal bowel movements do not always occur daily
- Not to use in presence of abdominal pain, nausea, vomiting
- To notify prescriber if constipation unrelieved or if symptoms of electrolyte imbalance occur: muscle cramps, pain, weakness, dizziness, excessive thirst
- Inform patient that product may take up to 3 days to soften stools
- Take oral prep with a full glass of water unless on fluid restrictions and increase fluid intake

dofetilide (℞)

Tikosyn

Func. class.: Antidysrhythmic (Class III)

Action: Blocks cardiac ion channel carrying the rapid component of delayed potassium current, no effect on sodium channels

Uses: Atrial fibrillation, flutter, maintenance of normal sinus rhythm

DOSAGE AND ROUTES

- *Adult:* **PO** 125-500 mcg bid depending on CCr, may be adjusted q2-3hr to get appropriate increase in QTc

Renal dose

- *Adult:* **PO** CCr >60 ml/min 500 mcg bid; CCr 40-60 ml/min 250 mcg bid; CCr 20-39 ml/min 125 mcg bid; CCr <20 ml/min do not use

Available forms: Caps 125, 250, 500 mcg

SIDE EFFECTS

CNS: Syncope, dizziness, headache

CV: Hypotension, postural hypotension, bradycardia, angina, PVCs, substernal pressure, transient hypertension, precipitation of angina, **QT prolongation**

GI: Nausea, vomiting, severe diarrhea, anorexia

RESP: Dyspnea, respiratory infections

Contraindications: Children, hypersensitivity, digoxin toxicity, aortic stenosis, pulmonary hypertension, severe renal disease

Black Box Warning: QT prolongation, torsade de pointes

Precautions: Pregnancy (C), breastfeeding, AV block, bradycardia, electrolyte imbalance

Black Box Warning: Renal disease, arrhythmias

PHARMACOKINETICS

Well absorbed, max plasma conc 2-3 hr, steady state 2-3 days, half-life 10 hr, metabolized by liver, excreted by kidneys

INTERACTIONS

- Do not use with cimetidine, ketoconazole, verapamil, prochlorperazine, trimethoprim-sulfamethizole, amiloride, metformin, megestrol, triamterene

Increase: hypokalemia—potassium-depleting diuretics

Drug/Herb

⚠ ***Increase:*** toxicity, death—aconite
Increase: serotonin effect—horehound
Increase: effect—aloe, broom, buckthorn (chronic use), cascara sagrada (chronic use), Chinese rhubarb, figwort, fumitory, goldenseal, kudzu, licorice
Decrease: effect—coltsfoot

Drug/Food

- Do not use with grapefruit or juice

NURSING CONSIDERATIONS

Assess:

- ECG continuously to determine product effectiveness, PVCs, other dysrhythmias; renal function, QTc and baseline q3mo; if QTc >440 msec or 500 msec if ventricular conduction disturbance, discontinue until QTc is at starting level; this product is only available to facilities that have been educated in this administration, patient must be hospitalized
- AF patients should receive anticoagulation prior to cardioversion
- Cardiac status: rate, rhythm, character, continuously; B/P

Administer:

- For 3 days hospitalized
- Give dofetilide after withholding class I or III antidysrhythmic for 3 half-lives of dofetilide

Perform/provide:

- Place patient in supine position unless otherwise ordered; assist with ambulation

Evaluate:

- Therapeutic response: control in atrial fibrillation

Teach patient/family:

- To make position changes slowly; orthostatic hypotension may occur
- Notify prescriber if fast heartbeats with fainting or dizziness occur
- Notify all prescribers of all medications and supplements taken
- That if dose is missed, do not double, take next dose at usual time
- Avoid breastfeeding

dolasetron (℞)

(do-la′se-tron)
Anzemet
Func. class.: Antiemetic
Chem. class.: 5-HT3 receptor antagonist

Action: Prevents nausea, vomiting by blocking serotonin peripherally, centrally, and in the small intestine
Uses: Prevention of nausea, vomiting associated with cancer chemotherapy, radiotherapy, and prevention of postoperative nausea, vomiting
Unlabeled uses: Radiotherapy-induced nausea/vomiting

DOSAGE AND ROUTES

Prevention of nausea/vomiting of cancer chemotherapy

- *Adult and child 2-16 yr:* **IV** 1.8 mg/kg as a single dose, ½ hr prior to chemotherapy
- *Adult:* **PO** 100 mg 1 hr prior to chemotherapy
- *Child 2-16 yr:* **PO** 1.8 mg/hr prior to chemotherapy; max 100 mg

Prevention of postoperative nausea/vomiting

- *Adult:* **IV** 12.5 mg as a single dose, 15 min before cessation of anesthesia; **PO** 100 mg 2 hr before surgery (prevention only)
- *Child 2-16 yr:* **IV** 0.35 mg/kg as a single dose, 15 min before cessation of anesthesia; **PO** 1.2 mg/kg 2 hr before surgery (prevention only)

Available forms: Tabs 50, 100 mg; inj 20 mg/ml (12.5 mg/0.625 ml)

SIDE EFFECTS

CNS: Headache, dizziness, fatigue, drowsiness
CV: **Dysrhythmias,** ECG changes, hypo/hypertension, tachycardia, bradycardia
GI: Diarrhea, constipation, increased AST, ALT, abdominal pain, anorexia
GU: Urinary retention, oliguria
MISC: Rash, **bronchospasm**

Contraindications: Hypersensitivity
Precautions: Pregnancy (B), breastfeeding, children, geriatric patients, hypokalemia, electrolyte imbalances; granisetron/ondansetron/palonosetron hypersensitivity, QT prolongation

PHARMACOKINETICS

Well absorbed, metabolized to active metabolite, half-life of active metabolite 8 hr, max concentrations after 1 hr

INTERACTIONS

Increase: dysrhythmias—antidysrhythmics
Increase: dolasetron levels—cimetidine
Increase: QT prolongation—thiazide, loop diuretics
Decrease: dolasetron levels—rifampin

NURSING CONSIDERATIONS

Assess:
• For absence of nausea, vomiting during chemotherapy
• For hypersensitivity reaction: rash, bronchospasm
• For cardiac conduction conditions, electrolyte imbalances, dysrhythmias, heart rate

Administer:
• By inj 100 mg/½ min or less or diluted in 50 ml compatible sol; give over 15 min
• Not to mix product for oral administration in juice until immediately before administration; apple or apple-grape diluted can be kept for 2 hr at room temperature

Perform/provide:
• Storage at room temperature 48 hr after dilution

Evaluate:
• Therapeutic response: absence of nausea, vomiting during cancer chemotherapy

Teach patient/family:
• To report diarrhea, constipation, nausea, vomiting, rash, or changes in respirations
• May cause headache, use analgesic

donepezil (℞)

(don-ep-ee′zill)
Aricept, Aricept ODT
Func. class.: Anti-Alzheimer agent
Chem. class.: Reversible cholinesterase inhibitor

D

Action: Elevates acetylcholine concentrations (cerebral cortex) by slowing degradation of acetylcholine released in cholinergic neurons; does not alter underlying dementia
Uses: Mild to severe dementia in Alzheimer's disease
Unlabeled uses: Subcortical, vascular dementia, dementia with Lewy bodies, Pick's disease

DOSAGE AND ROUTES

• *Adult:* **PO** 5 mg/day at bedtime; may increase to 10 mg/day after 4-6 wk

Available forms: Tabs 5, 10 mg; orally disintegrating tabs (Aricept ODT) 5, 10 mg; oral sol 1 mg/ml

SIDE EFFECTS

CNS: Dizziness, ***insomnia,*** somnolence, ***headache,*** fatigue, abnormal dreams, syncope, **seizures,** drowsiness, agitation, depression
CV: **Atrial fibrillation,** hypo/hypertension, **sinus bradycardia, AV block**
GI: ***Nausea, vomiting,*** anorexia, ***diarrhea,*** abdominal pain, **GI bleeding,** weight loss
GU: Urinary frequency, UTI, incontinence
INTEG: Rash, flushing, diaphoresis, bruising
MS: Cramps, arthritis, arthralgia
RESP: Rhinitis, URI, cough, pharyngitis

Contraindications: Hypersensitivity to this product or piperidine derivatives
Precautions: Pregnancy (C), breastfeeding, children, sick sinus syndrome, history of ulcers, GI bleeding, hepatic disease, bladder obstruction, asthma, seizures, COPD

PHARMACOKINETICS

Well absorbed PO; metabolized by CYP2D6, CYP3A4; elimination half-life 10 hr single dose, 70 hr multiple dosing; protein binding 96%

INTERACTIONS

Increase: donepezil effects—CYP2D6, CYP3A4 inhibitors
Increase: synergistic effect—succinylcholine, cholinesterase inhibitors, cholinergic agonists
Increase: gastric acid secretions—NSAIDs
Decrease: donepezil effects—CYP2D6, CYP3A4 inducers
Decrease: action of anticholinergics
Decrease: donepezil effect—carbamazepine, dexamethasone, phenytoin, phenobarbital, rifampin
Drug/Herb
Decrease: donepezil—St. John's wort

NURSING CONSIDERATIONS

Assess:
- B/P: hypo/hypertension, heart rate
- Mental status: affect, mood, behavioral changes, depression, complete suicide assessment
- GI status: nausea, vomiting, anorexia, diarrhea
- GU status: urinary frequency, incontinence, I&O

Administer:
- Between meals; may be given with meals for GI symptoms
- Dosage adjusted to response no more than q4-6wk
- Oral solution: measure with calibrated oral syringe or other calibrated device
- Orally disintegrating tabs: allow to dissolve on tongue before swallowing

Perform/provide:
- Assistance with ambulation during beginning therapy; dizziness, ataxia may occur

Evaluate:
- Therapeutic response: decrease in confusion, improved mood

Teach patient/family:
- To report side effects: twitching, nausea, vomiting, sweating, dizziness; indicates cholinergic crisis or overdose
- To use product exactly as prescribed
- To notify prescriber of nausea, vomiting, diarrhea (dose increase or beginning treatment), or rash
- Not to increase or abruptly decrease dose; serious consequences may result
- That product is not a cure, relieves symptoms

⚠ High Alert

*DOPamine (℞)

(doe′pa-meen)
DOPamine HCl, Revimine ♣
Func. class.: Adrenergic
Chem. class.: Catecholamine

Do not confuse:
DOPamine/DOBUTamine

Action: Causes increased cardiac output; acts on β_1- and α-receptors, causing vasoconstriction in blood vessels; low dose causes renal and mesenteric vasodilation; β_1 stimulation produces inotropic effects with increased cardiac output

Uses: Shock, increased perfusion, hypotension, cardiogenic/septic shock

Unlabeled uses: Bradycardia, cardiac arrest, CPR, acute renal failure, cirrhosis, barbiturate intoxication

DOSAGE AND ROUTES

Shock
- *Adult:* **IV INF** 1-20 mcg/kg/min, not to exceed 50 mcg/kg/min, titrate to patient's response
- *Child:* **IV** 1-20 mcg/kg/min adjust depending on response

COPD
- *Adult:* **IV** 4 mcg/kg/min

CHF
- *Adult:* **IV** 3-10 mcg/kg/min

RDS
- *Infant:* **IV** 5 mcg/kg/min

Bradycardia (unlabeled)

• *Adult:* **IV** 2-10 mcg/kg/min, titrate as needed

Available forms: Inj 40 mg, 80 mg, 160 mg/ml; conc for IV inf 0.8, 1.6, 3.2 mg/ml in 250, 500 ml D_5W

SIDE EFFECTS

CNS: Headache, anxiety

CV: Palpitations, tachycardia, hypertension, ectopic beats, angina, wide QRS complex, peripheral vasoconstriction, hypotension

GI: Nausea, vomiting, diarrhea

INTEG: Necrosis, tissue sloughing with extravasation, **gangrene**

RESP: Dyspnea

Contraindications: Hypersensitivity, ventricular fibrillation, tachydysrhythmias, pheochromocytoma, hypovolemia

Precautions: Pregnancy (C), breastfeeding, geriatric patients, arterial embolism, peripheral vascular disease, sulfite hypersensitivity, acute MI

Black Box Warning: Extravasation

PHARMACOKINETICS

IV: Onset 5 min; duration <10 min; metabolized in liver, kidney, plasma; excreted in urine (metabolites); half-life 2 min

INTERACTIONS

• Do not use within 2 wk of MAOIs; hypertensive crisis may result

Increase: bradycardia, hypotension—phenytoin

Increase: dysrhythmias—general anesthetics

Increase: severe hypertension—ergots

Increase: B/P—oxytocics

Increase: pressor effect—tricyclics, MAOIs

Decrease: DOPamine action—β-blockers, α-blockers

Drug/Lab Test

Increase: urinary catecholamine, serum glucose

NURSING CONSIDERATIONS

Assess:

• Hypovolemia; if present, correct first

• Oxygenation/perfusion deficit (check B/P, chest pain, dizziness, loss of consciousness)

• Heart failure: S_3 gallop, dyspnea, neck vein distention, bibasilar crackles in patients with CHF, cardiomyopathy, palpate peripheral pulses

• I&O ratio: if urine output decreases, without decrease in B/P, product may need to be reduced

• ECG during administration continuously; if B/P increases, product should be decreased; PCWP, CVP during inf

• B/P and pulse q5min

• Paresthesias and coldness of extremities; peripheral blood flow may decrease

• Inj site: tissue sloughing; if this occurs, administer phentolamine mixed with NS

Administer:

IV route

• IV after diluting 200-400 mg/250-500 ml of D_5W, D_5 0.45% NaCl, D_5 0.9% NaCl, D_5LR, LR; use large vein

• After reconstituting, use inf pump; give at rate of 0.5-5 mcg/kg/min, increase by 1-4 mcg/kg/min at 10-30 min intervals, until desired response

Y-site compatibilities: Aldesleukin, amifostine, amiodarone, amrinone, atracurium, aztreonam, cefpirome, ciprofloxacin, cisatracurium, cladribine, diltiazem, DOBUTamine, DOXOrubicin liposome, enalaprilat, epinephrine, esmolol, famotidine, fentanyl, fluconazole, foscarnet, granisetron, haloperidol, heparin, hydrocortisone, hydromorphone, labetalol, lidocaine, lorazepam, meperidine, methylPREDNISolone, metronidazole, midazolam, milrinone, morphine, niCARdipine, nitroglycerin, norepinephrine, ondansetron, pancuronium, piperacillin/tazobactam, potassium chloride, propofol, ranitidine, remifentanil, sargramostim, sodium nitroprusside, streptokinase, tacrolimus, theophylline, thiotepa, tolazoline, vecuronium, verapamil, vit B/C, warfarin, zidovudine

Perform/provide:

• Storage of reconstituted sol for up to 24 hr if refrigerated

• Do not use discolored sol; protect from light

Evaluate:

• Therapeutic response: increased B/P with stabilization; increased urine output

Teach patient/family:

• The reason for product administration

Treatment of overdose: Discontinue IV, may give a short-acting α-adrenergic blocker

doripenem (℞)

(dore-i-pen′em)

Doribax

Func. class.: Antiinfective—miscellaneous

Chem. class.: Carbapenem

Action: Bactericidal, interferes with cell wall replication of susceptible organisms; osmotically unstable cell wall swells, bursts from osmotic pressure

Uses: Serious infections caused by *Acinetobacter baumannii, Bacteroides caccae, Bacteroides fragilis, Bacteroides thetaiotaomicron, Bacteroides uniformis, Bacteroides vulgatus, Escherichia coli, Klebsiella pneumoniae, Peptostreptococcus micros, Proteus mirabilis, Pseudomonas aeruginosa, Streptococcus constellatus, Streptococcus intermedius*; complicated urinary tract infections, pyelonephritis, complicated intraabdominal infections

DOSAGE AND ROUTES

• *Adult:* **IV** 500 mg q8hr × 5-14 days; if improvement occurs after 3 days, switch to an appropriate oral product

Available forms: Powder for inj 500 mg

SIDE EFFECTS

CNS: **Seizures,** headache

GI: Diarrhea, nausea, vomiting, **pseudomembranous colitis, hepatitis**

HEMA: **Neutropenia, leukopenia**

INTEG: *Rash,* urticaria, phlebitis, erythema at inj site, **Stevens-Johnson syndrome, toxic epidermal necrolysis,** pruritus

SYST: **Anaphylaxis**

Contraindications: Hypersensitivity to carbapenems (meropenem, doripenem, imipenem), penicillin, beta-lactam; viral infection

Precautions: Pregnancy (B), breastfeeding, geriatric patients, renal disease, seizure disorder, pseudomembranous colitis

PHARMACOKINETICS

IV: Distributed to most body fluids/tissue, excreted mainly unchanged in urine, 70% recovered in 48 hr, half-life 1 hr, half-life extended in renal disease

INTERACTIONS

Increase: doripenem plasma levels—probenecid

Decrease: effect of valproic acid, divalproex sodium

Drug/Herb

• Do not use acidophilus with antiinfectives; separate by several hours

Drug/Lab Test

Increase: AST, ALT, LDH, BUN, alk phos, bilirubin, creatinine

False positive: Direct Coombs' test

NURSING CONSIDERATIONS

Assess:

• Sensitivity to carbapenem antibiotics, penicillins

• Renal disease: lower dose may be required

• Bowel pattern daily; if severe diarrhea occurs, product should be discontinued; may indicate pseudomembranous colitis

• For infection: temp; sputum; characteristics of wound, before, during, and after treatment

⚠ Allergic reactions, anaphylaxis: rash, urticaria, pruritus; may occur few days after therapy begins

• Overgrowth of infection: perineal itching, fever, malaise, redness, pain, swelling, drainage, rash, diarrhea, change in cough, sputum

Administer:

- After C&S is taken
- 500-mg dose: constitute vial with 10 ml of sterile water for inj or NaCl 0.9%; gently shake; (50 mg/ml); the solution must be further diluted using a 21G needle; withdraw susp and add to 100 ml infusion bag of D_5W; gently shake until clear
- 250-mg dose: constitute vial with 10 ml of sterile water for inj or NaCl 0.9%; gently shake; (50 mg/ml); the solution must be further diluted using a 21G needle; withdraw susp and add to 100-ml inf bag of D_5W; gently shake; remove 55 ml of solution; discard; the remaining solution contains 250 mg doripenem (4.5 mg/ml)

Solution compatibilities: D_5W, 0.9% NaCl, sterile water for inj

Evaluate:

- Therapeutic response: negative C&S; absence of symptoms and signs of infection

Teach patient/family:

- To report severe diarrhea; may indicate pseudomembranous colitis
- To report sore throat, bruising, bleeding, joint pain; may indicate blood dyscrasias (rare)
- To report overgrowth of infection: black, furry tongue; vaginal itching; foul-smelling stools
- To avoid breastfeeding; product is excreted in breast milk

Treatment of hypersensitivity: Epinephrine, antihistamines; resuscitate if needed (anaphylaxis)

dorzolamide ophthalmic

See Appendix B

doxapram (℞)

(dox'a-pram)

Dopram

Func. class.: Analeptic

Action: Respiratory stimulation through activation of peripheral carotid chemoreceptor; with higher doses, medullary respiratory centers are stimulated; with progressive CNS stimulation

Uses: Chronic obstructive pulmonary disease (COPD), postanesthesia respiratory depression, prevention of acute hypercapnia, product-induced CNS depression

Unlabeled uses: Neonatal apnea

DOSAGE AND ROUTES

Postanesthesia

- *Adult:* **IV** inj 0.5-1 mg/kg, not to exceed 1.5 mg/kg total as a single inj; **IV INF** 250 mg in 250 ml sol, not to exceed 4 mg/kg; run at 1-3 mg/min

Drug-induced CNS depression

- *Adult:* **IV** Priming dose of 2 mg/kg, repeated in 5 min; repeat q1-2hr until patient awakes; **IV INF** priming dose 2 mg/kg at 1-3 mg/min, not to exceed 3 g/day

COPD (hypercapnia)

- *Adult:* **IV INF** 1-2 mg/min, not to exceed 3 mg/min for no longer than 2 hr

Apnea of premature infant (unlabeled)

- *Infant:* **IV** 1-1.5 mg/kg/hr loading dose followed by inf of 0.5-2.5 mg/kg/hr

Available forms: Inj 20 mg/ml

SIDE EFFECTS

CNS: **Seizures,** (clonus/generalized), *headache,* restlessness, dizziness, confusion, paresthesias, flushing, sweating, bilateral Babinski's sign, rigidity, depression

CV: Chest pain, hypertension, change in heart rate, lowered T waves, tachycardia, **dysrhythmias**

EENT: Pupil dilation, sneezing

GI: Nausea, vomiting, diarrhea, desire to defecate

GU: Retention, incontinence, elevation of BUN, albuminuria
INTEG: Pruritus, irritation at inj site
RESP: **Laryngospasm, bronchospasm,** rebound hypoventilation, dyspnea, cough, tachypnea, hiccups

Contraindications: Hypersensitivity, seizure disorders, severe hypertension, severe bronchial asthma, severe dyspnea, severe cardiac disorders, flail chest, pneumothorax, PE, severe respiratory disease

Precautions: Pregnancy (B), breastfeeding, children, bronchial asthma, pheochromocytoma, severe tachycardia, dysrhythmias, hypertension, hyperthyroidism

PHARMACOKINETICS

IV: Onset 20-40 sec, peak 1-2 min, duration 5-10 min, metabolized by liver, excreted by kidneys (metabolites), half-life 2.5-4 hr

INTERACTIONS

- Synergistic pressor effect: MAOIs, sympathomimetics
- Cardiac dysrhythmias: halothane, cyclopropane, enflurane; delay use of doxapram for at least 10 min after inhalation anesthetics

NURSING CONSIDERATIONS

Assess:

- BP, heart rate, deep tendon reflexes, ABGs, LOC before administration, q30min
- Po_2, Pco_2, O_2 saturation during treatment
- Hypertension, dysrhythmias, tachycardia, dyspnea, skeletal muscle hyperactivity; may indicate overdosage; discontinue product
- Respiratory stimulation: increased rate, abnormal rhythm
- Extravasation; change IV site q48hr
- Patient closely for ½-1 hr

Administer:

IV route

- Undiluted or diluted with equal parts of sterile H_2O for inj; may be diluted 250 mg/250 ml of D_5W, $D_{10}W$ and run as inf; rapid inf may cause hemolysis
- IV undiluted over 5 min; IV inf at 1-3 mg/min; adjust for desired respiratory response, using inf pump IV; if an inf is used after initial dose, start at 1-3 mg/min depending on patient response; D/C after 2 hr; wait 1-2 hr and repeat
- Only after adequate airway is established
- After O_2, IV barbiturates, resuscitative equipment available

Syringe compatibilities: Amikacin, bumetadine, chlorproMAZINE, cimetidine, cisplatin, cyclophosphamide, DOPamine, doxycycline, epinephrine, hydrOXYzine, imipramine, isoniazid, lincomycin, methotrexate, netilmicin, phytonadione, pyridoxine, terbutaline, thiamine, tobramycin, vinCRIStine

Perform/provide:

- Placing patient in Sims' position to prevent aspiration of vomitus
- Discontinue infusion if side effects occur; narrow margin of safety

Evaluate:

- Therapeutic response: increased breathing capacity

Teach patient/family:

- Purpose of medication

doxazosin (℞)

(dox-ay′zoe-sin)

Cardura, Cardura XL

Func. class.: Peripheral α_1-adrenergic receptor blocker

Chem. class.: Quinazoline

Do not confuse:
Cardura/Coumadin/Cardene/Ridaura

Action: Peripheral blood vessels are dilated, peripheral resistance lowered; reduction in B/P results from peripheral α_1-adrenergic receptors being blocked

Uses: Hypertension, urinary outflow obstruction, symptoms of benign prostatic hyperplasia

Unlabeled uses: BPH with finasteride, CHF

DOSAGE AND ROUTES

BPH

• *Adult:* **PO** 1 mg/day, increase in stepwise manner to 2, 4, 8 mg/day as needed at 1-2 wk intervals, max 8 mg

Hypertension

• *Adult:* **PO** 1 mg/day, increasing up to 16 mg/day if required; usual range 4-16 mg/day

• *Geriatric:* **PO** 0.5 mg nightly, gradually increase

Available forms: Tabs 1, 2, 4, 8 mg; ext rel tabs 4, 8 mg

SIDE EFFECTS

CNS: Dizziness, headache, drowsiness, anxiety, depression, vertigo, weakness, fatigue, asthenia

CV: Palpitations, *orthostatic hypotension*, tachycardia, edema, **dysrhythmias,** chest pain

EENT: Epistaxis, tinnitus, dry mouth, red sclera, pharyngitis, rhinitis

GI: Nausea, vomiting, diarrhea, constipation, abdominal pain

GU: Incontinence, polyuria, priapism

Contraindications: Hypersensitivity to quinazolines

Precautions: Pregnancy (C), breastfeeding, children, hepatic disease

PHARMACOKINETICS

PO: Onset 2 hr, peak 2-6 hr, duration 6-12 hr, half-life 22 hr, metabolized in liver, excreted via bile/feces (<63%) and in urine (9%), extensively protein bound (98%)

INTERACTIONS

Increase: hypotensive effects—alcohol, other antihypertensives, sildenafil, vardenafil, nitrates

Decrease: antihypertensive effects of clonidine

Drug/Herb

• Toxicity: yohimbe

Increase: doxazosin effect—angelica, hawthorn

Decrease: doxazosin effect—butcher's broom, capsicum peppers

NURSING CONSIDERATIONS

Assess:

• B/P (lying, standing) and pulse 2-6 hr after each dose and with each increase; postural effects may occur, crackles, dyspnea, orthopnea with B/P; pulse; jugular venous distention during beginning treatment

• BUN, uric acid if on long-term therapy

• I&O, weight daily

• Edema in feet, legs daily

• Skin turgor, dryness of mucous membranes for hydration status

Administer:

• Tabs broken, crushed, or chewed; if chewed, will be bitter; do not break, crush, or chew XL tabs

Perform/provide:

• Storage in tight container in cool environment

Evaluate:

• Therapeutic response: decreased B/P; decreased symptoms of BPH

Teach patient/family:

• That fainting occasionally occurs after first dose; do not drive or operate machinery for 4 hr after first dose or after dosage increase or take first dose at bedtime

• To take 1st dose at bedtime to decrease orthostatic B/P changes, may take 1-2 wk to respond in BPH

Treatment of overdose: Administer volume expanders or vasopressors; discontinue product; place in supine position

doxepin (℞)

(dox′e-pin)

doxepin HCl, Novo-Doxepin ♣, Prudoxin Cream, Triadapin ♣, Zonalon Topical Cream

Func. class.: Antidepressant, tricyclic, antihistamine (topical)

Chem. class.: Dibenzoxepin, tertiary amine

Action: Blocks reuptake of norepinephrine, serotonin into nerve endings, increasing action of norepinephrine, serotonin in nerve cells

Uses: Major depression, anxiety; *topical:* lichen simplex, atopic dermatitis, eczema

Unlabeled uses: Topical pruritus, insomnia, migraine prophylaxis

DOSAGE AND ROUTES

Depression/anxiety

• *Adult:* **PO** 25-75 mg/day, may increase to 300 mg/day for severely ill, give in divided doses if >150 mg/day

• *Geriatric:* **PO** 10-25 mg at bedtime, increase q wk by 10-25 mg to desired dose, max 150 mg/day

Pruritus

• *Adult:* **PO** 10 mg at bedtime, may increase to 25 mg at bedtime; **TOP** apply thin film qid at least 3 hr apart

Available forms: Caps 10, 25, 50, 75, 100, 150 mg; oral conc 10 mg/ml; cream 5%

SIDE EFFECTS

CNS: Dizziness, drowsiness, confusion, headache, anxiety, tremors, stimulation, weakness, insomnia, nightmares, EPS (geriatric patients), increased psychiatric symptoms, paresthesia, **suicidal ideation**

CV: Orthostatic hypotension, ECG changes, tachycardia, **hypertension,** palpitations, **dysrhythmias**

EENT: Blurred vision, tinnitus, mydriasis, ophthalmoplegia, glossitis

GI: Diarrhea, dry mouth, nausea, vomiting, **paralytic ileus,** increased appetite, cramps, epigastric distress, jaundice, **hepatitis,** stomatitis, constipation

GU: Urinary retention, **acute renal failure**

HEMA: **Agranulocytosis, thrombocytopenia, eosinophilia, leukopenia,** pancytopenia, purpuric disorder

INTEG: Rash, urticaria, sweating, pruritus, photosensitivity

Contraindications: Hypersensitivity to tricyclics, urinary retention, closed-angle glaucoma, prostatic hypertrophy

Precautions: Pregnancy (C) (PO) (B) (topical), breastfeeding, geriatric patients, seizures

Black Box Warning: Children, suicidal patients

PHARMACOKINETICS

PO: Steady state 2-8 days, metabolized by liver, excreted by kidneys, crosses placenta, excreted in breast milk, half-life 8-24 hr

INTERACTIONS

Increase: hyperpyretic crisis, seizures, hypertensive episode—MAOIs

Increase: hypertensive action—epinephrine, norepinephrine

Increase: hypertensive crisis—clonidine, do not use together

Increase: doxepin effect—cimetidine, fluoxetine, fluvoxamine, paroxetine, sertraline

Increase: CNS depression—barbiturates, benzodiazepines, sedative/hypnotics, alcohol, other CNS depressants

Increase: QT interval: class 1C antiarrhythmics (propafenone, flecainide), quinolones

Increase: toxicity—SSRIs

Drug/Herb

• Serotonin syndrome: SAM-e, St. John's wort

Increase: anticholinergic effect—belladonna, corkwood, henbane, jimsonweed

Increase: doxepin action—evening primrose oil, hops, kava, lavender, scopolia

Increase: hypertension—yohimbe

Drug/Lab Test

Increase: serum bilirubin, blood glucose, alk phos, LFTs

NURSING CONSIDERATIONS

Assess:

• B/P (lying, standing), pulse q4hr; if systolic B/P drops 20 mm Hg, hold product, notify prescriber; VS q4hr in patients with CV disease

- Blood studies: CBC, leukocytes, differential, cardiac enzymes if patient is receiving long-term therapy
- Hepatic studies: AST, ALT, bilirubin
- Weight weekly; appetite may increase with product
- ECG for flattening of T wave, bundle branch block, AV block, dysrhythmias in cardiac patients; product should be discontinued gradually several days before surgery
- EPS primarily in geriatric patients: rigidity, dystonia, akathisia
- Mental status: mood, sensorium, affect, suicidal tendencies, increase in psychiatric symptoms: depression, panic
- Urinary retention, constipation; constipation most likely in children, geriatric patients
- Withdrawal symptoms: headache, nausea, vomiting, muscle pain, weakness; not usual unless product is discontinued abruptly
- Alcohol consumption; if alcohol is consumed, hold dose until morning

Administer:

- Oral conc should be diluted with 120 ml of water, milk, orange, grapefruit, tomato, prune, or pineapple juice; do not mix with grape juice
- Increased fluids, bulk in diet for constipation
- With food, milk for GI symptoms, do not give with carbonated beverages
- Dosage at bedtime for oversedation during day; may take entire dose at bedtime; geriatric patients may not tolerate daily dosing
- Gum, hard candy, or frequent sips of water for dry mouth
- Topically by applying to affected area; rub slightly

Perform/provide:

- Storage in tight container protected from direct sunlight
- Assistance with ambulation during beginning therapy, since drowsiness/dizziness occurs
- Safety measures primarily for geriatric patients
- Checking to see PO medication swallowed

Evaluate:

- Therapeutic response: decreased anxiety, depression

Teach patient/family:

- That therapeutic effect (depression) may take 2-3 wk, antianxiety effects sooner
- To use caution in driving, other activities requiring alertness, because of drowsiness, dizziness, blurred vision
- To avoid alcohol ingestion, other CNS depressants, may potentiate effects
- Not to discontinue medication abruptly after long-term use; may cause nausea, headache, malaise
- To wear sunscreen or large hat, since photosensitivity occurs
- That clinically worsening and suicide may occur
- To report immediately urinary retention

Treatment of overdose: ECG monitoring; lavage, activated charcoal; administer anticonvulsant, sodium bicarbonate

doxercalciferol (℞)

Hectorol

Func. class.: Parathyroid agent (calcium regulator)

Chem. class.: Vit D hormone

Action: Synthetic vit D analog, reduces parathyroid hormone

Uses: To lower high parathyroid hormone levels in patients undergoing chronic kidney dialysis and those in stages 3 or 4 of chronic renal disease prior to dialysis

Unlabeled uses: Renal osteodystrophy

DOSAGE AND ROUTES

- *Adult:* **PO** iPTH level >400 pg/ml 10 mcg 3×/wk at dialysis; dose titration iPTH level decreased by <50% and >300 pg/ml increase by 2.5 mcg at 8 wk intervals as necessary; iPTH level 150-300 pg/ml maintain; iPTH levels <100 pg/ml suspend for 1 wk, then resume at a dose that is at least 2.5 mcg lower

• *Adult:* **IV BOL** Initial iPTH level >400 pg/ml 4 mcg 3×/wk at the end of dialysis, or approximately every other day; dose titration iPTH level decreased by <50% and >300 pg/ml increase by 1-2 mcg at 8 wk intervals; iPTH level 150-300 pg/ml maintain; iPTH level <100 pg/ml suspend for 1 wk, then resume at a dose that is at least 1 mcg lower

Available forms: Caps 2.5 mcg; inj 2 mcg/ml

SIDE EFFECTS

CNS: Drowsiness, headache, lethargy
GI: Nausea, diarrhea, vomiting, anorexia, dry mouth, constipation, cramps, metallic taste
GU: Polyuria, hypercalciuria, hyperphosphatemia, hematuria
MS: Myalgia, arthralgia, decreased bone development
RESP: SOB

Contraindications: Hypersensitivity, hyperphosphatemia, hypercalcemia, vit D toxicity

Precautions: Pregnancy (C), breastfeeding, renal calculi, CV disease, hepatic disease

PHARMACOKINETICS

Peak 11-12 hr, metabolized in liver, terminal half-life 32-37 hr

INTERACTIONS

Decrease: absorption of doxercalciferol—cholestyramine, magnesium antacids, mineral oil, do not use together

NURSING CONSIDERATIONS

Assess:

• BUN, urinary calcium, AST, ALT, cholesterol, creatinine, albumin, uric acid, chloride, magnesium, electrolytes, urine pH, phosphate; may increase calcium, should be kept at 9-10 mg/dl, vit D 50-135 international units/dl, phosphate 70 mg/dl
• Alk phos; may be decreased
• For increased product level, since toxic reactions may occur rapidly
• For dry mouth, metallic taste, polyuria, bone pain, muscle weakness, headache, fatigue, change in LOC, dysrhythmias, increased respirations, anorexia, nausea, vomiting, cramps, diarrhea, constipation; may indicate hypercalcemia
• Renal status: decreased urinary output (oliguria, anuria), edema in extremities, weight gain 5-7 lb, periorbital edema
• Nutritional status, diet for sources of vit D (milk, some seafood); calcium (dairy products, dark green vegetables), phosphates (dairy products) must be avoided

Administer:

• Do not break, crush, or chew caps

Perform/provide:

• Storage protected from light, heat, moisture
• Restriction of sodium, potassium if required
• Restriction of fluids if required for chronic renal failure

Evaluate:

• Therapeutic response: calcium 9-10 mg/dl, decreasing symptoms of hypocalcemia, hypoparathyroidism

Teach patient/family:

• The symptoms of hypercalcemia
• About foods rich in calcium
• To avoid products with sodium in chronic renal failure: cured meats, dairy products, cold cuts, olives, beets, pickles, soups, meat tenderizers
• To avoid products with potassium in chronic renal failure: oranges, bananas, dried fruit, peas, dark green leafy vegetables, milk, melons, beans
• To avoid OTC products containing calcium, potassium, sodium, or antacids in chronic renal failure
• To avoid all preparations containing vit D
• To monitor weight weekly

High Alert

*DOXOrubicin (℞)

(dox-oh-roo′bi-sin)

Adriamycin PFS, Adriamycin RDF, Rubex

*DOXOrubicin liposome (℞)

Doxil

Func. class.: Antineoplastic, antibiotic

Chem. class.: Anthracycline glycoside

Do not confuse:
DOXOrubicin/Idamycin/DAUNOrubicin
Adriamycin/Aredia/Idamycin

Action: Inhibits DNA synthesis primarily; derived from *Streptomyces peucetius;* replication is decreased by binding to DNA, which causes strand splitting; active throughout entire cell cycle; a vesicant

Uses: Wilms' tumor; bladder, breast, liver, lung, ovarian, stomach, testicular, thyroid cancer; Hodgkin's disease; acute lymphoblastic leukemia; myeloblastic leukemia; neuroblastomas; lymphomas; sarcomas; *Doxil:* AIDS-related Kaposi's sarcoma, metastatic ovarian carcinoma

Unlabeled uses: Colorectal hepatocellular, pancreatic cancer, desmoid tumor, malignant melanoma, multiple myeloma

DOSAGE AND ROUTES

DOXOrubicin

- *Adult:* **IV** 60-75 mg/m^2 q3wk, or 30 mg/m^2 on days 1-3 of 4-wk cycle, not to exceed 550 mg/m^2 cumulative dose
- *Child:* **IV** 30 mg/m^2/day × 3 days, may repeat q4wk

Hepatic dose

- *Adult:* **IV** Bilirubin 1.2-3 mg/dl give 50% of dose; bilirubin 3.1-5 mg/dl give 25% of dose

DOXOrubicin liposome

Kaposi's sarcoma

- *Adult:* **IV** 20 mg/m^2 q3wk

Ovarian cancer

- *Adult:* **IV** 50 mg/m^2 (DOXOrubicin equivalent) given 1 mg/min, if no adverse reactions, may increase to finish inf in 1 hr

Gastric/pancreatic cancer (unlabeled)

- *Adult:* **IV** 30 mg/m^2/dose on days 1 and 29 q8wk given with fluorouracil/mitomycin

Multiple myeloma (unlabeled)

- *Adult:* **IV** 9 mg/m^2/day as a **CONT IV** × 4 days with vinCRIStine/dexamethasone (VAD regimen)

Available forms: Inj 10, 20, 50, 100, 150 mg; liposomal dispersion for inj: (Doxil) 20 mg/10 ml, 50 mg/30 ml

SIDE EFFECTS

CV: Increased B/P, **sinus tachycardia, PVCs,** chest pain, **bradycardia, extrasystoles**

GI: Nausea, vomiting, anorexia, *mucositis,* **hepatotoxicity**

GU: Impotence, sterility, amenorrhea, gynecomastia, hyperuricemia

HEMA: **Thrombocytopenia, leukopenia, anemia**

INTEG: Rash, necrosis at inj site, dermatitis, reversible *alopecia,* cellulitis, thrombophlebitis at inj site

Contraindications: Pregnancy (D) 1st trimester, breastfeeding, hypersensitivity, systemic infections, cardiac disorders

Precautions: Cardiac/renal disease, gout

Black Box Warning: Hepatic disease, bone marrow depression (severe), extravasation, heart failure, secondary malignancy

PHARMACOKINETICS

Triphasic pattern of elimination; half-life 12 min, 3⅓ hr, 29⅔ hr; metabolized by liver; crosses placenta; excreted in urine, bile, breast milk

INTERACTIONS

Increase: hypersensitivity—mercaptopurine

Increase: toxicity—other antineoplastics or radiation, mercaptopurine
Increase: hemorrhagic cystitis risk, cardiac toxicity—cyclophosphamide
Decrease: antibody response—live virus vaccine
Drug/Lab Test
Increase: uric acid

NURSING CONSIDERATIONS

Assess:

- CBC, differential, platelet count weekly; withhold product if WBC is <4000/mm^3 or platelet count is <75,000/mm^3; notify prescriber of these results
- Blood, urine uric acid levels
- Renal studies: BUN, serum uric acid, urine CCr, electrolytes before, during therapy
- I&O ratio; report fall in urine output to <30 ml/hr
- Monitor temp q4hr; fever may indicate beginning infection
- Hepatic studies before, during therapy: bilirubin, AST, ALT, alk phos as needed or monthly; check for jaundice of skin and sclera, dark urine, clay-colored stools, itchy skin, abdominal pain, fever, diarrhea
- ECG; watch for ST-T wave changes, low QRS and T, possible dysrhythmias (sinus tachycardia, heart block, PVCs); signs of irreversible cardiomyopathy
- Bleeding: hematuria, guaiac, bruising, or petechiae, mucosa or orifices q8hr
- Effects of alopecia on body image; discuss feelings about body changes; almost total alopecia is expected
- Inflammation of mucosa, breaks in skin
- Buccal cavity q8hr for dryness, sores, ulceration, white patches, oral pain, bleeding, dysphagia
- Alkalosis if severe vomiting is present
- Local irritation, pain, burning at inj site
- GI symptoms: frequency of stools, cramping
- Acidosis, signs of dehydration: rapid respirations, poor skin turgor, decreased urine output, dry skin, restlessness, weakness
- Cardiac status: B/P, pulse, character, rhythm, rate, ABGs, ECG

Administer:

- Antiemetic 30-60 min before giving product to prevent vomiting
- Allopurinol or sodium bicarbonate to maintain uric acid levels, alkalinization of urine
- Topical or systemic analgesics for pain
- Transfusion for anemia
- Antispasmodic for GI symptoms

IV route

- Using cytotoxic handling procedures

⚠ Do not interchange DOXOrubicin with DOXOrubicin liposome

- Hydrocortisone, dexamethasone, or sodium bicarbonate (1 mEq/1 ml) for extravasation; apply ice compresses
- IV after diluting 10 mg/5 ml of NaCl for inj; another 5 ml of diluent/10 mg is recommended; shake; give over 3-5 min; give through Y-tube of free-flowing 5% dextrose INF or NS
- IV liposome inj (Doxil): dilute dose up to 90 mg/250 ml D_5W, give over ½ hr; do not admix with other sol or meds
- Dose modifications for toxicity: Grade 1, redose unless patient has experienced previous grade 3 or 4; Grade 2, delay dosing up to 2 wk or until resolved to grades 0 or 1; Grade 3 delay dosing up to 2 wk or until resolved to grades 0 or 1, resume dose at 25% decrease, return to original dosing after interval; Grade 4 delay dosing up to 2 wk or until grade 0 or 1, resume dose at 25% decrease then return to original dose, if after 2 wk there is no resolution, discontinue

Additive compatibilities: Ondansetron

Syringe compatibilities: Bleomycin, cisplatin, cyclophosphamide, droperidol, leucovorin, methotrexate, metoclopramide, mitomycin, vinCRIStine

Y-site compatibilities: Amifostine, aztreonam, bleomycin, chlorproMAZINE, cimetidine, cisplatin, cladribine, cyclophosphamide, dexamethasone, diphenhydrAMINE, droperidol, famotidine, filgrastim, fludarabine, fluorouracil, granisetron, hydromorphone, leucovorin, lorazepam, melphalan, methotrexate, methylPRED-NISolone, metoclopramide, mitomycin, morphine, ondansetron, paclitaxel, prochlorperazine, promethazine, propofol, ranitidine, sargramostim, sodium bicarbonate, teniposide, thiotepa, vinBLAStine, vinCRIStine, vinorelbine

Perform/provide:

- Liquid diet: carbonated beverages, gelatin may be added if patient is not nauseated or vomiting
- Increased fluid intake to 2-3 L/day to prevent urate, calculi formation
- Rinsing of mouth tid-qid with water, club soda; brushing of teeth bid-tid with soft brush or cotton-tipped applicators for stomatitis; use unwaxed dental floss
- Storage at room temperature for 24 hr after reconstituting or 48 hr refrigerated

Evaluate:

- Therapeutic response: decreased tumor size, spread of malignancy

Teach patient/family:

- To add 2-3 L of fluids unless contraindicated prior to and for 24-48 hr after, to decrease possible hemorrhagic cystitis
- To report any complaints, side effects to nurse or prescriber
- That hair may be lost during treatment and wig or hairpiece may make patient feel better; tell patient that new hair may be different in color, texture
- To avoid foods with citric acid, hot or rough texture
- To report any bleeding, white spots, ulcerations in mouth to prescriber; tell patient to examine mouth daily
- That urine and other body fluids may be red-orange for 48 hr
- To avoid crowds and persons with infections when granulocyte count is low
- That barrier contraceptive measures are recommended during therapy and 4 mo after; avoid breastfeeding
- To avoid vaccinations; reactions may occur; avoid alcohol

doxycycline (℞)

(dox-i-sye'kleen)

Adoxa, Apo-Doxy ♣, Doryx, Doxy, Doxycaps, Doxycin ♣, doxycycline, Monodox, Novodoxylin ♣, Periostat, Vibramycin, Vibra-Tabs

Func. class.: Antiinfective

Chem. class.: Tetracycline

Do not confuse:
doxycycline/doxepin

Action: Inhibits protein synthesis, phosphorylation in microorganisms by binding to 30S ribosomal subunits, reversibly binding to 50S ribosomal subunits; bacteriostatic

Uses: Syphilis, *Chlamydia trachomatis,* gonorrhea, *Rickettsia*, lymphogranuloma venereum, uncommon gram-negative/positive organisms, malaria prophylaxis, chronic periodontitis, acne, anthrax, Lyme disease

Unlabeled uses: Traveler's diarrhea, prevention of chronic bronchitis, leptospirosis, pleural effusion

DOSAGE AND ROUTES

Most infections

- *Adult:* **PO/IV** 100 mg q12hr on day 1, then 100 mg/day; **IV** 200 mg in 1-2 inf on day 1, then 100-200 mg/day
- *Child >8 yr:* **PO/IV** 2.2-4.4 mg/kg/day in divided doses q12hr

Gonorrhea (uncomplicated) in patients allergic to penicillin

- *Adult:* **PO** 100 mg q12hr × 7 days or 300 mg followed 1 hr later by another 300 mg

Malaria prophylaxis

- *Adult:* **PO** 100 mg/day 1-2 days prior to travel, daily during travel, and 4 wk after return

C. trachomatis

- *Adult:* **PO** 100 mg bid × 7 days

Syphilis

- *Adult:* **PO** 100 mg bid × 14 days

Anthrax

- *Adult and child >8 yr:* **IV** 100 mg q12hr; change to **PO** when able × 60 days

• *Child ≤8 yr:* **PO** 2.2 mg/kg q12hr × 60 days; **IV** 100 mg q12hr, change to **PO** when able × 60 days

Lyme disease

• *Adult:* **PO** 100 mg bid × 14-21 days

Periodontitis

• *Adult:* 20 mg bid after scaling and root planing for ≤9 mo; give close to meal time AM or PM

Pleural effusion (unlabeled)

• *Adult:* **INTRACAVITARY** 500 mg diluted with 250 ml 0.9% NaCl given by chest tube lavage and drainage

Available forms: Tabs 100 mg; caps 50, 75, 100 mg; syr 50 mg/5 ml; inj 100, 200 mg; powder for oral susp 25 mg/5 ml; tabs for mouth products 20 mg; inj 42.5 mg

SIDE EFFECTS

CNS: Fever

CV: Pericarditis

EENT: Dysphagia, glossitis, decreased calcification of deciduous teeth, oral candidiasis, tooth discoloration

GI: Nausea, abdominal pain, vomiting, diarrhea, anorexia, enterocolitis, **hepatotoxicity,** flatulence, abdominal cramps, gastric burning, stomatitis

GU: Increased BUN

HEMA: **Eosinophilia, neutropenia, thrombocytopenia, hemolytic anemia**

INTEG: Rash, urticaria, photosensitivity, increased pigmentation, **exfoliative dermatitis,** pruritus

SYST: **Stevens-Johnson syndrome, angioedema**

Contraindications: Pregnancy (D), children <8 yr, hypersensitivity to tetracyclines, esophageal ulceration

Precautions: Breastfeeding, hepatic disease, pseudomembranous colitis, ulcerative colitis

PHARMACOKINETICS

PO: Well absorbed; widely distributed; peak 1½-4 hr; half-life 14-17 hr; excreted in urine, feces, bile; 90% protein bound; crosses placenta; enters breast milk

INTERACTIONS

Increase: effect—anticoagulants

Decrease: doxycycline effect—antacids, $NaHCO_3$, dairy products, alkali products, iron, kaolin/pectin, barbiturates, carbamazepine, phenytoin, cimetidine sucralfate, cholestyramine, colestipol, rifampin, bismuth

Decrease: effects—penicillins, oral contraceptives, digoxin

Drug/Herb

• Do not use acidophilus with antiinfectives; separate by several hours

Increase: action—bromelain

Drug/Lab Test

Increase: BUN, alk phos, bilirubin, amylase, ALT, AST

False increase: urinary catecholamines

NURSING CONSIDERATIONS

Assess:

• I&O ratio

• Blood studies: PT, CBC, AST, ALT, BUN, creatinine

• Signs of infection

• Allergic reactions: rash, itching, pruritus, angioedema

• Nausea, vomiting, diarrhea; administer antiemetic, antacids as ordered

• Overgrowth of infection: fever, malaise, redness, pain, swelling, drainage, perineal itching, diarrhea, changes in cough or sputum

• IV site for phlebitis/thrombosis; product is highly irritating

Administer:

• Do not break, crush, or chew caps

• After C&S

• An empty stomach, or with a full glass of water 2 hr before or after meals; avoid dairy products, antacids, laxatives, iron-containing products; if these must be taken, give 2 hr before or after this agent

IV route

• After diluting 100 mg or less/10 ml of sterile H_2O or NS for inj; further dilute with 100-1000 ml of NaCl, D_5, Ringer's LR D_5LR, Normosol-M, Normosol-R in D_5W; run 100 mg or less over 1-4 hr; do

not give IM/SUBCUT; inf must be completed in 6 hr, when diluted in LR sol, or 12 hr in other sol
Additive compatibilities: Ranitidine
Syringe compatibilities: Doxapram
Y-site compatibilities: Acyclovir, amifostine, amiodarone, aztreonam, cisatracurium, cyclophosphamide, diltiazem, filgrastim, fludarabine, granisetron, hydromorphone, magnesium sulfate, melphalan, meperidine, morphine, ondansetron, perphenazine, propofol, remifentanil, sargramostim, tacrolimus, teniposide, theophylline, thiotepa, vinorelbine
Perform/provide:
- Storage in tight, light-resistant container at room temperature; IV stable for 12 hr at room temperature, 72 hr refrigerated; discard if precipitate forms

Evaluate:
- Therapeutic response: decreased temp, absence of lesions, negative C&S

Teach patient/family:
- To avoid sun, since burns may occur; sunscreen does not seem to decrease photosensitivity
- That all prescribed medication must be taken to prevent superinfection
- That if children ≤8 yr old are undergoing tooth development, teeth will be permanently discolored

⚠ High Alert

dronedarone (℞)
(drone′da′rone)
Multaq
Func. class.: Antidysrhythmic (class III)
Chem. class.: Iodinated benzofuran derivative

Action: Prolongs duration of action potential and effective refractory period, noncompetitive α- and β-adrenergic inhibition; increases RR and QT intervals, decreases sinus rate, decreases peripheral vascular resistance
Uses: Atrial fibrillation, atrial flutter

DOSAGE AND ROUTES
- *Adult:* **PO** 400 mg bid, discontinue class I, III antidysrhythmics, or strong CYP3A4 inhibitors prior to beginning treatment, max 800 mg/day

Available forms: Tabs 400 mg

D

SIDE EFFECTS
CV: Bradycardia, **heart failure, QT prolongation, torsade de pointes**
ENDO: Hypo/hyperthyroidism
GI: Nausea, vomiting, diarrhea, abdominal pain
INTEG: Rash, photosensitivity
Contraindications: Pregnancy (X), breastfeeding, 2nd-, 3rd-degree AV block, bradycardia, severe sinus node dysfunction, hypersensitivity, heart failure, hepatic disease, QT prolongation
Precautions: Children, electrolyte imbalances, elderly, Asian patients, females

PHARMACOKINETICS
Peak 3-6 hr, half-life 13-19 hr, metabolized by liver, excreted by feces (84%), kidneys (6%), protein binding >98%

INTERACTIONS
Increase: dronedarone levels: CYP3A inhibitors/2D6 inhibitors
Decrease: dronedarone levels: 3A/2D6 inducers
Increase: 3A/2D6 substrate levels
Increase: bradycardia—β-blockers, calcium channel blockers
Increase: levels of cycloSPORINE, dextromethorphan, digoxin, disopyramide, flecainide, methotrexate, phenytoin, procainamide, quinidine, theophylline
Increase: anticoagulant effects—warfarin
Drug/Herb
Increase: dronedarone effect—aloe, broom, buckthorn, cascara sagrada, Chinese rhubarb, figwort, fumitory, goldenseal, kudzu, licorice, rhubarb, senna
Decrease: dronedarone effect—coltsfoot
Drug/Food:
- Avoid grapefruit

Increase: dronedarone effect

Drug/Lab Test
Increase: T_4

NURSING CONSIDERATIONS

Assess:

• ECG To determine product effectiveness; measure PR, QRS, QT intervals; check for PVCs, other dysrhythmias, B/P continuously for hypo/hypertension; report dysrhythmias, slowing heart rate
• Serum creatinine, potassium, magnesium
• I&O ratio; electrolytes (potassium, creatinine, magnesium)
• For dehydration or hypovolemia
• For rebound hypertension after 1-2 hr
• Hypothyroidism: lethargy, dizziness, constipation, enlarged thyroid gland, edema of extremities, cool, pale skin
• Hyperthyroidism: restlessness, tachycardia, eyelid puffiness, weight loss, frequent urination, menstrual irregularities, dyspnea; warm, moist skin
• Cardiac rate, respiration: rate, rhythm, character, chest pain; start with patient hospitalized and monitored up to 1 wk

Administer:

PO route

• Give bid with morning, evening meals
• Give MedGuide, should be dispensed with each prescription/refill

Evaluate:

• Therapeutic response: atrial fibrillation/flutter

Teach patient/family:

• To take this product as directed; avoid missed doses; do not use with grapefruit juice
• To report side effects immediately

Treatment of overdose: O_2, artificial ventilation, ECG, administer DOPamine for circulatory depression, administer diazepam or thiopental for seizures, isoproterenol

⚠ High Alert

droperidol (℞)

(droe-per′i-dole)
droperidol, Inapsine
Func. class.: Sedative/hypnotic
Chem. class.: Butyrophenone

Action: Acts on CNS at subcortical levels, produces tranquilization, sleep; antiemetic; mild α-blockade

Uses: Premedication for surgery; induction, maintenance in general anesthesia; postoperatively for nausea, vomiting

Unlabeled uses: Anxiety, general anesthesia induction/maintenance, preanesthesia, sedation induction

DOSAGE AND ROUTES

Induction, adjunct

• *Adult:* **IV/IM** 1.25-2.5 mg, may give additional 1.25 mg
• *Child 2-12 yr:* **IV** 0.05-0.1 mg/kg, titrate to response

Premedication

• *Adult:* **IM** 2.5 mg ½-1 hr before surgery, may give 1.25-2.5 mg additionally
• *Child 2-12 yr:* **IM** 0.05-0.1 mg/kg

Available forms: Inj 2.5 mg/ml

SIDE EFFECTS

CNS: EPS (dystonia, akathisia, flexion of arms, fine tremors); dizziness, anxiety, drowsiness, restlessness, hallucination, depression, **seizures, neuroleptic malignant syndrome**

CV: Tachycardia, hypotension, **prolonged QT, torsade de pointes**

EENT: Upward rotation of eyes, oculogyric crisis

INTEG: Chills, facial sweating, shivering

RESP: **Laryngospasm, bronchospasm**

Contraindications: Breastfeeding, children <2 yr, hypersensitivity

Precautions: Pregnancy (C), geriatric patients, CV disease (hypotension, bradydysrhythmias), renal/hepatic disease, Parkinson's disease, pheochromocytoma,

CHF, hypokalemia, hypomagnesemia, cardiac hypertrophy

Black Box Warning: QT prolongation, torsade de pointes

PHARMACOKINETICS

IM/IV: Onset 3-10 min, peak ½ hr, duration 3-6 hr, metabolized in liver, excreted in urine as metabolites, crosses placenta, half-life 2-3 hr

INTERACTIONS

Increase: CNS depression—alcohol, opiates, barbiturates, antihistamines, antipsychotics, or other CNS depressants
Increase: hypotension—nitrates, antihypertensives
Increase: side effects of lithium
Increase: QT prolongation—class IA/III antiarrhythmics, some phenothiazines, tricyclics, some quinolones, and others
Drug/Herb
Increase: action—kava

NURSING CONSIDERATIONS

Assess:

- VS q10min during IV administration, q30min after IM dose
- EPS: dystonia, akathisia

⚠ For increasing heart rate or decreasing B/P, notify prescriber at once; do not place patient in Trendelenburg position, or sympathetic blockade may occur, causing respiratory arrest

- ECG prior to and 2-3 hr after administration for serious arrhythmias

Administer:

- Protect solution from light
- Anticholinergics (benztropine, diphenhydrAMINE) for EPS
- Only with crash cart, resuscitative equipment nearby
- IM deep in large muscle mass

IV, direct route

- Undiluted; give through Y-tube at 10 mg or less/min; titrate to patient response

Intermittent IV INF route

- May be given as an inf by adding dose to 250 ml LR, D_5W, 0.9% NaCl; give slowly, titrate to patient response

Syringe compatibilities: Atropine, bleomycin, butorphanol, chlorproMAZINE, cimetidine, cisplatin, cyclophosphamide, dimenhyDRINATE, diphenhydrAMINE, DOXOrubicin, fentanyl, glycopyrrolate, hydrOXYzine, meperidine, metoclopramide, midazolam, mitomycin, morphine, nalbuphine, pentazocine, perphenazine, prochlorperazine, promazine, promethazine, scopolamine, vinBLAStine, vinCRIStine

Y-site compatibilities: Amifostine, aztreonam, bleomycin, cisatracurium, cisplatin, cladribine, cyclophosphamide, cytarabine, DOXOrubicin, DOXOrubicin liposome, famotidine, filgrastim, fluconazole, fludarabine, granisetron, hydrocortisone, idarubicin, melphalan, meperidine, metoclopramide, mitomycin, ondansetron, paclitaxel, potassium chloride, propofol, remifentanil, sargramostim, teniposide, thiotepa, vinBLAStine, vinCRIStine, vinorelbine, vit B/C

Evaluate:

- Therapeutic response: decreased anxiety, absence of vomiting during and after surgery

Teach patient/family:

- To rise slowly from sitting or standing to minimize orthostatic hypotension
- To avoid ambulation without assistance

D

drotrecogin alfa (℞)

(droh'treh-koh-jin al'fah)

Xigris

Func. class.: Thrombolytic
Chem. class.: Recombinant human activated protein C

Action: Activated protein C exerts an antithrombotic effect by inhibiting factor Va/VIIIa

Uses: Severe sepsis associated with organ dysfunction

DOSAGE AND ROUTES

- *Adult:* **IV INF** 24 mcg/kg/hr × 96 hr; based on actual body weight

Available forms: Powder for inj, lyophilized, 5, 20 mg

SIDE EFFECTS

HEMA: Decreased Hct, **bleeding**

SYST: **GI, GU, intracranial, intraabdominal, intrathoracic, retroperitoneal bleeding; surface bleeding**

Contraindications: Hypersensitivity, internal active bleeding, intraspinal surgery, CNS neoplasms, ulcerative colitis, hypocoagulation, within 3 mo of hemorrhagic stroke, epidural catheter in place, cerebral embolism/thrombosis/ hemorrhage, within 2 mo of major surgery, trauma

Precautions: Pregnancy (C), breastfeeding, children, within 6 wk of GI bleeding, PT–INR >3, use >96 hr, hepatic disease, within 3 mo of ischemic stroke

PHARMACOKINETICS

Inactivated by endogenous plasma protease inhibitors, half-life 1.6 hr

INTERACTIONS

- Bleeding potential: aspirin, indomethacin, phenylbutazone, anticoagulants, thrombolytics, glycoprotein IIb/IIIa inhibitors, cilostazol, clopidogrel, dipyridamole, ticlopidine, other NSAIDs

NURSING CONSIDERATIONS

Assess:

⚠ For bleeding during treatment; hematuria, hematemesis, bleeding from mucous membranes, epistaxis, ecchymosis; may require transfusion (rare), continue to assess for bleeding

- Blood studies (Hct, platelets, PTT, PT, TT, aPTT) before starting therapy; PT or aPTT must be less than 2× control before starting therapy; PTT or PT q3-4hr during treatment
- VS, B/P, pulse, respirations, neurologic signs, temp at least q4hr; temp >104° F (40° C) indicates internal bleeding; systolic pressure increase >25 mm Hg should be reported to prescriber

⚠ For neurologic changes that may indicate intracranial bleeding

⚠ Retroperitoneal bleeding: back pain, leg weakness, diminished pulses

Administer:

IV route

- Reconstitute 5-mg vial/2.5 ml; 20-mg vial/10 ml sterile water for inj to a concentration of 2 mg/ml; slowly add sterile water for inj, do not shake or invert, gently swirl until dissolved
- Further dilute with 0.9% NaCl, slowly withdraw prescribed amount and add to bag of 0.9% NaCl, direct stream to side of bag, gently invert bag; do not transport inf bag between locations using mechanical delivery systems
- Use immediately after reconstituting, may be held for only 3 hr at controlled room temperature 59° F-86° F; must complete inf within 12 hr after preparation
- Do not use if discolored or if particulate is present
- If using an inf pump, usual concentration is 100-200 mcg/ml; if using a syringe pump, usual concentration is 100-1000 mcg/ml
- Use a dedicated IV line, or dedicated lumen of central venous catheter; may use only 0.9% NaCl, LR, dextrose, or dextrose/ saline mixtures through same line
- Do not expose to heat or direct sunlight
- Discontinue 2 hr prior to invasive surgery or procedures introducing risk of bleeding; may be reinstated 12 hr after invasive procedures if hemostasis achieved; may restart immediately after less invasive procedures

Perform/provide:

- Refrigerated storage at 2° C to 8° C (36° F to 46° F); do not freeze
- Protect unreconstituted vials from light; keep in carton until time of use

Evaluate:

- Therapeutic response: Decreasing symptoms of sepsis, lack of mortality

Teach patient/family:

- Reason for therapy and expected results
- That bleeding may occur for up to 1 mo after therapy; signs, symptoms of bleeding

duloxetine (℞)

(du-lox'uh-teen)

Cymbalta

Func. class.: Antidepressant—miscellaneous

Chem. class.: Serotonin-norepinephrine reuptake inhibitor (SNRI)

Action: May potentiate serotonergic, noradrenergic activity in the CNS; in studies duloxetine is a potent inhibitor of neuronal serotonin and norepinephrine reuptake

Uses: Major depressive disorder (MDD), neuropathic pain associated with diabetic neuropathy, generalized anxiety disorder, fibromyalgia

Unlabeled uses: Urinary incontinence

DOSAGE AND ROUTES

Depression

- *Adult:* **PO** 40-60 mg/day as a single dose or 2 divided doses

Diabetic neuropathy

- *Adult:* **PO** 60 mg/day

Generalized anxiety disorder

- *Adult:* **PO** 60 mg/day, may start with 30 mg/day × 1 wk then increase to 60 mg/day

Fibromyalgia

- *Adult:* **PO** 30 mg/day × 1 wk, then 60 mg/day

Renal dose

- *Adult:* **PO** Start with 20 mg, gradually increase, avoid use in severe renal disease

Available forms: Caps 20, 30, 60 mg

SIDE EFFECTS

CNS: Insomnia, anxiety, dizziness, tremor, somnolence, fatigue, decreased appetite, decreased weight, agitation, diaphoresis, hallucinations, **malignant neuroleptic-like syndrome reaction,** aggression, **seizures**

CV: **Thrombophlebitis,** peripheral edema, hypertension, palpitations, **supraventricular dysrhythmia**

EENT: Abnormal vision

ENDO: Hypoglycemia

GI: Constipation, diarrhea, dysphagia, *nausea,* vomiting, anorexia, dry mouth, colitis, gastritis, abdominal pain, **hepatic failure**

GU: Abnormal ejaculation, urinary hesitation/retention/frequency, ejaculation delayed, erectile dysfunction, gynecologic bleeding

INTEG: Photosensitivity, bruising, sweating, **Stevens-Johnson syndrome**

MS: Gait disturbance, muscle spasm, restless leg syndrome

SYST: **Anaphylaxis, angioedema**

Contraindications: Alcohol intoxication, alcoholism, closed-angle glaucoma, hepatic disease, hepatitis, jaundice, hypersensitivity

Precautions: Pregnancy (C), breastfeeding, geriatric patients, mania, hypertension, renal/cardiac disease, seizures, increased intraocular pressure, anorexia nervosa, bleeding, dehydration, diabetes, hyponatremia, hypotension, hypovolemia, orthostatic hypotension, abrupt drug withdrawal

Black Box Warning: Children, suicidal ideation

PHARMACOKINETICS

Well absorbed; extensively metabolized (CYP2D6, CYP1A2) in the liver to an active metabolite; 70% of product recovered in urine, 20% in feces; 90% protein binding; half-life 12 hr

INTERACTIONS

- Narrow therapeutic index: CYP2D6 extensively metabolized products (flecainide, phenothiazines, propafenone, tricyclics, thioridazine)

⚠ Hyperthermia, rigidity, rapid fluctuations of vital signs, mental status changes, neuroleptic malignant syndrome—MAOIs, coadministration is contraindicated or within 14 days of MAOI use

Increase: CNS depression—opioids, antihistamines, sedative/hypnotics

Increase: serotonin syndrome—SSRIs

Increase: action of duloxetine—CYP1A2 inhibitors (fluvoxamine, quinolone anti-infectives); CYP2D6 inhibitors (fluoxetine, quinidine, paroxetine)
Increase: ALT, bilirubin—alcohol

Drug/Herb

• Serotonin syndrome: SAM-e, St. John's wort
Increase: CNS depression—chamomile, hops, kava, lavender, skullcap, valerian
Increase: anticholinergic effect—corkwood, jimsonweed
Increase: hypertension—yohimbe

NURSING CONSIDERATIONS

Assess:

• B/P lying, standing; pulse q4hr; if systolic B/P drops 20 mm Hg, hold product, notify prescriber; take VS q4hr in patients with CV disease
• Hepatic studies: AST, ALT, bilirubin
• Weight q wk; weight loss or gain; appetite may increase; peripheral edema may occur
• Sugarless gum, hard candy, frequent sips of water for dry mouth
⚠ Mental status: mood, sensorium, affect, suicidal tendencies, increase in psychiatric symptoms; depression, panic
• Withdrawal symptoms: headache, nausea, vomiting, muscle pain, weakness; not usual unless product is discontinued abruptly
⚠ For malignant neuroleptic-like syndrome reaction

Administer:

• Swallow cap whole; do not break, crush, or chew; do not sprinkle on food or mix with liquid
• Without regard to food

Perform/provide:

• Storage in tight container at room temperature; do not freeze
• Assistance with ambulation during beginning therapy since drowsiness, dizziness occur
• Checking to see if PO medication swallowed

Evaluate:

• Therapeutic response: decreased depression

Teach patient/family:

• To report urinary retention
• To use with caution when driving or other activities requiring alertness because of drowsiness, dizziness, blurred vision
• To avoid alcohol ingestion, MAOIs, other CNS depressants
• Not to discontinue medication quickly after long-term use; may cause nausea, headache, malaise; taper
• That clinically worsening and suicide risk may occur
• To wear sunscreen or large hat, since photosensitivity may occur
• To notify prescriber if pregnancy is planned or suspected, or if breastfeeding
• Improvement may occur in 4-8 wk

dutasteride (℞)

(doo-tass'ter-ide)
Avodart
Func. class.: 5α-reductase inhibitor
Chem. class.: Synthetic 4-azasteroid compound

Action: Inhibits both types 1 and 2 forms of a steroid enzyme that converts testosterone to 5α-dihydrotestosterone (DHT), which is responsible for the initial growth of prostatic tissue
Uses: Treatment of benign prostatic hyperplasia (BPH) in men with an enlarged prostate gland, may be used in combination with tamsulosin
Unlabeled uses: Alopecia

DOSAGE AND ROUTES

• *Adult:* **PO** 0.5 mg/day

Alopecia (unlabeled)

• *Adult:* **PO** 0.5-2.5 mg/day

Available form: Caps 0.5 mg

SIDE EFFECTS

GU: Decreased libido, impotence, gynecomastia, ejaculation disorders (rare), mastalgia, teratogenesis
INTEG: **Serious skin infections**

Contraindications: Pregnancy (X), breastfeeding, women, children, hypersensitivity
Precautions: Hepatic disease

PHARMACOKINETICS

Peak 2-3 hr, protein binding 99%, metabolized in liver by CYP3A4, excreted in feces, half-life 5 wk at steady state

INTERACTIONS

Increase: dutasteride concentrations—ritonavir, ketoconazole, verapamil, diltiazem, cimetidine, ciprofloxacin, antiretroviral protease inhibitors, or other products metabolized by the CYP3A4 pathway
Drug/Lab Test
Increase: TSH
Decrease: PSA

NURSING CONSIDERATIONS

Assess:
- For decreasing symptoms in BPH: decreasing urinary retention, frequency, urgency, nocturia
- PSA levels, digital rectal, urinary obstruction; determine the absence of urinary cancer before starting treatment
- Blood studies: ALT, AST, bilirubin, CBC with differential, serum creatinine, serum electrolytes

Administer:
- Swallow caps whole; do not break, crush, or chew
- Without regard to meals

Evaluate:
- Therapeutic response: Decreasing symptoms of BPH—decreased urinary retention/frequency/urgency, nocturia

Teach patient/family:
- To read patient information leaflet before starting therapy and reread it upon prescription renewal
- To notify prescriber if therapeutic response decreases; if edema occurs
- Not to discontinue product abruptly
- About changes in sex characteristics
- That men taking dutasteride should not donate blood for at least 6 mo after last dose, to prevent blood administration to pregnant female
- That caps should not be handled by a pregnant woman because this product can be absorbed through the skin
- That ejaculate volume may decrease during treatment; that product rarely interferes with sexual function

dyphylline (℞)

(dye'fi-lin)
Dylix, dyphylline, Lufyllin
Func. class.: Bronchodilator
Chem. class.: Xanthine, theophylline derivative

Action: Relaxes smooth muscle of respiratory system by blocking phosphodiesterase, which increases cyclic AMP; cyclic AMP results in positive inotropic, chronotropic effects, bronchodilation, stimulation of CNS
Uses: Bronchial asthma, bronchospasm in chronic bronchitis and emphysema, COPD

DOSAGE AND ROUTES

- *Adult and child >6 yr:* **PO** up to 15 mg/kg/dose, max 60 mg/kg/day

Renal dose
- *Adult:* **PO** CCr 50-80 ml/min 75% of original dose; CCr 10-50 ml/min 50% of original dose; CCr <10 ml/min 25% of original dose

Available forms: Tabs 200, 400 mg; elix 33.3 mg, 53.3 mg/5 ml

SIDE EFFECTS

CNS: Anxiety, restlessness, insomnia, dizziness, **seizures,** headache, lightheadedness, muscle twitching
CV: Palpitations, **circulatory failure,** *sinus tachycardia,* hypotension, flushing, **dysrhythmias**
GI: Nausea, diarrhea, *vomiting, anorexia,* dyspepsia, epigastric pain, rectal irritation, bleeding, reflux
INTEG: Flushing, urticaria

OTHER: Fever, dehydration, **albuminuria,** hyperglycemia, increased diuresis
RESP: Tachypnea, **respiratory arrest**
Contraindications: Hypersensitivity to xanthines
Precautions: Pregnancy (C), breastfeeding, children, geriatric patients, CHF, cor pulmonale, diabetes mellitus, hypertension, renal/hepatic disease, glaucoma, hyperthyroidism, seizure disorder, peptic ulcer

PHARMACOKINETICS

Well absorbed, peak 1 hr, duration 6 hr, half-life 2 hr, excreted in urine (85%) unchanged and in breast milk

INTERACTIONS

- Cardiotoxicity: β-blockers

Increase: action of dyphylline—cimetidine, propranolol, erythromycin, probenecid
Increase: dyphylline metabolism—barbiturates, phenytoin
Decrease: dyphylline elimination—uricosurics
Decrease: phenytoin levels

NURSING CONSIDERATIONS

Assess:

- Dyphylline blood levels; toxicity may occur with small increase above 20 mcg/ml; assess for product toxicity: nausea, vomiting, anorexia, cramping, diarrhea, confusion, dysrhythmias, seizures, diuresis, flushing, headache
- Monitor I&O; diuresis occurs; dehydration may be the result in geriatric patients or children
- Whether theophylline was given recently
- Auscultate lung fields bilaterally; notify prescriber of abnormalities, monitor pulmonary function studies baseline and periodically
- Allergic reactions: rash, urticaria; product should be discontinued

Administer:

- Give around the clock to maintain blood levels, give daily dose each AM
- PO after meals to decrease GI symptoms; absorption may be affected

Perform/provide:

- Storage protected from light, at room temperature

Evaluate:

- Therapeutic response: decreased dyspnea, respiratory rate, rhythm

Teach patient/family:

- To check OTC medications, current prescription medications for ephedrine; will increase stimulation; not to drink alcohol, caffeine, or other xanthine products; not to change brands
- To avoid hazardous activities; dizziness, drowsiness, blurred vision may occur
- For GI upset, to take product with 8 oz water and food
- To avoid smoking, condition may worsen
- To obtain blood levels 6-12 mo

econazole topical

See Appendix B

ecothiophate ophthalmic

See Appendix B

Rarely Used

eculizumab (℞)

(e-kue-liz′oo-mab)
Soliris
Func. class.: Monoclonal antibody

Uses: Proximal nocturnal hemoglobinuria (PNH), a rare genetic form of hemolytic anemia

DOSAGE AND ROUTES

- *Adult:* **IV INF** 600 mg q7 days × 4 wk, then a single dose of 900 mg q7days by IV INF after the 4th dose, then 900 mg q14days by IV INF

Contraindications: Hypersensitivity, discontinuing product rapidly (serious hemolysis)

Black Box Warning: Infection

Rarely Used

edetate calcium disodium (℞)

(ee′de-tate)

calcium disodium versenate, calcium EDTA, edathamil calcium disodium, sodium calcium edetate

Func. class.: Heavy metal antagonist (antidote)

Do not confuse:
edetate calcium disodium/edetate disodium

Uses: Lead poisoning, acute lead encephalopathy

DOSAGE AND ROUTES

Lead mobilization test

• *Adult:* **IV** 25-30 mg/kg (up to 2 g) in 250-1000 ml D_5W over 1-6 hr

Acute lead encephalopathy (blood levels 20-70 mcg/dl)

• *Adult:* **IM** 1 g/m^2/day divided q8-12hr × 5 days, may repeat course, max 75 mg/kg/day

Acute lead poisoning (blood levels 20-70 mcg/dl)

• *Adult:* **IV INF** 1 g/m^2/day over 8-12 hr × 5 days, may repeat as needed, max 75 mg/kg/day

Chronic lead poisoning (blood levels 20-70 mcg/dl)

• *Adult:* **IV INF** 1 g/m^2/day over 8-12 hr × 5 days, may repeat as needed

Contraindications: Hypersensitivity, anuria, poisoning of other metals, severe renal disease, hepatitis

Black Box Warning: Children <3 yr

Rarely Used

edetate disodium (℞)

(ee′de-tate)

Disodium EDTA, Endrate

Func. class.: Heavy metal antagonist (chelator)

Do not confuse:
edetate disodium/edetate calcium disodium

Uses: Hypercalcemic crisis, control of ventricular dysrhythmias associated with digoxin toxicity

DOSAGE AND ROUTES

Digitalis glycoside toxicity/ventricular dysrhythmias/hypercalcemia crisis

• *Adult:* **IV** 50 mg/kg/day given over 3 hr or more/day × 5 days; skip 2 days; repeat as needed up to 15 doses; max 3 g/day

Contraindications: Children <3 yr, hypersensitivity, anuria, hepatic insufficiency, poisoning of other metals, severe renal disease, seizure disorders, active/inactive TB

efavirenz (℞)

(ef-ah-veer′enz)

Sustiva

Func. class.: Antiretroviral

Chem. class.: Nonnucleoside reverse transcriptase inhibitor (NNRTI)

Action: Binds directly to reverse transcriptase and blocks RNA, DNA polymerase, causing a disruption of the enzyme's site

Uses: HIV-1 in combination with other antivirals

Unlabeled uses: HIV prophylaxis

DOSAGE AND ROUTES

Given in combination with protease inhibitor or nucleoside analog reverse transcriptase inhibitors (NARTIs)

• *Adult and child >40 kg:* **PO** 600 mg/day at bedtime
• *Child 10-15 kg:* **PO** 200 mg/day at bedtime
• *Child 15-20 kg:* **PO** 250 mg/day at bedtime
• *Child 20-25 kg:* **PO** 300 mg/day at bedtime
• *Child 25-32.5 kg:* **PO** 350 mg/day at bedtime
• *Child 32.5-40 kg:* **PO** 400 mg/day at bedtime

Available forms: Caps 50, 100, 200 mg; 600-mg tabs

SIDE EFFECTS

CNS: Fatigue, impaired cognition, insomnia, abnormal dreams, depression, headache, dizziness, anxiety, drowsiness
GI: *Diarrhea,* abdominal pain, *nausea,* hyperlipidemia, constipation, increased LFTs
GU: Hematuria, kidney stones
INTEG: Rash, **erythema multiforme, Stevens-Johnson syndrome, toxic epidermal necrolysis**

Contraindication: Pregnancy (D), hypersensitivity

Precautions: Breastfeeding, children <3 yr, renal/hepatic disease, myelosuppression, depression, seizures

PHARMACOKINETICS

Peak 3–5 hr, well absorbed, metabolized by liver, terminal half-life 52-76 hr, >99% protein binding, excreted in urine/feces

INTERACTIONS

• Do not give together with benzodiazepines, ergots, midazolam, triazolam, cisapride
Increase: CNS depression—alcohol, antidepressants, antihistamines, opioids
Increase: levels of both products—ritonavir, estrogens, anticonvulsants
Increase: levels of warfarin, ergots, midazolam, triazolam, statins (except pravastatin, fluvastatin)
Decrease: levels of indinavir, saquinavir, clarithromycin, methadone
Decrease: efavirenz metabolism—CYP3A4 inhibitors (conivaptan, ambrisentan, sorafenib)
Decrease: efavirenz effect—CYP3A4 inducers (carbamazepine, rifamycins)

Drug/Herb
Decrease: efavirenz level—St. John's wort, do not use together

Drug/Food
Increase: absorption—high-fat foods

Drug/Lab Test
Increase: ALT
False positive: cannibinoids

NURSING CONSIDERATIONS

Assess:
• Signs of infection, anemia
• Hepatic studies: ALT, AST; renal studies
• Bowel pattern before, during treatment; if severe abdominal pain with bleeding occurs, product should be discontinued; monitor hydration
• Skin eruptions; rash, urticaria, itching
• Allergies before treatment, reaction to each medication
• CBC, blood chemistry, plasma HIV RNA, absolute CD4+/CD8+ cell counts/%, serum β_2 microglobulin, serum ICD+24 antigen levels, cholesterol, hepatic enzymes
• Signs of toxicity: severe nausea/vomiting, maculopapular rash

Administer:
• Give on empty stomach; at bedtime to decrease CNS side effects

Evaluate:
• Therapeutic response: increased CD4 cell counts; decreased viral load; slowing progression of HIV

Teach patient/family:
• To take as prescribed; if dose is missed, take as soon as remembered; do not double dose; take with water, juice; taken on empty stomach at bedtime
• To make sure health care provider knows all the medications, supplements, or OTC products taken
• That if severe rash occurs, to notify health care provider; that adverse reac-

tions (rash, dizziness, abnormal dreams, insomnia) lessen after a month
- Not to breastfeed or become pregnant if taking this product, use nonhormonal contraception, serious birth defects have occurred
- To avoid hazardous activities if dizziness/drowsiness occur
- That product does not cure disease, but controls symptoms, HIV can be transmitted to others even while taking this product, to continue with safe-sex practices

eletriptan (℞)
(el-ee-trip'tan)
Relpax
Func. class.: Antimigraine agent, abortive
Chem. class.: 5-HT_1-1B/1D receptor agonist, triptan

Action: Binds selectively to the vascular 5-HT_1-receptor subtype; causes vasoconstriction in cranial arteries
Uses: Acute treatment of migraine with or without aura

DOSAGE AND ROUTES
- *Adult:* **PO** 20 mg, may increase if needed, max 40 mg (single dose); may repeat in 2 hr if headache improves but returns, max 80 mg/24 hr

Available forms: Tabs 20, 40 mg

SIDE EFFECTS
CNS: Dizziness, headache, anxiety, paresthesia, asthenia, somnolence, flushing, fatigue, hot/cold sensation, chills, vertigo, hypertonia
CV: Chest pain, palpitations, hypertension
GI: Nausea, dry mouth
MS: Weakness, back pain
RESP: Chest tightness, pressure
Contraindications: Hypersensitivity, coronary artery vasospasm, peripheral vascular disease, hemiplegic/basilar migraine, concurrent use of ergotamine-containing preparations, uncontrolled hypertension; ischemic bowel, heart disease; severe renal/hepatic disease
Precautions: Pregnancy (C), breastfeeding, children, geriatric patients, postmenopausal women, men >40 yr, risk factors of CAD, MI, or other cardiac disease, hypercholesterolemia, obesity, diabetes, impaired renal/hepatic function

PHARMACOKINETICS
Onset of pain relief 2 hr, metabolized in the liver, 70% excreted in urine and feces

INTERACTIONS
Increase: plasma concentration of eletriptan—CYP3A4 inhibitors (clarithromycin, erythromycin, itraconazole, ketoconazole, nelfinavir, ritonavir), propranolol
Drug/Herb
Increase: effect—butterbur

NURSING CONSIDERATIONS
Assess:
- For symptoms of migraine: pain location, character, intensity, nausea, vomiting, aura
- B/P; signs/symptoms of coronary vasospasms
- Tingling, hot sensation, burning, feeling of pressure, numbness, flushing
- For stress level, activity, recreation, coping mechanisms
- Neurologic status: LOC, blurring vision, nausea, vomiting, tingling in extremities preceding headache
- Ingestion of tyramine foods (pickled products, beer, wine, aged cheese), food additives, preservatives, colorings, artificial sweeteners, chocolate, caffeine, which may precipitate these types of headaches
- Urine output; monitor kidney function
- Patients with CAD risk factors; first dose should be administered in prescriber's office or medical facility

Administer:
- Swallow tabs whole; do not break, crush, or chew
- At beginning of headache; if headache returns, repeat dose after 2 hr of first dose if first dose is ineffective

Perform/provide:
• Quiet, calm environment with decreased stimulation from noise, bright light, excessive talking

Evaluate:
• Therapeutic response: decrease in frequency, severity of migraine

Teach patient/family:
• To report any side effects to prescriber
• To use contraception while taking product; inform prescriber if pregnant or intend to become pregnant
• To provide dark, quiet environment
• That product does not prevent or reduce number of migraine attacks

Rarely Used

eltrombopag
(el-trom′boe-pag)
Promacta
Func. class: Hemostatic
Chem. class.: Thrombopoietin receptor agonist

Uses: Idiopathic thrombocytopenic purpura that have not responded to conventional treatment. Available on a limited basis.

DOSAGES AND ROUTES
• *Adult:* **IV** 50 mg daily on empty stomach, Asian patients should be started on 25 mg daily

Contraindications: Hypersensitivity

emedastine ophthalmic
See Appendix B

emtricitabine (℞)
(em-tri-sit′uh-bean)
Emtriva
Func. class.: Antiretroviral
Chem. class.: Nucleoside reverse transcriptase inhibitor (NRTI)

Action: A synthetic nucleoside analog of cytosine. Inhibits replication of HIV virus by competing with the natural substrate and then becoming incorporated into cellular DNA by viral reverse transcriptase, thereby terminating cellular DNA chain

Uses: HIV-1 infection with other antiretroviral

Unlabeled uses: HBV (hepatitis B virus) infection, HIV prophylaxis

DOSAGE AND ROUTES
Oral cap and solution are not interchangeable
• *Adult:* **PO** Caps 200 mg/day; oral sol 240 mg (24 ml)/day
• *Child 3 mo-17 yr:* **PO** Caps 200 mg/day; oral sol 6 mg/kg/day, max 240 mg (24 ml)

Renal dose
• *Adult:* **PO** Caps CCr 30-49 ml/min 200 mg q48hr; oral sol 120 mg q24hr; caps CCr 15-29 ml/min 200 mg q72hr; oral sol 80 mg q24hr; caps CCr <15 ml/min 200 mg q96hr; oral sol 60 mg q24hr

Available forms: Cap 200 mg; oral sol 10 mg/ml

SIDE EFFECTS
CNS: Headache, abnormal dreams, *depression,* dizziness, *insomnia,* neuropathy, paresthesia, *asthenia*
GI: Nausea, vomiting, diarrhea, anorexia, abdominal pain, dyspepsia, **hepatomegaly with steatosis (may be fatal)**
INTEG: Rash, skin discolorization
MS: Arthralgia, myalgia
RESP: Cough
SYST: Change in body fat distribution, **lactic acidosis**

Contraindications: Hypersensitivity

Black Box Warning: Lactic acidosis

Precautions: Pregnancy (B), breastfeeding, children, geriatric patients, renal disease

Black Box Warning: Hepatic insufficiency, chronic hepatitis B virus (HPV)

PHARMACOKINETICS
Rapidly, extensively absorbed; peak 1-2 hr; protein binding <4%; excreted unchanged in urine (86%), feces (14%); half-life 10 hr

NURSING CONSIDERATIONS

Assess:

- Renal/hepatic function tests: AST, ALT, bilirubin, amylase, lipase, triglycerides periodically during treatment

⚠ For lactic acidosis, severe hepatomegaly with steatosis; if lab reports confirm these conditions, discontinue treatment; may be fatal

Administer:

- Give without regard to meals
- Oral cap and solution are not interchangeable

Perform/provide:

- Storage (caps) at 25° C (77° F); (oral sol) refrigerated, use within 3 mo

Evaluate:

- Therapeutic response: Decrease in signs/symptoms of HIV

Teach patient/family:

- That GI complaints resolve after 3-4 wk of treatment
- Not to breastfeed while taking this product
- That product must be taken at same time of day to maintain blood level
- That product will control symptoms, but is not a cure for HIV; patient is still infectious, may pass HIV virus on to others
- That other products may be necessary to prevent other infections
- That changes in body fat distribution may occur

enalapril/ enalaprilat (℞)

(e-nal'a-pril)/(e-nal'a-pril-at)
Vasotec

Func. class.: Antihypertensive
Chem. class.: Angiotensin-converting enzyme (ACE) inhibitor

Do not confuse:
enalapril/ramipril/Anafranil/Eldepryl

Action: Selectively suppresses renin-angiotensin-aldosterone system; inhibits ACE; prevents conversion of angiotensin I to angiotensin II, dilation of arterial, venous vessels

Uses: Hypertension, CHF, left ventricular dysfunction

Unlabeled uses: Diabetic nephropathy, hypertensive emergency/urgency, post-MI, proteinuria, renal crisis in scleroderma

DOSAGE AND ROUTES

Hypertension

- *Adult:* **PO** 2.5-5 mg/day, may increase or decrease to desired response, range 10-40 mg/day; **IV** 0.625-1.25 mg q6hr over 5 min
- *Child:* **PO** 0.08 mg/kg/day in 1-2 divided doses, max 0.58 mg/kg/day
- *Child:* **IV** 5-10 mcg/kg/dose q8-24hr

Patients on diuretics

- *Adult:* **IV** 0.625 mg over 5 min, may give additional doses of 1.25 mg q6hr

Renal impairment

- *Adult:* **PO** 2.5 mg/day (CCr <30 ml/min) increase gradually; **IV** CCr >30 ml/min 1.25 mg q6hr; CCr <30 ml/min 0.625 mg as one-time dose, increase as per B/P

CHF

- *Adult:* **PO** 2.5-20 mg/day in 2 divided doses, max 40 mg/day in divided doses

Hypertensive emergency/urgency (unlabeled)

- *Adult:* **PO** 2.5 mg bid, gradually titrate up to 20 mg bid

Available forms: *Enalapril:* tabs 2.5, 5, 10, 20 mg; *enalaprilat:* inj 1.25 mg/ml

SIDE EFFECTS

CNS: Insomnia, dizziness, paresthesias, headache, fatigue, anxiety

CV: Hypotension, chest pain, tachycardia, **dysrhythmias,** syncope, angina, **MI,** orthostatic hypotension

EENT: Tinnitus; visual changes; sore throat; double vision; dry, burning eyes

GI: Nausea, vomiting, colitis, cramps, diarrhea, constipation, flatulence, dry mouth, loss of taste

GU: **Proteinuria, renal failure,** increased frequency of polyuria or oliguria

HEMA: **Agranulocytosis, neutropenia**

INTEG: Rash, purpura, alopecia, hyperhidrosis, photosensitivity
META: Hyperkalemia
RESP: Dyspnea, dry cough, crackles, **angioedema**

Contraindications: Hypersensitivity, history of angioedema

Black Box Warning: Pregnancy (D)

Precautions: Breastfeeding, renal disease, hyperkalemia, hepatic failure, dehydration, bilateral renal artery stenosis

PHARMACOKINETICS

Enalapril:
PO: Onset 1 hr, peak 4-6 hr, duration ≥24 hr, half-life 1½ hr, metabolized by liver to active metabolite, excreted in urine
Enalaprilat:
IV: Onset 5-15 min, peak up to 4 hr

INTERACTIONS

Increase: hypersensitivity—allopurinol
Increase: hypotension—diuretics, other antihypertensives, phenothiazines, nitrates, acute alcohol ingestion, general anesthesia
Increase: potassium levels—salt substitutes, potassium-sparing diuretics, potassium supplements, cycloSPORINE, indomethacin
Increase: levels of lithium, digoxin
Decrease: effects of enalapril—antacids, rifampin

Drug/Herb

• Severe photosensitivity: St. John's wort
⚠ Fatal hypokalemia: arginine
Increase: effect—pill-bearing spurge
Decrease: effect—pineapple, yohimbe

Drug/Lab Test

Increase: ALT, AST, bilirubin, alk phos, glucose, uric acid
False positive: ANA titer

NURSING CONSIDERATIONS

Assess:

• Blood studies: neutrophils, decreased platelets; WBC with differential baseline and q3mo, if neutrophils <1000/mm^3, discontinue treatment (recommended in collagen-vascular disease)
• B/P, peak/trough level, orthostatic hypotension, syncope when used with diuretic, pulse q4hr; note rate, rhythm, quality
• Electrolytes: K, Na, Cl during 1st 2 wk of therapy
• Baselines in renal, hepatic studies before therapy begins and 1 wk into therapy
• Edema in feet, legs daily
• Skin turgor, dryness of mucous membranes for hydration status
• Symptoms of CHF: edema, dyspnea, wet crackles

Administer:

• Prepare in sterile environment using aseptic technique
• Dilute each dose with ≤50 ml of compatible sol
• For a 25 mcg/ml dilution often used in neonatal or pediatric patients, combine 1 ml of enalaprilat 1.25 mg/ml and 49 ml of compatible sol for IV

IV, direct/Intermittent IV INF route

• Undiluted over 5 min, use diluent provided or 50 ml D_5W, 0.9% NaCl, 0.9% NaCl in D_5W or LR, Isolyte E, give through Y-tube of free-flowing inf of 0.9% NaCl, D_5W, LR, Isolyte E

Additive compatibilities: DOBUTamine, DOPamine, heparin, meropenem, nitroglycerin, nitroprusside, potassium chloride

Y-site compatibilities: Allopurinol, amifostine, amikacin, aminophylline, ampicillin, ampicillin/sulbactam, aztreonam, butorphanol, calcium gluconate, cefazolin, cefoperazone, ceftazidime, ceftizoxime, chloramphenicol, cimetidine, cisatracurium, cladribine, clindamycin, dextran 40, DOBUTamine, DOPamine, DOXOrubicin liposome, erythromycin, esmolol, famotidine, fentanyl, filgrastim, ganciclovir, gentamicin, granisetron, heparin, hetastarch, hydrocortisone, labetalol, lidocaine, magnesium sulfate, melphalan, meropenem, methylPREDNISolone, metronidazole, morphine, nafcillin, niCARdipine, nitroprusside, penicillin G potassium, phenobarbital, piperacillin, piperacillin/tazobactam, potassium chloride, potassium phosphate, propofol, ranitidine, remifentanil, teniposide, thiotepa, tobramycin, trimethoprim-sulfamethoxazole, vancomycin, vinorelbine

Evaluate:

- Therapeutic response: decreased B/P

Teach patient/family:

- Not to use OTC (cough, cold, or allergy) products unless directed by prescriber; to avoid potassium, salt substitutes
- To avoid sunlight or wear sunscreen for photosensitivity
- To comply with dosage schedule, even if feeling better
- To notify prescriber of mouth sores, sore throat, fever, swelling of hands or feet, irregular heartbeat, chest pain, signs of angioedema
- That excessive perspiration, dehydration, vomiting, diarrhea may lead to fall in blood pressure; consult prescriber if these occur
- That product may cause dizziness, fainting; light-headedness may occur during 1st few days of therapy
- That product may cause skin rash, impaired perspiration or angioedema; discontinue if angioedema occurs
- Not to discontinue product abruptly
- That CV adverse reactions may reoccur
- To rise slowly to sitting or standing position to minimize orthostatic hypotension

Treatment of overdose: Lavage, IV atropine for bradycardia, IV theophylline for bronchospasm, digoxin, O_2, diuretic for cardiac failure

enfuvirtide (℞)

(en-fyoo′vir-tide)

Fuzeon

Func. class.: Antiretroviral

Chem. class.: Fusion Inhibitor

Action: Inhibitor of the fusion of HIV-1 with CD4+ cells

Uses: Treatment of HIV-1 infection in combination with other antiretrovirals

Unlabeled uses: HIV prophylaxis following occupational exposure

DOSAGE AND ROUTES

- *Adult:* **SUBCUT** 90 mg (1 ml) bid
- *Child 6-16 yr and <42.6 kg:* **SUBCUT** 2 mg/kg bid, max 90 mg bid; 11-15.5 kg 27 mg/0.3 ml bid; 15.6-20 kg 36 mg/0.4 ml bid; 20.1-24.5 kg 45 mg/0.5 ml bid; 24.6-29 kg 54 mg/0.6 ml bid; 29.1-33.5 kg 63 mg/0.7 ml bid; 33.6-38 kg 72 mg/0.8 ml bid; 38.1-42.5 kg 81 mg/0.9 ml bid

HIV prophylaxis (unlabeled)

- *Adult:* **SUBCUT** 90 mg bid added to PEP regimen

Available forms: Powder for inj, lyophilized 108 mg (90 mg/ml when reconstituted)

SIDE EFFECTS

CNS: Anxiety, peripheral neuropathy, taste disturbance, **Guillain-Barré syndrome,** insomnia, depression

GI: Abdominal pain, anorexia, constipation, pancreatitis

GU: **Glomerulonephritis, renal failure**

HEMA: **Thrombocytopenia, neutropenia**

INTEG: Inj site reactions

MISC: Influenza, cough, conjunctivitis, lymphadenopathy, myalgia, hyperglycemia, pneumonia, rhinitis, fatigue

Contraindications: Breastfeeding, hypersensitivity

Precautions: Pregnancy (B), children <6 yr, liver disease, myelosuppression, infections

PHARMACOKINETICS

Peak 8 hr, terminal half-life 3.8 hr, well absorbed, undergoes catabolism, 92% protein binding

NURSING CONSIDERATIONS

Assess:

- Signs of infection, inj site reactions
- Renal studies: BUN, creatinine, renal failure may occur
- Bowel pattern before, during treatment; if severe abdominal pain or constipation occurs, notify prescriber; monitor hydration
- Skin eruptions, rash, urticaria, itching
- Allergies before treatment, reaction to each medication
- CBC, blood chemistry, plasma HIV RNA, absolute CD4+/CD8+ cell counts/%, serum β_2 microglobulin, serum ICD+24 antigen levels, cholesterol

Administer:

- Reconstitute vial with 1.1 ml of sterile water for inj; tap and roll to mix; allow to stand until completely dissolved
- Do not mix with other medications
- SUBCUT, give bid, rotate sites; preferred sites are upper arm, anterior thigh, abdomen

Evaluate:

- Therapeutic response: increased CD4 cell counts; decreased viral load; slowing progression of HIV-1 infection

Teach patient/family:

- To notify prescriber if pregnancy is suspected, or if breastfeeding
- That pneumonia may occur, to contact prescriber if cough, fever occur
- That hypersensitive reactions may occur, rash, pruritus; stop product, contact prescriber
- That this product is not a cure for HIV-1 infection but controls symptoms, HIV-1 can still be transmitted to others
- This product is to be used in combination only with other antiretrovirals

⚠ High Alert

enoxaparin (℞)

(ee-nox′a-par-in)

Lovenox

Func. class.: Anticoagulant, antithrombotic

Chem. class.: Low-molecular-weight heparins (LMWH)

Do not confuse:

enoxaparin/enoxacin

Lovenox/Lotronex

Action: Binds to antithrombin III inactivating factors Xa/IIa resulting in higher ratio of anti–factor Xa to IIa

Uses: Prevention of DVT (inpatient or outpatient), PE (inpatient) in hip and knee replacement, abdominal surgery at risk for thrombosis; unstable angina/non–Q-wave MI

Unlabeled uses: Antiphospholipid antibody syndrome, arterial thromboembolism prophylaxis, cerebral thromboembolism, percutaneous coronary intervention

DOSAGE AND ROUTES

DVT prevention before hip/knee surgery

- *Adult:* **SUBCUT** 30 mg bid given 12-24 hr postop for 7-10 days, until DVT risk is diminished

DVT prevention before hip replacement

- *Adult:* **SUBCUT** 40 mg/day started 9-15 hr preop or 30 mg bid, started 12-24 hr postop, continued until DVT risk is diminished or is adequately on anticoagulant

DVT prophylaxis before abdominal surgery

- *Adult:* **SUBCUT** 40 mg/day starting 24 hr prior to surgery × 7-10 days to prevent thromboembolic complications

Treatment of DVT/PE

- *Adult:* **SUBCUT** 1 mg/kg q12hr (without PE-outpatient); 1 mg/kg q12hr or 1.5 mg/kg/day (with or without PE-inpatient); warfarin should be started within 72 hr and continued until INR is 2-3 (usually 7 days)

Prevention of ischemic complications in unstable angina/non–Q-wave MI

• *Adult:* **SUBCUT/IV** 1 mg/kg q12hr until stable with aspirin 100-325 mg/day × ≥2 days

Available forms: Prefilled syringes/inj 30 mg/0.3 ml, 40 mg/0.4 ml, 60 mg/0.6 ml, 80 mg/0.8 ml, 100 mg/1 ml, 120 mg/0.8 ml, 150 mg/ml; multidose vials 100 mg/ml (3 ml)

SIDE EFFECTS

CNS: Fever, confusion

GI: Nausea

HEMA: **Hemorrhage, hypochromic anemia, thrombocytopenia, bleeding**

INTEG: Ecchymosis, inj site hematoma

META: Hyperkalemia in renal failure

SYST: Edema, peripheral edema

Contraindications: Hypersensitivity to this product, benzyl alcohol, heparin, or pork; active major bleeding, hemophilia, leukemia with bleeding, peptic ulcer disease, thrombocytopenic purpura, heparin-induced thrombocytopenia

Precautions: Pregnancy (B), breastfeeding, children, geriatric patients, low weight men (<57 kg), women (<45 kg), severe renal/hepatic disease, blood dyscrasias, severe hypertension, subacute bacterial endocarditis, acute nephritis, recent burn, spinal surgery, indwelling catheters

Black Box Warning: Lumbar puncture, epidural anesthesia, spinal anesthesia

PHARMACOKINETICS

SUBCUT: 90% absorbed, maximum antithrombin activity (3-5 hr), elimination half-life 4½ hr, excreted in urine

INTERACTIONS

Increase: enoxaparin action—anticoagulants, salicylates, NSAIDs, antiplatelets, thrombolytics

Drug/Herb

Increase: risk of bleeding—agrimony, alfalfa, angelica, anise, basil, bay, bilberry, black currant, black haw, bogbean, bromelain, buchu, cat's claw, chondroitin, cinchona bark, dong quai, evening primrose, fenugreek, feverfew, fish oils, garlic, ginger, ginkgo, ginseng, horse chestnut, Irish moss, kava, kelp, kelpware, khella, licorice, lovage, lungwort, meadowsweet, motherwort, mugwort, nettle, papaya, parsley (large amts), pau d'arco, pineapple, poplar, prickly ash, red clover, safflower, saw palmetto, skullcap, tonka bean, turmeric, wintergreen, yarrow

Decrease: anticoagulant effect—chamomile, coenzyme Q10, flax, glucomannan, goldenseal, guar gum

Drug/Lab Test

Increase: AST, ALT

Decrease: platelet count

NURSING CONSIDERATIONS

Assess:

• Blood studies (Hct, CBC, coagulation studies, platelets, occult blood in stools), anti–factor Xa (should be checked 4 hr after inj); thrombocytopenia may occur

• For bleeding: gums, petechiae, ecchymosis, black tarry stools, hematuria; notify prescriber

• For neurologic symptoms in patients who have received spinal anesthesia

Administer:

• Only after screening patient for bleeding disorders

• Do not mix with other products or infusion fluids

⚠ Only this product when ordered; not interchangeable with heparin or other LMWHs

• At same time each day to maintain steady blood levels

• Avoid all IM inj that may cause bleeding

• Prepare in a sterile environment using aseptic technique

• Dilution may be stored for up to 4 wk in glass vial at room temperature, up to 2 wk in TB syringes with rubber stoppers at room temperature or refrigerated

SUBCUT route

• Do not give IM; begin 1 hr prior to surgery; do not aspirate; rotate sites; do not expel bubble from syringe before administration

• To recumbent patient, give SUBCUT; rotate inj sites (left/right anterolateral, left/right posterolateral abdominal wall)

• Insert whole length of needle into skin fold held with thumb and forefinger

• If withdrawing from multidose vial, use TB syringe for proper measurement

• Prefilled syringes (30, 40 mg) are not graduated; do not use for partial doses

• Do not administer if particulate is present

IV route

• Use multidose vial for IV administration; use TB syringe or other graduated syringe to measure dose; give IV BOL through IV line, flush after

Perform/provide:

• Storage at 77° F (25° C); do not freeze

Evaluate:

• Therapeutic response: prevention of DVT

Teach patient/family:

• To use soft-bristle toothbrush to avoid bleeding gums, to use electric razor

• To report any signs of bleeding: gums, under skin, urine, stools

• To avoid OTC products containing aspirin unless approved by prescriber

Treatment of overdose: Protamine SO_4 1% sol; dose should equal dose of enoxaparin

entacapone (℞)

(en′ta-kah-pone)

Comtan

Func. class.: Antiparkinson agent

Chem. class.: COMT inhibitor

Action: Inhibits COMT (catechol *O*-methyltransferase) and alters the plasma pharmacokinetics of levodopa. Given with levodopa/carbidopa

Uses: Parkinson's disease in those experiencing end of dose, decreased effect as adjunct to levodopa/carbidopa

DOSAGE AND ROUTES

• *Adult:* **PO** 200 mg given with carbidopa/levodopa, max 1600 mg/day

Available forms: Tabs, film coated 200 mg

SIDE EFFECTS

CNS: Involuntary choreiform movements, hand tremors, fatigue, headache, anxiety, twitching, numbness, dyskinesia, hypokinesia, hyperkinesia, weakness, confusion, agitation, nightmares, psychosis, hallucination, hypomania, severe depression, dizziness, **neuroleptic malignant syndrome**

CV: Orthostatic hypotension

GI: Nausea, vomiting, anorexia, abdominal distress, dry mouth, flatulence, bitter taste, diarrhea, constipation, dyspepsia, gastritis, GI disorder

INTEG: Rash, sweating, alopecia

MISC: Dark urine and other body fluids, back pain, dyspnea, purpura, fatigue, asthenia, bacterial infection, **rhabdomyolysis**

Contraindications: Hypersensitivity

Precautions: Pregnancy (C), breastfeeding, children, renal/hepatic disease, affective disorders, psychosis

PHARMACOKINETICS

Duration up to 8 hr; excreted in urine, feces; well absorbed; protein binding 98%; metabolized in liver extensively; enters breast milk; half-life of levodopa is extended, half-life 0.5 hr initial, 2.5 hr second

INTERACTIONS

• Prevents catecholamine metabolism, do not use together—nonselective MAOIs

Increase: B/P, tachycardia, dysrhythmias, avoid use—bitolterol, DOPamine, DOBUTamine, epinephrine, methyldopa, isoetharine, norepinephrine

Decrease: excretion of entacapone—ampicillin, chloramphenicol, probenecid, erythromycin, rifampin

Drug/Herb

Increase: B/P—ma huang

Decrease: effect—kava

NURSING CONSIDERATIONS

Assess:

⚠ Neuroleptic malignant syndrome: high temp, increased CPK, rigidity, change in LOC

- Involuntary movements in Parkinson's disease: akinesia, tremors, staggering gait, muscle rigidity, drooling when given with levodopa/carbidopa
- B/P, respiration during initial treatment
- Mental status: affect, mood, behavioral changes, depression; complete suicide assessment

Administer:

- Only after MAOIs have been discontinued for 2 wk
- Give with a dose of levodopa/carbidopa; this product has no effect on its own

Perform/provide:

- Assistance with ambulation during beginning therapy

Evaluate:

- Therapeutic response: decrease in akathisia, increased mood when given with levodopa/carbidopa

Teach patient/family:

- That hallucinations, mental changes, nausea, dyskinesia can occur and may mean patient is overmedicated
- To change positions slowly to prevent orthostatic hypotension; not to drive or operate machinery until stabilized on medication and mental performance is not affected
- To use product exactly as prescribed
- That urine, sweat may darken
- To notify prescriber if pregnancy is suspected; or if lactating, product is excreted in breast milk

entecavir (℞)

(en-te'ka-veer)

Baraclude

Func. class.: Antiviral

Chem. class.: Guanosine nucleoside analog

Action: Inhibits hepatitis B virus DNA polymerase by competing with natural substrates and by causing DNA termination after its incorporation into viral DNA; causes viral DNA death

Uses: Chronic hepatitis B (HBV)

DOSAGE AND ROUTES

Chronic hepatitis B (nucleoside treatment–naive)

- *Adult and adolescent ≥16 yr:* **PO** 0.5 mg/day

Chronic hepatitis B while receiving lamivudine or known lamivudine-resistant mutations

- *Adult and adolescent ≥16 yr:* **PO** 1 mg/day

Renal dose

- *Adult:* **PO** CCr ≥50 ml/min 0.5 mg/day; CCr 30-49 ml/min 0.25 mg/day, 0.5 mg/day for lamivudine-refractory patient; CCr 10-29 ml/min 0.15/day, 0.3 for lamivudine-refractory patient; CCr <10 ml/min 0.05 mg PO/day, 0.1 mg for lamivudine-refractory patient

Available forms: Tabs, film coated 0.5, 1 mg; oral sol 0.05 mg/ml

SIDE EFFECTS

CNS: Headache, fatigue, dizziness, insomnia

ENDO: Hyperglycemia

GI: Dyspepsia, nausea, vomiting, diarrhea, elevated liver function enzymes

INTEG: Alopecia, rash

SYST: **Lactic acidosis, severe hepatomegaly with stenosis**

Contraindications: Hypersensitivity

Precautions: Pregnancy (C), breastfeeding, children, geriatric patients, severe renal disease

Black Box Warning: Hepatic disease, hepatitis, HIV, lactic acidosis

PHARMACOKINETICS

Peak 0.5-1.5 hr, steady state 6-10 days, 100% bioavailability, extensively distributed to tissues, protein binding 13%, terminal half-life 128-149 hr, excreted unchanged (62%-73%) via kidneys

INTERACTIONS

Drug/Food

Decrease: absorption—high-fat meal

Drug/Lab Test

Increase: ALT, AST, total bilirubin, amylase, lipase, creatinine, blood glucose, urine glucose

Decrease: platelets, albumin

NURSING CONSIDERATIONS

Assess:

- For nephrotoxicity: increasing CCr, BUN
- For HIV before beginning treatment, because HIV resistance may occur in chronic hepatitis B patients
- ⚠ For lactic acidosis, severe hepatomegaly with stenosis
- Geriatric patients more carefully; may develop renal, cardiac symptoms more rapidly
- For exacerbations of hepatitis (jaundice, pruritus, fatigue) after discontinuing treatment, monitor LFTs

Administer:

- By mouth on empty stomach 2 hr before or after food
- After hemodialysis

Perform/provide:

- Storage in cool environment; protect from light

Evaluate:

- Therapeutic response: decreased symptoms of chronic hepatitis B, improving LFTs

Teach patient/family:

- Not to take with food
- To take exactly as prescribed
- Do not stop medication without approval of prescriber
- That optimal duration of treatment is unknown
- To avoid use with other medications unless approved by prescriber
- To notify prescriber of decreased urinary output, blood in urine
- Symptoms of lactic acidosis: muscle pain, severe tiredness, weakness, trouble breathing, stomach pain with nausea/vomiting, coldness in arms/legs, fast/irregular heartbeat, dizziness
- Symptoms of hepatotoxicity: eyes/skin turns yellow, dark urine, light bowel movements, no appetite for days, nausea, stomach pain
- That product does not cure, but lowers the amount of HBV in body
- That product does not stop you from spreading HBV to others by sex, sharing needles, or being exposed to blood
- Not to breastfeed

⚠ High Alert

ephedrine (℞)

(e-fed′rin)

ephedrine sulfate, Pretz-D (OTC)

Func. class.: Bronchodilator, nonselective adrenergic, mixed direct and indirect effects

Chem. class.: Phenylisopropylamine

Do not confuse:

ephedrine/epinephrine

Action: Causes increased contractility and heart rate by acting on β-receptors in the heart; also acts on α-receptors, causing vasoconstriction in blood vessels

Uses: Shock; increased perfusion; hypotension, bronchodilation

Unlabeled uses: Orthostatic hypotension

DOSAGE AND ROUTES

Hypotension

• *Adult:* **PO** 25 mg daily-qid; **IM/SUBCUT** 25-50 mg; **IV** 10-25 mg, max 150 mg/24 hr
• *Child:* **SUBCUT/IV** 25-100 mg/m^2/day in 4-6 divided doses

Bronchodilator

• *Adult and child >12 yr:* **PO** 12.5-50 mg q3-4hr prn, max 150 mg/24 hr; **NASAL** 2-3 sprays in each nostril q4hr
• *Child 2-12 yr:* **PO** 2-3 mg/kg or 100 mg/m^2/day in 4-6 divided doses

Available forms: Inj 25, 30, 50 mg/ml; caps 25, 50 mg

SIDE EFFECTS

CNS: Tremors, anxiety, insomnia, sweating, headache, dizziness, confusion, hallucinations, **seizures, CNS depression, cerebral hemorrhage,** weakness, drowsiness
CV: Palpitations, tachycardia, hypertension, chest pain, **dysrhythmias**
GI: Anorexia, nausea, vomiting
GU: Dysuria, urinary retention
RESP: **Dyspnea**

Contraindications: Hypersensitivity to sympathomimetics, closed-angle glaucoma, nonanaphylactic shock during general anesthesia, hypertension

Precautions: Pregnancy (C), breastfeeding, cardiac disorders, hyperthyroidism, diabetes mellitus, prostatic hypertrophy, angina

PHARMACOKINETICS

Metabolized in liver; excreted in urine (unchanged), breast milk; crosses blood-brain barrier, placenta; half-life 3-6 hr

PO: Onset 15-60 min, duration 2-4 hr
IM: Onset 10-20 min, duration 1 hr
IV: Onset 5 min, duration 2 hr

INTERACTIONS

• Dysrhythmia: halothane anesthetics, cardiac glycosides, levodopa

Increase: severe hypertension—oxytocics
Increase: hypertensive crisis—ergots, MAOIs
Increase: effect of ephedrine—urinary alkalizers
Decrease: effect of guanethidine
Decrease: effect of ephedrine—methyldopa, urinary acidifiers, rauwolfia alkaloids, α-adrenergic blockers, diuretics, tricyclics

NURSING CONSIDERATIONS

Assess:

• I&O ratio
• ECG continuously during administration; if B/P increases, product is decreased; B/P and pulse q5min after parenteral route; CVP or PWP during infusion if possible
• For paresthesias and coldness of extremities; peripheral blood flow may decrease; long-term use may produce a pseudoanxiety state requiring sedative; increased lactic acid with severe metabolic acidosis can occur
• Inj site: tissue sloughing; if this occurs, administer phentolamine mixed with 0.9% NaCl

Administer:

IV, direct route

• Through Y-tube or 3-way stopcock; give 10-25 mg slowly; may repeat in 5-10 min, protect from light

Additive compatibilities: Chloramphenicol, lidocaine, metaraminol, nafcillin, penicillin G potassium

Solution compatibilities: D_5W, $D_{10}W$, LR, 0.9% NaCl, 0.45% NaCl, Ringer's

Syringe compatibilities: Pentobarbital

Y-site compatibilities: Etomidate, propofol

Perform/provide:

• Storage of reconstituted sol refrigerated no longer than 24 hr
• Do not use discolored sol

Evaluate:

• Therapeutic response: increased B/P with stabilization

Teach patient/family:
- The reason for product administration
- To avoid use with OTC medications unless approved by prescriber

ephedrine nasal agent
See Appendix B

epinastine ophthalmic
See Appendix B

⚠ High Alert

epinephrine (℞)
(ep-i-nef′rin)

Adrenalin Ana-Guard, AsthmaHaler Mist, AsthmaNefrin (racepinephrine), Bronitin Mist, Bronkaid Mist, Epinal, epinephrine, Epinephrine Pediatric, EpiPen, EpiPen Jr., Epitrate, Eppy/N, Medihaler microNefrin, Nephron, Primatene Mist, S-2, Sus-Phrine, Vaponefrin (racepinephrine)

Func. class.: Bronchodilator nonselective adrenergic agonist, vasopressor

Chem. class.: Catecholamine

Do not confuse:
epinephrine/ephedrine

Action: β_1- and β_2-agonist causing increased levels of cAMP producing bronchodilation, cardiac, and CNS stimulation; high doses cause vasoconstriction via α-receptors; low doses can cause vasodilation via β_2-vascular receptors

Uses: Acute asthmatic attacks, hemostasis, bronchospasm, anaphylaxis, allergic reactions, cardiac arrest, adjunct in anesthesia, shock

Unlabeled uses: Bradycardia, chloroquine overdose

DOSAGE AND ROUTES

Asthma
- *Adult and child:* **INH** 1-2 puffs of 1:100 or 2.25% racemic q15min

Bronchodilator
- *Adult:* **SUBCUT/IM** 0.3-0.5 mg (1:1000 sol) q10-15min-4hr, max 1 mg/dose

Anaphylactic reaction/asthma
- *Adult:* **SUBCUT/IM** 0.3-0.5 mg, repeat q10-15min, max 1 mg/dose; epinephrine susp 0.5 mg **SUBCUT,** may repeat 0.5-1.5 mg q6hr
- *Child:* **SUBCUT** 0.01 mg/kg, repeat q15min, × 2 doses, then q4hr, max 0.5 mg/dose; epinephrine susp 0.025 mg/kg **SUBCUT,** may repeat q6hr, max 0.75 mg in child ≤30 kg

Cardiac arrest (ACLS)
- *Adult:* **IV** 1 mg q3-5min; **ENDOTRACHEAL** 2-2.5 mg; **INTRACARDIAC** 0.3-0.5 mg

Symptomatic bradycardia/pulseless arrest (PALS)
- *Child:* **IV** 0.01 mg/kg, may repeat q3-5min up to 0.1-0.2 mg/kg; **ENDOTRACHEAL** give 2-10 × **IV** dose diluted to a volume of 3-5 ml of 0.9% NaCl, followed by positive pressure ventilation

Available forms: Aerosol 0.16 mg/spray, 0.2 mg/spray, 0.25 mg/spray; inj 1:1000 (1 mg/ml), 1:200 (5 mg/ml), 0.01 mg/ml (1:100,000), 0.1 mg/ml (1:10,000), 0.5 mg/ml (1:2000); sol for nebulization 1:100, 1.25%, 2.25% (base)

SIDE EFFECTS

CNS: Tremors, anxiety, insomnia, headache, *dizziness,* confusion, hallucinations, **cerebral hemorrhage**, weakness, drowsiness

CV: Palpitations, tachycardia, hypertension, *dysrhythmias,* increased T wave

GI: Anorexia, nausea, vomiting

MISC: Sweating, dry eyes

RESP: Dyspnea

Contraindications: Hypersensitivity to sympathomimetics, closed-angle glaucoma, nonanaphylactic shock during general anesthesia

Precautions: Pregnancy (C), breastfeeding, cardiac disorders, hyperthyroidism, diabetes mellitus, prostatic hypertrophy, hypertension, organic brain syndrome, local anesthesia of certain areas, labor, cardiac dilation, coronary insufficiency, cerebral arteriosclerosis, organic heart disease

PHARMACOKINETICS

Crosses placenta, metabolized in liver

SUBCUT: Onset 5-15 min, duration 20 min-4 hr

INH: Onset 1-5 min, duration 1-3 hr

INTERACTIONS

- Do not use with MAOIs or tricyclics; hypertensive crisis may occur
- Toxicity: other sympathomimetics

Decrease: hypertensive effects—α-adrenergic blockers

NURSING CONSIDERATIONS

Assess:

- ECG during administration continuously; if B/P increases, decrease dose; B/P and pulse q5min after parenteral route; CVP, ISVR, PCWP during inf if possible; inadvertent high arterial B/P can result in angina, aortic rupture, cerebral hemorrhage
- Inj site: tissue sloughing; administer phentolamine with NS
- Sulfite sensitivity, which may be life-threatening
- Cardiac status, I&O; blood glucose in diabetes

Administer:

- Increased dose of insulin in diabetic patients if glucose is elevated
- Check for correct concentration, route, dosage before administering

IM/SUBCUT route

- Rotate inj sites, massage after inj, shake before using

Endotracheal route

- Give directly via endrotracheal tube, use 1:10,000 sol; for small dose further dilute dose prior to administration, follow with quick insufflations

Inhalation route

- Place in nebulizer (10 gtt of a 1% base sol)
- Dilute racepinephrine 2.25% sol

IV route

- Parenteral dose slowly, after reconstituting 1 mg (1:1000 sol)/10 ml or more 0.9% NaCl; to prepare a 1:10,000 sol for maintenance, may be further diluted in 500 ml D_5W; give 1 mg or less over 1 min or more through Y-tube or 3-way stopcock; 1 mg = 1 ml of 1:1000 or 10 ml of 1:10,000; protect from light, use large vein

Additive compatibilities: Cimetidine, DOBUTamine, floxacillin, furosemide, metaraminol, ranitidine, verapamil

Syringe compatibilities: Doxapram, heparin, milrinone

Y-site compatibilities: Atracurium, calcium chloride, calcium gluconate, cisatracurium, diltiazem, DOBUTamine, DOPamine, famotidine, fentanyl, furosemide, heparin, hydrocortisone sodium succinate, hydromorphone, labetalol, lorazepam, midazolam, milrinone, morphine, niCARdipine, nitroglycerin, norepinephrine, pancuronium, phytonadione, potassium chloride, propofol, ranitidine, remifentanil, vecuronium, vit B/C, warfarin

Perform/provide:

- Storage of reconstituted sol refrigerated no longer than 24 hr
- Do not use discolored sol

Evaluate:

- Therapeutic response: increased B/P with stabilization or ease of breathing

Teach patient/family:

- The reason for product administration and how to administer
- To rinse mouth after use to prevent dryness after inhalation
- Not to take OTC preparations

Treatment of overdose: Administer an α-blocker and a β-blocker

epinephrine/ epinephryl borate ophthalmic

See Appendix B

epinephrine nasal agent

See Appendix B

⚠ High Alert

epirubicin (℞)

(ep-ih-roo′bi-sin)

Ellence

Func. class.: Antineoplastic, antibiotic

Chem. class.: Anthracycline

Action: Inhibits DNA synthesis primarily; replication is decreased by binding to DNA, which causes strand splitting; maximum cytotoxic effects at S and for G_2 phases, a vesicant

Uses: Adjuvant therapy for breast cancer with axillary node involvement following resection

Unlabeled uses: Used in combination for treatment of advanced forms of cancer: bladder, gastric, head and neck, hepatocellular, lung, ovarian, multiple myeloma, soft tissue sarcoma

DOSAGE AND ROUTES

• *Adult:* **IV INF** 100-120 mg/m^2 initially, given with other antineoplastics (cyclophosphamide, 5-fluorouracil); given in repeated cycles; 3-4 wk cycles

Epirubicin dosage adjustments

• *Adult:* **IV** 100 mg/m^2 on day 1 of each cycle; toxicity nadir platelet counts <50,000 mm^3, ANC 250 mm^3, neutropenic fever or grade 3 or 4 nonhematologic toxicity; next cycle give 75% of day 1 dose; delay next cycle until platelets are ≥100,000 mm^3, ANC ≥1500 mm^3, and nonhematologic toxicities have recovered to < grade 1

Hepatic dose

• *Adult:* **IV** Bilirubin 1.2-3 mg/dl or AST 2-4 × normal upper limit 50% of starting dose; bilirubin >3 mg/dl or AST >4 × normal upper limit 25% of starting dose

Available forms: Inj (2 mg/ml) 10 mg/5 ml, 50 mg/25 ml, 150 mg/75 ml, 200 mg/100 ml

SIDE EFFECTS

CV: Increased B/P, **sinus tachycardia, PVCs,** chest pain, **bradycardia, extrasystoles**

GI: Nausea, vomiting, anorexia, mucositis, diarrhea

GU: Amenorrhea, hot flashes, hyperuricemia

HEMA: **Thrombocytopenia, leukopenia, anemia, neutropenia, secondary AML**

INTEG: Rash, **necrosis,** *pain at inj site, reversible alopecia*

MISC: Infection, febrile neutropenia, lethargy, fever, conjunctivitis, **tumor lysis syndrome**

Contraindications: Pregnancy (D), breastfeeding, hypersensitivity to this product, anthracyclines, anthracenediones, baseline neutrophil count <1500 cell/mm^3, severe myocardial insufficiency, recent MI, systemic infections

Black Box Warning: Severe hepatic disease

Precautions: Children, geriatric patients, cardiac/renal/hepatic disease; gout, previous anthracycline use

Black Box Warning: Bone marrow depression (severe), heart failure, extravasation, secondary malignancy

PHARMACOKINETICS

Triphasic pattern of elimination; half-life 3 min, 2.5 hr, 33 hr; metabolized by liver; crosses placenta; excreted in urine, bile, breast milk

INTERACTIONS

Increase: toxicity—other antineoplastics or radiation, cimetidine

Decrease: antibody response—live virus vaccine

NURSING CONSIDERATIONS

Assess:

- Bone marrow depression, infection: increased temp
- CBC, differential, platelet count weekly; withhold product if baseline neutrophil ≤1500/mm^3; leukocyte nadir occurs 10-14 days after administration, recovery by 21st day; notify prescriber of these results
- Blood, urine uric acid levels; swelling, joint pain primarily in extremities, patient should be well hydrated to prevent urate deposits
- Renal studies: BUN, serum uric acid, urine CCr, electrolytes before, during therapy; I&O ratio; report fall in urine output to <30 ml/hr; dosage adjustment is needed if serum creatinine >5 mg/dl
- Hepatic studies before, during therapy: bilirubin, AST, ALT, alk phos as needed or monthly
- Cardiac status: B/P, pulse, character, rhythm, rate, ABGs, ECG, LVEF, MUGA scan, or ECHO; watch for ST-T wave changes, low QRS and T, possible dysrhythmias (sinus tachycardia, heart block, PVCs)
- Bleeding: hematuria, guaiac, bruising, or petechiae, mucosa or orifices q8hr
- Effects of alopecia on body image; discuss feelings about body changes
- Local irritation, pain, burning, necrosis at inj site
- GI symptoms: frequency of stools, cramping

Administer:

- Antiemetic 30-60 min before giving product to prevent vomiting
- Allopurinol or sodium bicarbonate to maintain uric acid levels, alkalinization of urine

IV route

- Using cytotoxic handling procedures; pregnant women must not handle product
- Hydrocortisone, dexamethasone, or sodium bicarbonate (1 mEq/1 ml) for extravasation; apply ice compresses
- Given into tubing of free-flowing IV infusion (0.9% NaCl or D_5) give over 3-5 min; do not mix with other products in syringe

Perform/provide:

- Strict hand-washing technique, gloves, protective clothing
- Liquid diet: carbonated beverages, gelatin may be added if patient is not nauseated or vomiting
- Increased fluid intake to 2-3 L/day to prevent urate, calculi formation

Evaluate:

- Therapeutic response: decreased tumor size, spread of malignancy

Teach patient/family:

- To report any complaints, side effects to nurse or prescriber
- That hair may be lost during treatment and wig or hairpiece may make patient feel better; tell patient that new hair may be different in color, texture
- To avoid crowds and persons with infections when granulocyte count is low
- That contraceptive measures are recommended during therapy and 4 mo thereafter for men and women
- To avoid vaccinations, reactions may occur; to avoid cimetidine during therapy
- That urine may appear red for 2 days
- To avoid OTC medications, supplements unless approved by prescriber
- That irreversible myocardial damage, leukopenia, menopause may occur

eplerenone (℞)

(ep-ler-ee'known)

Inspra

Func. class.: Antihypertensive

Chem. class.: Selective aldosterone receptor antagonist

Action: Binds to mineralocorticoid receptor and blocks the binding of aldosterone, a component of the renin-angiotensin aldosterone system (RAAS)

Uses: Hypertension, alone or in combination with thiazide diuretics, CHF, post-MI

DOSAGE AND ROUTES

• *Adult:* **PO** 50 mg/day, initially, may increase to 50 mg bid after 4 wk; start dose at 25 mg/day if patient is taking CYP3A4 inhibitors

CHF/post-MI

• *Adult:* **PO** 25 mg/day initially, may increase to 50 mg/day max

Available forms: Tabs 25, 50, 100 mg

SIDE EFFECTS

CNS: Headache, dizziness, fatigue

CV: Angina, **MI**

GI: Increased GGT diarrhea, abdominal pain, increased ALT

GU: Increased BUN, creatinine, gynecomastia, mastodynia (males), abnormal vaginal bleeding

META: Hyperkalemia, hyponatremia, hypercholesteremia, hypertriglyceridemia, increased uric acid

RESP: Cough

Contraindications: Breastfeeding, children, hypersensitivity, increased serum creatinine >2 mg/dl (male), >1.8 mg/dl (female), potassium >5.5 mEq/L, type 2 diabetes with microalbuminuria, hepatic disease, CCr <30 ml/min; CCr <50 ml/min in hypertension

Precautions: Pregnancy (B), breastfeeding, geriatric patients, impaired renal/hepatic function, hyperkalemia

PHARMACOKINETICS

Peak 1½ hr, serum protein binding 50%, half-life 4-6 hr, metabolized by liver (CYP3A4 inhibitor), excreted in urine

INTERACTIONS

Increase: hyperkalemia—ACE inhibitors, angiotensin II antagonists, NSAIDs, potassium supplements, potassium-sparing diuretics

Increase: serum levels of lithium

Increase: levels of eplerenone—CYP3A4 inhibitors (ketoconazole, itraconazole, saquinavir, erythromycin, verapamil, fluconazole), reduce dose of eplerenone

Decrease: antihypertensive effect—NSAIDs

Drug/Herb

Increase: toxicity, death—aconite

Increase: antihypertensive effect—barberry, betony, black catechu, black cohosh, bloodroot, broom, burdock, cat's claw, dandelion, goldenseal, hawthorn, Irish moss, Jamaican dogwood, kelp, khella, mistletoe, parsley

Increase or decrease: antihypertensive effect—astragalus, cola tree

Decrease: antihypertensive effect—coltsfoot, guarana, khat, licorice, yohimbe

Decrease: levels of eplerenone—St. John's wort

Drug/Food

• Grapefruit juice increased product level by 25%

NURSING CONSIDERATIONS

Assess:

• B/P at peak/trough level of product, orthostatic hypotension, syncope when used with diuretic; monitor lithium level in those also taking lithium

• Renal studies: protein, BUN, creatinine; increased LFTs, uric acid may be increased

• Potassium levels, hyperkalemia may occur

Perform/provide:

• Storage in tight container at 86° F (30° C) or less

Evaluate:

- Therapeutic response: decreased B/P

Teach patient/family:

- Not to discontinue product abruptly
- Not to use OTC products (cough, cold, allergy) unless directed by prescriber; do not use salt substitutes containing potassium without consulting prescriber
- Important to comply with dosage schedule, even if feeling better
- That product may cause dizziness, fainting, light-headedness; may occur during first few days of therapy
- How to take B/P, and normal readings for age-group

epoetin (℞)

(ee-poe′e-tin)

EPO, Epogen, Eprex ♣, Procrit

Func. class.: Antianemic, biologic modifier, hormone

Chem. class.: Amino acid polypeptide

Action: Erythropoietin is one factor controlling rate of red cell production; product is developed by recombinant DNA technology

Uses: Anemia caused by reduced endogenous erythropoietin production, primarily end-stage renal disease; to correct hemostatic defect in uremia; anemia due to AZT treatment in HIV patients or chemotherapy; reduction of allogenic blood transfusion in surgery patients

Unlabeled uses: Anemia in premature preterm infants

DOSAGE AND ROUTES

Anemia related to chemotherapy (nonmyeloid malignancies)

- *Adult:* **SUBCUT** 150 units/kg 3×/wk, may increase after 2 mo up to 300 units/kg 3×/wk

Anemia in chronic renal failure

- *Adult:* **SUBCUT/IV** 50-100 units/kg 3×/wk, then adjust to maintain target Hct of 30%-36%
- *Child:* **IV/SUBCUT** 50 units/kg 3×/wk

Anemia secondary to zidovudine treatment

- *Adult:* **SUBCUT/IV** 100 units/kg 3×/wk × 2 mo, may increase by 50-100 units/kg q1-2mo, up to 300 units/kg 3×/wk

Surgery

- *Adult:* **SUBCUT** 300 units/kg/day × 10 days prior to surgery, the day of surgery, and for 4 days postsurgery or 600 units/kg at 3 wk, 2 wk, 1 wk, prior to and on day of surgery

Available forms: Inj 2000, 3000, 4000, 10,000, 20,000, 40,000 units/ml

SIDE EFFECTS

CNS: **Seizures,** coldness, sweating, headache

CV: *Hypertension,* **hypertensive encephalopathy, CHF,** edema, **DVT**

INTEG: Pruritus, rash, inj site reaction

MISC: Iron deficiency

MS: Bone pain

RESP: Cough

Contraindications: Hypersensitivity to mammalian cell–derived products, or human albumin, uncontrolled hypertension

Precautions: Pregnancy (C), breastfeeding, children <1 mo, seizure disorder, multidose preserved formulation contains benzyl alcohol and should not be used in premature infants, porphyria, CV disease, hemodialysis, latex allergy, hypertension, history of CABG

Black Box Warning: Hgb >12 g/dl, surgery

PHARMACOKINETICS

IV: Metabolized in body, extent of metabolism unknown, onset of increased reticulocyte count 2-6 wk, peak immediate

INTERACTIONS

- Need for increased heparin during hemodialysis

NURSING CONSIDERATIONS

Assess:

• Renal studies: urinalysis, protein, blood, BUN, creatinine; I&O, report drop in output <50 ml/hr

⚠ Blood studies: ferritin, transferrin monthly; transferrin sat ≥20%, ferritin ≥100 ng/ml; Hct 2×/wk until stabilized in target range (30%-36%) then at regular intervals; those with endogenous erythropoietin levels of <500 units/L respond to this agent; monitor Hct 2×/wk in chronic renal failure; patients treated with zidovudine or cancer patients should be monitored weekly, then periodically after stabilization; death may occur in Hgb >12 g/dl

• B/P; check for rising B/P as Hct rises, antihypertensives may be needed; hypertension may occur rapidly leading to hypertensive encephalopathy

• CNS symptoms: coldness, sweating, pain in long bones; for seizures if Hct is increased within 2 wk by 4 pts

• For hypersensitivity reactions: skin rashes, urticaria (rare), antibody development does not occur

⚠ For pure cell aplasia (PRCA) in absence of other causes, evaluate by testing sera for recombinant erythropoetin antibodies; any loss of response to epoetin should be evaluated

• Dialysis patients: thrill, bruit of shunts, monitor for circulation impairment

Administer:

• Do not shake vial

SUBCUT route

• Before injecting preservative free-, single-dose formulation may be admixed using 0.9% NaCl with benzyl alcohol 0.9% at a 1:1 ratio to reduce inj site discomfort

IV route

• Additional heparin to lower chance of clots

• By direct inj or bolus into IV tubing or venous line at end of dialysis

• Decrease dose by 25 units/kg, if Hct increases by 4% in 2 wk; increase dose if Hct does not increase by 5-6 pts after 8 wk of therapy, suggested target Hct range 30%–36%

Solution compatibilities: Do not dilute or administer with other solutions

Evaluate:

• Therapeutic response: increase in reticulocyte count in 2-6 wk, Hgb/Hct; increased appetite, enhanced sense of well-being

Teach patient/family:

• To avoid driving or hazardous activity during beginning of treatment

• To monitor B/P

• To take iron supplements, vit B_{12}, folic acid as directed

eprosartan (℞)

(ep-roh-sar'tan)

Teveten

Func. class.: Antihypertensive

Chem. class.: Angiotensin II–receptor antagonist (Subtype AT_1)

Action: Blocks the vasoconstrictor and aldosterone-secreting effects of angiotensin II; selectively blocks the binding of angiotensin II to the AT_1 receptor found in tissues

Uses: Hypertension, alone or with other antihypertensives

DOSAGE AND ROUTES

• *Adult:* **PO** 600 mg/day; dose may be divided and given bid with total daily doses from 400-800 mg

Available forms: Tabs 400, 600 mg

SIDE EFFECTS

CNS: *Dizziness*, depression, fatigue, headache

CV: Chest pain

EENT: Sinusitis

GI: *Diarrhea, dyspepsia,* abdominal pain

GU: UTI

META: Hypertriglyceridemia

MS: Myalgia, arthralgia

RESP: *Cough, upper respiratory infection,* rhinitis, pharyngitis, viral infection

SYST: **Anaphylaxis**

Contraindications: Hypersensitivity

Black Box Warning: Pregnancy (D) 2nd/3rd trimesters

Precautions: Pregnancy (C) 1st trimester, breastfeeding, children, geriatric patients, hypersensitivity to ACE inhibitors; renal/hepatic disease, angioedema

PHARMACOKINETICS

Peak 1-2 hr, food delays absorption, protein binding 98%, moderate renal impairment increases product levels by 30%, hepatic impairment increases levels by 40%, excreted in urine and feces, half-life 5-9 hr

INTERACTIONS

Decrease: antihypertensive effect—NSAIDs, salicylates

Drug/Herb

Increase: toxicity, death—aconite

Increase: antihypertensive effect—barberry, betony, black catechu, black cohosh, bloodroot, broom, burdock, cat's claw, dandelion, goldenseal, hawthorn, Irish moss, Jamaican dogwood, kelp, khella, mistletoe, parsley

Increase or decrease: antihypertensive effect—astragalus, cola tree

Decrease: antihypertensive effect—coltsfoot, guarana, khat, licorice, yohimbe

Drug/Lab Test

Increase: ALT, AST, alk phos

Decrease: Hgb

NURSING CONSIDERATIONS

Assess:

- B/P with position changes, pulse q4hr; note rate, rhythm, quality
- Electrolytes (K, Na, Cl)
- Baselines in renal, hepatic studies before therapy begins
- Edema in feet, legs daily
- Skin turgor, dryness of mucous membranes for hydration status

Administer:

- Without regard to meals

Evaluate:

- Therapeutic response: Decrease B/P

Teach patient/family:

- To comply with dosage schedule, even if feeling better
- To notify prescriber of fever; chest pain; swelling of hands, feet, face, lip, or tongue
- That excessive perspiration, dehydration, diarrhea may lead to fall in blood pressure; consult prescriber if these occur
- That product may cause dizziness, avoid hazardous activities until effect is known
- Not to take this medication if pregnant or breastfeeding, or have had an allergic reaction to this product
- To take missed dose as soon as possible, unless within 1 hr before next dose
- That therapeutic effect may take 2-3 wk

⚠ High Alert

eptifibatide (℞)

(ep-tih-fib'ah-tide)

Integrilin

Func. class.: Antiplatelet agent

Chem. class.: Glycoprotein IIb/IIIa inhibitor

Action: Platelet glycoprotein antagonist; this agent reversibly prevents fibrinogen, von Willebrand's factor from binding to the glycoprotein IIb/IIIa receptor, inhibiting platelet aggregation

Uses: Acute coronary syndrome including those undergoing percutaneous coronary intervention (PCI)

DOSAGE AND ROUTES

Acute coronary syndrome

- *Adult:* **IV BOL** 180 mcg/kg as soon as diagnosed, max 22.6 mg, then **IV CONT** 2 mcg/kg/min until discharge or CABG up to 72 hr, max 15 mg/hr

PCI in patients without acute coronary syndrome

- *Adult:* **IV BOL** 180 mcg/kg given immediately before PCI; then 2 mcg/kg/min × 18 hr and a second 180-mcg/kg bolus, 10 min after 1st bolus; continue inf for up to 18-24 hr at rate of 1 mcg/kg/min

Renal dose

• *Adult:* **IV BOL** CCr <50 ml/min: 2-4 mg/dl same loading dose, then ½ usual inf dose

Available forms: Sol for inj 2 mg/ml (10 ml), 0.75 mg/ml (100 ml)

SIDE EFFECTS

CV: **Stroke,** hypotension

GU: Hematuria

HEMA: **Thrombocytopenia**

SYST: **Bleeding, anaphylaxis**

Contraindications: Hypersensitivity, active internal bleeding; history of bleeding, stroke within 2 yr; major surgery with severe trauma, severe hypertension, history of intracranial bleeding, current or planned use of another parenteral GP IIb/IIIa inhibitor, dependence on renal dialysis, coagulopathy, AV malformation, aneurysm

Precautions: Pregnancy (B), breastfeeding, children, geriatric patients, bleeding, impaired renal function

PHARMACOKINETICS

Onset within 1 hr, protein binding 25%, half-life 1.5-2 hr, steady state 4-6 hr, metabolism limited, excretion via kidneys

INTERACTIONS

• Do not give with glycoprotein inhibitors IIb, IIIa

Increase: bleeding—aspirin, heparin, NSAIDs, anticoagulants, ticlopidine, clopidogrel, dipyridamole, thrombolytics, valproate, abciximab

Drug/Herb

Increase: Bleeding risk—arnica, chamomile, clove, dong quai, feverfew, garlic, ginger, ginkgo, Panax ginseng

NURSING CONSIDERATIONS

Assess:

⚠ Platelets, Hgb, Hct, creatinine, PT/APTT baseline INR within 6 hr of loading dose and daily therafter, patients undergoing PCI should have ACT monitored; maintain APTT 50-70 sec unless PCI is to be performed; during PCI, ACT should be 200-300 sec; if platelets drop <100,000/mm^3, obtain additional platelet counts; if thrombocytopenia is confirmed, discontinue product; also, draw Hct, Hgb, serum creatinine

⚠ For bleeding: gums, bruising, ecchymosis, petechiae; from GI, GU tract, cardiac cath sites, IM inj sites

Administer:

• Aspirin and heparin may be given with this product; check for bleeding

• D/C heparin before removing femoral artery sheath, after PCI

IV route

• After withdrawing bolus dose from 10-ml vial, give IV push over 1-2 min; follow bolus dose with continuous inf using pump, give product undiluted directly from 100-ml vial, spike 100-ml vial with vented inf set, use caution when centering spike on circle of stopper top

Y-site compatabilities: alteplase, atropine, DOBUTamine, heparin, lidocaine, meperidine, metoprolol, midazolam, morphine, nitroglycerin, verapamil

Solution compatibilities: 0.9% NaCl, D_5/0.9% NaCl

Perform/provide:

• Do not give discolored solutions or those with particulates, discard unused amount

• Discontinue product prior to CABG

• All medications PO if possible, avoid IM inj and all catheters

Teach patient/family:

• Reason for medication and expected results

• To report bruising, bleeding, chest pain immediately

ergonovine (℞)

(er-goe-noe′veen)

ergonovine, Ergotrate

Func. class.: Oxytocic

Chem. class.: Ergot alkaloid

Action: Stimulates uterine contractions and vascular smooth muscle, decreases bleeding

Uses: Postpartum or postabortion hemorrhage

Unlabeled uses: Variant angina diagnosis

DOSAGE AND ROUTES

Oxytocic

- *Adult:* **PO/SL** 0.2-0.4 mg q6-12hr; **IM** 0.2 mg q2-4hr, not to exceed 5 doses; **IV** 0.2 mg given over 1 min

Variant angina diagnosis (unlabeled)

- *Adult:* **IV** 50 mcg q5min up to 400 mcg or when chest pain occurs

Available forms: Inj 0.2, 0.25 ✤ mg/ml; tabs 0.2 mg

SIDE EFFECTS

CNS: Headache, dizziness, fainting

CV: Hypertension, chest pain

EENT: Tinnitus

GI: Nausea, vomiting, diarrhea

GU: Cramping

INTEG: Sweating

RESP: Dyspnea

Contraindications: Hypersensitivity to ergot medication, augmentation of labor, before delivery of placenta, spontaneous abortion (threatened), PID

Precautions: Cardiac/renal/hepatic disease, asthma, anemia, seizure disorders, hypertension, glaucoma, obliterative vascular disease

PHARMACOKINETICS

Metabolized in liver, excreted in urine

IM: Onset 2-5 min, duration 3 hr

IV: Onset immediate, duration 45 min

INTERACTIONS

- Hypertension: sympathomimetics, ergots

Drug/Herb

Increase: serotonin effect—horehound

NURSING CONSIDERATIONS

Assess:

- Ergotism: nausea, vomiting, weakness, muscular pain, insensitivity to cold, paresthesias of extremities; product should be discontinued
- B/P, pulse; watch for change that may indicate hemorrhage
- Respiratory rate, rhythm, depth; notify prescriber of abnormalities
- Fundal tone, nonphasic contractions; check for relaxation

Administer:

- IM inj deep in large muscle mass; rotate inj sites if additional doses are given
- With emergency equipment available

IV, direct route

- Dilute with 5 ml 0.9% NaCl, give through Y-tube or 3-way stopcock over 1 min

Additive compatibilities: Amikacin, cephapirin, sodium bicarbonate

Evaluate:

- Therapeutic response: decreased blood loss, severe cramping

Teach patient/family:

- To report increased blood loss, increased temp, or foul-smelling lochia; that cramping is normal
- The importance of pad count
- To avoid nicotine products

Treatment of overdose: Stop product, give vasodilators, heparin, dextran

ergotamine (℞)

(er-got′a-meen)

Ergomar, Ergostat, Gynergen ✤

dihydroergotamine

(dye-hye-droe-er-got′a-meen)

DHE45, Dihydroergotamine-Sandoz ✤, Migranal

Func. class.: α-Adrenergic blocker, vascular headache suppressant

Chem. class.: Ergot alkaloid—amino acid

Action: Constricts smooth muscle in peripheral, cranial blood vessels, relaxes uterine muscle; blocks serotonin release

Uses: Vascular headache (migraine, cluster histamine)

DOSAGE AND ROUTES

Ergotamine

• *Adult:* **SL** 1 tab (2 mg), may use q30min, max 3 tabs (6 mg)/24 hr or 10 mg/wk

Dihydroergotamine

• *Adult:* **SUBCUT/IM** 1 mg, may repeat in 1 hr to 3 mg, max 3 mg/day or 6 mg/wk; **IV** 0.5-1 mg, may repeat in 1 hr, max 2 mg/day or 6 mg/wk; **INTRANASAL** 1 spray in each nostril, repeat in 15 min, max 3 mg/24 hr, 4 mg/wk

• *Child ≥6 yr:* **SUBCUT/IM** 0.5 mg, may repeat in 1 hr; **IV:** 0.25 mg, may repeat in 1 hr

Severe acute migraine

• *Child 12-16 yr:* **IV** 0.25-0.5 mg, may repeat q20min for 1-2 doses

Available forms: *Ergotamine:* SL tabs 2 mg; tabs 1 mg; *dihydroergotamine:* inj 1 mg/ml; nasal spray 4 mg/ml

SIDE EFFECTS

CNS: Numbness in fingers, toes, headache, weakness

CV: Transient tachycardia, chest pain, bradycardia, edema, claudication, increase or decrease in B/P, **MI,** peripheral vascular ischemia

GI: Nausea, vomiting, diarrhea, abdominal cramps

MS: Muscle pain

Contraindications: Pregnancy (X), hypersensitivity to ergot preparations, occlusion (peripheral, vascular), renal/hepatic disease, peptic ulcer, intermittent claudication, glaucoma, CVA

Black Box Warning: Coronary artery disease, hypertension, Raynaud's disease, peripheral vascular disease, angina

Precautions: Breastfeeding, children, anemia, geriatric patients, basilar/hemiplagic migraine

Black Box Warning: MI, stroke, Buerger's disease, cardiac disease

PHARMACOKINETICS

Metabolized in liver, excreted as metabolites in feces, crosses blood-brain barrier, excreted in breast milk, protein binding 90%-93%, half-life 2 hr

PO: Peak 30 min-3 hr, duration up to 48 hr

IM/SUBCUT: Peak (IM) 15-30 min, (SUBCUT) 30-60 min; duration (IM) 3-4 hr, (SUBCUT) 8 hr

IV: Peak 3 min, duration 8 hr

INTERACTIONS

Increase: toxicity—CYP4503A4 inhibitors (protease inhibitors, some macrolides, azole antifungals); do not use together

Increase: vasoconstriction—β-blockers, oral contraceptives, nicotine, vasoconstrictors, other migraine agents

Drug/Herb

Increase: serotonin effect—horehound

NURSING CONSIDERATIONS

Assess:

• Migraine characteristics: duration, nausea, vomiting, change in vision, frequency before and at least 1 hr after administration

• Ergotism: nausea, vomiting, weakness, muscular pain, insensitivity to cold, paresthesia of extremities; product should be discontinued

• Toxicity: dyspnea; hypo/hypertension; rapid, weak pulse; delirium; nausea; vomiting

• For peripheral ischemia, GI side effects

Administer:

• At beginning of headache; dose must be titrated to patient response

• Not to pregnant women; harm to fetus may occur

Intranasal route

• Prime nasal sprayer 4× before dose, use 1 spray in each nostril, wait 15 min, use another spray in each nostril, use nasal applicator for 4 treatments only, discard

IV route

• Give dihydroergotamine undiluted over 1 min

Perform/provide:
- Quiet, calm environment with decreased stimulation for noise, bright light, or excessive talking

Evaluate:
- Therapeutic response: decrease in frequency, severity of headache

Teach patient/family:
- Not to use OTC medications; serious product interactions may occur
- To maintain dose at approved level; not to increase even if product does not relieve headache
- To report side effects including increased vasoconstriction starting with cold extremities, then paresthesia, weakness
- That an increase in headaches may occur when this product is discontinued after long-term use

⚠ To keep product out of reach of children; death may occur

Treatment of overdose: Induce emesis or gastric lavage if orally ingested; administer saline cathartic; keep warm

erlotinib (℞)

(er-loe'tye-nib)

Tarceva

Func. class.: Antineoplastic—miscellaneous

Chem. class.: Epidermal growth factor receptor inhibitor

Action: Not fully understood; inhibits intracellular phosphorylation of cell surface receptors associated with epidermal growth factor receptors

Uses: Non–small cell lung cancer (NSCLC), pancreatic cancer

Unlabeled uses: Squamous cell head and neck cancer

DOSAGE AND ROUTES

Non–small cell lung cancer (NSCLC)
- *Adult:* **PO** 150 mg/day

Pancreatic cancer
- *Adult:* **PO** 100 mg/day in combination with gemcitabine

CYP3A4 inducers concurrently (such as rifampin or phenytoin)
- Dosage increase is advised

CYP3A4 inhibitors (atazanavir, clarithromycin, indinavir, itraconazole, ketoconazole, telithromycin, ritonavir, saquinavir, troleandomycin, nelfinavir)
- Dosage reduction may be needed

Head/neck cancer (unlabeled)
- *Adult:* **PO** 150 mg daily

Available forms: Tabs 25, 100, 150 mg

SIDE EFFECTS

CNS: **CVA,** anxiety, depression, headache, rigors

CV: **MI/ischemia**

EENT: Ocular changes, *conjunctivitis, eye pain*

GI: Nausea, diarrhea, vomiting, anorexia, mouth ulceration, **hepatic failure, GI perforation**

GU: **Renal impairment/failure**

HEMA: **Deep vein thrombosis**

INTEG: Rash, **Stevens-Johnson–like skin reaction, toxic epidermal necrolysis**

MISC: Fatigue, infection

RESP: **Interstitial lung disease,** *cough, dyspnea,* **ARDs, pulmonary fibrosis**

SYST: **Hepatorenal syndrome**

Contraindications: Pregnancy (D), breastfeeding, hypersensitivity

Precautions: Children, geriatric patients, ocular/pulmonary/renal/hepatic disorders

PHARMACOKINETICS

Slowly absorbed (60%); peak 3-7 hr; excreted in feces (86%), urine (<4%); metabolized by CYP3A4; terminal half-life 36 hr; protein binding 93%

INTERACTIONS

Increase: erlotinib concentrations—CYP3A4 inhibitors (ketoconazole, itraconazole, erythromycin, clarithromycin, telithromycin)

Increase: plasma concentration of warfarin, metoprolol

Decrease: erlotinib levels—CYP3A4 inducers (phenytoin, rifampin, carbamazepine, phenobarbital)

Drug/Herb

Decrease: erlotinib levels—St. John's wort

NURSING CONSIDERATIONS

Assess:

⚠ For MI/ischemia, CVA in pancreatic cancer patients

⚠ Pulmonary changes: lung sounds, cough, dyspnea; interstitial lung disease may occur, may be fatal; discontinue therapy if confirmed

- Ocular changes: eye irritation, corneal erosion/ulcer, aberrant eyelash growth
- GI symptoms: frequency of stools; if diarrhea is poorly tolerated, therapy may be discontinued for up to 14 days
- Blood studies: INR, LFTs, PT

Administer:

- 1 hr before or 2 hr after food
- Interrupt dosing if severe changes to liver function occur (total bilirubin >3× ULN and/or transaminases >5× ULN when normal pretreatment LFTs)

Evaluate:

- Therapeutic response: decrease NSCLC cells, pancreatic cancer cells

Teach patient/family:

⚠ To report adverse reactions immediately: SOB, severe abdominal pain, persistent diarrhea or vomiting, ocular changes, skin eruptions

- Reason for treatment, expected results
- Use reliable contraception during treatment, pregnancy (D), avoid breastfeeding

ertapenem (℞)

(er-tah-pen′em)

Invanz

Func. class.: Antiinfective—miscellaneous

Chem. class.: Carbapenem

Do not confuse:

Invanz/Avinza

Action: Interferes with cell wall replication of susceptible organisms; osmotically unstable cell wall swells, bursts from osmotic pressure

Uses: Adult patients with moderate to severe infections caused by the following organisms: intraabdominal infections—*Escherichia coli, Clostridium clostridioforme, Eubacterium lentum, Peptostreptococcus* sp., *Bacteroides fragilis, Bacteroides distasonis, Bacteroides ovatus, Bacteroides thetaiotaomicron, Bacteroides uniformis;* complicated skin/skin structure infections—*Staphylococcus aureus* (methicillin-susceptible), *Streptococcus pyogenes, E. coli, Peptostreptococcus* sp.; community-acquired pneumonia—*Streptococcus pneumoniae* (penicillin-susceptible), *Haemophilus influenzae* (β-lactamase–negative), *Moraxella catarrhalis;* complicated UTI—*E. coli, Klebsiella pneumoniae;* acute pelvic infections—*Streptococcus agalactiae, E. coli, B. fragilis, Porphyromonas asaccharolytica, Peptostreptococcus* sp., *Prevotella bivia,* infection prophylaxis prior to elective colorectal surgery

DOSAGE AND ROUTES

Complicated intraabdominal infections

- *Adult:* **IM/IV** 1 g/day × 5-14 days
- *Child 3 mo-12 yr:* **IM/IV** 15 mg/kg bid × 5-14 days

Complicated skin/skin structure infections

- *Adult:* **IM/IV** 1 g/day × 7-14 days
- *Child 3 mo-12 yr:* **IM/IV** 15 mg/kg bid × 7-14 days

Community-acquired pneumonia

- *Adult:* **IM/IV** 1 g/day × 10-14 days
- *Child 3 mo-12 yr:* **IM/IV** 15 mg/kg bid × 10-14 days

Complicated UTI

- *Adult:* **IM/IV** 1 g/day × 10-14 days
- *Child 3 mo-12 yr:* **IM/IV** 15 mg/kg bid × 10-14 days

Acute pelvic infections

- *Adult:* **IM/IV**1 g/day × 3-10 days
- *Child 3 mo-12 yr:* **IM/IV** 15 mg/kg bid 3-10 days

Surgical infection prophylaxis (unlabeled)

• *Adult:* **IV** 1 g as a single dose 1 hr prior to surgical incision

Available form: Powder, lyophilized, 1 g

SIDE EFFECTS

CNS: Insomnia, **seizures,** dizziness, *headache*

CV: **Tachycardia**

GI: Diarrhea, nausea, vomiting, **pseudomembranous colitis**

GU: Vaginitis

INTEG: Rash, urticaria, *pruritus,* pain at inj site, *infused vein complication, phlebitis/thrombophlebitis,* erythema at inj site

RESP: Dyspnea, cough, pharyngitis, crackles, respiratory distress

SYST: **Anaphylaxis**

Contraindications: Hypersensitivity to this product or its components, to amide-type local anesthetics (IM only); anaphylactic reactions to β-lactams

Precautions: Pregnancy (B), breastfeeding, children, geriatric patients, GI/renal/hepatic disease

PHARMACOKINETICS

IV: Onset immediate; peak dose dependent; half-life 4 hr; metabolized by liver; excreted in urine, feces, breast milk

INTERACTIONS

Increase: ertapenem levels—probenecid; do not coadminister

Drug/Herb

• Do not use acidophilus with antiinfectives; separate by several hours

Drug/Lab Test

Increase: hepatic enzymes

NURSING CONSIDERATIONS

Assess:

• Sensitivity to carbapenem antibiotics, other β-lactam antibiotics, penicillins

• Renal disease: lower dose may be required

• Bowel pattern daily: if severe diarrhea occurs, product should be discontinued; may indicate pseudomembranous colitis

• For infection: temp, sputum, characteristics of wound before, during, after treatment

⚠ Allergic reactions, anaphylaxis; rash, urticaria, pruritus; may occur a few days after therapy begins

• Overgrowth of infection: perineal itching, fever, malaise, redness, pain, swelling, drainage, rash, diarrhea, change in cough or sputum

Administer:

• By IV or IM

• After C&S is taken

IM route

• Reconstitute 1-g vial of ertapenem with 3.2 ml of 1% lidocaine HCl without epinephrine, shake well

• Withdraw contents, administer deep IM in large muscle mass, use within 1 hr

IV route

• Do not confuse or mix with other medications; do not use diluents containing dextrose

• Reconstitute 1-g vial of ertapenem with either 10 ml of water for inj, 0.9% NaCl, or bacteriostatic water for inj

• Shake well to dissolve, transfer contents of reconstituted vial to 50 ml 0.9% NaCl inj

• Complete inf within 6 hr

Evaluate:

• Therapeutic response: negative C&S, absence of signs and symptoms of infection

Teach patient/family:

• To report severe diarrhea; may indicate pseudomembranous colitis; CNS side effects

• To report overgrowth of infection: black, furry tongue, vaginal itching, foul-smelling stools

• To avoid breastfeeding; product is excreted in breast milk

Treatment of overdose: Epinephrine, antihistamines; resuscitate if needed (anaphylaxis)

erythromycin base (℞)
(eh-rith-roh-my'sin)
Apo-Erythro ✦, E-Mycin, Eramycin, Erybid ✦, Eryc, Ery-Tab, E-Base, Erythromid ✦, Erythromycin Base Filmtab, Erythromycin Delayed-Release, Novo-Rythro Encap ✦, PCE

erythromycin estolate (℞)
Ilosone, Novo-Rythro ✦

erythromycin ethylsuccinate (℞)
Apo-Erythro-Es ✦, E.E.S., Ery Ped, Novo-Rythro ✦

erythromycin gluceptate (℞)

erythromycin lactobionate (℞)
Erythrocin

erythromycin stearate (℞)
Apo-Erythro-S ✦, Novo-Rythro ✦

Func. class.: Antiinfective
Chem. class.: Macrolide

Do not confuse:
erythromycin/azithromycin

Action: Binds to 50S ribosomal subunits of susceptible bacteria and suppresses protein synthesis

Uses: Infections caused by *Neisseria gonorrhoeae;* mild to moderate respiratory tract, skin, soft tissue infections caused by *Bordetella pertussis, Borrelia burgdorferi, Chlamydia trachomatis; Corynebacterium diphtheriae, Haemophilus influenzae* (when used with sulfonamides); *Legionella pneumophila,* Legionnaire's disease, *Listeria monocytogenes; Mycoplasma pneumoniae, Streptococcus pneumoniae,* syphilis: *Treponema pallidum*

Unlabeled uses: Facilitation of GI motility

DOSAGE AND ROUTES

Soft tissue infections

- *Adult:* **PO** (base, estolate, stearate) 250-500 mg q6hr; **PO** (ethylsuccinate) 400-800 mg q6hr; **IV INF** (lactobionate) 15-20 mg/kg/day divided q6hr
- *Child:* **PO** (salts) 30-50 mg/kg/day in divided doses q6hr; **IV** (lactobionate) 20-40 mg/kg/day in divided doses q6hr, max adult dose

Neisseria gonorrhoeae/PID

- *Adult:* **IV** (gluceptate, lactobionate) 500 mg q6hr × 3 days, then **PO** (base, estolate, stearate) 250 mg or 400 mg (ethylsuccinate) q6hr × 1 wk

Syphilis

- *Adult:* **PO** 500 mg qid × 14 days

Chlamydia

- *Adult:* **PO** 500 mg q6hr × 1 wk or 250 mg qid × 2 wk
- *Infant:* **PO** 50 mg/kg/day in 4 divided doses × 3 wk or more
- *Newborn:* **PO** 50 mg/kg/day in 4 divided doses × 2 wk or more

Intestinal amebiasis

- *Adult:* **PO** (base, estolate, stearate) 250 mg q6hr × 10-14 days
- *Child:* **PO** (base, estolate, stearate) 30-50 mg/kg/day in divided doses q6hr × 10-14 days

GI motility facilitation (unlabeled)

- *Adult:* **PO** 150-250 mg tid-qid, 30 min before meals

Available forms: *Base:* enteric-coated tabs 250, 333, 500 mg; film-coated tabs 250, 500 mg; enteric-coated caps 250, 333 mg; *estolate:* tabs 500 mg; caps 125, 250 mg; drops 100 mg/ml; susp 125, 250 mg/5 ml; *stearate:* film-coated tabs 250 mg; *ethylsuccinate:* chewable tabs 200 mg; susp 100 mg/2.5 ml, 200, 400 mg/5 ml; powder for inj 500 mg and 1 g (lactobionate), 1 g (as gluceptate)

SIDE EFFECTS

CNS: **Seizures**
CV: **Dysrhythmias, QT prolongation**
EENT: Hearing loss, tinnitus
GI: Nausea, vomiting, diarrhea, **hepatotoxicity,** abdominal pain, stomatitis,

heartburn, anorexia, pruritus ani, **pseudomembranous colitis**
GU: Vaginitis, moniliasis
INTEG: Rash, urticaria, pruritus, thrombophlebitis (IV site)
SYST: **Anaphylaxis**
Contraindications: Hypersensitivity, preexisting hepatic disease (estolate)
Precautions: Pregnancy (B), breastfeeding, geriatric patients, hepatic disease, GI disease, QT prolongation, seizure disorder, myasthenia gravis

PHARMACOKINETICS

Peak 4 hr (base); ½–2½ hr (ethylsuccinate); half-life 1-2 hr; metabolized in liver; excreted in bile, feces; protein binding 75%-90%; inhibitor of CYP3A4 and P-glycoprotein

INTERACTIONS

⚠ Serious dysrhythmias—diltiazem, itraconazole, ketoconazole, nefazodone, pimozide, protease inhibitors, sparfloxacin, verapamil
Increase: action, toxicity of alfentanil, alprazolam, bromocriptine, busPIRone, carbamazepine, cilostazol, clindamycin, clozapine, cycloSPORINE, diazepam, digoxin, disopyramide, ergots, felodipine, HMG-CoA reductase inhibitors, methylPREDNISolone, midazolam, quinidine, rifabutin, sildenafil, tacrolimus, tadalafil, theophylline, triazolam, vardenafil, vinBLAStine, warfarin

Drug/Herb

- Do not use acidophilus with antiinfectives; separate by several hours

Drug/Lab Test

Increase: AST/ALT
Decrease: folate assay
False increase: 17-OHCS/17-KS

NURSING CONSIDERATIONS

Assess:

- For infection: temp, characteristics of wounds, urine, stools, sputum, WBCs, baseline and periodically
- I&O ratio; report hematuria, oliguria in renal disease
- Hepatic studies: AST, ALT, if patient is on long-term therapy
- Cardiac status: dysrhythmias, QT prolongation
- Hearing baseline and after treatment
- Renal studies: urinalysis, protein, blood
- C&S before product therapy; product may be given as soon as culture is taken; C&S may be repeated after treatment
- Bowel pattern before, during treatment
- Skin eruptions, itching
- Respiratory status: rate, character, wheezing, tightness in chest; discontinue product if these occur
- Allergies before treatment, reaction of each medication

Administer:

- Do not break, crush, or chew time-rel cap or tab; chew only chewable tabs
- Do not give by IM or IV push
- Enteric-coated tablets may be given with food
- Oral product with full glass of water; do not give with fruit juice
- Oral product with food for GI symptoms

IV route

- After diluting 500 mg or less/10 ml sterile H_2O without preservatives; dilute further in 80-250 ml of 0.9% NaCl, LR, Normosol-R; may be further diluted to 1 mg/ml and given as cont inf; run 1 g or less/100 ml over ½-1 hr; cont inf over 6 hr, may require buffers to neutralize pH if dilution is <250 ml, use inf pump

Gluceptate

Additive compatibilities: Calcium gluconate, hydrocortisone, methicillin, penicillin G potassium, potassium chloride, sodium bicarbonate

Lactobionate

Additive compatibilities: Aminophylline, ampicillin, cimetidine, diphenhydrAMINE, hydrocortisone, lidocaine, methicillin, penicillin G potassium or sodium, pentobarbital, polymyxin B, potassium chloride, prednisoLONE, prochlorperazine, promazine, ranitidine, sodium bicarbonate, verapamil
Syringe compatibilities: Methicillin

Y-site compatibilities: Acyclovir, amiodarone, cyclophosphamide, diltiazem, enalaprilat, esmolol, famotidine, foscarnet, heparin, hydromorphone, idarubicin, labetalol, lorazepam, magnesium sulfate, meperidine, midazolam, morphine, multivitamins, perphenazine, tacrolimus, theophylline, vit B/C, zidovudine

Perform/provide:

- Storage at room temperature; store susp in refrigerator
- Adequate intake of fluids (2 L) during diarrhea episodes

Evaluate:

- Therapeutic response: decreased symptoms of infection

Teach patient/family:

- To report sore throat, fever, fatigue (could indicate superinfection), rhythm changes in the heart, hearing loss
- To notify nurse of diarrhea stools, dark urine, pale stools, jaundice of eyes or skin, and severe abdominal pain
- To take at evenly spaced intervals; complete dosage regimen; take without food unless formulation

Treatment of hypersensitivity: Withdraw product; maintain airway; administer epinephrine, aminophylline, O_2, IV corticosteroids

erythromycin ophthalmic

See Appendix B

erythromycin topical

See Appendix B

escitalopram (℞)

(es-sit-tal'oh-pram)

Lexapro

Func. class.: Antidepressant, SSRI (selective serotonin reuptake inhibitor)

Action: Inhibits CNS neuron uptake of serotonin but not of norepinephrine

Uses: General anxiety disorder; major depressive disorder in adults/adolescents

Unlabeled uses: Panic disorder, social phobia

DOSAGE AND ROUTES

- *Adult:* **PO** 10 mg/day in AM or PM; after 1 wk if no clinical improvement is noted, dose may be increased to 20 mg/day PM; maintenance 10-20 mg/day, reassess to determine need for treatment

Hepatic dose/geriatric

- *Adult:* **PO** 10 mg/day

Available forms: Tabs 5, 10, 20 mg; oral sol 5 mg (as base)/5 ml (contains sorbitol)

SIDE EFFECTS

CNS: Headache, nervousness, insomnia, drowsiness, anxiety, tremor, dizziness, fatigue, sedation, poor concentration, abnormal dreams, agitation, **seizures,** apathy, euphoria, hallucinations, delusions, psychosis, **malignant neuroleptic-like syndrome reactions**

CV: Hot flashes, palpitations, angina pectoris, **hemorrhage,** hypertension, **tachycardia,** 1st-degree AV block, **bradycardia, MI, thrombophlebitis,** postural hypotension

EENT: Visual changes, ear/eye pain, photophobia, tinnitus

GI: Nausea, diarrhea, dry mouth, anorexia, dyspepsia, constipation, cramps, vomiting, taste changes, flatulence, decreased appetite

GU: Dysmenorrhea, decreased libido, urinary frequency, UTI, amenorrhea, cystitis, impotence, urine retention

INTEG: Sweating, rash, pruritus, acne, alopecia, urticaria, photosensitivity
MS: Pain, arthritis, twitching
RESP: Infection, pharyngitis, nasal congestion, sinus headache, sinusitis, cough, dyspnea, bronchitis, asthma, hyperventilation, pneumonia
SYST: Asthenia, viral infection, fever, allergy, chills
Contraindications: Hypersensitivity
Precautions: Pregnancy (C), breastfeeding, geriatric patients, renal/hepatic disease, history of seizures

Black Box Warning: Children/adolescents ≤12 yr, suicidal ideation

PHARMACOKINETICS

PO: Metabolized in liver; excreted in urine; 56% protein binding; metabolized by CYP2C19, 3A4, half-life 27-32 hr; half-life increased by 50% in geriatric patients

INTERACTIONS

• Paradoxical worsening of OCD: busPIRone
• Serotonin syndrome: tryptophan, amphetamines, antidepressants, busPIRone, lithium, amantadine, bromocriptine
⚠ Do not use MAOIs with or 14 days before escitalopram
Increase: CNS depression—alcohol, antidepressants, opioids, sedatives
Increase: side effects of escitalopram—highly protein-bound products
Increase: effect—haloperidol
Increase: half-life of diazepam
Increase: levels or toxicity of carbamazepine, lithium, warfarin, phenytoin, antipsychotics, antidysrhythmics
Increase: levels of tricyclics, phenothiazines
Increase: bleeding risk—NSAIDs, salicylates
Decrease: escitalopram effect—cyproheptadine

Drug/Herb
• SAM-e, St. John's wort: do not use together
Increase: anticholinergic effect—corkwood, jimsonweed
Increase: CNS effect—hops, kava, lavender
Increase: hypertension—yohimbe

Drug/Lab Test
Increase: serum bilirubin, blood glucose, alk phos
Decrease: VMA, 5-HIAA
False increase: urinary catecholamines

NURSING CONSIDERATIONS

Assess:
• Mental status: mood, sensorium, affect, suicidal tendencies, increase in psychiatric symptoms, depression, panic
• Appetite in bulemia nervosa, weight daily, increase nutritious foods in diet, watch for bingeing and vomiting
• Allergic reactions: itching, rash urticaria, product should be discontinued, may need to give antihistamine
• B/P (lying/standing), pulse q4hr; if systolic B/P drops 20 mm Hg, hold product, notify prescriber
• Blood studies: CBC, leukocytes, differential, cardiac enzymes if patient is receiving long-term therapy; check platelets; bleeding can occur
• Hepatic studies: AST, ALT, bilirubin, creatinine; thyroid function studies
• Weight q wk; appetite may decrease with product
• ECG for flattening of T wave, bundle branch, AV block, dysrhythmias in cardiac patients
• Alcohol consumption; if alcohol is consumed, hold dose until AM

Administer:
• With food or milk for GI symptoms, give with full glass of water
• Crushed if patient is unable to swallow medication whole
• Dosage at bedtime if oversedation occurs during the day
• Gum, hard candy, frequent sips of water for dry mouth
• Oral sol: measure with calibrated device

Perform/provide:

- Storage at room temperature; do not freeze
- Assistance with ambulation during therapy, since drowsiness, dizziness occur
- Safety measures primarily in geriatric patients
- Checking to see if PO medication swallowed

Evaluate:

- Therapeutic response: decreased depression

Teach patient/family:

- That therapeutic effect may take 1-4 wk
- To use caution in driving, other activities requiring alertness because of drowsiness, dizziness, blurred vision
- To use sunscreen to prevent photosensitivity
- To avoid alcohol ingestion, other CNS depressants
- To notify prescriber if pregnant or plan to become pregnant or breastfeed
- To change positions slowly, orthostatic hypotension may occur
- To avoid all OTC products unless approved by prescriber
- To report immediately signs of urinary retention
- That clinical worsening and suicide risk may occur
- Using MedGuide provided
- About drug interactions

Treatment of overdose: Activated charcoal, supportive care

esmolol (℞)

(ez′moe-lole)

Brevibloc

Func. class.: β-Adrenergic blocker (antidysrhythmic II)

Do not confuse:

esmolol/Osmitrol

Brevibloc/Brevital

Action: Competitively blocks stimulation of β_1-adrenergic receptors in the myocardium; produces negative chronotropic, inotropic activity (decreases rate of SA node discharge, increases recovery time), slows conduction of AV node, decreases heart rate, decreases O_2 consumption in myocardium; also decreases renin-aldosterone-angiotensin system at high doses; inhibits β_2-receptors in bronchial system at higher doses

Uses: Supraventricular tachycardia, noncompensatory sinus tachycardia, hypertensive crisis, intraoperative and postoperative tachycardia and hypertension

Unlabeled uses: Acute MI, ECT, thyroid storm, pheochromocytoma

DOSAGE AND ROUTES

- *Adult:* **IV** Loading dose 500 mcg/kg/min over 1 min; maintenance 50 mcg/kg/min for 4 min; if no response in 5 min, give 2nd loading dose; then increase inf to 100 mcg/kg/min for 4 min; if no response, repeat loading dose, then increase maintenance inf by 50 mcg/kg/min (max of 200 mcg/kg/min), titrate to patient response
- *Child:* **IV** a total loading dose of 600 mcg/kg over 2 min, maintenance **IV INF** 200 mcg/kg/min, titrate upward by 50-100 mcg/kg/min q5-10min until B/P, heart rate reduced by >10%

Available forms: Inj 10 mg, 20 mg/ml

SIDE EFFECTS

CNS: Confusion, light-headedness, paresthesia, somnolence, fever, dizziness, fatigue, headache, depression, anxiety, **seizures**

CV: Hypotension, bradycardia, chest pain, peripheral ischemia, SOB, **CHF**, conduction disturbances, 1st-, 2nd-, 3rd-degree heart block

GI: Nausea, vomiting, anorexia, gastric pain, flatulence, constipation, heartburn, bloating

GU: Urinary retention, impotence, dysuria

INTEG: Induration, inflammation at site, discoloration, edema, erythema, burning pallor, flushing, rash, pruritus, dry skin, alopecia

RESP: **Bronchospasm**, dyspnea, cough, wheeziness, nasal stuffiness, **pulmonary edema**

Contraindications: 2nd- or 3rd-degree heart block, cardiogenic shock, CHF, cardiac failure, hypersensitivity, severe bradycardia

Precautions: Pregnancy (C), breastfeeding, geriatric patients, hypotension, peripheral vascular disease, diabetes, hypoglycemia, thyrotoxicosis, renal disease, atrial fibrillation, bronchospasms, hyperthyroidism

Black Box Warning: Abrupt discontinuation

PHARMACOKINETICS

Onset very rapid, duration short, half-life 9 min, metabolized by hydrolysis of the ester linkage, excreted via kidneys

INTERACTIONS

- Avoid use with MAOIs

Increase: digoxin levels—digoxin

Increase: α-adrenergic stimulation—ephedrine, epinephrine, amphetamine, norepinephrine, phenylephrine, pseudoephedrine

Decrease: action of thyroid hormones

Decrease: action of esmolol—thyroid hormone

Drug/Herb

- Potassium deficiency: aloe, buckthorn, cascara sagrada, senna

Increase: β-blocking effect—betel palm, butterbur, cola tree, figwort, fumitory, guarana, hawthorn, lily of the valley, motherwort, plantain

Increase: CV reactions—jaborandi tree

Decrease: β-blocking effect—coenzyme Q10, yohimbe

Drug/Lab Test

Interference: glucose/insulin tolerance test

NURSING CONSIDERATIONS

Assess:

- I&O ratio, weight daily, watch for signs of CHF (jugular vein distention, weight gain, crackles, edema)
- B/P, pulse q4hr; note rate, rhythm, quality; rapid changes can cause shock; if systolic <100 or diastolic <60, notify prescriber before giving product
- ECG continuously during inf, hypotension is common
- Baselines in renal/hepatic studies, blood glucose before therapy begins
- Breath sounds and respiratory pattern: wheezing from bronchospasm

Administer:

- Reduced dosage in cool environment, not to discontinue product suddenly

IV route

- IV diluted 5 g/20 ml of D_5W, D_5R, D_5 0.9% NaCl, 0.45% NaCl, LR, D_5 0.45% NaCl, 0.9% NaCl further dilute in the remaining 480 ml (10 mg/ml) and give as infusion; give loading dose over 1 min, then maintenance over 4 min; may repeat loading dose q5min with increased maintenance dose; maintenance dose should not be >200 mcg/kg/min and be given up to 48 hr; dose should be tapered at 25 mcg/kg/min; use inf pump

Additive compatibilities: Aminophylline, atracurium, bretylium, heparin

Y-site compatibilities: Amikacin, aminophylline, amiodarone, ampicillin, atracurium, butorphanol, calcium chloride, cefazolin, cefoperazone, ceftazidime, ceftizoxime, chloramphenicol, cimetidine, cisatracurium, clindamycin, diltiazem, DOPamine, enalaprilat, erythromycin, famotidine, fentanyl, gentamicin, heparin, hydrocortisone, insulin (regular), labetalol, magnesium sulfate, methyldopate, metronidazole, midazolam, morphine, nafcillin, nitroglycerin, nitroprusside, norepinephrine, pancuronium, penicillin G potassium, phenytoin, piperacillin, polymyxin B, potassium chloride, potassium phosphate, propofol, ranitidine, remifentanil, streptomycin, tacrolimus, tobramycin, trimethoprim-sulfamethoxazole, vancomycin, vecuronium

Perform/provide:

- Storage protected from light, moisture; in cool environment

Evaluate:

- Therapeutic response: lower B/P immediately, lower heart rate

Teach patient/family:

- To notify prescriber if chest pain, SOB, wheezing, hypotension, bradycardia, pain, swelling occurs at IV site

Treatment of overdose: Discontinue product

esomeprazole (℞)

(es'oh-mep'rah-zohl)

Nexium

Func. class.: Antiulcer

Chem. class.: Proton pump inhibitor, benzimidazole

Action: Suppresses gastric secretion by inhibiting hydrogen/potassium ATPase enzyme system in gastric parietal cell; characterized as gastric acid pump inhibitor, because it blocks final step of acid production

Uses: Gastroesophageal reflux disease (GERD), adult/child; severe erosive esophagitis, adult/child; treatment of active duodenal ulcers in combination with antiinfectives for *Helicobacter pylori* infection; long-term use in hypersecretory conditions

DOSAGE AND ROUTES

***Active duodenal ulcers associated with* H. pylori**

- *Adult:* **PO** 40 mg/day × 10 days in combination with clarithromycin 500 mg bid × 10 days and amoxicillin 1000 mg bid × 10 days

Hepatic dose

- *Adult:* **PO/IV** Max 20 mg/day (severe hepatic disease)

GERD/erosive esophagitis

- *Adult:* **PO** 20 or 40 mg/day × 4-8 wk; no adjustment needed in renal/liver failure, geriatric patients; **IV** 20 or 40 mg/day up to 10 days
- *Adolescent and child 12-17 yr:* **PO** 20 or 40 mg/day 1 hr before meals, up to 8 wk
- *Child 1-11 yr:* **PO** 10 mg/day 1 hr before meals for up to 8 wk

Available forms: Delayed rel caps 20, 40 mg; powder for IV inj 20, 40 mg/vial; delayed rel powder for oral susp 20, 40 mg

SIDE EFFECTS

CNS: Headache, dizziness

GI: Diarrhea, flatulence, abdominal pain, constipation, dry mouth, **hepatic failure, hepatitis**

INTEG: Rash, dry skin

MISC: **Heart failure**

RESP: Cough, **pneumonia**

SYST: **Stevens-Johnson syndrome, toxic epidermal necrolysis, exfoliative dermatitis**

Contraindications: Hypersensitivity

Precautions: Pregnancy (B), breastfeeding, children, geriatric patients

PHARMACOKINETICS

Well absorbed 90%; protein binding 97%; extensively metabolized liver (CYP2C19); terminal half-life 1-1.5 hr; eliminated in urine as metabolites and in feces; in geriatric patients, elimination rate decreased, bioavailability increased

INTERACTIONS

Increase: effect, toxicity of diazepam, digoxin, penicillins

Decrease: effect—dapsone, iron, itraconazole, ketoconazole, indinavir, calcium carbonate, vitamin B_{12}

NURSING CONSIDERATIONS

Assess:

- GI system: bowel sounds q8hr, abdomen for pain, swelling, anorexia
- Hepatic enzymes: AST, ALT, alk phos during treatment

Administer:

- Swallow caps whole; do not crush or chew; cap may be opened and sprinkled over tbsp of applesauce
- Same time daily, before or with a meal

IV, direct route

• Reconstitute each vial with 5 ml 0.9% NaCl, D_5W, LR; give over 3 min

Intermittent IV INF route

• Dilute reconstituted sol to 50 ml, give over 30 min, do not admix, flush line with D_5W, 0.9% NaCl, LR after inf

Evaluate:

• Therapeutic response: absence of epigastric pain, swelling, fullness

Teach patient/family:

• To report severe diarrhea; abdominal pain; black, tarry stools; product may have to be discontinued

• That diabetic patient should know hypoglycemia may occur

• To avoid hazardous activities; dizziness may occur

• To avoid alcohol, salicylates, NSAIDs; may cause GI irritation

estradiol (℞)
(es-tra-dye′ole)
Estrace

estradiol cypionate (℞)
depGynogen, Depo-Estradiol, Depogen, Dura-Estrin, E-Cypionate, Estragyn LA5, Estro-Cyp, Estrofem, Estroject-LA, Estrol-L.A.

estradiol gel (℞)
Divigel, Elestrin

estradiol spray (℞)
Evamist

estradiol topical emulsion (℞)
Estrasorb

estradiol valerate (℞)
Clinigen LA, Delestrogen, Dioval, Duragen, Estra-L, Estro-span, Femogex ♣, Gynogen LA, Menaval, Valergen

estradiol transdermal system (℞)
Alora, Climara, Esclim, Estraderm, FemPatch, Vivelle

estradiol vaginal tablet (℞)
Vagifem

estradiol vaginal ring (℞)
Estring

Func. class.: Estrogen, progestins

Action: Needed for adequate functioning of female reproductive system; affects release of pituitary gonadotropins, inhibits ovulation, adequate calcium use in bone

Uses: Vasomotor symptoms (menopause), inoperable breast cancer (selected cases), prostatic cancer, atrophic vaginitis, kraurosis vulvae, hypogonadism, primary ovarian failure, prevention of osteoporosis, castration

DOSAGE AND ROUTES

Hormone replacement/menopause symptoms

• *Adult:* **TRANSDERMAL** 0.05-0.1 mg/24 hr, apply 2×/wk; **GEL** apply entire unit dose packet to 5- × 7-inch area of upper thigh/day, alternate thighs; **SPRAY** (Evamist) 1 spray to inner surface of forearm/day in AM

Menopause/hypogonadism/castration/ovarian failure

• *Adult:* **PO** 1-2 mg/day, 3 wk on, 1 wk off or 5 days on, 2 days off; **IM** (cypionate) 1-5 mg q3-4wk; (valerate) 10-20 mg q4wk

• *Adult:* **TOP** (Estraderm) 0.05 mg/24 hr applied 2×/wk; (Climara) 0.05 mg/hr applied 1×/wk in a cyclic regimen; women with hysterectomy may use continuously

Prostatic cancer

• *Adult:* **IM** (valerate) 30 mg q1-2wk; **PO** (oral estradiol) 1-2 mg tid

Breast cancer

• *Adult:* **PO** 10 mg tid × 3 mo or longer

Atropic vaginitis/kraurosis vulvae

• *Adult:* **VAG CREAM** 2-4 g/day × 1-2 wk, then 1 g 1-3×/wk cycled; vag tab 1/day × 2 wk, maintenance 1 tab 2×/wk; **VAG RING** inserted and left in place continuously for 3 mo

Vasomotor symptoms

• *Adult:* **TOP** After cleaning and drying skin on left thigh, calf, rub in contents of pouch using both hands until completely absorbed; wash hands

Available forms: *Estradiol:* tabs 0.5, 1, 2 mg; *valerate:* inj 10, 20, 40 mg/ml; *transdermal:* 0.025, 0.0375, 0.05, 0.075, 0.1 mg/24 hr release rate; *vag cream:* 100 mcg/g; *vag tab:* 25 mcg; *vag ring:* 2 mg/90 days; *topical emulsion:* 2.5 mg; *gel* (Divigel) 0.1%; *spray* (Evamist) 1.53 mg/acuation

SIDE EFFECTS

CNS: Dizziness, headache, migraines, depression, **seizures**

CV: Hypotension, thrombophlebitis, edema, **thromboembolism, stroke, pulmonary embolism, myocardial infarction,** chest pain

EENT: Contact lens intolerance, increased myopia, astigmatism, throat swelling, eyelid edema

GI: Nausea, vomiting, diarrhea, anorexia, pancreatitis, cramps, constipation, increased appetite, increased weight, **cholestatic jaundice, hepatic adenoma**

GU: Amenorrhea, cervical erosion, breakthrough bleeding, dysmenorrhea, vaginal candidiasis, breast changes, *gynecomastia, testicular atrophy, impotence,* **increased risk of breast cancer, endometrial cancer,** changes in libido; **toxic shock, vaginal wall ulceration/erosion (vag ring)**

INTEG: Rash, urticaria, acne, hirsutism, alopecia, oily skin, seborrhea, purpura, melasma

META: Folic acid deficiency, hypercalcemia, hyperglycemia

Contraindications: Pregnancy (X), breastfeeding, reproductive cancer, genital bleeding (abnormal, undiagnosed)

Black Box Warning: Breast/endometrial cancer, thromboembolic disorders, MI, stroke

Precautions: Hypertension, asthma, blood dyscrasias, gallbladder/bone/renal/hepatic disease, CHF, diabetes mellitus, depression, migraine headache, seizure disorders, family history of cancer of breast or reproductive tract, smoking, uterine fibroids, vaginal irritation/infection

Black Box Warning: Cardiac disease, dementia

PHARMACOKINETICS

PO/INJ/TRANSDERMAL: Degraded in liver, excreted in urine, crosses placenta, excreted in breast milk

INTERACTIONS

Increase: action of corticosteroids

Increase: toxicity—cycloSPORINE, dantrolene

Decrease: action of anticoagulants, oral hypoglycemics, tamoxifen
Decrease: estradiol action—anticonvulsants, barbiturates, phenylbutazone, rifampin, calcium

Drug/Herb

- Altered estrogen effect: black cohosh, DHEA

Increase: estrogen effect—alfalfa, hops
Decrease: estrogen effect—saw palmetto, St. John's wort

Drug/Food

Increase: estrogen level—grapefruit juice

Drug/Lab Test

Increase: BSP retention test, PBI, T_4, serum sodium, platelet aggregation, thyroxine-binding globulin (TBG), prothrombin, factors VII, VIII, IX, X, triglycerides
Decrease: serum folate, serum triglyceride, T_3 resin uptake test, glucose tolerance test, antithrombin III, pregnanediol, metyrapone test
False positive: LE prep, ANA

NURSING CONSIDERATIONS

Assess:

- Blood glucose of diabetic patient, hyperglycemia may occur
- Weight daily, notify prescriber of weekly weight gain >5 lb; if increase, diuretic may be ordered
- B/P q4hr, watch for increase caused by H_2O and sodium retention
- I&O ratio; decreasing urinary output, increasing edema, report changes
- Hepatic studies, including AST, ALT, bilirubin, alk phos baseline, periodically; periodic folic acid level
- Hypertension, cardiac symptoms, jaundice, hypercalcemia
- Mental status: affect, mood, behavioral changes, aggression
- Female patient for intact uterus, if so, progesterone should be added to estrogen therapy to decrease risk of endometrial cancer

Administer:

- Titrated dose; use lowest effective dose
- IM inj deeply in large muscle mass

PO route

- With food or milk to decrease GI symptoms

Transdermal route

- Apply to trunk of body 2×/wk; press firmly and hold in place for 10 sec to ensure good contact
- On intermittent cycle schedule: 3 wk on, then 1 wk off; if patch falls off, reapply

Topical route

- Use Evamist daily; spray to inner upper arm; may increase to 2-3×/day based on response; allow to dry for 2 min

Vaginal route

- Use applicator provided

Evaluate:

- Therapeutic response: reversal of menopause symptoms or decrease in tumor size in prostatic, breast cancer

Teach patient/family:

- To weigh weekly, report gain >5 lb
- ⚠ To report breast lumps, vaginal bleeding, edema, jaundice, dark urine, clay-colored stools, dyspnea, headache, blurred vision, abdominal pain, numbness or stiffness in legs, chest pain, tenderness, redness, and swelling in extremities; male to report impotence or gynecomastia; dermal rash with transdermal patch

Rarely Used

estramustine (℞)
(ess-tra-muss'teen)
Emcyt
Func. class.: Antineoplastic alkylating agent

Uses: Metastatic prostate cancer

DOSAGE AND ROUTES

- *Adult:* **PO** 10-16 mg/kg/day or 600 mg/m^2/day in 3-4 divided doses; treatment may continue for ≥3 mo

Contraindications: Pregnancy (D), hypersensitivity to estradiol, thromboembolic disorders, stroke, thrombophlebitis

estrogens, conjugated (℞)

Cenestin, C.E.S. ✱, Congest, Premarin, Premphase

estrogens, conjugated synthetic B (℞)

Enjuvia

Func. class.: Estrogen, hormone

Do not confuse:
Premarin/Provera

Action: Needed for adequate functioning of female reproductive system; affects release of pituitary gonadotropins, inhibits ovulation, adequate calcium use in bone

Uses: Vasomotor symptoms (menopause), inoperable breast cancer, prostatic cancer, abnormal uterine bleeding, hypogonadism, primary ovarian failure, prevention of osteoporosis, castration

Unlabeled uses: Gender identity disorder

DOSAGE AND ROUTES

Estrogens conjugated

Vasomotor symptoms (menopause)

• *Adult:* **PO** 0.3-1.25 mg/day 3 wk on, 1 wk off

Prevention of osteoporosis

• *Adult:* **PO** 0.625 mg/day or in cycle

Atrophic vaginitis

• *Adult:* **VAG CREAM** 2-4 g/day × 21 days, off 7 days, repeat

Prostatic cancer

• *Adult:* **PO** 1.25-2.5 mg tid

Advanced inoperable breast cancer

• *Adult:* **PO** 10 mg tid × 3 mo or longer

Abnormal uterine bleeding

• *Adult:* **IV/IM** 25 mg, repeat in 6-12 hr

Castration/primary ovarian failure

• *Adult:* **PO** 1.25 mg/day, 3 wk on, 1 wk off

Hypogonadism

• *Adult:* **PO** 2.5-7.5 mg/day × 20 days/mo

Estrogens conjugated synthetic B

Vasomotor symptoms (menopause)

• *Adult:* **PO** 0.625 mg/day initially; may increase based on response

Available forms: Tabs 0.3, 0.45, 0.625, 0.9, 1.25, 2.5 mg; inj 25 mg/vial; vag cream 0.625 mg/g; *synthetic B:* tabs 0.625, 1.25 mg

SIDE EFFECTS

CNS: Dizziness, headache, migraine, depression, **seizures,** mood disturbances

CV: Hypotension, thrombophlebitis, edema, **thromboembolism, stroke, pulmonary embolism, MI,** chest pain

EENT: Contact lens intolerance, increased myopia, astigmatism

GI: Nausea, vomiting, diarrhea, anorexia, pancreatitis, cramps, constipation, increased appetite, **cholestatic jaundice, hepatic adenoma,** weight gain/loss

GU: Amenorrhea, cervical erosion, breakthrough bleeding, dysmenorrhea, vaginal candidiasis, breast changes, *gynecomastia, testicular atrophy, impotence,* **increased risk of breast cancer, endometrial cancer,** libido changes

INTEG: Rash, urticaria, acne, hirsutism, alopecia, oily skin, seborrhea, purpura, melasma

META: Folic acid deficiency, hypercalcemia, hyperglycemia

Contraindications: Pregnancy (X), breastfeeding, thromboembolic disorders, reproductive cancer, genital bleeding (abnormal, undiagnosed), hypersensitivity

Black Box Warning: Endometrial cancer

Precautions: Hypertension, asthma, blood dyscrasias, CHF, diabetes mellitus, depression, migraine headache, seizure disorders, gallbladder/bone/hepatic/renal disease, family history of cancer of breast or reproductive tract, smoking, dementia, hypothyroidism, obesity, SLE

Black Box Warning: Cardiac disease, dementia

PHARMACOKINETICS

PO/IM/IV: Degraded in liver, excreted in urine, crosses placenta, excreted in breast milk

INTERACTIONS

Increase: toxicity—cycloSPORINE, dantrolene

Increase: action of corticosteroids

Decrease: action of estrogens—anticonvulsants, barbiturates, phenylbutazone, rifampin

Decrease: action of anticoagulants, oral hypoglycemics, tamoxifen

Drug/Herb

- Altered estrogen effect—black cohosh, DHEA

Increase: estrogen effect—alfalfa, hops

Decrease: estrogen effect—saw palmetto, St. John's wort

Drug/Food

Increase: estrogen level—grapefruit juice

Drug/Lab Test

Increase: BSP retention test, PBI, T_4, serum sodium, platelet aggregation, thyroxine-binding globulin (TBG), prothrombin, factors VII, VIII, IX, X, triglycerides

Decrease: serum folate, serum triglyceride, T_3 resin uptake test, glucose tolerance test, antithrombin III, pregnanediol, metyrapone test

False positive: LE prep, antinuclear antibodies

NURSING CONSIDERATIONS

Assess:

- Blood glucose if diabetic patient, hyperglycemia may occur
- Weight daily; notify prescriber of weekly weight gain >5 lb; if increase, diuretic may be ordered
- B/P q4hr; watch for increase caused by H_2O and Na retention
- I&O ratio; be alert for decreasing urinary output, increasing edema
- Hepatic studies: AST, ALT, bilirubin, alk phos
- Hypertension, cardiac symptoms, jaundice, hypercalcemia
- Mental status: affect, mood, behavioral changes, aggression
- Female patient for intact uterus; if so, progesterone should be added to estrogen therapy to decrease risk of endometrial cancer; abnormal uterine bleeding, breast exam

Administer:

- Titrated dose, use lowest effective dose

IM route

- IM reconstitute after withdrawing >5 ml of air from container and inject sterile diluent on vial side, rotate to dissolve; give inj deep in large muscle mass
- With food or milk to decrease GI symptoms (PO)

Vaginal route

- Use applicator provided

IV, direct route

- IV, after reconstituting as for IM, inject into distal port of running IV line of D_5W, 0.9% NaCl, LR at 5 mg/min or less

Y-site compatibilities: Heparin/hydrocortisone, potassium chloride, vit B/C

Evaluate:

- Therapeutic response: absence of breast engorgement, reversal of menopause symptoms, or decrease in tumor size in prostatic cancer

Teach patient/family:

- To avoid breastfeeding, since product is excreted in breast milk
- To weigh weekly, report gain >5 lb

⚠ To report breast lumps, vaginal bleeding, edema, jaundice, dark urine, clay-colored stools, dyspnea, headache, blurred vision, abdominal pain, leg pain and redness, numbness or stiffness in legs, chest pain; male to report impotence or gynecomastia

- To avoid sunlight or wear sunscreen; burns may occur
- To notify prescriber if pregnancy is suspected
- That vasomotor symptoms improve in 2 wk, max relief in 8 wk

eszopiclone (℞)

(es-zop′i-klone)

Lunesta

Func. class.: Sedative/hypnotic, nonbenzodiazepine

Chem. class.: Cyclopyrrolone

Controlled Substance Schedule IV

Action: Interacts with GABA receptors

Uses: Insomnia

DOSAGE AND ROUTES

• *Adult:* **PO** 2 mg immediately before bed, may increase to 3 mg if needed

Hepatic dose/CYP3A4 inhibitors

• *Adult:* **PO** 1 mg immediately before bed in severe hepatic disease

Available forms: Tabs 1, 2, 3 mg

SIDE EFFECTS

CNS: Worsening depression, hallucinations, headache, daytime drowsiness, **suicidal thoughts/actions,** migraine, restlessness, anxiety, sleep driving, sleepwalking

CV: Peripheral edema, chest pain

GI: Dry mouth, bitter taste (dysgeusia)

GU: Gynecomastia, dysmenorrhea

INTEG: Rash, **angioedema**

Contraindications: Hypersensitivity, ethanol intoxication

Precautions: Pregnancy (C), breastfeeding, children, geriatric patients, severe hepatic disease

PHARMACOKINETICS

Onset rapid; peak 1 hr; duration 6 hr; extensively metabolized in the liver by CYP3A4, CYP2E1; excreted via kidneys; half-life 6 hr, elderly 9 hr, protein binding 52%-59%

INTERACTIONS

Increase: CNS depression—CNS depressants

Increase: toxicity due to decreased eszopiclone elimination—CYP3A4 inhibitors (clarithromycin, itraconazole, ketoconazole, nefazodone, nelfinavir, ritonavir, troleandomycin)

Drug/Food

Decrease: drug action—high fat meal

NURSING CONSIDERATIONS

Assess:

• Sleep pattern: ability to go to sleep, stay asleep, early morning awakenings, conservative methods used

• For abuse of this or other products

Administer:

• Do not break, crush, or chew tab

• Immediately before bedtime

• Avoid use with a high fat meal

Evaluate:

• Therapeutic response: ability to sleep and stay asleep throughout the night

Teach patient/family:

• That daytime drowsiness may occur; not to engage in hazardous activities until effect is known

• That all other medications and supplements should be avoided unless approved by prescriber

• To notify prescriber if suspected or planned pregnancy

etanercept (℞)

(eh-tan′er-sept)

Enbrel

Func. class.: Antirheumatic agent (disease modifying) (DMARDs)

Chem. class.: Anti-TNF agent

Action: Binds tumor necrosis factor (TNF), which is involved in immune and inflammatory reactions

Uses: Acute, chronic rheumatoid arthritis that has not responded to other disease-modifying agents, polyarticular course juvenile rheumatoid arthritis (JRA), ankylosing spondylitis, plaque psoriasis, psoriatic arthritis

Unlabeled uses: Crohn's disease; plaque psoriasis (child ≥4 yr)

DOSAGE AND ROUTES

Rheumatoid/psoriatic arthritis, ankylosing spondylitis

- *Adult:* **SUBCUT** 50 mg q wk
- *Child 2-17 yr:* **SUBCUT** 0.8 mg/kg/wk, max 50 mg/wk

Plaque psoriasis

- *Adult:* **SUBCUT** 50 mg 2×/wk × 3 mo
- *Adolescent and child 4-17 yr (unlabeled):* **SUBCUT** 0.8 mg/kg/wk, max 50 mg/wk

Juvenile rheumatoid arthritis (JRA)

- *Adolescent and child 2-17 yr:* **SUBCUT** 0.8 mg/kg/wk, max 50 mg/wk

Available forms: Powder for inj 25 mg; inj 50 mg/ml; autoinjector, single use

SIDE EFFECTS

CNS: *Headache,* asthenia, dizziness

GI: Abdominal pain, dyspepsia, vomiting

HEMA: **Pancytopenia, anemia, thrombocytopenia, leukopenia, neutropenia**

INTEG: Rash, *inj site reaction,* keratoderma blenorrhagicum

RESP: *Pharyngitis, cough, URI, non-URI,* sinusitis, *rhinitis*

SYST: **Serious infections, sepsis, death, malignancies**

Contraindications: Sepsis, active infections

Black Box Warning: Hypersensitivity to this product, latex, benzyl alcohol

Precautions: Pregnancy (B), breastfeeding, children <4 yr, geriatric patients, malignancies, CHF

Black Box Warning: Infection

PHARMACOKINETICS

Elimination half-life 102 hr, 60% absorbed (SUBCUT)

INTERACTIONS

- Do not give concurrently with vaccines, immunizations should be brought up to date before treatment
- Avoid use with anakinra, cyclophosphamide

NURSING CONSIDERATIONS

Assess:

- Pain, stiffness, ROM, swelling of joints before, during, and after treatment
- For inj site pain, swelling, usually occurs after 2 inj (4-5 days)

Administer:

- After reconstituting 1 ml of supplied diluent, slowly inject diluent into vial, swirl contents, do not shake, sol should be clear/colorless, do not use if cloudy or discolored
- Do not admix with other sol or medications, do not use filter
- May be injected SUBCUT into upper arm, abdomen, or thigh, rotate inj sites

Evaluate:

- Therapeutic response: decreased inflammation, pain in joints

Teach patient/family:

- That product must be continued for prescribed time to be effective
- To use caution when driving; dizziness may occur
- Not to receive live vaccinations during treatment
- About self-administration if appropriate: inj should be made in thigh, abdomen, upper arm; rotate sites at least 1 in from old site
- To notify prescriber of possible infection (upper respiratory or other)

ethambutol (℞)

(e-tham′byoo-tole)

Etibi ✦, Myambutol

Func. class.: Antitubercular

Chem. class.: Diisopropylethylene diamide derivative

Do not confuse:

ethambutol/Ethmozine

Action: Inhibits RNA synthesis, decreases tubercle bacilli replication

Uses: Pulmonary TB, as an adjunct, other mycobacterial infections

DOSAGE AND ROUTES

- *Adult and child >13 yr:* **PO** 15-25 mg/kg/day as a single dose or 50 mg/kg 2×/wk or 25-30 mg/kg 3×/wk

Renal disease

- CCr 10-50 ml/min dose q24-36hr; CCr <10 ml/min dose q48hr

Retreatment

- *Adult:* **PO** 25 mg/kg/day as single dose × 2 mo with at least 1 other product, then decrease to 15 mg/kg/day as single dose, max 2.5 g/day
- *Child:* **PO** 15 mg/kg/day

Available forms: Tabs 100, 400 mg

SIDE EFFECTS

CNS: Headache, confusion, fever, malaise, dizziness, *disorientation,* hallucinations

EENT: Blurred vision, optic neuritis, photophobia, decreased visual acuity

GI: Abdominal distress, anorexia, nausea, vomiting

INTEG: Dermatitis, pruritus, **toxic epidermal necrolysis,** erythema multiforme

META: Elevated uric acid, acute gout, impaired hepatic function

MISC: **Thrombocytopenia,** joint pain, bloody sputum, **anaphylaxis**

Contraindications: Children <13 yr, hypersensitivity, optic neuritis

Precautions: Pregnancy (B), breastfeeding, renal disease, diabetic retinopathy, cataracts, ocular defects, hepatic and hematopoietic disorders

PHARMACOKINETICS

Peak 2-4 hr, half-life 3 hr, metabolized in liver, excreted in urine (unchanged product/inactive metabolites, unchanged product in feces)

INTERACTIONS

- Delayed absorption of ethambutol: aluminum salts
- Neurotoxicity: other neurotoxics

Increase: adverse reactions—ethionamide

NURSING CONSIDERATIONS

Assess:

- Hepatic studies q wk × 2 wk, then q2mo: ALT, AST, bilirubin
- Signs of anemia: Hct, Hgb, fatigue
- Mental status often: affect, mood, behavioral changes; psychosis may occur
- Hepatic status: decreased appetite, jaundice, dark urine, fatigue
- C&S, including sputum, before treatment
- Visual status: decreased activity, altered color perception

Administer:

- With meals to decrease GI symptoms
- Antiemetic if vomiting occurs
- After C&S is completed; q mo to detect resistance
- 2 hr before antacids

Evaluate:

- Therapeutic response: decreased symptoms of TB, decrease in acid-fast bacteria

Teach patient/family:

- To avoid alcohol products
- That compliance with dosage schedule, duration is necessary
- That scheduled appointments must be kept or relapse may occur
- To report any visual changes, rash, hot, swollen, painful joints, numbness or tingling of extremities to prescriber

etidronate (℞)

(eh-tih-droe′nate)

Didronel

Func. class.: Bone resorption inhibitor

Chem. class.: Bisphosphonate

Do not confuse:

etidronate/etretinate/etomidate

Action: Decreases bone resorption and new bone development (accretion)

Uses: Paget's disease, heterotopic ossification, hypercalcemia of malignancy

Unlabeled uses: Osteoporosis/osteoporosis prophylaxis

DOSAGE AND ROUTES

Paget's disease

• *Adult:* **PO** 5-10 mg/kg/day, 2 hr before meals with water, not to exceed 20 mg/kg/day, max 6 mo or 11-20 mg/kg/day for max of 3 mo

Heterotopic ossification

• *Adult:* **PO** 20 mg/kg/day × 2 wk, then 10 mg/kg/day for 10 wk, total 12 wk

Hypercalcemia

• *Adult:* **PO** 20 mg/kg/day × 30 days

Heterotopic ossification/hip replacement

• *Adult:* **PO** 20 mg/kg/day × 4 wk before and 3 mo after surgery (4 mo total)

Available forms: Tabs 200, 400 mg

SIDE EFFECTS

CNS: Headache

CV: **Atrial fibrillation**

GI: Nausea, constipation, diarrhea, gastritis, esophagitis

GU: **Nephrotoxicity**

MISC: Dyspnea, low magnesium, phosphorus, alopecia, **Stevens-Johnson syndrome, angioedema**

MS: Bone pain, hypocalcemia, decreased mineralization of nonaffected bones, osteonecrosis of the jaw, arthralgia, leg cramps

Contraindications: Clinically overt osteomalacia

Precautions: Pregnancy (C), breastfeeding, children, renal disease, restricted vit D, calcium, colitis, vit D deficiency, anemia, esophagitis, pathologic fractures, severe renal disease with creatinine >5 mg/dl, poor dentition, asthma, coagulopathy, dental disease or work, GERD, hiatal hernia, hyperthyroidism, infection, phosphate hypersensitivity

PHARMACOKINETICS

Absorbed poorly (PO), not metabolized, excreted in urine/feces, therapeutic response 1-3 mo

INTERACTIONS

Increase: protime—warfarin

Decrease: absorption—calcium, aluminum, magnesium antacids/supplements, iron products

Drug/Food

Decrease: absorption—dairy products

NURSING CONSIDERATIONS

Assess:

• I&O ratio; check for decreased output in renal patients

• Dental health

• BUN, creatinine, phosphate calcium, alk phos; calcium should be kept at 9-10 mg/dl, vit D 50-135 international units/dl

• For bone pain, weakness during treatment

• Muscle spasm, laryngospasm, paresthesias, facial twitching, colic; may indicate hypocalcemia

• Nutritional status, diet for sources of vit D (milk, some seafood), calcium (dairy products, dark green vegetables), phosphates—adequate intake is necessary

• Persistent nausea or diarrhea

Administer:

PO route

• On empty stomach with water 2 hr before meals; avoid simultaneous vitamins/mineral/antacids with calcium, iron, magnesium, or aluminum

Evaluate:

• Therapeutic response: management of bone deficiencies, Paget's disease

Teach patient/family:

• To avoid OTC products

• That therapeutic response may take 1-3 mo; effects persist for months after product is discontinued

• That adequate intake of calcium, vit D is necessary

• To report sudden onset of unexplained pain, restricted mobility, heat over bone; hypercalcemic relapse

• To continue good oral hygiene

Rarely Used

etomidate (℞)

(e-tom′i-date)

Amidate

Func. class.: General anesthetic

Uses: Induction of general anesthesia

DOSAGE AND ROUTES

- *Adult and child >10 yr:* **IV** 0.2-0.6 mg/kg over ½-1 min

Contraindications: Hypersensitivity, labor/delivery

⚠ High Alert

etoposide (℞)

(e-toe-poe′side)

Toposar, VP-16

etoposide phosphate (℞)

Etopophos

Func. class.: Antineoplastic—miscellaneous

Chem. class.: Semisynthetic podophyllotoxin

Action: Inhibits mitotic activity through metaphase to mitosis; also inhibits cells from entering mitosis, depresses DNA, RNA synthesis, cell cycle specific S and G_2; binds to a complex of DNA and topoisomerase II

Uses: Leukemias, testicular cancer, small cell carcinoma of the lung

Unlabeled uses: Lymphomas

DOSAGE AND ROUTES

Testicular cancer

- *Adult:* **IV** 50-100 mg/m^2/day × 5 days given q3-5wk or 200-250 mg/m^2/wk, or 125-140 mg/m^2/day 3 × wk, q5wk

Small cell carcinoma of the lung

- *Adult:* **PO** 70 mg/m^2/day × 4 days, given q3-4wk, **IV** 35 mg/m^2/day × 4 days, up to 50 mg/m^2/day × 5 day q3-4wk

Available forms: Inj 20 mg/ml; caps 50 mg

SIDE EFFECTS

CNS: Headache, *fever,* peripheral neuropathy, paresthesias, confusion

CV: Hypotension, **MI, dysrhythmias**

GI: Nausea, vomiting, anorexia, **hepatotoxicity,** dyspepsia, diarrhea, constipation

GU: **Nephrotoxicity**

HEMA: **Thrombocytopenia, leukopenia, myelosuppression, anemia**

INTEG: Rash, alopecia, phlebitis at IV site, radiation recall, **Stevens-Johnson syndrome**

RESP: **Bronchospasm,** pleural effusion

SYST: **Anaphylaxis**

Contraindications: Pregnancy (D), breastfeeding, hypersensitivity, severe renal/hepatic disease

Precautions: Children, renal/hepatic disease, gout

Black Box Warning: Bone marrow depression, infection, bleeding

PHARMACOKINETICS

Half-life 7 hr, metabolized in liver, excreted in urine, crosses placental barrier

INTERACTIONS

Increase: bone marrow depression—other antineoplastics, radiation

Increase: adverse reactions—live virus vaccines

NURSING CONSIDERATIONS

Assess:

- CBC, differential, platelet count weekly; withhold product if WBC is <1000 or platelet count is <50,000; notify prescriber
- Renal studies: BUN; serum uric acid; urine CCr; electrolytes before, during therapy
- I&O ratio; report fall in urine output to <30 ml/hr; check B/P bid and report any significant decrease
- Monitor temp q4hr; may indicate beginning infection

• Hepatic studies before, during therapy (bilirubin, AST, ALT, LDH) as needed or monthly
• Bleeding: hematuria, guaiac stools, bruising or petechiae, mucosa or orifices q8hr
• Effects of alopecia on body image; discuss feelings about body changes
• Jaundice of skin and sclera, dark urine, clay-colored stools, itchy skin, abdominal pain, fever, diarrhea
• B/P q15min during infusion; if systolic reading <90 mm Hg, discontinue inf and notify prescriber
• Buccal cavity q8hr for dryness, sores or ulceration, white patches, oral pain, bleeding, dysphagia
• Local irritation, pain, burning, discoloration at inj site
⚠ Symptoms indicating severe allergic reaction: rash, pruritus, urticaria, purpuric skin lesions, itching, flushing
⚠ Symptoms of anaphylaxis: flushing, restlessness, coughing, difficulty breathing
• Frequency of stools, characteristics: cramping, acidosis; signs of dehydration: rapid respirations, poor skin turgor, decreased urine output, dry skin, restlessness, weakness

Administer:
• Antiemetic 30-60 min before giving product and prn to prevent vomiting
• Allopurinol or sodium bicarbonate to maintain uric acid levels, alkalinization of urine
• Antispasmodic, epinephrine, corticosteroids, antihistamines for reactions

IV route (VePesid)
• Using cytotoxic handling procedures
• After diluting 100 mg/250 ml or more D_5W or NaCl to 0.2-0.4 mg/ml, infuse over 30-60 min; phosphate may be given over 5 min-3½ hr; may dilute further to 0.1 mg/ml in 0.9% NaCl, D_5W

Additive compatibilities: Carboplatin, cisplatin, cytarabine, floxuridine, fluorouracil, hydrOXYzine, ifosfamide, ondansetron

Y-site compatibilities: Allopurinol, amifostine, aztreonam, cladribine, DOXOrubicin liposome, fludarabine, granisetron, melphalan, ondansetron, paclitaxel, piperacillin/tazobactam, sargramostim, sodium bicarbonate, teniposide, thiotepa, vinorelbine

Intermittent IV INF route (Etopophos)
• Reconstitute each vial with 5 or 10 ml of D_5W, 0.9% NaCl for a concentration of 20 mg/ml or 10 mg/ml, respectively; may give diluted or undiluted to concentration of as little as 0.1 mg/ml

Perform/provide:
• Liquid diet: carbonated beverages, Jell-O; dry toast or crackers may be added if patient is not nauseated or vomiting
• Increase fluid intake to 2-3 L/day to prevent urate deposits, calculi formation
• Diet low in purines: organ meats (kidney, liver), dried beans, peas to maintain alkaline urine
• Nutritious diet with iron, vitamin supplements

Evaluate:
• Therapeutic response: decreased tumor size, spread of malignancy

Teach patient/family:
• To report any complaints or side effects to nurse or prescriber
• To report any changes in breathing or coughing
• That hair may be lost during treatment; a wig or hairpiece may make patient feel better; tell patient that new hair may be different in color, texture
• That metallic taste may occur
• To report symptoms of infection
• Avoid immunizations
• Avoid crowds or persons with known infections
• Use reliable contraception; avoid breastfeeding

etravirine (℞)

(e-tra'veer-een)

Intelence

Func. class.: Antiretroviral

Chem. class.: Nonnucleoside reverse transcriptase inhibitor (NNRTI)

Action: Binds directly to reverse transcriptase blocking the RNA- and DNA-dependent DNA polymerase action causing a disruption of the enzyme's catalytic site

Uses: In combination with other antiretroviral agents for HIV infection in treatment-experienced patients with evidence of HIV replication despite ongoing antiretroviral therapy

DOSAGE AND ROUTES

• *Adult:* **PO** 200 mg bid after a meal, max 400 mg/day; not established in naïve patients

Available forms: Tabs 100 mg

SIDE EFFECTS

CNS: ***Headache, insomnia,*** amnesia, anxiety, confusion, fatigue, nightmares, peripheral neuropathy, **seizures, stroke,** tremor

CV: **Atrial fibrillation,** hypertension, MI

EENT: Blurred vision

GI: ***Nausea, vomiting, diarrhea, anorexia,*** abdominal pain, increased AST/ALT, constipation, flatulence, gastritis, GERD, **hematemesis, hepatitis,** hepatomegaly, **pancreatitis**

GU: **Renal failure**

HEMA: **Hemolytic anemia, neutropenia, thrombocytopenia, anemia**

INTEG: ***Rash,*** erythema multiforme, **angioedema, Stevens-Johnson syndrome**

OTHER: Diabetes mellitus, gynecomastia, hyperamylasemia, hypercholesterolemia, hyperglycemia, hyperlipidemia

RESP: Dyspnea, **bronchospasm**

Contraindications: Breastfeeding, hypersensitivity

Precautions: Pregnancy (B), children, geriatric patients, impaired hepatic function, antimicrobial resistance, hepatitis, hypercholesterolemia, hypertriglycerides, immune reconstitution syndrome

PHARMACOKINETICS

99.9% plasma protein binding; metabolized by CYP3A4, 2C9, 2C19; half-life 21-61 hr; excreted in feces

INTERACTIONS

• Do not use concurrently with atazanavir, carbamazepine, delavirdine, fosamprenavir, fosphenytoin, phenytoin, phenobarbital, rifapentine, rifampin, tipranavir

• Altered effect of cycloSPORINE, tacrolimus, sirolimus

Increase: myopathy, rhabdomyolysis—HMG-CoA reductase inhibitors

Increase: etravirine levels—fluconazole, itraconazole, ketoconazole, lopinavir, posaconazole, ritonavir, voriconazole

Increase: withdrawal symptoms—methadone

Increase: levels of diazepam, rifampin, voriconazole, warfarin

Decrease: levels of amiodarone, atazanavir, clarithromycin, flecainide, fosamprenavir, lidocaine, mexiletine, propafenone, quinidine, sildenafil, tadalafil, vardenafil

Decrease: etravirine levels—bepridil, darunavir, dexamethasone, disopyramide, efavirenz, nevirapine, ritonavir, saquinavir, tipranavir

Drug/Herb

Decrease: etravirine—St. John's wort

NURSING CONSIDERATIONS

Assess:

• For symptoms of HIV and for possible infections; increased temp

⚠ For fatal hypersensitivity reactions: fever, rash, nausea, vomiting, fatigue, cough, dyspnea, diarrhea, abdominal discomfort; treatment should be discontinued and not restarted

• For blood dyscrasias (anemia, granulocytopenia): bruising, fatigue, bleeding, poor healing
• Renal studies: BUN, serum uric acid, CCr before, during therapy; these may be elevated throughout treatment
• Hepatic studies before and during therapy: bilirubin, AST, ALT, amylase, alk phos, creatine phosphokinase, creatinine, q mo
• Blood counts q2wk; monitor viral load and CD4 counts during treatment; watch for decreasing granulocytes, Hgb; if low, therapy may have to be discontinued and restarted after hematologic recovery; blood transfusions may be required
• Cholesterol/lipid profile during treatment

Administer:

• Give in combination with other antiretrovirals with food

Perform/provide:

• Storage in cool environment; protect from light

Evaluate:

• Therapeutic response: increased CD4 count, decreased viral load

Teach patient/family:

• That product is not a cure but will control symptoms; patient is still infective, may pass AIDS virus to others
• To notify prescriber of sore throat, swollen lymph nodes, malaise, fever; other infections may occur; to stop product and notify prescriber immediately if skin rash, fever, cough, shortness of breath, GI symptoms; advise all health care providers that allergic reaction has occurred with etravirine
• That follow-up visits must be continued since serious toxicity may occur; blood counts must be done
• To use contraception during treatment; still able to transmit disease
• Give patient Medication Guide and Warning Card, discuss points on guide
• That other products may be necessary to prevent other infections
• To take medication following a meal

everolimus (℞)

(e-ve-ro'-li-mus)

Afinitor

Func. class.: Antineoplastic—miscellaneous

Chem. class.: Immunosuppressant, macrolide

Action: Proliferation signal inhibitor that inhibits mammalian target of rapamycin (mTOR). This pathway is dysregulated in cancer

Uses: Renal cell cancer in those with failed treatment with suritinib or sorafenib

DOSAGE AND ROUTES

• *Adult:* **PO** 10 mg daily as long as clinically beneficial; with strong 3A4 inducers 10 mg daily, then may increase by 5 mg increments to 20 mg daily

Hepatic dose

• *Adult:* **PO** (Child-Pugh B) 5 mg daily, not to be used in (Child-Pugh C)

Available forms: Tabs 5, 10 mg

SIDE EFFECTS

CNS: *Headache, insomnia, paresthesia,* chills, fever

CV: Hypertension, *CHF,* peripheral edema

EENT: Blurred vision, photophobia

GI: Nausea, vomiting, diarrhea

GU: **Renal failure**

HEMA: **Anemia, leukopenia, thrombocytopenia**

INTEG: *Rash, acne*

META: Hyperglycemia, increased creatinine, *hyperlipemia,* hyperphosphatemia, weight loss

RESP: **Pleural effusion,** *dyspnea*

Contraindications: Breastfeeding, hypersensitivity to this product, rapamine, torisel

Precautions: Pregnancy (D), children <13 yr, renal/hepatic disease; diabetes mellitus, infection, hyperlipidemia, plural effusion

PHARMACOKINETICS

Rapidly absorbed; peak 1-2 hr, protein binding 74%; extensively metabolized by CYP3A4 enzyme system, half-life 30 hr, reduced by high-fat meal

INTERACTIONS

Increase: blood levels—antifungals, calcium channel blockers, cimetidine, danazol, erythromycin, cycloSPORINE, HIV-protease inhibitors
Decrease: blood levels of everolimus—carbamazepine, phenobarbital, phenytoin, rifamycin, rifapentine
Decrease: effect of vaccines

Drug/Herb

- St. John's wort: may decrease the effect of everolimus

Drug/Food

- Alters bioavailability; use consistently with or without food; do not use with grapefruit juice

NURSING CONSIDERATIONS

Assess:

- Lipid profile: cholesterol, triglycerides, a lipid-lowering agent may be needed; blood glucose

⚠ Blood studies: Hgb, WBC, platelets during treatment q mo; if leukocytes $<3000/mm^3$ or platelets $<100,000/mm^3$, product should be discontinued or reduced; decreased hemoglobulin level may indicate bone marrow suppression

- Hepatic studies: alk phos, AST, ALT, amylase, bilirubin, and for hepatotoxicity: dark urine, jaundice, itching, light-colored stools; product should be discontinued

Administer:

- Swallow tabs whole with a full glass of water; do not chew, crush, or break
- Take at same time of day
- Follow procedure for proper handling of antineoplastics
- All medications PO if possible, avoiding IM inj; bleeding may occur
- Store protected from light, at room temperature

Evaluate:

- Therapeutic response

Teach patient/family:

- To report fever, rash, severe diarrhea, chills, sore throat, fatigue; serious infections may occur; clay-colored stools, cramping (hepatotoxicity)
- To avoid crowds, persons with known infections to reduce risk of infection
- To use contraception before, during, and 12 wk after product has been discontinued, avoid breastfeeding
- Not to use with grapefruit juice
- To avoid vaccines
- To take up to 6 hr after normally scheduled time if dose is missed
- That product may decrease male/female fertility
- That drinking alcohol is not recommended

exemestane (℞)

(ex-em′eh-stane)
Aromasin
Func. class.: Antineoplastic
Chem. class.: Aromatase inhibitor

Action: Lowers serum estradiol concentrations; many breast cancers have strong estrogen receptors
Uses: Advanced breast carcinoma not responsive to other therapy (postmenopausal)

DOSAGE AND ROUTES

- *Adult:* **PO** 25 mg/day after meals; may need 50 mg/day if taken with a potent CYP3A4 inhibitor

Available forms: Tabs 25 mg

SIDE EFFECTS

CNS: Headache, depression, insomnia, anxiety, fatigue, hot flashes
CV: Hypertension
GI: Nausea, vomiting, diarrhea, constipation, abdominal pain, increased appetite
HEMA: Lymphopenia
MS: Fracture, bone loss
RESP: Cough, *dyspnea*

Contraindications: Pregnancy (D), breastfeeding, premenopausal women, hypersensitivity
Precautions: Children, geriatric patients, renal/hepatic disease

PHARMACOKINETICS

Half-life 24 hr; excreted in feces, urine

INTERACTIONS

Decrease: exemestane action—CYP3A4 inducers, estrogens

NURSING CONSIDERATIONS

Assess:
- B/P, hypertension may occur

Administer:
- With meals at same time of day

Perform/provide:
- Liquid diet, if needed, including cola, gelatin; dry toast or crackers may be added if patient is not nauseated or vomiting
- Nutritious diet with iron, vitamin supplements as ordered

Evaluate:
- Therapeutic response: decreased tumor size, spread of malignancy

Teach patient/family:
- To report any complaints, side effects to prescriber
- That hot flashes are reversible after discontinuing treatment
- To use reliable contraception; do not breastfeed
- That vit D, calcium may be used for bone loss

exenatide (℞)

(ex-en′a-tide)
Byetta
Func. class.: Antidiabetic
Chem. class.: Incretin mimetic

Action: Binds and activates known human GLP-1 receptor, mimics natural physiology for self-regulating glycemic control

Uses: Type 2 diabetes mellitus given in combination with metformin, a sulfonylurea, or a thiazolidinedione
Unlabeled uses: Once-weekly dosing

DOSAGE AND ROUTES

- *Adult:* **SUBCUT** 5 mcg bid 1 hr before morning and evening meal; may increase to 10 mcg bid after 1 mo of therapy
- *Adult (unlabeled):* **SUBCUT** (sustained-release formulation) 2 mg q wk

Available forms: Inj 5, 10 mcg

SIDE EFFECTS

CNS: Headache, dizziness, feeling jittery, restlessness, weakness
ENDO: **Hypoglycemia**
GI: Nausea, vomiting, diarrhea, dyspepsia, anorexia, gastroesophageal reflux, weight loss
Contraindications: Hypersensitivity
Precautions: Pregnancy (C), geriatric patients, severe renal/hepatic/GI disease

PHARMACOKINETICS

Peak 2.1 hr, elimination by glomerular filtration

INTERACTIONS

- May increase the effect of acetaminophen
- Do not use with erythromycin, metoclopramide

Increase: hypoglycemia—ACE inhibitors, corticosteroids, disopyramide, sulfonylureas, anabolic steroids, androgens, fibric acid derivatives, alcohol
Increase: hyperglycemia—phenothiazines
Decrease: action of digoxin, lovastatin, acetaminophen (elixir)
Decrease: hypoglycemia—niacin, dextrothyroxine, thiazide diuretics, triamterene, estrogens, progestins, oral contraceptives, MAOIs

NURSING CONSIDERATIONS

Assess:
- Fasting blood, glucose, A1c levels, postprandial glucose during treatment to determine diabetes control

• Hypo/hyperglycemic reaction that can occur soon after meals; for severe hypoglycemia give IV $D_{50}W$, then IV dextrose solution
• For nausea/vomiting, ability to tolerate product

Administer:
• Subcutaneous only, do not give IV/IM
• Pen needles must be purchased separately, pen needles must be compatible
• Prime prior to use
• Inject into thigh, abdomen, upper arm; rotate sites
• Product 1 hr before meals; if patient is NPO, may need to hold dose to prevent hypoglycemia

Perform/provide:
• Storage in refrigerator for unopened pen; may store at room temperature after opening for up to 30 days

Evaluate:
• Therapeutic response: decrease in polyuria, polydipsia, polyphagia, clear sensorium, improving A1c, weight; absence of dizziness, stable gait

Teach patient/family:
• The symptoms of hypo/hyperglycemia, what to do about each; to have glucagon emergency kit available; to carry a glucose source (candy, sugar cube) to treat hypoglycemia
• That product must be continued on daily basis; explain consequences of discontinuing product abruptly
• That diabetes is a lifelong illness; product will not cure disease
• That all food in diet plan must be eaten to prevent hypoglycemia
• To carry emergency ID with prescriber and medications
• To continue weight control, dietary restrictions, exercise, hygiene
• That regular blood glucose monitoring and A1c testing is needed
• To notify prescriber if pregnant or intend to become pregnant
• To read "Information for the Patient" and "Pen User Manual"; provide education on self-injection

ezetimibe (℞)

(ehz-eh-tim′bee)

Zetia

Func. class.: Antilipemic; cholesterol absorption inhibitor

Action: Inhibits absorption of cholesterol by the small intestine

Uses: Hypercholesterolemia, homozygous familial hypercholesterolemia (HoFH), homozygous sitosterolemia

DOSAGE AND ROUTES

• *Adult/adolescent/child >10 yr:* **PO** 10 mg/day; may be given with HMG-CoA reductase inhibitor at same time; may be given with bile acid sequestrant; give ezetimibe 2 hr before or 4 hr after the bile acid sequestrant

Available forms: Tabs 10 mg

SIDE EFFECTS

CNS: Fatigue, dizziness, headache
GI: Diarrhea, abdominal pain
MISC: Chest pain
MS: Myalgias, arthralgias, back pain
RESP: Pharyngitis, sinusitis, cough, URI

Contraindications: Hypersensitivity, severe hepatic disease

Precautions: Pregnancy (C), breastfeeding, children, hepatic disease

PHARMACOKINETICS

Metabolized in small intestine, liver; excreted in feces 78%, urine 11%

INTERACTIONS

Increase: action of ezetimibe—fibric acid derivatives, cycloSPORINE
Decrease: action of ezetimibe—antacids, cholestyramine

Drug/Herb
Increase: effect—glucomannan
Decrease: effect—gotu kola

NURSING CONSIDERATIONS

Assess:

- Lipid levels, LFTs baseline and periodically during treatment; CPK if muscle pain is present

Administer:

- Without regard to meals

Evaluate:

- Therapeutic response: decreased cholesterol

Teach patient/family:

- That compliance is needed
- That risk factors should be decreased: high-fat diet, smoking, alcohol consumption, absence of exercise
- To notify prescriber if pregnancy is suspected or planned
- To notify prescriber if unexplained weakness or muscle pain is present

⚠ High Alert

factor VIIa, recombinant (℞)

Niastase ♣, NovoSeven, NovoSevenRT

Func. class.: Antihemophilic

Action: Promotes hemostasis by activating the intrinsic pathway of coagulation

Uses: Bleeding in hemophilia A or B, with inhibitors to factor VIII or IX , factor VII deficiency, acquired hemophilia

Unlabeled uses: Coumarin toxicity, von Willebrand's disease

DOSAGE AND ROUTES

Bleeding prophylaxis or hemophilia with inhibitors to factor VIII/IX

- *Adult:* **IV BOL** 90 mcg/kg q2hr until hemostasis occurs, or until therapy is deemed to be inadequate; posthemostatic doses q3-6hr may be required

Bleeding prophylaxis factor VII deficiency

- *Adult:* **IV BOL** 15-30 mcg/kg over 2-5 min q4-6hr

Acquired hemophilia

- *Adult/adolescent/child:* **IV BOL** 70-90 mcg/kg q2-3hr

Available forms: Lyophilized powder 1.2 mg/vial (1200 mcg/vial), 2.4 mg/vial (2400 mcg/vial), 4.8 mg/vial (4800 mcg/vial) recombinant human coagulation factor VIIa (rFVIIa); *NovoSevenRT:* 1 mg, 2, 5 mg powder for inj

SIDE EFFECTS

CNS: Fever, headache, **cerebral artery occlusion**

CV: **Ischemic heart disease, MI,** hypertension

INTEG: Pain, redness at inj site, pruritus, purpura, rash

SYST: **Hemorrhage NOS, hemarthrosis, fibrinogen plasma decreased,** hypertension, bradycardia, **DIC, coagulation disorder, thrombosis, acute renal failure**

Contraindications: Hypersensitivity to this product or mouse, hamster, or bovine products

Precautions: Pregnancy (C), breastfeeding, children, DIC, septicemia, intracranial hemorrhage

PHARMACOKINETICS

Half-life 2.3 hr

INTERACTIONS

- Do not use with activated prothrombin complex concentrates or prothrombin complex concentrate

NURSING CONSIDERATIONS

Assess:

- VS, B/P, pulse, respirations, neurologic signs, temp at least q4hr, temp 104° F (40° C) or indicators of internal bleeding, cardiac rhythm
- PT, aPTT, plasma FVII clotting, clotting inhibitor titers
- For thrombosis, dose should be reduced or stopped

Administer:

IV route (NovoSeven)

- Bring to room temperature; for 1.2 mg vial/2.2 ml sterile water for inj; 4.8 mg vial/8.5 ml sterile water for inj

- Remove caps from stop, cleanse stopper with alcohol, allow to dry, draw back plunger of sterile syringe and allow air into syringe, insert needle of syringe into sterile water for inj, inject the air and withdraw amount required, insert syringe needle with diluent into product vial, aim to side so liquid runs down vial wall, gently swirl until dissolved, use within 3 hr, give by bol over 3-5 min
- Do not admix, keep refrigerated until ready to use, avoid sunlight

IV route (NovoSevenRT)

- May be stored in refrigerator or room temperature prior to reconstitution
- Reconstitute with hisitidine diluent 1.1 ml for 1 mg vial, 2.1 ml for 2 mg vial, 5.2 ml for 5 mg vial; allow diluent to run down side of vial; gently swirl until powder is dissolved (1 mg/ml)

Evaluate:

- Therapeutic response: hemostasis

⚠ High Alert

factor IX complex (human) (℞)

Alpha-Nine SD, BeneFIX, Konyne 80, Mononine, Profilnine/Alpha Nine, Proplex SX-T, Proplex T

Func. class.: Hemostatic
Chem. class.: Factors II, VII, IX, X

Action: Causes an increase in blood levels of clotting factors II, VII, IX, X; factor IX (human) has IX activity

Uses: Hemophilia B (Christmas disease), factor IX deficiency, anticoagulant reversal, control of bleeding in patients with factor VIII inhibitors, reversal of overdose of anticoagulants in emergencies

DOSAGE AND ROUTES

Factor IX complex (human) bleeding in hemophilia B

- *Adult and child:* **IV** Establish 25% of normal factor IX or 60-75 units/kg, then 10-20 units/kg/day 1-2×/wk

Prophylaxis for bleeding in hemophilia B

- *Adult and child:* **IV** 10-20 units/kg 1-2×/wk

Bleeding in hemophilia A/inhibitors of factor VIII (Proplex T, Konyne 80)

- *Adult and child:* **IV** 75 units/kg, repeat in 12 hr

Oral anticoagulant reversal

- *Adult and child:* **IV** 15 units/kg

Factor VII deficiency (use Proplex T only)

- *Adult and child:* **IV** 0.5 units/kg × weight (kg) × desired factor IX increase (% of normal); repeat q4-6hr if needed

Factor IX (human) minor-moderate hemorrhage

Use only Alpha Nine, Alpha-Nine SD

- *Adult and child:* **IV** Dose to increase factor IX level to 20%-30% in one dose

Serious hemorrhage

- *Adult and child:* **IV** Dose to increase factor IX to 30%-50% as daily inf

Minor hemorrhage (mononine only)

- *Adult and child:* **IV** Dose to increase factor IX to 15%-25% (20-30 units/kg), repeat in 24 hr if needed

Major hemorrhage

- *Adult and child:* **IV** Dose to increase factor IX to 25%-50% (75 units/kg) q18-30hr × 10 days or less

Available forms: Inj (number of units noted on label)

SIDE EFFECTS

CNS: Headache, dizziness, malaise, paresthesia, *lethargy, chills, fever, flushing*

CV: Hypotension, tachycardia, *MI,* **venous thrombosis, pulmonary embolism**

GI: Nausea, vomiting, abdominal cramps, jaundice, **viral hepatitis**

HEMA: **Thrombosis, hemolysis, AIDS, DIC**

INTEG: Rash, flushing, *urticaria*

RESP: **Bronchospasm**

Contraindications: Hypersensitivity to mouse/hamster protein, hepatic disease,

DIC, elective surgery, mild factor IX deficiency

Precautions: Pregnancy (C), neonates/infants

PHARMACOKINETICS

IV: Half-life factor VII–3-6 hr, factor IX–24-36 hr; rapidly cleared from plasma

INTERACTIONS

- Incompatible with protein products

⚠ ***Increase:*** thrombosis risk—aminocaproic acid; do not administer

Decrease: effect of warfarin

NURSING CONSIDERATIONS

Assess:

- Blood studies (coagulation factors assays by % normal: 5% prevents spontaneous hemorrhage, 30%-50% for surgery, 80%-100% for severe hemorrhage)
- Increased B/P, pulse
- For bleeding q15-30min, immobilize and apply ice to affected joints
- I&O; if urine becomes orange or red, notify prescriber
- Allergic or pyrogenic reaction: fever, chills, rash, itching, slow inf rate if not severe

⚠ DIC: bleeding, ecchymosis, hypersensitivity, changes in coagulation tests

- For tingling sensation; if present, rate should be reduced

Administer:

- Hepatitis B vaccine before administration
- IV after warming to room temperature 3 ml/min or less, with plastic syringe only; do not admix
- After dilution with provided diluent, 50 units/ml or 25 units/ml; do not exceed 10 ml/min; decrease rate if fever, headache, flushing, tingling occur
- After crossmatch if patient has blood type A, B, AB, to determine incompatibility with factor

BeneFIX

- Allow vials of concentrate/diluent to warm to room temperature
- After removing flip top cap from vial, wipe top of vial with alcohol swab; allow to dry
- Peel back cover from vial adapter package; do not remove
- Place vial adapter over vial; press firmly until snaps; attach plunger rod to diluent syringe and break plastic tip cap from diluent syringe
- Lift the package away from the adapter and connect diluent syringe; depress plunger; swirl contents

Perform/provide:

- Storage of reconstituted sol for 3 hr at room temperature or up to 2 yr refrigeration (powder); check expiration date

Evaluate:

- Therapeutic response: prevention of hemorrhage

Teach patient/family:

- To report any signs of bleeding: gums, under skin, urine, stools, emesis
- The risk of viral hepatitis, AIDS; to be tested q2-3mo for HIV, even though risk is low
- That immunization for hepatitis B may be given first
- To carry emergency ID identifying disease; avoid salicylates, NSAIDs; inform other health professionals of condition

F

famciclovir (℞)

(fam-cy′clo-veer)

Famvir

Func. class.: Antiviral

Chem. class.: Guanosine nucleoside

Action: Inhibits DNA polymerase and viral DNA synthesis by conversion of this guanosine nucleoside to penciclovir

Uses: Treatment of acute herpes zoster (shingles), genital herpes; recurrent mucocutaneous herpes simplex virus (HSV) in HIV patients; initial episodes of herpes genitalis; herpes labialis in the immunocompromised

Unlabeled uses: Bell's palsy, herpes labialis prophylaxis, postherpetic neuralgia prophylaxis

DOSAGE AND ROUTES

Herpes zoster

• *Adult:* **PO** 500 mg q8hr for 7 days

Renal dose

• *Adult:* **PO** CCr ≥60 ml/min, 500 mg q8hr; CCr 40-59 ml/min, 500 mg q12hr; CCr 20-39 ml/min, 500 mg q24hr; CCr <20 ml/min 250 mg q24hr

Recurrent herpes simplex virus

• *Adult:* **PO** 125 mg q12hr × 5 days

Renal dose

• *Adult:* **PO** CCr <39 ml/min 125 mg q24hr × 5 days

Suppression of recurrent herpes simplex virus

• *Adult:* **PO** 250 mg q12hr up to 1 yr

Renal dose

• *Adult:* **PO** CCr 20-39 ml/min 125 mg q12hr × 5 days; CCr <20 ml/min 125 mg q24hr × 5 days

Genital herpes/herpes labialis (recurrent)

• *Adult:* **PO** 125 mg bid × 5 days or 1000 mg bid for 1 day; begin treatment at first sign of recurrence

Suppression of recurrent genital herpes

• *Adult:* **PO** 250 mg bid for up to a year

Herpes genitalis initial episodes

• *Adult:* **PO** 250 mg tid × 7-10 days

Bell's palsy (unlabeled)

• *Adult:* **PO** 750 mg tid × 7 days with predniSONE

Varicella-zoster virus (shingles); chickenpox (unlabeled)

• *Adult:* **PO** 500 mg q8hr × 7 days preferably within 48 hr of onset

Herpes zoster in HIV (unlabeled)

• *Adult:* **PO** 500 mg tid × 7-10 days

Available forms: Tabs 125, 250, 500 mg

SIDE EFFECTS

CNS: Headache, fatigue, dizziness, paresthesia, somnolence, fever

GI: Nausea, vomiting, diarrhea, constipation, abdominal pain, anorexia

GU: Decreased sperm count

INTEG: Pruritus

MS: Back pain, arthralgia

RESP: Pharyngitis, sinusitis

Contraindications: Hypersensitivity to this product, penciclovir, acyclovir, ganciclovir, valacyclovir, valganciclovir

Precautions: Pregnancy (B), breastfeeding, renal disease

PHARMACOKINETICS

Bioavailability 77%, 20% protein binding, 73% excreted via kidneys, terminal plasma half-life 2-3 hr

INTERACTIONS

Decrease: renal excretion—theophylline, probenecid, digoxin

Decrease: metabolism—cimetidine

NURSING CONSIDERATIONS

Assess:

• For number, distribution of lesions; burning, itching, pain, which are early symptoms of herpes infection; assess daily during therapy

• Renal studies: urine CCr, BUN before and during treatment if decreased renal function; dose may have to be lowered

• Bowel pattern before, during treatment; diarrhea may occur

• Posttherapeutic neuralgia during and after treatment

Administer:

• With or without meals; absorption does not appear to be lowered when taken with food

• As soon as diagnosed; in herpes zoster within 72 hr

Evaluate:

• Therapeutic response: decreased size, spread of lesions

Teach patient/family:

• How to recognize beginning infection

• How to prevent spread of infection; that this medication does not prevent the spread to others, that condoms should be used

• The reason for medication, expected results

• That women with genital herpes should have yearly Pap smears, cervical cancer is more likely

famotidine (OTC, ℞)

(fa-moe'ti-deen)

Maximum Strength Pepcid, Mylanta AR, Pepcid, Pepcid AC, Pepcid AC Acid Controller, Pepcid RPD

Func. class.: H_2-histamine receptor antagonist

Action: Competitively inhibits histamine at histamine H_2-receptor site, decreasing gastric secretion while pepsin remains at a stable level

Uses: Short-term treatment of active duodenal ulcer, maintenance therapy for duodenal ulcer, Zollinger-Ellison syndrome, multiple endocrine adenomas, gastric ulcers; gastroesophageal reflux disease, heartburn

Unlabeled uses: GI disorders in those taking NSAIDs; urticaria; prevention of stress ulcers, aspiration pneumonitis, inactivation of oral pancreatic enzymes in pancreatic disorders; paclitaxel hypersensitivity reactions

DOSAGE AND ROUTES

Active ulcer

• *Adult:* **PO** 40 mg/day at bedtime × 4-8 wk, then 20 mg/day at bedtime if needed (maintenance); **IV** 20 mg q12hr if unable to take **PO**

• *Child 1-16 yr:* **PO** 0.5 mg/kg/day at bedtime or divided bid, max 40 mg/day

Hypersecretory conditions

• *Adult:* **PO** 20 mg q6hr; may give 160 mg q6hr if needed; **IV** 20 mg q12hr if unable to take **PO**

Heartburn relief/prevention

• *Adult:* **PO** 10 mg with water or 15 min-1 hr before eating

Paclitaxel hypersensitivity reactions

• *Adult:* **IV** 20 mg ½ hr prior to infusion

Renal disease

• *Adult:* **PO** CCr <50 ml/min, decrease dose by 50% or extend interval to 36-48 hr

Available forms: Tabs 10, 20, 40 mg; gel cap 10 mg; powder for oral susp 40 mg/5 ml; inj 10 mg/ml, 20 mg/50 ml 0.9% NaCl; orally disintegrating tabs (RPD) 20, 40 mg; chew tabs 10 mg

F

SIDE EFFECTS

CNS: Headache, dizziness, paresthesia, depression, anxiety, somnolence, insomnia, fever, **seizures in renal disease**

CV: **Dysrhythmias**

EENT: Taste change, tinnitus, orbital edema

GI: Constipation, nausea, vomiting, anorexia, cramps, abnormal hepatic enzymes, diarrhea

HEMA: **Thrombocytopenia, aplastic anemia**

INTEG: Rash, **toxic epidermal necrolysis, Stevens-Johnson syndrome**

MS: Myalgia, arthralgia

RESP: **Pneumonia**

Contraindications: Hypersensitivity

Precautions: Pregnancy (B), breastfeeding, children <12 yr, geriatric patients, severe renal/hepatic disease

PHARMACOKINETICS

Plasma protein-binding 15%-20%, metabolized in liver 30% (active metabolites), 70% excreted by kidneys, half-life 2½-3½ hr

PO: Onset 30-60 min, duration 6-12 hr, peak 1-3 hr, absorption 50%

IV: Onset immediate, peak 30-60 min, duration 8-15 hr

INTERACTIONS

Decrease: absorption—ketoconazole

Decrease: famotidine absorption—antacids

NURSING CONSIDERATIONS

Assess:

• For epigastric pain, adominal pain, frank or occult blood in emesis, stools

• Blood counts during therapy; watch for

decreasing platelets; if low, therapy may have to be discontinued and restarted after hematologic recovery
• For bleeding, hematuria, hematuresis, occult blood in stools; abdominal pain
• Blood dyscrasias (thrombocytopenia): bruising, fatigue, bleeding, poor healing

Administer:
• Antacids 1 hr before or 2 hr after famotidine; may be given with foods or liquids
• After shaking oral suspension

IV, direct route
• After diluting 2 ml of product (10 mg/ml) in 0.9% NaCl to total volume of 5-10 ml; inject over 2 min to prevent hypotension

Intermittent IV INF route
• After diluting 20 mg (2 ml) of product in 100 ml of LR, 0.9% NaCl, D_5W, $D_{10}W$; run over 15-30 min

Additive compatibilities: Cefazolin, flumazenil, vancomycin

Y-site compatibilities: Acyclovir, allopurinol, amifostine, aminophylline, amphotericin, ampicillin, ampicillin/sulbactam, amrinone, amsacrine, atropine, aztreonam, bretylium, calcium gluconate, cefazolin, cefoperazone, cefotaxime, cefotetan, cefoxitin, ceftazidime, ceftizoxime, ceftriaxone, cefuroxime, cephalothin, cephapirin, chlorproMAZINE, cisatracurium, cisplatin, cladribine, cyclophosphamide, cytarabine, dexamethasone, dextran 40, digoxin, diphenhydrAMINE, DOBUTamine, DOPamine, DOXOrubicin, DOXOrubicin liposome, droperidol, enalaprilat, epinephrine, erythromycin, esmolol, filgrastim, fluconazole, fludarabine, folic acid, gentamicin, granisetron, haloperidol, heparin, hydrocortisone, hydromorphone, hydrOXYzine, imipenem/cilastatin, insulin (regular), isoproterenol, labetalol, lidocaine, lorazepam, magnesium sulfate, melphalan, meperidine, methotrexate, methylPREDNISolone, metoclopramide, mezlocillin, midazolam, morphine, nafcillin, nitroglycerin, nitroprusside, norepinephrine, ondansetron, oxacillin, paclitaxel, perphenazine, phenylephrine, phenytoin, phytonadione, piperacillin, potassium chloride/phosphate, procainamide, propofol, remifentanil, sargramostim, sodium bicarbonate, teniposide, theophylline, thiamine, thiotepa, ticarcillin, ticarcillin/clavulanate, verapamil, vinorelbine

Perform/provide:
• Storage in cool environment (oral); IV sol is stable for 48 hr at room temperature; do not use discolored sol; discard unused oral sol after 1 mo
• Increase in bulk and fluids in the diet to prevent constipation

Evaluate:
• Therapeutic response: decreased abdominal pain

Teach patient/family:
• That product must be continued for prescribed time in prescribed method to be effective; do not double dose
• To report bleeding, bruising, fatigue, malaise, since blood dyscrasias occur
• About possibility of decreased libido, reversible after discontinuing therapy
• To avoid irritating foods, alcohol, aspirin, and extreme temperature of foods that may irritate GI system
• That smoking should be avoided; diminishes effectiveness of product
• To avoid tasks requiring alertness; dizziness, drowsiness may occur

fat emulsions (℞)

Intralipid 10%, Intralipid 20%, Liposyn II 10%, Liposyn II 20%, Liposyn III 10%, Liposyn III 20%, Soyacal 20%

Func. class.: Caloric

Chem. class.: Fatty acid, long chain; nutritional supplement

Action: Needed for energy, heat production; consist of neutral triglycerides, primarily unsaturated fatty acids

Uses: Increase calorie intake, fatty acid deficiency, prevention

DOSAGE AND ROUTES

Deficiency
• *Adult and child:* **IV** 8%-10% of required calorie intake (intralipid)

Adjunct to TPN

• *Adult:* **IV** 1 ml/min over 15-30 min (10%) or 0.5 ml/min over 15-30 min (20%); may increase to 500 ml over 4-8 hr if no adverse reactions occur; max 2.5 g/kg

• *Child:* **IV** 0.1 ml/min over 10-15 min (10%) or 0.05 ml/min over 10-15 min (20%); may increase to 1 g/kg over 4 hr if no adverse reactions occur; max 4 g/kg

Prevention of deficiency

• *Adult:* **IV** 500 ml 2×/wk (10%), given 1 ml/min for 30 min, max 500 ml over 6 hr

• *Child:* **IV** 5-10 ml/kg/day (10%), given 0.1 ml/min for 30 min, max 100 ml/hr

Available forms: Inj 10% (50, 100, 200, 250, 500 ml), 20% (50, 100, 200, 250, 500 ml)

SIDE EFFECTS

CNS: Dizziness, headache, drowsiness, **focal seizures**

CV: **Shock**

GI: Nausea, vomiting, **hepatomegaly**

HEMA: **Hyperlipemia, hypercoagulation, thrombocytopenia, leukopenia, leukocytosis**

RESP: Dyspnea, **fat in lung tissue**

Contraindications: Hypersensitivity to this product or eggs, soybeans, legumes; hyperlipemia, lipid necrosis, acute pancreatitis accompanied by hyperlipemia, hyperbilirubinemia of the newborn; renal insufficiency, hepatic damage

Precautions: Pregnancy (C), premature/term newborns, severe hepatic disease, diabetes mellitus, thrombocytopenia, gastric ulcers, sepsis

PHARMACOKINETICS

Completely absorbed, distributed to intravascular space, converted to triglycerides then to free fatty acids

NURSING CONSIDERATIONS

Assess:

• Triglycerides, free fatty acid levels, platelet counts daily to prevent fat overload, thrombocytopenia

• Hepatic studies: AST, ALT, Hct, Hgb; notify prescriber if abnormal

• Nutritional status: calorie count by dietitian; monitor weight daily

Administer:

Intermittent IV INF route

• At 10% (1 ml/min); 20% (0.5 ml/min) initially × 15-30 min, may increase 10% (120 ml/hr); 20% (62.5 ml/hr) if no adverse reaction; do not give more than 500 ml on first day

• After changing IV tubing at each inf: infection may occur with old tubing

• With inf pump at prescribed rate; do not use in-line filter sized for lipid emulsion; clogging will occur

Additive compatibilities: Chloramphenicol, cimetidine, cycloSPORINE, diphenhydrAMINE, famotidine, heparin, hydrocortisone, multivitamins, nizatidine, penicillin G potassium

Y-site compatibilities: Ampicillin, cefamandole, cefazolin, cefoxitin, cephapirin, clindamycin, digoxin, DOPamine, erythromycin, furosemide, gentamicin, IL-2, isoproterenol, kanamycin, lidocaine, norepinephrine, oxacillin, penicillin G potassium, ticarcillin, tobramycin

Perform/provide:

• Do not use mixed sol if separated or oily looking

Evaluate:

• Therapeutic response: increased weight

Teach patient/family:

• The reason for use of lipids

febuxostat (℞)

(feb-ux′oh-stat)

Uloric

Func. class.: Antigout drug, antihyperuricemic

Chem. class.: Xanthene oxidase inhibitor

Action: Inhibits the enzyme xanthine oxidase, reducing uric acid synthesis, more selective for xanthine oxidase than allopurinol

Uses: Chronic gout, hyperuricemia

DOSAGE AND ROUTES

• *Adult:* **PO** 40 mg daily, may increase to 80 mg daily if uric acid levels are > 6 mg/dl after 2 wk of therapy

Available forms: Tabs 40, 80 mg

SIDE EFFECTS

CNS: Weakness, flushing

CV: **MI, atrial fibrillation, atrial flutter, AV block,** bradycardia, hyper/hypotension, palpitations, **sinus tachycardia, stroke,** angina

EENT: Retinopathy, cataracts, epistaxis

GI: Nausea, vomiting, anorexia, constipation, diarrhea, dyspepsia, hematemesis, hepatitis, hepatomegaly, weight gain/loss, cholecystitis, cholelithiasis, melena

GU: Renal failure, urinary urgency/frequency/incontinence, nephrolithiasis, hemateria

HEMA: **Thrombocytopenia, anemia, pancytopenia, leukopenia, bone marrow suppression**

INTEG: Rash

MISC: Arthralgia, gout flare

Contraindications: Hypersensitivity

Precautions: Pregnancy (C), breastfeeding, children, renal/hepatic/cardiac/neoplastic disease, stroke, MI, organ transplant, Lesch-Nyhan syndrome

PHARMACOKINETICS

Peak 1-1.5 hr; excreted in feces, urine; half-life 5-8 hr; protein binding 99.2%

INTERACTIONS

Increase: toxicity—azathioprine

Increase: xanthine nephropathy, calculi—rasburicase, antineoplastics

Increase: myelosuppression—mercaptopurine, theophylline

NURSING CONSIDERATIONS

Assess:

• Uric acid levels q2wk; uric acid levels should be 6 mg/dl or less

• CBC, AST, BUN, creatinine before starting treatment, periodically

• I&O ratio; increase fluids to 2 L/day to prevent stone formation and toxicity

• For rash, hypersensitivity reactions, discontinue

• For gout: joint pain, swelling; may use with NSAIDs for acute gouty attacks and gout flare

Administer:

PO route

• With meals to prevent GI symptoms; may crush and add to foods or fluids

• A few days before antineoplastic therapy

Evaluate:

• Therapeutic response: decreased pain in joints, decreased stone formation in kidneys, decreased uric acid levels

Teach patient/family:

• That tabs may be crushed

• To take as prescribed; if dose is missed, take as soon as remembered; do not double dose

• To increase fluid intake to 2 L/day unless contraindicated

• To avoid alcohol, caffeine; will increase uric acid levels

• To report cardiovascular events to prescriber

Rarely Used

felbamate (℞)

(fell'ba-mate)

Felbatol

Func. class.: Anticonvulsant

Uses: Partial seizures, with or without generalization in adults; partial and generalized seizures in children with Lennox-Gastaut syndrome

DOSAGE AND ROUTES

Adjunctive therapy

• *Adult and child >14 yr:* **PO** Add 1.2 g/day in 3-4 divided doses; reduce other anticonvulsants (valproic acid, phenytoin, carbamazepine and derivatives) by 20%-33% to control plasma concentrations; may increase felbamate 1.2 g/day increments q wk, up to 3.6 g/day

Monotherapy

• *Adult:* **PO** 1.2 g/day in 3-4 divided doses; titrate with close supervision; increase dose by 600-mg increments q2wk to 3.6 g/day if needed

Lennox-Gastaut syndrome adjunctive therapy

• *Child 2-14 yr:* **PO** Add 15 mg/kg/day in 3-4 divided doses; reduce other anticonvulsants (valproic acid, phenytoin, carbamazepine, and derivatives) by 20%-33% to control plasma concentrations; may increase felbamate 15 mg/kg/day q wk up to 45 mg/kg/day, max 3600 mg/day

Contraindications: Hypersensitivity to this product, other carbamates

Black Box Warning: Aplastic anemia, hepatic disease, anemia, agranulocytosis, bone marrow suppression, hematologic disease, hepatitis, leukopenia, neutropenia, thrombocytopenia

felodipine (℞)

(fe-loe′-di-peen)

Renedil ♣

Func. class.: Antihypertensive, calcium channel blocker, antianginal

Chem. class.: Dihydropyridine

Do not confuse:

Plendil/pindolol/Pletal/Prilosec/Prinivil

Action: Inhibits calcium ion influx across cell membrane, resulting in inhibition of excitation/contraction

Uses: Essential hypertension, alone or with other antihypertensives; angina pectoris; Prinzmetal's angina (vasospastic)

Unlabeled uses: Hypertension in adolescents and children

DOSAGE AND ROUTES

• *Adult:* **PO** 5 mg/day initially, usual range 2.5-10 mg/day; max 10 mg/day; do not adjust dosage at intervals of <2 wk

• *Geriatric:* **PO** 2.5 mg/day

Hepatic disease

• **PO** 2.5-5 mg, max 10 mg/day

Hypertension in adolescent/child (unlabeled)

• *Adolescent and child:* **PO** 2.5 mg initially, titrate upward, max 10 mg/day

Available forms: Ext rel tabs 2.5, 5, 10 mg

SIDE EFFECTS

CNS: Headache, fatigue, drowsiness, dizziness, anxiety, depression, nervousness, insomnia, light-headedness, paresthesia, tinnitus, psychosis, somnolence

CV: **Dysrhythmia,** edema, **CHF,** hypotension, palpitations, **MI, pulmonary edema,** tachycardia, syncope, AV block, angina

GI: Nausea, vomiting, diarrhea, gastric upset, constipation, increased LFTs, dry mouth

GU: Nocturia, polyuria

HEMA: Anemia

INTEG: Rash, pruritus

MISC: Flushing, sexual difficulties, cough, nasal congestion, shortness of breath, wheezing, epistaxis, respiratory infection, chest pain, **Stevens-Johnson syndrome,** gingival hyperplasia

Contraindications: Hypersensitivity, sick sinus syndrome, 2nd- or 3rd-degree heart block, hypotension <90 mm Hg systolic

Precautions: Pregnancy (C), breastfeeding, children, geriatric patients, CHF, hepatic injury, renal disease

PHARMACOKINETICS

Peak plasma levels 2.5-5 hr, highly protein bound, >99% metabolized in liver, 0.5% excreted unchanged in urine, elimination half-life 11-16 hr

INTERACTIONS

Increase: bradycardia, CHF—β-blockers, digoxin, phenytoin, disopyramide

Increase: toxicity—ketoconazole, erythromycin, itraconazole, propranolol

Increase: hypotension—fentanyl, nitrates, alcohol, quinidine

Decrease: antihypertensive effects—NSAIDs

Drug/Herb

Increase: toxicity, death—aconite

Increase: antihypertensive effect—barberry, betony, black catechu, black cohosh, bloodroot, broom, burdock, cat's claw, dandelion, ginseng, ginkgo, goldenseal, Irish moss, Jamaican dogwood, kelp, khella, mistletoe, parsley

Increase or decrease: antihypertensive effect—astragalus, cola tree

Decrease: antihypertensive effect—coltsfoot, guarana, khat, licorice, St. John's wort, yohimbe

Drug/Food

Increase: felodipine level—grapefruit juice

NURSING CONSIDERATIONS

Assess:

- I&O, weight daily; for CHF: weight gain, crackles, dyspnea, edema, jugular venous distention
- Renal, hepatic studies
- Cardiac status: B/P, pulse, respiration; ECG periodically
- For angina pain: location, duration, intensity; ameliorating, aggravating factors

Administer:

- Swallow whole; do not break, crush, or chew ext rel products
- Once daily without regard to meals

Evaluate:

- Therapeutic response: decreased B/P, decreased anginal attacks, increase in activity tolerance

Teach patient/family:

- To avoid hazardous activities until stabilized on product, dizziness is no longer a problem
- To avoid OTC products, alcohol, unless directed by a prescriber, to limit caffeine consumption
- The importance of complying with all areas of medical regimen: diet, exercise, stress reduction, product therapy
- That tablets may appear in stools, but are insignificant
- To report dyspnea, palpitations, irregular heart beat, swelling of extremities, nausea, vomiting, severe dizziness, severe headache
- To change positions slowly to prevent orthostatic hypotension
- To obtain correct pulse, to contact prescriber if pulse is <50 bpm
- To use protective clothing, sunscreen to prevent photosensitivity

Treatment of overdose: Atropine for AV block, vasopressor for hypotension

fenofibrate (℞)

(fen-oh-fee'brate)

Antara, Lipofen, Lofibra, Tricor, Triglide

Func. class.: Antilipemic

Chem. class.: Fibric acid derivative

Action: Increases lipolysis and elimination of triglyceride-rich particles from plasma by activating lipoprotein lipase, resulting in triglyceride change in size and composition of LDL leading to rapid breakdown of LDL; mobilizes triglycerides from tissue; increases excretion of neutral sterols

Uses: Hypercholesterolemia, types IV, V hyperlipidemia that do not respond to other treatment and are at risk for pancreatitis, Fredrickson type IIa, IIb, hypertriglyceridemia

Unlabeled uses: Polymetabolic syndrome X

DOSAGE AND ROUTES

Hypertriglyceridemia

- *Adult:* **PO** (Antara) 43-130 mg/day; (Lofibra) 67-200 mg/day; (Tricor) 48-145 mg/day; (Triglide) 50-160 mg/day

Primary hypercholesterolemia/ mixed hyperlipidemia

- *Adult:* **PO** (Antara) 130 mg/day; (Lofibra) 200 mg/day; (Tricor) 145 mg/day; (Triglide) 160 mg/day

Renal dose (geriatric)

- *Adult:* **PO** (Tricor) CCr 30-80 ml/min 48 mg/day; CCr <30 ml/min, contraindicated
- *Adult:* **PO** CCr 11-49 ml/min 50 mg/ day (Triglide, Liprofen), 43 mg/day (An-

tara), 67 mg/day (Lofibra); CCr <10 ml/min contraindicated (Antara, Lipofen, Lofibra, Triglide)

Available forms: Tabs (Triglide) 50, 160 mg; (Tricor) 48, 145 mg; micronized cap (Antara) 45, 87, 130 mg; (Lofibra) 67, 134, 200 mg; cap (Lipofen) 50, 150 mg

SIDE EFFECTS

CNS: Fatigue, weakness, drowsiness, dizziness, insomnia, depression, vertigo
CV: Angina, **dysrhythmias,** hypertension
GI: *Nausea,* vomiting, dyspepsia, increased liver enzymes, flatulence, hepatomegaly, gastritis
GU: Dysuria, proteinuria, oliguria, urinary frequency
HEMA: Anemia, leukopenia, ecchymosis, **thrombosis/pulmonary embolism**
INTEG: *Rash,* urticaria, pruritus
MISC: Polyphagia, weight gain
MS: *Myalgias, arthralgias,* myopathy
RESP: Pharyngitis, bronchitis, cough

Contraindications: Hypertensivity, severe renal/hepatic disease, primary biliary cirrhosis, preexisting gallbladder disease

Precautions: Pregnancy (C), breastfeeding, geriatric patients, peptic ulcer, pancreatitis, renal/hepatic disease

PHARMACOKINETICS

Peak 6-8 hr, protein binding 99%, converted to fenofibric acid, metabolized in liver, excreted in urine (60%), half-life 20 hr

INTERACTIONS

• Nephrotoxicity: cycloSPORINE
• Avoid use with HMG-CoA reductase inhibitors, rhabdomyolysis may occur

Increase: anticoagulant effects—oral anticoagulants

Decrease: absorption of fenofibrate—bile acid sequestrants

Drug/Herb

Increase: effect—glucomannan

Decrease: effect—gotu kola

Drug/Food

Increase: absorption

NURSING CONSIDERATIONS

Assess:

• Lipid levels, LFTs baseline and periodically during treatment, CPK if muscle pain occurs, CBC, Hct, Hgb; PT with anticoagulant therapy
• Pancreatitis, cholelithiasis renal failure, rhabdomyolyis (when combined with HMG Co-A reductase inhibitors), myositis, product should be discontinued

Administer:

• Product with meals; may increase q4-8wk

Evaluate:

• Therapeutic response: decreased triglycerides

Teach patient/family:

• That compliance is needed
• That risk factors should be decreased: high-fat diet, smoking, alcohol consumption, absence of exercise
• To notify prescriber if pregnancy is suspected or planned
• To report GU symptoms: decreased libido, impotence, dysuria, proteinuria, oliguria, hematuria
• To notify prescriber of muscle pain, weakness, fever, fatigue; epigastric pain

fenofibric acid (℞)

(fen′oh-fye′brick)

TriLipix, Fibricor

Func. class.: Antilipemic

Chem. class.: Fibric acid derivative

Action: An active metabolite of fenofibrate; increases lipolysis and elimination of triglyceride-rich particles from plasma by activating lipoprotein lipase, resulting in triglyceride change in size and composition of LDL leading to rapid breakdown of LDL; mobilizes triglycerides from tissue; increases excretion of neutral sterols

Uses: Hyperlipoproteinemia, hypertriglyceridemia

DOSAGE AND ROUTES

Combination with HMG-COA reductase inhibitors to reduce triglycerides and increase HDL-C in those with mixed dyslipidemia or coronary heart disease

• *Adult:* del rel cap **PO** 135 mg daily

Severe hypertriglyceridemia

• *Adult:* del rel cap **PO** 45-135 daily; tabs 35-105 mg daily

Available forms: Tabs, 35, 105 mg; caps, gastro-resistant pellet 45, 135 mg

SIDE EFFECTS

CNS: Fatigue, weakness, drowsiness, dizziness, insomnia, depression, vertigo, asthenia, headache

CV: Hypertension

EENT: Blurred vision

GI: *Nausea,* vomiting, dyspepsia, increased liver enzymes, abdominal pain, cholecystitis, cholelithiasis, constipation, diarrhea, hepatitis, jaundice, pancreatitis

GU: Impotence, decreased libido

HEMA: Anemia, leukopenia, **thrombosis/pulmonary embolism,** agranulocytosis, eosinophilia

INTEG: *Rash,* urticaria, pruritus, **Stevens-Johnson syndrome**

MISC: Infection

MS: *Myalgias, arthralgias,* myopathy, back pain, ms pain

RESP: Pharyngitis, cough

Contraindications: Breastfeeding, hypertensivity, severe renal/hepatic disease, primary biliary cirrhosis, preexisting gallbladder disease

Precautions: Pregnancy (C), geriatric patients, pancreatitis, thromboembolic disease

PHARMACOKINETICS

Peak (del rel cap) 4-5 hr, tabs 2.5 hr, protein binding 99%, converted to fenofibric acid, metabolized in liver, excreted in urine (60%), halflife 20 hr

INTERACTIONS

• Nephrotoxicity: cycloSPORINE

• Monitor use with HMG-CoA reductase inhibitors, rhabdomyolysis may occur

Increase: anticoagulant effects—oral anticoagulants

Decrease: absorption of fenofibrate—bile acid sequestrants

Drug/Herb

Increase: effect—glucomannan

Decrease: effect—gotu kola

Drug/Food

Increase: absorption

NURSING CONSIDERATIONS

Assess:

• Lipid levels, LFTs baseline and periodically during treatment, CBC with differential, CPK, serum bilirubin (direct/indirect)

• Pancreatitis, cholelithiasis renal failure, rhabdomyolyis (when combined with HMG-COA reductase inhibitors), myositis, product should be discontinued

Administer:

• Product with meals; may increase q4-8wk

Evaluate:

• Therapeutic response: decreased triglycerides

Teach patient/family:

• That compliance is needed

• That risk factors should be decreased: high-fat diet, smoking, alcohol consumption, absence of exercise

• To notify prescriber if pregnancy is suspected or planned

• To report GU symptoms: decreased libido, impotence

• To notify prescriber of muscle pain, weakness, fever, fatigue; epigastric pain

fenoldopam (℞)

(feh-nahl′doh-pam)

Corlopam

Func. class.: Antihypertensive, vasodilator

Action: Agonist at D_1-like DOPamine receptors; binds to α_2-adrenoceptors; increases renal blood flow

Uses: Hypertensive crisis, malignant hypertension

Unlabeled uses: Prevention of contrast agent–associated nephrotoxicity

DOSAGE AND ROUTES

- *Adult:* **IV** 0.1-1.6 mcg/kg/min
- *Child:* **CONT IV** 0.2 mcg/kg/min with effects within 5 min; may increase dose to 0.3-0.5 mcg/kg/min q20-30min depending on response

Available forms: Inj conc 10 mg/ml in single-use ampules; inj 10 mg/ml

SIDE EFFECTS

CNS: Headache, anxiety, dizziness, insomnia
CV: **Hypotension,** ST-T-wave changes, angina pectoris, tachycardia, palpitations, **MI, ischemic heart disease, flushing**
GI: Nausea, vomiting, constipation, diarrhea
HEMA: **Leukocytosis,** bleeding
INTEG: Sweating
META: Increased BUN, glucose, LDH, creatinine, hypokalemia

Contraindications: Hypersensitivity, sulfite sensitivity

Precautions: Pregnancy (B), breastfeeding, children, tachycardia, intraocular pressure, hypokalemia

PHARMACOKINETICS

Adult: Onset 5 min, duration 15-30 min, elimination half-life 5 min, steady state 20 min, crosses placenta, conjugated in the liver

Child 1 mo-12 yr: Elimination half-life 3-5 min

INTERACTIONS

Increase: hypotension—avoid use with β-blockers

Drug/Herb

Increase: toxicity, death—aconite

Increase: antihypertensive effect—barberry, betony, black catechu, black cohosh, bloodroot, broom, burdock, cat's claw, dandelion, goldenseal, Irish moss, Jamaican dogwood, kelp, khella, mistletoe, parsley

Increase or decrease: antihypertensive effect—astragalus, cola tree

Decrease: antihypertensive effect—coltsfoot, guarana, khat, licorice

NURSING CONSIDERATIONS

Assess:

- B/P, HR q5min until stabilized, then q1hr × 2 hr, then q4hr, pulse, jugular venous distention q4hr ECG; expect tachycardia (dose-dependent)
- Electrolytes, blood studies: K, Na, C1, CO_2, CBC, serum glucose
- IV site for extravasation

Administer:

- To patient in recumbent position; keep in that position for 1 hr after administration

Adult

- After diluting contents of ampules in 0.9% NaCl, or 5% dextrose inj (40 mcg/ml); then add 4 ml of conc (40 mg of product/1000 ml); 2 ml of conc (20 mg of product/500 ml); 1 ml of conc (10 mg of product/250 ml); do not admix

Child

- Use inf pump
- After dilution 3 ml (30 mg)/500 ml (60 mcg/ml); 1.5 ml (15 mg)/250 ml (60 mcg/ml); 0.6 ml (6 mg)/100 ml (60 mcg/ml)

Perform/provide:

- Diluted sol is stable in normal light/temperature for 24 hr

Evaluate:

- Therapeutic response: decreased B/P

Teach patient/family:

- To report dyspnea, chest pain, bleeding, pain at inj site
- Reason for medication and expected results

F

⚠ High Alert

fentanyl (℞)

(fen'ta-nill)

Actig, Fentanyl, Fentora, Onsolis, Sublimaze

fentanyl transdermal (℞)

Duragesic

Func. class.: Opioid analgesic

Chem. class.: Synthetic phenylpiperidine

Controlled Substance Schedule II

Do not confuse:

fentanyl/Sufenta

Action: Inhibits ascending pain pathways in CNS, increases pain threshold, alters pain perception by binding to opiate receptors

Uses: Controls moderate to severe pain; preoperatively, postoperatively; adjunct to general anesthetic, adjunct to regional anesthesia; *Fentanyl:* anesthesia as premedication, conscious sedation; *Actiq:* breakthrough cancer pain

DOSAGE AND ROUTES

Fentanyl

Anesthetic

- *Adult:* **IV** 25-100 mcg (0.7-2 mcg/kg) q2-3min prn

Anesthesia supplement

- *Adult and child >12 yr:* **IM/IV** 2-20 mcg/kg **IV INF** 0.025-0.25 mcg/kg/min

Induction and maintenance

- *Adult:* **IV BOL** 5-40 mcg/kg
- *Child 2-12 yr:* **IV** 2-3 mcg/kg

Preoperatively

- *Adult and child >12 yr:* **IM/IV** 0.05-0.1 mg q30-60min before surgery

Postoperatively

- *Adult and child >12 yr:* **IM/IV** 0.05-0.1 mg q1-2hr prn

Sedation/analgesia

- *Adult and child >12 yr:* **IV** 0.5-1 mcg/kg/dose; may repeat after 30-60 min
- *Child 1-12 yr:* **IV BOL** 1-2 mcg/kg/dose; may repeat after 30-60 min intervals; **CONT IV** 1-5 mcg/kg/hr after IV bol dose
- *Neonate:* **IV BOL** 0.5-3 mcg/kg/dose; **CONT IV** 0.5-2 mcg/kg/hr after IV bol

Actiq

- *Adult:* **TRANSMUCOSAL** 200 mcg, redose if needed 15 min after completion of 1st dose, do not give more than 2 doses during titration period

Fentora

- *Adult:* **BUCCAL** 100 mcg placed above rear molar between upper cheek and gum

Onsolis

- *Adult:* **TRANSMUCOSAL** 200 mcg, titrate, max 1200 mcg/dose or 4 doses/day

Fentanyl transdermal

- *Adult:* 25 mcg/hr; may increase until pain relief occurs; apply patch to flat surface on upper torso and wear for 72 hr; apply new patch on different site for continued relief

Available forms: Inj 0.05 mg/ml; lozenges 100, 200, 300, 400 mcg; lozenges on a stick 200, 400, 600, 800, 1200, 1600 mcg; buccal tab 100, 200, 400, 600, 800 mcg; oral dissolving film (Onsolis) 120, 200, 400, 600, 800 mcg; *transdermal:* patch 12, 25, 50, 75, 100 mcg/hr

SIDE EFFECTS

CNS: Dizziness, delirium, euphoria, sedation

CV: **Bradycardia, arrest,** hypo/hypertension

EENT: Blurred vision, miosis

GI: Nausea, vomiting, constipation

GU: Urinary retention

INTEG: Rash, diaphoresis

MS: Muscle rigidity

RESP: **Respiratory depression, arrest, laryngospasm**

Contraindications: Hypersensitivity to opiates, myasthenia gravis

Precautions: Pregnancy (C), breastfeeding, geriatric patients, increased intracranial pressure, seizure disorders, severe respiratory disorders, cardiac dysrhythmias

Black Box Warning: Children, accidental exposure, ambient temperature increase, fever, opioid-naive patients, skin abrasion (TD patch), substance abuse, respiratory depression

PHARMACOKINETICS

Metabolized by liver, excreted by kidneys, crosses placenta, excreted in breast milk, half-life 1½-6 hr, 80% bound to plasma proteins

IM: Onset 7-8 min, peak 30 min, duration 1-2 hr

IV: Onset 1 min, peak 3-5 min, duration ½-1 hr

INTERACTIONS

Increase: fentanyl effect with other CNS depressants—alcohol, opioids, sedative/hypnotics, antipsychotics, skeletal muscle relaxants

Decrease: fentanyl effect—CYP3A4 inducers (carbamazepine, phenytoin, phenobarbital, rifampin)

Drug/Herb

Increase: anticholinergic effect—corkwood

Increase: action—Jamaican dogwood, gotu kola, kava, lavender, mistletoe, nettle, pokeweed, poppy, senega, St. John's wort, valerian

Drug/Lab Test

Increase: amylase, lipase

NURSING CONSIDERATIONS

Assess:

- VS after parenteral route; note muscle rigidity, drug history, hepatic and renal function tests
- CNS changes: dizziness, drowsiness, hallucinations, euphoria, LOC, pupil reaction
- Allergic reactions: rash, urticaria
- Respiratory dysfunction: respiratory depression, character, rate, rhythm; notify prescriber if respirations are <10/min

Administer:

- By inj (IM, IV); give slowly to prevent rigidity
- Must have emergency equipment available, opioid antagonists, O_2; to be used by only those trained; (IV) products to be used in OR, ER, ICU

Transmucosal route

- Remove foil just before administration; instruct patient to place between cheek and lower gum, moving it back and forth and suck, not chew (Actiq); place above rear molar (Fentora); place film on the inside of the cheek (Onsolis); all products not used or partially used should be flushed down the toilet

Transdermal route

- q72hr for continuous pain relief; dosage is adjusted after at least two applications, apply to clean, dry skin, press firmly
- Give short-acting analgesics until patch takes effect (8-24 hr); when reducing dosage or switching to alternative IV treatment, withdraw gradually; serum levels drop gradually, give ½ the equianalgesic dose of new analgesic 12-18 hr after removal as ordered

IV route

- IV undiluted by anesthesiologist or diluted with 5 ml or more sterile H_2O or 0.9% NaCl given through Y-tube or 3-way stopcock at 0.1 mg or less/1-2 min

Additive compatibilities: Bupivacaine, caffeine citrate, clonidine, droperidol, epinephrine, ketamine, lidocaine, ziconotide

Solution compatibilities: D_5W, 0.9% NaCl

Syringe compatibilities: Alprostadil, atracurium, atropine, bupivacaine/ketamine, butorphanol, chlorproMAZINE, cimetidine, clonidine/lidocaine, diphenhyDRINATE, diphenhydrAMINE, droperidol, heparin, hydromorphone, hydrOXYzine, meperidine, metoclopramide, midazolam, morphine, pentazocine, perphenazine, prochlorperazine, promazine, promethazine, ranitidine, scopolamine

Y-site compatibilities: Amphotericin B cholesteryl, atracurium, cisatracurium, diltiazem, DOBUTamine, DOPamine, enalaprilat, epinephrine, esmolol, etomidate, furosemide, heparin, hydrocortisone, hydromorphone, labetalol, lorazepam, midazolam, milrinone, morphine, nafcillin, niCARdipine, nitroglycerin, norepinephrine, pancuronium, potassium chloride, propofol, ranitidine, remifentanil, sargramostim, thiopental, vecuronium, vit B/C

Perform/provide:

- Storage in light-resistant area at room temperature

Evaluate:

- Therapeutic response: induction of anesthesia, relief of breakthrough cancer pain, pain relief
- Cancer pain, general pain relief

Teach patient/family:

- Coughing, turning, deep breathing for postoperative patients
- Safety measures: side rails, night-light, call bell within reach
- CNS changes: physical dependence; not to use with alcohol, other CNS depressants

Transdermal route

- That excessive heat may increase absorption
- That excessive perspiration may alter adhesiveness
- To dispose of patch by placing sticky sides together and flushing in toilet
- That patient may need to clip hair before applying to ensure adhesion

ferrous fumarate (℞)

Femiron, Feostat, Feostat Drops, Hemocyte, Ircon, Nephro-Fer, Novofumar ✦, Palafer ✦, Span-FF

ferrous gluconate (℞)

Fergon, Fertinic ✦, Novoferrogluc ✦

ferrous sulfate (℞)

Apo-Ferrous Sulfate ✦, ED-IN-SOL, Feosol, Fer-gen-sol, Fer-Iron Drops, Fero-Grad, Mol-Iron

ferrous sulfate, dried (℞)

Fe^{50}, Feosol, Feratab, Novoferrosulfa ✦, PMS-Ferrous Sulfate, Slow Fe

ferric gluconate complex (℞)

Ferrlecit

carbonyl iron (OTC)

(kar′bo-nil)

Feosol

iron polysaccharide (OTC)

Hytinic, Niferex, Nu-Iron, Nu-Iron 150

Func. class.: Hematinic

Chem. class.: Iron preparation

Action: Replaces iron stores needed for red blood cell development, energy and O_2 transport, utilization; fumarate contains 33% elemental iron; gluconate, 12%; sulfate, 20%; iron, 30%; ferrous sulfate exsiccated

Uses: Iron deficiency anemia, prophylaxis for iron deficiency in pregnancy, nutritional supplementation

DOSAGE AND ROUTES

Fumarate

- *Adult:* **PO** 50-100 mg tid
- *Child:* **PO** 3 mg/kg/day (elemental iron) tid-qid

• *Infant:* **PO** 10-25 mg/day (elemental iron) in 3-4 divided doses, max 15 mg/day

Gluconate

• *Adult:* **PO** 200-600 mg daily-tid

• *Child 6-12 yr:* **PO** 300-900 mg/day

• *Child <6 yr:* **PO** 100-300 mg/day

Sulfate

• *Adult:* **PO** 0.75-1.5 g/day in divided doses tid

• *Child 6-12 yr:* **PO** 600 mg/day in divided doses

Pregnancy

• *Adult:* **PO** 300-600 mg/day in divided doses

Complex

• *Adult:* **IV INF** (125 mg) 10 ml/100 ml of NaCl for inj given over 1 hr

Iron polysaccharide

• *Adult:* **PO** 100-200 mg tid

• *Child:* **PO** 4-6 mg/kg/day in 3 divided doses

Available forms: *Fumarate:* tabs 63, 195, 200, 324, 325 mg; chewable tabs 100 mg; cont rel tabs 300 mg; oral susp 100 mg/5 ml, 45 mg/0.6 ml; *gluconate:* tabs 300, 320, 325 mg; caps 86, 325, 435 mg; film-coated tabs 300 mg; elix 300 mg/5 ml; *sulfate:* tabs 195, 300, 325 mg; enteric-coated tabs 325 mg; ext rel tabs, time-rel caps, 525 mg; *dried:* tabs 200 mg; ext rel tabs 160 mg; ext rel caps 160 mg; *complex:* inj 62.5 mg/5 ml (12.5 mg/ml); *iron polysaccharide:* tabs 50 mg; caps 150 mg; sol 100 mg/5 ml

SIDE EFFECTS

GI: Nausea, constipation, epigastric pain, black and red tarry stools, vomiting, diarrhea

INTEG: Temporarily discolored tooth enamel and eyes

SYST: **Hypersensitivity reactions (Ferrlecit)**

Contraindications: Hypersensitivity, ulcerative colitis/regional enteritis, hemosiderosis/hemochromatosis, peptic ulcer disease, hemolytic anemia, cirrhosis

Precautions: Pregnancy (B) (ferric gluconate complex), (C) (iron dextran, oral products), anemia (long term)

Black Box Warning: Accidental exposure

PHARMACOKINETICS

PO: Excreted in feces, urine, skin, breast milk; enters bloodstream; bound to transferrin; crosses placenta

F

INTERACTIONS

Increase: action of iron preparation—ascorbic acid, chloramphenicol

Decrease: absorption of penicillamine, levodopa, methyldopa, fluoroquinolones, L-thyroxine, tetracycline

Decrease: absorption of iron preparations—antacids, H_2-antagonists, proton pump inhibitors, cholestyramine, vit E

Drug/Herb

• Forms insoluble complex: black catechu

Increase: iron effect—anise

Decrease: iron absorption—allspice, bilberry, condurango, elderberry, eyebright (PO), gentian, ground ivy, hawthorn, horse chestnut, lady mantle, lemon balm, marshmallow, meadowsweet, mistletoe, motherwort, nettle, oak bark, plantain, poplar, prickly ash, raspberry, sage, tea made with artichoke, valerian

Drug/Food

Decrease: absorption—dairy products, caffeine, eggs

Drug/Lab Test

False positive: occult blood

NURSING CONSIDERATIONS

Assess:

• Blood studies: Hct, Hgb, reticulocytes, bilirubin before treatment, at least monthly; iron studies (Fe, TIBC, ferritin)

⚠ Toxicity: nausea, vomiting, diarrhea (green, then tarry stools), hematemesis, pallor, cyanosis, shock, coma

• Elimination; if constipation occurs, increase water, bulk, activity

• Nutrition: amount of iron in diet (meat, dark green leafy vegetables, dried beans, dried fruits, eggs)
• Cause of iron loss or anemia, including salicylates, sulfonamides, antimalarials, quinidine

Administer:

• Swallow tabs whole; not to break, crush, or chew unless labeled as chewable
• Between meals for best absorption; may give with juice; do not give with antacids or milk, delay at least 1 hr; if GI symptoms occur, give after meals even if absorption is decreased; eggs, milk products, chocolate, caffeine interfere with absorption
• Liquid through plastic straw to avoid discoloration of tooth enamel; dilute thoroughly
• At least 1 hr before bedtime, since corrosion may occur in stomach; ferrous gluconate is less GI irritating than ferrous sulfate
• For <6 mo for anemia

Perform/provide:

• Storage in tight, light-resistant container

Evaluate:

• Therapeutic response: improvement in Hct, Hgb, reticulocytes; decreased fatigue, weakness

Teach patient/family:

• That iron will change stools black or dark green
• That iron poisoning may occur if increased beyond recommended level
• To keep out of reach of children
• Not to substitute one iron salt for another; elemental iron content differs (e.g., 300 mg ferrous fumarate contains about 100 mg elemental iron; 300 mg ferrous gluconate contains only about 30 mg elemental iron)
• To avoid reclining position for 15-30 min after taking product to avoid esophageal corrosion
• To follow diet high in iron; to avoid taking iron, dairy products, calcium supplements and vit C together, they compete for absorption

Treatment of overdose: Induce vomiting; give eggs, milk until lavage can be done

ferumoxytol (℞)

(fer'ue-mox'i-tol)
Feraheme
Func. class.: Hematinic

Action: Iron is carried by transferrin to the bone marrow, where it is incorporated into hemoglobin

Uses: Iron deficiency anemia in chronic kidney disease

Unlabeled uses: MRI

DOSAGE AND ROUTES

• *Adult:* **IV** 510 mg of elemental iron followed by a second dose 3-8 days later; if giving during dialysis, give after B/P is stable and after 1 hr of hemodialysis

Available forms: 510 mg/17 ml solution for inj

SIDE EFFECTS

CNS: Headache, dizziness
CV: Chest pain, hyper/hypotension, hypervolemia, edema
GI: Nausea, vomiting, abdominal pain, constipation, diarrhea
INTEG: Rash, pruritus, urticaria, fever
MS: Back pain
OTHER: **Anaphylaxis**
RESP: Dyspnea, cough

Contraindications: Hypersensitivity, hemochrometosis

Precautions: Pregnancy (B), breastfeeding, children, geriatric patients, all anemias excluding iron deficiency anemia, iron overload, dialysis, hepatic disease, hypotension, MRI, siderblastic anemia, thalassemia

PHARMACOKINETICS

Half-life 15 hr

INTERACTIONS

Increase: toxicity—oral iron; do not use

NURSING CONSIDERATIONS

Assess:

- Blood studies: Hct, Hgb, reticulocytes, transferrin, plasma iron concentrations, ferritin, total iron-binding, bilirubin before treatment, at least monthly
- Allergy: anaphylaxis, rash, pruritus, fever, wheezing; notify prescriber immediately, keep emergency equipment available
- Cardiac status: hyper/hypotension, hypervolemia
- Toxicity: nausea, vomiting, diarrhea, fever, abdominal pain (early symptoms), cyanotic-looking lips, nailbeds, seizures, CV collapse (late symptoms)

Administer:

- Only with epinephrine, Solu-medrol available in case of anaphylactic reaction during dose

IV route

- Give directly in dialysis line by slow inj or inf; give by slow inj at 1 ml/min (5 min/vial); inf dilute each vial exclusively in a maximum of 100 ml of 0.9% NaCl, give at rate of 100 mg of iron/15 min, discard unused portions

Perform/provide:

- Storage at room temperature in cool environment, do not freeze

Evaluate:

- Therapeutic response: increased serum iron levels, Hct, Hgb

Teach patient/family:

- To report itching, rash, chest pain, headache, vertigo, nausea, vomiting, abdominal pain, joint/muscle pain, numbness, tingling
- That iron poisoning may occur if increased beyond recommended level; not to take oral iron preparation
- May alter MRI studies

Treatment of overdose: Discontinue product, treat allergic reaction, give diphenhydrAMINE or epinephrine as needed, give iron-chelating product in acute poisoning

fesoterodine (℞)

(fess′oh-ter-oh-deen)

Toviaz

Func. class.: Overactive bladder product

Chem. class.: Muscarinic receptor antagonist

Action: Relaxes smooth muscles in urinary tract by inhibiting acetylcholine at postganglionic sites

Uses: Overactive bladder (urinary frequency, urgency), urinary incontinence

F

DOSAGE AND ROUTES

- *Adult and geriatric:* **PO EXT REL** 4 mg/day, may increase to 8 mg/day based on response, max 4 mg/day in those taking potent CYP3A4 inhibitors

Renal dose

- *Adult:* **PO EXT REL** Max 4 mg/day in severe renal impairment

Available forms: Ext rel tabs 4, 8 mg

SIDE EFFECTS

CV: Chest pain, angina, QT prolongation

EENT: Xerophthalmia

GI: Nausea, vomiting, abdominal pain, constipation, dry mouth

GU: Dysuria, urinary retention

INTEG: Rash

MISC: Peripheral edema

MS: Back pain

RESP: Cough

SYST: Infection

Contraindications: GI obstruction, ileus, pyloric stenosis, urinary retention, gastric retention, hypersensitivity

Precautions: Pregnancy (C), breastfeeding, children, renal/hepatic disease, closed-angle glaucoma, urinary tract obstruction, ambient temperature increase, autonomic neuropathy, constipation, contact lenses, hazardous activity, GERD, gastroparesis, myasthenia gravis, prostatic hypertrophy, toxic megacolon, ulcerative colitis

PHARMACOKINETICS

Rapidly absorbed, protein binding 50%, excreted in urine/feces, half-life 7 hr

INTERACTIONS

Increase: action of fesoterodine—antiretroviral protease inhibitors, macrolide antiinfectives, azole antifungals

Increase: anticholinergic effect—antimuscarinics, anticholinergics

Increase: urinary frequency—diuretics

Drug/Herb

Decrease: fesoterodine—caffeine, green tea, guarana

Drug/Food

Increase: fesoterodine level—grapefruit juice

Decrease: fesoterodine level—cola, coffee, tea

Drug/Lab Test

Increase: LFTs

NURSING CONSIDERATIONS

Assess:

- Urinary patterns: distention, nocturia, frequency, urgency, incontinence
- Allergic reactions: rash; if this occurs, product should be discontinued

Administer:

- Do not break, crush, or chew ext rel product
- Give without regard to meals

Perform/provide:

- Storage at room temperature; protect from moisture

Evaluate:

- Therapeutic response: absence of urinary frequency, urgency, incontinence

Teach patient/family:

- Not to drink liquids before bedtime
- The importance of bladder maintenance

fexofenadine (℞)

(fex-oh-fi′na-deen)

Allegra

Func. class.: Antihistamine—2nd generation

Chem. class.: Piperidine, peripherally selective

Do not confuse:

Allegra/Viagra

Action: Acts on blood vessels, GI, respiratory system by competing with histamine for H_1-receptor site; decreases allergic response by blocking pharmacologic effects of histamine, less sedating

Uses: Rhinitis, allergy symptoms, chronic idiopathic urticaria

DOSAGE AND ROUTES

- *Adult and child >12 yr:* **PO** 60 mg bid or 180 mg/day
- *Child 6-11 yr:* **PO** 30 mg bid; **ORALLY DISINTEGRATING TAB** 30 mg bid dissolved on tongue

Renal dose

- *Adult and child ≥12 yr:* **PO** CCr <80 ml/min 60 mg/day

Available forms: Tabs 30, 60, 180 mg; caps 60 mg; oral suspension 6 mg/ml, orally disintegrating tab 30 mg

SIDE EFFECTS

CNS: Headache, stimulation, drowsiness, sedation, fatigue, confusion, blurred vision, tinnitus, restlessness, tremors, paradoxical excitation in children or geriatric patients

CV: Hypotension, palpitations, bradycardia, tachycardia, **dysrhythmias** (rare)

GI: Nausea, diarrhea, abdominal pain, vomiting, constipation

GU: Frequency, dysuria, urinary retention, impotence

HEMA: **Hemolytic anemia, thrombocytopenia, leukopenia, agranulocytosis, pancytopenia**

INTEG: Rash, eczema, photosensitivity, urticaria

RESP: Thickening of bronchial secretions, dry nose, throat

Contraindications: Breastfeeding, newborn or premature infants, hypersensitivity, severe hepatic disease

Precautions: Pregnancy (C), children, geriatric patients, respiratory disease, closed-angle glaucoma, prostatic hypertrophy, bladder neck obstruction, asthma

PHARMACOKINETICS

Well absorbed; onset 1 hr; peak 2-3 hr; duration 12-24 hr; 80% excreted in urine; half-life 14.5 hr, increased in renal disease

INTERACTIONS

Decrease: effect—magnesium-aluminum-containing antacids

Drug/Herb

Increase: anticholinergic effect—corkwood, henbane leaf

Increase: sedation—hops, Jamaican dogwood, khat, senega, St. John's wort

Drug/Food

Decrease: absorption of product—apple, orange, grapefruit, pomegranate juice

Drug/Lab Test

False negative: skin allergy tests

NURSING CONSIDERATIONS

Assess:

- Allergy: itchy, runny, watery eyes; congested nose; before and during treatment
- I&O ratio: be alert for urinary retention, frequency, dysuria, especially geriatric patients; product should be discontinued if these occur
- Respiratory status: rate, rhythm, increase in bronchial secretions, wheezing, chest tightness

Administer:

- With food or milk to decrease GI symptoms; caps/tabs should not be given with juice
- Orally disintegrating tab: allow to dissolve, swallow

Perform/provide:

- Storage in tight, light-resistant container

Evaluate:

- Therapeutic response: absence of running or congested nose or rashes

Teach patient/family:

- All aspects of product use; to notify prescriber if confusion, sedation, hypotension occur
- To avoid driving, other hazardous activity if drowsiness occurs
- To avoid alcohol, other CNS depressants
- Not to exceed recommended dose; dysrhythmias may occur

Treatment of overdose: Lavage, diazepam, vasopressors, IV phenytoin

F

Rarely Used

fibrinogen, concentrate, human (℞)

(fi-brin-o-gen)

RiaSTAP

Func. class.: Hemostatic, orphan

Uses: Hemorrage, afibrinogen, hypofibrinogenemia

DOSAGES AND ROUTES

When fibrinogen concentrate is not known

- *Adult/adolescent/child:* **IV** 70 mg/kg, max 5 ml/min, maintain fibrinogen level of 100 mg/dl until hemostasis is obtained

When fibrinogen is known

- *Adult/adolescent/child:* **IV** individualized

Contraindications: Hypersensitivity

filgrastim (℞)

(fill-grass'stim)

G-CSF, granulocyte colony stimulator, Neupogen

Func. class.: Biologic modifier

Chem. class.: Granulocyte colony-stimulating factor

Action: Stimulates proliferation and differentiation of neutrophils

Uses: To decrease infection in patients receiving antineoplastics that are myelosuppressive; to increase WBC in patients with product-induced neutropenia; bone marrow transplantation

Unlabeled uses: Neutropenia in HIV infection, aplastic anemia, ganciclovir-induced neutropenia, zidovudine-induced neutropenia

DOSAGE AND ROUTES

After myelosuppressive chemotherapy

• *Adult and child:* **IV/SUBCUT** 5 mcg/kg/day in a single dose × 14 days; may increase by 5 mcg/kg in each cycle

After bone marrow transplantation

• *Adult:* **IV/SUBCUT** 10 mcg/kg/day as an **INF (IV)** over 4 hr or 24 hr, begin 24 hr after chemotherapy and 24 hr after bone marrow transplantation

Peripheral blood progenitor cell collection/therapy

• *Adult:* 10 mcg/kg/day as a bolus or **CONT INF** × 4 days or more before leukapheresis, continue to last leukapheresis; may alter dose if WBC >100,000 cells/mm^3

Severe neutropenia (chronic), idiopathic/cyclical

• *Adult:* **SUBCUT** 5 mcg/kg daily

Available forms: Inj 300 mcg/ml, 480 mcg/1.6 ml, 480 mcg/0.8 ml, 3000 mcg/0.5 ml

SIDE EFFECTS

CNS: Fever, headache

GI: *Nausea,* vomiting, diarrhea, mucositis, anorexia

HEMA: **Thrombocytopenia,** excessive leukocytosis

INTEG: Alopecia, exacerbation of skin conditions, urticaria, cutaneous vasculitis

MS: Osteoporosis, skeletal pain

OTHER: Chest pain, hypotension

RESP: **Acute respiratory distress syndrome,** wheezing, **alveolar hemorrhage**

Contraindications: Hypersensitivity to proteins of *Escherichia coli*

Precautions: Pregnancy (C), breastfeeding, cardiac conditions, children, myeloid malignancies, radiation therapy, sepsis, sickle cell disease, chemotherapy, respiratory disease

PHARMACOKINETICS

SUBCUT: Onset 5-60 min, peak 2-8 hr, duration up to a week

IV: Onset 5-60 min, peak 24 hr, duration up to a week

INTERACTIONS

Increase: adverse reactions—do not use this product concomitantly with antineoplastics, lithium

Drug/Lab Test

Increase: uric acid, LDH, alk phos

NURSING CONSIDERATIONS

Assess:

• Blood studies: CBC, platelet count before treatment and twice weekly; neutrophil counts may be increased for 2 days after therapy

• B/P, respirations, pulse before and during therapy

• Bone pain, give mild analgesics

• CBC with differential platelets

Administer:

• Using single-use vials; after dose is withdrawn, do not reenter vial

• No earlier than 24 hr after antineoplastics, bone marrow infusion

• Do not shake; may warm to room temperature before using; discard any product left out for >24 hr

• For 2 wk or until ANC is 10,000/mm^3 after the expected chemotherapy neutrophil nadir

SUBCUT route

• May divide into 2 inj if amount to be given is >1 ml

IV route

• Dilute in D_5W to a conc of 5-15 mcg/ml, vial is for one-time use; give over 15-30 min (chemotherapy); over 4-24 hr (bone marrow transplantation); do not use 0.9% NaCl to dilute product

Y-site compatibilities: Acyclovir, allopurinol, amikacin, aminophylline, ampicillin, ampicillin/sulbactam, aztreonam, bleomycin, bumetanide, buprenorphine, butorphanol, calcium gluconate, carboplatin, carmustine, cefazolin, cefotetan, ceftazidime, chlorproMAZINE, cimetidine, cisplatin, cyclophosphamide, cytarabine, dacarbazine, DAUNOrubicin, dexamethasone, diphenhydrAMINE, DOXOrubicin, doxycycline, droperidol, enalaprilat, famotidine, floxuridine, fluconazole, fludarabine, gallium, ganciclovir, granisetron, haloperidol, hydrocortisone, hydromorphone, hydrOXYzine, idarubicin, ifosfamide, leucovorin, lorazepam, mechlorethamine, melphalan, meperidine, mesna, methotrexate, metoclopramide, miconazole, minocycline, mitoxantrone, morphine, nalbuphine, netilmicin, ondansetron, plicamycin, potassium chloride, promethazine, ranitidine, sodium bicarbonate, streptozocin, ticarcillin, ticarcillin/clavulanate, tobramycin, trimethoprim-sulfamethoxazole, vancomycin, vinBLAStine, vinCRIStine, vinorelbine, zidovudine

Perform/provide:

• Storage in refrigerator; do not freeze; may store at room temperature up to 24 hr

Evaluate:

• Therapeutic response: absence of infection

Teach patient/family:

• The technique for self-administration: dose, side effects, disposal of containers and needles; provide instruction sheet

finasteride (℞)

(fin-ass′te-ride)

Propecia, Proscar

Func. class.: Hormone, androgen inhibitor, hair stimulant

Chem. class.: 5-α-Reductase inhibitor

Do not confuse:

finasteride/furosemide

Proscar/ProSom/Prozac

Action: Inhibits 5-α-reductase and reduction in DHT; DHT induces androgenic effects by binding to androgen receptors in the cell nuclei of the prostate gland, liver, skin; prevents development of BHP

Uses: Symptomatic benign prostatic hyperplasia (Proscar); male-pattern baldness (Propecia)

Unlabeled uses: Hirsutism, prostate cancer prophylaxis

F

DOSAGE AND ROUTES

BPH

• *Adult:* **PO** 5 mg/day × 6-12 mo

Male pattern baldness

• *Adult:* **PO** 1 mg/day for 3 mo or more for results

Hirsutism (unlabeled)

• *Adult (non-pregnant):* **PO** 5 mg/day alone or in combination with oral contraceptives

Prostate cancer prophylaxis (unlabeled)

• *Adult (male):* **PO** 5 mg/day

Available forms: Tabs (Propecia) 1 mg, (Proscar) 5 mg

SIDE EFFECTS

GU: Impotence, decreased libido, decreased volume of ejaculate

INTEG: Rash

MISC: Breast tenderness

Contraindications: Pregnancy (X), breastfeeding, children, women who are pregnant or may become pregnant should not handle tabs, hypersensitivity

Precautions: Large residual urinary volume, severely diminished urinary flow, hepatic function abnormalities

PHARMACOKINETICS

Bioavailability 63%; readily absorbed from GI tract; plasma protein binding 90%; metabolized in the liver; excreted in urine (metabolites) 39%, feces (57%); crosses blood-brain barrier; peak 1-2 hr; duration 24 hr

INTERACTIONS

Decrease: finasteride effect—theophylline, adrenergic bronchodilators, anticholinergics

Drug/Lab Test

Decrease: PSA levels (finasteride)

NURSING CONSIDERATIONS

Assess:

- BPH: urinary patterns, residual urinary volume, severely diminished urinary flow
- PSA levels and digital rectal exam prior to initiating therapy and periodically thereafter
- Hepatic studies prior to treatment; extensively metabolized in liver

Administer:

- Without regard to meals
- For a minimum of 6 mo; not all patients will respond

Perform/provide:

- Storage <86° F (30° C); protect from light; keep container tightly closed

Evaluate:

- Therapeutic response: increased urinary flow; decreased postvoiding dribbling, frequency, nocturia or hair growth within 3-6 mo; regression of prostate size

Teach patient/family:

⚠ Pregnant women or women who may become pregnant should not touch crushed tabs or come into contact with semen of a patient taking this product; may adversely affect developing male fetus

- That volume of ejaculate may be decreased during treatment; impotence and decreased libido may also occur
- Propecia results may not occur for 3 mo
- Proscar results may not occur for 6-12 mo

flavocoxid (℞)

(flav-uh-kox′id)

Limbrel

Func. class.: Analgesic, nonopioid

Chem. class.: Flavanoid

Action: Exhibits antiinflammatory, analgesic properties, thought to be due to inhibition of prostaglandin synthesis via inhibition of cyclooxygenase

Uses: For dietary management of osteoarthritis

DOSAGE AND ROUTES

- *Adult:* **PO** 250-500 mg q12hr

Available forms: Cap 250 mg

SIDE EFFECTS

MISC: Hypertension, increase in varicose veins, psoriasis

MS: Fluid accumulation in the knees

Contraindications: Hypersensitivity

Precautions: Pregnancy (UK), breastfeeding, children <18 yr, history of stomach ulcers, angina, CAD, edema, geriatric patients, GI disease, rheumatoid arthritis, stroke, tachycardia/MI

PHARMACOKINETICS

Metabolism primarily via glucuronidation and sulfation

NURSING CONSIDERATIONS

Assess:

- For pain of rheumatoid arthritis, osteoarthritis; check ROM, inflammation of joints, characteristics of pain

Administer:

- 1 hr before or after meals, food increases absorption

Evaluate:

- Therapeutic response: decreased pain, inflammation in arthritic conditions

Teach patient/family:

- That product does not take the place of other products, including corticosteroids for osteoarthritis
- To notify prescriber if pregnancy is planned or suspected

Rarely Used

flavoxate (℞)

(fla-vox′ate)

Func. class.: Spasmolytic

Uses: Relief of nocturia, incontinence, suprapubic pain, dysuria, frequency associated with urologic conditions (symptomatic only)

DOSAGE AND ROUTES

• *Adult and child >12 yr:* **PO** 100-200 mg tid-qid

Contraindications: Hypersensitivity, GI obstruction, GI hemorrhage, GU obstruction, achalasia, ileus

flecainide (℞)

(flek-ay′nide)

Tambocor

Func. class.: Antidysrhythmic (Class IC)

Action: Decreases conduction in all parts of the heart, with greatest effect on His-Purkinje system, which stabilizes cardiac membrane

Uses: Life-threatening ventricular dysrhythmias, sustained ventricular tachycardia, supraventricular tachydysrhythmias, paroxysmal atrial fibrillation/flutter associated with disabling symptoms

Unlabeled uses: Atrial fibrillation, single dose

DOSAGE AND ROUTES

PSVTT/PAF

• *Adult:* **PO** 50 mg q12hr; may increase q4days by 50 mg q12hr to desired response, max 300 mg/day

Life-threatening ventricular dysrhythmias

• *Adult:* **PO** 100 mg q12hr; may increase by 50 mg q12hr q4days, max 400 mg/day

Renal dose

• *Adult:* **PO** CCr <35 ml/min 100 mg daily or 50 mg bid, initially

Available forms: Tabs 50, 100, 150 mg

SIDE EFFECTS

CNS: Headache, dizziness, involuntary movement, confusion, psychosis, restlessness, irritability, paresthesias, ataxia, flushing, somnolence, depression, anxiety, malaise, fatigue, asthenia, tremors

CV: Hypotension, bradycardia, angina, PVCs, **heart block, cardiovascular collapse, arrest,** dysrhythmias, **CHF, fatal ventricular tachycardia**

EENT: Tinnitus, *blurred vision,* hearing loss, corneal deposits, dry eyes

GI: Nausea, vomiting, anorexia, constipation, abdominal pain, flatulence, change in taste, diarrhea

GU: Impotence, decreased libido, polyuria, urinary retention

HEMA: **Leukopenia, thrombocytopenia**

INTEG: Rash, urticaria, edema, swelling

RESP: Dyspnea, **respiratory depression**

Contraindications: Hypersensitivity, severe heart block, cardiogenic shock, nonsustained ventricular dysrhythmias, frequent PVCs, non–life-threatening dysrhythmias

Precautions: Pregnancy (C), breastfeeding, children, geriatric patients, renal/hepatic disease, CHF, respiratory depression, myasthenia gravis, electrolyte abnormalities

Black Box Warning: MI, cardiac arrhythmias

PHARMACOKINETICS

Peak 3 hr, half-life 12-27 hr, metabolized by liver, excreted unchanged by kidneys (10%), excreted in breast milk

INTERACTIONS

Increase: of both products—propranolol

Increase: CV depressant action—β-blockers, disopyramide, verapamil

Increase: flecainide level—amiodarone, cimetidine, ritonavir
Increase: digoxin level—digoxin
Increase or decrease: effect—urinary, alkalinizing agents, acidifying agents
Drug/Herb
Increase: toxicity, death—aconite
Increase: effect—aloe, broom, chronic buckthorn use, cascara sagrada (chronic use), Chinese rhubarb, figwort, fumitory, goldenseal, kudzu, licorice
Increase: serotonin effect—horehound
Decrease: effect—coltsfoot
Drug/Lab Test
Increase: CPK

NURSING CONSIDERATIONS

Assess:
- I&O, daily weight

⚠ CHF: edema, weight gain, dyspnea, jugular vein distention, crackles
- For hypokalemia, hyperkalemia before administration; correct electrolytes
- Blood levels: trough (0.2-1 mcg/ml)
- B/P, ECG or Holter monitor continuously for fluctuations; watch for QRS widening, prolongation of QT and PR
- CNS effects: dizziness, confusion, psychosis, paresthesias, seizures; product should be discontinued
- Increased respiration, increased pulse; product should be discontinued

Administer:
- Reduced dosage as soon as dysrhythmia is controlled
- May give with meals for GI upset
- May adjust dose q4days

Evaluate:
- Therapeutic response: decreased dysrhythmias

Teach patient/family:
- To change position slowly from lying or sitting to standing to minimize orthostatic hypotension
- To take as prescribed, not to skip or double dose
- To avoid hazardous activities that require alertness until response is known
- To carry emergency ID with disorder, medications taken
- To notify all health care providers of treatment
- To report new or worsening cardiac symptoms

Treatment of overdose: O_2, artificial ventilation, ECG, DOPamine for circulatory depression, diazepam or thiopental for seizures, treat ventricular dysrhythmias

Rarely Used

floxuridine (℞)

(flox-yoor′i-deen)
FUDR
Func. class.: Antineoplastic, antimetabolite

Uses: Hepatocellular; colorectal cancer metastatic to liver

DOSAGE AND ROUTES

- *Adult:* **INTRAARTERIAL** by cont inf 0.1-0.6 mg/kg/day × 1-6 wk; **HEPATIC ARTERY INJ** 0.4-0.6 mg/kg/day × 1-6 wk

Contraindications: Pregnancy (D), breastfeeding; hypersensitivity, poor nutritional status, serious infections

Black Box Warning: Myelosuppression, GI bleeding

fluconazole (℞)

(floo-kon′a-zole)
Diflucan
Func. class.: Antifungal, systemic
Chem class: Triazole derivative

Do not confuse:
Diflucan/Diprivan
Action: Inhibits ergosterol biosynthesis, causes direct damage to fungal membrane phospholipids
Uses: Oropharyngeal candidiasis, chronic mucocutaneous candidiasis, systemic, vaginal, urinary candidiasis, cryptococcal meningitis, prevention of candidiasis in bone marrow transplant in those who receive chemotherapy and/or radiation therapy

Unlabeled uses: Prophylaxis, systemic candidiasis in very-low-birthweight premature infants

DOSAGE AND ROUTES

Vaginal candidiasis
- *Adult:* **PO** 150 mg as a single dose

Serious fungal infections
- *Adult:* **PO/IV** 50-400 mg initially, then 200 mg/day for 4 wk
- *Child:* 6-12 mg/kg/day

Oropharyngeal candidiasis
- *Adult:* **PO/IV** 200 mg initially, then 100 mg/day for at least 2 wk
- *Child:* **PO/IV** 6 mg/kg initially, then 3 mg/kg/day for ≥2 wk

Prevention of candidiasis in bone marrow transplant
- *Adult:* **PO/IV** 400 mg/day

Renal disease
- *Adult:* **PO/IV** CCr ≤50 ml/min, after loading dose, give 50% of usual dose

Available forms: Tabs 50, 100, 150, 200 mg; inj 2 mg/ml; powder for oral susp 50, 200 mg/ml

SIDE EFFECTS

CNS: Headache

GI: Nausea, vomiting, diarrhea, cramping, flatus, increased AST, ALT, **hepatotoxicity**

INTEG: **Stevens-Johnson syndrome**

Contraindications: Hypersensitivity to this product or azoles

Precautions: Pregnancy (C), breastfeeding, renal/hepatic disease

PHARMACOKINETICS

Peak 2-4 hr, bioavailability (PO) >90%, excreted unchanged in urine 80%, metabolized by CYP3A enzyme system at dose >200 mg/day

INTERACTIONS

Increase: hypoglycemia—oral antidiabetics

Increase: anticoagulation—warfarin

Increase: plasma concentrations—cycloSPORINE, phenytoin, theophylline, rifabutin, tacrolimus

Increase: effect of zidovudine

Decrease: effect of oral contraceptives

Drug/Herb

Increase: nephrotoxicity—gossypol

NURSING CONSIDERATIONS

Assess:
- For infection: clearing of CSF and other culture during treatment, obtain C&S baseline and throughout, product may be started as soon as culture is taken

⚠ For hepatotoxicity: increasing AST, ALT, periodically alk phos, bilirubin

Administer:

PO route
- Shake oral susp before each use

IV route
- After diluting according to package directions; run at 200 mg/hr or less; do not use plastic containers in connections; check for bag leaks
- Using an inf pump check for extravasation and necrosis q2hr
- Do not use if cloudy or precipitated
- Do not admix; do not refrigerate

Y-site compatibilities: Acyclovir, aldesleukin, allopurinol, amifostine, amikacin, aminophylline, ampicillin/sulbactam, aztreonam, benztropine, cefazolin, cefepime, cefotetan, cefoxitin, chlorproMAZINE, cimetidine, cisatracurium, dexamethasone, diphenhydrAMINE, DOBUTamine, DOPamine, DOXOrubicin liposome, droperidol, famotidine, filgrastim, fludarabine, foscarnet, gallium, ganciclovir, gentamicin, granisetron, heparin, hydrocortisone, immune globulin, leucovorin, lorazepam, melphalan, meperidine, meropenem, metoclopramide, metronidazole, midazolam, morphine, nafcillin, nitroglycerin, ondansetron, oxacillin, paclitaxel, pancuronium, penicillin G potassium, phenytoin, piperacillin/tazobactam, prochlorperazine, promethazine, propofol, ranitidine, remifentanil, sargramostim, tacrolimus, teniposide, theophylline, thiotepa, ticarcillin/clavulanate, tobramycin, vancomycin, vecuronium, vinorelbine, zidovudine

Perform/provide:

- Storage protected from moisture and light, diluted sol is stable 24 hr, do not freeze

Evaluate:

- Therapeutic response: decreasing oral candidiasis, fever, malaise, rash; negative C&S for infection organism

Teach patient/family:

- That long-term therapy may be needed to clear infection
- That medication may be taken with food to reduce GI effects
- To notify prescriber of nausea, vomiting, diarrhea, jaundice, anorexia, clay-colored stools, dark urine
- Use alternative method of contraception while taking this product

Rarely Used

fludarabine (℞)

(floo-dar′a-been)

Fludara, Oforta

Func. class.: Antineoplastic, antimetabolite

Uses: Chronic lymphocytic leukemia, non-Hodgkin's lymphoma

DOSAGE AND ROUTES

- *Adult:* **IV** 25 mg/m^2 over 30 min/day × 5 days, may repeat q28days; reconstitute with 2 ml of sterile water for inj; dissolution should occur in <15 sec, adjust dose based on toxicity

Contraindications: Pregnancy (D), breastfeeding, hypersensitivity

Black Box Warning: Hemolytic anemia, bone marrow suppression, coma, seizures, visual disturbances

fludrocortisone (℞)

(floo-droe-kor′ti-sone)

Func. class.: Corticosteroid, synthetic

Chem. class.: Mineralocorticoid

Action: Promotes increased reabsorption of sodium and loss of potassium, water, hydrogen from distal renal tubules

Uses: Adrenal insufficiency, salt-losing adrenogenital syndrome, Addison's disease

Unlabeled uses: Renal tubular acidosis (type IV), idiopathic orthostatic hypotension

DOSAGE AND ROUTES

- *Adult:* **PO** 100-200 mcg/day
- *Child:* **PO** 50-100 mcg/day

Idiopathic hypotension (unlabeled)

- *Adult:* **PO** 50-100 mcg/day

Available forms: Tabs 100 mcg (0.1 mg)

SIDE EFFECTS

CNS: Flushing, sweating, headache, paralysis, dizziness, **seizures**

CV: Hypertension, **circulatory collapse, thrombophlebitis, embolism,** tachycardia, **CHF,** *edema*

ENDO: Weight gain, adrenal suppression, hyperglycemia

META: Hypokalemia

MISC: Hypersensitivity, cataracts, GI ulcers, **anaphylaxis**

MS: Fractures, osteoporosis, weakness

Contraindications: Children <2 yr, hypersensitivity, acute glomerulonephritis, amebiasis, psychoses, Cushing's syndrome, fungal infections

Precautions: Pregnancy (C), breastfeeding, children >2 yr, osteoporosis, CHF, hypertension, diabetes

PHARMACOKINETICS

Peak 1.5 hr, half-life 18-36 hr, metabolized by liver, excreted in urine

INTERACTIONS

Increase: B/P—sodium-containing food or medication
Decrease: fludrocortisone action—barbiturates, rifampin, phenytoin
Decrease: potassium levels—thiazides, potassium-wasting products, loop diuretics, amphotericin B, piperacillin, mezlocillin

Drug/Herb

Increase: hypokalemia—aloe, buckthorn, cascara sagrada, Chinese rhubarb, senna
Increase: corticosteroid effect—aloe, licorice, perilla

Drug/Lab Test

Increase: potassium, sodium
Decrease: Hct

NURSING CONSIDERATIONS

Assess:

- Weight daily; notify prescriber of weekly gain >5 lb
- I&O ratio; be alert for decreasing urinary output, increasing edema
- B/P q4hr, pulse; notify prescriber if chest pain occurs
- Potassium depletion: paresthesias, fatigue, nausea, vomiting, depression, polyuria, dysrhythmias, weakness
- Electrolytes: sodium, potassium, chloride, hypokalemia is common

Administer:

- Titrated dose; use lowest effective dose
- With food or milk to decrease GI symptoms

Perform/provide:

- Assistance with ambulation in patient with bone tissue disease to prevent fractures

Evaluate:

- Therapeutic response: correction of adrenal insufficiency

Teach patient/family:

- That emergency ID as steroid user should be carried
- Not to discontinue this medication abruptly
- To notify health care provider of muscle cramps, weight gain, edema, nausea, infection, trauma, stress
- Not to breastfeed while taking this medication
- Avoid exposure to disease, trauma

flumazenil (℞)

(flu-maz′e-nill)
Anexate ✦, Romazicon
Func. class.: Antidote: Benzodiazepine receptor antagonist
Chem. class.: Imidazobenzodiazepine derivative

Action: Antagonizes actions of benzodiazepines on CNS, competitively inhibits activity at benzodiazepine recognition site on GABA/benzodiazepine receptor complex

Uses: Reversal of sedative effects of benzodiazepines

DOSAGE AND ROUTES

Reversal of conscious sedation or in general anesthesia

- *Adult:* **IV** 0.2 mg given over 15 sec; wait 45 sec, then give 0.2 mg if consciousness does not occur; may be repeated at 60-sec intervals prn (max 3 mg/hr) or 1 mg/5 min
- *Child:* **IV** 10 mcg (0.01 mg)/kg; cumulative dose of 1 mg or less

Management of suspected benzodiazepine overdose

- *Adult:* **IV** 0.2 mg given over 30 sec; wait 30 sec, then give 0.3 mg over 30 sec if consciousness does not occur; further doses of 0.5 mg can be given over 30 sec at intervals of 1 min up to cumulative dose of 3 mg
- *Child:* **IV** 10 mcg (0.01 mg/kg), cumulative dose of <1 mg

Available forms: Inj 0.1 mg/ml

SIDE EFFECTS

CNS: Dizziness, agitation, emotional lability, confusion, **seizures**, somnolence, panic attacks

CV: Hypertension, palpitations, cutaneous vasodilation, **dysrhythmias,** bradycardia, tachycardia, chest pain
EENT: Abnormal vision, blurred vision, tinnitus
GI: Nausea, vomiting, hiccups
SYST: Headache, inj site pain, increased sweating, fatigue, rigors

Contraindications: Hypersensitivity to this product or benzodiazepines, serious cyclic antidepressant overdose, patients given benzodiazepine for control of life-threatening condition

Precautions: Pregnancy (C), breastfeeding, children, geriatric patients, status epilepticus, head injury, labor/delivery, renal/hepatic disease, hypoventilation, panic disorder, drug and alcohol dependency, ambulatory patients

Black Box Warning: Benzodiazepine dependence, seizures

PHARMACOKINETICS

Terminal half-life 41-79 min, metabolized in liver, onset 1-2 min

INTERACTIONS

- Toxicity: mixed product overdosage
- Antagonize action of benzodiazepines, zaleplon, zolpidem

NURSING CONSIDERATIONS

Assess:

- Cardiac status using continuous monitoring
- For seizures; protect patient from injury; most likely those that have withdrawals from sedatives
- GI symptoms: nausea, vomiting; place in side-lying position to prevent aspiration
- Allergic reactions: flushing, rash, urticaria, pruritus

Administer:

- Check airway and IV access before administration
- Using large vein

IV, direct route

- Give undiluted or diluted with 0.9% NaCl, D_5W, LR, give over 15 sec into running IV
- Stable for 24 hr if drawn into a syringe or mixed with other solutions

Additive compatibilities: Aminophylline, cimetidine, DOBUTamine, DOPamine, famotidine, heparin, lidocaine, procainamide, ranitidine

Solution compatibilities: D_5W

Evaluate:

- Therapeutic response: decreased sedation, respiratory depression, toxicity

Teach patient/family:

- That amnesia may continue
- Not to engage in hazardous activities for 18-24 hr after discharge
- Not to take any alcohol or nonprescription products for 18-24 hr

flunisolide nasal agent

See Appendix B

fluocinolone ophthalmic

See Appendix B

fluocinolone topical

See Appendix B

fluoride (PO) (℞)

(floor′ide)

Fluor-A-Day ♣, Fluoride Loz, Fluoritab, Flura-Loz, Karidium, Luride, Pediaflor, Pharmaflur, Phos-Flur, Solu-Flur ♣

fluoride (Topical) (℞)

ACT, Fluorigard, Fluorinse, Gel Kam, Gel-Tin, Karigel, MouthKote, Stop, Thera-Flur

Func. class.: Trace elements

Chem. class.: Fluoride ion

Action: Needed for hard tooth enamel and for resistance to periodontal disease; reduces acid production by dental bacteria

Uses: Prevention of dental caries, osteoporosis

DOSAGE AND ROUTES

Prevention of dental caries

• *Adult and child >12 yr:* **TOP** 10 ml 0.2% sol/day after brushing teeth, rinse mouth for >1 min with sol

• *Child 6-12 yr:* **TOP** 5 ml 0.2% sol

• *Child 4-8 yr:* 1.1 mg/day

• *Child 1-3 yr:* 0.7 mg/day

Mild-moderate osteoporosis

• *Adult:* **PO** Slow rel fluoride 25 mg, given as calcium citrate 400 mg bid

Available forms: Chew tabs 0.5, 1 mg; tabs 1 mg, effervescent tabs 10 mg; drops 0.125, 0.25, 0.5 mg/drop; rinse supplements 0.2 mg/ml, rinse 0.01%, 0.02%, 0.04%, 0.09%; gel 0.1%, 0.5%; lozenges 1 mg; sol 0.2 mg/ml; honey-wax, slow rel sodium fluoride tab

SIDE EFFECTS

ACUTE OVERDOSE: **Black tarry stools, bloody vomit, diarrhea, decreased respiration, increased salivation, watery eyes**

CHRONIC OVERDOSE: **Hypocalcemia and tetany, respiratory arrest, sores in mouth, constipation, loss of appetite, nausea, vomiting, weight loss, discoloration of teeth** (white, black, brown)

Contraindications: Pregnancy (UK), hypersensitivity to this product or tartrazine

Precautions: Children <6 yr

PHARMACOKINETICS

PO: Excreted in urine and feces; crosses placenta, breast milk

INTERACTIONS

• Avoid use with calcium products

Drug/Food

• Avoid use with dairy products

NURSING CONSIDERATIONS

Assess:

• For mottling of teeth during treatment

Administer:

• Drops after meals with fluids or undiluted tabs; may be chewed; do not swallow whole; may be given with water or juice; avoid milk

Evaluate:

• Therapeutic response: absence of dental caries

Teach patient/family:

• To monitor children using gel or rinse; not to be swallowed

• Not to drink, eat, or rinse mouth for at least ½ hr

• Not to use during pregnancy

• To apply after brushing and flossing at bedtime

• To store out of children's reach

fluorometholone ophthalmic

See Appendix B

⚠ High Alert

fluorouracil (℞)

(flure-oh-yoor′a-sil)

Adrucil, Carac, Efudex, Fluoroplex, 5-FU

Func. class.: Antineoplastic, antimetabolite

Chem. class.: Pyrimidine analog

Do not confuse:
fluorouracil/flucytosine

Action: Inhibits DNA, RNA synthesis; interferes with cell replication by competitively inhibiting thymidylate production, S phase of cell cycle–specific, a vesicant

Uses: *Systemic:* cancer of breast, colon, rectum, stomach, pancreas; *topical:* multiple actinic keratoses, superficial basal cell carcinomas

DOSAGE AND ROUTES

Doses vary widely.

Advanced colorectal cancer

• *Adult:* **IV** 370 mg/m^2 given after leucovorin or 425 mg/m^2 given after leucovorin daily × 5 days; repeat q4-5wk

Other cancer

• *Adult:* **IV** 12 mg/kg/day × 4 days, not to exceed 800 mg/day; may repeat with 6 mg/kg on days 6, 8, 10, 12; maintenance is 10-15 mg/kg/wk as a single dose, not to exceed 1 g/wk

Actinic/solar keratoses

• *Adult:* **TOP** 1% cream/sol 1-2×/day or 2-5% sol for hands

Superficial basal cell carcinoma

• *Adult:* **TOP** 5% sol or cream 2×/day × 3-12 wk

Available forms: Inj 50 mg/ml; cream 1%, 5%; sol 1%, 2%, 5%

SIDE EFFECTS

Systemic use

CNS: Lethargy, malaise, weakness, acute cerebellar dysfunction

CV: Myocardial ischemia, angina

EENT: Epistaxis, light intolerance, lacrimation

GI: Anorexia, stomatitis, diarrhea, nausea, vomiting, **hemorrhage,** enteritis glossitis

HEMA: **Thrombocytopenia, leukopenia, myelosuppression, anemia, agranulocytosis**

INTEG: Rash, fever, photosensitivity

Contraindications: Pregnancy (X), breastfeeding, hypersensitivity, poor nutritional status, serious infections, major surgery within 1 month

Black Box Warning: Myelosuppression

Precautions: Children, renal/hepatic disease, angina

Black Box Warning: GI bleeding

PHARMACOKINETICS

Half-life 20 hr terminal; metabolized in the liver; excreted in the urine; crosses blood-brain barrier

INTERACTIONS

Increase: toxicity, bone marrow depression—radiation or other antineoplastics

Decrease: antibody response—live virus vaccines

Drug/Lab Test

Increase: AST, ALT, LDH, serum bilirubin, Hct, Hgb, WBC, platelets, 5-HIAA

Decrease: albumin

NURSING CONSIDERATIONS

Assess:

• CBC, differential, platelet count daily (IV); withhold product if WBC is <3500/mm^3 or platelet count is <100,000/mm^3; notify prescriber of these results; product should be discontinued; nadir of leukopenia within 2 wk, recovery 1 mo

• Renal studies: BUN, serum uric acid, urine CCr, electrolytes before, during therapy

• Hepatic studies before, during therapy: bilirubin, alk phos, AST, ALT, LDH; before and during therapy

• Bleeding: hematuria, guaiac, bruising or petechiae, mucosa or orifices q8hr

• Inflammation of mucosa, breaks in skin; buccal cavity q8hr for dryness, sores or ulceration, white patches, oral pain, bleeding, dysphagia
• GI symptoms: frequency of stools, cramping, intractable vomiting, stomatitis

Administer:

• Antiemetic 30-60 min before giving product to prevent vomiting and for several days thereafter

Topical route

• Wear gloves when applying; may use with a loose dressing; use a plastic or wooden applicator

IV route

• Prepared in biologic cabinet using gloves, gown, mask; use cytoxic handling procedures
• Undiluted; may inject through Y-tube or 3-way stopcock; give over 1-3 min; may be diluted in NS, D_5W, given over 2-8 hr as IV INF

Additive compatibilities: Bleomycin, cephalothin, cyclophosphamide, etoposide, floxuridine, hydromorphone, ifosfamide, methotrexate, mitoxantrone, prednisoLONE, vinCRIStine

Solution compatibilities: Amino acids 4.25%/D_{25}, D_5/LR, $D_{3.3}$/0.3 NaCl, D_5W, 0.9% NaCl, TPN #23

Syringe compatibilities: Bleomycin, cisplatin, cyclophosphamide, furosemide, heparin, leucovorin, methotrexate, metoclopramide, mitomycin, vinBLAStine, vinCRIStine

Y-site compatibilities: Allopurinol, amifostine, aztreonam, bleomycin, cefepime, cisplatin, cyclophosphamide, DOXOrubicin, DOXOrubicin liposome, fludarabine, furosemide, granisetron, heparin, hydrocortisone, leucovorin, mannitol, melphalan, methotrexate, metoclopramide, mitomycin, paclitaxel, piperacillin/tazobactam, potassium chloride, propofol, sargramostim, teniposide, thiotepa, vinBLAStine, vinCRIStine, vit B/C

Perform/provide:

• Strict asepsis, protective isolation if WBC levels are low
• Changing of IV site q48hr
• Rinsing of mouth tid-qid with water, club soda; brushing of teeth bid-tid with soft brush or cotton-tipped applicator for stomatitis; use unwaxed dental floss, give ice chips for mucositis
• Nutritious diet with iron, vitamin supplements, low fiber, few dairy products, especially when combined with radiotherapy as ordered

Evaluate:

• Therapeutic response: decreased tumor size, spread of malignancy

Teach patient/family:

• To avoid crowds, persons with known infections
• To avoid foods with citric acid, hot or rough texture if stomatitis is present; to drink adequate fluids
• To report stomatitis: any bleeding, white spots, ulcerations in mouth; tell patient to examine mouth daily, report symptoms; viscous lidocaine may be used
• To report signs of infection: fever, sore throat, flulike symptoms
• To report signs of anemia: fatigue, headache, faintness, shortness of breath, irritability
• To report bleeding: avoid use of razors, commercial mouthwash
• To avoid use of aspirin products or NSAIDs
• To use contraception during therapy (men and women); avoid breastfeeding (topical use)
• Not to receive vaccinations during therapy
• To use sunscreen or stay out of the sun to prevent photosensitivity
• About hair loss, explore use of wigs or other products until hair regrowth occurs
• To apply topically only to affected areas, being careful around mouth, nose, eyes

F

fluoxetine (℞)

(floo-ox′eh-teen)

Prozac, Prozac Weekly, Sarafem

Func. class.: Antidepressant, SSRI (selective serotonin reuptake inhibitor)

Do not confuse:

Prozac/Proscar/ProSom/Prilosec

Sarafem/Serophene

Action: Inhibits CNS neuron uptake of serotonin but not of norepinephrine

Uses: Major depressive disorder, obsessive-compulsive disorder (OCD), bulimia nervosa; *Sarafem:* premenstrual dysphoric disorder (PMDD), panic disorder

Unlabeled uses: Alcoholism, anorexia nervosa, ADHD, bipolar II affective disorder, borderline personality disorder, cataplexy, narcolepsy, kleptomania, migraine, obesity, posttraumatic stress disorder, schizophrenia, Tourette's syndrome, trichotillomania, levodopa-induced dyskinesia, social phobia

Bulimia nervosa

• *Adult:* **PO** 60 mg/day in AM

Depression/obsessive-compulsive disorder

• *Adult:* **PO** 20 mg/day in AM; after 4 wk if no clinical improvement is noted, dose may be increased to 20 mg bid in AM, PM, not to exceed 80 mg/day; **PO** 90 mg/wk

• *Geriatric:* **PO** 5-10 mg/day, increase as needed

• *Child 5-18 yr:* **PO** 5-10 mg/day, max 20 mg/day

Premenstrual dysphoric disorder (Sarafem)

• *Adult:* **PO** 20 mg/day, may be taken daily 14 days before menses

ADHD (unlabeled)

• *Adult:* **PO** 20-60 mg/day

Alcoholism (unlabeled)

• *Adult:* **PO** 20-80 mg/day

Anorexia nervosa (unlabeled)

• *Adult:* **PO** 10 mg every other day-20 mg/day

Bipolar II affective disorder (unlabeled)

• *Adult:* **PO** 10 mg every other day-20 mg/day

Borderline personality disorder (unlabeled)

• *Adult:* **PO** 20 mg/day

Kleptomania (unlabeled)

• *Adult:* **PO** 60-80 mg/day

Migraine, chronic daily headaches (unlabeled)

• *Adult:* **PO** 10-80 mg/day

Narcolepsy (unlabeled)

• *Adult:* **PO** 20-40 mg/day

Posttraumatic stress disorder (unlabeled)

• *Adult:* **PO** 10-80 mg/day

Schizophrenia (unlabeled)

• *Adult:* **PO** 20-60 mg/day

Available forms: Caps 10, 20, 40 mg; tabs 10, 20 mg; oral sol 20 mg/5 ml; del rel caps (Prozac Weekly) 90 mg

SIDE EFFECTS

CNS: Headache, nervousness, insomnia, drowsiness, anxiety, tremor, dizziness, fatigue, sedation, poor concentration, abnormal dreams, agitation, **seizures,** apathy, euphoria, hallucinations, delusions, psychosis, **suicidal ideation, neuroleptic malignant syndrome–like reactions**

CV: Hot flashes, palpitations, angina pectoris, **hemorrhage,** hypertension, **tachycardia,** first-degree AV block, **bradycardia, MI, thrombophlebitis**

EENT: Visual changes, ear/eye pain, photophobia, tinnitus

GI: Nausea, diarrhea, dry mouth, anorexia, dyspepsia, constipation, cramps, vomiting, taste changes, flatulence, decreased appetite

GU: Dysmenorrhea, decreased libido, urinary frequency, UTI, amenorrhea, cystitis, impotence, urine retention

INTEG: Sweating, rash, pruritus, acne, alopecia, urticaria

META: Hyponatremia

MS: Pain, arthritis, twitching

RESP: Infection, pharyngitis, nasal congestion, sinus headache, sinusitis,

cough, dyspnea, bronchitis, asthma, hyperventilation, pneumonia
SYST: *Asthenia, viral infection, fever, allergy, chills,* hyponatremia
Contraindications: Hypersensitivity
Precautions: Pregnancy (C), breastfeeding, geriatric patients, diabetes mellitus

Black Box Warning: Children, suicidal ideation

PHARMACOKINETICS

PO: Peak 6-8 hr, metabolized in liver, excreted in urine, terminal half-life 2-3 days, norfluoxetine active metabolite half-life 9.3 days, steady state 28-35 days, protein binding 94%

INTERACTIONS

- Paradoxical worsening of OCD: busPIRone
- Do not use with thioridazine, or within 5 wk of discontinuing fluoxetine
- Do not use with serotonin precursors (tryptophan)

⚠ Do not use MAOIs with or 14 days prior to fluoxetine
Increase: side effects—highly protein-bound products
Increase: effect—haloperidol
Increase: half-life of diazepam
Increase: levels or toxicity of carbamazepine, lithium, digoxin, warfarin, phenytoin
Increase: levels of tricyclics, phenothiazines
Increase: CNS depression—alcohol, antidepressants, opioids, sedatives
Decrease: fluoxetine effect—cyproheptadine

Drug/Herb

⚠ Do not use together; increased risk of serotonin syndrome: St. John's wort, SAM-e
Increase: anticholinergic effect—corkwood, jimsonweed
Increase: CNS effect—hops, kava, lavender

Drug/Lab Test

Increase: serum bilirubin, blood glucose, alk phos
Decrease: VMA, 5-HIAA
False increase: urinary catecholamines

NURSING CONSIDERATIONS

Assess:

- Mental status: mood, sensorium, affect, suicidal tendencies, increase in psychiatric symptoms, depression, panic; monitor for seizures, seizure potential is increased
- Appetite in bulimia nervosa, weight daily, increase nutritious foods in diet, watch for bingeing and vomiting
- Allergic reactions: itching, rash urticaria, product should be discontinued, may need to give antihistamine
- B/P (lying/standing), pulse q4hr; if systolic B/P drops 20 mm Hg, hold product, notify prescriber; take vital signs q4hr in patients with CV disease
- Blood studies: CBC, leukocytes, differential, cardiac enzymes if patient is receiving long-term therapy; check platelets; bleeding can occur
- Hepatic studies: AST, ALT, bilirubin, creatinine
- Weight q wk; appetite may decrease with product
- ECG for flattening of T wave, bundle branch, AV block, dysrhythmias in cardiac patients
- Alcohol consumption; if alcohol is consumed, hold dose until AM

Administer:

- With food or milk for GI symptoms
- Crushed if patient is unable to swallow medication whole (tab only)
- Dosage at bedtime if oversedation occurs during the day; may take entire dose at bedtime; geriatric patients may not tolerate once/day dosing
- Gum, hard candy, frequent sips of water for dry mouth
- Prozac weekly on the same day each week

Perform/provide:

- Storage at room temperature; do not freeze

F

• Assistance with ambulation during therapy, since drowsiness, dizziness occur
• Safety measures primarily in geriatric patients
• Checking to see if PO medication swallowed

Evaluate:
• Therapeutic response: decreased depression, symptoms of OCD

Teach patient/family:
• That therapeutic effect may take 1-4 wk
• To use caution in driving, other activities requiring alertness because of drowsiness, dizziness, blurred vision
• To use sunscreen to prevent photosensitivity
• To avoid alcohol ingestion, other CNS depressants
• To notify prescriber if pregnant or plan to become pregnant or breastfeed
• To change positions slowly, orthostatic hypotension may occur
• To avoid all OTC products unless approved by prescriber
• That suicidal thoughts, behavior may occur in young adults, children

Treatment of overdose: Activated charcoal, supportive care

fluoxymesterone (℞)
(floo-oks-i-mes′te-rone)
Androxy
Func. class.: Hormone-androgen
Chem. class.: Alkylated derivative of testosterone

Controlled Substance Schedule C-III

Action: Androgens are responsible for sexual maturation, suppression of gonadotropin-releasing hormones, LH, FSH, by a negative feedback mechanism

Uses: Inoperable female breast cancer, male hypogonadism, delayed male puberty

DOSAGE AND ROUTES

Androgen replacement in male hypogonadism
• *Adult:* **PO** 5 mg 1-4 ×/day, may increase dose, max 40 mg/day

Delayed male puberty
• *Adult and adolescent:* **PO** 2.5-10 mg/day × 4-6 mo, max 20 mg/day

Inoperable female breast cancer
• *Adult:* **PO** 10-40 mg/day in divided doses, continue for ≥2-3 mo

Available forms: Tabs 10 mg

SIDE EFFECTS

CV: **Heart failure**
GI: **Hepatitis**
GU: Amenorrhea, feminization, virilization, prostatic hypertrophy, priapism, oligospermia, oligomenorrhea, gynecomastia
HEMA: Coagulation disorders (clotting factors II, V, VII, X)
INTEG: Alopecia, acne, hirsutism, seborrhea
MISC: Edema, hypercalcemia

Contraindications: Pregnancy (X), breastfeeding, prostate cancer, male breast cancer

Precautions: Diabetes mellitus, CV/hepatic/renal disease, geriatric patients, hypercalcemia, hypothyroidism

PHARMACOKINETICS

Metabolized in liver; excreted in urine, breast milk; crosses placenta; half-life 9.2 hr

INTERACTIONS

• Edema: corticosteroids
Increase: nephrotoxicity—cycloSPORINE
Increase: erythropoiesis—darbepoetin, epoetin; avoid concurrent administration
Increase: PT—warfarin
Increase: hepatotoxicity—other hepatotoxic agents
Decrease: glucose levels may alter need for oral antidiabetics, insulin
Decrease: androgen effect—5-α reductase inhibitors (dutasteride, finasteride)

Drug/Herb
Decrease: fluoxymesterone effect—saw palmetto
Drug/Food
Decrease: fluoxymesterone effect—soy

NURSING CONSIDERATIONS

Assess:
- Weight daily; notify prescriber if weekly weight gain is >5 lb
- I&O ratio; be alert for decreasing urinary output, increasing edema
- Growth rate in children; growth rate may be uneven (linear/bone growth) with extended use
- Electrolytes: K, Na, Cl, Ca; cholesterol
- Hepatic studies: ALT, AST, bilirubin
- Edema, hypertension, cardiac symptoms
- Signs of masculinization in female: increased libido, deepening of voice, decreased breast tissue, enlarged clitoris, menstrual irregularities; male: gynecomastia, impotence, testicular atrophy
- Hypercalcemia: lethargy, polyuria, polydipsia, nausea, vomiting, constipation; product may have to be decreased
- Hypoglycemia in diabetics; oral antidiabetic action is increased

Administer:
- As a single dose or up to 4×/day

Perform/provide:
- Storage at controlled room temperature (68°-77° F)

Evaluate:
- Therapeutic response: decreased advance of inoperable female breast cancer, male puberty

Teach patient/family:
- To notify prescriber if therapeutic response decreases; if edema occurs
- About changes in sex characteristics
- That women should report menstrual irregularities, voice changes, acne, facial hair growth
- To notify prescriber if pregnancy is planned or suspected; use contraception while taking product
- That 2-3 mo course is necessary to determine objective treatment in breast cancer
- To report signs/symptoms of hepatic disorder

fluphenazine decanoate (℞)
(floo-fen′a-zeen)
Modecate ✦, Modecate Concentrate ✦, Prolixin Decanoate

fluphenazine enanthate (℞)
Moditen Enanthate ✦, Prolixin Enanthate

fluphenazine hydrochloride (℞)
Apo-Fluphenazine ✦, Moditen HCl ✦, Moditen HCl-H.P. ✦, Permitil ✦, Prolixin

Func. class.: Antipsychotic
Chem. class.: Phenothiazine, piperazine

Do not confuse:
Prolixin/Proloid

Action: Depresses cerebral cortex, hypothalamus, limbic system, which control activity and aggression; blocks neurotransmission produced by DOPamine at synapse; exhibits strong α-adrenergic and anticholinergic blocking action; mechanism for antipsychotic effects is unclear

Uses: Psychotic disorders, schizophrenia

DOSAGE AND ROUTES

Decanoate
- *Adult and child >16 yr:* **IM/SUBCUT** 12.5-25 mg q1-3wk, may increase slowly
- *Child 12-16 yr:* **IM/SUBCUT** 6.25-18.75 mg, then repeat q1-3wk, then increase slowly, max 25 mg
- *Child 5-12 yr:* **IM/SUBCUT** 3.125-12.5 mg, then repeat q1-3wk, increase slowly

Enanthate
- *Adult:* **IM/SUBCUT** 25 mg q1-3wk, max 100 mg/dose

HCl
- *Adult:* **PO** 2.5-10 mg, in divided doses q6-8hr, max 40 mg/day; **IM** initially 1.25

mg, then 2.5-10 mg in divided doses q6-8hr

• *Child:* **PO** 0.25-3.5 mg/day in divided doses q4-6hr, max 10 mg/day

Available forms: *Decanoate:* inj 25 mg/ml; *enanthate:* inj 25 mg/ml; *HCl:* tabs 1, 2.5, 5, 10 mg; elix 2.5 mg/5 ml; inj 2.5 ml

SIDE EFFECTS

CNS: EPS: pseudoparkinsonism, akathisia, dystonia, tardive dyskinesia, drowsiness, headache, **seizures, neuroleptic malignant syndrome**

CV: Orthostatic hypotension, hypertension, **cardiac arrest,** ECG changes, **tachycardia**

EENT: Blurred vision, glaucoma, dry eyes

GI: Dry mouth, nausea, vomiting, anorexia, constipation, diarrhea, jaundice, weight gain, **paralytic ileus, hepatitis,** cholecystic jaundice

GU: Urinary retention, urinary frequency, enuresis, impotence, amenorrhea, gynecomastia

HEMA: Anemia, **leukopenia, leukocytosis, agranulocytosis, aplastic anemia, thrombocytopenia**

INTEG: Rash, photosensitivity, dermatitis

RESP: **Laryngospasm,** dyspnea, **respiratory depression**

Contraindications: Hypersensitivity, circulatory collapse, hepatic damage, cerebral arteriosclerosis, coronary disease, severe hypo/hypertension, blood dyscrasias, coma, brain damage, closed-angle glaucoma, bone marrow depression, alcohol and barbiturate withdrawal

Precautions: Pregnancy (C), breastfeeding, children <12 yr, geriatric patients, seizure disorders, hypertension, cardiac/hepatic disease

Black Box Warning: Dementia

PHARMACOKINETICS

Metabolized by liver, excreted in urine (metabolites), crosses placenta, enters breast milk, protein binding >90%, not dialyzable

PO/IM (HCl): Onset 1 hr, peak 2-4 hr, duration 6-8 hr, half-life 3.5-4 days

IM/SUBCUT (enanthate): Onset 24-72 hr, duration 1-3 wk

IM/SUBCUT (decanoate): Onset 1-3 days; peak 1-2 days, duration over 4 wk, single-dose half-life 6.8-9.6 days, multiple dose 14.3 days

INTERACTIONS

Increase: sedation—other CNS depressants, alcohol, barbiturate anesthetics

Increase: toxicity—epinephrine

Increase: anticholinergic effects—anticholinergics

Decrease: effects of levodopa, lithium

Decrease: fluphenazine effects—smoking, barbiturates

Drug/Herb

Increase: EPS—betel palm, kava

Increase: anticholinergic effect—henbane leaf

Increase: action—cola tree, hops, kava, nettle, nutmeg

Drug/Lab Test

Increase: LFTs, cardiac enzymes, cholesterol, blood glucose, prolactin, bilirubin, cholinesterase

Decrease: hormones (blood and urine)

False positive: pregnancy tests, PKU urinary steroids, 17-OHCS

NURSING CONSIDERATIONS

Assess:

• Swallowing of PO medication; check for hoarding, giving of medication to other patients

• I&O ratio; palpate bladder if low urinary output occurs, urinary retention may be the cause

• Bilirubin, CBC, LFTs monthly

• Urinalysis is recommended before and during prolonged therapy

• Affect, orientation, LOC, reflexes, gait, coordination, sleep pattern disturbances

• B/P standing and lying; take pulse and respirations q4hr during initial treatment; establish baseline before starting treatment; report drops of 30 mm Hg

• Dizziness, faintness, palpitations, tachycardia on rising
• EPS including akathisia (inability to sit still, no pattern to movements), tardive dyskinesia (bizarre movements of jaw, mouth, tongue, extremities), pseudoparkinsonism (rigidity, tremors, pill rolling, shuffling gait)
• Constipation, urinary retention daily; if these occur, increase bulk, H_2O in diet

Administer:

• Elixir with juice, milk, or uncaffeinated drinks
• Anticholinergic agent if EPS occur
• IM inj into large muscle mass; to minimize postural hypotension, give inj and have patient remain seated or recumbent for ½ hr
• Use dry needle, or solution will become cloudy; use 21G or larger due to viscosity

Syringe compatibilities: Benztropine, diphenhydrAMINE, hydrOXYzine

Perform/provide:

• Decreased sensory input by dimming lights, avoiding loud noises
• Supervised ambulation until stabilized on medication; do not involve in strenuous exercise; fainting is possible; patient should not stand still for long periods
• Increased fluids to prevent constipation
• Sips of water, candy, gum for dry mouth
• Storage in tight, light-resistant container in cool environment

Evaluate:

• Therapeutic response: decrease in emotional excitement, hallucinations, delusions, paranoia, reorganization of patterns of thought, speech

Teach patient/family:

• That orthostatic hypotension occurs often; to rise from sitting or lying position gradually; avoid hazardous activities until stabilized on medication
• To avoid hot tubs, hot showers, tub baths, since hypotension may occur; that in hot weather, heat stroke may occur; take extra precautions to stay cool
⚠ To avoid abrupt withdrawal of this product, or EPS may result; product should be withdrawn slowly
• To avoid OTC preparations (cough, hay fever, cold) unless approved by prescriber; serious product interactions may occur; avoid use with alcohol, CNS depressants; increased drowsiness may occur
• To use a sunscreen to prevent burns
• About importance of compliance with product regimen
• About EPS and necessity for meticulous oral hygiene, since oral candidiasis may occur
• To report sore throat, malaise, fever, bleeding, mouth sores; if these occur, CBC should be drawn and product discontinued
• That urine may turn pink to reddish-brown

Treatment of overdose: Lavage; if orally ingested, provide an airway; *do not induce vomiting*

flurandrenolide topical

See Appendix B

flurazepam (℞)

(flure-az′e-pam)
Apo-Flurazepam ♣, flurazepam, Novoflupam ♣, Somnol ♣
Func. class.: Sedative/hypnotic
Chem. class.: Benzodiazepine, long-acting

Controlled Substance Schedule IV (USA), Targeted (CDSA IV) (Canada)

Do not confuse:
flurazepam/temazepam

Action: Produces CNS depression at the limbic, thalamic, hypothalamic levels of CNS; may be mediated by neurotransmitter γ-aminobutyric acid (GABA); results are sedation, hypnosis, skeletal muscle relaxation, anticonvulsant activity, anxiolytic action

Uses: Insomnia, short term

Unlabeled uses: Anxiety

DOSAGE AND ROUTES

• *Adult:* **PO** 15-30 mg at bedtime; may repeat dose once if needed

• *Geriatric:* **PO** 15 mg at bedtime; may increase if needed

Hepatic dose

• *Adult:* **PO** 5 mg at bedtime

Available forms: Caps 15, 30 mg

SIDE EFFECTS

CNS: Lethargy, drowsiness, daytime sedation, dizziness, confusion, lightheadedness, headache, anxiety, irritability, complex sleep-related reactions: sleep driving, sleep eating

CV: Chest pain, pulse changes, palpitations

GI: Nausea, vomiting, diarrhea, heartburn, abdominal pain, constipation

HEMA: **Leukopenia, granulocytopenia** (rare)

MISC: Physical, psychological dependence, blurred vision, **apnea**

Contraindications: Pregnancy (X), breastfeeding, hypersensitivity to benzodiazepines, intermittent porphyria, uncontrolled pain, sleep apnea

Precautions: Children <15 yr, geriatric patients, anemia, renal/hepatic disease, suicidal individuals, drug abuse, psychosis, angioedema, pulmonary disease, suicidal ideation

PHARMACOKINETICS

PO: Onset 15-45 min, duration 7-8 hr, metabolized by liver, excreted by kidneys (inactive/active metabolites), crosses placenta, excreted in breast milk, half-life 47-100 hr, 97% protein binding

INTERACTIONS

Increase: flurazepam effects—cimetidine, disulfiram, probenicid, isoniazid, oral contraceptives, fluoxetine, ketoconazole, propranolol, valproic acid, CYP3A4 inhibitors

Increase: CNS depression—alcohol, CNS depressants

Decrease: flurazepam effect—rifampin, barbiturates, theophylline

Drug/Herb

Increase: sedative effect—catnip, chamomile, clary, cowslip, kava, lavender, mistletoe, nettle, pokeweed, poppy, Queen Anne's lace, senega, valerian

Increase: hypotension—black cohosh

Decrease: flurazepam effect—St. John's wort

Drug/Lab Test

Increase: AST, ALT, serum bilirubin

Decrease: RAI uptake

False increase: urinary 17-OHCS

NURSING CONSIDERATIONS

Assess:

• Mental status: mood, sensorium, affect, memory (long, short), physical, psychological dependence or tolerance

• Type of sleep problem: falling asleep, staying asleep

• Withdrawal signs if discontinued abruptly

• For excessive sedation, impaired coordination especially in geriatric patients

Administer:

• ½-1 hr before bedtime for sleeplessness

• Caps may be opened and mixed with food

• Best to avoid in geriatric patients; long half-life

Perform/provide:

• Assistance with ambulation after receiving dose

• Safety measures: night-light, call bell within easy reach

• Checking to see if PO medication has been swallowed

• Storage in tight container in cool environment

Evaluate:

• Therapeutic response: ability to sleep at night, decreased amount of early morning awakening if taking product for insomnia

Teach patient/family:

• To avoid driving or other activities requiring alertness until product is stabilized

• To avoid alcohol ingestion or CNS depressants; serious CNS depression may result

• That effects may take 2 nights for benefits to be noticed, limit to 7-10 days continuous use

• Alternative measures to improve sleep: reading, exercise several hours before bedtime, warm bath, warm milk, TV, self-hypnosis, deep breathing

• That hangover is common in geriatric patients

• To use contraceptives; pregnancy category (X)

Treatment of overdose: Lavage, activated charcoal; monitor electrolytes, VS

flurbiprofen ophthalmic

See Appendix B

flutamide (℞)

(floo′-ta-mide)

Apo-Flutamide ♣, Novo-Flutamide ♣

Func. class.: Antineoplastic, hormone

Chem. class.: Antiandrogen

Action: Interferes with androgen uptake in the nucleus or androgen activity in target tissues; arrests tumor growth in androgen-sensitive tissue (i.e., prostate gland)

Uses: Metastatic prostatic carcinoma, stage D_2 in combination with LHRH agonistic analogs (leuprolide), B_2-C in combination with goserelin and radiation

DOSAGE AND ROUTES

• *Adult:* **PO** 250 mg q8hr, for a daily dosage of 750 mg

Available forms: Caps 125, 250 ♣mg

SIDE EFFECTS

CNS: Hot flashes, drowsiness, confusion, depression, anxiety, paresthesia

GI: Diarrhea, nausea, vomiting, increased levels in hepatic studies, **hepatitis,** anorexia, **hepatotoxicity**

GU: Decreased libido, impotence, gynecomastia

HEMA: **Leukopenia, thrombocytopenia, hemolytic anemia**

INTEG: Irritation at site, rash, photosensitivity

MISC: Edema, neuromuscular and pulmonary symptoms, hypertension

Contraindications: Pregnancy (D), hypersensitivity

Black Box Warning: Severe hepatic disease

Precautions: G6PD deficiency, hemoglobinopathy, lactase deficiency, polycystic ovary syndrome, tobacco smoking

PHARMACOKINETICS

Rapidly and completely absorbed; excreted in urine and feces as metabolites; half-life 6 hr, geriatric half-life 8 hr; 94% bound to plasma proteins

INTERACTIONS

Increase: PT—warfarin

Decrease: flutamide action—LHRH analog (leuprolide)

NURSING CONSIDERATIONS

Assess:

⚠ Hepatic studies: AST, ALT, alk phos, which may be elevated; if LFTs are elevated, product may need to be discontinued; monitor CBC, bilirubin, creatinine

• For CNS symptoms, including drowsiness, confusion, depression, anxiety

Administer:

• Do not break, crush, or chew caps

• Flutamide must be taken with leuprolide; do not change dosing

F

Evaluate:
• Therapeutic response: decrease in prostatic tumor size, decrease in spread of cancer

Teach patient/family:
• To report side effects: decreased libido, impotence, breast enlargement, hot flashes, diarrhea
• To report nausea, vomiting, yellow eyes or skin, dark urine, clay-colored stools, hepatotoxicity may be the cause
• Notify of yellow, green urine discoloration
• Avoid sun exposure, tanning beds
• To use contraception during treatment; pregnancy category (D)

fluticasone (℞)

(floo-tic'a-sone)
Flovent HFA, Flovent Diskus ♣
Func. class: Corticosteroids, inhalation; antiasthmatic

Action: Decreases inflammation by inhibiting mast cells, macrophages, and leukotrienes; antiinflammatory, and vasoconstrictor properties

Uses: Prevention of chronic asthma during maintenance treatment in those requiring oral corticosteroids; nasal symptoms of seasonal/perennial, and allergic/nonallergic rhinitis

DOSAGE AND ROUTES

Prevention of chronic asthma during maintenance treatment in those requiring oral corticosteroids

Flovent HFA
• *Adult and child ≥12 yr:* **INH** 88-660 mcg bid (in those previously taking bronchodilators, alone); **INH** 88-220 mcg bid, max 440 mcg bid (in those previously taking inhaled corticosteroids); **INH** 440 mcg bid, max 880 mcg bid (in those previously taking oral corticosteroids)

Flovent Diskus ♣
• *Adult and child ≥12 yr:* **INH** 100 mcg bid, max 500 mcg (in those previously taking bronchodilators, alone); **INH** 100-250 mcg bid, max 500 mcg bid (in those previously taking inhaled corticosteroids); **INH** 500-1000 mcg bid, max 1000 mcg bid (in those previously taking oral corticosteroids)
• *Child 4-11 yr:* **INH** Initially 50 mcg bid, max 100 mcg bid (in those previously taking bronchodilators alone or inhaled corticosteroids)

Available forms: Nasal spray 50 mcg/metered spray; oral inhalation aerosol 44, 110, 220 mcg; oral inhalation powder 50, 100, 250 mcg

SIDE EFFECTS

CNS: Fever, headache, nervousness, dizziness, migraines, numbness in fingers
EENT: ***Pharyngitis***, sinusitis, rhinitis, laryngitis, hoarseness, dry eyes, cataracts, nasal discharge, epistaxis
GI: Diarrhea, abdominal pain, nausea, vomiting, ***oral candidiasis***, gastroenteritis
GU: UTI
INTEG: Urticaria, dermatitis
META: Hyperglycemia, growth retardation in children, cushingoid features
MISC: Influenza, **eosinophilic conditions, angioedema, Churg-Strauss syndrome,** adrenal insufficiency (high doses)
MS: Osteoporosis, muscle soreness, joint pain
RESP: ***Upper respiratory infection***, dyspnea, cough, bronchitis, **bronchospasm**

Contraindications: Hypersensitivity, primary treatment in status asthmaticus

Precautions: Pregnancy (C), breastfeeding, active infections, glaucoma, diabetes, immunocompromised patients

PHARMACOKINETICS

Absorption 30% aerosol, 13.5% powder; protein binding 91%; metabolized in the liver after absorption in lung; half-life 7.8 hr; <5% excreted in urine and feces

Nasal INH: Onset 12 hr, peak several days, duration 1-2 wk

Oral INH: Onset 24 hr, peak several days, duration 1-2 wk

INTERACTIONS

Increase: fluticasone levels—CYP450 3A4 inhibitors (ketoconazole)

Drug/Lab Test

Increase: urine/serum glucose

NURSING CONSIDERATIONS

Assess:

- Respiratory status: lung sounds, pulmonary function tests during and several months after change from systemic to inhalation corticosteroids
- Withdrawal symptoms from oral corticosteroids: depression, pain in joints, fatigue

⚠ Adrenal insufficiency: nausea, weakness, fatigue, hypotension, hypoglycemia, anorexia; may occur when changing from systemic to inhalation corticosteroids; may be life-threatening

- Growth rate in children
- Adrenal function tests periodically: hypothalamic–pituitary-adrenal axis suppression in long-term treatment

Administer:

- Give at 1 min intervals
- Decrease dose to lowest effective dose after desired effect, decrease dose at 2-4 wk intervals

Inhalation route (aerosol)

- In general, child <4 yr requires a face mask with spacer/VHC device for delivery; allow 3-5 INH per actuation

Evaluate:

- Therapeutic response: decreased severity of asthma

Teach patient/family:

- To use bronchodilator first before using inhalation, if taking both
- Not to use for acute asthmatic attack; for acute asthma, may require oral corticosteroids
- To avoid smoking, smoke-filled rooms, those with URIs, those not immunized against chickenpox or measles
- To rinse mouth after inhaled product to decrease risk of oral candidiasis

fluticasone nasal agent

See Appendix B

fluticasone topical

See Appendix B

fluvastatin (℞)

(flu'vah-stay-tin)

Lescol, Lescol XL

Func. class.: Antilipidemic

Chem. class.: HMG-CoA reductase inhibitor

Action: Inhibits HMG-CoA reductase enzyme, which reduces cholesterol synthesis

Uses: As an adjunct in primary hypercholesterolemia (types Ia, Ib), coronary atherosclerosis in CAD; to reduce the risk for undergoing coronary revascularization in patients with CAD

DOSAGE AND ROUTES

- *Adult:* **PO** 20-40 mg/day in PM initially, usual range 20-80 mg, max 80 mg; may be given in 2 doses (40 mg AM, 40 mg PM); dosage adjustments may be made in 4 wk intervals or more

Available forms: Caps 20, 40 mg; ext rel tab 80 mg

SIDE EFFECTS

CNS: Headache, dizziness, insomnia, **Lou Gehrig's disease (ALS)**

EENT: Lens opacities

GI: Abdominal pain, cramps, nausea, constipation, diarrhea, dyspepsia, flatus, **hepatic dysfunction,** pancreatitis

HEMA: **Thrombocytopenia, hemolytic anemia, leukopenia**

INTEG: Rash, pruritus

MISC: Fatigue, influenza, photosensitivity

MS: Myalgia, **myositis, rhabdomyolysis,** *arthritis, arthralgia*

RESP: Upper respiratory infection, rhinitis, cough, pharyngitis, sinusitis

Contraindications: Pregnancy (X), breastfeeding, hypersensitivity, active hepatic disease

Precautions: Past hepatic disease, alcoholism, severe acute infections, trauma, hypotension, uncontrolled seizure disorders, severe metabolic disorders, electrolyte imbalance, myopathy, rhabdomyolysis

PHARMACOKINETICS

Peak response 3-4 wk, metabolized in liver, highly protein bound, excreted primarily in feces, half-life 1-6 days, steady state 4-5 wk

INTERACTIONS

Increase: effects of warfarin, digoxin

Increase: myalgia, myositis—cycloSPORINE, gemfibrozil, niacin, erythromycin, clofibrate; azole antiinfectives

Increase: effects of fluvastatin—alcohol, lithium, cimetidine, ranitidine, omeprazole, saquinavir

Increase: levels of clozapine, methadone, propranolol, theophylline, tricyclics

Increase: serotonin syndrome—MAOIs, tramadol

Increase: QT interval—pimozide, thioridazine; avoid concurrent use

Drug/Herb

Increase: effect—glucomannan

Decrease: effect—gotu kola, St. John's wort

Drug/Food

- Grapefruit juice: possible increased toxicity

Decrease: absorption—oat bran, high fat

NURSING CONSIDERATIONS

Assess:

- Fasting lipid profile (cholesterol, LDL, HDL, TG) q8wk, then q3-6mo when stable
- Hepatic studies q1-2mo during the first 1½ yr of treatment; AST, ALT, LFTs may be increased
- Renal studies in patients with compromised renal system: BUN, I&O ratio, creatinine

⚠ For muscle pain, tenderness; obtain baseline CPK if elevated; if these occur, product should be discontinued

Administer:

- Do not break, crush, or chew ext rel tabs
- Bile acid sequestrant should be given at least 2 hr before or after fluvastatin

Perform/provide:

- Storage in cool environment in tight container protected from light

Evaluate:

- Therapeutic response: decrease in LDL, VLDL, total cholesterol; increased HDL, decreased triglycerides

Teach patient/family:

- That blood work will be necessary during treatment, to take as prescribed
- To report severe GI symptoms, headache, muscle pain, weakness, tenderness
- That previously prescribed regimen will continue: low-cholesterol diet, exercise program, smoking cessation
- To report suspected pregnancy, not to use during pregnancy
- To use sunscreen or stay out of sun to prevent photosensitivity
- To notify all health care providers of products taken

fluvoxamine (℞)

(flu-vox'a-meen)

Luvox CR

Func. class.: Antidepressant SSRI (selective serotonin reuptake inhibitor)

Do not confuse:

Luvox/Levoxyl

Action: Inhibits CNS neuron uptake of serotonin but not of norepinephrine

Uses: Obsessive-compulsive disorder, social phobia

Unlabeled uses: Depression, bulimia nervosa, panic disorder, autism, anxiety, posttraumatic stress disorder (PTSD), premenstrual dysphoric disorder (PMDD)

DOSAGE AND ROUTES

Obsessive-compulsive disorder (OCD)

• *Adult:* **PO** 50 mg at bedtime, increase by 50 mg at 4-7 day intervals, max 300 mg; doses over 100 mg should be divided; **EXT REL** 100 mg at bedtime, may titrate upward by 50 mg/wk, max 300 mg/day

• *Child 8-17 yr:* **PO** 25 mg at bedtime, increase by 25 mg/day q4-7days, max 200 mg/day; doses over 50 mg should be divided

Social anxiety disorder

• *Adult:* **PO EXT REL CAP** (Luvox CR) 100 mg at bedtime, initially, titrate as needed by 50 mg/wk to 100-300 mg/day; **PO** 50 mg at bedtime, titrate as needed by 50 mg q4-7days to 50-300 mg/day

• *Child/adolescent 12-17 yr:* **PO** 25 mg at bedtime, titrate by 25-50 mg q4-7days, max 300 mg/day, if total daily dose >50 mg, divide equally

Hepatic dose/geriatric

• *Adult:* **PO** 25 mg at bedtime, may titrate upward slowly

Autism (unlabeled)

• *Adult:* **PO** up to 150 mg/day

Bulimia nervosa, depression (unlabeled)

• *Adult:* **PO** 50 mg at bedtime × 4-7 days, titrate by 25-50 mg/dose q4-7days as needed

Premenstrual dysphoric disorder (unlabeled)

• *Adult:* **PO** 50 mg/day, may titrate to 100 mg/day

Schizophrenia (unlabeled)

• *Adult:* **PO** 100 mg daily in combination with other agents

Available forms: Tabs 25, 50, 100 mg; ext rel cap 100, 150 mg

SIDE EFFECTS

CNS: Headache, drowsiness, dizziness, seizures, sleep disorders, insomnia, **suicidal ideation (children/adolescents), neuroleptic malignant syndrome–like reactions**

GI: Nausea, anorexia, constipation, **hepatotoxicity**, *vomiting, diarrhea,* dry mouth

GU: Decreased libido, anorgasmia

INTEG: Rash, sweating

Contraindications: Hypersensitivity

Precautions: Pregnancy (C), breastfeeding, geriatric patients, hepatic/cardiac disease, abrupt discontinuation, dehydration, ECT, hyponatremia, hypovolemia, bipolar disorder, seizure disorder

Black Box Warning: Children <8 yr, suicidal ideation

PHARMACOKINETICS

Crosses blood-brain barrier, 77% protein binding, metabolism by the liver, terminal half-life 15.6 hr, peak 2-8 hr

INTERACTIONS

⚠ Fatal reaction—MAOIs

Increase: CNS depression—alcohol, barbiturates, benzodiazepines

Increase: fluvoxamine, toxicity levels—tricyclics, clozapine, alosetron, tizanidine; do not use together

Increase: metabolism, decrease effects—smoking

Decrease: metabolism, increase action of propranolol, diazepam, lithium, theophylline, carbamazepine, warfarin

Drug/Herb

⚠ ***Increase:*** effect, possible fatal reaction—St. John's wort

Increase: anticholinergic effect—corkwood, jimsonweed

Increase: CNS effect—hops, kava, lavender

NURSING CONSIDERATIONS

Assess:

• Hepatic studies: AST, ALT, bilirubin

• Mental status: mood, sensorium, affect, suicidal tendencies; increase in psychiatric symptoms: depression, panic, obsessive-compulsive symptoms

• Constipation; most likely in geriatric patients

⚠ For toxicity: nausea, vomiting, diarrhea, syncope, increased pulse, seizures

Administer:

- Do not break, crush, or chew ext rel product
- With food, milk for GI symptoms

Perform/provide:

- Storage at room temperature; do not freeze

Evaluate:

- Therapeutic response: decrease in depression

Teach patient/family:

- That therapeutic effects may take 2-3 wk
- To use caution in driving, other activities requiring alertness because of drowsiness, dizziness that may occur
- Not to use other CNS depressants, alcohol, barbiturates, benzodiazepines, St. John's wort, kava
- To notify prescriber if pregnancy is suspected or planned
- To notify prescriber of allergic reaction
- To increase bulk in diet if constipation occurs, especially geriatric patients
- That suicidal behaviors, thoughts may occur
- To stop taking MAOIs at least 14 days before starting this product

Treatment of overdose: Activated charcoal, gastric lavage

folic acid (vit B_9) (OTC)

(foe'lik a'sid)

Apo-Folic ✱, Folate, Folvite, Novofolacid ✱, Vitamin B_9

Func. class.: Vit B complex group, water-soluble vitamin

Action: Needed for erythropoiesis; increases RBC, WBC, platelet formation in megaloblastic anemias

Uses: Megaloblastic or macrocytic anemia caused by folic acid deficiency; hepatic disease, alcoholism, hemolysis, intestinal obstruction, pregnancy to reduce risk of neural tube defect

Unlabeled uses: Reduce risk of heart disease, stroke, methotrexate toxicity prophylaxis

DOSAGE AND ROUTES

RDA

- *Adult and child ≥14 yr:* **PO** 400 mcg
- *Adult (pregnant/lactating):* **PO** 600 mcg/day
- *Child 9-13 yr:* **PO** 300 mcg
- *Child 4-8 yr:* **PO** 200 mcg
- *Child 1-3 yr:* **PO** 150 mcg
- *Infant 6 mo-1 yr:* **PO** 80 mcg
- *Neonates and infants <6 mo:* **PO** 65 mcg

Megaloblastic/macrocytic anemia due to folic acid or nutritional deficiency

- *Pregnant/lactating:* **PO** 800-1000 mcg

Therapeutic dose

- *Adult and child:* **PO/IM/SUBCUT/IV** up to 1 mg/day

Maintenance dose

- *Adult and child >4 yr:* **PO/IM/SUBCUT/IV** 0.4 mg/day
- *Pregnant and lactating:* **PO/IM/SUBCUT/IV** 0.8-1 mg/day
- *Child <4 yr:* **PO/IM/SUBCUT/IV** up to 0.3 mg/day
- *Infant:* **PO/IM/SUBCUT/IV** up to 0.1 mg/day

Prevention of neural tube defects during pregnancy

- *Adult:* **PO** 0.6 mg/day

Prevention of megaloblastic anemia during pregnancy

- *Adult:* **PO/IM/SUBCUT** up to 1 mg/day during pregnancy

Tropical sprue

- *Adult:* **PO** 3-15 mg/day

Available forms: Tabs 0.1, 0.4, 0.8, 1, 5 mg; inj 5, 10 mg/ml

SIDE EFFECTS

INTEG: Flushing

RESP: **Bronchospasm**

Contraindications: Hypersensitivity, anemias other than megaloblastic/macrocytic anemia, vit B_{12} deficiency anemia, uncorrected pernicious anemia

Precautions: Pregnancy (A)

PHARMACOKINETICS

PO: Peak ½-1 hr, bound to plasma proteins, excreted in breast milk, metabolized by liver, excreted in urine (small amounts)

INTERACTIONS

Increase: need for folic acid—estrogen, hydantoins, carbamazepine, glucocorticoids
Decrease: folate levels—methotrexate, sulfonamides, sulfasalazine, trimethoprim
Decrease: phenytoin levels, fosphenytoin, may increase seizures

NURSING CONSIDERATIONS

Assess:
- For fatigue, dyspnea, weakness, dyspnea that are signs of megaloblastic anemia
- Hgb, Hct, and reticulocyte count
- Nutritional status: bran, yeast, dried beans, nuts, fruits, fresh vegetables, asparagus
- Products currently taken: estrogen, carbamazepine, glucocorticoids, hydantoins; these products may cause increased folic acid use by body and contribute to a deficiency if taking other neurotoxic products

Administer:

IV route
- Direct undiluted 5 mg or less/1 min or more; or may be added to most IV sol or TPN

Solution compatibilities: $D_{20}W$
Y-site compatibilities: Famotidine

Perform/provide:
- Storage in light-resistant container

Evaluate:
- Therapeutic response: increased weight, oriented, well-being; absence of fatigue; increase in reticulocyte count within 5 days of beginning treatment, absence of neural tube defect

Teach patient/family:
- To take product exactly as prescribed; periodic lab work is required
- To alter nutrition to include high–folic-acid foods: organ meats, vegetables, fruit
- That urine will turn bright yellow
- To notify prescriber of allergic reaction
- To avoid breastfeeding

⚠ High Alert

fondaparinux (℞)

(fon-dah-pair′ih-nux)

Arixtra

Func. class.: Anticoagulant, antithrombotic
Chem. class.: Synthetic, selective factor Xa inhibitor

Do not confuse:
Arixtra/Anti-Xa

Action: Acts by antithrombin III (ATIII)-mediated selective inhibition of factor Xa; neutralization of factor Xa interrupts blood coagulation and inhibits thrombin formation; does not inactivate thrombin (activated factor II) or affect platelets

Uses: Prevention/treatment of deep-vein thrombosis, PE in hip and knee replacement, hip fracture or abdominal surgery

Unlabeled uses: Acute coronary syndrome

DOSAGE AND ROUTES

Deep vein thrombosis/PE
- *Adult <50 kg:* **SUBCUT** 5 mg/day × 5 days or more until INR is 2-3; may give warfarin within 72 hr of fondaparinux
- *Adult 50-100 kg:* **SUBCUT** 7.5 mg/day × 5 days or more until INR is 2-3; may give warfarin within 72 hr of fondaparinux
- *Adult >100 kg:* **SUBCUT** 10 mg/day × 5 days or more until INR is 2-3; may give warfarin within 72 hr of fondaparinux

Prevention of deep vein thrombosis
- *Adult:* **SUBCUT** 2.5 mg/day, given 6 hr after surgery; continue for 5-9 days; hip surgery up to 32 days; abdominal surgery up to 24 days

Coronary artery thrombosis prophylaxis/acute coronary syndrome (unlabeled)

• *Adult:* **SUBCUT** 2.5 mg until hospital discharge or for up to 8 days with standard treatment

Available forms: Inj 2.5 mg/0.5 ml, 5 mg/0.4 ml, 7.5 mg/0.6 ml, 10 mg/0.8 ml prefilled syringes

SIDE EFFECTS

CNS: Fever, confusion, headache, dizziness, *insomnia*

GI: Nausea, vomiting, diarrhea, dyspepsia, *constipation,* increased AST, ALT

GU: UTI, urinary retention

HEMA: Anemia, minor bleeding, purpura, hematoma, **thrombocytopenia, major bleeding (intracranial, cerebral, retroperitoneal hemorrhage), postoperative hemorrhage, heparin-induced thrombocytopenia**

INTEG: Increased wound drainage, bullous eruption, local reaction—*rash,* pruritus, inj site bleeding

META: Hypokalemia

OTHER: Hypotension, pain, *edema*

Contraindications: Hypersensitivity to this product; hemophilia, leukemia with bleeding, peptic ulcer disease, hemorrhagic stroke, surgery, thrombocytopenic purpura, weight <50 kg, severe renal disease (CCr <30 ml/min), active major bleeding, bacterial endocarditis

Precautions: Pregnancy (B), breastfeeding, children, geriatric patients, alcoholism, hepatic disease (severe), blood dyscrasias, heparin-induced thrombocytopenia, uncontrolled, severe hypertension, subacute bacterial endocarditis, acute nephritis, mild to moderate renal disease

Black Box Warning: Spinal/epidural anesthesia, lumbar puncture

PHARMACOKINETICS

Rapidly, completely absorbed; peak steady state 3 hr; distributed primarily in blood; does not bind to plasma proteins except 94% to ATIII; metabolism unknown; eliminated unchanged in urine in 72 hr in normal renal function; terminal half-life 17-21 hr

INTERACTIONS

• Do not mix with other products or infusion fluids

Increase: bleeding risk—salicylates, NSAIDs, abciximab, eptifibatide, tirofiban, clopidogrel, dipyridamole, quinidine, valproic acid

Drug/Herb

Increase: bleeding risk—agrimony, alfalfa, angelica, anise, basil, bay, bilberry, black haw, bogbean, bromelain, buchu, chondroitin, cinchona bark, dong quai, fenugreek, feverfew, garlic, ginger, ginkgo, ginseng, horse chestnut, Irish moss, kelp, kelpware, khella, lovage, lungwort, meadowsweet, motherwort, mugwort, nettle, papaya, parsley (large amounts), pau d'arco, pineapple, poplar, prickly ash, safflower, saw palmetto, tonka bean, turmeric, wintergreen, yarrow

Decrease: anticoagulant effect—chamomile, coenzyme Q10, flax, glucomannan, goldenseal, guar gum

NURSING CONSIDERATIONS

Assess:

• Blood studies (Hct, CBC, coagulation studies, platelets, occult blood in stools), thrombocytopenia may occur; if platelets <100,000/mm^3, treatment should be discontinued

• For bleeding: gums, petechiae, ecchymosis, black tarry stools, hematuria; decreased Hct, notify prescriber

• For neurologic symptoms in patients who have received spinal anesthesia

• For risk of hemorrhage if coadministering with other products that may cause bleeding

• For hypersensitivity: rash, fever, chills; notify prescriber

Administer:

• Alone; do not mix with other products or solutions; cannot be used interchangeably (unit to unit) with other anticoagulants

- For 5-9 days
- Only after screening patient for bleeding disorders
- SUBCUT only; do not give IM; do not give earlier than 6 hr after surgery

SUBCUT route

- Check for discolored sol or sol with particulate; if present, do not give
- Administer 6-8 hr after surgery
- Administer to recumbent patient, rotate inj sites (left/right anterolateral, left/right posterolateral abdominal wall)
- Wipe surface of inj site with alcohol swab, twist plunger cap and remove, remove rigid needle guard by pulling straight off needle, do not aspirate, do not expel air bubble from surface
- Insert whole length of needle into skinfold held with thumb and forefinger
- When product is injected, a soft click may be felt or heard
- Give at same time each day to maintain steady blood levels; observe inj site
- Avoid all IM inj that may cause bleeding

⚠ Administer only this product when ordered; not interchangeable with heparin

Perform/provide:

- Storage at 25° C (77° F); do not freeze

Evaluate:

- Therapeutic response: Prevention of DVT

Teach patient/family:

- To use soft-bristle toothbrush to avoid bleeding gums, to use electric razor
- To report any signs of bleeding: gums, under skin, urine, stools
- To avoid OTC products containing aspirin

formoterol (℞)

(for-moh′ter-ahl)

Foradil Aerolizer, Perforomist

Func. class.: Bronchodilator

Chem. class.: β-Adrenergic agonist

Do not confuse:

Foradil/Toradol

Action: Has β_1 and β_2 action; relaxes bronchial smooth muscle and dilates the trachea and main bronchi by increasing levels of cAMP, which relaxes smooth muscles; causes increased contractility and heart rate by acting on β-receptors in heart

Uses: Maintenance, treatment of asthma, COPD, prevention of exercise-induced bronchospasm

DOSAGE AND ROUTES

Maintenance, treatment of asthma

- *Adult and child ≥5 yr:* **INH** AM and PM long-term 1 cap (12 mcg) q12hr using aerolizer inhaler

Maintenance of COPD

- *Adult:* **INH** 12 mcg q12hr

Prevention of exercise-induced bronchospasm

- *Adult and child ≥12 yr:* **INH** prn occasionally 1 cap (12 mcg) at least 15 min before exercise

Available form: INH powder in cap 12 mcg

SIDE EFFECTS

CNS: Tremors, anxiety, insomnia, headache, dizziness, stimulation

CV: Palpitations, tachycardia, hypertension

GI: Nausea, vomiting, xerostomia

RESP: Bronchial irritation, dryness of oropharynx, **bronchospasms** (overuse), infection, inflammatory reaction (child)

Contraindications: Hypersensitivity to sympathomimetics, closed-angle glaucoma

Precautions: Pregnancy (C), geriatric patients, cardiac disorders, hyperthyroidism, diabetes mellitus, prostatic hypertrophy, hypertension

Black Box Warning: Respiratory insufficiency

PHARMACOKINETICS

Onset 15 min; peak 1-3 hr; duration 12 hr; metabolized in liver, lungs, GI tract; half-life 10 hr

INTERACTIONS

⚠ ***Increase:*** serious dysrhythmias—MAOIs, tricyclics

Increase: effects of both products—other sympathomimetics

Decrease: action when used with β-blockers

NURSING CONSIDERATIONS

Assess:

- Respiratory function: B/P, pulse, lung sounds; note sputum color, character; respiratory function tests prior to and during treatment
- I&O ratio; check for urinary retention, frequency, hesitancy
- Cardiac status: hypertension, palpitations, tachycardia
- For paresthesias and coldness of extremities; peripheral blood flow may decrease

Administer:

- Place cap in aerolizer inhaler; the cap is punctured; do not wash aerolizer inhaler
- Pull off cover, twist mouthpiece to open, push buttons in; make sure the four pins are visible; remove cap from blister pack, place cap in chamber; twist to close, press (a click will be heard), release, patient should exhale, place inhaler in mouth, inhale rapidly

Perform/provide:

- Storage at room temperature, protection from heat, moisture

Evaluate:

- Therapeutic response: ease of breathing

Teach patient/family:

- To rinse mouth after use
- Correct use of inhaler; review package insert with patient; to avoid getting aerosol in eyes
- About all aspects of product; to avoid smoking, smoke-filled rooms, persons with respiratory infections

Treatment of overdose: Administration of a β-blocker

fosamprenavir (℞)

(fos-am-pren′a-veer)

Lexiva

Func. class.: Antiretroviral

Chem. class.: Protease inhibitor

Action: A prodrug of amprenavir; inhibits human immunodeficiency virus (HIV) protease, which prevents maturation of the infectious virus

Uses: HIV-1 infection in combination with antiretrovirals

DOSAGE AND ROUTES

Therapy-naïve patients

- *Adult:* **PO** 1400 mg bid without ritonavir or fosamprenavir 1400 mg/day and ritonavir 200 mg/day or fosamprenavir 700 mg bid and ritonavir 100 mg bid

Protease experienced patients (PI)

- *Adult:* **PO** 700 mg bid and ritonavir 100 mg bid

Combination with efavirenz

- *Adult:* **PO** Add another 100 mg/day of ritonavir for a total of 300 mg/day when all three products are given

Hepatic dose

- *Adult:* **PO** (Child-Pugh 5-6) 700 mg bid without ritonavir (treatment-naive patients) or 700 mg bid with ritonavir 100 mg daily (treatment-naive or experienced patients); (Child-Pugh 7-9) 700 mg bid without ritonavir (treatment-naive patients) or 450 mg bid with ritonavir 100 mg daily (treatment-naive or experienced patients); (Child-Pugh 10-15) 350 mg bid without ritonavir (treatment-naive patients) or 300 mg bid with ritonavir 100 mg daily (treatment-naive or experienced patients)

Available forms: Tabs 700 mg (equivalent to 600 mg amprenavir)

SIDE EFFECTS

CNS: Headache, fatigue, depression, oral paresthesia

GI: Nausea, diarrhea, vomiting, abdominal pain

INTEG: Rash, pruritus
MISC: Redistribution or accumulation of body fat, hyperglycemia, **Stevens-Johnson syndrome**
Contraindications: Hypersensitivity to protease inhibitors
Precautions: Pregnancy (C), breastfeeding, geriatric patients, hepatic disease, hemolytic anemia, diabetes, sulfa sensitivity

PHARMACOKINETICS

A prodrug of amprenavir, peak 1½-4 hr; 90% protein binding; metabolized in the liver by cytochrome P4503AY (CYP3A4); excretion of unchanged product is minimal; half-life 7.7 hr

INTERACTIONS

- May affect coagulation: warfarin
- Avoid use with rifampin, delavirdine, H_2 receptor antagonists, estrogens, oral contraceptives, proton-pump inhibitors, carbamazepine, phenobarbital, phenytoin because may lose virologic response and possibly lead to resistance to fosamprenavir

⚠ Serious life-threatening reactions: amiodarone, calcium channel blockers, lidocaine, pimozide, ergots, midazolam, triazolam, flecainide, propafenone
Increase: effect—rifbutin, ketoconazole, itraconazole, sildenafil, vardenafil
Increase: toxicity—HMG-CoA reductase inhibitors
Decrease: effect of oral contraceptives, methadone
Decrease: fosamprenavir levels—nevirapine, antacids, efavirenz, saquinavir, ranitidine, carbamazepine, phenytoin, lopinavir/ritonavir, barbiturates, proton-pump inhibitors, H_2 receptor antagonists
Drug/Herb
- Avoid use with—St. John's wort

Drug/Lab Test
Increase: serum glucose, AST, ALT, triglycerides

NURSING CONSIDERATIONS

Assess:
- Bowel pattern before, during treatment, monitor hydration
- Skin eruptions, rash, urticaria, itching; allergy to sulfonamides, cross sensitivity may occur
- Viral load, CD4 cell counts baseline and throughout treatment

⚠ Stevens-Johnson syndrome; skin reactions, report immediately
Administer:
- Without regard to food

Teach patient/family:
- To avoid taking with other medications unless directed by provider
- That product does not cure, but does manage symptoms and does not prevent transmission of HIV to others
- To use nonhormonal form of birth control while taking this product
- If dose is missed, take as soon as remembered up to 1 hr before next dose; do not double dose
- Not to alter dose or stop therapy without talking to physician
- Advise physician if they have sulfa allergy
- To report all medications, including herbal supplements, to physician
- That patients receiving phosphodiesterase type 5 inhibitors may be at increased risk for PDE5 inhibitor adverse effects

fosaprepitant (℞)
(phos-a-prep′ih-tant)
Emend
Func. class.: Antiemetic
Chem. class.: Miscellaneous

Action: A selective antagonist of human substance P/neurokinin 1 (NK_1) receptors decreasing emetic reflex, prodrug of aprepitant
Uses: Prevention of nausea/vomiting associated with cancer chemotherapy (highly emetogenic/moderately emetogenic) including high-dose cisplatin, used

in combination with other antiemetics; postoperative nausea/vomiting

DOSAGE AND ROUTES

• *Adult:* **IV INF** 115 mg over 15 min, 30 min prior to chemotherapy as an alternative to the 1st dose of aprepitant on day 1 of the aprepitant-CINV regimen

Available forms: Powder for inj 115 mg

SIDE EFFECTS

CNS: Headache, dizziness, insomnia, anxiety, depression, confusion, peripheral neuropathy

CV: Bradycardia, tachycardia, DVT, hypo/hypertension

GI: Diarrhea, constipation, abdominal pain, anorexia, gastritis, increased AST/ALT, *nausea,* vomiting, heartburn

GU: Increased BUN, serum creatine, proteinuria, dysuria

HEMA: Anemia, **thrombocytopenia, neutropenia**

INTEG: Pruritus, rash, urticaria, **anaphylaxis**

MISC: Asthenia, fatigue, dehydration, fever, hiccups, tinnitus, **Stevens-Johnson syndrome**

Contraindications: Hypersensitivity to this product or polysorbate 80

Precautions: Pregnancy (B), breastfeeding, children, geriatric patients, hepatic disease, continuous use for nausea and vomiting not recommended

PHARMACOKINETICS

Rapidly converted to aprepitant (within 30 min), metabolized in liver by CYP3A4 enzymes to an active metabolite, half-life 13 hr, 95% protein bound

INTERACTIONS

Increase: aprepitant action—CYP3A4 inhibitors (ketoconazole, itraconazole, nefazodone, troleandomycin, clarithromycin, ritonavir, nelfinavir, diltiazem)

Increase: action of CYP3A4 substrates (pimozide, cisapride, dexamethasone, terfenadine, astemizole, methylPREDNISolone, midazolam, alprazolam, triazolam, docetaxel, paclitaxel, etoposide, irinotecan, imatinib, ifosfamide, vinorelbine, vinBLAStine, vinCRIStine)

Decrease: aprepitant action—CYP3A4 inducers (rifampin, carbamazepine, phenytoin)

Decrease: action of CYP2C9 substrates (warfarin, tolbutamide, phenytoin), hormonal contraceptives

Decrease: action of both products—paroxetine

Drug/Food

Decrease: effect—grapefruit juice

NURSING CONSIDERATIONS

Assess:

• CV status: hyper/hypotension, bradycardia, tachycardia, DVT

• For absence of nausea, vomiting during chemotherapy

• LFTs

Administer:

IV INF route

• Give IV route

• Only approved as a substitute for the 1st dose of aprepitant in 3-day regimen

• Reconstitution: use aseptic technique; inject 5 ml 0.9% NaCl into the vial, directing stream to wall of vial to prevent foam; swirl; do not shake

• Prepare inf bag with 110 ml NS; do not dilute or reconstitute with any divalent cations such as calcium, magnesium, including LR, Hartmann's sol

• Withdraw the entire volume from vial and transfer to infusion bag; total volume 115 ml (1 mg/1 ml)

• Gently invert bag 2-3 times; reconstituted sol is stable for 24 hr at lower room temperature or <25° C

• Visually inspect for particulates and discoloration

• Infuse over 15 min

Evaluate:

• Therapeutic response: absence of nausea, vomiting during cancer chemotherapy

Teach patient/family:

• To report diarrhea, constipation

• To report all medications and herbals

to prescriber prior to taking this medication
- To use nonhormonal form of contraception while taking this agent; oral contraceptive effect may be decreased
- To have clotting monitored closely during 2 wk period following administration of aprepitant if on warfarin
- To avoid breastfeeding

foscarnet (℞)
(foss-kar′net)
Foscavir
Func. class.: Antiviral
Chem. class.: Inorganic pyrophosphate organic analog

Action: Antiviral activity is produced by selective inhibition at the pyrophosphate binding site on virus-specific DNA polymerases and reverse transcriptases at concentrations that do not affect cellular DNA polymerases
Uses: Treatment of CMV retinitis, HSV infections, used with ganciclovir for relapsing patients

DOSAGE AND ROUTES
CMV retinitis
- *Adult:* **IV INF** 60 mg/kg given over at least 1 hr, q8hr × 2-3 wk or 90 mg/kg q12hr; usually give with at least 750-1000 ml **NS** daily

HSV
- *Adult:* **IV** 40 mg/kg q8-12hr × 2-3 wk

Renal dose
- *Adult:* **IV**

Male:

$$\frac{140 - \text{age}}{\text{serum creatinine} \times 72} = \text{CCr}$$

Female: 0.85 × above value
Dose based on table provided in package insert
Available forms: Inj 6000 mg/250 ml, 12,000 mg/500 ml (24 mg/ml)

SIDE EFFECTS
CNS: *Fever*, dizziness, *headache*, **seizures,** *fatigue*, neuropathy, tremor, ataxia, dementia, stupor, EEG abnormalities, vertigo, **coma,** abnormal gait, hypertonia, EPS, hemiparesis, **paralysis,** hyperreflexia, paraplegia, **tetany,** hyporeflexia, neuralgia, neuritis, **cerebral edema,** *paresthesia*, depression, *confusion*, *anxiety*, insomnia, somnolence, amnesia, hallucinations, agitation
CV: Hypertension, palpitations, ECG abnormalities, 1st-degree AV block, nonspecific ST-T segment changes, hypotension, cerebrovascular disorder, cardiomyopathy, **cardiac arrest,** bradycardia, dysrhythmias
EENT: Visual field defects, vocal cord paralysis, speech disorders, taste perversion, eye pain, conjunctivitis, tinnitus, otitis
GI: *Nausea*, *vomiting*, *diarrhea*, *anorexia*, abdominal pain, constipation, dysphagia, rectal hemorrhage, dry mouth, melena, flatulence, ulcerative stomatitis, pancreatitis, enteritis, enterocolitis, glossitis, proctitis, stomatitis, increased amylases, gastroenteritis, **pseudomembranous colitis,** duodenal ulcer, **paralytic ileus, esophageal ulceration,** abnormal A-G ratio, increased AST, ALT, cholecystitis, **hepatitis,** dyspepsia, tenesmus, hepatosplenomegaly, jaundice
GU: **Acute renal failure,** decreased CCr and increased serum creatinine, **glomerulonephritis, toxic nephropathy, nephrosis, renal tubular disorders, pyelonephritis, uremia, hematuria, albuminuria,** dysuria, polyuria
HEMA: *Anemia*, **granulocytopenia, leukopenia, thrombocytopenia,** platelet abnormalities, **thrombosis, pulmonary embolism, coagulation disorders, decreased prothrombin, hypochromic anemia, pancytopenia, hemolysis, leukocytosis,** lymphadenopathy, epistaxis, lymphopenia
INTEG: *Rash*, sweating, pruritus, skin ulceration, seborrhea, skin discoloration, alopecia, acne, dermatitis, pain/inflammation at inj site, facial edema, dry skin, urticaria
MS: Arthralgia, myalgia

RESP: Coughing, dyspnea, pneumonia, sinusitis, pharyngitis, **pulmonary infiltration,** stridor, **pneumothorax, hemoptysis, bronchospasm,** bronchitis, **respiratory depression, pleural effusion, pulmonary hemorrhage,** rhinitis

SYST: Hypokalemia, hypocalcemia, hypomagnesemia; increased alk phos, LDH, BUN; acidosis, hypophosphatemia, hyperphosphatemia, dehydration, glycosuria, increased CPK, hypervolemia, infection, **sepsis, death, ascites,** hyponatremia, hypochloremia, hypercalcemia

Contraindications: Hypersensitivity, CCr <0.4 ml/min/kg

Precautions: Pregnancy (C), breastfeeding, children, geriatric patients, seizure disorders, severe anemia

Black Box Warning: Renal disease, electrolyte/mineral imbalances

PHARMACOKINETICS

14%-17% protein bound, half-life 18-88 hr in normal renal function, 79%-92% excreted via kidneys

INTERACTIONS

Increase: nephrotoxicity—aminoglycosides, amphotericin B, NSAIDs, lithium, cycloSPORINE

Increase: hypocalcemia—pentamidine

NURSING CONSIDERATIONS

Assess:

General

- Renal, hepatic studies: BUN, creatinine, AST, ALT
- I&O ratio, urine pH, serum creatinine baseline, 3×/wk during initial therapy, then 2×/wk thereafter; CCr baseline, throughout treatment; if CCr <0.4 ml/min/kg, discontinue
- Blood counts q2wk; watch for decreasing granulocytes, Hgb; if low, therapy may have to be discontinued and restarted after hematologic recovery; blood transfusions may be required
- Lesions in HSV
- Electrolytes and minerals (Ca, P, Mg, Na, K); watch closely for tetany during first administration
- GI symptoms: nausea, vomiting, diarrhea; severe symptoms may necessitate discontinuing product
- ⚠ Blood dyscrasias (anemia, granulocytopenia); bruising, fatigue, bleeding, poor healing
- Allergic reactions: flushing, rash, urticaria, pruritus

CMV retinitis

- Culture should be done prior to treatment (blood, urine, throat); a negative culture does not rule out CMV
- Ophthalmic exam should confirm diagnosis

Administer:

- Increased fluids before and during product administration to induce diuresis and minimize renal toxicity

Intermittent IV INF route

- Using inf device, at no more than 1 mg/kg/min; do not give by rapid or bolus IV; give by CVP or peripheral vein; standard 24 mg/ml sol may be used without dilution if using by CVP; dilute the 24 mg/ml sol to 12 mg/ml with D_5W or NS if using peripheral vein

Y-site compatibilities: Aldesleukin, amikacin, aminophylline, ampicillin, aztreonam, benzquinamide, cefazolin, cefoperazone, cefoxitin, ceftazidime, ceftizoxime, ceftriaxone, cefuroxime, chloramphenicol, cimetidine, clindamycin, dexamethasone, DOPamine, erythromycin, fluconazole, flucytosine, furosemide, gentamicin, heparin, hydrocortisone, hydromorphone, hydrOXYzine, imipenem-cilastatin, metoclopramide, metronidazole, miconazole, morphine, nafcillin, oxacillin, penicillin G potassium, phenytoin, piperacillin, ranitidine, ticarcillin/clavulanate, tobramycin

Perform/provide:

- Regular ophthalmologic exams
- Close monitoring during therapy for tingling, numbness, paresthesias; if these occur, stop inf, obtain lab sample for electrolytes

Evaluate:
- Therapeutic response: improvement in CMV retinitis

Teach patient/family:
- To call prescriber if sore throat, swollen lymph nodes, malaise, fever occur, since other infections may occur
- To report perioral tingling, numbness in extremities, and paresthesias
- That serious product interactions may occur if OTC products are ingested; check first with prescriber
- That product is not a cure but will control symptoms

fosinopril (℞)

(foss'in-oh-pril)
Monopril
Func. class.: Antihypertensive
Chem. class.: Angiotensin-converting enzyme (ACE) inhibitor

Do not confuse:
Monopril/minoxidil/Accupril/Monoket

Action: Selectively suppresses renin-angiotensin-aldosterone system; inhibits ACE; prevents conversion of angiotensin I to angiotensin II; results in dilation of arterial, venous vessels

Uses: Hypertension, alone or in combination with thiazide diuretics, systolic CHF

DOSAGE AND ROUTES

CHF
- *Adult:* **PO** 10 mg/day, then up to 40 mg/day increased over several weeks; use lower dose in those diuresed before fosinopril

Hypertension
- *Adult:* **PO** 10 mg/day initially, then 20-40 mg/day divided bid or daily, max 80 mg/day

Available forms: Tabs 10, 20, 40 mg

SIDE EFFECTS

CNS: Insomnia, paresthesia, headache, dizziness, fatigue, memory disturbance, tremor, mood change

CV: Hypotension, chest pain, palpitations, angina, orthostatic hypotension, dysrhythmias, tachycardia

GI: Nausea, constipation, vomiting, diarrhea

GU: **Proteinuria,** increased BUN, creatinine, decreased libido

HEMA: Decreased Hct, Hgb; **eosinophilia, leukopenia, neutropenia**

INTEG: **Angioedema,** rash, flushing, sweating, photosensitivity, pruritus

META: Hyperkalemia

MS: Arthralgia, myalgia

RESP: Cough, sinusitis, dyspnea, **bronchospasm**

Contraindications: Breastfeeding, children, hypersensitivity to ACE inhibitors

Black Box Warning: Pregnancy (D)

Precautions: Geriatric patients, impaired hepatic function, hypovolemia, blood dyscrasias, CHF, COPD, asthma, angioedema, hyperkalemia, renal artery stenosis, renal disease

PHARMACOKINETICS

Peak 3 hr, serum protein binding 97%, half-life 11.5-14 hr, metabolized by liver (metabolites excreted in urine, feces)

INTERACTIONS

Increase: hypersensitivity reactions—allopurinol

Increase: hypotension—diuretics, other antihypertensives, ganglionic blockers, adrenergic blockers, phenothiazines, nitrates, acute alcohol ingestion

Increase: toxicity—vasodilators, hydrALAZINE, prazosin, potassium-sparing diuretics, sympathomimetics, digoxin, lithium

Decrease: absorption—antacids

Decrease: antihypertensive effect—indomethacin, NSAIDs, salicylates

Drug/Herb

⚠ ***Increase:*** fatal hypokalemia—arginine

Increase: severe photosensitivity—St. John's wort

Increase: antihypertensive effect—hawthorn, pill-bearing spurge
Decrease: antihypertensive effect—pineapple, yohimbe
Drug/Lab Test
Increase: AST, ALT, alk phos, glucose, bilirubin, uric acid
False positive: urine acetone
Positive: ANA titer

NURSING CONSIDERATIONS

Assess:

- Blood studies: neutrophils, decreased platelets; obtain WBC with differential baseline and q mo × 6 mo, then q2-3mo × 1 yr; if neutrophils <1000/mm^3, discontinue (recommended in collagen-vascular disease)
- B/P, orthostatic hypotension, syncope
- Renal studies: protein, BUN, creatinine; increased levels may indicate nephrotic syndrome
- Baselines in renal, hepatic studies before therapy begins
- Potassium levels, although hyperkalemia rarely occurs
- Edema in feet, legs daily; weigh daily in CHF
- Allergic reactions: rash, fever, pruritus, urticaria; product should be discontinued if antihistamines fail to help

Administer:

- May be taken without regard to meals

Perform/provide:

- Storage in tight container at 86° F (30° C) or less
- Supine position for severe hypotension

Evaluate:

- Therapeutic response: decrease in B/P

Teach patient/family:

- Not to discontinue product abruptly; take at same time of day
- Not to use OTC products (cough, cold, allergy) unless directed by prescriber; not to use salt substitutes containing potassium without consulting prescriber
- The importance of complying with dosage schedule, even if feeling better
- To rise slowly to sitting or standing position to minimize orthostatic hypotension
- To notify prescriber of mouth sores, sore throat, fever, swelling of hands or feet, irregular heartbeat, chest pain, nonproductive cough
- To report excessive perspiration, dehydration, vomiting, diarrhea; may lead to fall in B/P
- That product may cause dizziness, fainting, light-headedness during first few days of therapy
- That product may cause skin rash or impaired perspiration
- How to take B/P; normal readings for age-group
- To notify prescriber if pregnancy is planned or suspected

Treatment of overdose: 0.9% NaCl IV inf, hemodialysis

fosphenytoin (℞)

(foss-fen′i-toy-in)
Cerebyx
Func. class.: Anticonvulsant
Chem. class.: Hydantoin, phosphate phenytoin ester

Action: Inhibits spread of seizure activity in motor cortex by altering ion transport; increases AV conduction, prodrug of phenytoin
Uses: Generalized tonic-clonic seizures, status epilepticus, partial seizures

DOSAGE AND ROUTES

All doses in PE (phenytoin sodium equivalent)

Status epilepticus

- *Adult and adolescent:* **IV** 15-20 mg PE/kg
- *Child <12 yr (unlabeled):* **IV** 15-20 mg PE/kg

Nonemergency/maintenance dosing

- *Adult and adolescent >16 yr:* **IM/IV** 10-20 mg PE/kg; 4-6 mg PE/kg/day (maintenance); start maintenance 12 hr after loading dose; give in 2-3 divided doses

Available forms: Inj 150 mg (100 mg phenytoin equiv), 750 mg (500 mg phenytoin equiv), 50-mg/ml vials

SIDE EFFECTS

CNS: Drowsiness, dizziness, insomnia, paresthesias, depression, **suicidal tendencies,** aggression, headache, confusion, paresthesia
CV: Hypo/hypertension, **ventricular fibrillation, CHF, shock**
EENT: Nystagmus, diplopia, blurred vision
GI: Nausea, vomiting, diarrhea, constipation, anorexia, weight loss, hepatitis, jaundice, gingival hyperplasia
HEMA: **Agranulocytosis, leukopenia, aplastic anemia, thrombocytopenia, megaloblastic anemia**
INTEG: Rash, lupus erythematosus, **Stevens-Johnson syndrome,** hirsutism, hypersensitivity, pruritus
SYST: Hyperglycemia, hypokalemia, SJS/TEN (Asian patients positive for HLA-B 1502)

Contraindications: Pregnancy (D), hypersensitivity, psychiatric conditions, bradycardia, SA and AV block, Stokes-Adams syndrome, absence seizures

Precautions: Breastfeeding, allergies, renal/hepatic disease, myocardial insufficiency, hypoalbuminemia, hypothyroidism, Asian patients positive for HLA-B 1502

PHARMACOKINETICS

Metabolized by liver, excreted by kidneys, protein binding 99%, converted to phenytoin

INTERACTIONS

Increase: fosphenytoin level—cimetidine, amiodarone, chloramphenicol, estrogens, H_2 antagonists, phenothiazines, salicylates, sulfonamides, tricyclics, CYP1A2 inhibitors

Decrease: fosphenytoin effects—alcohol (chronic use), antihistamines, antacids, tramadol, antineoplastics, rifampin, folic acid, carbamazepine, theophylline, CYP1A2 inducers

Drug/Herb

Increase: anticonvulsant effect—ginkgo

Decrease: anticonvulsant effect—ginseng, santonica, valerian

Drug/Lab Test

Increase: glucose, alk phos

Decrease: dexamethasone, metyrapone test serum, PBI, urinary steroids

NURSING CONSIDERATIONS

Assess:

- Product level: therapeutic level 10-20 mcg/ml, toxic level 30-50 mcg/ml, wait at least 2 hr after dose before testing, 4 hr after IM dose
- Blood studies: CBC, platelets q2wk until stabilized, then q mo × 12 mo, then q3mo; discontinue product if neutrophils <1600/mm^3; serum calcium, albumin, phosphorus
- ⚠ Mental status: mood, sensorium, affect, memory (long, short), suicidal thoughts/behaviors
- Seizure activity including type, location, duration, and character; provide seizure precaution
- Renal studies: urinalysis, BUN, urine creatinine
- Hepatic studies: ALT, AST, bilirubin, creatinine
- Allergic reaction: red, raised rash; if this occurs, product should be discontinued
- For toxicity: bone marrow depression, nausea, vomiting, ataxia, diplopia, cardiovascular collapse, slurred speech, confusion
- Respiratory depression; rate, depth, character of respirations
- ⚠ Blood dyscrasias: fever, sore throat, bruising, rash, jaundice
- Continuous monitoring of ECG, B/P, respiratory function
- Rash, discontinue as soon as rash develops, serious adverse reactions such as Stevens-Johnson syndrome can occur

Administer:

IV, direct route

- Dilute product in D_5W or 0.9% NaCl (1.5-25 mg PE/ml); give at a rate of <150 mg PE/min (adult) or <3 mg PE/kg/min (child)

Y-site compatibilities: Esmolol, famotidine, foscarnet, lorazepam

Additive compatibilities: Potassium chloride

Solution compatibilities: D_5W, $D_{10}W$, amino acid inj 10%, D_5LR, D_5/0.9% NaCl, Plasmalyte A, LR, sterile water for inj

Evaluate:

- Therapeutic response: decrease in severity of seizures

Teach patient/family:

- The reason for and expected outcome of treatment
- Not to use machinery or engage in hazardous activity, as drowsiness, dizziness may occur
- To carry emergency ID denoting product use, name of prescriber
- To notify prescriber of rash, bleeding, bruising, slurred speech, jaundice of skin or eyes, joint pain, nausea, vomiting, severe headaches
- To keep all medical appointments, including lab work, physical assessment
- To notify prescriber if pregnancy is planned, suspected
- To use contraception while using this product

fospropofol

See Appendix A—Selected New Drugs

frovatriptan (℞)

(froh-vah-trip′tan)

Frova

Func. class.: Antimigraine agent

Chem. class.: 5-HT_1-Receptor agonist

Action: Binds selectively to the vascular 5-HT_{1B}, 5-HT_{1D} receptor subtypes, exerts antimigraine effect; binds to benzodiazepine receptor sites, causes vasoconstriction in cranium

Uses: Acute treatment of migraine with or without aura

DOSAGE AND ROUTES

- *Adult:* **PO** 2.5 mg, a 2nd dose may be taken after ≥2 hr; max 3 tabs (7.5 mg/day)

Available form: Tabs 2.5 mg

SIDE EFFECTS

CNS: Hot/cold sensation, paresthesia, *dizziness,* headache, fatigue, insomnia, anxiety, somnolence, **seizures**

CV: Flushing, chest pain, palpitation

GI: Dry mouth, dyspepsia, abdominal pain, diarrhea, vomiting, nausea

MS: Skeletal pain

Contraindications: Hypersensitivity, angina pectoris, history of MI, documented silent ischemia, Prinzmetal's angina, ischemic heart disease; concurrent ergotamine-containing preparations; uncontrolled hypertension; basilar or hemiplegic migraine; ischemic bowel disease; peripheral vascular disease, severe hepatic disease, prophylactic migraine treatment

Precautions: Pregnancy (C), breastfeeding, children, geriatric patients, postmenopausal women, men >40 yr, risk factors for CAD, hypercholesterolemia, obesity, diabetes, impaired hepatic function, seizure disorder

PHARMACOKINETICS

Onset of pain relief 2-3 hr, terminal half-life 25-29 hr, protein binding 15%, metabolized liver CYP450 1A2 enzyme system

INTERACTIONS

Increase: frovatriptan levels—CYP1A2 inhibitors (cimetidine, ciprofloxacin, erythromycin), estrogen, propranolol, oral contraceptives

Increase: toxicity—SSRIs, other serotonin agonists (dextromethorphan, tramadol, antidepressants)

Drug/Herb

Increase: effect—butterbur

NURSING CONSIDERATIONS

Assess:

- Migraine symptoms: aura, unable to view light
- B/P; signs/symptoms of coronary vasospasms
- For stress level, activity, recreation, coping mechanisms
- Ingestion of tyramine-containing foods (pickled products, beer, wine, aged cheese), food additives, preservatives, colorings, artificial sweeteners, chocolate, caffeine, which may precipitate these types of headaches

Administer:

- Swallow tabs whole; do not break, crush, or chew
- With fluids
- 2 days/wk or less; rebound headache may occur

Perform/provide:

- Quiet, calm environment with decreased stimulation from noise, bright light, excessive talking

Evaluate:

- Therapeutic response: decrease in frequency, severity of migraine

Teach patient/family:

- To report any side effects to prescriber
- To use contraception while taking product; inform prescriber if pregnant or intend to become pregnant
- Consult prescriber if breastfeeding

fulvestrant (℞)

(full-vess′trant)

Faslodex

Func. class.: Antineoplastic

Chem. class.: Estrogen-receptor antagonist

Action: Inhibits cell division by binding to cytoplasmic estrogen receptors, downregulates estrogen receptors

Uses: Advanced breast carcinoma in estrogen-receptor-positive patients (usually postmenopausal)

Unlabeled uses: Loading dose in metastatic breast cancer

DOSAGE AND ROUTES

- *Adult:* **IM** 250 mg q mo

Available forms: Inj 50 mg/ml

SIDE EFFECTS

CNS: Headache, depression, dizziness, insomnia, paresthesia, anxiety

GI: Nausea, vomiting, anorexia, constipation, diarrhea, abdominal pain

HEMA: **Anemia**

INTEG: Rash, sweating, hot flashes, inj site pain

MS: Bone pain, arthritis, back pain

RESP: Pharyngitis, dyspnea, cough

SYST: **Angioedema**

Contraindications: Pregnancy (D), breastfeeding, children, hypersensitivity

Precautions: Hepatic disease

PHARMACOKINETICS

Half-life 40 days, metabolized by CYP3A4, excretion feces 90%

NURSING CONSIDERATIONS

Assess:

- For side effects, report to prescriber

Administer:

IM route

- IM 5 ml as a single inj or 2, 2.5 ml inj; give slowly in buttock
- Antiemetic 30-60 min before giving product to prevent vomiting prn

Perform/provide:

- Liquid diet, if needed, including cola, gelatin; dry toast or crackers may be added if patient is not nauseated or vomiting
- Nutritious diet with iron, vitamin supplements as ordered
- Store in refrigerator, protect from light

Evaluate:

- Therapeutic response: decreased tumor size, spread of malignancy

Teach patient/family:

- To report any complaints, side effects to prescriber
- To report vaginal bleeding immediately
- That tumor flare—increase in size of tumor, increased bone pain—may occur and will subside rapidly; may take analgesics for pain

• That premenopausal women must use mechanical birth control because ovulation may be induced; do not breastfeed
• To use contraception to prevent pregnancy; pregnancy category (D)

furosemide (℞)

(fur-oh'se-mide)
Apo-Furosemide ♣, Furoside ♣, Lasix, Lasix Special ♣, Myrosemide ♣, Novosemide ♣, Uritol ♣

Func. class.: Loop diuretic
Chem. class.: Sulfonamide derivative

Do not confuse:
furosemide/torsemide
Lasix/Luvox/Lomotil/Lanoxin

Action: Inhibits reabsorption of sodium and chloride at proximal and distal tubule and in the loop of Henle

Uses: Pulmonary edema; edema in CHF, hepatic disease, nephrotic syndrome, ascites, hypertension

Unlabeled uses: Hypercalcemia in malignancy, hypertensive emergency/urgency, pulmonary edema or prevention of hemodynamic effects associated with blood product transfusion

DOSAGE AND ROUTES

Edema

• *Adult:* **PO** 20-80 mg/day in AM; may give another dose in 6 hr up to 600 mg/day; **IM/IV** 20-40 mg, increased by 20 mg q2hr until desired response
• *Child:* **PO/IM/IV** 2 mg/kg; may increase by 1-2 mg/kg/q6-8hr up to 6 mg/kg

Acute pulmonary edema

• *Adult:* **IV** 40 mg given over several min, repeated in 1 hr; increase to 80 mg if needed

Hypertensive crisis/acute renal failure

• *Adult:* **IV** 100-200 mg over 1-2 min

Antihypercalcemia

• *Adult:* **IM/IV** 80-100 mg q1-4hr or **PO** 120 mg/day or divided bid
• *Child:* **IM/IV** 25-50 mg, repeat q4hr if needed

Hypertensive emergency/urgency (unlabeled)

• *Adult:* **IV** 40-80 mg

Pulmonary edema/prevention of adverse hemodynamic effects associated with blood product transfusion (unlabeled)

• *Adult:* **IV** 40 mg injected slowly, then 80 mg injected slowly in 2 hr if needed
• *Child:* **IM/IV** 1-2 mg/kg q6-12hr
• *Premature neonate >32 wk postconceptional age:* **IM/IV** 1-2 mg/kg q12-24hr
• *Premature neonate ≤32 wk postconceptional age:* **IM/IV** Max 1 mg/kg q≤24hr

Available forms: Tabs 20, 40, 80 mg; oral sol 8 mg/ml, 10 mg/ml; inj 10 mg/ml

SIDE EFFECTS

CNS: Headache, fatigue, weakness, vertigo, paresthesias
CV: Orthostatic hypotension, chest pain, ECG changes, **circulatory collapse**
EENT: Loss of hearing, ear pain, tinnitus, blurred vision
ELECT: Hypokalemia, hypochloremic alkalosis, hypomagnesemia, hyperuricemia, hypocalcemia, hyponatremia, metabolic alkalosis
ENDO: Hyperglycemia
GI: Nausea, diarrhea, dry mouth, vomiting, anorexia, cramps, oral, gastric irritations, pancreatitis
GU: Polyuria, **renal failure,** glycosuria
HEMA: **Thrombocytopenia, agranulocytosis, leukopenia, neutropenia, anemia**
INTEG: Rash, pruritus, purpura, **Stevens-Johnson syndrome,** sweating, photosensitivity, urticaria
MS: Cramps, stiffness

Contraindications: Breastfeeding, infants, hypersensitivity to sulfonamides, anuria, hypovolemia, electrolyte depletion

Precautions: Pregnancy (C), diabetes mellitus, dehydration, severe renal disease, cirrhosis, ascites

PHARMACOKINETICS

PO: Onset 1 hr, peak 1-2 hr, duration 6-8 hr, absorbed 70%
IV: Onset 5 min; peak ½ hr; duration 2 hr (metabolized by the liver 30%); excreted in urine, some as unchanged product, feces; crosses placenta; excreted in breast milk; half-life ½-1 hr

INTERACTIONS

Increase: toxicity—lithium, nondepolarizing skeletal muscle relaxants, digoxin
Increase: hypotensive action of antihypertensives, nitrates
Increase: ototoxicity—aminoglycosides, cisplatin, vancomycin
Increase: effects of anticoagulants, salicylates
Decrease: furosemide effect—probenecid

Drug/Herb

- Severe photosensitivity: St. John's wort

Increase: diuretic effect—aloe, cucumber, dandelion, khella, horsetail, pumpkin, Queen Anne's lace

Drug/Lab Test

Interference: GTT
Increase: LDL

NURSING CONSIDERATIONS

Assess:

- Signs of metabolic alkalosis: drowsiness, restlessness
- Signs of hypokalemia: postural hypotension, malaise, fatigue, tachycardia, leg cramps, weakness
- Rashes, temp elevation daily
- Confusion, especially in geriatric patients; take safety precautions if needed
- Hearing, including tinnitus and hearing loss, when giving high doses for extended periods
- Weight, I&O daily to determine fluid loss; effect of product may be decreased if used daily
- Rate, depth, rhythm of respiration, effect of exertion, lung sounds
- B/P lying, standing; postural hypotension may occur
- Electrolytes (K, Na, Cl); include BUN, blood glucose, CBC, serum creatinine, blood pH, ABGs, uric acid, calcium, magnesium
- Skin turgor, edema, condition of mucous membranes in mouth and nose
- Glucose in urine if patient is diabetic
- Allergies to sulfonamides, thiazides

Administer:

- In AM to avoid interference with sleep if using product as a diuretic
- Potassium replacement if potassium <3 mg/dl
- PO with food if nausea occurs; absorption may be decreased slightly; tabs may be crushed

IV route

- Undiluted; may be given through Y-tube or 3-way stopcock; give 20 mg or less/min; may be added to NS or D_5W if large doses are required and given as IV inf, max 4 mg/min; use inf pump

Additive compatibilities: Amikacin, aminophylline, ampicillin, atropine, bumetanide, calcium gluconate, cefamandole, cefoperazone, cefuroxime, cimetidine, cloxacillin, dexamethasone, diamorphine, digoxin, epinephrine, heparin, isosorbide, kanamycin, lidocaine, meropenem, morphine, nitroglycerin, penicillin G, potassium chloride, ranitidine, scopolamine, sodium bicarbonate, theophylline, tobramycin, verapamil

Syringe compatibilities: Bleomycin, cisplatin, cyclophosphamide, fluorouracil, heparin, leucovorin, methotrexate, mitomycin

Y-site compatibilities: Allopurinol, amifostine, amikacin, amphotericin B cholesteryl, aztreonam, bleomycin, cefepime, cisplatin, cladribine, cyclophosphamide, cytarabine, docetaxel, DOXOrubicin liposome, epinephrine, fentanyl, fludarabine, fluorouracil, foscarnet, granisetron, heparin, hydrocortisone, hydromorphone, indomethacin, kanamycin, leucovorin, linezolid, lorazepam, melphalan, meropenem, methotrexate, mitomycin, nitroglycerin, norepinephrine, paclitaxel, piperacillin/tazobactam, potassium chloride, propofol, ranitidine, remifentanil, sargramostim, tacrolimus, teniposide, thiotepa, tobramycin, tolazoline, vit B/C

Perform/provide:

• Increased fluid intake 2-3 L/day unless contraindicated

Evaluate:

• Therapeutic response: improvement in edema of feet, legs, sacral area (CHF); increase urine output, decreased B/P; decreased calcium levels (hypercalcemia)

Teach patient/family:

• To discuss the need for a high-potassium diet or potassium replacement with prescriber

• To rise slowly from lying or sitting position; orthostatic hypotension may occur

• To recognize adverse reactions that may occur: muscle cramps, weakness, nausea, dizziness

• Regarding entire regimen, including exercise, diet, stress relief for hypertension

• To take with food or milk for GI symptoms

• To use sunscreen or protective clothing to prevent photosensitivity

• To take early in day to prevent sleeplessness

• To avoid OTC medication unless directed by prescriber

Treatment of overdose: Lavage if taken orally; monitor electrolytes; administer dextrose in saline; monitor hydration, CV, renal status

gabapentin (℞)

(gab'a-pen-tin)

Neurontin

Func. class.: Anticonvulsant

Do not confuse:

Neurontin/Noroxin/Neoral

Action: Mechanism unknown; may increase seizure threshold; structurally similar to GABA; gabapentin binding sites in neocortex, hippocampus

Uses: Adjunct treatment of partial seizures, with or without generalization in patients >12 yr; adjunct in partial seizures in children 3-12 yr, postherpetic neuralgia

Unlabeled uses: Tremors in multiple sclerosis, neuropathic pain, bipolar disorder, migraine prophylaxis, diabetic neuropathy, nystagmus, pruritus, spasticity, menopause, hot flashes

DOSAGE AND ROUTES

• *Adult and child >12 yr:* **PO** 900-1800 mg/day in 3 divided doses; may titrate by giving 300 mg on first day, 300 mg bid on second day, 300 mg tid on third day; may increase to 1800-2400 mg/day by adding 300 mg on subsequent days

• *Child 5-12 yr:* **PO** 10-15 mg/kg/day in 3 divided doses, initially titrate dose upward over approximately 3 days; 25-35 mg/kg/day; all given in 3 divided doses

• *Child 3-4 yr:* **PO** 10-15 mg/kg/day in 3 divided doses, initially titrate dose upward over approximately 3 days; 40 mg/kg/day; all given in 3 divided doses

Postherpetic neuralgia

• *Adult:* **PO** 300 mg on day 1, 600 mg/day divided bid on day 2, 900 mg/day divided tid, may titrate to 1800-3600 mg divided tid if needed

Renal dose

• *Adult and child >12 yr:* CCr 30-60 ml/min 300 mg bid, CCr 15-30 ml/min 400-1400 mg/day divided, CCr <15 ml/min 125 mg/day; CCr 15-30 ml/min 200-700 mg daily; CCr <15 ml/min 100-300 mg daily

Uremic pruritus in hemodialysis (unlabeled)

• *Adult:* **PO** 300 mg 3×/wk

Brachioradical pruritus (unlabeled)

• *Adult:* **PO** 300-1800 mg/day

Available forms: Caps 100, 300, 400 mg; tabs 600, 800 mg; oral sol 250 mg/5 ml

SIDE EFFECTS

CNS: Drowsiness, confusion, dizziness, fatigue, anxiety, somnolence, ataxia, amnesia, abnormal thinking, unsteady gait, *depression;* children 3-12 yr old, emotional lability, aggression, thought disorder, hyperkinesia, hostility, **seizures, suicidal ideation**

CV: Vasodilation, peripheral edema, hypotension

EENT: Dry mouth, blurred vision, *diplopia,* nystagmus

GI: Constipation, increased appetite, dental abnormalities, nausea, vomiting
GU: Impotence, bleeding, *UTI*
HEMA: **Leukopenia,** decreased WBC
INTEG: Pruritus, abrasion, **Stevens-Johnson syndrome**
MS: Myalgia
RESP: ***Rhinitis,*** pharyngitis, cough
Contraindications: Hypersensitivity to this product
Precautions: Pregnancy (C), breastfeeding, children <12 yr, geriatric patients, renal disease, hemodialysis

PHARMACOKINETICS

Largely unbound to plasma proteins; not metabolized; excreted in urine (unchanged); elimination half-life 5-7 hr; prolonged to 130 hr in ESRD

INTERACTIONS

Increase: CNS depression—alcohol, sedatives, antihistamines, all other CNS depressants
Decrease: gabapentin levels—antacids, sevelamar, ketorolac
Drug/Herb
Increase: CNS depression—chamomile, hops, kava, skullcap, valerian
Drug/Lab Test
False positive: urinary protein using Ames N-multistix SG

NURSING CONSIDERATIONS

Assess:
- Seizures: aura, location, duration, activity at onset
- Pain: location, duration, characteristics if using for chronic pain
- Renal studies: urinalysis, BUN, urine creatinine q3mo
- Description of seizures; location, duration, characteristics

⚠ Mental status: mood, sensorium, affect, behavioral changes, suicidal thoughts/behaviors; if mental status changes, notify prescriber
- Eye problems, need for ophthalmic exam before, during, after treatment (slit lamp, funduscopy, tonometry)

Administer:
- Do not crush or chew caps; caps may be opened and contents put in applesauce or dissolved in juice
- 2 hr apart when giving antacids
- Give without regard to meals
- Gradually withdraw over 7 days, abrupt withdrawal may precipitate seizures

Perform/provide:
- Storage at room temperature away from heat and light
- Hard candy, frequent rinsing of mouth, gum for dry mouth
- Assistance with ambulation during early part of treatment; dizziness occurs
- Seizure precautions: padded side rails; move objects that may harm patient
- Increased fluids, bulk in diet for constipation

Evaluate:
- Therapeutic response: decreased seizure activity; decrease in chronic pain

Teach patient/family:
- To carry emergency ID stating patient's name, products taken, condition, prescriber's name and phone number
- To avoid driving, other activities that require alertness: dizziness, drowsiness may occur
- Not to discontinue medication quickly after long-term use, taper over ≥1 wk; withdrawal-precipitated seizures may occur, not to double doses if dose is missed, take if 2 hr or more before next dose
- To notify prescriber if pregnancy planned or suspected, avoid breastfeeding

Treatment of overdose: Lavage, VS

galantamine (℞)

(gah-lan'tah-meen)
Razadyne, Razadyne ER
Func. class.: Anti-Alzheimer agent, centrally acting cholinesterase inhibitor

Action: Enhances cholinergic functioning by increasing acetylcholine in cerebral cortex

Uses: Mild to moderate dementia of Alzheimer's disease

Unlabeled uses: Vascular dementia, dementia with Lewy bodies, Pick's disease

DOSAGE AND ROUTES

• *Adult:* **PO** 4 mg bid with morning and evening meals; after 4 wk or more may increase to 8 mg bid; may increase to 12 mg bid after another 4 wk, usual dose 16-24 mg/day in 2 divided doses; **EXT REL** 8 mg/day in AM; may increase to 16 mg/day after 4 wk, and 24 mg/day after another 4 wk

Hepatic dose

• *Adult:* **PO** (Child-Pugh 7-9) Max 16 mg/day; (Child-Pugh 10-15) avoid use

Renal dose

• *Adult:* **PO** CCr 10-70 ml/min, max 16 mg/day; CCr <9 ml/min, avoid use

Available forms: Tabs 4, 8, 12 mg; ext rel tabs 8, 16, 24 mg; oral sol 4 mg/ml

SIDE EFFECTS

CNS: Tremors, insomnia, depression, dizziness, headache, somnolence, fatigue

CV: Bradycardia, chest pain

GI: Nausea, vomiting, anorexia, abdominal distress, flatulence, diarrhea

GU: Urinary incontinence, bladder outflow obstruction, hematuria

HEMA: Anemia

META: Weight decrease

MS: Asthenia

RESP: Upper respiratory tract infection, rhinitis

Contraindications: Hypersensitivity to this product, GI bleeding, jaundice, renal failure, breastfeeding, children

Precautions: Pregnancy (B), respiratory/renal/hepatic/cardiac disease, seizure disorder, peptic ulcer, asthma, bradycardia, heart block, geriatric patients, surgery, urinary tract obstruction

PHARMACOKINETICS

Rapidly and completely absorbed; metabolized by CYP2D6, 3A4; excreted via kidneys; clearance is lower in geriatric patients, hepatic disease; clearance is 20% lower in females; elimination half-life 7 hr, 18% protein binding

INTERACTIONS

• Synergistic effect: cholinomimetics, other cholinesterase inhibitors

Increase: galantamine effect—CYP3A4 inhibitors (anti-retroviral protease inhibitors, ketoconazole, erythromycin, conivaptan, delaviridine, diltiazem, efavirenz, fluconazole, fluroxamine, imatinib, itraconazole, clarithromycin, troleandomycin, nefazodone, nicardipine, verapamil, voriconazole, zafirlukast), St. John's wort

Increase: GI effects—NSAIDs

Decrease: galantamine effect—CYP3A4 inducers (bosentan, carbamazepine, nevirapine, oxcarbazepine, phenytoin, fosphenytoin/rifabutin, rifampin, rifapentine, troglitazone)

Drug/Herb

• Cholinergic antagonism: jimsonweed, scopolia

Increase: effect—pill-bearing spurge

NURSING CONSIDERATIONS

Assess:

• Hepatic studies: AST, ALT, alk phos, LDH, bilirubin, CBC

• For severe GI effects: nausea, vomiting, anorexia, weight loss

• B/P, heart rate, respiration during initial treatment

• Mental status: affect, mood, behavioral changes, depression, memory, attention, confusion

Administer:

• With meals; take with morning and evening meal (immediate rel); morning (ext rel)

• Dose increase after minimum of 4 wk at prior dose; if dose is interrupted for 3 days or more, restart at lower dose, titrate to current dose

• Ext rel product can be opened and sprinkled on food, do not crush or chew

• Measure oral sol with calibrated device

Perform/provide:
- Assistance with ambulation during beginning therapy
- Complete suicide assessment

Evaluate:
- Therapeutic response: decreased confusion

Teach patient/family:
- Correct procedure for giving oral solution, using instruction sheet provided
- To notify prescriber of severe GI effects
- To report hypo/hypertension, slow heart rate
- This product is not a cure, but relieves symptoms

gallium (℞)

(gal′ee-um)

Ganite

Func. class.: Electrolyte modifier

Chem. class.: Hypocalcemic product

Action: Lowers serum calcium levels by inhibiting calcium resorption from bone

Uses: Cancer-related hypercalcemia

DOSAGE AND ROUTES

- *Adult:* **IV** 100-200 mg/m^2/day × 5 days; infuse over 24 hr, rest period of 2-4 wk between courses, discontinue earlier if serum calcium is in normal range

Available forms: Inj 25 mg/ml

SIDE EFFECTS

CNS: Confusion, hallucinations, vivid dreams, encephalopathy, lethargy

CV: Tachycardia, hypotension

EENT: Blurred vision, optic neuritis, hearing loss

GI: Nausea, vomiting, diarrhea, constipation, mucositis, metallic taste

GU: **Nephrotoxicity,** increased BUN, creatinine

HEMA: **Anemia, leukopenia, thrombocytopenia**

META: *Hypophosphatemia,* hypocalcemia, decreased serum bicarbonate, hypomagnesemia

RESP: Dyspnea, **pleural effusion**

Contraindications: Hypersensitivity, hypocalcemia

Black Box Warning: Renal failure, severe renal disease (specific gravity >2.5 mg/dl)

Precautions: Pregnancy (C), breastfeeding, children, mild renal disease, dehydration

PHARMACOKINETICS

IV: Onset 12-48 hr, peak 5 days, duration 4-14 days, excreted by kidneys

INTERACTIONS

Increase: nephrotoxicity—aminoglycosides, amphotericin B, cisplatin, foscarnet, ganciclovir, vancomycin, vaccines, toxoids

NURSING CONSIDERATIONS

Assess:
- Renal status: BUN, creatinine, urine output; if creatinine level is 2.5 mg/dl or more, product should be discontinued
- Monitor calcium, phosphate, bicarbonate, since all levels may be decreased and supplements of phosphate may be needed
- For hypercalcemia: nausea, vomiting, fatigue, weakness, thirst, dehydration, dysrhythmias, change in mental status
- For hypocalcemia: dysrhythmias; paresthesia; twitching; colic; laryngospasm; Trousseau's, Chvostek's sign; tremors
- For hypophosphatemia: confusion, decreased reflexes, joint stiffness and pain, portal hypotension

Administer:

IV route
- Adequate hydration with IV saline, 2 L/day during treatment
- After dilution of dose/1 L 0.9% NaCl or D_5W, run over 24 hr, use inf pump

Y-site compatibilities: Acyclovir, allopurinol, amifostine, aminophylline, ampicillin/sulbactam, aztreonam, cefazolin, ceftazidime, ceftriaxone, cimetidine, ciprofloxacin, cladribine, cyclophosphamide, dexamethasone, diphenhydrAMINE, filgrastim, fluconazole, furosemide, granisetron, heparin, hydrocortisone, ifosfamide, magnesium sulfate, mannitol, melphalan, meperidine, mesna, methotrexate, metoclopramide, ondansetron, piperacillin, piperacillin/tazobactam, potassium chloride, ranitidine, sodium bicarbonate, teniposide, thiotepa, ticarcillin/clavulanate, trimethoprim-sulfamethoxazole, vancomycin, vinorelbine

Perform/provide:

• Storage of solution 48 hr at room temperature, 1 wk in refrigerator

Evaluate:

• Therapeutic response: decreased serum calcium levels

Teach patient/family:

• Signs of low calcium, phosphorous

• To report changes in urinary output

• To follow dietary guidelines given by prescriber, including avoiding calcium (dairy products, broccoli) and vit D (fortified milk, grain products, fish oil)

ganciclovir (℞)

(gan-sye'kloe-vir)

Cytovene, Vitrasert

Func. class.: Antiviral

Chem. class.: Synthetic nucleoside analog

Do not confuse:

Cytovene/Cytosar

Action: Inhibits replication of herpesviruses, competitively inhibits human CMV DNA polymerase and is incorporated resulting in termination of DNA elongation

Uses: Cytomegalovirus (CMV) retinitis in immunocompromised persons, including those with AIDS, after indirect ophthalmoscopy confirms diagnosis, prophylaxis CVM in transplantation

Unlabeled uses: CMV pneumonia in organ transplant patients; CMV gastroenteritis, esophagitis, colitis; CMV pneumonitis, congenital CMV disease; Epstein-Barr virus; herpes simplex types 1, 2; varicella-zoster, hepatitis B

DOSAGE AND ROUTES

Prevention of CMV

• *Adult:* **IV** 5 mg/kg/dose over 1 hr q12hr × 1-2 wk, then 5 mg/kg/day 7 day/wk, then 6 mg/kg/day × 5 days/wk; **PO** 1000 mg tid starting 10 days post-transplant × 14 wks

Induction treatment

• *Adult:* **IV** 5 mg/kg/dose given over 1 hr, q12hr × 2-3 wk

Maintenance treatment

• *Adult:* **IV INF** 5 mg/kg given over 1 hr, daily × 7 days/wk; or 6 mg/kg/day × 5 days/wk; **PO** 1000 mg tid with food or 500 mg q3hr while awake for 6 doses; **INTRAVITREAL** 4.5 mg implant

Renal dose

• *Adult:* **PO/IV** Reduce dose in CCr <70 ml/min

Available forms: Powder for inj 500 mg/vial; caps 250, 500 mg; implant, intraviteral 4.5 mg

SIDE EFFECTS

CNS: *Fever,* chills, **coma,** *confusion*, abnormal thoughts, dizziness, bizarre dreams, *headache*, psychosis, tremors, somnolence, *paresthesia*, *weakness,* **seizures,** peripheral neuropathy

CV: Dysrhythmia, hypo/hypertension

EENT: Retinal detachment in CMV retinitis, ocular hypertension, ocular pain, conjunctival scarring, cataracts

GI: Abnormal LFTs, nausea, vomiting, anorexia, diarrhea, abdominal pain, **hemorrhage, perforation, pancreatitis**

GU: **Hematuria,** *increased creatinine,* BUN

HEMA: **Granulocytopenia, thrombocytopenia, irreversible neutropenia, anemia, eosinophilia, pancytopenia**

INTEG: Rash, alopecia, *pruritus*, urticaria, pain at site, phlebitis, **Stevens-Johnson syndrome**

RESP: Dyspnea

Contraindications: Hypersensitivity to acyclovir, ganciclovir, famciclovir, penciclovir, valacyclovir, valganciclovir

Black Box Warning: Absolute neutrophil count <500, platelet count <25,000 (intravitreal)

Precautions: Pregnancy (C), breastfeeding, children <6 mo, geriatric patients, preexisting cytopenias, renal function impairment, radiation therapy

Black Box Warning: Secondary malignancy, bone marrow suppression, anemia, infertility, neutropenia

PHARMACOKINETICS

Half-life 3-4½ hr; excreted by kidneys (unchanged); crosses blood-brain barrier, CSF, increased bioavailability with fatty foods

INTERACTIONS

⚠ Severe granulocytopenia: zidovudine, antineoplastics, radiation; do not give together

Increase: ganciclovir toxicity—adriamycin, amphotericin B, cycloSPORINE, dapsone, DOXOrubicin, flucytosine, pentamidine, probenecid, trimethoprim-sulfamethoxazole combinations, vinBLAStine, vinCRIStine, or other nucleoside analogs, mycophenolate

Increase: seizures—imipenem/cilastatin

Increase: tenofovir effect—ganciclovir

Decrease: ganciclovir renal clearance—probenecid

Decrease: didanosine effect—ganciclovir

NURSING CONSIDERATIONS

Assess:

- CMV retinitis: culture should be completed before starting treatment (urine, blood, throat), ophthalmic exam
- Infection: increased temp, sore throat, chills, fever; report to prescriber
- For leukopenia/neutropenia/thrombocytopenia: WBCs, platelets q2days during 2×/day dosing and then q1wk
- For leukopenia with daily WBC count in patients with prior leukopenia with other nucleoside analogs or for whom leukopenia counts are <1000 cells/mm^3 at start of treatment
- Serum creatinine or CCr ≥q2wk
- For seizures, dysrhythmias

Administer:

PO route

- With food

IV route

- Mixed in biologic cabinet, using gown, gloves, mask; use cytotoxic handling procedures

Intermittent IV INF route

- IV after diluting 500 mg/10 ml sterile H_2O for inj (50 mg/ml); shake; further dilute in 100 ml D_5W, 0.9% NaCl, LR, Ringer's and run over 1 hr; use inf pump, in-line filter
- Slowly; do not give by bolus IV, IM, SUBCUT inj
- Using reconstituted sol within 12 hr; do not refrigerate or freeze; inf solution is stable for 14 days when refrigerated

Y-site compatibilities: Allopurinol, amphotericin B cholesteryl, cisplatin, cyclophosphamide, DOXOrubicin liposome, enalaprilat, etoposide, filgrastim, fluconazole, gatifloxacin, granisetron, linezolid, melphalan, methotrexate, paclitaxel, propofol, remifentanil, tacrolimus, teniposide, thiotepa

Evaluate:

- Therapeutic response: decreased symptoms, or prevention of CMV

Teach patient/family:

- That product does not cure condition, that regular blood tests, ophthalmologic exams are necessary
- That major toxicities may necessitate discontinuing product
- To use contraception during treatment and that infertility may occur; should use barrier contraception for 90 days after treatment
- To take PO with food
- ⚠ To report infection: fever, chills, sore throat; blood dyscrasias: bruising, bleeding, petechiae
- To avoid crowds, persons with respiratory infections
- To use sunscreen to prevent burns

ganciclovir ophthalmic

See Appendix B

ganirelix (℞)

Orgalutran 🍁

Func. class.: Gonadotropin-releasing hormone antagonist

Chem. class.: Synthetic decapeptide

Action: Inhibitor of pituitary gonadotropin secretion; initially increases LH and FSH, induces a rapid suppression of gonadotropin secretion

Uses: For inhibition of premature LH surges in women undergoing controlled ovarian hyperstimulation

DOSAGE AND ROUTES

• *Adult:* **SUBCUT** 250 mcg/day during early to mid-follicular phase, continue until the day of hCG administration

Available forms: Inj 250 mcg/0.5 ml

SIDE EFFECTS

CNS: Headache

ENDO: Ovarian hyperstimulation syndrome, abdominal pain (GYN)

GI: Nausea

GU: *Spotting, breakthrough bleeding,* decreased urine, **fetal death**

INTEG: Pain on inj

SYST: **Fetal death**

Contraindications: Pregnancy (X), breastfeeding, hypersensitivity, latex allergy

PHARMACOKINETICS

Excreted in feces/urine, half-life 13-16 hr, metabolized to metabolites, protein binding 82%

NURSING CONSIDERATIONS

Assess:

• For suspected pregnancy, product should not be used

• For latex allergy, product should not be used

• Reproductive tests: serum progesterone, LH, estradiol, ovarian ultrasound, pelvic exam; baseline and during treatment

Administer:

• SUBCUT using abdomen, around navel or upper thigh; swab inj area with disinfectant; clean a 2-in circle and allow to dry; pinch up area between thumb and finger; insert needle at 45 degrees to 90 degrees to surface; if positioned correctly, no blood will be drawn back into syringe; if blood is drawn into syringe, reposition needle without removing it; inject slowly

Perform/provide:

• Protection from light

Evaluate:

• Therapeutic response: pregnancy

Teach patient/family:

• To report abdominal pain, vaginal bleeding

gatifloxacin ophthalmic

See Appendix B

gefitinib (℞)

(ge-fi′tye-nib)

Iressa

Func. class.: Antineoplastic—miscellaneous

Chem. class.: Epidermal growth factor receptor inhibitor

Action: Not fully understood; inhibits intracellular phosphorylation of cell surface receptors associated with epidermal growth factor receptors

Uses: Advanced/metastatic non–small cell lung cancer (NSCLC) in those who have not responded to platinum or docetaxel products

DOSAGE AND ROUTES

• *Adult:* **PO** 250 mg/day

CYP3A4 inducers concurrently (such as rifampin or phenytoin)

• *Adult:* **PO** 500 mg/day

Available forms: Tabs 250 mg

SIDE EFFECTS

EENT: Amblyopia, conjunctivitis, eye pain, corneal erosion/ulcer
GI: *Nausea, diarrhea, vomiting,* anorexia, **pancreatitis,** mouth ulceration, **hepatotoxicity**
INTEG: *Rash,* pruritus, *acne, dry skin,* **toxic epidermal neurolysis, angioedema**
MISC: Peripheral edema, **hemorrhage**
RESP: **Interstitial lung disease,** cough, dyspnea, pneumonia

Contraindications: Pregnancy (D), breastfeeding, children, hypersensitivity
Precautions: Geriatric patients, ocular/pulmonary/renal/hepatic disorders

PHARMACOKINETICS

Slowly absorbed; excreted in feces (86%), urine (<4%); elimination half-life 48 hr; metabolism by CYP3A4

INTERACTIONS

Increase: gefitinib concentrations—ketoconazole, itraconazole, erythromycin, clarithromycin
Increase: bone marrow suppression—clozapine
Increase: plasma concentration of warfarin, metoprolol
Decrease: gefitinib levels—phenytoin, rifampin, cimetidine, ranitidine, sodium bicarbonate

Drug/Herb
Decrease: gefitinib levels—St. John's wort

NURSING CONSIDERATIONS

Assess:
⚠ Pulmonary changes: lung sounds, cough, dyspnea; interstitial lung disease may occur, may be fatal; discontinue therapy if confirmed
• Ocular changes: eye irritation, corneal erosion/ulcer, aberrant eyelash growth
⚠ Pancreatitis: abdominal pain, levels of amylase, lipase
⚠ Toxic epidermal necrosis, angioedema
• GI symptoms: frequency of stools, if diarrhea is poorly tolerated, therapy may be discontinued for up to 14 days

Administer:
• Without regard to food; avoid grapefruit juice

Evaluate:
• Therapeutic response: decreased NSCLC

Teach patient/family:
⚠ To report adverse reactions immediately: shortness of breath, severe abdominal pain, ocular changes, skin eruptions
• Reason for treatment, expected results
• Use contraception during treatment; avoid breastfeeding
• Avoid persons with infections

G

gemcitabine (℞)

(jem-sit'a-been)
Gemzar
Func. class.: Antineoplastic—miscellaneous
Chem. class.: Nucleoside analog

Do not confuse:
Gemzar/Zinecard

Action: Exhibits antitumor activity by killing cells undergoing DNA synthesis (S-phase) and blocking G1/S-phase boundary

Uses: Adenocarcinoma of the pancreas (nonresectable stage II, III, or metastatic stage IV); in combination with cisplatin for inoperable, advanced, or metastatic non–small cell lung cancer; advanced breast cancer in combination with paclitaxel; with carboplatin for ovarian cancer; biliary tract cancer

Unlabeled uses: Bladder cancer, mesothelioma, adjuvant treatment in pancreatic cancer, ovarian cancer single agent

DOSAGE AND ROUTES

Pancreatic carcinoma (nonresectable stage II, III, IV)
• *Adult:* **IV** 1000 mg/m^2 given over ½ hr q wk × 7 wk, then 1 wk rest period; subsequent cycles should be infused once q wk × 3 wk out of every 4 wk depending on hematologic toxicity

Non–small cell lung cancer

• *Adult:* **IV** (4-wk schedule) 1000 mg/m² given over ½ hr on days 1, 8, 15, of each 28-day cycle; give cisplatin **IV** 100 mg/m² on day 1 after gemcitabine

• *Adult:* **IV** (3-wk schedule) 1250 mg/m² given over ½ hr on days 1, 8 of each 21-day cycle; give cisplatin **IV** 100 mg/m² after the inf of gemcitabine on day 1

Advanced breast cancer

• *Adult:* **IV** 1250 mg/m² over ½ hr on days 1 and 8 of a 21-day cycle; give paclitaxel 175 mg/m² over 3 hr prior to gemcitabine on day 1

Recurrent ovarian cancer (single agent) (unlabeled)

• *Adult:* **IV** 1 g/m², days 1, 8, 15 of a 28-day cycle

Adjuvant treatment of pancreatic cancer (unlabeled)

• *Adult:* **IV** 1000 mg/m² over 30 min on days 1, 8, 15 q28days × 6 cycles

Available forms: Lyophilized powder for inj 20 mg/ml

SIDE EFFECTS

GI: Diarrhea, nausea, vomiting, anorexia, constipation, stomatitis

GU: Proteinuria, hematuria

HEMA: **Leukopenia, anemia, neutropenia, thrombocytopenia**

INTEG: Irritation at site, rash, alopecia

OTHER: Dyspnea, fever, **hemorrhage**, infection, flulike symptoms, paresthesia, peripheral edema

Contraindications: Pregnancy (D), breastfeeding, hypersensitivity

Precautions: Children, geriatric patients, myelosuppression, irradiation, renal/hepatic disease

PHARMACOKINETICS

Half-life 42-379 min, crosses placenta

INTERACTIONS

Increase: bleeding—NSAIDs, alcohol, salicylates, anticoagulants

Increase: myelosuppression, diarrhea—other antineoplastics, radiation

Decrease: antibody response—live virus vaccines

Drug/Lab Test

Increase: BUN, AST, ALT, alk phos, bilirubin, creatinine

NURSING CONSIDERATIONS

Assess:

• CBC, differential, platelet count before each dose; absolute granulocyte count >1000, platelets >100,000, give complete dose; absolute granulocyte count 500-1000, platelets 50,000-100,000, give 75%; absolute granulocyte count <500, platelets <50,000, do not give

• Blood dyscrasias: bruising, bleeding, petechiae

• I&O, nutritional intake; food preferences: list likes, dislikes

• Renal, hepatic studies before and during treatment; may increase AST, ALT, alk phos, bilirubin, BUN, creatinine

• Buccal cavity for dryness, sores/ulceration, white patches, oral pain, bleeding, dysphagia

• GI symptoms: frequency of stools; cramping

• Signs of dehydration: rapid respirations, poor skin turgor, decreased urine output, dry skin, restlessness, weakness

Administer:

IV route

• Prepare in biologic cabinet using gown, mask, gloves; use cytotoxic handling procedures

• After reconstituting with 0.9% NaCl 5-ml/200-mg vial of product or 25 ml/1 g of product, shake = 40 mg/ml may be further diluted with 0.9% NaCl to conc as low as 0.1 mg/ml; discard unused portions, give over ½ hr, do not admix

Y-site compatibilities: Amifostine, amikacin, aminophylline, ampicillin, aztreonam, bleomycin, bumetanide, butorphanol, calcium gluconate, cefoxitin, ceftazidime, ceftizoxime, ceftriaxone, chlorproMAZINE, cimetidine, ciprofloxacin, cisplarin, clindamycin, cyclophosphamide, cytarabine, dactinomycin, DAUNOrubicin, diphenhydrAMINE, DOBUTamine, docetaxel, DOPamine, DOXOrubicin, droperidol, enalaprilat, etoposide, famotidine, floxuridine, fluconazole, fludarabine, fluorouracil, gentamicin, granisetron, haloperidol, heparin, hydrocortisone, hydromorphone, idarubicin, ifosfamide, leucovorin, linezolid, lorazepam, mannitol, meperidine, mesna, metoclopramide, metronidazole, minocycline, mitoxantrone, morphine, nalbuphine, ondansetron, paclitaxel, promethazine, ranitidine, streptozocin, teniposide, thiotepa, ticarcillin, tobramycin, topotecan, trimethoprim/sulfamethoxazole, vancomycin, vinBLAStine, vinCRIStine, vinorelbine, zidovudine

Perform/provide:

- Increased fluid intake to 2-3 L/day to prevent dehydration, unless contraindicated
- Rinsing of mouth tid-qid with water, club soda; brushing of teeth bid-tid with soft brush or cotton-tipped applicator for stomatitis; use unwaxed dental floss
- Nutritious diet with iron, low fiber, few dairy products
- Antiemetic agents

Evaluate:

- Therapeutic response: decrease in tumor size; decrease in spread of cancer; symptom relief

Teach patient/family:

- To avoid foods with citric acid or hot or rough texture if stomatitis is present; to drink adequate fluids
- To avoid use with NSAIDs, alcohol, salicylates
- To report stomatitis; any bleeding, white spots, ulcerations in mouth; tell patient to examine mouth daily, report symptoms
- To report signs of anemia: fatigue, headache, faintness, SOB, irritability; hematuria, dysuria
- To use contraception during therapy and for 4 mo after
- Not to receive vaccinations during treatment
- About possible hair loss and what can be done
- To report flulike symptoms, swelling of feet/legs
- To report bruising, bleeding: gums, blood in urine, stool, emesis
- To avoid crowds, persons with known upper respiratory infections
- To avoid use of hard-bristle toothbrush, electric razor

gemfibrozil (℞)

(jem-fi′broe-zil)

gemfibrozil, Lopid

Func. class.: Antilipemic

Chem. class.: Fibric acid derivative

Do not confuse:

Lopid/Levbid/Slo-bid

Action: Inhibits biosynthesis of VLDL, decreases triglycerides, increases HDL

Uses: Type IIb, IV, V hyperlipidemia as adjunct with diet therapy

DOSAGE AND ROUTES

- *Adult:* **PO** 600 mg bid 30 min before AM, PM meal

Available forms: Tabs 600 mg; caps 300 mg ♣

SIDE EFFECTS

CNS: Fatigue, vertigo, headache, paresthesia, dizziness, somnolence

GI: Dyspepsia, diarrhea, abdominal pain, nausea, vomiting

HEMA: **Leukopenia, anemia, eosinophilia, thrombocytopenia**

INTEG: Rash, urticaria, pruritus

MISC: Taste perversion

Contraindications: Severe renal/hepatic disease, preexisting gallbladder disease, primary biliary cirrhosis, hypersensitivity

Precautions: Pregnancy (C), breastfeeding, monitor hematologic and hepatic function

PHARMACOKINETICS

Peak 1-2 hr; plasma protein binding >90%; half-life 1½ hr; 70% excreted in urine as conjugate, <2% excreted unchanged; metabolized in liver (minimal)

INTERACTIONS

Increase: hypoglycemic effect—sulfonylureas
Increase: anticoagulant properties—oral anticoagulants
Increase: risk of myositis, myalgia—HMG-CoA reductase inhibitors
Decrease: effect of cycloSPORINE

Drug/Herb

Increase: effect—glucomannan
Decrease: effect—gotu kola

Drug/Lab Test

Increase: LFTs, CPK, BSP, thymol turbidity, glucose
Decrease: Hgb, Hct, WBC

NURSING CONSIDERATIONS

Assess:

- Triglycerides, cholesterol; if lipids increase, product should be discontinued; LDL, VLDL baseline and periodically
- Renal, hepatic studies, CBC, blood glucose if patient is on long-term therapy; if LFTs increase, therapy should be discontinued
- Bowel pattern daily; watch for increasing diarrhea (common)

Administer:

- 30 min before morning and evening meals

Evaluate:

- Therapeutic response: decreased cholesterol, triglyceride levels, HDL, cholesterol ratios improved

Teach patient/family:

- That compliance is needed for positive results; do not double or skip dose
- That risk factors should be decreased: high-fat diet, smoking, alcohol consumption, absence of exercise
- To notify prescriber of diarrhea, nausea, vomiting, chills, fever, sore throat, muscle cramps, abdominal cramps, severe flatulence
- That product may be discontinued if no improvement in 3 mo

gemifloxacin (℞)

(gem-ah-flox′a-sin)
Factive
Func. class.: Antiinfective
Chem. class.: Fluoroquinolone

Action: Inhibits DNA gyrase, which is an enzyme involved in replication, transcription, and repair of bacterial DNA

Uses: Acute bacterial exacerbation of chronic bronchitis caused by *Streptococcus pneumoniae, Haemophilus influenzae, Haemophilus parainfluenzae, Moraxella catarrhalis*; community-acquired pneumonia caused by *Streptococcus pneumoniae* including multiproduct resistant strains, *H. influenzae, M. catarrhalis, Mycoplasma pneumoniae, Chlamydia pneumoniae, Klebsiella pneumoniae*

Unlabeled uses: *Actinetobacter iwoffii,* cystitis, *Klebsiella oxytoca, Legionella pneumophilia, Proteus vulgaris,* pyelonephritis, sinusitis, *Streptococcus Pyogenes* (group A beta-hemolytic streptococci), urinary tract infection

DOSAGE AND ROUTES

- *Adult:* **PO** 320 mg/day × 5-10 days depending on type of infection

Renal dose

- *Adult:* **PO** CCr ≤40 ml/min 160 mg q24hr

Available forms: Tabs 320 mg

SIDE EFFECTS

CNS: Dizziness, headache, somnolence, depression, insomnia, nervousness, confusion, agitation, **seizures**
CV: QT prolongation, vasodilation
EENT: Visual disturbances
GI: Diarrhea, *nausea,* vomiting, anorexia, flatulence, heartburn, dry mouth; increased AST, ALT; constipation, abdominal pain, oral thrush, glossitis, stomatitis, **pseudomembranous colitis**
HEMA: **Thrombocytopenia, neutropenia**

INTEG: Rash, pruritus, urticaria, *photosensitivity*
MS: Tendinitis, **tendon rupture**
SYST: **Anaphylaxis, Stevens-Johnson syndrome**

Contraindications: Hypersensitivity to quinolones

Precautions: Pregnancy (C), breastfeeding, children, geriatric patients, hypokalemia, hypomagnesium, renal disease, seizure disorders, excessive exposure to sunlight, psychosis, increased intracranial pressure, history of QT interval prolongation, dysrhythmias

Black Box Warning: Tendon pain/rupture, tendinitis

PHARMACOKINETICS

Rapidly absorbed; bioavailability 71%; peak 1-2 hr; half-life 4-12 hr; excreted in urine as active product, metabolites

INTERACTIONS

Increase: toxicity of gemifloxacin—probenecid

Increase: QT prolongation—drugs that increase QT prolongation

⚠ ***Decrease:*** effect of antidysrhythmias (amiodarone, procainamide, quinidine, sotalol, disopyramide), tricyclics; result in life-threatening arrhythmias, QT prolongation

Decrease: absorption antacids containing aluminum, magnesium, sucralfate, zinc, iron, give 2 hr before or 3 hr after meals

Drug/Herb

- Do not use acidophilus with antiinfectives; separate by several hours

NURSING CONSIDERATIONS

Assess:

- Renal, hepatic studies: BUN, creatinine, AST, ALT; I&O ratio
- CNS symptoms: insomnia, vertigo, headache, agitation, confusion

⚠ Allergic reactions and anaphylaxis: rash, flushing, urticaria, pruritus, chills, fever, joint pain; may occur a few days after therapy begins; epinephrine and resuscitation equipment should be available for anaphylactic reaction

- Bowel pattern daily, if severe diarrhea occurs, product should be discontinued
- For overgrowth of infection: perineal itching, fever, malaise, redness, pain, swelling, drainage, rash, diarrhea, change in cough, sputum

⚠ For tendon pain, if present, discontinue use

Administer:

- 2 hr before or 3 hr after aluminum/magnesium antacids, iron, zinc products, or buffered 2 hr before sucralfate

Evaluate

- Therapeutic response: negative C&S, absence of signs/symptoms of infection

Teach patient/family:

- May take with or without food
- That fluids must be increased to 2 L/day to avoid crystallization in kidneys
- That if dizziness or light-headedness occurs, perform activities with assistance
- To complete full course of product therapy
- To contact prescriber if adverse reactions occur
- To avoid iron- or mineral-containing supplements or aluminum/magnesium antacids, buffered products within 2 hr before and 3 hr after dosing; 2 hr before sucralfate
- That photosensitivity may occur and sunscreen should be used
- To use frequent rinsing of mouth, sugarless candy or gum for dry mouth
- To avoid other medication unless approved by prescriber

⚠ High Alert

gemtuzumab (℞)

(gem-tue-zue'mab)
Mylotarg
Func. class.: Antineoplastic—miscellaneous
Chem. class.: Monoclonal antibody

Action: Composed of recombinant humanized IgG_4 kappa antibody, binds to

CD33 antigen that is released in myeloid cells

Uses: Acute myeloid leukemia (AML) in patients with first relapse who are 60 yr or older

DOSAGE AND ROUTES

• *Adult:* **IV** 9 mg/m^2 as a 2 hr inf; before giving inf, give diphenhydrAMINE 50 mg **PO**, acetaminophen 650-1000 mg **PO** 1 hr prior to inf; then use acetaminophen 650-1000 mg q4hr for additional 2 doses

Available forms: Powder for inj, lyophilized 5 mg

SIDE EFFECTS

CNS: Dizziness, insomnia, depression, headache

CV: Hypo/hypertension, hemorrhage, tachycardia

GI: Anorexia, diarrhea, constipation, nausea, stomatitis, vomiting, **fatal liver toxicity**

GU: Hematuria, **vaginal hemorrhage**

HEMA: **Prolonged neutropenia, thrombocytopenia**

INTEG: Rash, herpes simplex, local reaction, petechiae, pruritus

META: Hypokalemia, hypomagnesemia

MISC: Fever, myalgias, headache, chills, peripheral edema

RESP: Cough, pneumonia, epistaxis, rhinitis, dyspnea

Contraindications: Pregnancy (D), breastfeeding

Black Box Warning: Hypersensitivity to this product or marine protein, severe myelosuppression

Precautions: Children, severe renal disease

Black Box Warning: Hepatic disease, pulmonary disease, infusion-related reactions

PHARMACOKINETICS

Half-life 45 and 100 hr, respectively

INTERACTIONS

Increase: bone marrow suppression—other antineoplastics, radiation

NURSING CONSIDERATIONS

Assess:

• For symptoms of infection; chills, fever, headache, may be masked by product fever

• For pulmonary symptoms: cough, dyspnea

• CNS reaction: LOC, mental status, dizziness, confusion

• Cardiac status: lung sounds; ECG before and during treatment, especially in those with cardiac disease

• Bone marrow depression: bruising, bleeding, blood in stools, urine, sputum, emesis

• Blood studies: BUN, creatinine, AST, ALT, electrolytes, bilirubin, CBC, uric acid

Administer:

• Do not give IV push or bolus

• Protect from light; use biologic safety hood; allow to come to room temperature

• Reconstitute each vial with 5 ml sterile water for inj using sterile syringes; swirl each vial; check for discoloration or particulate matter; give over 2 hr; use a separate line with 1.2-micron terminal filter

• May be premedicated with methylPREDNISolone and antiemetics

Perform/provide:

• Storage of reconstituted sol for ≤8 hr in refrigerator

Evaluate:

• Therapeutic response: improvement in blood counts

Teach patient/family:

• To take acetaminophen for fever

• To avoid hazardous tasks, since confusion, dizziness may occur; avoid prolonged sunlight, use sunscreen

• To report signs of infection: sore throat, fever, diarrhea, vomiting

• To avoid immunizations

• To avoid crowds, people with known infections

• That product is very toxic

gentamicin (℞)

(jen-ta-mye'sin)

Cidomycin ✤, Garamycin, gentamicin sulfate, G-Mycin, Jenamicin

Func. class.: Antiinfective

Chem. class.: Aminoglycoside

Do not confuse:
Garamycin/kanamycin

Action: Interferes with protein synthesis in bacterial cell by binding to ribosomal subunit, causing misreading of genetic code; inaccurate peptide sequence forms in protein chain, causing bacterial death

Uses: Severe systemic infections of CNS, respiratory, GI, urinary tract, bone, skin, soft tissues caused by susceptible strains of *Pseudomonas aeruginosa, Proteus, Klebsiella, Serratia, Escherichia coli, Enterobacter, Citrobacter, Staphylococcus, Shigella, Salmonella, Acinetobacter, Bacillus anthracis,* acute PID

DOSAGE AND ROUTES

Severe systemic infections

• *Adult:* **IV INF** 3-6 mg/kg/day in divided doses q8hr; dilute in 50-200 ml 0.9% NaCl or D_5W given over 30 min-1 hr; **IV** (pulse dosing, once daily dosing) (unlabeled) 5-7 mg/kg; **IM** 3 mg/kg/day in divided doses q8hr

• *Child:* **IM/IV** 2-2.5 mg/kg q8hr; **IV** (pulse dosing, once daily dosing) (unlabeled) 5 mg/kg

• *Neonate and infant:* **IM/IV** 2.5 mg/kg q8-12hr

• *Neonate <1 wk:* **IV** 2.5 mg/kg q12-24hr

Renal dose

• *Adult:* **IM/IV** 1-1.7 mg/kg initially, then adjust according to renal function studies

Available forms: Inj 10, 40 mg/ml; premixed inj 40, 60, 70, 80, 100 mg/50 ml; 40, 60, 80, 90, 100, 120, 160, 180 mg/ml

SIDE EFFECTS

CNS: Confusion, depression, numbness, tremors, **seizures**, muscle twitching, **neurotoxicity**, dizziness, vertigo

CV: Hypo/hypertension, palpitations, edema

EENT: **Ototoxicity**, *deafness*, visual disturbances, tinnitus

GI: Nausea, vomiting, anorexia; increased ALT, AST, bilirubin; hepatomegaly, **hepatic necrosis**, splenomegaly

GU: **Oliguria, hematuria, renal damage, azotemia, renal failure, nephrotoxicity**, proteinuria

HEMA: **Agranulocytosis, thrombocytopenia, leukopenia, eosinophilia**, anemia

INTEG: Rash, burning, urticaria, dermatitis, alopecia, photosensitivity

Contraindications: Hypersensitivity to this or other aminoglycosides, fungal/viral/mycobacterial infection

Black Box Warning: Pregnancy (D), severe renal disease

Precautions: Breastfeeding, neonates, geriatric patients

Black Box Warning: Mild renal disease, hearing deficits, myasthenia gravis, Parkinson's disease

PHARMACOKINETICS

Not metabolized, excreted unchanged in urine, crosses placental barrier

IM: Onset rapid, peak 1-2 hr

IV: Onset immediate; peak 1-2 hr; plasma half-life 1-2 hr, infants 6-7 hr; duration 6-8 hr

INTERACTIONS

Increase: ototoxicity, neurotoxicity, nephrotoxicity—other aminoglycosides, amphotericin B, polymyxin, vancomycin, ethacrynic acid, furosemide, mannitol, methoxyflurane, cisplatin, cephalosporins, penicillins, cidofovir, acyclovir

Increase: effects—nondepolarizing neuromuscular blockers

Drug/Herb

• Do not use acidophilus with antiinfectives; separate by several hours

NURSING CONSIDERATIONS

Assess:

- Weight before treatment; calculation of dosage is usually based on ideal body weight, but may be calculated on actual body weight
- I&O ratio, urinalysis daily for proteinuria, cells, casts; report sudden change in urine output; toxicity is increased in patients with decreased renal function if high doses are given
- VS during inf; watch for hypotension, change in pulse
- IV site for thrombophlebitis, including pain, redness, swelling, q30min, change site if needed; discontinue, apply warm compresses to site
- Serum peak, drawn at 30-60 min after IV inf or 60 min after IM inj, and trough level drawn just before next dose; blood level should be 2-4 times bacteriostatic level; peak = 4-10 mcg/ml, trough = 0.5-2 mcg/ml
- Urine pH if product is used for UTI; urine should be kept alkaline
- Renal impairment by securing urine for CCr testing, BUN, serum creatinine; lower dosage should be given in renal impairment (CCr <80 ml/min)
- Eighth cranial nerve dysfunction by audiometric testing; also ringing, roaring in ears, vertigo; assess hearing before, during, after treatment
- Dehydration: high specific gravity, decrease in skin turgor, dry mucous membranes, dark urine
- Overgrowth of infection including fever, malaise, redness, pain, swelling, perineal itching, diarrhea, stomatitis, change in cough or sputum
- C&S before starting treatment to identify infecting organism
- Vestibular dysfunction: nausea, vomiting, dizziness, headache; product should be discontinued if severe
- Inj sites for redness, swelling, abscesses; use warm compresses at site

Administer:

- IM inj in large muscle mass; rotate inj sites
- Product in evenly spaced doses to maintain blood level

IV route

- After diluting in 50-200 ml NS or D_5W; sol concentration should be 1 mg/ml or less; decrease vol of diluent in child; maintain 0.1% sol run over ½-1 hr (adults) or up to 2 hr (children); flush IV line with NS or D_5W after administration

Additive compatibilities: Atracurium, aztreonam, bleomycin, cefoxitin, cimetidine, ciprofloxacin, fluconazole, meropenem, methicillin, metronidazole, ofloxacin, penicillin G sodium, ranitidine, verapamil

Syringe compatibilities: Clindamycin, methicillin, penicillin G sodium

Y-site compatibilities: Acyclovir, amifostine, amiodarone, amsacrine, atracurium, aztreonam, cefpirome, ciprofloxacin, cyclophosphamide, cytarabine, diltiazem, enalaprilat, esmolol, famotidine, filgrastim, fluconazole, fludarabine, foscarnet, granisetron, hydromorphone, IL-2, insulin, labetalol, lorazepam, magnesium sulfate, melphalan, meperidine, meropenem, midazolam, morphine, multivitamins, ondansetron, paclitaxel, pancuronium, perphenazine, sargramostim, tacrolimus, teniposide, theophylline, thiotepa, tolazine, vecuronium, vinorelbine, vit B/C, zidovudine

Perform/provide:

- Adequate fluids of 2-3 L/day, unless contraindicated, to prevent irritation of tubules
- Supervised ambulation, other safety measures with vestibular dysfunction

Evaluate:

- Therapeutic response: absence of fever, draining wounds, negative C&S after treatment

Teach patient/family:

- To report headache, dizziness, symptoms of overgrowth of infection, renal impairment
- To report loss of hearing, ringing, roaring in ears, or feeling of fullness in head

gentamicin ophthalmic
See Appendix B

gentamicin topical
See Appendix B

glatiramer (℞)
(glah-tear′a-meer)
Copaxone
Func. class.: Multiple sclerosis agent

Action: Unknown, may modify the immune responses responsible for multiple sclerosis (MS)

Uses: Reduction of the frequency of relapses in patients with relapsing-remitting MS, after first clinical episode with MRI results consistent with MS

DOSAGE AND ROUTES

- *Adult:* **SUBCUT** 20 mg/day

Available forms: Inj, premixed 20 mg/ml

SIDE EFFECTS

CNS: Anxiety, hypertonia, tremor, vertigo, speech disorder, *agitation,* confusion

CV: Migraine, palpitations, syncope, tachycardia, vasodilation, chest pain, hypertension

EENT: Ear pain, blurred vision

GI: Nausea, vomiting, diarrhea, anorexia, gastroenteritis

GU: Urinary urgency, dysmenorrhea, vaginal moniliasis

HEMA: Ecchymosis, lymphadenopathy

INTEG: Pruritus, rash, sweating, urticaria, erythema, inj site reaction

META: Edema, weight gain

MS: Arthralgia, back pain, neck pain, increased muscle tone

RESP: Bronchitis, dyspnea, laryngismus, rhinitis

Contraindications: Hypersensitivity to this product or mannitol

Precautions: Pregnancy (B), breastfeeding, children <18 yr, immune disorders, renal disease

PHARMACOKINETICS

May be hydrolyzed locally, may reach regional lymph nodes

NURSING CONSIDERATIONS

Assess:

- Blood, renal, hepatic studies: prior to treatment
- For CNS symptoms: anxiety, confusion, vertigo
- GI status: diarrhea, vomiting, abdominal pain, gastroenteritis
- Cardiac status: tachycardia, palpitations, vasodilation, chest pain

Administer:

SUBCUT route

- Using a sterile syringe/needle to transfer the supplied diluent into the vial; rotate vial gently; do not shake; withdraw medication using a syringe with 27G needle; administer SUBCUT into hip, thigh, arm; discard unused portion
- Use SUBCUT route only; do not give IM or IV
- Do not use sol that contains precipitate or is discolored
- Use immediately

Evaluate:

- Therapeutic response: decreased symptoms of MS

Teach patient/family:

- Give written, detailed instructions about the product; provide initial and return demonstrations on inj procedure; give information on use and disposal of product, inj site reaction (hives, rash, irritation, severe pain, flushing, chest pain)
- That blurred vision, sweating may occur
- That irregular menses, dysmenorrhea, or metrorrhagia as well as breast pain may occur; use contraception during treatment
- That if pregnancy is suspected, or if nursing, notify prescriber

- Not to change dosing or to stop taking product without advice of prescriber
- Immediate post inj reaction: flushing, chest pain, palpitations, anxiety, dyspnea, laryngeal constriction, urticaria, does not usually require treatment

glimepiride (℞)
(glye-me'pi-ride)
Amaryl
*glipiZIDE (℞)
(glip-i'zide)
Glucotrol, Glucotrol XL
Func. class.: Antidiabetic
Chem. class.: Sulfonylurea (2nd generation)

Do not confuse:
glipiZIDE/Glucotrol/glyBURIDE

Action: Causes functioning β-cells in pancreas to release insulin, leading to drop in blood glucose levels; may improve insulin binding to insulin receptors or increase the number of insulin receptors with prolonged administration; may also reduce basal hepatic glucose secretion; not effective if patient lacks functioning β-cells

Uses: Type 2 diabetes mellitus

DOSAGE AND ROUTES

Glimepiride
- *Adult:* **PO** 1-2 mg/day with breakfast, then increase q1-2wk, max 8 mg/day
- *Geriatric:* **PO** 1 mg/day; may increase if needed

Renal dose
- *Adult:* **PO** CCr <20 ml/min, 1 mg/day with breakfast, may titrate upward as needed

GlipiZIDE
- *Adult:* **PO** 5 mg initially before breakfast, then increase to desired response; max 40 mg/day in divided doses or 15 mg/dose; **PO** (XL) 5 mg/day with breakfast, may increase to 10 mg/day, max 20 mg/day
- *Geriatric:* **PO** 2.5 mg/day; may increase if needed

Hepatic disease
- *Adult:* **PO** 2.5 mg initially, then increase to desired response; max 40 mg/day in divided doses or 15 mg/dose

Available forms: *Glimepiride:* tabs 1, 2, 4 mg; *glipiZIDE:* tabs, scored 5, 10 mg; ext rel tab (XL) 2.5, 5, 10 mg

SIDE EFFECTS

CNS: ***Headache, weakness, dizziness, drowsiness,*** tinnitus, fatigue, vertigo
ENDO: **Hypoglycemia**
GI: **Hepatotoxicity, cholestatic jaundice,** nausea, vomiting, diarrhea, heartburn
HEMA: **Leukopenia, thrombocytopenia, agranulocytosis, aplastic anemia;** increased AST, ALT, alk phos; **pancytopenia, hemolytic anemia**
INTEG: Rash, allergic reactions, pruritus, urticaria, eczema, photosensitivity, erythema, allergic vasculitis

Contraindications: Hypersensitivity to sulfonylureas, type 1 diabetes, diabetic ketoacidosis

Precautions: Pregnancy (C), geriatric patients, cardiac disease, severe renal/hepatic disease, G6PD deficiency

PHARMACOKINETICS

PO: Completely absorbed by GI route, onset 1-1½ hr, peak 1-3 hr, duration 10-24 hr, half-life 2-4 hr, metabolized in liver, excreted in urine, 90%-95% is plasma protein bound

INTERACTIONS

- May mask symptoms of hypoglycemia: β-blockers

Increase: action of digoxin, glycosides
Increase: hypoglycemic effects—insulin, MAOIs, cimetidine, chloramphenicol, guanethidine, methyldopa, NSAIDs, salicylates, probenecid, androgens, anticoagulants, clofibrate, fenfluramine, fluconazole, gemfibrozil, histamine H_2 antagonists, magnesium salts, phenylbutazone, sulfinpyrazone, sulfonamides, tricyclics, urinary acidifiers

Decrease: hypoglycemic effect—thiazide diuretics, rifampin, isoniazid, cholestyramine, diazoxide, hydantoins, urinary alkalinizers, charcoal

Drug/Herb

Increase: antidiabetic effect—alfalfa, aloe, basil, bay, bilberry, bitter melon, black catechu, buchu, burdock, coriander, dandelion, eyebright (po), garlic, glucomannan, glucosamine, goat's rue, gymnema, horehound, horse chestnut, jambul, myrrh, myrtle

Increase: glucose tolerance—karela

Increase or decrease: hypoglycemic effect—chromium, fenugreek, ginseng, coenzyme Q10

Decrease: hypoglycemic effect—broom, buchu, dandelion, glucosamine, juniper

Decrease: antidiabetic effect—bee pollen, blue cohosh, broom, chromium, elecampane, eucalyptus, gotu kola

Drug/Lab Test

Increase: AST, ALT, LDH, BUN, creatinine

NURSING CONSIDERATIONS

Assess:

• Hypo/hyperglycemic reaction that can occur soon after meals; for severe hypoglycemia give IV $D_{50}W$, then IV dextrose solution

• Blood, A1c levels during treatment to determine diabetes control

• CBC baseline and throughout treatment

Administer:

• Do not break, crush, or chew ext rel tabs; may crush tabs and mix with fluids if unable to swallow whole

• Product 30 min before meals; if patient is NPO, may need to hold dose to prevent hypoglycemia

Perform/provide:

• Storage in tight, light-resistant container at room temperature

Evaluate:

• Therapeutic response: decrease in polyuria, polydipsia, polyphagia; clear sensorium; absence of dizziness; stable gait; improved serum glucose, A1c

Teach patient/family:

• Not to drink alcohol; explain disulfiram reaction (nausea, headache, cramps, flushing, hypoglycemia)

• To check for symptoms of cholestatic jaundice: dark urine, pruritus, yellow sclera; prescriber should be notified

• The symptoms of hypo/hyperglycemia, what to do about each; to have glucagon emergency kit available, carry sugar packets

• That product must be continued on daily basis; explain consequences of discontinuing product abruptly

• To take product in morning to prevent hypoglycemic reactions at night

• To use sunscreen or stay out of the sun to prevent photosensitivity

• To avoid OTC medications unless ordered by prescriber

• That diabetes is a lifelong illness; product will not cure disease

• That all food in diet plan must be eaten to prevent hypoglycemia

• To carry emergency ID with prescriber and medications

• To test using blood glucose meter while on this product

• To continue weight control, dietary restrictions, exercise, hygiene

• Ext rel tab may appear in stool

Treatment of overdose: Glucose 25 g IV via dextrose 50% solution 50 ml, 1 mg glucagon or carbohydrate depending on severity

*glyBURIDE (℞)

(glye'byoor-ide)

Apo-Glyburide ✤, DiaBeta ✤, Euglucon ✤, Gen-Glybe ✤, Glynase PresTab, Micronase, Novo-Glyburide ✤, Nu-Glyburide ✤

Func. class.: Antidiabetic

Chem. class.: Sulfonylurea (2nd generation)

Do not confuse:

glyBURIDE/Glucotrol/glipiZIDE

DiaBeta/Zebeta

Action: Causes functioning β-cells in pancreas to release insulin, leading to drop in blood glucose levels; may improve insulin binding to insulin receptors and increase number of insulin receptors with prolonged administration; may also reduce basal hepatic glucose secretion; not effective if patient lacks functioning β-cells

Uses: Type 2 diabetes mellitus

DOSAGE AND ROUTES

DiaBeta/Micronase

- *Adult:* **PO** 1.25-5 mg initially, then increased to desired response at weekly intervals up to 20 mg/day; may be given as a single or divided dose
- *Geriatric:* **PO** 1.25 mg initially, then increased to desired response; max 20 mg/day, maintenance 1.25-20 mg/day

Glynase PresTab (micronized)

- *Adult:* **PO** 1.5-3 mg/day initially, may increase by 1.5 mg/wk, max 12 mg/day
- *Geriatric:* **PO** 0.75-3 mg/day, may increase by 1.5 mg/wk

Available forms: Tabs (DiaBeta) 1.25, 2.5, 5 mg; (Glynase PresTab) 1.5, 3, 6 mg

SIDE EFFECTS

CNS: *Headache, weakness,* paresthesia, tinnitus, fatigue, vertigo

ENDO: **Hypoglycemia**

GI: Nausea, fullness, heartburn, **hepatotoxicity, cholestatic jaundice,** vomiting, diarrhea

HEMA: **Leukopenia, thrombocytopenia, agranulocytosis, aplastic anemia,** increased AST, ALT, alk phos

INTEG: Rash, allergic reactions, pruritus, urticaria, eczema, photosensitivity, erythema

MS: Joint pain

Contraindications: Hypersensitivity to sulfonylureas, type 1 diabetes, diabetic ketoacidosis, renal failure

Precautions: Pregnancy (C), geriatric patients, cardiac/thyroid disease, severe renal/hepatic disease, severe hypoglycemic reactions

PHARMACOKINETICS

PO: Completely absorbed by GI route; onset 2-4 hr; peak 4 hr; duration 24 hr; half-life 10 hr; metabolized in liver; excreted in urine, feces (metabolites); crosses placenta; 99% is plasma protein bound

INTERACTIONS

- Mask symptoms of hypoglycemia: β-blockers

Increase: level—digoxin

Increase: hypoglycemic effects—insulin, MAOIs, oral anticoagulants, chloramphenicol, guanethidine, methyldopa, NSAIDs, salicylates, probenecid, androgens, fenfluramine, fluconazole, gemfibrozil, histamine H_2 antagonists, magnesium salts, phenylbutazone, sulfinpyrazone, sulfonamides, tricyclics, urinary acidifiers

Decrease: both products' effect—diazoxide

Decrease: glyBURIDE action—thiazide diuretics, rifampin, isoniazid, cholestyramine, hydantoins, urinary alkalinizers, charcoal

Drug/Herb

Increase: antidiabetic effect—alfalfa, aloe, basil, bay, bilberry, bitter melon, black catechu, buchu, burdock, coriander, dandelion, eyebright (po), garlic, glu-

comannan, glucosamine, goat's rue, gymnema, horehound, horse chestnut, jambul, myrrh, myrtle
Increase: glucose tolerance: karela
Increase or decrease: hypoglycemic effect—chromium, coenzyme Q10, fenugreek, ginseng
Decrease: antidiabetic effect—bee pollen, blue cohosh, broom, chromium, elecampane, eucalyptus, gotu kola
Decrease: hypoglycemic effect—broom, buchu, dandelion, glucosamine, juniper
Drug/Lab Test
Increase: AST, ALT, LDH, BUN, creatinine

NURSING CONSIDERATIONS

Assess:
- Hypo/hyperglycemic reaction that can occur soon after meals; for severe hypoglycemia, give IV $D_{50}W$, then IV dextrose sol
- Blood glucose; A1c levels during treatment
- CBC baseline and throughout treatment

Administer:
- With breakfast, hold dose if NPO to avoid hypoglycemia

Perform/provide:
- Storage in tight container in cool environment

Evaluate:
- Therapeutic response: decrease in polyuria, polydipsia, polyphagia; clear sensorium; absence of dizziness; stable gait; improved serum glucose, A1c

Teach patient/family:
- To check for symptoms of cholestatic jaundice: dark urine, pruritus, jaundiced sclera; if these occur, notify prescriber
- To use a blood glucose meter for testing while on this product
- The symptoms of hypo/hyperglycemia, what to do about each
- That product must be continued on daily basis; explain consequences of discontinuing product abruptly
- To take product in morning to prevent hypoglycemic reactions at night
- To avoid OTC medications unless ordered by prescriber
- That diabetes is a lifelong illness; product will not cure disease
- That all food included in diet plan must be eaten to prevent hypoglycemia; to have glucagon emergency kit, sugar packets available
- To use sunscreen or stay out of the sun to prevent photosensitivity
- To carry an emergency ID with prescriber and medications

Treatment of overdose: Glucose 25 g IV via dextrose 50% sol, 50 ml, 1 mg glucagon, or carbohydrate depending on severity

G

Rarely Used

glycerin (OTC)

(gli'ser-in)
Colace Glycerin Suppositories, Fleet Babylax, Glycerin USP, Glycerol, Osmoglyn, Sani-Supp
Func. class.: Laxative, hyperosmotic

Uses: Constipation, intraocular pressure reduction

DOSAGE AND ROUTES

Laxative
- *Adult and child >6 yr:* **RECT SUPP** 3 g; **ENEMA** 5-15 ml
- *Child <6 yr:* **RECT SUPP** 1-1.5 g; **ENEMA** 2-5 ml

Intraocular pressure reduction
- *Adult:* **PO** 1-1.8 g/kg once, then may be given 500 mg/kg q6hr
- *Child:* **PO** 1-1.5 g/kg once, then 500 mg/kg 4-8 hr after first dose

Contraindications: Hypersensitivity

glycopyrrolate (℞)

(glye-koe-pye'roe-late)
glycopyrrolate, Robinul, Robinul-Forte
Func. class.: Cholinergic blocker, antispasmodic
Chem. class.: Quaternary ammonium compound

Action: Inhibits the action of acetylcholine at receptor sites in parasympathetic nervous system, which controls secretions, free acids in stomach

Uses: Decreased secretions before surgery, reversal of neuromuscular blockade, peptic ulcer disease, irritable bowel syndrome, bradycardia, drooling

DOSAGE AND ROUTES

Preoperatively

- *Adult:* **IM** 4 mcg/kg ½-1 hr before surgery, max 0.1 mg
- *Child >2 yr (unlabeled):* **IM** 4 mcg/kg 30-60 min before procedure
- *Child <2 yr (unlabeled):* **IM** 4-9 mcg/kg

Intraoperative

- *Adult:* **IV** 0.1 mg; may repeat q2-3min prn
- *Child:* **IM/IV** 4 mcg/kg q2-3min prn; max 0.1 mg/dose

Reversal of neuromuscular blockade

- *Adult and child:* **IV** 200 mcg for each 1 mg of neostigmine or 5 mg **IV** of pyridostigmine simultaneously

GI disorders

- *Adult:* **PO** 1-2 mg bid-tid, max 6 mg/day; **IM/IV** 100-200 mcg tid-qid, titrated to patient response

Antidysrhythmic

- *Adult:* **IV** 100 mcg, may repeat q2min
- *Child:* **IV** 4.4 mcg/kg, may repeat q2min, max 100 mcg

Secretion control

- *Child:* **PO** 40-100 mcg/kg/dose tid-qid; **IM/IV** 4-10 mcg/kg/dose q3-4hr; max 0.2 mg/dose or 0.8 mg/24 hr

Available forms: Tabs 1, 2 mg; inj 200 mcg (0.2 mg)/ml

SIDE EFFECTS

CNS: Confusion, anxiety, restlessness, irritability, delusions, hallucinations, headache, sedation, depression, incoherence, dizziness, lethargy, flushing, weakness, **seizures**
CV: Palpitations, tachycardia, postural hypotension, paradoxical bradycardia
EENT: Blurred vision, photophobia, dilated pupils, difficulty swallowing, increased intraocular pressure, mydriasis, cycloplegia
GI: *Dryness of mouth, constipation,* nausea, vomiting, abdominal distress, paralytic ileus, altered taste perception
GU: Urinary hesitancy, retention, impotence
INTEG: Urticaria, allergic reactions
MISC: Suppression of lactation, nasal congestion, decreased sweating, **malignant hyperthermia**
SYST: **Anaphylaxis**

Contraindications: Children <3 yr, hypersensitivity, closed-angle glaucoma, myasthenia gravis, GI/GU obstruction, tachycardia, myocardial ischemia, hepatic disease, ulcerative colitis, toxic megacolon, prostatic hypertrophy

Precautions: Pregnancy (B), breastfeeding, geriatric patients, pulmonary/renal disease, CHF, hyperthyroidism, CAD, Down syndrome, hiatal hernia, hypertension

PHARMACOKINETICS

Excreted in urine (>80% unchanged), half-life 1-2 hr
PO: Peak 1 hr, duration 8-12 hr
IM: Peak 30-45 min, duration 2-7 hr
IV: Peak 10-15 min, duration 2-7 hr

INTERACTIONS

Increase: anticholinergic effect—alcohol, antihistamines, phenothiazines, amantadine, tricyclics
Decrease: glycopyrrolate absorption—antacids, antidiarrheals

NURSING CONSIDERATIONS

Assess:

- I&O ratio; retention commonly causes decreased urinary output
- Urinary hesitancy, retention: palpate bladder if retention occurs
- Constipation; increase fluids, bulk, exercise if this occurs
- Mental status: affect, mood, CNS depression, worsening of mental symptoms during early therapy

Administer:

- Parenteral dose with patient recumbent to prevent postural hypotension
- Parenteral dose slowly; keep in bed for at least 1 hr after dose; monitor VS
- After checking dose carefully; even slight overdose may lead to toxicity
- With or after meals to prevent GI upset; may give with fluids other than water

IV route

- Undiluted, give through a Y-tube or 3-way stopcock; give 0.2 mg or less over 1-2 min

Syringe compatibilities: Atropine, benzquinamide, chlorproMAZINE, cimetidine, codeine, diphenhydrAMINE, droperidol, droperidol/fentanyl, hydromorphone, hydrOXYzine, levorphanol, lidocaine, meperidine, meperidine/promethazine, midazolam, morphine, nalbuphine, neostigmine, oxymorphone, procaine, prochlorperazine, promazine, promethazine, pyridostigmine, ranitidine, scopolamine, triflupromazine, trimethobenzamide

Solution compatibilities: D_5W, 0.9% NaCl, Ringer's, D_5/0.45% NaCl

Perform/provide:

- Storage at room temperature

Evaluate:

- Therapeutic response: decreased secretions; decreased pain in GI disorders; reversal of neuromuscular blockers

Teach patient/family:

- Hard candy, frequent drinks, sugarless gum to relieve dry mouth, use good oral hygiene
- Not to discontinue this product abruptly; to taper off over 1 wk; to take PO ½-1 hr before meals
- To avoid driving, other hazardous activities; drowsiness, blurred vision may occur
- To avoid OTC medication: cough, cold preparations with alcohol, antihistamines unless directed by prescriber
- To avoid hot temperatures, since sweating is decreased, heat stroke is possible
- To change positions slowly to prevent orthostatic hypotension
- To notify prescriber of eye pain, blurred vision, light sensitivity; cardiac dysrhythmias

golimumab (℞)

(goal-lim'yu-mab)

Simponi

Func. class.: Antirheumatic agent (disease modifying), immunomodulator

Chem. class.: Monoclonal antibody, DMARDs, Tumor necrosis factor (TNF-α) modifier

Action: Monoclonal antibody specific for human tumor necrosis factor (TNF); elevated levels of TNF are found in patients with rheumatoid arthritis

Uses: Rheumatoid arthritis (RA), ankylosing spondylitis, psoriatic arthritis

DOSAGE AND ROUTES

- *Adult:* **SUBCUT** 50 mg q month, for RA; give with methotrexate

Available form: Inj 50 mg/0.5 ml prefilled syringe, SmartJect Auto Injector

SIDE EFFECTS

CNS: Dizziness, paresthesia

CV: Hypertension

GI: **Hepatitis**

HEMA: **Agranulocytosis, aplastic anemia, leukopenia, polycythemia, thrombocytopenia, pancytopenia**

INTEG: Psoriasis

MISC: **Increased cancer risk,** antibody development to this drug; **risk of infection (TB, invasive fungal infections, other opportunistic infections), may be fatal,** inj site reactions

Contraindications: Hypersensitivity, active infections

Precautions: Pregnancy (B), breastfeeding, children, geriatric patients, CNS demyelinating disease, latent TB, CHF, hepatitis B carriers, blood dyscrasias, surgery, MS, neurological disease, diabetes, immunosuppression

PHARMACOKINETICS

Terminal half-life 2 wk, lower

INTERACTIONS

- Do not give concurrently with vaccines; immunizations should be brought up to date before treatment

Increase: infection—abatacept, etanercept, rilonacept, rituximab, adalimumab, anakinra, immunosuppressants, infliximab

NURSING CONSIDERATIONS

Assess:

- Pain, stiffness, ROM, swelling of joints during treatment
- For inj site pain, swelling; usually occur after 2 inj (4-5 days)
- ⚠ For infections (fever, flulike symptoms, dyspnea, change in urination, redness/swelling around any wounds), stop treatment if present; some serious infections including sepsis may occur, may be fatal; patients with active infections should not be started on this product

Administer:

SUBCUT route

- Do not admix with other sol or medications; do not use filter; protect from light; give at 45-degree angle using abdomen, thighs; rotate inj sites; discard unused portions
- Other DMARDs should be continued during this therapy

Evaluate:

- Therapeutic response: decreased inflammation, pain in joints, decreased joint destruction

Teach patient/family:

- About self-administration if appropriate: inj should be made in thigh, abdomen, upper arm; rotate sites at least 1 inch from old site, do not inject in areas that are bruised, red, hard
- That if medication is not taken when due, inject next dose as soon as remembered and inject next dose as scheduled
- Not to take any live virus vaccines during treatment
- To report signs/symptoms of infection, allergic reaction, or lupus-like syndrome

goserelin (℞)

(goe'se-rel-lin)

Zoladex

Func. class.: Gonadotropin-releasing hormone, antineoplastic (hormone)

Chem. class.: Synthetic decapeptide analog of LHRH

Action: Inhibitor of pituitary gonadotropin secretion; initially increases LH and FSH, with increases in testosterone, reduction in sex steroid levels (substitute serum testosterone levels)

Uses: Advanced prostate cancer stage B2-C (10.8 mg), endometriosis, advanced breast cancer, endometrial thinning (3.6 mg)

DOSAGE AND ROUTES

- *Adult:* **SUBCUT** 3.6 mg q28days or 10.8 mg q12wk

Endometrial thinning

- *Adult:* **SUBCUT** 1-2 depot inj, usually 1 depot, surgery performed at 4 wk; if 2 depots, surgery performed 2-4 wk after 2nd depot

Available forms: Depot inj 3.6, 10.8 mg

SIDE EFFECTS

CNS: Headaches, **spinal cord compression,** *anxiety, depression, dizziness, in-*

somnia, lethargy, hot flashes, emotional lability
CV: **Dysrhythmia, cerebrovascular accident,** hypertension, **MI,** chest pain, **CHF**
ENDO: Gynecomastia, breast tenderness, hot flashes
GI: Nausea, vomiting, constipation, diarrhea, ulcer
GU: Spotting, breakthrough bleeding, decreased libido, renal insufficiency, urinary obstruction, urinary tract infection, *impotence*
INTEG: Rash, pain on inj, diaphoresis
MS: Osteoneuralgia
RESP: COPD, URI
Contraindications: Pregnancy (D) (breast cancer), (X) (endometriosis), breastfeeding, children, nondiagnosed vaginal bleeding; hypersensitivity to LHRH, LHRH-agonist analogs; 10.8 mg dose contraindicated in women
Precautions: Spinal cord decompression, renal disease, bone mineral density loss

PHARMACOKINETICS

Peak serum concentrations in 14-28 days; half-life 4½ hr

INTERACTIONS

Drug/Lab Test

Increase: alk phos, estradiol, FSH, LH, testosterone levels
Decrease: testosterone levels, progesterone

NURSING CONSIDERATIONS

Assess:

- Pregnancy test prior to therapy
- I&O ratios; palpate bladder for distention in urinary obstruction
- For relief of bone pain (back pain), change in motor function
- Acid phosphatase PSA baseline and periodically

Administer:

Depot

- SUBCUT using implant, inserted by qualified person into upper subcutaneous tissue in abdominal wall q28days or q12wk (10.8 mg), do not attempt to remove air bubbles from syringe

Evaluate:

- Therapeutic response: more normal levels of PSA, acid phosphatase, alk phos; testosterone level of <25 ng/dl

Teach patient/family:

- That gynecomastia and postmenopausal symptoms may occur but will decrease after treatment is discontinued
- That bone pain may increase, then decrease
- To notify prescriber of difficulty urinating, hot flashes
- To keep appointments
- Not to breastfeed, use effective nonhormonal contraception

G

granisetron (℞)

(grane-iss'e-tron)
Kytril, Sancuso
Func. class.: Antiemetic
Chem. class.: 5-HT_3 receptor antagonist

Action: Prevents nausea, vomiting by blocking serotonin peripherally, centrally, and in the small intestine
Uses: Prevention of nausea, vomiting associated with cancer chemotherapy including high-dose cisplatin, radiation
Unlabeled uses: Acute nausea, vomiting following surgery

DOSAGE AND ROUTES

Nausea, vomiting in chemotherapy

- *Adult and child ≥2 yr:* **IV** 10 mcg/kg over 5 min, 30 min before the start of cancer chemotherapy; **TD** apply 1 patch (3.1 mg/24 hr) to upper outer arm 24-48 hr before chemotherapy
- *Adult:* **PO** 1 mg bid, give first dose 1 hr before chemotherapy and next dose 12 hr after first

Nausea, vomiting in radiation therapy

- *Adult:* **PO** 2 mg/day 1 hr prior to radiation

Available forms: Inj 1 mg/ml; tab 1 mg; oral sol 2 mg/10 ml; patch TD 3.1 mg/24 hr

SIDE EFFECTS

CNS: ***Headache, asthenia,*** anxiety, dizziness

CV: Hypertension

GI: Diarrhea, ***constipation,*** increased AST, ALT, ***nausea***

HEMA: **Leukopenia**, anemia, **thrombocytopenia**

MISC: Rash, **bronchospasm**

Contraindications: Hypersensitivity to this product or benzyl alcohol

Precautions: Pregnancy (B), breastfeeding, children, geriatric patients, ondansetron hypersensitivity

PHARMACOKINETICS

Metabolized in liver to an active metabolite, half-life 10-12 hr, protein binding 65%

INTERACTIONS

Increase: EPS—antipsychotics

NURSING CONSIDERATIONS

Assess:

• For absence of nausea, vomiting during chemotherapy

• Hypersensitive reaction: rash, bronchospasm

Administer:

IV route

• May give undiluted over 30 sec via Y-site

IV, intermittent infusion

• Dilute in 0.9% NaCl for inj or D_5W (20-50 ml); give over 5-15 min; ½ hr before chemotherapy

Additive compatibilities: Dexamethasone, methylPREDNISolone

Solution compatibilities: D_5W, 0.9% NaCl

Y-site compatibilities: Acyclovir, allopurinol, amifostine, amikacin, aminophylline, amphotericin B cholesteryl, ampicillin, ampicillin/sulbactam, amsacrine, aztreonam, bleomycin, bumetanide, buprenorphine, butorphanol, calcium gluconate, carboplatin, carmustine, cefazolin, cefepime, cefonicid, cefoperazone, cefotaxime, cefotetan, cefoxitin, ceftazidime, ceftizoxime, ceftriaxone, cefuroxime, chlorproMAZINE, cimetidine, ciprofloxacin, cisplatin, cladribine, clindamycin, cyclophosphamide, cytarabine, dacarbazine, dactinomycin, DAUNOrubicin, dexamethasone, diphenhydrAMINE, DOBUTamine, DOPamine, DOXOrubicin, DOXOrubicin liposome, doxycycline, droperidol, enalaprilat, etoposide, famotidine, filgrastim, fluconazole, fluorouracil, floxuridine, fludarabine, furosemide, gallium, ganciclovir, gentamicin, haloperidol, heparin hydrocortisone, hydromorphone, hydrOXYzine, idarubicin, ifosfamide, imipenem-cilastatin, leucovorin, lorazepam, magnesium sulfate, melphalan, meperidine, mesna, methotrexate, methylPREDNISolone, metoclopramide, metronidazole, mezlocillin, miconazole, minocycline, mitomycin, mitoxantrone, morphine, nalbuphine, netilmicin, ofloxacin, paclitaxel, piperacillin, piperacillin/tazobactam, plicamycin, potassium chloride, prochlorperazine, promethazine, propofol, ranitidine, sargramostim, sodium bicarbonate, streptozocin, teniposide, thiotepa, ticarcillin, ticarcillin/clavulanate, tobramycin, trimethoprim-sulfamethoxazole, vancomycin, vinBLAStine, vinCRIStine, vinorelbine, zidovudine

Perform/provide:

• Storage at room temperature for 24 hr after dilution

Evaluate:

• Therapeutic response: absence of nausea, vomiting during cancer chemotherapy

Teach patient/family:

• To report diarrhea, constipation, rash, changes in respirations

• That headache requiring an analgesic is common

guaifenesin (OTC, ℞)

(gwye-fen'e-sin)

AllFen Jr., Altarussin, Benylin-E ♣, Diabetic Tussin Expectorant, Ganidin NR, guaifenesin, Guaifenesin NR, Guiatuss, Humibid, Mucinex, Naldecon Senior EX, Organidin NR, Refenesen, Robitussin Chest Congestion, Scot-Tussin Expectorant, Siltussin DAS, Siltussin SA

Func. class.: Expectorant

Action: Increases the volume and reduces viscosity of secretions in the trachea and bronchi to facilitate secretion removal

Uses: Productive and nonproductive cough

DOSAGE AND ROUTES

- *Adult and child ≥12 yr:* **PO** 200-400 mg q4hr; **EXT REL** 600-1200 mg q12hr, max 2.4 g/day
- *Child 6-12 yr:* **PO** 100-200 mg q4hr; **EXT REL** 600 mg q12hr, max 1.2 g/day
- *Child 2-6 yr:* **PO** 50-100 mg q4hr; max 600 mg/day

Available forms: Tabs 200, 400 mg; oral sol 100 mg/5 ml; ext rel tabs 600, 1200 mg; syrup 100 mg/5 ml; oral granules 50, 100 mg/packet

SIDE EFFECTS

CNS: Drowsiness, headache, dizziness

GI: Nausea, anorexia, vomiting, diarrhea

Contraindications: Hypersensitivity; chronic, persistent cough

Precautions: Pregnancy (C), breastfeeding, CHF, asthma, emphysema, fever

PHARMACOKINETICS

Half-life 1 hr, excreted urine (metabolites)

NURSING CONSIDERATIONS

Assess:

- Cough: type, frequency, character, including sputum; fluids should be increased to 2 L/day

Administer:

- Do not break, crush, chew ext rel tabs

Perform/provide:

- Storage at room temperature
- Increased fluids, room humidification to liquefy secretions

Evaluate:

- Therapeutic response: productive cough, thinner secretions

Teach patient/family:

- To avoid driving, other hazardous activities if drowsiness occurs (rare)
- To avoid smoking, smoke-filled room, perfumes, dust, environmental pollutants, cleansers
- To consult health provider if cough lasts >7 days

Rarely Used

guanfacine (℞)

(gwahn'fa-seen)

Intuniv, Tenex

Func. class.: Antihypertensive

Uses: Hypertension in individual using a thiazide diuretic or other antihypertensive

Unlabeled uses: Heroin withdrawal, ADHD

DOSAGE AND ROUTES

- *Adult:* **PO** 1 mg/day at bedtime; may increase dose in 3-4 wk to 2 mg/day, max 4 mg daily

Contraindications: Hypersensitivity

halcinonide topical

See Appendix B

H

haloperidol (℞)
(hal-oh-pehr′ih-dol)
Apo-Haloperidol ♣, Haldol, Novo-Peridol ♣, Peridol ♣

haloperidol decanoate (℞)
Haldol Decanoate, Haldol LA ♣

haloperidol lactate (℞)
Haldol, Haldol Concentrate, Haloperidol Intensol

Func. class.: Antipsychotic, neuroleptic

Chem. class.: Butyrophenone

Do not confuse:
haloperidol/Halotestin
Haldol/Stadol

Action: Depresses cerebral cortex, hypothalamus, limbic system, which control activity and aggression; blocks neurotransmission produced by DOPamine at synapse; exhibits strong α-adrenergic, anticholinergic blocking action; mechanism for antipsychotic effects unclear

Uses: Psychotic disorders, control of tics, vocal utterances in Gilles de la Tourette's syndrome, short-term treatment of hyperactive children showing excessive motor activity, prolonged parenteral therapy in chronic schizophrenia, organic mental syndrome with psychotic features, hiccups (short-term), emergency sedation of severely agitated or delirious patients

Unlabeled uses: Nausea, vomiting in surgery; autism; migraine headache

DOSAGE AND ROUTES

Psychosis

• *Adult:* **PO** 0.5-5 mg bid or tid initially depending on severity of condition; dose is increased to desired dose, max 100 mg/day; **IM** (lactate) 2-5 mg q4-8hr or bid-tid

• *Geriatric:* **PO/IM** 0.25-0.5 mg daily-bid, titrate q3-4days by 0.25-0.5 mg/dose

• *Child 3-12 yr:* **PO/IM** (lactate) 0.05-0.15 mg/kg/day

• *Adult:* **IM** (decanoate) initial dose is 10-15 mg × daily oral dose at 4 wk interval; do not administer **IV**; not to exceed 100 mg

Chronic schizophrenia

• *Adult:* **IM** (decanoate) 50-100 mg q4wk

• *Child 3-12 yr:* **PO/IM** 0.05-0.15 mg/kg/day

Tics/vocal utterances

• *Adult:* **PO** 0.5-5 mg bid or tid, increased until desired response occurs

• *Child 3-12 yr:* **PO** 0.05-0.075 mg/kg/day

Hyperactive children

• *Child 3-12 yr:* **PO** 0.05-0.075 mg/kg/day

Available forms: Tabs 0.5, 1, 2, 5, 10, 20 mg; *lactate:* conc 2 mg/ml; inj 5 mg/ml, *decanoate:* 50 mg/ml, 100 mg /ml

SIDE EFFECTS

CNS: EPS: pseudoparkinsonism, akathisia, dystonia, tardive dyskinesia, drowsiness, headache, **seizures, neuroleptic malignant syndrome,** confusion

CV: Orthostatic hypotension, hypertension, **cardiac arrest,** ECG changes, **tachycardia, QT prolongation, sudden death**

EENT: Blurred vision, glaucoma, dry eyes

GI: Dry mouth, nausea, vomiting, anorexia, constipation, diarrhea, jaundice, weight gain, **ileus, hepatitis**

GU: Urinary retention, dysuria, urinary frequency, enuresis, impotence, amenorrhea, gynecomastia

INTEG: Rash, photosensitivity, dermatitis

RESP: **Laryngospasm,** dyspnea, **respiratory depression**

SYST: **Risk for death (dementia)**

Contraindications: Children <3 yr, hypersensitivity, blood dyscrasias, coma, brain damage, bone marrow depression, alcohol and barbiturate withdrawal states, Parkinson's disease, angina, epilepsy, urinary retention, closed-angle glaucoma

Precautions: Pregnancy (C), breastfeeding, geriatric patients, seizure disorders, hypertension, pulmonary/cardiac/hepatic disease

Black Box Warning: Dementia

PHARMACOKINETICS

Metabolized by liver; excreted in urine, bile; crosses placenta; enters breast milk; protein binding 92%, terminal half-life 12-36 hr (metabolites)

PO: Onset erratic, peak 2-6 hr, half-life 24 hr

IM: Onset 15-30 min, peak 15-20 min, half-life 21 hr

IM (Decanoate): Peak 4-11 days, half-life 3 wk

INTERACTIONS

Increase: oversedation—other CNS depressants, alcohol, barbiturate anesthetics

Increase: toxicity—epinephrine, lithium

Increase: both drugs effects—β-adrenergic blockers, alcohol

Increase: anticholinergic effects—anticholinergics

Decrease: effects—lithium, levodopa

Decrease: haloperidol effects—phenobarbital, carbamazepine

Drug/Herb

• Antagonist action: jimsonweed, scopolia

Increase: action—chamomile, cola tree, hops, kava, nettle, nutmeg, skullcap, valerian

Increase: EPS—betel palm, kava

Drug/Lab Test

Increase: LFTs, cardiac enzymes, cholesterol, blood glucose, prolactin, bilirubin, PBI, cholinesterase, alk phos

Decrease: hormones (blood, urine), PT

False positive: pregnancy tests, PKU

False negative: urinary steroids

NURSING CONSIDERATIONS

Assess:

• Swallowing of PO medication; check for hoarding or giving of medication to other patients

• I&O ratio; palpate bladder if low urinary output occurs

• Bilirubin, CBC, LFTs monthly

• Urinalysis is recommended before and during prolonged therapy

• Affect, orientation, LOC, reflexes, gait, coordination, sleep pattern disturbances

• B/P standing and lying; take pulse and respirations q4hr during initial treatment; establish baseline before starting treatment; report drops of 30 mm Hg

• Dizziness, faintness, palpitations, tachycardia on rising

• EPS including akathisia (inability to sit still, no pattern to movements), tardive dyskinesia (bizarre movements of jaw, mouth, tongue, extremities), pseudoparkinsonism (rigidity, tremors, pill rolling, shuffling gait)

• Skin turgor daily

⚠ For neuroleptic malignant syndrome: hyperthermia, muscle rigidity, altered mental status, increased CPK, seizures, hypo/hypertension, tachycardia, notify prescriber immediately

• Constipation, urinary retention daily; if these occur, increase bulk, water in diet

Administer:

• Reduced dose to geriatric patients

• Antiparkinsonian agent, to be used if EPS occurs

• Avoid use with CNS depressants

PO route

• Oral liquid: use calibrated dropper; do not mix in coffee or tea

• PO with food or milk

IM route

• IM inj into large muscle mass, use 21G, 2-in needle; give no more than 3 ml/inj site; patient should remain recumbent for ½ hr

IV route

• Give undiluted for psychotic episode at 5 mg/min

• Give by intermittent inf after dilution in 30-50 ml of D_5W, run over ½ hr

Solution compatibilities: D_5W

Syringe compatibilities: Hydromorphone, sufentanil

Y-site compatibilities: Amifostine, amsacrine, aztreonam, cimetidine, cisatracurium, cladribine, DOBUTamine, DOPamine, DOXOrubicin liposome, famotidine, filgrastim, fludarabine, granisetron, lidocaine, lorazepam, melphalan, midazolam, nitroglycerin, norepinephrine, ondansetron, paclitaxel, phenylephrine, propofol, remifentanil, sufentanil, tacrolimus, teniposide, theophylline, thiotepa, vinorelbine

Perform/provide:

- Decreased sensory input by dimming lights, avoiding loud noises
- Supervised ambulation until stabilized on medication; do not involve in strenuous exercise program because fainting is possible; patient should not stand still for long periods
- Increased fluids, fiber to prevent constipation
- Sips of water, sugarless candy, gum for dry mouth
- Storage in tight, light-resistant container

Evaluate:

- Therapeutic response: decrease in emotional excitement, hallucinations, delusions, paranoia, reorganization of patterns of thought, speech, improvement in specific behaviors

Teach patient/family:

- That orthostatic hypotension occurs often and to rise from sitting or lying position gradually
- To avoid hazardous activities until stabilized on medication
- To remain lying down after IM inj for at least 30 min
- To avoid hot tubs, hot showers, tub baths, since hypotension may occur
- To avoid abrupt withdrawal of this product, or EPS may result; product should be withdrawn slowly
- To avoid OTC preparations (cough, hay fever, cold) unless approved by prescriber, since serious product interactions may occur; avoid use with alcohol; increased drowsiness may occur
- To use a sunscreen to prevent burns
- Regarding compliance with product regimen
- About EPS and necessity for meticulous oral hygiene, since oral candidiasis may occur
- To report impaired vision, jaundice, tremors, muscle twitching
- That in hot weather, heat stroke may occur; take extra precautions to stay cool

Treatment of overdose: Activated charcoal, lavage if orally ingested; provide an airway; do not induce vomiting

⚠ High Alert

heparin (℞)

(hep′a-rin)

Calcilean ♣, Calciparine ♣, Hepalean ♣, Heparin Leo ♣, heparin sodium, Hep-Lock, Hep-Lock U/P

Func. class.: Anticoagulant, antithrombotic

Do not confuse:

heparin/Hespan

Action: Prevents conversion of fibrinogen to fibrin and prothrombin to thrombin by enhancing inhibitory effects of antithrombin III

Uses: Prevention of deep-vein thrombosis, PE, MI, open heart surgery, disseminated intravascular clotting syndrome, atrial fibrillation with embolization, as an anticoagulant in transfusion and dialysis procedures, prevention of DVT/PE, to maintain patency of indwelling venipuncture devices; diagnosis, treatment of DIC

DOSAGE AND ROUTES

Deep vein thrombosis/MI

- *Adult:* **IV BOL** 5000-7000 units q4hr then titrated to PTT or ACT level; **IV INF** after bolus dose, then 1000 units/hr titrated to PTT or ACT level
- *Child:* **IV INF** 50 units/kg, maintenance 100 units/kg q4hr or 20,000 units/m^2 daily

Anticoagulation

- *Adult:* **SUBCUT** 5000 units IV then 10,000-20,000 units, then 8000-10,000 units q8hr or 15,000-20,000 units q12hr **INTERMITTENT IV BOL** 10,000 units, then 5000-10,000 units q4-6hr; **CONT IV**

INF 5000 units (35-70 units/kg), then 20,000-40,000 units given over 24 hr

- *Child >1 yr:* **INTERMITTENT IV BOL** 50-100 units/kg, then 50-100 units/kg q4hr; **CONT INF** 75 units/kg, then 20 units/kg/hr, adjust to maintain aPTT at 60-85 sec
- *Neonate and infant <1 yr:* **CONT IV INF** 75 units/kg, then 28 units/kg/hr, adjust to maintain aPTT at 60-85 sec

Cardiovascular surgery

- *Adult:* **IV INF** 150-300 units/kg
- *Child/infant/neonate:* **IA** 100 units/kg in artery prior to cardiac catheter

Prophylaxis for DVT/PE

- *Adult:* **SUBCUT** 5000 units q8-12hr

Heparin flush

- *Adult and child:* **IV** 10-100 units/ml

Arterial line patency

- *Neonate:* **IA** 0.5-2 units/ml

Available forms: Sol for inj 10, 100, 1000, 5000, 7500, 10,000, 20,000, 40,000 units/ml; premixed 1000 units/500 ml, 2000 units/1000 ml, 12,500 units/250 ml, 25,000 units/250 ml, 25,000 units/500 ml; lock flush preparations 10 units/ml

SIDE EFFECTS

CNS: Fever, chills, headache
GU: **Hematuria**
HEMA: **Hemorrhage, thrombocytopenia, anemia**
INTEG: Rash, dermatitis, urticaria, pruritus, delayed transient alopecia, hematoma, cutaneous necrosis (SUBCUT)
SYST: **Anaphylaxis**

Contraindications: Hypersensitivity, hemophilia, leukemia with bleeding, peptic ulcer disease, severe thrombocytopenic purpura, severe renal/hepatic disease, blood dyscrasias, severe hypertension, subacute bacterial endocarditis, acute nephritis

Precautions: Pregnancy (C), children, geriatric patients, alcoholism, hyperlipidemia, diabetes, renal disease

PHARMACOKINETICS

Half-life 1½ hr; excreted in urine; 95% bound to plasma proteins; does not cross placenta or alter breast milk; removed from the system via the lymph and spleen; partially metabolized in kidney, liver; excreted in urine (<50% unchanged)

SUBCUT: Onset 20-60 min, duration 8-12 hr, well absorbed

IV: Peak 5 min, duration 2-6 hr

INTERACTIONS

- Resistance to heparin: streptokinase

Increase: diazepam action

Increase: heparin action—oral anticoagulants, salicylates, dextran, NSAIDs, platelet inhibitors, cephalosporins, penicillins, ticlopidine, dipyridamole

Decrease: corticosteroids action

Decrease: heparin action—digoxin, tetracyclines, antihistamines

Drug/Herb

Increase: risk of bleeding—agrimony, alfalfa, angelica, anise, basil, bay, bilberry, black haw, bogbean, bromelain, buchu, chamomile, chondroitin, cinchona bark, dong quai, fenugreek, feverfew, garlic, ginger, ginkgo, ginseng, horse chestnut, Irish moss, kelp, kelpware, khella, lovage, lungwort, meadowsweet, motherwort, mugwort, nettle, papaya, parsley (large amts), pau d'arco, pineapple, poplar, prickly ash, safflower, saw palmetto, tonka bean, turmeric, wintergreen, yarrow

Decrease: anticoagulant effect—coenzyme Q10, flax, glucomannan, goldenseal, guar gum

Drug/Lab Test

Increase: ALT, AST, INR, PT, PTT, potassium

Decrease: platelets, triglycerides, cholesterol, plasma free fatty acids

NURSING CONSIDERATIONS

Assess:

⚠ Bleeding: gums, petechiae, ecchymosis, black tarry stools, hematuria, epistaxis, decrease in Hct, B/P; may indicate

H

bleeding, hemorrhage; HIT may occur after product discontinuation

• Blood studies (Hct, occult blood in stools) q3mo

• Partial prothrombin time, which should be 1.5-2.5 × control; for continuous IV inf, check aPTT baseline 6 hr after initiation and 6 hr after any dose change; use aPTT for dosing adjustments; once 2 therapeutic aPTT has been measured, check aPTT daily

• Platelet count q2-3days; thrombocytopenia may occur on 4th day of treatment

• Hypersensitivity: rash, chills, fever, itching; report to prescriber

Administer:

• Cannot be used interchangeably (unit for unit) with LMWHs or heparinoids

• At same time each day to maintain steady blood levels

• Do not mistake heparin sodium inj 10,000 units/ml and Hep-Lock U/P 10 units/ml; they have similar blue labeling

• SUBCUT deep with 25G ⅜-in needle; do not massage area or aspirate when giving SUBCUT inj; give in abdomen between pelvic bones, rotate sites; do not pull back on plunger, leave in for 10 sec; apply gentle pressure for 1 min

• Changing needles is not recommended

• Avoiding all IM inj that may cause bleeding, hematoma

IV route

• Diluted in 0.9% NaCl, dextrose, Ringer's sol and given by direct, intermittent, or continuous inf; give 1000 units or less over 1 min; then 5000 units or less over 1 min; inf may run from 4-24 hr; use inf pump

• When product is added to inf sol for cont IV, invert container at least 6 times to ensure adequate mixing

• Blood after adding 7500 units/100 ml NaCl inj, add 6-8 ml of this sol/100 ml of whole blood

Additive compatibilities: Aminophylline, amphotericin, ascorbic acid, bleomycin, calcium gluconate, cefepime, chloramphenicol, clindamycin, colistimethate, dimenhyDRINATE, DOPamine, enalaprilat, esmolol, floxacillin, fluconazole, flumazenil, furosemide, hydrocortisone, isoproterenol, lidocaine, lincomycin, magnesium sulfate, meropenem, methyldopate, methylPREDNISolone, metronidazole/sodium bicarbonate, nafcillin, norepinephrine, octreotide, penicillin G, potassium chloride, promazine, ranitidine, sodium bicarbonate, verapamil, vit B/C

Syringe compatibilities: Aminophylline, amphotericin B, ampicillin, atropine, azlocillin, bleomycin, cefamandole, cefazolin, cefoperazone, cefotaxime, cefoxitin, chloramphenicol, cimetidine, cisplatin, clindamycin, cyclophosphamide, diazoxide, digoxin, dimenhyDRINATE, DOBUTamine, DOPamine, epinephrine, fentanyl, fluorouracil, furosemide, leucovorin, lidocaine, lincomycin, methotrexate, metoclopramide, mitomycin, moxalactam, nafcillin, naloxone, neostigmine, nitroglycerin, norepinephrine, pancuronium, penicillin G, phenobarbital, piperacillin, sodium nitroprusside, succinylcholine, trimethoprim-sulfamethoxazole, verapamil, vinCRIStine

Y-site compatibilities: Acyclovir, aldesleukin, allopurinol, amifostine, aminophylline, ampicillin, ampicillin/sulbactam, atracurium, atropine, aztreonam, betamethasone, bleomycin, calcium gluconate, cefazolin, cefotetan, ceftazidime, ceftriaxone, chlordiazepoxide, chlorproMAZINE, cimetidine, cisplatin, cladribine, clindamycin, conjugated estrogens, cyanocobalamin, cyclophosphamide, cytarabine, dexamethasone, digoxin, diphenhydrAMINE, DOPamine, DOXOrubicin liposome, edrophonium, enalaprilat, epinephrine, esmolol, ethacrynate, etoposide, famotidine, fentanyl, fluconazole, fludarabine, fluorouracil, foscarnet, furosemide, gallium, gemcitabine, granisetron, hydrALAZINE, hydrocortisone, hydromorphone, insulin (regular), isoproterenol, kanamycin, leucovorin, linezolid, lidocaine, lorazepam, magnesium sulfate, melphalan, menadiol, meperidine, meropenem, methotrexate, methoxamine, methyldopate, methylergonovine, metoclopramide, metronidazole, midazolam, milrinone, minocycline, mitomycin, morphine, nafcillin, neostigmine, nitroglycerin, nitroprusside, norepinephrine, ondansetron, oxacillin, oxytocin, paclitaxel, pancuronium, penicillin G potassium, pentazocine, phytonadione, piperacillin, piperacillin/tazobactam, potassium chloride, prednisoLONE, procainamide, prochlorperazine, propofol, propranolol, pyridostigmine, ranitidine, remifentanil, sargramostim, scopolamine, sodium bicarbonate, streptokinase, succinylcholine, tacrolimus, theophylline, thiopental, thiotepa, ticarcillin, ticarcillin/clavulanate, tirofiban, trimethobenzamide, trimethaphan, vecuronium, vinBLAStine, vinorelbine, warfarin, zidovudine

Perform/provide:

• Storage at room temperature

Evaluate:

• Therapeutic response: decrease of DVT, PTT 1.5-2.5 × control, free-flowing IV

Teach patient/family:

• To avoid OTC preparations that may cause serious product interactions unless directed by prescriber

• That product may be held during active bleeding (menstruation), depending on condition

• To use soft-bristle toothbrush to avoid bleeding gums, avoid contact sports, use electric razor, avoid IM inj

• To carry emergency ID identifying product taken

• To report to prescriber any signs of bleeding: gums, under skin, urine, stools

• To report to prescriber any signs of hypersensitivity: rash, chills, fever, itching

Treatment of overdose: Withdraw product, protamine 1 mg protamine/100 units heparin

hepatitis B immune globulin (℞)

BayHep B, Nabi-HB

Func. class.: Immune globulin

Action: Provides passive immunity to hepatitis B

Uses: Prevention of hepatitis B virus in exposed patients, including passive immunity in neonates born to HBsAg-positive mother

DOSAGE AND ROUTES

• *Adult and child:* **IM** 0.06 ml/kg (usual 3-5 ml) within 7 days of exposure; repeat 28 days after exposure, if patient wishes not to receive the hepatitis B vaccine

Neonates born to hepatitis B surface antigen—positive persons

• *Neonate:* **IM** 0.5 ml within 12 hr of birth

Available forms: Inj 1-, 4-, 5-ml vials; neonatal syringe 0.5 ml

SIDE EFFECTS

CNS: Headache, dizziness, fever

GI: Nausea, vomiting

INTEG: Soreness at inj site, urticaria, erythema, swelling

SYST: Induration, **anaphylaxis, angioedema**

Contraindications: Hypersensitivity to immune globulins, coagulation disorders

Precautions: Pregnancy (C), breastfeeding, children, geriatric patients, hemophilia, active infection, IgA deficiency

INTERACTIONS

• Do not use within 3 months of hepatitis B immune globulin, MMR, varicella, or rotavirus vaccines even after discontinuing product

NURSING CONSIDERATIONS

Assess:

• For history of allergies, skin conditions (eczema, psoriasis, dermatitis), reactions to vaccinations

• For skin reactions: rash, induration, urticaria

⚠ For anaphylaxis: inability to breathe, bronchospasm, hypotension, wheezing, diaphoresis, fever, flushing

Administer:

• After rotating vial; do not shake

• Only with epinephrine 1:1000 on unit to treat laryngospasm

• In deltoid for better absorption (adult)

Perform/provide:
- Written record of immunization
- Comfort measures

Evaluate:
- Prevention of hepatitis B

Teach patient/family:
- That discomfort may occur at site
- To report any rash, wheezing, inability to breathe immediately

homatropine ophthalmic
See Appendix B

*hydrALAZINE (℞)
(hye-dral'a-zeen)
Apresoline, hydrALAZINE HCl, Novo-Hylazin ♣
Func. class.: Antihypertensive, direct-acting peripheral vasodilator
Chem. class.: Phthalazine

Do not confuse:
hydrALAZINE/hydrOXYzine
Apresoline/allopurinol

Action: Vasodilates arteriolar smooth muscle by direct relaxation; reduction in blood pressure with reflex increases in heart rate, stroke volume, cardiac output

Uses: Essential hypertension; severe essential hypertension

Unlabeled uses: CHF

DOSAGE AND ROUTES

Hypertension
- *Adult:* **PO** 10 mg qid 2-4 days, then 25 mg for rest of first wk, then 50 mg qid individualized to desired response, max 300 mg/day
- *Child:* **PO** 0.75-1 mg/kg/day in 4 divided doses, max 25 mg/dose

Hypertensive crisis
- *Adult:* **IV BOL** 10-20 mg q4-6hr, administer **PO** as soon as possible; **IM** 10-50 mg q4-6hr
- *Child:* **IV BOL** 0.1-0.6 mg/kg q4-6hr; **IM** 0.1-0.6 mg/kg q4-6hr

CHF
- *Adult:* **PO** 10-25 mg tid, max 75 mg tid

Available forms: Inj 20 mg/ml; tabs 10, 25, 50, 100 mg

SIDE EFFECTS

CNS: Headache, tremors, dizziness, anxiety, peripheral neuritis, depression, fever, chills

CV: Palpitations, reflex tachycardia, angina, **shock,** rebound hypertension

GI: Nausea, vomiting, anorexia, diarrhea, constipation, paralytic ileus

GU: Urinary retention

HEMA: **Leukopenia, agranulocytosis,** anemia, **thrombocytopenia**

INTEG: Rash, pruritus, urticaria

MISC: Nasal congestion, muscle cramps, *lupuslike symptoms,* flushing, edema, dyspnea

Contraindications: Hypersensitivity to hydrALAZINEs, mitral valvular rheumatic heart disease, dissecting aortic aneurysm

Precautions: Pregnancy (C), breastfeeding, geriatric patients, CVA, advanced renal disease, CAD, hepatic disease, SLE

PHARMACOKINETICS

Half-life 2-8 hr, metabolized by liver, 12%-14% excreted in urine, protein binding 89%

PO: Onset 20-30 min, peak 1-2 hr, duration 6-12 hr

IM: Onset 10-30 min, peak 1 hr, duration 2-12 hr

IV: Onset 5-30 min, peak 10-80 min, duration 2-12 hr

INTERACTIONS

Increase: severe hypotension—MAOIs

Increase: tachycardia, angina—sympathomimetics (epinephrine, norepinephrine)

Increase: hypotension—other antihypertensives, alcohol

Increase: effects of β-blockers

Decrease: hydrALAZINE effects—indomethacin

Drug/Herb

Increase: toxicity, death—aconite

Increase: antihypertensive effect—barberry, betony, black catechu, black cohosh, bloodroot, broom, burdock, cat's claw, dandelion, goldenseal, hawthorn, Irish moss, Jamaican dogwood, kelp, khella, mistletoe, parsley

Increase or decrease: antihypertensive effect—astragalus, cola tree

Decrease: antihypertensive effect—coltsfoot, guarana, khat, licorice, yohimbe

NURSING CONSIDERATIONS

Assess:

- Cardiac status: B/P q5min × 2 hr, then q1hr × 2 hr, then q4hr; pulse, jugular venous distention q4hr
- Electrolytes, blood studies: K, Na, Cl, CO_2, CBC, serum glucose
- Weight daily, I&O
- LE prep, ANA titer before starting therapy and during treatment; assess for fever, joint pain, rash, sore throat (lupus-like symptoms); notify prescriber
- Edema in feet, legs daily
- Skin turgor, dryness of mucous membranes for hydration status
- Crackles, dyspnea, orthopnea
- IV site for extravasation, rate
- Fever, joint pain, tachycardia, palpitations, headache, nausea
- Mental status: affect, mood, behavior, anxiety; check for personality changes

Administer:

- Give with meals (PO) to enhance absorption
- To recumbent patient, keep for 1 hr after administration

IV route

- IV undiluted; give through Y-tube or 3-way stopcock, give each 10 mg over 1 min or more

Additive compatibilities: DOBUTamine

Y-site compatibilities: Heparin, hydrocortisone, potassium chloride, verapamil, vit B/C

Solution compatibilities: D_5LR, D_5W, $D_{10}W$, $D_{10}LR$ 0.45% NaCl, 0.9% NaCl, Ringer's, LR

Evaluate:

- Therapeutic response: decreased B/P

Teach patient/family:

- To take with food to increase bioavailability (PO)
- To avoid OTC preparations unless directed by prescriber
- To notify prescriber if chest pain, severe fatigue, fever, muscle or joint pain occurs
- To rise slowly to prevent orthostatic hypotension
- To notify prescriber if pregnancy is suspected

Treatment of overdose: Administer vasopressors, volume expanders for shock; if PO, lavage or give activated charcoal, digitalization

H

hydrochlorothiazide (℞)

(hye-droe-klor-oh-thye′a-zide)

Apo-Hydrol ✦, Esidrix, HCTZ, Hydro-Chlor, hydrochlorothiazide, Hydro-D, HydroDIURIL, Microzide, Neo-Codema ✦, Novohydrazide ✦, Oretic, Urozide ✦

Func. class.: Thiazide diuretic, antihypertensive

Chem. class.: Sulfonamide derivative

Action: Acts on distal tubule and ascending limb of loop of Henle by increasing excretion of water, sodium, chloride, potassium

Uses: Edema, hypertension, diuresis, CHF; edema in corticosteroid, estrogen, NSAIDs, idiopathic lower extremity edema therapy

DOSAGE AND ROUTES

- *Adult:* **PO** 12.5-100 mg/day
- *Geriatric:* **PO** 12.5 mg/day, initially
- *Child >6 mo:* **PO** 2 mg/kg/day in divided doses
- *Child <6 mo:* **PO** up to 2-4 mg/kg/day in divided doses

Available forms: Tabs 25, 50, 100 mg; caps 12.5 mg; oral sol 10 mg/5 ml, 100 mg/ml

SIDE EFFECTS

CNS: Drowsiness, paresthesia, depression, headache, *dizziness, fatigue, weakness,* fever

CV: Irregular pulse, orthostatic hypotension, palpitations, volume depletion, allergic myocarditis

EENT: Blurred vision

ELECT: *Hypokalemia,* hypercalcemia, hyponatremia, hypochloremia, hypomagnesemia

GI: *Nausea, vomiting, anorexia,* constipation, diarrhea, cramps, pancreatitis, GI irritation, **hepatitis**

GU: *Urinary frequency,* polyuria, **uremia, glucosuria,** hyperuricemia

HEMA: **Aplastic anemia, hemolytic anemia, leukopenia, agranulocytosis, thrombocytopenia, neutropenia**

INTEG: *Rash,* urticaria, purpura, photosensitivity, alopecia, erythema multiforme

META: *Hyperglycemia, hyperuricemia,* increased creatinine, BUN

Contraindications: Hypersensitivity to thiazides or sulfonamides, anuria, renal decompensation, hypomagnesemia

Precautions: Pregnancy (B), breastfeeding, hypokalemia, renal/hepatic disease, gout, COPD, LE, diabetes mellitus, hyperlipidemia, CCr <25 ml/min

PHARMACOKINETICS

PO: Onset 2 hr, peak 4 hr, duration 6-12 hr, half-life 6-15 hr, excreted unchanged by kidneys, crosses placenta, enters breast milk

INTERACTIONS

Increase: hyperglycemia, hyperuricemia, hypotension—diazoxide

Increase: hypokalemia—glucocorticoids, amphotericin B

Increase: toxicity—lithium, nondepolarizing skeletal muscle relaxants, cardiac glycosides

Increase: renal failure risk—NSAIDs

Increase: effects—loop diuretics

Decrease: antidiabetics effects

Decrease: thiazides absorption—cholestyramine, colestipol

Drug/Herb

- Severe photosensitivity: St. John's wort

Increase: hypokalemia—aloe, buckthorn, cascara sagrada, Chinese rhubarb, gossypol, licorice, nettle, senna

Increase: diuretic effect—cucumber, dandelion, ginkgo, horsetail, khella, licorice, nettle, pumpkin, Queen Anne's lace

Drug/Lab Test

Increase: BSP retention, amylase, parathyroid test

Decrease: PBI, PSP

NURSING CONSIDERATIONS

Assess:

- Weight, I&O daily to determine fluid loss; effect of product may be decreased if used daily
- Rate, depth, rhythm of respiration, effect of exertion
- B/P lying, standing; postural hypotension may occur
- Electrolytes: K, Mg, Na, Cl; include BUN, blood glucose, CBC, serum creatinine, blood pH, ABGs, uric acid, Ca; renal function
- Glucose in urine if patient is diabetic
- Signs of metabolic alkalosis: drowsiness, restlessness
- Signs of hypokalemia: postural hypotension, malaise, fatigue, tachycardia, leg cramps, weakness, dehydration
- Rashes, temp daily
- Confusion, especially in geriatric patients; take safety precautions if needed

Administer:

- In AM to avoid interference with sleep if using product as a diuretic
- Potassium replacement if potassium <3 mg/dl
- With food; if nausea occurs, absorption may be decreased slightly

Evaluate:

- Therapeutic response: improvement in edema of feet, legs, sacral area daily, decreased B/P

Teach patient/family:

- To increase fluid intake to 2-3 L/day unless contraindicated; to rise slowly from lying or sitting position
- To notify prescriber of muscle weakness, cramps, nausea, dizziness; hypokalemia is common
- That product may be taken with food or milk
- To use sunscreen for photosensitivity
- That blood glucose may be increased in diabetics
- To take early in day to avoid nocturia
- To avoid alcohol; avoid OTC meds unless approved by prescriber

Treatment of overdose: Lavage if taken orally; monitor electrolytes; administer dextrose in saline; monitor hydration, CV, renal status

hydrocodone (℞)

(hye-droe-koe′done)

Hycodan, Robidone ✦, Tussigon

hydrocodone/acetaminophen (℞)

Anexsia, Bancap HC, Ceta-Plus, Co-Gesic, Duocet, Hydrocet, Hydrogesic, Lorcet, Lortab, Maxidone, Norco, Panlor, Polygesic, Stagesic, T-Gesic, Vanacet, Vicodin, Vicodin ES, Vicodin HP, Xodol, Zamicet, Zydone

hydrocodone/ibuprofen (℞)

Ibudone, Reprexain, Vicoprofen

Func. class.: Antitussive opioid analgesic/nonopioid analgesic

Controlled Substance Schedule III

Do not confuse:

hydrocodone/hydrocortisone

Hycodan/Vicodin

Action: Acts directly on cough center in medulla to suppress cough; binds to opiate receptors in CNS to reduce pain

Uses: Hyperactive and nonproductive cough, mild-moderate pain

DOSAGE AND ROUTES

Analgesic

- *Adult:* **PO** 2.5-10 mg q3-6hr prn

Antitussive

- *Adult:* **PO** 5 mg q4-6hr prn, max 30 mg/24 hr

Available forms: *Hydrocodone:* tabs 5 mg (Hycodan); syr 5 mg/ml (Hycodan, Robidone ✦); *hydrocodone/acetaminophen:* tabs 2.5 mg hydrocodone/500 mg acetaminophen (Lortab 2.5/500), 5 mg hydrocodone/400 mg acetaminophen (Zydone), 5 mg hydrocodone/500 mg acetaminophen (Anexsia 5/500, Co-Gesic, Dolacet, Hydrocet, Hydrogesic, Hy-Phen, Lorcet, Lortab 5/500, Maragesic-H, Panacet 5/500, Stagesic, T-Gesic, Vicodin); 7.5 mg hydrocodone/400 mg acetaminophen (Zydone), 7.5 mg hydrocodone/500 mg acetaminophen (Lortab 7.5/500), 7.5 mg hydrocodone/650 mg acetaminophen (Anexsia 7.5/650, Lorcet Plus), 7.5 mg hydrocodone/750 mg acetaminophen (Vicodin ES), 10 mg hydrocodone/325 acetaminophen (Norco), 10 mg hydrocodone/500 mg acetaminophen (Lortab 10/500), 10 mg hydrocodone/650 mg acetaminophen (Lorcet 10/650, Vicodin HP), 10 mg hydrocodone/660 acetaminophen (Anexsia 10/660, Vicodin HP); caps 5 mg hydrocodone/500 mg acetaminophen (Bancap HC, Dolacet, Hydrocet, Hydrogesic, Lorcet-HD, Maragesic-H, Stagesic, T-Gesic, Zydone); elixir or oral solution 2.5 mg hydrocodone/167 mg acetaminophen/5 ml; *hydrocodone/aspirin:* tabs 5 mg hydrocodone/500 mg aspirin (Alor 5/500, Azdone, Damason-P, Lortab ASA, Panasal 5/500); *hydrocodone/ibuprofen:* tabs 7.5 mg hydrocodone/200 mg ibuprofen (Vicoprofen)

SIDE EFFECTS

CNS: *Drowsiness*, dizziness, lightheadedness, confusion, headache, sedation, euphoria, dysphoria, weakness,

hallucinations, disorientation, mood changes, dependence, **seizures**
CV: Palpitations, tachycardia, bradycardia, change in B/P, **circulatory depression**, syncope; **cardiac arrest (children)**
EENT: Tinnitus, blurred vision, miosis, diplopia
GI: Nausea, vomiting, anorexia, constipation, cramps, dry mouth, ulcers
GU: Increased urinary output, dysuria, urinary retention
INTEG: Rash, urticaria, flushing, pruritus
RESP: **Respiratory depression; pulmonary edema, bronchopneumonia, respiratory arrest (children)**

Contraindications: Acne rosacea/vulgaris, Cushing's, measles, perioral dermatitis, varicella, abrupt discontinuation, hypersensitivity to this product or benzyl hypersensitivity

Precautions: Pregnancy (C), breastfeeding, neonates, addictive personality, increased intracranial pressure, MI (acute), severe heart disease, respiratory depression, renal/hepatic disease, bowel impaction, urinary retention, viral infection, ulcerative colitis, seizures, sulfite hypersensitivity, psychosis, hypertension, hyperthyroidism

PHARMACOKINETICS

Onset 10-20 min, duration 4-6 hr, half-life 3½-4½ hr, metabolized in liver, excreted in urine, crosses placenta

INTERACTIONS

Increase: CNS depression—alcohol, opioids, sedative/hypnotics, phenothiazines, skeletal muscle relaxants, general anesthetics, tricyclics
Increase: severe reactions—MAOIs

Drug/Herb
Increase: CNS depression—Jamaican dogwood, lavender, mistletoe, nettle, pokeweed, poppy, senega, valerian
Increase: anticholinergic effect—corkwood

Drug/Lab Test
Increase: amylase, lipase

NURSING CONSIDERATIONS

Assess:
- Pain: intensity, type, location, and other characteristics
- CNS changes: dizziness, drowsiness, hallucinations, euphoria, LOC, pupil reaction
- Allergic reactions: rash, urticaria
- Cough and respiratory dysfunction: respiratory depression, character, rate, rhythm; notify prescriber if respirations are <10/min
- Need for pain medication, physical dependence
- History of ulcers if using the ibuprofen combination product

Administer:
- Do not break, crush, or chew tabs; only scored tabs can be broken
- With antiemetic after meals if nausea or vomiting occurs
- Do not exceed 4 g acetaminophen with combination product

Perform/provide:
- Storage in light-resistant area at room temperature
- Assistance with ambulation
- Safety measures: night-light, call bell within easy reach

Evaluate:
- Therapeutic response: decrease in pain or cough

Teach patient/family:
- To report any symptoms of CNS changes, allergic reactions
- That physical dependency may result when used for extended periods
- That withdrawal symptoms may occur: nausea, vomiting, cramps, fever, faintness, anorexia
- To avoid driving, other hazardous activities, drowsiness occurs
- To avoid other CNS depressants, will enhance sedating properties of this product

Treatment of overdose: Naloxone HCl (Narcan) 0.2-0.8 mg IV, O_2, IV fluids, vasopressors

hydrocortisone (℞)

(hy-dro-kor'tih-sone)

Cortef, Cortenema, Hydrocortone

hydrocortisone acetate (℞)

Cortifoam, Hydrocortone Acetate

hydrocortisone cypionate (℞)

Cortef

hydrocortisone sodium phosphate (℞)

Hydrocortone Phosphate

hydrocortisone sodium succinate (℞)

A-hydroCort, Solu-Cortef

Func. class.: Corticosteroid

Chem. class.: Short-acting glucocorticoid

Do not confuse:
hydrocortisone/hydrocodone

Action: Decreases inflammation by suppression of migration of polymorphonuclear leukocytes, fibroblasts, reversal of increased capillary permeability, and lysosomal stabilization

Uses: Severe inflammation, septic shock, adrenal insufficiency, ulcerative colitis, collagen disorders

Unlabeled uses: Carpal tunnel syndrome, Churg-Strauss syndrome, endophthalmitis, mixed connective tissue disease, multiple myeloma, polyarteritis nodosa, polychondritis, pulmonary edema, temporal arteritis, Wegener's granulomatosis

DOSAGE AND ROUTES

Adrenal insufficiency/inflammation

• *Adult:* **PO** 5-30 mg bid-qid; **IM/IV** 100-250 mg (succinate), then 50-100 mg **IM** as needed; **IM/IV** (phosphate) 15-240 mg q12hr

Shock prevention

• *Adult:* **IM/IV** (succinate) 500 mg-2 g q2-6hr

• *Child:* **IM/IV** (succinate) 0.16-1 mg/kg or 6-30 mg/m² given daily or bid

Colitis

• *Adult:* **PO** 20-240 mg (base)/day in 2-4 divided doses; **ENEMA** 100 mg nightly for 21 days

• *Child:* **PO** 2-8 mg (base)/kg/day or 60-240 mg (base)/m²/day in 3-4 divided doses

Available forms: Tabs 5, 10, 20 mg; inj 25, 50 mg/ml; enema 100 mg/60 ml; *acetate:* inj 25 ♣, 50 mg/ml ♣, enema 10% aerosol foam; supp 25 mg; *cypionate:* oral susp 10 mg/5 ml; *phosphate:* inj 50 mg/ml; *succinate:* inj 100 mg ♣, 250 mg ♣, 500 mg ♣, 1000 mg/vial ♣

SIDE EFFECTS

CNS: Depression, flushing, sweating, headache, mood changes

CV: Hypertension, **circulatory collapse, thrombophlebitis, embolism,** tachycardia, edema

EENT: Fungal infections, increased intraocular pressure, blurred vision

GI: Diarrhea, nausea, abdominal distention, **GI hemorrhage,** increased appetite, **pancreatitis**

HEMA: **Thrombocytopenia**

INTEG: Acne, poor wound healing, ecchymosis, petechiae

MS: Fractures, osteoporosis, weakness

Contraindications: Children <2 yr, psychosis, hypersensitivity, idiopathic thrombocytopenia (IM), acute glomerulonephritis, amebiasis, fungal infections, nonasthmatic bronchial disease, AIDS, TB, recent MI (associated with left ventricular rupture)

Precautions: Pregnancy (C), breastfeeding, diabetes mellitus, glaucoma, osteoporosis, seizure disorders, ulcerative colitis, CHF, myasthenia gravis, renal disease, esophagitis, peptic ulcer, metastatic carcinoma

PHARMACOKINETICS

Metabolized by liver, excreted in urine (17-OHCS, 17-KS), crosses placenta

PO: Peak 1-2 hr, duration 1-1½ days

H

IM/IV: Onset 20 min, peak 4-8 hr, duration 1-1½ days
RECT: Onset 3-5 days

INTERACTIONS

Increase: GI bleeding risk—salicylates, NSAIDs
Increase: side effects—alcohol, amphotericin B, digoxin, cycloSPORINE, diuretics
Decrease: hydrocortisone action—cholestyramine, colestipol, barbiturates, rifampin, ephedrine, phenytoin, theophylline
Decrease: anticoagulant effects, anticonvulsants, antidiabetics, calcium supplements, toxoids, vaccines

Drug/Herb

Increase: hypokalemia—aloe, buckthorn, cascara sagrada, cat's claw, Chinese rhubarb, echinacea, senna, St. John's wort
Increase: corticosteroid effect—aloe, licorice, perilla

Drug/Lab Test

Increase: cholesterol, sodium, blood glucose, uric acid, calcium, urine glucose
Decrease: Ca, K, T_4, T_3, thyroid ^{131}I uptake test, urine 17-OHCS, 17-KS
False negative: skin allergy tests

NURSING CONSIDERATIONS

Assess:

- Potassium, blood glucose, urine glucose while on long-term therapy; hypokalemia and hyperglycemia
- Weight daily, notify prescriber of weekly gain >5 lb
- B/P q4hr, pulse; notify prescriber of chest pain
- I&O ratio; be alert for decreasing urinary output, increasing edema
- Plasma cortisol levels during long-term therapy (normal level: 138-635 nmol/L SI units when drawn at 8 AM)
- Infection: increased temp, WBC, even after withdrawal of medication; product masks infection
- Potassium depletion: paresthesias, fatigue, nausea, vomiting, depression, polyuria, dysrhythmias, weakness
- Edema, hypertension, cardiac symptoms
- Mental status: affect, mood, behavioral changes, aggression

Administer:

- Daily dose in AM for better results
- IM inj deep in large muscle mass; rotate sites; avoid deltoid; use 21G needle
- In one dose in AM to prevent adrenal suppression; avoid SUBCUT administration; may damage tissue
- With food or milk for GI symptoms (PO)
- Rectal: telling patient to retain for 20 min if possible

IV route

- Phosphate: IV undiluted or added to dextrose or saline inj and given by inf; give 25 mg or less/min
- Succinate: IV in mix-o-vial, or reconstitute 250 mg or less/2 ml bacteriostatic H_2O for inj; mix gently; give direct IV over 1 min or more; may be further diluted in 100, 250, 500, or 1000 ml of D_5W, D_5 0.9%, NaCl 0.9% given over ordered rate

Sodium phosphate preparations

Additive compatibilities: Amikacin, amphotericin B, bleomycin, cephapirin, metaraminol, sodium bicarbonate, verapamil

Syringe compatibilities: Metoclopramide

Y-site compatibilities: Allpurinol, amifostine, aztreonam, cefepime, cladribine, famotidine, filgrastim, fluconazole, fludarabine, granisetron, melphalan, ondansetron, paclitaxel, piperacillin/tazobactam, teniposide, thiotepa, vinorelbine

Sodium succinate preparations

Additive compatibilities: Amikacin, aminophylline, amphotericin B, calcium chloride, calcium gluconate, cephalothin, cephapirin, chloramphenicol, clindamycin, cloxacillin, corticotropin, DAUNOrubicin, diphenhydrAMINE, DOPamine, erythromycin, floxacillin, lidocaine, magnesium sulfate, mephentermine, metronidazole/sodium bicarbonate, mitomycin, mitoxantrone, netilmicin,

netilmicin/potassium chloride, norepinephrine, penicillin G potassium/sodium, piperacillin, polymyxin B, potassium chloride, sodium bicarbonate, theophylline, thiopental, vancomycin, verapamil, vit B/C

Syringe compatibilities: Metoclopramide, thiopental

Y-site compatibilities: Acyclovir, allopurinol, amifostine, aminophylline, amphotericin B cholesteryl, ampicillin, amrinone, amsacrine, atracurium, atropine, aztreonam, betamethasone, calcium gluconate, cefepime, cefmetazole, cephalothin, cephapirin, chlordiazepoxide, chlorproMAZINE, cisatracurium, cladribine, cyanocobalamin, cytarabine, dexamethasone, digoxin, diphenhydrAMINE, DOPamine, DOXOrubicin liposome, droperidol, edrophonium, enalaprilat, epinephrine, esmolol, estrogens conjugated, ethacrynate, famotidine, fentanyl, fentanyl/droperidol, filgrastim, fludarabine, fluorouracil, foscarnet, furosemide, gallium, granisetron, heparin, hydrALAZINE, insulin (regular), isoproterenol, kanamycin, lidocaine, lorazepam, magnesium sulfate, melphalan, menadiol, meperidine, methicillin, methoxamine, methylergonovine, minocycline, morphine, neostigmine, norepinephrine, ondansetron, oxacillin, oxytocin, paclitaxel, pancuronium, penicillin G potassium, pentazocine, phytonadione, piperacillin/tazobactam, prednisolone, procainamide, prochlorperazine, propofol, propranolol, pyridostigmine, remifentanil, scopolamine, sodium bicarbonate, succinylcholine, tacrolimus, teniposide, theophylline, thiotepa, trimethaphan, trimethobenzamide, vecuronium, vinorelbine

Perform/provide:

- Assistance with ambulation in patient with bone tissue disease to prevent fractures

Evaluate:

- Therapeutic response: decreased inflammation, GI symptoms

Teach patient/family:

- That emergency ID as corticosteroid user should be carried
- To notify prescriber if therapeutic response decreases; dosage adjustment may be needed; of signs of infection
- Not to discontinue abruptly, or adrenal crisis can result; product should be tapered off
- That product can mask infection and cause hypoglycemia (diabetic)
- To avoid OTC products: salicylates, alcohol in cough products, cold preparations unless directed by prescriber
- About cushingoid symptoms of adrenal insufficiency: nausea, anorexia, fatigue, dizziness, dyspnea, weakness, joint pain
- To avoid live-virus vaccines if using steroids long term

hydrocortisone topical

See Appendix B

⚠ High Alert

hydromorphone (℞)

(hye-droe-mor′fone)

Dilaudid, Dilaudid HP, hydromorphone HCl, Hydrostat IR, PMS-Hydromorphone

Func. class.: Opiate analgesic

Chem. class.: Semisynthetic phenanthrene

Controlled Substance Schedule II

Do not confuse:

hydromorphone/meperidine/morphine

Dilaudid/Demerol

Action: Inhibits ascending pain pathways in CNS, increases pain threshold, alters pain perception

Uses: Moderate to severe pain, nonproductive cough

DOSAGE AND ROUTES

Analgesic

- *Adult:* **PO** (oral solution) 2.5-10 mg q3-6hr or (tabs) 2-4 mg q4-6hr; **IM/**

SUBCUT/IV 1-2 mg q4-6hr prn, may be increased; **RECT** 3 mg q6-8hr prn

- *Geriatric:* **PO** 1-2 mg q4-6hr
- *Child >50 kg (unlabeled):* **PO** 2-4 mg q3-4hr in opioid-naive patients, titrate
- *Infant >6 mo/child <50 kg (unlabeled):* **PO** 0.04-0.08 mg/kg q3-4hr in opioid-naive patients, titrate

Available forms: Inj 1, 2, 4, 10 mg/ml; tabs 2, 4, 8 mg; supp 3 mg; oral sol 5 mg/5 ml

SIDE EFFECTS

CNS: Drowsiness, dizziness, confusion, headache, sedation, euphoria, mood changes, **seizures**

CV: Palpitations, bradycardia, change in B/P, hypotension, tachycardia, peripheral vasodilation

EENT: Tinnitus, blurred vision, miosis, diplopia

GI: Nausea, vomiting, anorexia, constipation, cramps, dry mouth, paralytic ileus

GU: Increased urinary output, dysuria, urinary retention

INTEG: Rash, urticaria, bruising, flushing, diaphoresis, pruritus

RESP: **Respiratory depression,** dyspnea

Contraindications: Hypersensitivity

Precautions: Pregnancy (C), breastfeeding, children <18 yr, addictive personality, increased intracranial pressure, MI (acute), severe heart disease, renal/hepatic disease, bowel impaction, abrupt discontinuation, COPD

Black Box Warning: Respiratory depression, opioid-naive patients, substance abuse

PHARMACOKINETICS

Onset 15-30 min, peak ½-1 hr, duration 4-5 hr, metabolized by liver, excreted by kidneys, crosses placenta, excreted in breast milk, half-life 2-3 hr

INTERACTIONS

Increase: effects—alcohol, opiates, sedative/hypnotics, antipsychotics, skeletal muscle relaxants

⚠ ***Increase:*** severe reactions—MAOIs

Drug/Herb

Increase: action—chamomile, hops, Jamaican dogwood, kava, lavender, mistletoe, nettle, pokeweed, poppy, senega, skullcap, St. John's wort, valerian

Increase: anticholinergic effect—corkwood

Drug/Lab Test

Increase: amylase

NURSING CONSIDERATIONS

Assess:

- Respiratory dysfunction: respiratory depression, character, rate, rhythm; notify prescriber if respirations are <10/min
- I&O ratio; check for decreasing output; may indicate urinary retention
- CNS changes: dizziness, drowsiness, hallucinations, euphoria, LOC, pupil reaction
- Bowel function, constipation
- Allergic reactions: rash, urticaria
- Need for pain medication, physical dependence
- Pain control, sedation by scoring on 0-10 scale, ATC dosing is best for pain control

Administer:

- With antiemetic if nausea, vomiting occur
- When pain is beginning to return; determine interval by response
- Rotate inj sites when giving SUBCUT

IV route

- Direct, diluted with 5 ml sterile H_2O or NS; give through Y-connector or 3-way stopcock; give 2 mg or less/3-5 min
- IV INF: Dilute each 0.1-1 mg/ml NS (0.1-1 mg/ml), deliver by opioid syringe infusor; may be diluted in D_5W, D_5/NaCl, 0.45% NaCl, or NS for larger amounts and delivery through an inf pump

Additive compatibilities: Bupivacaine, clonidine, fluorouracil, heparin, midazolam, ondansetron, potassium chloride, promethazine, verapamil, ziconotide

Solution compatibilities: D_5W, D_5/0.45% NaCl, D_5/0.9% NaCl, D_5/LR, D_5/Ringer's sol, 0.45% NaCl, 0.9% NaCl, Ringer's and lactated Ringer's sol

Syringe compatibilities: Atropine, bupivacaine, ceftazidime, chlorproMAZINE, cimetidine, dimenhyDRINATE, diphenhydrAMINE, fentanyl, glycopyrrolate, haloperidol, hydrOXYzine, lorazepam, midazolam, pentazocine, pentobarbital, prochlorperazine, promethazine, ranitidine, scopolamine, tetracaine, thiethylperazine, trimethobenzamide

Y-site compatibilities: Acyclovir, allopurinol, amifostine, amikacin, amsacrine, aztreonam, cefamandole, cefazolin, cefepime, cefmetazole, cefoperazone, cefotaxime, cefoxitin, ceftazidime, ceftizoxime, cefuroxime, cephalothin, cephapirin, chloramphenicol, cisatracurium, cisplatin, cladribine, clindamycin, cyclophosphamide, cytarabine, diltiazem, DOBUTamine, DOPamine, DOXOrubicin, DOXOrubicin liposome, doxycycline, epinephrine, erythromycin lactobionate, famotidine, fentanyl, filgrastim, fludarabine, foscarnet, furosemide, gentamicin, granisetron, heparin, kanamycin, labetalol, lorazepam, magnesium sulfate, melphalan, methotrexate, metronidazole, mezlocillin, midazolam, milrinone, morphine, moxalactam, nafcillin, niCARdipine, nitroglycerin, norepinephrine, ondansetron, oxacillin, paclitaxel, penicillin G potassium, piperacillin, piperacillin/tazobactam, propofol, ranitidine, remifentanil, teniposide, thiotepa, ticarcillin, tobramycin, trimethoprim-sulfamethoxazole, vancomycin, vecuronium, vinorelbine

Perform/provide:

- Storage in light-resistant area at room temperature
- Assistance with ambulation
- Safety measures: side rails, night-light, call bell within easy reach

Evaluate:

- Therapeutic response: decrease in pain

Teach patient/family:

- To report any symptoms of CNS changes, allergic reactions
- That physical dependency may result when used for extended periods
- That withdrawal symptoms may occur: nausea, vomiting, cramps, fever, faintness, anorexia
- To avoid driving, other hazardous activities, drowsiness occurs

Treatment of overdose: Naloxone HCl (Narcan) 0.2-0.8 mg IV, O_2, IV fluids, vasopressors

hydroxychloroquine (℞)

(hye-drox-ee-klor′oh-kwin)

Plaquenil, Quineprox

Func. class.: Antimalarial, antirheumatic (DMARDs)

Chem. class.: 4-Aminoquinoline derivative

Action: Inhibits parasite replications, transcription of DNA to RNA by forming complexes with DNA in parasite

Uses: Malaria caused by *Plasmodium vivax, P. malariae, P. ovale, P. falciparum* (some strains); SLE, rheumatoid arthritis

Unlabeled uses: SLE in children

DOSAGE AND ROUTES

Malaria

- *Adult:* **PO** Suppression or prevention 200 mg q wk, begin 1-2 wk before travel, continue 4 wk after returning; treatment 400 mg, then 200 mg at 6, 24, 48 hr after 1st dose
- *Child:* **PO** Suppression or prevention 5 mg/kg q wk, begin 1-2 wk before travel, continue 4 wk after returning; treatment 10 mg/kg, then 5 mg/kg at 6, 18, 24 hr after 1st dose

Lupus erythematosus

- *Adult:* **PO** 400 mg daily-bid; length depends on patient response; maintenance 200-400 mg/day

• *Child (unlabeled):* **PO** 5 mg/kg/day, max 400 mg/day, long-term therapy is contraindicated

Rheumatoid arthritis

• *Adult:* **PO** 400-600 mg/day for 4-12 wk; then 200-300 mg/day after good response

• *Child:* **PO** 3-5 mg/kg/day max 400 mg/day

Available forms: Tabs 200 mg

SIDE EFFECTS

CNS: Headache, stimulation, fatigue, irritability, **seizures,** bad dreams, dizziness, confusion, psychosis, decreased reflexes

CV: Hypotension, heart block, **asystole with syncope**

EENT: Blurred vision, corneal changes, retinal changes, difficulty focusing, tinnitus, vertigo, deafness, photophobia, corneal edema

GI: Nausea, vomiting, anorexia, diarrhea, cramps

HEMA: **Thrombocytopenia, agranulocytosis, leukopenia, aplastic anemia**

INTEG: Pruritus, pigmentation changes, skin eruptions, lichen planus–like eruptions, eczema, **exfoliative dermatitis,** alopecia, **Stevens-Johnson syndrome**

Contraindications: Hypersensitivity, retinal field changes

Black Box Warning: Children (long term), ocular disease

Precautions: Pregnancy (C), breastfeeding, blood dyscrasias, severe GI disease, neurologic disease, alcoholism, hepatic disease, G6PD deficiency, psoriasis, eczema

PHARMACOKINETICS

Peak 1-2 hr; half-life 3-5 days; terminal half-life 32-50 days; metabolized in liver; excreted in urine, feces, breast milk; crosses placenta

INTERACTIONS

Increase: digoxin levels

Increase: antibody titer—rabies vaccine

Decrease: hydroxychloroquine action—Mg or Al compounds

NURSING CONSIDERATIONS

Assess:

• For SLE, malaria symptoms before and daily

• For rheumatoid arthritis: pain, swelling, ROM, temperature of joints

• Ophthalmic exam baseline and q6mo if long-term treatment or product dosage >150 mg/day

• Hepatic studies q wk: AST, ALT, bilirubin, if on long-term treatment

• Blood studies: CBC, platelets; WBC, RBC, platelets may be decreased; if severe, product should be discontinued

• For decreased reflexes: knee, ankle

• ECG during therapy: watch for depression of T waves, widening of QRS complex

• Allergic reactions: pruritus, rash, urticaria

• Blood dyscrasias: malaise, fever, bruising, bleeding (rare)

• For ototoxicity (tinnitus, vertigo, change in hearing); audiometric testing should be done before, after treatment

⚠ For toxicity: blurring vision, difficulty focusing, headache, dizziness, knee, ankle reflexes; product should be discontinued immediately

Administer:

• Tabs may be crushed and mixed with food, fluids

• Take with food or milk; at same time each day to maintain product level

• For malaria prophylaxis should be started 2 wk prior to exposure and 4-6 wk after leaving exposure area

Perform/provide:

• Storage in tight, light-resistant container at room temperature; keep inj in cool environment

Evaluate:

• Therapeutic response: decreased symptoms of malaria, SLE, rheumatoid arthritis

Teach patient/family:

• To use sunglasses in bright sunlight to decrease photophobia

• That urine may turn rust or brown

• To report hearing, visual problems, fever, fatigue, bruising, bleeding, which may indicate blood dyscrasias

Treatment of overdose: Induce vomiting; gastric lavage; administer barbiturate (ultrashort acting), vasopressor, ammonium chloride; tracheostomy may be necessary

Rarely Used

hydroxyethyl starch (℞)

Voluven

Func. class.: Hematologic agent

Chem. class.: Plasma volume expander

Uses: Treatment, prevention of hypovolemia

DOSAGE AND ROUTES

• *Adult and child >12 yr:* **IV INF** 50 ml/kg/day; infuse the first 10-20 ml slowly; monitor for anaphylaxis

Contraindications: Hypervolemic, renal failure with oliguria, anuria not related to hypovolemia, dialysis, severe hypernatremia/hyperchloremia, intracranial bleeding, hypersensitivity to this agent

hydroxyurea (℞)

(hye-drox′ee-yoo-ree-ah)

Droxia, Hydrea

Func. class.: Antineoplastic, antimetabolite

Chem. class.: Synthetic urea analog

Action: Acts by inhibiting DNA synthesis without interfering with RNA or protein synthesis; incorporates thymidine into DNA, causing direct damage to DNA strands; S phase specific of cell cycle

Uses: Melanoma, chronic myelogenous leukemia, recurrent or metastatic ovarian cancer, squamous cell carcinoma of the head and neck, sickle cell anemia

Unlabeled uses: Psoriasis, acute myelogenous leukemia (AML), astrocytoma, HIV, lung cancer, malignant glioma, polycythemia vera, thrombocytosis

DOSAGE AND ROUTES

Solid tumors

• *Adult:* **PO** 80 mg/kg as a single dose q3days or 20-30 mg/kg as a single dose daily

In combination with radiation

• *Adult:* **PO** 80 mg/kg as a single dose q3days; should be started 7 days before irradiation

Resistant chronic myelogenous leukemia

• *Adult:* **PO** 10-30 mg/kg/day as a single daily dose

Sickle cell anemia

• *Adult:* **PO** 15 mg/kg/day, may increase by 5 mg/kg/day q12wk, max 35 mg/kg/day

Renal disease

• CCr 10-50 ml/min dose 50%; CCr <10 ml/min dose 20%

Available forms: Caps 200, 300, 400, 500 mg

SIDE EFFECTS

CNS: Headache, confusion, hallucinations, dizziness, **seizures**

CV: Angina, ischemia

GI: Nausea, vomiting, anorexia, diarrhea, stomatitis, constipation, **hepatotoxicity**

GU: Increased BUN, uric acid, creatinine, temporary renal function impairment

HEMA: **Leukopenia, anemia, thrombocytopenia, megaloblastic erythropoiesis**

INTEG: *Rash,* urticaria, pruritus, dry skin, facial erythema

META: Hyperphosphatemia, hyperuricemia, hypocalcemia

MISC: Fever, chills, malaise, **secondary cancers,** tumor lysis syndrome

Contraindications: Pregnancy (D), breastfeeding, hypersensitivity

Black Box Warning: Leukopenia (<2500/mm^3), thrombocytopenia (<100,000/mm^3), anemia (severe)

Precautions: Renal disease (severe)

PHARMACOKINETICS

Readily absorbed when taken orally; peak level in 1-4 hr; degraded in liver; excreted in urine, almost totally eliminated in 24 hr; readily crosses blood-brain barrier; eliminated as CO_2; terminal half-life 3.5-4.5 hr

INTERACTIONS

Increase: toxicity—radiation or other antineoplastics

Increase: bleeding risk—NSAIDs, anticoagulants

Drug/Lab Test

Increase: renal studies

NURSING CONSIDERATIONS

Assess:

- CBC, differential, platelet count q wk; withhold product if WBC is <2500/mm^3 or platelet count is <100,000/mm^3; notify prescriber; product should be discontinued
- Renal studies: BUN, serum uric acid, urine CCr, electrolytes before, during therapy

⚠ Tumor lysis syndrome

- I&O ratio; report fall in urine output to <30 ml/hr
- Monitor temp q4hr; fever may indicate beginning infection
- Hepatic studies before, during therapy: bilirubin, alk phos, AST, ALT, LDH; prn or q mo
- B/P q3-4hr; check for chest pain; angina, ischemia may occur
- Bleeding: hematuria, guaiac, bruising or petechiae, mucosa or orifices q8hr
- Inflammation of mucosa, breaks in skin
- Buccal cavity for dryness, sores or ulceration, white patches, oral pain, bleeding, dysphagia
- Symptoms indicating severe allergic reaction: rash, urticaria, itching, flushing
- Neurotoxicity: headaches, hallucinations, seizures, dizziness

Administer:

- Do not crush or chew caps; caps can be opened and contents mixed with water
- Antiemetic 30-60 min before giving product and prn

Perform/provide:

- Rinsing of mouth tid-qid with water, club soda; brushing of teeth bid-tid with soft brush or cotton-tipped applicators for stomatitis; use unwaxed dental floss

Evaluate:

- Therapeutic response: decreased tumor size, spread of malignancy

Teach patient/family:

- To report signs of infection: elevated temp, sore throat, flulike symptoms
- To report signs of anemia: fatigue, headache, faintness, SOB, irritability
- To report bleeding: avoid use of razors, commercial mouthwash
- To avoid use of aspirin products, ibuprofen (thrombocytopenia)
- To avoid foods with citric acid, hot or rough texture if stomatitis is present
- To report stomatitis: any bleeding, white spots, ulcerations in the mouth; tell patient to examine mouth daily, report symptoms
- That contraceptive measures are recommended during therapy
- To notify prescriber of fever, chills, sore throat, nausea, vomiting, anorexia, diarrhea, bleeding, bruising; may indicate blood dyscrasias

*hydrOXYzine (℞)

(hye-drox′i-zeen)

ANX, Apo-Hydroxyzine ♣, Atarax, hydroxyzine, Hyzine-50, Multi-pax ♣, Novohydroxyzine ♣, Vistaril

Func. class.: Antianxiety/antihistamine/sedative-hypnotic, antiemetic

Chem. class.: Piperazine derivative

Do not confuse:

hydrOXYzine/hydrALAZINE

Atarax/amoxicillin/Ativan

Vistaril/Versed

Action: Depresses subcortical levels of CNS, including limbic system, reticular formation; competes with H_1-receptor sites

Uses: Anxiety preoperatively, postoperatively to prevent nausea, vomiting, to potentiate opioid analgesics; sedation; pruritus, ethanol withdrawal

DOSAGE AND ROUTES

Anxiety

- *Adult:* **PO** 25-100 mg tid-qid, max 600 mg/day; **IM** 50-100 mg q4-6hr
- *Geriatric:* **PO** max 50 mg/day
- *Child >6 yr:* **PO** 50-100 mg/day in divided doses
- *Child <6 yr:* **PO** 50 mg/day in divided doses

Alcohol withdrawal

- *Adult:* **IM** 50-100 mg, then q4-6hr

Preoperatively/postoperatively

- *Adult:* **IM** 25-100 mg q4-6hr
- *Child:* **IM** 0.5-1.1 mg/kg q4-6hr

Pruritus

- *Adult:* **PO** 25 mg tid-qid; **IM** 50-100 mg then q4-6hr prn, switch to **PO** as soon as feasible
- *Geriatric:* **PO** 10 mg tid-qid, max 50 mg/day
- *Child:* **PO** 50-100 mg/day in divided doses; **IM** 0.5-1 mg/kg/dose q4-6hr prn, use **PO** when possible

Antiemetic

- *Adult:* **IM** 25-100 mg/dose q4-6hr prn

Renal dose

- *Adult:* **PO** CCr <50 ml/min give 50% of dose

Available forms: Tabs 10, 25, 50, 100 mg; caps 10, 25, 50, 100 mg; oral susp 5 mg/5 ml; inj 25, 50 mg/ml

SIDE EFFECTS

CNS: Dizziness, drowsiness, confusion, headache, tremors, fatigue, depression, **seizures**

CV: Hypotension

GI: Dry mouth, increased appetite, nausea, diarrhea, weight gain

Contraindications: Pregnancy (1st trimester), breastfeeding, hypersensitivity to this product or cetirizine, acute asthma

Precautions: Pregnancy (C) (2nd/3rd trimester), geriatric patients, debilitated, renal/hepatic disease, closed-angle glaucoma, COPD, prostatic hypertrophy, asthma

PHARMACOKINETICS

PO: Onset 15-60 min, duration 4-6 hr, half-life 3 hr, metabolized by liver, excreted by kidneys

INTERACTIONS

Increase: CNS depressant effect—barbiturates, opioids, analgesics, alcohol, sedative/hypnotics, other CNS depressants

Increase: anticholinergic effects—phenothiazines, quinidine, disopyramide, antihistamines, antidepressants, atropine, haloperidol, MAOIs

Drug/Herb

Increase: anticholinergic effect—corkwood, henbane leaf, jimsonweed, scopolia

Increase: sedative action—chamomile, cowslip, hops, Jamaican dogwood, kava, khat, Queen Anne's lace, senega, skullcap, valerian

NURSING CONSIDERATIONS

Assess:

- B/P (lying, standing), pulse; if systolic B/P drops 20 mm Hg, hold product, notify prescriber
- Mental status: mood, sensorium, affect, anxiety, behavior, increased sedation

Administer:

PO route

- With food or milk for GI symptoms (PO)
- Crushed if patient is unable to swallow medication whole
- Gum, hard candy, frequent sips of water for dry mouth

IM route

- By Z-track inj in large muscle for IM to decrease pain, chance of necrosis, never give IV/SUBCUT

Additive compatibilities: Cisplatin, cyclophosphamide, cytarabine, dimenhyDRINATE, etoposide, lidocaine, mesna, methotrexate, nafcillin

H

Syringe compatibilities: Atropine, atropine/meperidine, benzquinamide, bupivacaine, butorphanol, chlorproMAZINE, cimetidine, codeine, diphenhydrAMINE, doxapram, droperidol, fentanyl, fluphenazine, glycopyrrolate, hydromorphone, lidocaine, meperidine, meperidine/atropine, methotrimeprazine, metoclopramide, midazolam, morphine, nalbuphine, oxymorphone, pentazocine, perphenazine, procaine, prochlorperazine, promazine, promethazine, scopolamine, sufentanil, thiothixene

Perform/provide:

- Assistance with ambulation during beginning therapy, since drowsiness/dizziness occurs
- Safety measures, including side rails
- Checking to see if PO medication has been swallowed

Evaluate:

- Therapeutic response: decreased anxiety

Teach patient/family:

- That medication is not to be used for everyday stress or used longer than 4 mo
- To avoid OTC preparations (cold, cough, hay fever) unless approved by prescriber
- To avoid driving, activities that require alertness
- To avoid alcohol ingestion, psychotropic medications
- Not to discontinue medication quickly after long-term use
- To rise slowly or fainting may occur

Treatment of overdose: Lavage if orally ingested; VS, supportive care; IV norepinephrine for hypotension

Rarely Used

hylan G-F 20

(hi'lan)

Synvisc, Synvisc One

Func. class.: Misc. agent

Uses: Osteoarthritis

DOSAGE AND ROUTES

- *Adult:* Intra-articular (Synvisc only) 2 ml (16 mg hylan polymers) q wk × 3 inj; (Synvisc One only) 6 ml (48 hylan polymers) as a single inj

Contraindications: Hypersensitivity to this product or hyaluronan; caution with allergies to avian proteins, feathers, egg products

hyoscyamine (℞)

(hye-oh-sye'a-meen)

Anaspaz, A-Spas S/L, Cystospaz, Donnamar, ED-SPAZ, Gastrosed, Levsin, Levsinex, NuLev Timecaps

Func. class.: Anticholinergic/antispasmodics

Chem. class.: Belladonna alkaloid

Action: Inhibits muscarinic actions of acetylcholine at postganglionic parasympathetic neuroeffector sites, reduces rigidity, tremors, hyperhidrosis of parkinsonism

Uses: Treatment of peptic ulcer disease in combination with other products; other GI disorders, other spastic disorders, IBS, urinary incontinence

DOSAGE AND ROUTES

- *Adult:* **PO/SL** 0.125-0.25 mg tid-qid before meals, at bedtime; **TIME REL** 0.375-0.75 mg q12hr; **IM/SUBCUT/IV** 0.25-0.5 mg q6hr
- *Geriatric:* Max 1.5 mg/day in divided doses or max 4 biphasic tabs

• *Child 2-12 yr:* **PO** individualized dose based on weight, max 0.75 mg/24 hr
• *Child <2 yr:* **PO** individualized dose based on weight

Available forms: Tabs 0.125, 0.15 mg; time rel caps 0.375 mg; time rel tabs 0.375 ml; sol 0.125 mg/ml; elix 0.125 mg/5 ml; inj 0.5 mg/ml

SIDE EFFECTS

CNS: ***Confusion, stimulation in geriatric patients,*** headache, insomnia, dizziness, drowsiness, anxiety, weakness, hallucination
CV: ***Palpitations,*** tachycardia
EENT: ***Blurred vision,*** photophobia, mydriasis, cycloplegia, increased ocular tension
GI: ***Dry mouth, constipation, paralytic ileus,*** heartburn, nausea, vomiting, dysphagia, absence of taste
GU: ***Urinary hesitancy, retention,*** impotence
INTEG: Urticaria, rash, pruritus, anhidrosis, fever, allergic reactions

Contraindications: Hypersensitivity to anticholinergics, closed-angle glaucoma, GI obstruction, myasthenia gravis, paralytic ileus, GI atony, toxic megacolon, prostatic hypertrophy

Precautions: Pregnancy (C), geriatric patients, hyperthyroidism, dysrhythmias, CHF, ulcerative colitis, hypertension, hiatal hernia, renal/hepatic disease, urinary retention, CAD

PHARMACOKINETICS

PO: Duration 4-6 hr, metabolized by liver, excreted in urine, half-life 3.5 hr

INTERACTIONS

Increase: anticholinergic effect—amantadine, tricyclics, MAOIs, H_1-antihistamines
Decrease: hyoscyamine effect—antacids
Decrease: effect of phenothiazines, levodopa, ketoconazole

Drug/Herb

Increase: constipation—black catechu
Increase: anticholinergic effect—butterbur, jimsonweed
Decrease: anticholinergic effect—jaborandi tree, pill-bearing spurge

NURSING CONSIDERATIONS

Assess:

• VS, cardiac status: checking for dysrhythmias, increased rate, palpitations
• I&O ratio; check for urinary retention or hesitancy
• GI complaints: pain, nausea, vomiting, anorexia

Administer:

• Do not break, crush, or chew time rel caps
• ½ hr before meals for better absorption
• Decreased dose to geriatric patients; metabolism may be slowed
• Gum, hard candy, frequent rinsing of mouth for dryness of oral cavity

Perform/provide:

• Storage in tight container protected from light
• Increased fluids, bulk, exercise to decrease constipation

Evaluate:

• Therapeutic response: absence of epigastric pain, bleeding, nausea, vomiting

Teach patient/family:

• To avoid driving, other hazardous activities until stabilized on medication
• To avoid alcohol or other CNS depressants; will enhance sedating properties of this product
• To avoid hot environments; heat stroke may occur; product suppresses perspiration
• To use sunglasses when outside to prevent photophobia; may cause blurred vision

H

ibandronate (℞)

(eye-ban'dro-nate)

Boniva

Func. class.: Bone-resorption inhibitor, electrolyte modifier

Chem. class.: Bisphosphonate

Action: Inhibits bone resorption, apparently without inhibiting bone formation and mineralization; absorbs calcium phosphate crystals in bone and may directly block dissolution of hydroxyapatite crystals of bone, more potent than other products

Uses: Osteoporosis and prophylaxis

Unlabeled uses: Hypercalcemia, osteolytic metastases, Paget's disease, osteoporosis (treatment/prevention) in those taking anastrozole

DOSAGE AND ROUTES

Postmenopausal osteoporosis

- *Adult:* **PO** 2.5 mg/day or 150 mg q mo; **IV BOL** 3 mg q3mo

Prophylaxis

- *Adult:* **PO** 2.5 mg/day or 150 mg q mo

Paget's disease (unlabeled)

- *Adult:* **IV** 2 mg as a single dose

Osteoporosis in those taking anastrozole (unlabeled)

- *Postmenopausal women:* **PO** 150 mg q mo

Osteolytic metastases (unlabeled)

- *Adult:* **IV** 6 mg over 1 hr × 3 days, repeat q4wk

Hypercalcemia (unlabeled)

- *Adult:* **IV INF** 2-4 mg over 2 hr

Renal dose

- *Adult:* **PO** CCr <30 ml/min, avoid use

Available forms: Tabs 2.5, 150 mg; sol for inj 1 mg/ml

SIDE EFFECTS

CNS: Fever, insomnia, dizziness, headache

CV: Hypertension, **atrial fibrillation**

EENT: Ocular pain/inflammation, uveitis

GI: Constipation, nausea, vomiting, diarrhea, dyspepsia

INTEG: Rash, inj site reaction

META: ***Hypomagnesemia, hypophosphatemia, hypocalcemia,*** hypercholesterolemia

MS: Bone pain, myalgia, osteonecrosis of the jaw

Contraindications: Achalasia, esophageal stricture, hypocalcemia, intraarterial administration, renal failure, vit D deficiency, hypersensitivity to bisphosphonates

Precautions: Pregnancy (C), breastfeeding, children, geriatric patients, anemia, chemotherapy, coagulopathy, dental disease, diabetes mellitus, dysphagia, GI/renal disease, GERD, hypertension, infection, multiple myeloma, phosphate hypersensitivity

PHARMACOKINETICS

Half-life 5-60 hr, 86%-99% protein binding, taken up mainly by bones, primarily in areas of high bone turnover, eliminated primarily by kidneys

INTERACTIONS

- Possible increased neurotoxicity: aminoglycosides, cycloSPORINE, tacrolimus, NSAIDs, radiopaque contrast agents

Increase: hypocalcemia—loop diuretics

Decrease: ibandronate effect—calcium, vit D

Drug/Food

- Do not take with food, calcium

NURSING CONSIDERATIONS

Assess:

- For atrial fibrillation
- Dental health; before dental extraction give antiinfectives
- Blood studies: electrolytes, Ca, P, Mg; creatinine/BUN
- For bone pain; use analgesics
- DEXA scan for bone mineral density

Administer:

PO route

- Give early AM with a glass of water; if q mo, give on same day of each month

IV route

- Using single-dose prefilled syringe; discard unused portion; give over 15-30 sec

Perform/provide:

- Storage at room temperature

Evaluate:

- Therapeutic response: increased bone mineral density

Teach patient/family:

- To report hypercalcemic relapse: nausea, vomiting, bone pain, thirst; unusual muscle twitching, muscle spasms, severe diarrhea, constipation
- To continue with dietary recommendations including calcium and vit D
- To obtain an analgesic from provider for bone pain
- That if nausea/vomiting occur, small, frequent meals may help
- To report vision symptoms: blurred vision, edema, inflammation; report to prescriber
- To report if pregnancy is planned or suspected or if planning to breastfeed
- To exercise regularly, to stop smoking, and decrease alcohol
- To take PO first thing in AM at least 60 min before other medications, food, beverages
- To sit upright for ≥60 min after PO

ibritumomab tiuxetan (℞)

(ee-brit-u-moe′mab)

Zevalin

Func. class.: Radiopharmaceutical

Chem. class.: Monoclonal antibody

Action: High affinity for indium-111, yttrium-90; induces CD20+ B-cell lines

Uses: Non-Hodgkin's lymphoma, B-cell NHL

DOSAGE AND ROUTES

- *Adult:* **IV** Ritaximab 250 mg/m^2 given first; within 4 hr, give 5 mCi (1.6 mg total) over 10 min, then repeat 7-9 days later

Available forms: Inj 3.2 mg/2 ml

SIDE EFFECTS

CV: **Cardiac dysrhythmias**

GI: Nausea, vomiting, anorexia, abdominal pain, diarrhea

GU: **Renal failure**

HEMA: **Leukopenia, neutropenia, thrombocytopenia,** anemia

INTEG: Irritation at site, rash, **fatal mucocutaneous infections (rare)**

OTHER: Fever, chills, asthenia, headache, **angioedema,** hypotension, myalgia, **bronchospasm, hemorrhage,** infections, cough, dyspnea, dizziness, anxiety

SYST: **Stevens-Johnson syndrome, secondary malignancies (AML, MDS), fatal infections**

Contraindications: Pregnancy (D), hypersensitivity to murine proteins, prior murine antibody exposure

Black Box Warning: Hypersensitivity to this agent, neutropenia, thrombocytopenia

Precautions: Breastfeeding, children, geriatric patients, cardiac conditions, immunizations after therapy

Black Box Warning: Altered biodistribution, infusion-related reaction

PHARMACOKINETICS

Half-life 30 hr

NURSING CONSIDERATIONS

Assess:

⚠ For signs of fatal inf reaction: hypoxia, pulmonary infiltrates, ARDS, MI, ventricular fibrillation, cardiogenic shock; most fatal inf reactions occur with first inf; potentially fatal

- Biodistribution: 1st image 2-24 hr, 2nd image 48-72 hr, 3rd image 90-120 hr (optimal)
- For infection; murine antibody titers

⚠ For signs of severe mucocutaneous reactions: Stevens-Johnson syndrome, lichenoid dermatitis, toxic epidermal lysis; occur 1-13 wk after product was given

⚠ Tumor lysis syndrome: acute renal failure requiring hemodialysis, hyperkale-

mia, hypocalcemia, hyperuricemia, hyperphosphatemia
• CBC, differential, platelet count weekly; withhold product if WBC is < 3500/mm^3, or platelet count <150,000/mm^3; notify prescriber of these results
• GI symptoms: frequency of stools
• Signs of dehydration: rapid respirations, poor skin turgor, decreased urine output, dry skin, restlessness, weakness

Administer:
• Do not use as bolus or IV direct
• See manufacturer's product labeling for preparation

Perform/provide:
• Increased fluid intake to 2-3 L/day to prevent dehydration, unless contraindicated
• Emergency equipment nearby with epinephrine, antihistamines, corticosteroids

Evaluate:
• Therapeutic response: improvement in blood counts, decreased evidence of disease

Teach patient/family:
• To report adverse reactions
• To use contraception during and for 12 months after therapy
• Radiation safety precautions, disposal of bodily fluids
• Symptoms of infections
• Neutropenia and bleeding precautions

ibuprofen (OTC, ℞)

(eye-byoo-proe'fen)
Actiprofen ♣, Advil, Advil Liqui-Gels, Advil Migraine, Apo-Ibuprofen ♣, Bayer Select Ibuprofen Pain Relief, Caldolor, Children's Advil, Children's Motrin, Excedrin IB, Genpril, Haltran, ibuprofen, IBU-TAB, Infant's Motrin, Junior Strength Advil, Medipren, Menadol, Midol Maximum Strength Cramp Formula, Motrin, Motrin IB, Motrin Junior Strength, Motrin Migraine Pain, Novoprofen ♣, Nu-Ibuprofen, Nuprin, PediaCare Children's Fever, Pediatric Advil drops, PediaCare Fever

ibuprofen lysine (℞)

NeoProfen

Func.class.: Nonsteroidal antiinflammatory, antipyretic, nonopioid analgesics
Chem. class.: Propionic acid derivative

Do not confuse:
Nuprin/Lupron

Action: Inhibits prostaglandin synthesis by decreasing enzyme needed for biosynthesis; analgesic, antiinflammatory, antipyretic

Uses: Rheumatoid arthritis, osteoarthritis, primary dysmenorrhea, gout, dental pain, musculoskeletal disorders, fever, migraine

Unlabeled uses: Ankylosing spondylitis, bone pain, cystic fibrosis, gouty arthritis, psoriatic arthritis

DOSAGE AND ROUTES

Self-treatment of minor aches/pains
• *Adult/adolescent:* **PO** (OTC product) 200 mg q4-6hr, may increase to 400 mg q4-6hr if needed, max 1200 mg/day

Analgesic
• *Adult:* **PO** 200-400 mg q4-6hr, max 3.2 g/day; OTC use max 1200 mg/day
• *Child:* **PO** 4-10 mg/kg/dose q6-8hr

Moderate to severe pain (hospitalized patients)

• *Adult:* **IV** 400-800 mg q6hr as an adjunct to opiate agonist therapy

Dysmenorrhea

• *Adult:* **PO** 400 mg q4hr, max 1200 mg/day

Antipyretic

• *Child 6 mo-12 yr:* **PO** 5 mg/kg (temp <102.5° F or 39.2° C), 10 mg/kg, (temp >102.5° F), may repeat q4-6hr, max 40 mg/kg/day

Antiinflammatory

• *Adult:* **PO** 300-800 mg tid-qid, max 3.2 g/day

• *Child:* **PO** 30-40 mg/kg/day in 3-4 divided doses, max 50 mg/kg/day

Patent ductus arteriosus (PDA) (NeoProfen)

• *Premature neonate ≤32 wk gestation who weighs 500-1500 g:* **IV** 10 mg/kg initially, then if needed, 2 doses 5 mg/kg at 24 hr intervals; if oliguria occurs, hold dose

Available forms: Tabs 100, 200, 400, 600, 800 mg; cap, liq gels 200 mg; oral susp 100 mg/5 ml; liq 100 mg/5 ml; chew tabs 50, 100 mg; drops 50 mg/1.25 ml; inj 10 mg/ml (NeoProfen); inj (Caldolor) 100 mg/ml

SIDE EFFECTS

CNS: *Headache,* dizziness, drowsiness, fatigue, tremors, confusion, insomnia, anxiety, depression

CV: Tachycardia, peripheral edema, palpitations, dysrhythmias, **CV thrombotic events, MI, stroke**

EENT: Tinnitus, hearing loss, blurred vision

GI: Nausea, *anorexia,* vomiting, diarrhea, jaundice, **hepatitis,** constipation, flatulence, cramps, dry mouth, peptic ulcer, **GI bleeding, ulceration, necrotizing enterocolitis, GI perforation**

GU: **Nephrotoxicity:** dysuria, hematuria, oliguria, azotemia

HEMA: **Blood dyscrasias,** increased bleeding time

INTEG: Purpura, rash, pruritus, sweating, urticaria, **nectrotizing fasciitis**

SYST: **Anaphylaxis, Stevens-Johnson syndrome**

Contraindications: Pregnancy (D) 3rd trimester, hypersensitivity, asthma, severe renal/hepatic disease

Black Box Warning: Perioperative pain in CABG

Precautions: Pregnancy (B) 1st and 2nd trimesters, breastfeeding, children, geriatric patients, bleeding disorders, GI disorders, cardiac disorders, hypersensitivity to other antiinflammatory agents, CHF, CCr <25 ml/min

Black Box Warning: GI bleeding, MI, stroke

PHARMACOKINETICS

PO: Onset ½ hr, peak 1-2 hr, half-life 1.8-2 hr, metabolized in liver (inactive metabolites), excreted in urine (inactive metabolites), 90%-99% plasma protein binding, does not enter breast milk, well absorbed

INTERACTIONS

Increase: bleeding risk—cefotetan, valproic acid, thrombolytics, antiplatelets, anticoagulants

Increase: blood dyscrasias possibility—antineoplastics, radiation

Increase: toxicity—digoxin, lithium, oral anticoagulants, cycloSPORINE, probenecid, methotrexate

Increase: GI reactions—aspirin, corticosteroids, NSAIDs, alcohol

Increase: hypoglycemia—oral antidiabetics, insulin

Decrease: effect of antihypertensives, thiazides, furosemide

Decrease: ibuprofen action—aspirin

Drug/Herb

Increase: bleeding risk—arnica, bogbean, chamomile, chondroitin, clove, dong quai, fenugreek, feverfew, garlic, ginger, ginkgo, ginseng *(Panax)*

Increase: gastric irritation—arginine, gossypol

Increase: NSAID effect—bearberry, bilberry

NURSING CONSIDERATIONS

Assess:

- Renal, hepatic, blood studies: BUN, creatinine, AST, ALT, Hgb, before treatment, periodically thereafter
- Pain: note type, duration, location, and intensity with ROM 1 hr after administration
- Audiometric, ophthalmic exam before, during, after long-term treatment; for eye, ear problems: blurred vision, tinnitus; may indicate toxicity
- For infection, may mask symptoms; fever: temp before and 1 hr after administration
- Cardiac status: edema (peripheral), tachycardia, palpitations; monitor B/P, pulse for character, quality, rhythm especially in patients with cardiac disease/ geriatric patients
- For history of peptic ulcer disorder; asthma, aspirin, hypersensitivity, check closely for hypersensitivity reactions

Administer:

PO route

- With food, milk, or antacid to decrease GI symptoms; however, taking on empty stomach best facilitates absorption; if nausea and vomiting occur/persist, notify prescriber
- Shake susp well before use

IV route

- Must be well hydrated prior to administration
- Dilute to ≤4 mg/ml (0.9% NaCl, LR, D_5) infuse over ≥30 min
- Discard unused portion
- Do not give IM
- Visually inspect for particulate
- Give within 30 min of preparation; give via IV port that is nearest insertion site; give over 15 min
- Check for extravasation; do not give in same line with TPN; interrupt TPN for 15 min before and after product administration

Perform/provide:

- Storage at room temperature

Evaluate:

- Therapeutic response: decreased pain, stiffness in joints; decreased swelling in joints; ability to move more easily; reduction in fever or menstrual cramping

Teach patient/family:

- To report blurred vision, ringing, roaring in ears; may indicate toxicity; eye and hearing tests should be done during long-term therapy
- To avoid driving, other hazardous activities if dizziness or drowsiness occurs
- ⚠ To report change in urinary pattern, increased weight, edema, increased pain in joints, fever, blood in urine; indicate nephrotoxicity
- That therapeutic inflammatory effects may take up to 1 mo
- ⚠ To avoid alcohol, NSAIDs, salicylates; bleeding may occur
- To use sunscreen to prevent photosensitivity
- To report use to all health care providers

Treatment of overdose: Lavage, activated charcoal, induce diuresis

⚠ High Alert

ibutilide (℞)

(eye-byoo'tih-lide)

Corvert

Func. class.: Antidysrhythmic (Class III)

Action: Prolongs duration of action potential and effective refractory period

Uses: For rapid conversion of atrial fibrillation/flutter including within 1 wk of coronary artery bypass or valve surgery

DOSAGE AND ROUTES

Atrial fibrillation flutter

- *Adult ≥60 kg:* **IV INF** 1 vial (1 mg) given over 10 min, may repeat same dose in 10 min
- *Adult <60 kg:* **IV INF** 0.01 mg/kg given over 10 min, may repeat same dose in 10 min

Atrial fibrillation/flutter after cardiac surgery

• *Adult ≥60 kg:* **IV INF** 0.5 mg; may repeat 1 time

• *Adult <60 kg:* **IV INF** 0.005 mg/kg; may repeat 1 time

Available forms: Inj 0.1 mg/ml

SIDE EFFECTS

CNS: Headache

CV: Hypotension, bradycardia, **sinus arrest, CHF, dysrhythmias, torsade de pointes,** hypertension, extrasystoles, ventricular tachycardia, bundle branch block, AV block, palpitations, supraventricular extrasystoles, syncope, **prolonged QT interval**

GI: Nausea

Contraindications: Hypersensitivity

Precautions: Pregnancy (C), breastfeeding, children <18 yr, geriatric patients, sinus node dysfunction, 2nd- or 3rd-degree AV block, electrolyte imbalances, bradycardia, renal/hepatic disease, CHF

Black Box Warning: QT prolongation, torsade de pointes, ventricular arrhythmias, ventricular tachycardia

PHARMACOKINETICS

Elimination half-life in 6 hr, metabolized by liver, excreted by kidneys

INTERACTIONS

• Prodysrhythmia: phenothiazines, tricyclics, tetracyclics, antidepressants, H_1-receptor antagonists, antihistamines

• Masking of cardiotoxicity: digoxin

• Do not use within 5 hr of ibutilide: Class Ia antidysrhythmics (disopyramide, quinidine, procainamide), Class III agents (amiodarone, sotalol)

Drug/Herb

Increase: toxicity, death—aconite

Increase: effect—aloe, broom, chronic buckthorn use, cascara sagrada (chronic use), Chinese rhubarb, figwort, fumitory, goldenseal, kudzu, licorice

Increase: serotonin effect—horehound

Decrease: effect—coltsfoot

NURSING CONSIDERATIONS

Assess:

• ECG continuously to determine product effectiveness, measure PR, QRS, QT intervals, check for PVCs, other dysrhythmias, discontinue if atrial fibrillation/flutter ceases

• I&O ratio; electrolytes: K, Na, Cl

• Hepatic studies: AST, ALT, bilirubin, alk phos

• For dehydration or hypovolemia

• For rebound hypertension after 1-2 hr

• Cardiac rate, respiration: rate, rhythm, character, chest pain

Administer:

IV route

• Undiluted or diluted in 50 ml 0.9% NaCl, or D_5W (0.017 mg/ml) give over 10 min

• Solution is stable for 48 hr refrigerated or 24 hr, room temperature

• Do not admix with other solution, products

• Reduce dosage slowly with ECG monitoring

Evaluate:

• Therapeutic response: decrease in atrial fibrillation/flutter

Teach patient/family:

• To report side effects immediately

• Reason for medication

⚠ High Alert

idarubicin (℞)

(eye-dah-roob′ih-sin)

Idamycin PFS

Func. class.: Antineoplastic, antibiotic

Chem. class.: Anthracycline glycoside

Do not confuse:

idarubicin/**DOXOrubicin/DAUNOrubicin/epirubicin**

Idamycin/**Adriamycin**

Action: Non–cell cycle specific; topoisomerase II inhibitor, a vesicant

Uses: Used in combination with other antineoplastics for acute myelocytic leukemia in adults

Unlabeled uses: Breast cancer, liquid tumors, non-Hodgkin's lymphoma, ALL, CLL, AML

DOSAGE AND ROUTES

• *Adult:* **IV** 8-12 mg/m^2/day × 3 days in combination with cytarabine (induction)

Renal/hepatic dose

• *Adult:* **IV** CCr >2.5 mg/dl reduce dose by 50%; bilirubin 2.6-5 mg/dl reduce dose by 50%; bilirubin >5 mg/dl do not use

Available forms: Inj 1 mg/ml

SIDE EFFECTS

CNS: Fever, chills, *headache,* **seizures**

CV: **Dysrhythmias, CHF, pericarditis, myocarditis,** peripheral edema, angina, **MI, myocardial toxicity**

GI: Nausea, vomiting, abdominal pain, mucositis, diarrhea, **hepatotoxicity**

GU: **Nephrotoxicity,** red urine

HEMA: **Thrombocytopenia, leukopenia, anemia**

INTEG: Rash, **extravasation,** dermatitis, *reversible alopecia,* urticaria, thrombophlebitis and tissue necrosis at inj site, radiation recall

SYST: **Infection,** tumor lysis syndrome

Contraindications: Pregnancy (D), breastfeeding, hypersensitivity

Black Box Warning: Myelosuppression, bilirubin >5 mg/dl

Precautions: Children, gout, bone marrow depression, preexisting CV disease

Black Box Warning: Renal/hepatic disease, heart failure

PHARMACOKINETICS

Half-life 22 hr; metabolized by liver; crosses placenta; excreted in bile, urine (primarily as metabolites); 97% protein binding

INTERACTIONS

Increase: toxicity—other antineoplastics or radiation

Decrease: antibody response—live virus vaccines

Drug/Lab Test

Increase: uric acid

NURSING CONSIDERATIONS

Assess:

• CBC, differential, platelet count weekly; withhold product if WBC is <4000/mm^3 or platelet count is <75,000/mm^3; notify prescriber of these results

• Renal studies: BUN, serum uric acid, urine CCr, electrolytes before, during therapy

• For tumor lysis syndrome: hyperkalemia, hyperphosphatemia, hyperuricemia, hypocalcemia

• I&O ratio; report fall in urine output to <30 ml/hr

• Monitor temp; fever may indicate beginning infection

• Hepatic studies before, during therapy: bilirubin, AST, ALT, alk phos prn or q mo; check for jaundice of skin, sclera, dark urine, clay-colored stools, itchy skin, abdominal pain, fever, diarrhea

• Cardiac toxicity: CHF, dysrythmias, cardiomyopathy; cardiac studies should be done before and periodically during treatment: ECG, chest x-ray, MUGA

• ECG: watch for ST-T wave changes, low QRS and T, possible dysrhythmias (sinus tachycardia, heart block, PVCs)

• Bleeding: hematuria, guaiac stools, bruising or petechiae, mucosa or orifices

• Effects of alopecia on body image; discuss feelings about body changes

• Inflammation of mucosa, breaks in skin

• Buccal cavity for dryness, sores, ulceration, white patches, oral pain, bleeding, dysphagia

⚠ Local irritation, pain, burning at inj site, extravasation, a vesicant

• GI symptoms: frequency of stools, cramping

Administer:

• Ice compress after stopping inf for extravasation

Intermittent IV INF route

- Do not give IM/SUBCUT
- Using cytotoxic handling procedures after preparing in biologic cabinet wearing gown, gloves, mask
- Antiemetic 30-60 min before giving product and 6-10 hr after treatment to prevent vomiting
- After reconstituting 5-mg vial with 5 ml 0.9% NaCl (1 mg/1 ml); give over 10-15 min through Y-tube or 3-way stopcock of inf of D_5 or NS; discard unused portion

Solution compatibilities: $D_{3.3}$/0.3% NaCl, D_5/0.9% NaCl, D_5W, LR, 0.9% NaCl

Y-site compatibilities: Amifostine, amikacin, aztreonam, cimetidine, cladribine, cyclophosphamide, cytarabine, diphenhydrAMINE, droperidol, erythromycin, filgrastim, granisetron, imipenem/cisplatin, magnesium sulfate, mannitol, melphalan, metoclopramide, potassium chloride, ranitidine, sargramostim, thiotepa, vinorelbine

Perform/provide:

- Strict hand washing technique, gloves, protective clothing
- Increase fluid intake to 2-3 L/day to prevent urate and calculi formation
- Rinsing of mouth tid-qid with water, club soda; brushing of teeth tid-qid with soft brush or cotton-tipped applicators for stomatitis; use unwaxed dental floss
- Storage at room temperature for 3 days after reconstituting or 7 days refrigerated

Evaluate:

- Therapeutic response: decreased liquid tumor, spread of malignancy

Teach patient/family:

- To report signs of CHF, cardiac toxicity, beginning infection
- That hair may be lost during treatment and wig or hairpiece may make patient feel better; tell patient that new hair may be different in color, texture
- To avoid foods with citric acid, hot or rough texture
- To avoid crowds, those with upper respiratory illness
- To report any bleeding, white spots, ulcerations in mouth; tell patient to examine mouth daily
- That urine may be red-orange for 48 hr
- To use contraception during treatment with this product and for ≥4 mo after treatment
- That all body fluids change color

⚠ High Alert

ifosfamide (℞)

(i-foss′fa-mide)

Ifex

Func. class.: Antineoplastic alkylating agent

Chem. class.: Nitrogen mustard

I

Do not confuse:
ifosfamide/cyclophosphamide

Action: Alkylates DNA, RNA, inhibits enzymes that allow synthesis of amino acids in proteins; also responsible for cross-linking DNA strands; activity is not cell cycle stage specific

Uses: Testicular cancer

Unlabeled uses: Soft tissue sarcoma, Ewing's sarcoma, non-Hodgkin's lymphoma, lung/pancreatic sarcoma

DOSAGE AND ROUTES

- *Adult:* **IV** 1.2-2 g/m^2/day × 5 days, repeat course q3wk, given with mesna

Renal dose

- *Adult:* **IV** CCr 31-60 ml/min, give 75% of dose; CCr 10-30 ml/min, give 50% of dose; CCr <10 ml/min, do not give

Available forms: Inj 1-, 3-g vials

SIDE EFFECTS

CNS: Facial paresthesia, fever, malaise, somnolence, confusion, depression, hallucinations, dizziness, disorientation, **seizures, coma,** cranial nerve dysfunction

GI: Nausea, vomiting, anorexia, **hepatotoxicity,** stomatitis, constipation, diarrhea

GU: **Hematuria, nephrotoxicity, hemorrhagic cystitis,** dysuria, urinary frequency

HEMA: **Thrombocytopenia, leukopenia, anemia**
INTEG: Dermatitis, alopecia, pain at inj site, hyperpigmentation
META: Metabolic acidosis

Contraindications: Pregnancy (D), hypersensitivity

Black Box Warning: Bone marrow suppression

Precautions: Breastfeeding, children, renal/hepatic disease

Black Box Warning: Coma, hemorrhagic cystitis

PHARMACOKINETICS

Metabolized by liver, saturation occurs at high doses, excreted in urine, half-life 7-15 hr, depends on dose

INTERACTIONS

Increase: myelosuppression—other antineoplastics, radiation
Increase: toxicity—CYP3A4 inducers, barbiturates, allopurinol
Increase: bleeding risk—NSAIDs, anticoagulants, salicylates, thrombolytics
Decrease: antibody response—live virus vaccines
Decrease: effect of ifosfamide—CYP3A4 inhibitors

NURSING CONSIDERATIONS

Assess:

- Hepatic studies before, during therapy (bilirubin, AST, ALT, LDH) monthly or as needed; jaundice of skin, sclera, dark urine, clay-colored stools, itchy skin, abdominal pain, fever, diarrhea

⚠ CBC, differential, platelet count weekly; withhold product if WBC <2000 or platelet count <50,000; notify prescriber; severe myelosuppression may occur

- Monitor temp (may indicate beginning infection)
- Blood dyscrasias (anemia, granulocytopenia); bruising, fatigue, bleeding, poor healing
- Allergic reactions: dermatitis, exfoliative dermatitis, pruritus, urticaria
- I&O ratio; monitor for hematuria; hemorrhagic cystitis can occur; increase fluids to 3 L/day

⚠ Neurologic symptoms: hallucinations, confusion, disorientation, product should be discontinued

- Bleeding: hematuria, guaiac, bruising or petechiae, mucosa or orifices

Administer:

- Antiemetic 30-60 min before giving product to prevent vomiting
- Always give with mesna to prevent ifosfamide-induced hemorrhagic cystitis, give hydration before and after inf

IV route

- After diluting 1 g/20 ml sterile or bacteriostatic H_2O for inj with parabens or benzyl only; shake; may be diluted further with D_5W, LR, NS, sterile H_2O for inj; 1 g/20 ml = 50 mg/ml; 1 g/50 ml = 20 mg/ml; 1 g/200 ml = 5 mg/ml; give over ≥30 min; may also give as continuous inf over 72 hr

Additive compatibilities: Carboplatin, cisplatin, etoposide, fluorouracil, mesna

Syringe compatibilities: Mesna

Y-site compatibilities: Allopurinol, amifostine, amphotericin B cholesteryl, aztreonam, DOXOrubicin liposome, filgrastim, fludarabine, gallium, granisetron, melphalan, ondansetron, paclitaxel, piperacillin/tazobactam, propofol, sargramostim, sodium bicarbonate, teniposide, thiotepa, vinorelbine

Perform/provide:

- Storage of powder at room temperature
- Increase fluid intake to ≥3 L/day to prevent hemorrhagic cystitis
- Warm compresses at inj site for inflammation

Evaluate:

- Therapeutic response: decrease in size and spread of tumor

Teach patient/family:

- To notify prescriber of sore throat, swollen lymph nodes, malaise, fever; other infections may occur

- Not to have vaccinations during or after treatment
- That hair may be lost during treatment; a wig or hairpiece may make the patient feel better; new hair may be different in color, texture
- To report signs of anemia: fatigue, headache, faintness, SOB, irritability
- To report bleeding; avoid use of razors, commercial mouthwash
- To avoid use of aspirin products, NSAIDs, ibuprofen, hemorrhage can occur
- To use contraceptive measures during therapy
- To avoid crowds, those with infections
- To report confusion, hallucinations, extreme drowsiness, numbness, tingling; avoid alcohol use for ≥4 mo after treatment

iloperidone (℞)

(ill-o-pehr′ih-dohn)

Fanapt

Func. class.: Antipsychotic

Chem. class.: Benzisoxazole derivative

Action: Unknown; may be mediated through both DOPamine type 2 (D2) and serotonin type 2 (5-HT2) antagonism

Uses: Schizophrenia

DOSAGE AND ROUTES

- *Adult:* **PO** 1 mg bid, 2 mg bid day 2, 4 mg bid day 3, 6 mg bid day 4, 8 mg bid day 5, 10 mg bid day 6, 12 mg bid day 7, max 24 mg/day in two divided doses

Available forms: Tabs 1, 2, 4, 6, 8, 10, 12 mg; titration pack

SIDE EFFECTS

CNS: EPS, pseudoparkinsonism, akathisia, dystonia, tardive dyskinesia; drowsiness, **seizures, neuroleptic malignant syndrome,** dizziness, delirium, depression, paranoia, fatigue, hostility, lethargy, restlessness, vertigo, tremor

CV: Orthostatic hypotension, **heart failure, AV block, QT prolongation,** tachycardia

EENT: Blurred vision, cataracts, nystagmus, tinnitus

GI: Nausea, vomiting, *anorexia, constipation,* jaundice, weight gain/loss, abdominal pain, stomatitis

GU: Hyperprolactinemia, urinary retention/incontinence, testicular pain, **renal failure**

HEMA: **Agranulocytosis, leukopenia, neutropenia**

MISC: **Renal artery occlusion**

Contraindications: Breastfeeding, hypersensitivity

Precautions: Pregnancy (C), children, geriatric patients, renal/hepatic disease, breast cancer, Parkinson's disease, dementia with Lewy bodies, seizure disorder, QT prolongation, bundle branch block, acute MI, ambient temperature increase, AV block, stroke, substance abuse, suicidal ideation, tardive dyskinesia, torsade de pointes, blood dyscrasias

PHARMACOKINETICS

PO: Extensively metabolized by liver to a major active metabolite by CYP2D6, CYP3A4, protein binding 95%, peak 2-4 hr, excreted urine and feces, terminal half-life 18 hr extensive metabolizers, 33 hr poor metabolizers

INTERACTIONS

Increase: sedation—other CNS depressants, alcohol

Increase: EPS—CYP2D6, 3A4 inhibitors (SSRIs)

Increase: EPS—other antipsychotics

Increase: QT prolongation—class IA/ III antidysrhythmics, some phenothiazines, β-agonists, local anesthetics, tricyclics, bepridil, haloperidol, methadone, chloroquine, clarithromycin, droperidol, erythromycin, grepafloxacin, halofantrine, pentamidine, probucol, sparfloxacin

Decrease: iloperidone action—CYP2D6, 3A4 inducers (carbamazepine, barbiturates, phenytoins, rifampin)

Drug/Herb

Increase: CNS depression—kava

Increase: action—cola tree, hops, nettle, nutmeg
Increase: EPS—betel palm, kava
Drug/Lab Test
Increase: prolactin levels

NURSING CONSIDERATIONS

Assess:

- Mental status before initial administration
- Swallowing of PO medication; check for hoarding or giving of medication to other patients
- I&O ratio; palpate bladder if urinary output is low
- Bilirubin, CBC, hepatic studies q mo
- Urinalysis before, during prolonged therapy
- Affect, orientation, LOC, reflexes, gait, coordination, sleep pattern disturbances
- B/P standing and lying; also pulse, respirations; take these q4hr during initial treatment; establish baseline before starting treatment; report drops of 30 mm Hg; watch for ECG changes; QT prolongation may occur
- Dizziness, faintness, palpitations, tachycardia on rising
- EPS, including akathisia, tardive dyskinesia (bizarre movements of the jaw, mouth, tongue, extremities), pseudoparkinsonism (rigidity, tremors, pill rolling, shuffling gait)
- For serious reactions in the geriatric patient: fatal pneumonia, heart failure, sudden death
- For neuroleptic malignant syndrome: hyperthermia, increased CPK, altered mental status, muscle rigidity
- Skin turgor daily
- Constipation, urinary retention daily; if these occur, increase bulk and water in diet
- Weight gain, hyperglycemia, metabolic changes in diabetes

Administer:

- Reduced dose in geriatric patients
- Anticholinergic agent on order from prescriber, to be used for EPS
- Avoid use with CNS depressants

Perform/provide:

- Decreased stimulus by dimming lights, avoiding loud noises
- Supervised ambulation until patient is stabilized on medication; do not involve in strenuous exercise program because fainting is possible; patient should not stand still for a long time
- Increased fluids to prevent constipation
- Sips of water, candy, gum for dry mouth
- Storage in tight, light-resistant container (PO); unopened vials in refrigerator, protect from light; do not freeze

Evaluate:

- Therapeutic response: decrease in emotional excitement, hallucinations, delusions, paranoia; reorganization of patterns of thought, speech

Teach patient/family:

- That orthostatic hypotension may occur and to rise from sitting or lying position gradually
- To avoid hot tubs, hot showers, tub baths; hypotension may occur
- To avoid abrupt withdrawal of this product; EPS may result; product should be withdrawn slowly
- To avoid OTC preparations (cough, hay fever, cold) unless approved by prescriber; serious product interactions may occur; avoid use of alcohol; increased drowsiness may occur
- To avoid hazardous activities if drowsy or dizzy
- To comply with product regimen
- To report impaired vision, tremors, muscle twitching
- That heat stroke may occur in hot weather; take extra precautions to stay cool
- To use contraception, inform prescriber if pregnancy is planned or suspected

Treatment of overdose: Lavage if orally ingested; provide airway; *do not induce vomiting*

imatinib (℞)

(im-ah-tin′ib)

Gleevec

Func. class.: Antineoplastic—miscellaneous

Chem. class.: Protein-tyrosine kinase inhibitor

Action: Inhibits Bcr-Abl tyrosine kinase created in chronic myeloid leukemia (CML)

Uses: Treatment of chronic myeloid leukemia (CML), Philadelphia chromosome positive in blast cell crisis or chronic failure after treatment failure with interferon alfa; gastrointestinal stromal tumors (GIST), positive for KIT; chronic eosinophilic leukemia, acute lymphocytic leukemia, dermatofibrosarcoma protuberans, myelodysplastic syndrome

DOSAGE AND ROUTES

CML, chronic phase

- *Adult:* **PO** 400-600 mg/day
- *Child:* **PO** 340 mg/m^2/day

CML, accelerated phase/blast crisis

- *Adult:* **PO** 600-800 mg/day

GIST

- *Adult:* **PO** 400 or 800 mg/day

Renal dose

- *Adult:* **PO** CCr 40-59 ml/min max 600 mg/day; CCr 20-39 ml/min decrease initial dose by 50%, max 400 mg/day; CCr <20 ml/min use with caution, 100 mg/day

Hepatic dose

- *Adult:* **PO** Total bilirubin 1.5-3 × ULN and any AST, decrease initial dose to 400 mg/day; total bilirubin >3 × ULN and any AST decrease initial dose to 300 mg/day

Available forms: Tabs 100, 400 mg

SIDE EFFECTS

CNS: **CNS hemorrhage,** headache, dizziness, insomnia

CV: **Hemorrhage, heart failure, cardiac tamponade, hypereosinophilia, cardiac toxicity**

EENT: Blurred vision, conjunctivitis

GI: *Nausea,* **hepatotoxicity, vomiting, dyspepsia,** GI hemorrhage, *anorexia, abdominal pain,* **GI perforation,** diarrhea

HEMA: **Neutropenia, thrombocytopenia, bleeding**

INTEG: *Rash, pruritus,* alopecia, photosensitivity

META: Fluid retention, hypokalemia, edema

MISC: Fatigue, epistaxis, pyrexia, night sweats, increased weight, flulike symptoms, hypothyroidism

MS: Cramps, pain, arthralgia, myalgia

RESP: Cough, dyspnea, nasopharyngitis, pneumonia, upper respiratory tract infection, pleural effusion, edema

Contraindications: Pregnancy (D), hypersensitivity

Precautions: Breastfeeding, children, geriatric patients, cardiac/renal/hepatic disease

PHARMACOKINETICS

Well absorbed (98%); protein binding 95%; metabolized by CYP3A4; excreted in feces, small amount in urine; peak 2-4 hr; duration 24 hr (imatinib), 40 hr (metabolite); half-life 18-40 hr

INTERACTIONS

Increase: hepatotoxicity—acetaminophen

Increase: imatinib concentrations—CYP3A4 inhibitors (ketoconazole, itraconazole, erythromycin, clarithromycin)

Increase: plasma concentrations of simvastatin, calcium channel blockers, ergots

Increase: plasma concentration of warfarin; avoid use with warfarin, use low-molecular-weight anticoagulants instead

Decrease: imatinib concentrations—CYP3A4 inducers (dexamethasone, phenytoin, carbamazepine, rifampin, phenobarbital)

Drug/Herb

Decrease: imatinib concentration—St. John's wort

NURSING CONSIDERATIONS

Assess:

- ANC and platelets; in chronic phase if ANC <1 × 10^9/L and/or platelets <50 × 10^9/L, stop until ANC >1.5 × 10^9/L and platelets >75 × 10^9/L; in accelerated phase/blast crisis if ANC <0.5 × 10^9/L and/or platelets <10 × 10^9/L, determine whether cytopenia is related to biopsy/aspirate, if not, reduce dose by 200 mg, if cytopenia continues, reduce dose by another 100 mg; if cytopenia continues for 4 wk, stop product until ANC ≥1 × 10^9/L
- For renal toxicity: if bilirubin >3 × IULN, withhold imatinib until bilirubin levels return to <1.5 × IULN
- For hepatotoxicity: monitor LFTs, before treatment and q mo; if liver transaminases >5 × IULN, withhold imatinib until transaminase levels return to <2.5 × IULN
- CBC, differential, platelet count weekly; withhold product if WBC is <3500/mm^3, or platelet count <100,000/mm^3; notify prescriber of these results; product should be discontinued
- Signs of fluid retention, edema: weigh, monitor lung sounds, assess for edema, some fluid retention is dose dependent

Administer:

- With meal and large glass of water, to decrease GI symptoms, doses of 800 mg should be given 400 mg bid

Perform/provide:

- Nutritious diet with iron, vitamin supplement, low fiber, few dairy products
- Storage at 25° C (77° F)

Evaluate:

- Therapeutic response: decrease in leukemic cells or size of tumor

Teach patient/family:

- To report adverse reactions immediately: shortness of breath, swelling of extremities, bleeding
- Reason for treatment, expected result
- That effect on male infertility is unknown

imipenem/cilastatin (℞)

(i-me-pen'em sye-la-stat'in)

Primaxin IM, Primaxin IV

Func. class.: Antiinfective—miscellaneous

Chem. class.: Carbapenem

Do not confuse:

imipenem/**Omnipen**

Primaxin/**Premarin**

Action: Interferes with cell wall replication of susceptible organisms; osmotically unstable cell wall swells, bursts from osmotic pressure; addition of cilastatin prevents renal inactivation that occurs with high urinary concentrations of imipenem

Uses: Serious infections caused by gram-positive: *Streptococcus pneumoniae,* group A β-hemolytic streptococci, *Staphylococcus aureus,* enterococcus; gram-negative: *Klebsiella, Proteus, Escherichia coli, Acinetobacter, Serratia, Pseudomonas aeruginosa, Salmonella, Shigella, Haemophilus influenzae, Listeria* sp.

DOSAGE AND ROUTES

- *Adult:* **IV** 250-500 mg q6-8hr; severe infections may require 1 g q6-8hr; may give **IM** q12hr (total daily **IM** dosage >1500 mg not recommended); mild to moderate infections
- *Child:* **IV** 60-100 mg/kg/day in divided doses, max 4 g/day; **IM** 10-15 mg/kg q6hr

Renal dose

- *Adult:* **IV** CCr 30-70 ml/min give 50% dose q6-8hr; CCr 20-30 ml/min give 40% dose q8-12hr; CCr 5-20 ml/min give 25% dose q12hr

Available forms: Inj (IV) 250, 500 mg; inj (IM) 500, 750 mg

SIDE EFFECTS

CNS: Fever, somnolence, **seizures,** confusion, dizziness, weakness, myoclonus

CV: Hypotension, palpitations, tachycardia

GI: Diarrhea, nausea, vomiting, **pseudomembranous colitis, hepatitis,** glossitis
GU: **Renal toxicity/failure**
HEMA: **Eosinophilia, neutropenia,** decreased Hgb, Hct
INTEG: Rash, urticaria, pruritus, pain at inj site, phlebitis, erythema at inj site
RESP: Chest discomfort, dyspnea, hyperventilation
SYST: **Anaphylaxis, Stevens-Johnson syndrome**

Contraindications: Hypersensitivity to this product or amide local anesthetics, or carbapenems, AV block, shock

Precautions: Pregnancy (C), breastfeeding, children, geriatric patients, seizure disorders, renal disease, head trauma, hypersensitivity to cephalosporins, penicillins, pseudomembranous colitis, ulcerative colitis

PHARMACOKINETICS

IV: Onset immediate, peak ½-1 hr, half-life 1 hr, 70%-80% excreted unchanged in urine

INTERACTIONS

Increase: imipenem plasma levels—probenecid
Increase: antagonistic effect—β-lactam antibiotics
Increase: seizure risk—ganciclovir, theophylline, aminophylline, cycloSPORINE
Decrease: effect of valproic acid

Drug/Herb

- Do not use acidophilus with antiinfectives; separate by several hours

Drug/Lab Test

Increase: AST, ALT, LDH, BUN, alk phos, bilirubin, creatinine
False-positive: direct Coombs' test

NURSING CONSIDERATIONS

Assess:

- For infection: increased temp, WBC, characteristics of wounds, sputum, urine culture or stool culture
- Sensitivity to penicillin—may have sensitivity to this product
- Renal disease: lower dose may be required
- Bowel pattern daily; if severe diarrhea occurs, product should be discontinued; may indicate pseudomembranous colitis

⚠ Allergic reactions, anaphylaxis: rash, urticaria, pruritus, wheezing, laryngeal edema; may occur few days after therapy begins; have epinephrine, antihistamine, emergency equipment available

- Overgrowth of infection: perineal itching, fever, malaise, redness, pain, swelling, drainage, rash, diarrhea, change in cough, sputum

Administer:

- After C&S is taken

IM route

- Reconstitute 500 mg/2 ml; or 750 mg/3 ml lidocaine without epinephrine; shake

IV route

- After reconstitution of 250 or 500 mg with 10 ml of diluent and shake; add to at least 100 ml of same inf sol
- 250-500 mg over 20-30 min; 1 g over 40-60 min; give through Y-tube or 3-way stopcock; do not give by IV bolus or if cloudy

Y-site compatibilities: Acyclovir, amifostine, aztreonam, cefepime, cisatracurium, diltiazem, famotidine, fludarabine, foscarnet, granisetron, idarubicin, insulin (regular), melphalan, methotrexate, ondansetron, propofol, remifentanil, tacrolimus, teniposide, thiotepa, vinorelbine, zidovudine

Evaluate:

- Therapeutic response: negative C&S; absence of signs and symptoms of infection

Teach patient/family:

⚠ To report severe diarrhea; may indicate pseudomembranous colitis

⚠ To report sore throat, bruising, bleeding, joint pain; may indicate blood dyscrasias (rare)

Treatment of anaphylaxis: Epinephrine, antihistamines; resuscitate if needed

I

imipramine (℞)

(im-ip'ra-meen)

Apo-Imipramine ✦, imipramine HCl ✦, Impril ✦, Novo Pramine ✦, Tipramine, Tofranil, Tofranil PM

Func. class.: Antidepressant, tricyclic

Chem. class.: Dibenzazepine, tertiary amine

Do not confuse:
imipramine/**desipramine**

Action: Blocks reuptake of norepinephrine, serotonin into nerve endings, increasing action of norepinephrine, serotonin in nerve cells

Uses: Depression, enuresis in children

Unlabeled uses: Chronic pain, migraine headaches, cluster headaches as adjunct, incontinence, ADHD, neuralgia, bulimia, neuropathic pain

DOSAGE AND ROUTES

• *Adult:* **PO** 75-100 mg/day in divided doses, may increase by 25-50 mg to 200 mg, max 300 mg/day; may give daily dose at bedtime

• *Geriatric:* **PO** 25-50 mg at bedtime, may increase to 100 mg/day in divided doses

• *Child ≥6 yr (unlabeled):* **PO** 1.5 mg/kg/day in divided doses, max 100 mg/day

Enuresis

• *Child 6-12 yr:* **PO** 10-25 mg at bedtime, max 75 mg

Neuropathic pain (unlabeled)

• *Adult:* **PO** 10-150 mg/day

Social phobia/panic disorder (unlabeled)

• *Adult:* **PO** 10 mg at betime, titrate q2-4days until 100-200 mg/day is reached

Overactive bladder (OAB) (unlabeled)

• *Adult:* **PO** 10-50 mg daily, may titrate to 150 mg/day

Cancer pain adjunct (unlabeled)

• *Child:* **PO** 0.2-0.4 mg/kg at bedtime, may increase by 50% q2-3days up to 1-3 mg/kg at bedtime

Available forms: Tabs 10, 25, 50 mg; caps 75, 100, 125, 150 mg

SIDE EFFECTS

CNS: Dizziness, drowsiness, confusion, **seizures,** headache, anxiety, tremors, stimulation, weakness, insomnia, nightmares, EPS (geriatric patients), increased psychiatric symptoms, paresthesia

CV: Orthostatic hypotension, ECG changes, tachycardia, hypertension, palpitations, **dysrhythmias**

EENT: Blurred vision, tinnitus, mydriasis

GI: Diarrhea, dry mouth, nausea, vomiting, **paralytic ileus;** increased appetite; cramps, epigastric distress, jaundice, **hepatitis,** stomatitis, constipation, taste change

GU: Retention, **acute renal failure**

HEMA: **Agranulocytosis, thrombocytopenia, eosinophilia, leukopenia**

INTEG: Rash, urticaria, sweating, pruritus, photosensitivity; hyperpigmentation (rare)

Contraindications: Pregnancy (D), hypersensitivity to tricyclics, AV block, bundle-branch block, ileus, QT prolongation

Precautions: Breastfeeding, geriatric patients, suicidal patients, severe depression, increased intraocular pressure, closed-angle glaucoma, urinary retention, cardiac/hepatic disease, hyperthyroidism, electroshock therapy, elective surgery, seizure disorders, prostatic hypertrophy, MI

Black Box Warning: Children

PHARMACOKINETICS

Steady state 2-5 days; metabolized by liver; excreted in urine, breast milk, feces; crosses placenta; half-life 6-20 hr

INTERACTIONS

⚠ Hyperpyretic crisis, seizures, hypertensive episode: MAOIs, clonidine

⚠ ***Increase:*** toxicity: SSRIs, avoid concurrent use
Increase: QT interval—tricyclics, gatifloxacin, levofloxacin, moxifloxacin, ziprasidone
Increase: effects of direct-acting sympathomimetics (epinephrine), alcohol, barbiturates, benzodiazepines, CNS depressants
Decrease: effects of guanethidine, clonidine, indirect-acting sympathomimetics (ephedrine)

Drug/Herb

Increase: anticholinergic effect—belladonna, corkwood, henbane, jimsonweed, scopolia
Increase: imipramine action—chamomile, hops, kava, lavender, skullcap, valerian
Increase: hypertension—yohimbe
Increase: serotonin syndrome—SAM-e, St. John's wort

Drug/Lab Test

Increase: serum bilirubin, alk phos, blood glucose
Decrease: 5-HIAA, VMA, urinary catecholamines

NURSING CONSIDERATIONS

Assess:

- B/P (lying, standing), pulse q4hr; if systolic B/P drops 20 mm Hg, hold product, notify prescriber; take vital signs q4hr in patients with CV disease
- Blood studies: CBC, leukocytes, differential, cardiac enzymes if patient is receiving long-term therapy
- Hepatic studies: AST, ALT, bilirubin
- Weight q wk; appetite may increase with product

⚠ ECG for flattening of T wave, bundle branch block, AV block, dysrhythmias in cardiac patients

- EPS primarily in geriatric patients: rigidity, dystonia, akathisia
- Mental status: mood, sensorium, affect, suicidal tendencies, increase in psychiatric symptoms: depression, panic
- Urinary retention, constipation; constipation is more likely to occur in children, geriatric patients

⚠ Withdrawal symptoms: headache, nausea, vomiting, muscle pain, weakness, diarrhea, insomnia, restlessness; not usual unless product is discontinued abruptly

- Alcohol consumption; if alcohol is consumed, hold dose until morning

Administer:

- Not to break, crush, or chew caps
- Increased fluids, bulk in diet for constipation, urinary retention
- With food or milk for GI symptoms
- Dosage at bedtime if oversedation occurs during day; may take entire dose at bedtime; geriatric patients may not tolerate once/day dosing
- Sugarless gum, hard candy, or frequent sips of water for dry mouth

Syringe compatibilities: Doxapram
Y-site compatibilities: Cladribine

Perform/provide:

- Storage in tight container at room temperature; do not freeze
- Assistance with ambulation during beginning therapy, since drowsiness/dizziness, orthostatic hypotension occurs
- Safety measures, primarily in geriatric patients

Evaluate:

- Therapeutic response: decreased depression, enuresis, pain

Teach patient/family:

- That therapeutic effects may take 2-3 wk
- That product is dispensed in small amounts because of suicide potential, especially in beginning of therapy
- To use caution in driving, other activities requiring alertness because of drowsiness, dizziness, blurred vision
- To report urinary retention immediately
- To avoid alcohol ingestion, other CNS depressants during treatment
- Not to discontinue medication quickly after long-term use; may cause nausea, headache, malaise
- To wear sunscreen or large hat, since photosensitivity occurs
- To rise slowly, orthostatic hypotension may occur

Treatment of overdose: ECG monitoring; lavage, activated charcoal; administer anticonvulsant

immune globulin IM (IMIG/IGIM) (℞)

Bay Gam 15%, Flebogamma 5%, Flebogamma DIF 5%, Gammagard Liquid 10%, Gamunex 10%, Privigen 10%, Vivaglobin 10%

immune globulin IV (IGIV, IVIG) (℞)

Bay Gam 15%, Flebogamma, 5%, Gammagard S/D, gamma globulin, Gammar-P IV, Iveegam EN, Polygam S/D, Privigen, Vivaglobin

immune globulin SC (SCIG/IGSC)

Bay Bam 15%, Flebogamma 5%, Flebogamma DIF 5%, Gammagard 10%, Gamunex 10%, Privigen 10%, Vivaglobin

Func. class.: Immune serum
Chem. class.: IgG

Action: Provides passive immunity to hepatitis A, measles, varicella, rubella, immune globulin deficiency; contains gamma globulin antibodies (IgG)

Uses: Immunodeficiency syndrome; B-cell chronic lymphocytic leukemia; Kawasaki syndrome; bone marrow transplantation; pediatric HIV infection; agammaglobulinemia; hepatitis A, B exposure; measles exposure; measles vaccine complications; purpura; rubella exposure; chickenpox exposure; chronic inflammatory demyelinating polyneuropathy

Unlabeled uses: IV posttransfusion purpura, Guillain-Barré syndrome, refractory pemphigus vulgaris, West Nile virus, meningitis, myasthenia gravis, thrombocytopenia encephalitis, HIV, cytomegalovirus, neonatal jaundice, RSV infection

DOSAGE AND ROUTES

Immune globulin IM (IMIG, IGIM)

Hepatitis A prophylaxis

- *Adult, geriatric, adolescent, child, infant (unlabeled):* **IM** 0.02 ml/kg for those who have not received hepatitis A vaccine and been exposed in the last 2 wk

Measles prophylaxis (exposed in last 6 days)

- *Adult:* **IM** 0.25 ml/kg (immunocompetent)
- *Child (unlabeled):* **IM** 0.5 ml/kg as a single dose, max 15 ml (immunocompromised)

Varicella prophylaxis

- *Adult:* **IM** 0.6-1.2 ml/kg as soon as possible and if varicella-zoster immune globulin is not available

Rubella prophylaxis in exposed/susceptible who will not consider a therapeutic abortion

- *Adult pregnant women:* **IM** 0.55 ml/kg

Immunoglobulin deficiency

- *Adult:* **IM** 1.32 ml/kg, then 0.66 ml/kg (at least 100 mg/kg) q3-4wk

Immune globulin IV (IVIG, IGIV)

Primary immunodeficiency

Gammagard S/D

- *Adult/adolescent/child:* **IV** 300-600 mg/kg q3-4wk

Polygam S/D

- *Adult/adolescent/child:* **IV** 100 mg/kg qmo, initially 200-400 mg/kg may be used

Gammar-P IV

- *Adult:* **IV** 200-400 mg/kg q3-4wk
- *Adolescent/child:* **IV** 200 mg/kg q3-4wk

Gamunex

- *Adult/adolescent/child:* **IV INF** 300-600 mg/kg (3-6 ml/kg) q3-4wk, initial inf rate 1 mg/kg/min (max 8 mg/kg/min)

Iveegam EN

- *Adult/adolescent/child:* **IV** 200 mg/kg q mo, max 800 mg/kg q mo

Panglobulin NF/Carimune NF

- *Adult/adolescent/child:* **IV** 200 mg/kg q mo

Octagam/Gamagard liquid/ Flebogamma 5%

- *Adult/adolescent/child:* **IV** 300-600 mg/kg q3-4wk

Privigen

- *Adult/adolescent/child ≥3 yr:* **IV** 200-800 mg q3wk

Idiopathic thrombocytopenic purpura (ITP)

Panglobulin NF/Carimune NF

- *Adult/child:* **IV** 400 mg/kg daily × 2-5 days, in acute ITP of childhood, only 2 of the 5 days are needed if initial platelets are 30,000-50,000 mcl after 2 doses

Gammagard S/D/Polygam S/D

- *Adult/adolescent/child:* **IV** 1000 mg/kg as a single dose, may give on alternate days for up to 3 doses

Gamunex

- *Adult/adolescent/child:* **IV INF** total dose of 2000 mg/kg, divided as 1000 mg/kg (10 ml/kg) give on 2 consecutive days, initial rate is 1 mg/kg/min (max 8 mg/kg/min), if after first dose adequate platelets are observed after 24 hr, may withhold second dose

Privigen

- *Adult/adolescent ≥15 yr:* **IV** 1 g/kg/day × 2 days

Kawasaki disease

Iveegam EN

- *Child:* **IV** 400 mg/kg daily × 4 consecutive days or a single dose of 2000 mg/kg over 10 hr, given with aspirin 100 mg/kg/day through 14th day of illness, then 3-5 mg/kg each day thereafter for 5 wk

Gammagard S/D/Polygam S/D

- *Infant/child:* **IV** 1000 mg/kg (single dose) or 400 mg/kg/day × 4 days beginning 7 days of fever onset, with aspirin 80-100 mg/kg/day × 4 divided doses

Immune globulin SC (SCIG/IGSC)

- *Adult/child >2 yr:* **SUBCUT INF** 100-200 mg/kg q wk, Vivaglobin brand of SCIG 160 mg IgG/ml, **SUBCUT** inj 15 ml/inj site, given at max of 20 ml/hr

Available forms: *IM:* Inj 2-, 10-ml v (Bay Gam); *IV:* 5%, 10% sol (Gamimu N, Venoglobulin-S); powder for inj 1-, 3 6-, 12-g vials (Carimune NF); 50 mg protein/ml in 2.5-, 5-, 10-g vials (Gammagard S/D); 1-, 2.5-, 5-, 10-g vials (Gammar-P IV); 500 mg, 1-, 2.5-, 5-g vials (Iveegam); 6-, 12-g vials (Panglobulin); 2.5-, 5-, 10-g vials (Polygam S/D); sol for inj 1-, 2.5-, 5-, 10-, 20-g vials (Gamunex)

SIDE EFFECTS

CNS: Headache, fatigue, malaise
GI: Abdominal pain
INTEG: Pain at inj site, rash, pruritus, chills
MS: Arthralgia, chest pain
SYST: Lymphadenopathy, **anaphylaxis**

Contraindications: Coagulopathy, hemophilia, IgA deficiency, thrombocytopenia

Precautions: Pregnancy (C), breastfeeding, children, agammaglobulinemia, bleeding, hypogammaglobulinemia, infection, IV, viral infection

INTERACTIONS

- Do not administer live virus vaccines within 3 mo of this product

Drug/Lab Test

Interference: glucose testing system

NURSING CONSIDERATIONS

Assess:

- For exposure date: this product should be given within 6 days of measles, 7 days of hepatitis B, 14 days of hepatitis A
- For anaphylaxis: diaphoresis, wheezing, chest tightness, hypotension

Administer:

- IM ≤3 ml in one site, use large muscle mass
- Only with epinephrine 1:1000, resuscitative equipment available
- Only within 2 wk of exposure to hepatitis A
- Immune globulin should not be given SUBCUT, IV, or intradermally

al
e

: N: IV undiluted or dilute ve 0.01 ml/kg/min; may in- .02-0.04 ml/kg/min
lobulin: IV diluted with provided give 0.5-1 ml/min × 15-30 min; crease to 1.5-2.5 ml/min
oglobulin-I: (50 mg/ml sol) give -0.02 ml/kg/min; if no adverse reac- n in ½ hr, increase to 0.04 ml/kg/min, ore at room temperature
- Gammagard: reconstitute with sterile H_2O for inj (50 mg protein/ml); give 0.5 ml/kg/hr, may increase to 4 ml/kg/hr, use inf set provided
- Gammar-IV: give 0.01 ml/kg/min (50 mg/ml sol) × 15-30 min, may increase to 0.02 ml/kg/min, may increase to 0.03-0.06 ml/kg/min

Y-site compatibilities: Fluconazole, sargramostim

Perform/provide:
- Storage at 36°-46° F (2°-8° C)

Evaluate:
- Prevention of infection, increased platelets

Teach patient/family:
- That passive immunity is temporary
- The treatment of anaphylaxis: epinephrine, diphenhydrAMINE, O_2, vasopressors, corticosteroids

⚠ High Alert

inamrinone (℞)

(in-am′rih-nohn)

Inocor

Func. class.: Inotropic

Chem. class.: Bipyrimidine derivative

Do not confuse:
inamrinone/amiodarone

Action: Positive inotropic agent with vasodilator properties; reduces preload and afterload by direct relaxation of vascular nooth muscle, increases cardiac output

es: Short-term management of CHF has not responded to other medication (diuretics, other vasodilators); can be used with digoxin

DOSAGE AND ROUTES

- *Adult and child:* **IV BOL** 0.75 mg/kg given over 2-3 min; start inf of 5-10 mcg/kg/min; may give another bol 30 min after start of therapy, max 10 mg/kg total daily dose
- *Infant:* **IV** 3-4.5 mg/kg in divided doses, then give by inf 10 mcg/kg/min
- *Neonate:* **IV** 3-4.5 mg/kg in divided doses, then give by inf 3-5 mcg/kg/min

Renal dose
- *Adult:* **IV** CCr >10 ml/min, 100% of dose; CCr <10 ml/min, 50%-75% of dose

Available forms: Inj 5 mg/ml

SIDE EFFECTS

CV: **Dysrhythmias,** *hypotension,* chest pain

GI: *Nausea, vomiting, anorexia,* abdominal pain, **hepatotoxicity (rare), ascites,** jaundice, hiccups

HEMA: **Thrombocytopenia**

INTEG: Allergic reactions, burning at inj site

RESP: Pleuritis, **pulmonary densities, hypoxemia**

Contraindications: Hypersensitivity to this product or bisulfites, severe aortic disease, severe pulmonic valvular disease, acute MI

Precautions: Pregnancy (C), breastfeeding, children, geriatric patients, renal/hepatic disease, atrial flutter/fibrillation, asthma

PHARMACOKINETICS

IV: Onset 2-5 min, peak 10 min, duration variable, half-life 4-6 hr, metabolized in liver, excreted in urine as product and metabolites 60%-90%

INTERACTIONS

- Excessive hypotension: antihypertensives, disopyramide
- Additive effect: cardiac glycosides

Drug/Herb
Increase: inamrinone action—aloe, buckthorn, cascara sagrada, senna
Drug/Lab Test
Increase: hepatic enzymes
Decrease: serum K

NURSING CONSIDERATIONS

Assess:
- B/P and pulse q5min during inf; if B/P drops 30 mm Hg, stop inf and call prescriber
- Electrolytes: K, S, Cl, Ca; renal studies: BUN, creatinine; blood studies: platelet count; monitor fluid status (CVP) in geriatric patients
- ALT, AST, bilirubin daily
- I&O ratio and weight daily; diuresis should increase with continuing therapy

⚠ If platelets are <150,000/mm^3, product is usually discontinued and another product started
- Extravasation; change site q48hr

Administer:
IV route
- Solution should be clear yellow
- Do not mix directly with dextrose solutions; chemical reaction occurs over 24 hr; precipitate forms if inamrinone and furosemide come in contact
- May give undiluted over 2-3 min or dilute with 0.9%, 0.45% NaCl to 1-3 mg/ml, run at prescribed rate by continuous inf
- By inf pump for doses other than bolus
- Potassium supplements if ordered for potassium levels <3.0, correct before using amrinone

Syringe compatibilities: Propranolol, verapamil

Y-site compatibilities: Aminophylline, atropine, bretylium, calcium chloride, cimetidine, cisatracurium, digoxin, DOBUTamine, DOPamine, epinephrine, famotidine, hydrocortisone, isoproterenol, lidocaine, metaraminol, methylPREDNISolone, nitroglycerin, nitroprusside, norepinephrine, phenylephrine, potassium chloride, propofol, propranolol, remifentanil, verapamil

Evaluate:
- Therapeutic response: increased ca[rdiac] output, decreased PCWP, adequa[te] CVP, decreased dyspnea, fatigue, edema[,] ECG

Teach patient/family:
- That burning may occur at IV site
- To report adverse reactions promptly
- Not to breastfeed unless approved by prescriber

Treatment of overdose: Discontinue product, support circulation

indapamide (℞)
(in-dap′a-mide)
indapamide, Lozide ✤
Func. class.: Diuretic—thiazide-like, antihypertensive
Chem. class.: Indoline

Action: Acts on proximal section of distal renal tubule by inhibiting reabsorption of sodium; may act by direct vasodilation caused by blocking of calcium channels

Uses: Edema of CHF, hypertension, diuresis

DOSAGE AND ROUTES

Edema
- *Adult:* **PO** 2.5 mg/day in AM; may be increased to 5 mg/day if needed

Antihypertensive
- *Adult:* **PO** 1.25-5 mg/day; may increase to 5 mg/day over 8 wk

Available forms: Tabs 1.25, 2.5 mg

SIDE EFFECTS

CNS: Headache, dizziness, fatigue, weakness, nervousness, agitation, extremity numbness, depression

CV: Orthostatic hypotension, volume depletion, palpitations, dysrhythmias, PVCs, vasculitis

EENT: Blurred vision, nasal congestion, increased intraocular pressure

ELECT: Hypochloremic alkalosis, hypomagnesemia, hyperuricemia, hypercalcemia, hyponatremia, hypokalemia, hyperglycemia

arrhea, dry mouth, vomit-
, cramps, constipation, ab-
n
ia, nocturia, urinary frequency,
ce
Rash, pruritus
amps
traindications: Hypersensitivity to product or sulfonamides, anuria, hetic coma
Precautions: Pregnancy (B), breastfeeding, hypokalemia, dehydration, ascites, hepatic disease, severe renal disease, CCr <25 ml/min (not effective)

PHARMACOKINETICS

Well absorbed (PO); widely distributed; metabolized by liver; excreted by kidney (small amounts); onset 1-2 hr; peak 2 hr; duration up to 36 hr; excreted in urine, feces; half-life 14-18 hr

INTERACTIONS

Increase: hyperglycemia—diazoxide
Increase: toxicity of muscle relaxants, steroids, lithium, digoxin
Decrease: hypokalemia—steroids, amphotericin B, other diuretics
Decrease: effects—antidiabetics, antigout agents, anticoagulants
Decrease: absorption—cholestyramine, colestipol
Decrease: hypotensive effect—indomethacin, NSAIDs

Drug/Herb

• Severe photosensitivity: St. John's wort
Increase: hypokalemia—aloe, buckthorn, cascara sagrada, Chinese cucumber, licorice, senna
Increase: diuretic effect—aloe, cucumber, dandelion, horsetail, pumpkin, ueen Anne's lace

ug/Lab Test

ease: calcium, parathyroid test glu- uric acid

NURSING CONSIDERATIONS

Assess:

• Weight daily, I&O daily to determine fluid loss; effect of product may be decreased if used daily
• Rate, depth, rhythm of respiration, effect of exertion
• B/P lying, standing; postural hypotension may occur
• Electrolytes: K, Mg, Na, Cl: include BUN, CBC, serum creatinine, blood pH, ABGs, uric acid, Ca, glucose
• Signs of metabolic alkalosis, hypokalemia
• Rashes, fever daily; allergy to sulfa products
• Confusion, especially in geriatric patients; take safety precautions if needed
• Hydration: skin turgor, thirst, dry mucous membranes

Administer:

• In AM to avoid interference with sleep
• With food, if nausea occurs; absorption may be decreased slightly

Evaluate:

• Therapeutic response: improvement in edema of feet, legs, sacral area daily, decreased B/P

Teach patient/family:

• Diet high in potassium; to rise slowly from lying or sitting position
• To recognize adverse reactions: muscle cramps, weakness, nausea, dizziness
• To take with food or milk for GI symptoms
• To take early in day to prevent nocturia
• To notify prescriber if urinary output decreases; daily weight

Treatment of overdose: Lavage if taken orally; monitor electrolytes, administer IV fluids; monitor hydration, CV, renal status

indinavir (℞)

(en-den′a-veer)

Crixivan

Func. class.: Antiretroviral

Chem. class.: Protease inhibitor

Do not confuse:
indinavir/Denavir

Action: Inhibits human immunodeficiency virus (HIV-1) protease; this prevents maturation of virus

Uses: HIV-1 in combination with other antiretrovirals

Unlabeled uses: Prevention of HIV-1 after exposure

DOSAGE AND ROUTES

• *Adult:* **PO** 800 mg q8hr; 400 mg bid with ritonavir 400 mg bid; or 800 mg bid with ritonavir 100-200 mg bid; decrease dose to 600 mg bid when given with lopinavir, ritonavir

Mild/moderate hepatic impairment

• *Adult:* **PO** 600 mg q8h

Available forms: Caps 100, 200, 333, 400 mg

SIDE EFFECTS

CNS: Headache, insomnia, dizziness, somnolence

GI: Diarrhea, abdominal pain, nausea, vomiting, anorexia, dry mouth

GU: Nephrolithiasis

INTEG: Rash

MS: Pain

OTHER: Asthenia, **insulin-resistant hyperglycemia,** hyperlipidemia, **ketoacidosis,** lipodystrophy

Contraindications: Hypersensitivity, breastfeeding

Precautions: Pregnancy (C), children, renal/hepatic disease, history of renal stones, diabetes, hypercholesterolemia, hemophilia

PHARMACOKINETICS

Terminal half-life 1-2 hr, 60% protein binding, metabolized liver, excreted 20% unchanged in urine

INTERACTIONS

⚠ Life-threatening dysrhythmias: ergots, midazolam, rifampin, triazolam

Increase: myopathy—statins (atorvastatin, lovastatin, simvastatin)

Increase: indinavir levels—CYP3A4 inhibitors (arepitant, protease inhibitors, azole antifungals, nefazodone, verapamil); phosphodiesterase 5 inhibitors (sildenafil, tadalafil, vardenafil)

Increase: levels of both products—clarithromycin, zidovudine

Increase: levels of isoniazid, oral contraceptives

Decrease: indinavir levels—CYP3A4 inducers (barbiturates, carbamazepine, non-nucleoside reverse transcriptase inhibitors, phenytoins, rifamycins, modafinil)

Decrease: of both products—anticonvulsants

Decrease: effect—CYP3A4 substrates (calcium channel blockers, immunosuppressants, benzodiazepines, azole antifungals, macrolides, SSRIs, statins)

Drug/Herb

Decrease: indinavir levels—St. John's wort; avoid concurrent use

Drug/Food

Decrease: indinavir absorption—grapefruit juice, high-fat, high-protein foods

Drug/Lab Test

Increase: AST, ALT, amylase, total bilirubin

NURSING CONSIDERATIONS

Assess:

• For complaints of lower back, flank pain, indicates kidney stones

• Signs of infection, anemia, the presence of other sexually transmitted diseases

• Hepatic studies: ALT, AST; total bilirubin, amylase, all may be elevated

• Viral load, CD4 during treatment

• Bowel pattern before, during treatment; if severe abdominal pain with bleeding occurs, product should be discontinued; monitor hydration

• Skin eruptions; rash, urticaria, itching
• Allergies before treatment, reaction of each medication; place allergies on chart

Administer:

• Do not break, crush, or chew caps
• With water, 1 hr before or 2 hr after meals; may be given with other liquids or small meal; do not give with high-fat, high-protein meals
• Dosage adjustment will need to be considered when given with efavirenz
• Water to 1.5 L/day minimum to prevent nephrolithiasis

Teach patient/family:

• To take as prescribed; if dose is missed, take as soon as remembered up to 1 hr before next dose; do not double dose
• That product must be taken in equal intervals around the clock to maintain blood levels for duration of therapy
⚠ That hyperglycemia may occur; watch for increased thirst; weight loss; hunger; dry, itchy skin; notify prescriber
• To increase fluids to prevent kidney stones, if stone formation occurs, treatment may need to be interrupted
• That product does not cure AIDS, only controls symptoms; not to donate blood

indomethacin (℞)

(in-doe-meth'a-sin)
Apo-Indomethacin ✦, Indameth ✦, Indocid ✦, Indocin, Indocin IV, Indocin PDA ✦, Indocin SR, indomethacin, Indomethacin Extended-Release, Indomethacin SR, Novomethacin ✦, Nu-Indo ✦

Func. class.: Nonsteroidal antiinflammatory product (NSAID), antirheumatic

Chem. class.: Propionic acid derivative

Do not confuse:
Indocin/Endocet

Action: Inhibits prostaglandin synthesis by decreasing enzyme needed for biosynthesis; analgesic, antiinflammatory, antipyretic

Uses: RA, ankylosing spondylitis, osteoarthritis, bursitis, tendinitis, acute gouty arthritis; closure of patent ductus arteriosus in premature infants (IV)

DOSAGE AND ROUTES

Arthritis/antiinflammatory

• *Adult:* **PO** 25-50 mg bid-qid; max 200 mg/day; **SUS REL** 75 mg/day, may increase to 75 mg bid

Acute gouty arthritis

• *Adult:* **PO** 100 mg intially, then 50 mg tid; use only for acute attack, then reduce dose

Patent ductus arteriosus

Longer or repeated treatment courses may be necessary for very premature infants
• *Infant <2 days:* **IV** 0.2 mg/kg, then 0.1 mg/kg × 2 doses after 12, 24 hr
• *Infant 2-7 days:* **IV** 0.2 mg/kg, then 0.2 mg/kg × 2 doses after 12, 24 hr
• *Infant >7 days:* **IV** 0.2 mg/kg, then 0.25 mg/kg × 2 doses after 12, 24 hr

Available forms: Caps 25, 50 mg; sus rel caps 75 mg; inj 1-mg vial; supp 50 mg; oral susp 5 mg/ml

SIDE EFFECTS

CNS: Dizziness, drowsiness, fatigue, tremors, confusion, insomnia, anxiety, depression, *headache*

CV: Tachycardia, peripheral edema, palpitations, dysrhythmias, hypertension, **CV thrombotic events, MI, stroke**

EENT: Tinnitus, hearing loss, blurred vision

GI: Nausea, anorexia, *vomiting,* diarrhea, jaundice, **cholestatic hepatitis,** *constipation,* flatulence, cramps, dry mouth, peptic ulcer, **ulceration, perforation, GI bleeding**

GU: **Nephrotoxicity: dysuria, hematuria, oliguria, azotemia**

HEMA: **Blood dyscrasias,** prolonged bleeding

INTEG: Purpura, rash, pruritus, sweating

Contraindications: Pregnancy (D) 3rd trimester, neonates, aortic coarctation, bleeding salicylate/NSAID hypersensitivity, ulcer disease

Black Box Warning: Perioperative pain in CABG

Precautions: Pregnancy (B) 1st trimester, breastfeeding, children, bleeding disorders, GI disorders, cardiac disorders, depression, renal/hepatic disease, asthma, diabetes, acute bronchospasm, ulcerative colitis, seizures, Parkinson's disease

Black Box Warning: Stroke, GI bleeding, MI

PHARMACOKINETICS

PO: Onset 1-2 hr; peak 3 hr; duration 4-6 hr; metabolized in liver, kidneys; excreted in urine, bile, feces; crosses placenta; excreted in breast milk; 99% protein binding; half-life 4.5 hr

INTERACTIONS

Increase: hyperkalemia—potassium-sparing diuretics

Increase: toxicity—lithium, methotrexate, cycloSPORINE, zidovudine, probenecid

Increase: effect of digoxin, penicillamine, phenytoin, aminoglycosides

Increase: bleeding risk—anticoagulants, abciximab, cefamandole, cefoperazone, cefotetan, clopidogrel, eptifibatide, plicamycin, ticlopidine, tirofiban, valproic acid, thrombolytics, aspirin, SSRIs, SNRIs

Decrease: effect of antihypertensives

Drug/Herb

Increase: bleeding risk—anise, arnica, bogbean, chamomile, chondroitin, clove, dong quai, feverfew, garlic, ginger, ginkgo, ginseng *(Panax)*

Increase: gastric irritation—arginine, gossypol

Increase: NSAIDs effect—bearberry, bilberry

NURSING CONSIDERATIONS

Assess:

- Arthritis symptoms: ROM, pain, swelling before and 2 hr after treatment
- For cardiac disease, CV, thrombotic events (MI, stroke) before administration
- Patent ductus arteriosus: respiratory rate, character, heart sounds
- Renal, hepatic, blood studies: BUN, creatinine, AST, ALT, Hgb, before treatment, periodically thereafter; if renal function has decreased, do not give subsequent doses
- For eye, ear problems: blurred vision, tinnitus; may indicate toxicity; audiometric, ophthalmic exam before, during, after treatment if on long-term therapy
- For confusion, mood changes, hallucinations, especially in geriatric patients
- For asthma, nasal polyps, aspirin sensitivity, may develop hypersensitivity to indomethacin

Administer:

PO route

- Do not break, crush, or chew sus rel cap or reg caps
- With food to decrease GI symptoms and prevent ulcerations
- Shake susp, do not mix with other liquids

IV route

- After diluting 1-2 mg/ml or more NS or sterile H_2O for inj without preservative; 5-10 sec to avoid dramatic shift in cerebral blood flow; do not inj/infuse via umbilical catheter

Y-site compatibilities: Furosemide, insulin (regular), potassium chloride, sodium bicarbonate, sodium nitroprusside

Perform/provide:

- Storage at room temperature

Evaluate:

- Therapeutic response: decreased pain, stiffness in joints, decreased swelling in joints, ability to move more easily

Teach patient/family:

- To report blurred vision, ringing, roaring in ears; may indicate toxicity
- To avoid driving, other hazardous activities if dizziness, drowsiness occurs
- To report change in urine pattern, increased weight, edema, increased pain in joints, fever, blood in urine; indicate nephrotoxicity; to report mood changes: anxiety, depression

• That therapeutic antiinflammatory effects may take up to 1 mo
• To avoid alcohol, NSAIDs, salicylates; bleeding may occur
• To report use to all health care providers

infliximab (℞)

(in-fliks'ih-mab)
Remicade
Func. class.: Biologic response modifiers
Chem. class.: Tumor necrosis factor modifiers

Action: Monoclonal antibody that neutralizes the activity of tumor necrosis factor alpha (TNF α) found in Crohn's disease; decreased infiltration of inflammatory cells
Uses: Crohn's disease, fistulizing (moderate-severe), RA given with methotrexate, plaque psoriasis, ankylosing spondylitis, ulcerative colitis, psoriasis
Unlabeled uses: Psoriatic arthritis, Behçet's syndrome, uveitis, juvenile arthritis

DOSAGE AND ROUTES

Crohn's disease (moderate-severe)/(fistulizing)
• *Adult:* **IV INF** 5 mg/kg initially, then at 2, 6 wk, q8wk thereafter. May increase to 10 mg/kg if needed
Rheumatoid arthritis
• *Adult:* **IV** 3 mg/kg initially, repeat at 2, 6 wk, thereafter q8wk
Available forms: Powder for inj 100 mg

SIDE EFFECTS

CNS: Headache, dizziness, depression, vertigo, fatigue, anxiety, fever, **seizures,** *chills, flulike symptoms,* demyelinating disease
CV: Chest pain, hyper/hypotension, **tachycardia,** CHF, **acute coronary syndrome**
GI: Nausea, vomiting, abdominal pain, stomatitis, constipation, dyspepsia, flatulence
GU: Dysuria, urinary frequency
HEMA: **Anemia, leukopenia, thrombocytopenia, pancytopenia**
INTEG: Rash, dermatitis, urticaria, dry skin, sweating, flushing, hematoma, pruritus, keratoderma blenorrhagicum
MS: Myalgia, back pain, arthralgia
RESP: URI, pharyngitis, bronchitis, cough, dyspnea, sinusitis
SYST: **Anaphylaxis, fatal infections, sepsis, malignancies, immunogenicity, Stevens-Johnson syndrome, toxic epidermal necrolysis**
Contraindications: Hypersensitivity to murines, moderate to severe CHF (NYHA Class III/IV)
Precautions: Pregnancy (B), breastfeeding, children, geriatric patients, COPD, hepatotoxicity, hemalologic abnormalities

Black Box Warning: Infection, neoplastic disease, TB

PHARMACOKINETICS

Distributed to vascular compartment, half-life 9.5 days

INTERACTIONS

• Do not administer live vaccines concurrently

NURSING CONSIDERATIONS

Assess:
• For RA, ROM, pain
• GI symptoms: nausea, vomiting, abdominal pain; monitor LFTs
• Periodic blood counts (CBC)
• CV status: B/P, pulse, chest pain
⚠ Allergic reaction, anaphylaxis: rash, dermatitis, urticaria, dyspnea, hypotension, fever, chills; discontinue if severe, administer epinephrine, corticosteroids, antihistamines; assess for allergies to murine proteins before starting therapy
⚠ Fatal infections: discontinue if infection occurs, do not administer to patients with active infections
• Identify TB before beginning treatment, a TB test should be obtained, if present,

TB should be treated prior to receiving infliximab

Administer:

Intermittent IV INF route

- Give immediately after reconstitution; reconstitute each vial with 10 ml of sterile water for inj; further dilute total dose/ 250 ml of 0.9% NaCl inj to a total conc of 0.4-4 mg/ml; use 21G or smaller needle for reconstitution; direct sterile water at glass wall of vial; gently swirl; do not shake; may foam; allow to stand for 5 min, give within 3 hr
- Give over ≥2 hr, use polyethylene-lined inf with in-line, sterile, low-protein-bind filter
- Do not admix

Perform/provide:

- Refrigerated storage, do not freeze

Evaluate:

- Therapeutic response: absence of fever, mucus in stools

Teach patient/family:

- Not to breastfeed while taking this product
- To notify prescriber of GI symptoms, hypersensitivity reactions, heart symptoms
- Not to operate machinery, drive if dizziness, vertigo occur
- Avoid live virus vaccinations

⚠ High Alert

INSULINS

Rapid Acting

insulin glulisine (℞)

Apidra

insulin aspart (℞)

Novolog, Novolog Flexpen, Novolog Pen Fill

insulin lispro (℞)

Humalog

Short Acting

insulin, regular (OTC)

Humulin R ✤, Novolin R, Novolin R Prefilled

insulin, regular concentrated (℞)

regular (concentrated)

Intermediate Acting

insulin, isophane suspension (NPH) (OTC)

Humulin N, Novolin N, Novolin N Prefilled

Long Acting

insulin detemir (℞)

Levemir

insulin glargine (℞)

Lantus

Mixtures

insulin, isophane suspension and regular insulin (℞)

Humulin 70/30, Humalin 30/70 ✤, Novolin 70/30, Novolin 70/30 Prefilled, Novolin ge 30/70 ✤

isophane insulin suspension (NPH) and insulin mixtures (℞)

Humulin 50/50

insulin lispro mixture (℞)

Humalog Mix 75/25, Humalog Mix 50/50

insulin aspart mixture (℞)

Novolog 70/30

Func.class.: Antidiabetic, pancreatic hormone

Chem. class.: Modified structures of endogenous human insulin

Do not confuse:
Lantus/lente
Novolin 70/30 PenFill/Novolin 70/30 Prefilled

Action: Decreases blood glucose; by transport of glucose into cells and the conversion of glucose to glycogen, indirectly increases blood pyruvate and lactate, decreases phosphate and potassium; insulin may be human (processed by recombinant DNA technologies)

Uses: Type 1 diabetes mellitus, type 2 diabetes mellitus, gestational diabetes, insulin lispro may be used in combination with sulfonylureas in children >3 yr

DOSAGE AND ROUTES

Insulin glulisine

• *Adult/adolescent/child ≥4 yr:* **SUBCUT** Dosage individualized, give within 15 min before or 20 min after starting a meal; *Adult* **IV** dilute to 1 unit/ml in inf systems with 0.9% NaCl, using PVC Viaflex inf bags and PVC tubing, use dedicated line

Insulin aspart

• *Adult/adolescent/child ≥6 yr:* **INTERMITTENT SUBCUT** Total daily dose is given as 2-4 inj/day just prior to beginning of a meal; in general, 50%-70% of total daily insulin may be given as insulin aspart, the remainder should be intermediate or long-acting insulin; **CONTINUOUS SUBCUT** Used with external insulin pump via cont SUBCUT insulin inf (CSII), the insulin dose should be based on the insulin dose from the previous regimen

Insulin lispro

• *Adult:* **SUBCUT** 15 min before meals

Human regular

• *Adult:* **SUBCUT** ½-1 before meals

Insulin, isophane suspension

• *Adult:* **SUBCUT** Dosage individualized by blood, urine glucose; usual dose 7-26 units; may increase by 2-10 units/day if needed

Insulin detemir

• *Adult:* **SUBCUT** 1 or 2 times/day; if 1 time, give with evening meal

Insulin glargine

• *Adult and child ≥6 yr:* **SUBCUT** 10 international units/day, range 2-100 international units/day

Regular insulin (ketoacidosis)

• *Adult:* **IV** 5-10 units, then 5-10 units/hr until desired response, then switch to **SUBCUT** dose; **IV/INF** 2-12 units (50 units/500 ml of normal saline)

• *Child:* **IV** 0.1 units/kg

Replacement

• *Adult and child:* **SUBCUT** 0.5-1 units/kg/day qid given 30 min before meals

• *Adolescent:* **SUBCUT** 0.8-1.2 mg/kg/day; this dosage is used during rapid growth

Available forms: *NPH* Inj 100 units/ml; *regular* inj 100 units/ml, cartridges 100 units/ml; *insulin analog* inj 100 units/ml; *isophane insulin* inj 100 units/ml, cartridges 100 units/ml; *insulin lispro* 100 units/ml, 1.5-ml cartridges, *insulin lispro* Humalog Pen sol for inj 100 units/ml; *insulin glulisine* inj 100 units/ml; *insulin glargine* inj 100 units/ml; *insulin detemir* inj 100 units/ml in 10 vials, 3-ml cartridges; *insulin aspart* inj 100 mg/ml (Flex Pen, Pen Fill)

SIDE EFFECTS

EENT: Blurred vision, dry mouth

INTEG: Flushing, rash, urticaria, warmth,

lipodystrophy, lipohypertrophy, swelling, redness
META: Hypoglycemia, rebound hyperglycemia (Somogyi effect 12-72 hr or longer)
MISC: Peripheral edema
SYST: **Anaphylaxis; possible cancer risk (insulin glargine)**
Contraindications: Hypersensitivity to protamine; creosol (aspart)
Precautions: Pregnancy (B) lispro, aspart, (C) all others

PHARMACOKINETICS

Rapid acting
Insulin glulisine: Onset 15-30 min, peak ½-1½ hr, duration, 3-4 hr
Insulin aspart: Onset 10-20 min, peak 1-3 hr, duration 3-5 hr
Insulin lispro: Onset 15-30 min, peak ½-1½ hr, duration 3-4 hr
Short acting
Insulin regular: Onset 30 min, peak 2.5-5 hr, duration up to 6 hr
Intermediate acting
Insulin, isophane suspension (NPH): Onset 1.5-4 hr, peak 4-12 hr, duration up to 24 hr
Long acting
Insulin detemir: Onset 0.8-2 hr, peak unknown, duration up to 24 hr (concentration dependent)
Insulin glargine: Onset 1.5 hr, no peak identified, duration ≥24 hr
Mixtures
Insulin, isophane suspension and regular insulin (70/30): Onset 10-20 min, peak 2.4 hr, duration up to 24 hr
Insophane insulin suspension (NPH) and insulin mixtures (50/50): Onset ½-1 hr, peak dual, duration 10-16 hr

INTERACTIONS

Increase: hypoglycemia—salicylate, alcohol, β-blockers, anabolic steroids, fenfluramine, phenylbutazone, sulfinpyrazone, guanethidine, oral hypoglycemics, MAOIs, tetracycline
Decrease: hypoglycemia—thiazides, thyroid hormones, oral contraceptives, corticosteroids, estrogens, DOBUTamine, epinephrine
Drug/Herb
Increase: antidiabetic effect—alfalfa, aloe, basil, bay, bilberry, bitter melon, black catechu, buchu, burdock, coriander, dandelion, eyebright (po), fenugreek, garlic, ginseng, glucomannan, glucosamine, goat's rue, gymnema, horehound, horse chestnut, jambul, myrrh, myrtle
Increase: glucose tolerance—karela
Increase: hypoglycemic—aceitilla, adiantum agrimony, aloe gel, banana flowers/roots, banyan stembark, bilberry, bitter melon, broom, bugleweed, burdock, carob, cumin, damiana, dandelion, eucalyptus, fenugreek, fo-ti, garlic, goat's rue, guar gum, horse chestnut, jambue, juniper, konjac, maitake, onion, psyllium, reishi
Decrease or increase: hypoglycemic effect—chromium
Decrease: hypoglycemic effect—annato, cocoa seeds, coffee seeds, cola seeds, guarana, ma huang, yerba maté, rosemary
Decrease: antidiabetic effect—bee pollen, blue cohosh, broom, chromium, elecampane, eucalyptus, gotu kola
Drug/Lab Test
Increase: VMA
Decrease: potassium, calcium
Interference: LFTs, thyroid function studies

NURSING CONSIDERATIONS

Assess:

- Fasting blood glucose; also A1c may be drawn to identify treatment effectiveness q3mo
- Urine ketones during illness; insulin requirements may increase during stress, illness, surgery

• For hypoglycemic reaction that can occur during peak time (sweating, weakness, dizziness, chills, confusion, headache, nausea, rapid weak pulse, fatigue, tachycardia, memory lapses, slurred speech, staggering gait, anxiety, tremors, hunger)
• For hyperglycemia: acetone breath; polyuria; fatigue; polydipsia; flushed, dry skin; lethargy

Administer:

SUBCUT route

• After warming to room temperature by rotating in palms to prevent injecting cold insulin; use only insulin syringes with markings or syringe matching units/ml; rotate inj sites within one area: abdomen, upper back, thighs, upper arm, buttocks; keep record of sites
• Increased dosages if tolerance occurs
• Premixed insulins and NPH are cloudy suspensions
• Regular human insulin, rapid-acting analogs, and long-acting analogs are clear; do not use if cloudy, thick, or discolored

CONT SUBCUT route (insulin infusion CSII)

• Do not mix with other insulins when using a pump
• Insulin lispro 3 ml cartridges are to be used in Disetronic H-TRON plus V100 pump using Disetronic rapid inf sets; the inf set and the cartridge adapter should be changed q3days; replace 3 ml cartridge q6days

IV route (insulin glulisine only)

• Dilute to 1 international unit/ml in inf systems with 0.9% NaCl using PVC viaflex inf bags and PVC tubing; use dedicated line; do not admix

IV route (regular only)

⚠ When regular insulin is administered IV, monitor glucose, potassium often to prevent fatal hypoglycemia, hypokalemia
• IV direct, undiluted via vein, Y-site, 3-way stopcock; give at 50 units/min or less
• By cont inf after diluting with IV sol and run at prescribed rate; use IV inf pump for correct dosing; give reduced dose at serum glucose level of 250 mg/100 ml

Additive compatibilities: Bretylium, cimetidine, lidocaine, meropenem, ranitidine, verapamil

Syringe compatibilities: Metoclopramide

Y-site compatibilities: Amiodarone, ampicillin, ampicillin/sulbactam, aztreonam, cefazolin, cefotetan, DOBUTamine, esmolol, famotidine, gentamicin, heparin, heparin/hydrocortisone, imipenem/cilastatin, indomethacin, magnesium sulfate, meperidine, meropenem, midazolam, morphine, nitroglycerin, oxytocin, pentobarbital, potassium chloride, propofol, ritodrine, sodium bicarbonate, sodium nitroprusside, tacrolimus, terbutaline, ticarcillin, ticarcillin/clavulanate, tobramycin, vancomycin, vit B/C

Perform/provide:

• Store at room temperature for <1 mo (some insulins); keep away from heat and sunlight; refrigerate all other supply; NPH, premixed insulins are cloudy; regular, rapid-acting analogs, long-acting analogs are clear; do not freeze—IV route, regular only

Evaluate:

• Therapeutic response: decrease in polyuria, polydipsia, polyphagia; clear sensorium; absence of dizziness; stable gait

Teach patient/family:

• That blurred vision occurs; not to change corrective lens until vision is stabilized 1-2 mo
• To keep insulin, equipment available at all times; carry a glucagon kit, candy, or lump of sugar to treat hypoglycemia
• That product does not cure diabetes but controls symptoms
• To carry emergency ID as diabetic
• To recognize hypoglycemia reaction: headache, tremors, fatigue, weakness
• To recognize hyperglycemia reaction: frequent urination, thirst, fatigue, hunger
• The dosage, route, mixing instructions, if any diet restrictions, disease process
• The symptoms of ketoacidosis: nausea; thirst; polyuria; dry mouth; decreased B/P; dry, flushed skin; acetone breath; drowsiness; Kussmaul respirations

- That a plan is necessary for diet, exercise; all food on diet should be eaten; exercise routine should not vary
- About blood glucose testing; make sure patient is able to determine glucose level
- To avoid OTC products unless directed by prescriber

Treatment of overdose: Glucose 25 g IV, via dextrose 50% sol, 50 ml or glucagon 1 mg

interferon alfa-2a (recombinant) (℞)

Roferon-A

interferon alfa-2b (recombinant) (℞)

a-2-interferon, Intron A

Func. class.: Antineoplastic—miscellaneous

Chem. class.: Protein product

Do not confuse:
Roferon-A/Imferon

Action: Antiviral action inhibits viral replication by reprogramming virus; antitumor action suppresses cell proliferation; immunomodulating action phagocytizes target cells; may also inhibit virus replication in virus-infested cells

Uses: Hairy cell leukemia in persons >18 yr; condylomata acuminata; chronic hepatitis C; 2a only chronic myelogenous leukemia; 2b only hepatitis B, malignant melanoma

Unlabeled uses: Bladder tumors, carcinoid tumors, non-Hodgkin's lymphoma, essential thrombocytopenia, cytomegaloviruses, herpes simplex, Kaposi's sarcoma, HPV-associated diseases, AIDS, renal cell cancer, hepatitis B virus, malignant melanoma, polio, mycosis fungoides, rhinovirus, smallpox, vesicular stomatitis virus

DOSAGE AND ROUTES

alfa-2a

Hairy cell leukemia

- *Adult:* **SUBCUT/IM** 3 million international units/day × 16-24 wk, then 3 million international units 3×/wk maintenance

Condylomata acuminata

- *Adult:* **INTRALESIONAL** 1 million international units/lesion 3×/wk × 3 wk

alfa-2b

Chronic hepatitis B

- *Adult:* 3 million international units/3×/wk × 18-24 mo **SUBCUT/IM** as 5 million international units/day or 10 million international units/3×/wk × 16 wk

Alfa-2b hairy cell leukemia

- *Adult:* **SUBCUT/IM** 2 million international units/m^2 3×/wk up to 6 mo

Condylomata acuminata

- *Adult:* **INTRALESIONAL** 1 million international units (0.1 ml) inj into each lesion 3×/wk on alternating days for 3 wk, treat ≤5 warts per course

Chronic hepatitis B

- *Adult:* **SUBCUT/IM** 30-35 million international units per/wk × 16 wk given 5 million international units/day or 10 million international units 3×/wk

Renal cell cancer (unlabeled)

- *Adult:* **SUBCUT** 5-18 million international units/m^2/day 3×/wk alone or in combination with interleukin-2, or 5-fluorouracil or vinBLASTine

Kaposi's sarcoma

- *Adult:* **SUBCUT/IM** 30 million international units/m^2 3×/wk

Available forms: *alfa-2a:* inj 3, 6, 36 million international units/ml; *alfa-2b:* inj 3, 5, 10, 18, 25 million units/vial, powder for inj 5, 10, 18, 25, 50 million units/vial

SIDE EFFECTS

CNS: Dizziness, confusion, numbness, paresthesias, hallucinations, **seizures, coma,** amnesia, anxiety, mood changes, depression, somnolence, paranoia, irritability, hostility, encephalopathy

CV: Edema, hypotension, hypertension, chest pain, palpitations, dysrhythmias, **CHF, MI, CVA,** tachycardia, syncope

GI: Weight loss, taste changes, nausea, anorexia, diarrhea, xerostomia

GU: Impotence

HEMA: **Neutropenia, thrombocytopenia**

INTEG: *Rash, dry skin, itching, alopecia,* flushing, photosensitivity, **serious skin infection**

MISC: *Flulike syndrome; fever, fatigue, myalgias, headache, chills,* optic neuritis, **anaphylaxis, angioedema**

Contraindications: Hypersensitivity

Precautions: Pregnancy (C), breastfeeding, children, severe hypotension, dysrhythmia, tachycardia, severe renal/hepatic disease, seizure disorder, optic neuritis, ocular/pulmonary/thyroid disease

Black Box Warning: Autoimmune disorders, cardiac disease, infection, depression

PHARMACOKINETICS

Half-life (interferon alfa-2a) 3.7-8.5 hr, peak 3-4 hr, half-life (interferon alfa-2b) 2-7 hr, peak 6-8 hr

INTERACTIONS

Increase: aminophylline levels—aminophylline

Increase: neutropenia—clozapine, warfarin, zidovudine

Drug/Lab Test

Interference: AST, ALT, LDH, alk phos, WBC, platelets, granulocytes, creatinine

NURSING CONSIDERATIONS

Assess:

- For symptoms of infection; chills, fever, headache; may be masked by product fever
- CNS reaction: LOC, mental status, dizziness, confusion, paresthesia, slurred speech, anxiety, depression, paranoia, hallucinations, suicidal thoughts
- Cardiac status: lung sounds; ECG before and during treatment, especially in those with cardiac disease; MI, CHF, CVA, hypo/hypertension may occur; LFTs, thyroid function tests
- Bone marrow depression: bruising, bleeding, blood in stools, urine, sputum, emesis
- CBC with differential before and during treatment, nadirs of leukopenia/thrombocytopenia occurs in 18-19 days (alfa-2a); recovery is in 3-4 wk; if granulocytes $<750/mm^3$ or platelets $<50,000/mm^2$, reduce by 50%; if granulocytes $<500/mm^3$ or platelets $<30,000/mm^2$ discontinue

Administer:

alfa-2a

- SUBCUT/IM after reconstituting 18 million units/3 ml of diluent provided (6 million units/ml)
- 36 million units/ml is used for Kaposi's sarcoma only

alfa-2b

- IM/SUBCUT after reconstituting 3-5 million international units/1 ml, 10 million international units/2 ml, 25 million international units/5 ml, of diluent provided, mix gently, do not shake
- Each brand has different dilution directions; check package insert
- Intralesional after reconstituting 10 million international units/1 ml bacteriostatic water for inj; ≤5 lesions can safely be treated at a time
- At bedtime to minimize side effects
- Acetaminophen as ordered to alleviate fever and headache

Perform/provide:

- Reconstituted sol must be used within 24 hr
- Increased fluid intake to 2-3 L/day

Evaluate:

- Therapeutic response: improved blood counts, disease progression or improvement

Teach patient/family:

- To take acetaminophen for fever
- To avoid hazardous tasks, since confusion, dizziness may occur; avoid prolonged sunlight, use sunscreen
- That brands of this product should not be changed; each form is different, with different doses
- That fatigue is common; activity may have to be altered; to take at bedtime to minimize flulike symptoms
- Not to become pregnant while taking product; possible mutagenic effects

- To report signs of infection: sore throat, fever, diarrhea, vomiting, sore or white patches in mouth
- That impotence may occur during treatment but is temporary
- That suicidal ideation is common; notify prescriber if severe or incapacitating

interferon alfacon-1

(℞)

(in-ter-feer′on al′fa-kon)

Infergen

Func. class.: Recombinant type 1 interferon

Action: Induces biologic responses and has antiviral, antiproliferative, and immunomodulatory effects

Uses: Chronic hepatitis C infections in those 18 yr and older with compensated liver disease who have anti-HCV antibodies or HCV RNA

Unlabeled uses: Hairy cell leukemia when used with G-CSF

DOSAGE AND ROUTES

- *Adult:* **SUBCUT** 9 mcg as a single inj 3×/wk × 24 wk; leave at least 48 hr between injections

Available forms: Inj 9 mcg/0.3 ml, 15 mcg/0.5 ml, 30 mcg/ml

SIDE EFFECTS

CNS: Depression, headache, fatigue, fever, rigors, insomnia, dizziness, agitation, nervousness, anxiety, lability, abnormal thinking

CV: Hypertension, palpitation, tachycardia

EENT: Tinnitus, earache, conjunctivitis, eye pain

GI: Abdominal pain, nausea, diarrhea, anorexia, dyspepsia, vomiting, constipation, flatulence, hemorrhoids, decreased salivation

GU: Dysmenorrhea, vaginitis, menstrual disorders

HEMA: **Granulocytopenia, thrombocytopenia, leukopenia,** ecchymosis, **aplastic anemia**

INTEG: Alopecia, pruritus, rash, erythema, dry skin

MISC: **Anaphylaxis, angioedema,** flu-like illness

MS: Back, limb, neck skeletal pain, rigors

RESP: Pharyngitis, upper respiratory infection, cough, sinusitis, rhinitis, respiratory tract congestion, epistaxis, dyspnea, bronchitis

Contraindications: Hypersensitivity to alpha interferons, or products from *Escherichia coli*

Precautions: Pregnancy (C), breastfeeding, children <18 yr, geriatric patients, thyroid disorders, myelosuppression, hepatic disease, seizure disorder, alcoholism, hepatitis

Black Box Warning: Cardiac disease, autoimmune disorder, infection, depression

PHARMACOKINETICS

Peak 24-36 hr

INTERACTIONS

Increase: myelosuppression—myelosuppressives

NURSING CONSIDERATIONS

Assess:

- For past or present history of depression, seizures; use with caution in these disorders
- Ophthalmologic status, report periodically
- CBC, LFTs, ECG, platelet counts, heme concentration, ANC, serum creatinine concentration, albumin, bilirubin, TSH, T_4, triglycerides, baseline and periodically
- For myelosuppression: hold dose if neutrophil count is $<500 \times 10^6$/L or if platelets are $<50 \times 10^9$/L
- For hypersensitivity: discontinue immediately if hypersensitivity occurs

Administer:
• Do not shake vial
• Use 1 dose per vial; discard unused portion
• Proper inj sites; rotate sites
• Do not miss doses

Evaluate:
• Therapeutic response: decreased chronic hepatitis C signs/symptoms

Teach patient/family:
• Provide patient or family member with written, detailed information about product
• To report signs/symptoms of infection, thyroid/liver dysfunction, changes in behavior

interferon alfa-n3 (℞)

(in-ter-feer′on)
Alferon N
Func. class.: Antineoplastic, antiviral
Chem. class.: Human interferon α-protein

Action: Binds interferon to membrane receptors on cell surface with high specificity; inhibition of virus replication, suppression of cell proliferation, increased phagocytosis

Uses: Condylomata acuminata (venereal/genital warts), papillomavirus

Unlabeled uses: Adenovirus, coronavirus, encephalomyocarditis virus, hepatitis B virus, hepatitis C infection/virus, hepatitis D, herpes simplex type 1 and 2, HIV, HTLV-I, poliovirus, rhinovirus, varicella-zoster virus, variola virus, vesicular stomatitis virus

DOSAGE AND ROUTES

External condylomata acuminata
• *Adult:* **INTRALESIONAL** 0.05 ml (250,000 international units) per wart, given 2×/wk × 8 wk; not to exceed 0.5 ml (2.5 million international units); inject into base of wart

Chronic hepatitis C (unlabeled)
• *Adult:* **SUBCUT/IM** 10 million international units 3×/wk × 6 mo (monotherapy); 3 million international units 3×/wk plus ribavirin 1000 mg **PO** daily × 6 mo (combination)

Available forms: Inj 5-m international units/L ml vial with 3.3 mg/ml phenol and 1 mg/ml human albumin

SIDE EFFECTS

CNS: Fever, headache, sweating, vasovagal reaction, chills, fatigue, dizziness, insomnia, sleepiness, depression, suicidal ideation
CV: Chest pain, hypotension
GI: Nausea, vomiting, heartburn, diarrhea, constipation, anorexia, stomatitis, dry mouth, taste disturbance
INTEG: Pain at inj site, pruritus, pyrosis
MISC: Flulike symptoms
MS: Myalgias, arthralgia, back pain

Contraindications: Hypersensitivity to this product, egg protein, IgG, neomycin, murine protein

Precautions: Pregnancy (C), breastfeeding, children, CHF, angina (unstable), COPD, diabetes mellitus with ketoacidosis, hemophilia, PE, thrombophlebitis, bone marrow depression, seizure disorder, hepatic/thyroid disease, suicidal ideation, albumin hypersensitivity, infection

PHARMACOKINETICS

Unable to detect

INTERACTIONS

Drug/Lab Test
Interference: AST, ALT, LDH, alk phos, WBC, platelets, granulocytes, creatinine

NURSING CONSIDERATIONS

Assess:
• For flulike symptoms; may be masked by drug fever
• CNS reaction: LOC, mental status, dizziness, confusion, insomnia, depression, suicidal ideation
• For body image disturbance

Administer:
• Acetaminophen to alleviate fever and headache

Perform/provide:
- Storage of reconstituted sol for 1 mo in refrigerator
- Increased fluid intake to 2-3 L/day

Evaluate:
- Therapeutic response: decrease in wart size

Teach patient/family:
- To avoid hazardous tasks, since confusion, dizziness may occur
- That brands of this product should not be changed; each form is different, with different doses
- That fatigue is common; activity may have to be altered
- Not to become pregnant while taking product; possible mutagenic effects
- To report signs of infection: sore throat, fever, diarrhea, vomiting
- To recognize the signs of hypersensitivity: liver, urticaria, wheezing, dyspnea; notify prescriber immediately
- That suicidal thoughts and behavior may occur

interferon beta-1a (℞)
(in-ter-feer'on)
Avonex, Rebif

interferon beta-1b (℞)
Betaseron, Extavia

Func. class.: Multiple sclerosis agent, immune modifier
Chem. class.: Interferon, *Escherichia coli* derivative

Action: Antiviral, immunoregulatory; action not clearly understood; biologic response modifying properties mediated through specific receptors on cells, inducing expression of interferon-induced gene products

Uses: Ambulatory patients with relapsing-remitting MS

Unlabeled uses: May be useful in treatment of AIDS, AIDS-related Kaposi's sarcoma, malignant melanoma, metastatic renal cell carcinoma, cutaneous T cell lymphoma, acute non-A/non-B hepatitis, chronic hepatitis C

DOSAGE AND ROUTES

Interferon beta-1a

Remitting-relapsing multiple sclerosis
- *Adult:* **IM** (Avonex) 30 mcg q wk
- *Adult:* **SUBCUT** (Rebif) 22 or 44 mcg 3×/wk with each dose 48 hr apart

Chronic hepatitis C (unlabeled)
- *Adult:* **SUBCUT** (Rebif) 44 mcg 3×/wk × 24 wk

Interferon beta-1b

Relapsing-remitting multiple sclerosis
- *Adult:* **SUBCUT** 0.0625 mg every other day for weeks 1 and 2, then 0.125 mg every other day for weeks 3 and 4, then 0.1875 mg every other day for weeks 5 and 6, then 0.25 mg every other day thereafter; higher doses should not be used

Available forms: *beta-1a:* (Avonex) 33 mcg (6.6 million international units/vial); (Rebif) 22 mcg, 44 mcg/0.5 ml; *beta-1b:* powder for inj 0.3 mg (9.6 m international units)

SIDE EFFECTS

CNS: Headache, fever, pain, chills, mental changes, depression, hypertonia, **suicide attempts, seizures**

CV: Migraine, palpitations, hypertension, tachycardia, peripheral vascular disorders

EENT: Conjunctivitis, blurred vision

GI: Diarrhea, constipation, vomiting, abdominal pain

GU: Dysmenorrhea, irregular menses, metrorrhagia, cystitis, breast pain

HEMA: **Decreased lymphocytes, ANC, WBC;** *lymphadenopathy,* anemia

INTEG: Sweating, inj site reaction

MS: Myalgia, **myasthenia**

RESP: Sinusitis, dyspnea

Contraindications: Hypersensitivity to natural or recombinant interferon-β or human albumin, hamster protein, rotovirus vaccine

Precautions: Pregnancy (C), breastfeeding, children <18 yr, chronic progressive MS, depression, mental disorders, seizure disorder, latex allergy, autoimmune disorders, bone marrow suppression, hepatotoxicity, cardiac disease, alcoholism, chickenpox, herpes zoster

PHARMACOKINETICS

beta-1a: Onset up to 12 hr, peak 48 hr, duration 4 days, half-life 8.6 hr
beta-1b: Onset rapid, peak 2-8 hr, duration unknown, half-life 8 min-4.3 hr

INTERACTIONS

Increase: myelosuppression—antineoplastics
Decrease: clearance of zidovudine
Drug/Herb
• Change in immunomodulation: astragalus, echinacea, melatonin
Drug/Lab Test
Interference: vaccines, toxoids; avoid concurrent use
Increase: LFTs

NURSING CONSIDERATIONS

Assess:
• Blood, thyroid, renal, hepatic studies: CBC, differential, platelet counts, BUN, creatinine ALT, urinalysis; if absolute neutrophil count <750/mm^3, or if AST/ALT is 10 × normal, product is discontinued
• CNS symptoms: headache, fatigue, depression
• GI status: diarrhea or constipation, vomiting, abdominal pain
• Cardiac status: increased B/P, tachycardia
• Mental status: depression, depersonalization, suicidal thoughts, insomnia
• For multiple sclerosis symptoms
Administer:
• Acetaminophen for fever, headache
• SUBCUT only; products are not interchangeable
Interferon beta-1a
• Reconstitute with 1.1-ml diluent, swirl, give within 6 hr, warm to room temperature before administration
Interferon beta-1b
• Reconstitute by injecting diluent provided (1.2 ml) into vial; swirl (8 m international units/ml); use 27G needle for inj
Perform/provide:
• Storage in refrigerator; do not freeze
Evaluate:
• Therapeutic response: decreased symptoms of multiple sclerosis
Teach patient/family:
• To provide patient or family member with written, detailed information about the product
• That blurred vision, sweating may occur
• That female patients may experience irregular menses, dysmenorrhea, or metrorrhagia as well as breast pain
• To use sunscreen to prevent photosensitivity
• To notify prescriber if pregnancy is suspected
• Inj technique and care of equipment
• To notify prescriber of increased temp, chills, muscle soreness, fatigue, depression, symptoms of nepatotoxicity

interferon gamma-1b (℞)

(in-ter-feer′on)
Actimmune
Func. class.: Biologic response modifier
Chem. class.: Lymphokine, interleukin type

Action: Species-specific protein synthesized in response to viruses, effects; can mediate killing of *Staphylococcus aureus, Toxoplasma gondii, Leishmania donovani, Listeria monocytogenes, Mycobacterium avium intracellulare;* enhances oxidative metabolism of macrophages, enhances antibody-dependent cellular cytotoxicity
Uses: Serious infections associated with chronic granulomatous disease, osteopetrosis
Unlabeled uses: *Mycobacterium avium* complex (MAC), ovarian cancer, pulmonary fibrosis

DOSAGE AND ROUTES

• *Adult:* **SUBCUT** 50 mcg/m^2 (1.5 million units/m^2) for patients with surface area >0.5 m^2; 1.5 mcg/kg/dose for patient with surface area <0.5 m^2; give Monday, Wednesday, Friday for 3×/wk dosing

Available forms: Inj 100 mcg (2 million units)/single-dose vial

SIDE EFFECTS

CNS: Headache, fatigue, depression, fever, chills

GI: Nausea, anorexia, abdominal pain, weight loss, diarrhea, vomiting, colitis

HEMA: **Leukopenia, thrombocytopenia, neutropenia**

INTEG: Rash, pain at inj site, **Stevens-Johnson syndrome**

MS: Myalgia, arthralgia

Contraindications: Hypersensitivity to interferon-γ, *Escherichia coli*–derived products

Precautions: Pregnancy (C), breastfeeding, children <1 yr, cardiac disease, seizure disorders, CNS disorders, myelosuppression

PHARMACOKINETICS

SUBCUT: Dose absorbed 89%, elimination half-life 5.9 hr, peak 7 hr

INTERACTIONS

• May interfere with fosphenytoin, phenytoin, warfarin, vaccines, toxoids

Increase: myelosuppression—other myelosuppressive agents

Increase: level of theophylline, aminophylline

Increase: liver toxicity—protease inhibitors, nucleoside reverse transcriptase inhibitors (NRTIs), non-nucleoside reverse transcriptase inhibitors (NNRTIs)

NURSING CONSIDERATIONS

Assess:

• Blood, renal, hepatic studies: CBC, differential, platelet counts, BUN, creatinine, ALT, urinalysis

• CNS symptoms: headache, fatigue, depression

Administer:

• At bedtime to minimize adverse reactions; administer acetaminophen for fever, headache

• 50% of dose if severe reactions occur or discontinue treatment until reactions subside

• In right and left deltoid and anterior thigh

• Warm to room temperature before use; do not leave at room temperature over 12 hr (unopened vial)

Perform/provide:

• Storage in refrigerator upon receipt; do not freeze; do not shake

Evaluate:

• Therapeutic response: decreased serious infections, improvement in existing infections and inflammatory conditions

Teach patient/family:

• The method of administration if family members will be giving medication

• Provide patient or family member with written, detailed information about product

ipratropium (℞)

(i-pra-troe′pee-um)

Atrovent HFA

Func. class.: Anticholinergic, bronchodilator

Chem. class.: Synthetic quaternary ammonium compound

Do not confuse:

Atrovent/Alupent

Action: Inhibits interaction of acetylcholine at receptor sites on the bronchial smooth muscle, resulting in decreased cGMP and bronchodilation

Uses: COPD; rhinorrhea in children 6-11 yr (nasal spray)

DOSAGE AND ROUTES

• *Adult:* 1-4 **INH** 4 × day, not to exceed 24 **INH**/24 hr; **SOL** 250-500 mcg (1 unit dose) given 3-4×/day

• *Child:* **INH** 1-2 inhalations q6-8hr; **NEB** 125-250 mcg q4-6hr

• *Child 5-12 yr:* **INTRANASAL** 1 spray in each nostril

Available forms: Aerosol 18 mcg/actuation; nasal spray 0.03%, 0.06%; sol for inh 0.0125% 🍁, 0.02%

SIDE EFFECTS

CNS: Anxiety, dizziness, headache, nervousness

CV: Palpitation

EENT: Dry mouth, blurred vision

GI: Nausea, vomiting, cramps

INTEG: Rash

RESP: Cough, worsening of symptoms, **bronchospasms**

Contraindications: Pregnancy (B); hypersensitivity to this product, atropine, bromide, soybean or peanut products

Precautions: Breastfeeding, children <12 yr, angioedema, heart failure, hepatic disease, hyperkalemia, hypotension, hypovolemia, renal artery, stenosis, surgery

PHARMACOKINETICS

Half-life 2 hr, does not cross blood-brain barrier

INTERACTIONS

Increase: toxicity—other bronchodilators (INH)

Increase: anticholinergic action—phenothiazines, antihistamines, disopyramide

Drug/Herb

Increase: constipation—black catechu

Increase: anticholinergic effect—butterbur, jimsonweed

Increase: bronchodilator effect—green tea (large amts), guarana

Decrease: anticholinergic effect—jaborandi tree, pill-bearing spurge

NURSING CONSIDERATIONS

Assess:

• For palpitations; if severe, product may have to be changed

• For tolerance over long-term therapy; dose may have to be increased or changed

• Atropine sensitivity; may also be sensitive to this product

• Respiratory status: rate, rhythm, auscultate breath sounds prior to and after administration

Administer:

Nebulizer route

• Use sol in nebulizer with a mouthpiece rather than a face mask

Intranasal route

• Priming pump initially requires 7 actuations of the pump, priming again is not necessary if used regularly

Perform/provide:

• Storage at room temperature

• Hard candy, frequent drinks, sugarless gum to relieve dry mouth

Evaluate:

• Therapeutic response: ability to breathe adequately

Teach patient/family:

• That compliance is necessary with number of inhalations/24 hr or overdose may occur; spacer device in the geriatric patients; max therapeutic effects may take 2-3 mo

• To shake before using

• The correct method of inhalation and cleaning of equipment daily

irbesartan (℞)

(er-be-sar′tan)

Avapro

Func. class.: Antihypertensive

Chem. class.: Angiotensin II receptor blocker (Type AT_1)

Do not confuse:

Avapro/Anaprox

Action: Blocks the vasoconstrictor and aldosterone-secreting effects of angiotensin II; selectively blocks the binding of angiotensin II to the AT_1 receptor found in tissues

Uses: Hypertension, alone or in combination; nephropathy in type 2 diabetic patients

Unlabeled uses: Heart failure

DOSAGES AND ROUTES

Hypertension

• *Adult:* **PO** 150 mg/day; may be increased to 300 mg/day

Nephropathy in type 2 diabetic patients

• *Adult:* **PO** Maintenance dose 300 mg/day, start 75 mg/day

Volume- and salt-depleted patients

• *Adult:* **PO** 75 mg/day

Available forms: Tabs 75, 150, 300 mg

SIDE EFFECTS

CNS: Dizziness, anxiety, headache, fatigue
CV: Hypotension
GI: Diarrhea, dyspepsia
MISC: Edema, chest pain, rash, tachycardia, UTI, **angioedema,** hyperkalemia
RESP: Cough, upper respiratory tract infection, sinus disorder, pharyngitis, rhinitis

Contraindications: Hypersensitivity

Black Box Warning: Pregnancy (D) 2nd/3rd trimester

Precautions: Pregnancy (C) 1st trimester, breastfeeding, children <6 yr, geriatric patients, hypersensitivity to ACE inhibitors; hepatic/renal disease; renal artery stenosis

PHARMACOKINETICS

Peak 1.5-2 hr, extensively metabolized, half-life 11-15 hr, highly bound to plasma proteins, excreted in urine and feces, protein binding 90%

INTERACTIONS

Increase: hyperkalemia: potassium-sparing diuretics, potassium salt substitutes

Increase: irbesartan level—CYP2C9 inhibitors

Decrease: antihypertensive effect—NSAIDs

Drug/Herb

Increase: toxicity, death—aconite

Increase: antihypertensive effect—barberry, betony, black catechu, black cohosh, bloodroot, broom, burdock, cat's claw, dandelion, goldenseal, hawthorn, Irish moss, Jamaican dogwood, kelp, khella, mistletoe, parsley

Increase or decrease: antihypertensive effect—astragalus, cola tree

Decrease: antihypertensive effect—coltsfoot, guarana, khat, licorice, yohimbe

NURSING CONSIDERATIONS

Assess:

• B/P, pulse q4hr; note rate, rhythm, quality
• Electrolytes: K, Na, Cl
• Baselines in renal, hepatic studies before therapy begins
• Edema in feet, legs daily
• Skin turgor, dryness of mucous membranes for hydration status

Administer:

• Without regard to meals

Evaluate:

• Therapeutic response: decreased B/P

Teach patient/family:

• To comply with dosage schedule, even if feeling better, max therapeutic effects may take 2-3 mo
• That product may cause dizziness, fainting; light-headedness may occur
• To rise slowly to sitting or standing position to minimize orthostatic hypotension
• To notify prescriber if pregnancy is suspected

⚠ High Alert

irinotecan (℞)

(ear-een-oh-tee'kan)

Camptosar

Func. class.: Antineoplastic hormone

Chem. class.: Topoisomerase inhibitor

Action: Cytotoxic by producing damage to single-strand DNA during DNA synthesis, binds to topoisomerase I

Uses: Metastatic carcinoma of the colon or rectum, or 1st-line treatment in combination with 5-FU and leucovorin for metastatic colon or rectal carcinomas

Unlabeled uses: Cervical, gastric, lung, ovarian, pancreatic cancer, malignant glioma

DOSAGE AND ROUTES

Single agent

• *Adult:* **IV** 125 mg/m^2 given over 1½ hr q wk × 4 wk, then 2-wk rest period, may be repeated; 4 wk or 2 wk off

Combination dosage schedules

• *Regimen 1:* Irinotecan 75-125 mg/m^2, leucovorin 20 mg/m^2, 5-FU 300-500 mg/m^2 depending on dosing levels

• *Regimen 2:* Irinotecan 120-180 mg/m^2, leucovorin 200 mg/m^2, 5-FU BOL 240-400 mg/m^2, 5-FU inf 360-600 mg/m^2

Hepatic dose

• *Adult:* **IV** 100 mg/m^2 q wk × 4 wk, then 2 wk rest, may repeat cycle or 300 mg/m^2 q3wk as tolerated (bilirubin 1-2 mg/dl and history of pelvic/abdominal radiation)

Available forms: Inj 20 mg/ml

SIDE EFFECTS

CNS: Fever, headache, chills, dizziness

CV: Vasodilation, edema, **thromboembolism**

GI: **Severe diarrhea,** *nausea, vomiting,* anorexia, constipation, cramps, flatus, stomatitis, dyspepsia, **hepatotoxicity**

HEMA: **Leukopenia, anemia, neutropenia**

INTEG: Irritation at site, rash, sweating, alopecia

MISC: Edema, asthenia, weight loss, back pain

RESP: Dyspnea, increased cough, rhinitis

Contraindications: Pregnancy (D), hypersensitivity

Precautions: Breastfeeding, children, geriatric patients, irradiation, hepatic disease

Black Box Warning: Myelosuppression, diarrhea

PHARMACOKINETICS

Rapidly and completely absorbed, excreted in urine and bile as metabolites, half-life 6-12 hr, bound to plasma proteins 30%-68%, increased risk for toxicity in those homozygous for UGT1A1 28

INTERACTIONS

Increase: toxicity—fluorouracil

Increase: bleeding risk—NSAIDs, anticoagulants

Increase: irinotecan levels—some CYP3A4 inhibitors (ketoconazole)

Increase: myelosuppression, diarrhea—other antineoplastics, radiation

Increase: lymphocytopenia, hyperglycemia—dexamethasone

Increase: akathisia—prochlorperazine

Increase: dehydration—diuretics

Decrease: irinotecan levels—CYP3A4 inducers (phenytoin, carbamazepine, phenobarbital)

Drug/Herb

Decrease: drug level—St. John's wort; avoid concurrent use

Drug/Lab Test

Increase: alk phos, AST

NURSING CONSIDERATIONS

Assess:

• For CNS symptoms: fever, headache, chills, dizziness

• CBC, differential, platelet count weekly; use colony-stimulating factor if WBC is <2000/mm^3, or platelet count <100,000/mm^3, Hgb ≤9 g/dl, neutrophil ≤1000/mm^3; notify prescriber of these results; product should be discontinued and colony-stimulating factor given

• Buccal cavity for dryness, sores or ulceration, white patches, oral pain, bleeding, dysphagia

⚠ GI symptoms: frequency of stools; cramping; severe life-threatening diarrhea may occur with fluid and electrolyte imbalances

• Signs of dehydration: rapid respirations, poor skin turgor, decreased urine output, dry skin, restlessness, weakness
• Bone marrow depression: bruising, bleeding, blood in stools, urine, sputum, emesis

Administer:
• Antiemetics and dexamethasone 10 mg at least ½ hr before antineoplastics
• Using cytotoxic handling procedures after preparing in biologic cabinet using gloves, mask, gown
• Early diarrhea and other cholinergic symptoms can be treated with atropine
• Late diarrhea must be treated promptly with loperimide; late diarrhea can be life-threatening

IV route
• By intermittent inf after diluting with 0.9% NaCl or D_5 (0.12-1.1 mg/ml); give over 1½ hr
• Do not admix with other solutions or medications
• Stable for 24 hr at room temperature; 48 hr, refrigerated

Perform/provide:
• Increased fluid intake to 2-3 L/day to prevent dehydration, unless contraindicated
• Rinsing of mouth tid-qid with water, club soda; brushing of teeth bid-tid with soft brush or cotton-tipped applicator for stomatitis; use unwaxed dental floss
• Nutritious diet with iron, low fiber, few dairy products; avoid raw fruits, vegetables, herbals

Evaluate:
• Therapeutic response: decrease in tumor size, decrease in spread of cancer

Teach patient/family:
• To avoid foods with citric acid or hot or rough texture if stomatitis is present; to drink adequate fluids
• To report stomatitis; any bleeding, white spots, ulcerations in mouth; tell patient to examine mouth daily, report symptoms
• To report signs of anemia: fatigue, headache, faintness, shortness of breath, irritability
• To use contraception during therapy
• To avoid salicylates, NSAIDs, alcohol; bleeding may occur
• About alopecia, that when hair grows back, it will be different texture, thickness
• To avoid vaccinations while taking this product
⚠ To report diarrhea that occurs 24 hr after administration, severe dehydration can occur rapidly

Treatment of overdose: Induce vomiting, provide supportive care, prevent dehydration

iron dextran (℞)

DexFerrum, INFeD
Func. class.: Hematinic
Chem. class.: Ferric hydroxide complex with dextran

Action: Iron is carried by transferrin to the bone marrow, where it is incorporated into hemoglobin

Uses: Iron deficiency anemia

DOSAGE AND ROUTES

• *Adult and child:* **IM** 0.5 ml as a test dose by Z-track, then no more than the following per day:
• *Adult <50 kg:* **IM** 100 mg
• *Adult >50 kg:* **IM** 250 mg
• *Child <5-9 kg:* **IM** 50 mg
• *Infant <5 kg:* **IM** 25 mg
• *Adult:* **IV** 0.5 ml (25 mg) test dose, then 100 mg/day after 2-3 days; give 25 mg test dose, wait 5 min, then infuse over 6-12 hr or use equation that follows:

$$\frac{0.3 \times \text{wt (lb)} \times 100\text{-Hgb (g/dl)} \times 100}{14.8} = \text{mg iron}$$

<30 lb (66 kg) should be given 80% of above formula dose

Available forms: Inj 50 mg/ml (2-ml, 10-ml vials)

SIDE EFFECTS

CNS: Headache, paresthesia, dizziness, shivering, weakness, **seizures**
CV: Chest pain, **shock,** hypotension, tachycardia
GI: *Nausea,* vomiting, metallic taste, abdominal pain
HEMA: **Leukocytosis**
INTEG: Rash, pruritus, urticaria, fever, sweating, chills, brown skin discoloration, pain at inj site, necrosis, sterile abscesses, phlebitis
OTHER: **Anaphylaxis**
RESP: Dyspnea

Contraindications:

Black Box Warning: Hypersensitivity

Precautions: Pregnancy (C), breastfeeding, neonates, infants <4 mo, children, acute renal disease, asthma, rheumatoid arthritis (IV), ankylosing spondylitis, lupus, hypotension, all anemias excluding iron deficiency anemia, hepatic/cardiac/renal disease

PHARMACOKINETICS

IM: Excreted in feces, urine, bile, breast milk; crosses placenta; most absorbed through lymphatics; can be gradually absorbed over weeks/months from fixed locations

INTERACTIONS

Increase: toxicity—oral iron; do not use
Decrease: reticulocyte response—chloramphenicol

Drug/Lab Test

False increase: serum bilirubin
False decrease: serum calcium
False positive: ^{99m}Tc diphosphate bone scan, iron test (large doses >2 ml)

NURSING CONSIDERATIONS

Assess:

- Observe for 1 hr after test dose
- Blood studies: Hct, Hgb, reticulocytes, transferrin, plasma iron concentrations, ferritin, total iron-binding, bilirubin before treatment, at least monthly
- Allergy: anaphylaxis, rash, pruritus, fever, chills, wheezing; notify prescriber immediately, keep emergency equipment available
- Cardiac status: anginal pain, hypotension, tachycardia
- Nutrition: amount of iron in diet (meat, dark green leafy vegetables, dried beans, dried fruits, eggs)
- Cause of iron loss or anemia, including use of salicylates, sulfonamides
- Toxicity: nausea, vomiting, diarrhea, fever, abdominal pain (early symptoms), cyanotic-looking lips, nailbeds, seizures, CV collapse (late symptoms)

Administer:

- D/C oral iron before parenteral; give only after test dose of 25 mg by preferred route; wait at least 1 hr before giving remaining portion
- IM deeply in large muscle mass; use Z-track method and a 19-20G 2-3-in needle; ensure needle is long enough to place product deep in muscle; change needles after withdrawing product and before injecting to prevent skin, tissue staining

⚠ Only with epinephrine available in case of anaphylactic reaction during dose

IV route

- IV after flushing with 10 ml 0.9% NaCl; give undiluted; may be diluted in 50-250 ml NS for inf; give 1 ml (50 mg) or less over 1 min or more; flush line after use with 10 ml 0.9% NaCl; patient should remain recumbent for ½-1 hr
- IV inj requires single-dose vial without preservative; verify on label IV use is approved

Additive compatibilities: Netilmicin
Solution compatibility: TPN No. 211

Perform/provide:

- Storage at room temperature in cool environment
- Recumbent position 30 min after IV inj to prevent orthostatic hypotension
- Therapeutic response: increased serum iron levels, Hct, Hgb

Teach patient/family:

- That iron poisoning may occur if increased beyond recommended level; not to take oral iron preparation or vitamins containing iron

- That delayed reaction may occur 1-2 days after administration and last 3-4 days (IV), 3-7 days (IM); report fever, chills, malaise, muscle, joint aches, nausea, vomiting, backache
- To avoid breastfeeding
- That stools may become dark

Treatment of overdose: Discontinue product, treat allergic reaction, give diphenhydrAMINE or epinephrine as needed, give iron-chelating product in acute poisoning

iron sucrose (℞)

Venofer

Func. class.: Hematinic

Chem. class.: Ferric hydroxide complex with dextran

Action: Iron is carried by transferrin to the bone marrow, where it is incorporated into hemoglobin

Uses: Iron deficiency anemia

Unlabeled uses: Dystrophic epidermolysis bullosa (DEB)

DOSAGE AND ROUTES

- *Adult:* **IV** 5 ml (100 mg of elemental iron) given during dialysis, most will need 1000 mg of elemental iron over 10 sequential dialysis sessions

Available forms: Inj 20 mg/ml

SIDE EFFECTS

CNS: Headache, dizziness

CV: Chest pain, hypo/hypertension, hypervolemia

GI: Nausea, vomiting, abdominal pain

INTEG: Rash, pruritus, urticaria, fever, sweating, chills

OTHER: **Anaphylaxis**

RESP: Dyspnea, pneumonia, cough

Contraindications: Hypersensitivity, all anemias excluding iron deficiency anemia, iron overload

Precautions: Pregnancy (B), breastfeeding, children, geriatric patients, abdominal pain, anaphylactic shock, arthralgia, chest pain, cough, diarrhea, dizziness, dyspnea, edema, increased LFTs, fever, headache, heart failure, hypo/hypertension, infection, MS pain nausea/vomiting, seizures, weakness

PHARMACOKINETICS

Excreted in urine, half-life 6 hr

INTERACTIONS

Increase: toxicity—oral iron, dimercaprol, do not use

Decrease: iron sucrose effect—chloramphenicol

NURSING CONSIDERATIONS

Assess:

- Blood studies: Hct, Hgb, reticulocytes, transferrin, plasma iron concentrations, ferritin, total iron-binding, bilirubin before treatment, at least monthly
- Allergy: anaphylaxis, rash, pruritus, fever, chills, wheezing; notify prescriber immediately, keep emergency equipment available
- Cardiac status: hypo/hypertension, hypervolemia
- Toxicity: nausea, vomiting, diarrhea, fever, abdominal pain (early symptoms), cyanotic-looking lips, nailbeds, seizures, CV collapse (late symptoms)

Administer:

⚠ Only with epinephrine, Solu-medrol available in case of anaphylactic reaction during dose

IV route

- Give directly in dialysis line by slow inj or inf; give by slow inj at 1 ml/min (5 min/vial); inf dilute each vial exclusively in a maximum of 100 ml of 0.9% NaCl, give at rate of 100 mg of iron/15 min, discard unused portions

Perform/provide:

- Storage at room temperature in cool environment, do not freeze

Evaluate:

- Therapeutic response: increased serum iron levels, Hct, Hgb

Teach patient/family:

- To report itching, rash, chest pain, headache, vertigo, nausea, vomiting, abdominal pain, joint/muscle pain, numbness, tingling

• That iron poisoning may occur if increased beyond recommended level; not to take oral iron preparation

Treatment of overdose: Discontinue product, treat allergic reaction, give diphenhydrAMINE or epinephrine as needed, give iron-chelating product in acute poisoning

isoflurophate ophthalmic

See Appendix B

isoniazid (℞)

(eye-soe-nye′a-zid)

INH, Isotamine ♣, Laniazid, Nydrazid, PMS-Isoniazid ♣

Func. class.: Antitubercular

Chem. class.: Isonicotinic acid hydrazide

Action: Bactericidal interference with lipid, nucleic acid biosynthesis

Uses: Treatment, prevention of TB

DOSAGE AND ROUTES

• *Adult:* **PO/IM** 5 mg/kg/day up to 300 mg/day or 15 mg/kg 2-3×/wk, max 900 mg 2-3×/wk

• *Child and infant:* **PO/IM** 10-15 mg/kg/day in 1-2 divided doses max 300 mg/day or 20-40 mg/kg, max 900 mg 2-3×/wk

Available forms: Tabs 50, 100, 300 mg; inj 100 mg/ml; powder, syr 50 mg/5 ml

SIDE EFFECTS

CNS: Peripheral neuropathy, dizziness, memory impairment, **toxic encephalopathy, seizures,** psychosis, slurred speech

EENT: Blurred vision, optic neuritis

GI: Nausea, vomiting, epigastric distress, **jaundice, fatal hepatitis**

HEMA: **Agranulocytosis, hemolytic, aplastic anemia, thrombocytopenia, eosinophilia, methemoglobinemia**

Hypersensitivity: Fever, skin eruptions, lymphadenopathy, vasculitis

MISC: Dyspnea, B_6 deficiency, pellagra, hyperglycemia, metabolic acidosis, gynecomastia, rheumatic syndrome, SLE-like syndrome

Contraindications: Hypersensitivity

Black Box Warning: Acute hepatic disease

Precautions: Pregnancy (C), children <13 yr, renal/hepatic disease, diabetic retinopathy, cataracts, ocular defects, IV drug users, people >35 yr, postpartum period, HIV, neuropathy

Black Box Warning: Alcoholism, females (Hispanics)

PHARMACOKINETICS

Metabolized in liver, excreted in urine (metabolites), crosses placenta, excreted in breast milk

PO: Peak 1-2 hr, duration 6-8 hr

IM: Peak 45-60 min

INTERACTIONS

Increase: toxicity—tyramine foods, alcohol, cycloSERINE, ethionamide, rifampin, carbamazepine, warfarin, phenytoin, benzodiazepines, meperidine

Decrease: absorption—aluminum antacids

Decrease: effectiveness of BCG vaccine, ketoconazole

Drug/Food

• Do not give with high-tyramine foods, alcohol

NURSING CONSIDERATIONS

Assess:

• Hepatic studies q wk: ALT, AST, bilirubin; increased test results may indicate hepatitis

• Mental status often: affect, mood, behavioral changes; psychosis may occur

• Hepatic status: decreased appetite, jaundice, dark urine, fatigue

• For paresthesia in hands, feet

Administer:

- PO with meals to decrease GI symptoms; better to take on empty stomach 1 hr before or 2 hr after meals
- Antiemetic if vomiting occurs
- After C&S is completed; q mo to detect resistance
- IM deep in large muscle mass; massage; rotate inj site; warm inj to room temperature to dissolve crystals

Evaluate:

- Therapeutic response: decreased symptoms of TB

Teach patient/family:

- That compliance with dosage schedule, duration is necessary, not to skip or double dose
- That scheduled appointments must be kept or relapse may occur

⚠ To avoid alcohol while taking product, may increase risk of hepatic injury

- That if diabetic, use blood glucose monitor to obtain correct result

⚠ To report weakness, fatigue, loss of appetite, nausea, vomiting, jaundice of skin or eyes, tingling/numbness of hands/feet

Treatment of overdose: Pyridoxine

isosorbide dinitrate (℞)

(eye-soe-sor′bide)

Apo-ISDN ♣, Cedocard-SR ♣, Coronex ♣, Dilatrate-SR, ISDN, Iso-Bid, Isonate, Isorbid, Isordil, Isosorbide dinitrate, Isotrate, Novosorbide ♣, Sorbitrate

isosorbide mononitrate (℞)

(eye-soe-sor′bide)

Imdur, ISMO, Isotrate ER, Monoket

Func. class.: Antianginal, vasodilator
Chem. class.: Nitrate

Do not confuse:
Monoket/Monopril
Imdur/Imuran/Inderal/K-Dur

Action: Relaxation of vascular smooth muscle, which leads to decreased preload, after-load, which is responsible for decreasing left ventricular end-diastolic pressure, systemic vascular resistance and reducing cardiac O_2 demand

Uses: Treatment, prevention of chronic stable angina pectoris, diffuse esophageal spasm

DOSAGE AND ROUTES

Dinitrate

- *Adult:* **PO** 5-40 mg qid; **SL,** buccal 2.5-5 mg, may repeat q5-10min × 3 doses; **CHEW TAB** 5-10 mg prn or q2-3hr as prophylaxis; **SUS REL** 40-80 mg q8-12hr

Mononitrate

- *Adult:* **PO** (ISMO, Monoket) 10-20 mg bid, 7 hr apart; (Imdur) initiate at 30-60 mg/day as a single dose, increase q3days as needed, may increase to 120 mg/day, max 240 mg/day

Available forms: *Dinitrate:* sus rel caps (SR) 40 mg; tabs 2.5, 5, 10, 20, 30 mg; SL tabs 2.5, 5, 10 mg; chew tabs 5, 10 mg; *mononitrate:* tabs (ISMO, Monoket) 10, 20 mg; ext rel (Imdur, ER) 30, 60, 120 mg

SIDE EFFECTS

CNS: Vascular headache, flushing, dizziness, weakness, faintness

CV: Postural hypotension, tachycardia, **collapse,** syncope, palpitations

GI: Nausea, vomiting, diarrhea

INTEG: Pallor, sweating, rash

MISC: Twitching, hemolytic anemia, **methemoglobinemia**

Contraindications: Hypersensitivity to this product or nitrates, severe anemia, increased intracranial pressure, cerebral hemorrhage, acute MI

Precautions: Pregnancy (C), breastfeeding, children, postural hypotension, MI, CHF, severe renal/hepatic disease

I

PHARMACOKINETICS

Mononitrate
SUS REL: Duration 6-8 hr
Dinitrate
Metabolized by liver, excreted in urine as metabolites (80%-100%)
PO: Onset 15-30 min, duration 4-6 hr
SUS REL: Onset up to 4 hr, duration 6-8 hr
SL: Onset 2-5 min, duration 1-4 hr
CHEW TAB: Onset 3 min, duration ½-3 hr

INTERACTIONS

⚠ Fatal hypotension: sildenafil, tadalafil, vardenafil
Increase: hypotension—β-blockers, diuretics, antihypertensives, alcohol, calcium channel blockers, phenothiazines
Drug/Herb
Decrease: antianginal effect—blue cohosh

NURSING CONSIDERATIONS

Assess:
- Pain: duration, time started, activity being performed, character
- B/P, pulse, respirations during beginning therapy
- Tolerance if taken over long period
- Headache, light-headedness, decreased B/P; may indicate a need for decreased dosage

Administer:
- Do not break, crush, or chew sus rel caps, SL tabs
- After checking expiration date
- PO with 8 oz H_2O on empty stomach
- SL tabs should be placed under the tongue until dissolved

Evaluate:
- Therapeutic response: decrease or prevention of anginal pain

Teach patient/family:
- To leave tabs in original container
- To avoid alcohol products
- That product may cause headache, but tolerance usually develops; taking with meals may reduce or eliminate headache
- That product may be taken before stressful activity (exercise, sexual activity)
- That SL may sting when product comes in contact with mucous membranes
- To avoid hazardous activities if dizziness occurs
- The importance of complying with complete medical regimen
- To make position changes slowly to prevent orthostatic hypotension

Rarely Used

isotretinoin (℞)

(eye-soe-tret′i-noyn)
Amnesteem, Claravis, Sotret
Func. class.: Antiacne agent, retinoid

Uses: Severe recalcitrant nodulocystic acne

DOSAGE AND ROUTES

- *Adult:* **PO** 0.5-2 mg/kg/day in 2 divided doses × 15-20 wk; if relapse occurs, repeat after 2 mo off product

Contraindications: Hypersensitivity, inflamed skin

Black Box Warning: Pregnancy (X)

isradipine (℞)

(is-ra′di-peen)
DynaCirc CR
Func. class.: Antihypertensive, antianginal (calcium channel blocker)
Chem. class.: Dihydropyridine

Do not confuse:
DynaCirc/Dynabac/Dynacin
Action: Inhibits calcium ion influx across cell membrane during cardiac depolarization; produces relaxation of coronary vascular smooth muscle, peripheral vascular smooth muscle; dilates coronary vascular arteries
Uses: Essential hypertension
Unlabeled uses: Angina pectoris

DOSAGE AND ROUTES

• *Adult:* **PO** 2.5 mg bid; increase at 2-4 wk intervals up to 10 mg bid or 5 mg/day; **CONT REL** 5 mg/day; increase q2-4wk; max 20 mg/day

Available forms: Caps 2.5, 5 mg, cont rel tabs (CR) 5, 10 mg

SIDE EFFECTS

CNS: Headache, fatigue, dizziness, fainting, sleep disturbances, weakness, depression, drowsiness

CV: Peripheral edema, tachycardia, hypotension, chest pain, **dysrhythmias,** syncope

GI: Nausea, vomiting, diarrhea, gastric upset, constipation, **hepatitis,** abdominal pain, distention, dry mouth

GU: Nocturia, urinary frequency

HEMA: **Leukopenia**

INTEG: Rash, pruritus, urticaria

MISC: Flushing

Contraindications: Sick sinus syndrome, 2nd- or 3rd-degree heart block, hypotension <90 mm Hg systolic, hypersensitivity to this product or dihydropyridines

Precautions: Pregnancy (C), breastfeeding, children, geriatric patients, CHF, hypotension, renal/hepatic disease

PHARMACOKINETICS

Metabolized in liver; metabolites excreted in urine, feces; secreted in breast milk; peak plasma levels at 1.5 hr immediate rel, 7-18 hr cont rel; half-life 8 hr; protein binding 95%

INTERACTIONS

Increase: additive/synergistic effect—β-blockers

Increase: bradycardia, conduction defects—disopyramide

Increase: hypotension—nitrates, fentanyl, other antihypertensives

Increase: serum concentration of isradipine—rifampin, ranitidine, CYP3A4 inducers

Decrease: serum concentration of isradipine—cimetidine, CYP3A4 inhibitors

Decrease: concentration—fluvastatin, lovastatin

Decrease: antihypertensive action—NSAIDs, salicylates

Drug/Herb

Increase: toxicity, death—aconite

Increase: antihypertensive effect—barberry, betony, black catechu, black cohosh, bloodroot, broom, burdock, cat's claw, dandelion, ginkgo, ginseng, goldenseal, hawthorn, Irish moss, Jamaican dogwood, kelp, khella, mistletoe, parsley

Increase or decrease: antihypertensive effect—astragalus, cola tree

Decrease: antihypertensive effect—coltsfoot, guarana, khat, licorice, St. John's wort, yohimbe

NURSING CONSIDERATIONS

Assess:

• I&O ratio, daily weight, watch for CHF: edema, dyspnea, weight gain, crackles, jugular vein distention

• Renal, hepatic studies, electrolytes prior to and during treatment

• Cardiac status: B/P, pulse, respiration, ECG; assess anginal pain, precipitating, ameliorating factors

Administer:

• Do not break, crush, or chew cont rel tabs

• Without regard to meals

Evaluate:

• Therapeutic response: decreased anginal pain, decreased B/P

Teach patient/family:

• To avoid hazardous activities until stabilized on product, dizziness is no longer a problem

• To limit caffeine consumption

• To avoid OTC products unless directed by prescriber

• The importance of compliance in all areas of regimen: diet, exercise, stress reduction

• To notify prescriber of irregular heartbeat, shortness of breath, swelling of feet and hands, pronounced dizziness, constipation, nausea, hypotension

Treatment of overdose: Defibrillation, β-agonists, IV calcium inotropic

I

agents, diuretics, atropine for AV block, vasopressor for hypotension

itraconazole (℞)

(it-ra-con′a-zol)

Sporanox

Func. class.: Antifungal, systemic

Chem. class.: Triazole derivative

Action: Alters cell membranes and inhibits several fungal enzymes

Uses: Systemic candidiasis, chronic mucocandidiasis, oral thrush, candiduria, histoplasmosis, chromomycosis, paracoccidioidomycosis, blastomycosis (pulmonary and extrapulmonary), aspergillosis onychomycosis

Unlabeled uses: Dermatomycosis, chromoblastomycosis, coccidioidomycosis, pityriasis versicolor, sebopsoriasis, vaginal candidiasis, cryptococcus, subcutaneous mycoses, dimorphic infections, leishmaniasis, fungal keratitis, alternariosis, zygomycosis

DOSAGE AND ROUTES

Dose varies with type of infection

- *Adult:* **PO** 200 mg/day with food; may increase to 400 mg/day if needed; life-threatening infections may require a loading dose of 200 mg tid × 3 days; **IV** 200 mg bid × 4 doses, then 200 mg/day, give each dose over 1 hr; maintenance **PO** 200-400 mg/day
- *Child:* **PO** 3-5 mg/kg/day

Available forms: Caps 100 mg; oral sol 10 mg/ml; inj 10 mg/ml

SIDE EFFECTS

CNS: Headache, dizziness, insomnia, somnolence, depression

CV: Hypertension

GI: Nausea, vomiting, anorexia, diarrhea, cramps, abdominal pain, flatulence, **GI bleeding, hepatotoxicity**

GU: Gynecomastia, impotence, decreased libido

INTEG: Pruritus, fever, *rash,* **toxic epidermal necrolysis**

MISC: Edema, fatigue, malaise, hypokalemia, tinnitus, **rhabdomyolysis**

Contraindications: Hypersensitivity, fungal meningitis, onychomycosis or dermatomycosis in cardiac dysfunction, females

Black Box Warning: Heart failure, ventricular dysfunction, coadministration with other products

Precautions: Pregnancy (C), breastfeeding, children, cardiac/hepatic disease, achlorhydria or hypochlorhydria (product-induced)

PHARMACOKINETICS

PO: Peak 3-5 hr; half-life 21 hr; metabolized in liver; excreted in bile, feces; requires acid pH for absorption; distributed poorly to CSF; highly protein bound; inhibits CYP4503A4

INTERACTIONS

⚠ Life-threatening CV reactions: pimozide, quinidine, dofetilide

Increase: tinnitus, hearing loss—quinidine

Increase: hepatotoxicity—other hepatotoxic products

Increase: edema—calcium channel blockers

Increase: severe hypoglycemia—oral hypoglycemics

Increase: sedation—triazolam, oral midazolam

Increase: levels, toxicity—busPIRone, busulfan, clarithromycin, cycloSPORINE, diazepam, digoxin, felodipine, fentanyl, indinavir, isradipine, niCARdipine, niFEDipine, nimodipine, phenytoin, quinidine, ritonavir, saquinavir, tacrolimus, warfarin

Decrease: effect of oral contraceptives

Decrease: itraconazole action—antacids, H_2-receptor antagonists, rifamycins, didanosine

Drug/Herb

- Nephrotoxicity: gossypol

Drug/Food

- Food increases absorption

NURSING CONSIDERATIONS

Assess:

- For type of infection, may begin treatment prior to obtaining results
- For infection: temp, WBC, sputum, baseline and periodically
- I&O ratio, potassium levels
- Hepatic studies (ALT, AST, bilirubin) if on long-term therapy
- For allergic reaction: rash, photosensitivity, urticaria, dermatitis

⚠ For hepatotoxicity: nausea, vomiting, jaundice, clay-colored stools, fatigue

Administer:

- In the presence of acid products only; do not use alkaline products or antacids within 2 hr of product; may give coffee, tea, acidic fruit juices

PO route

- Swallow caps whole; do not break, crush, or chew caps
- Give caps after full meal to ensure absorption
- Oral sol: patient should swish in mouth vigorously, use on empty stomach
- Oral sol and caps are not interchangeable on an mg/mg basis

IV route

- After adding full contents 25-50 ml bag of 0.9% NaCl mix, use inf pump, give at a rate of 1 ml/min, flush line with 0.9% NaCl after infusion; do not use by bolus

Perform/provide:

- Storage in tight container at room temperature, do not freeze

Evaluate:

- Therapeutic response: decreased fever, malaise, rash, negative C&S for infecting organism

Teach patient/family:

- That long-term therapy may be needed to clear infection (1 wk-6 mo depending on infection)
- To avoid hazardous activities if dizziness occurs
- To take 2 hr before administration of other products that increase gastric pH (antacids, H_2-blockers, omeprazole, sucralfate, anticholinergics); to notify health care provider of all medications taken; to take after a full meal (caps), on empty stomach (oral sol)
- The importance of compliance with product regimen, to use alternative method of contraceptive
- To notify prescriber of GI symptoms, signs of hepatic dysfunction (fatigue, nausea, anorexia, vomiting, dark urine, pale stools)

ixabepilone (℞)

(ix-ab-ep′i-lone)

Ixempra

Func. class.: Antineoplastic—miscellaneous

Chem. class.: Epothilone

Action: Microtubule stabilizing agent; microtubules are needed for cell division

Uses: Breast cancer

DOSAGE AND ROUTES

Breast cancer, metastatic or locally advanced given with capecitabine and resistant to anthracycline, taxane

- *Adult:* **IV INF** 40 mg/m^2 over 3 hr, q3wk plus capecitabine **PO** 2000 mg/m^2/day in 2 divided doses on days 1-14 q21days; in those with BSA >2.2 m^2, dose should be calculated for a BSA of 2.2 m^2

Breast cancer, metastatic or locally advanced resistant/refractory to anthracycline, taxane, capecitabine

- *Adult:* **IV INF** 40 mg/m^2 over 3 hr q3wk; in those with BSA >2.2 m^2, dose should be calculated for a BSA of 2.2 m^2

Dosage reduction in those taking a strong CYP3A4 inhibitor

- *Adult:* **IV INF** 20 mg/m^2 over 3 hr q3wk

Available forms: Powder for inj 15, 45 mg

SIDE EFFECTS

CNS: Peripheral neuropathy, impaired cognition, chills, fatigue, fever, flushing, headache, insomnia, *asthenia*

CV: Bradycardia, ***hypotension,*** abnormal ECG, angina, atrial flutter, cardiomyopathy, chest pain, edema, MI, vasculitis
GI: ***Nausea, vomiting, diarrhea,*** abdominal pain, anorexia, colitis, constipation, gastritis, jaundice, GERD, hepatic failure, trismus
GU: **Renal failure**
HEMA: **Neutropenia, thrombocytopenia, anemia,** infections, coagulopathy
INTEG: ***Alopecia,*** rash, hot flashes
META: Hypokalemia, metabolic acidosis
MS: ***Arthralgia, myalgia***
RESP: Bronchospasm, cough, dyspnea
SYST: ***Hypersensitivity reactions,*** **anaphylaxis,** dehydration

Contraindications: Pregnancy (D), breastfeeding, hypersensitivity to products with polyoxyethylated castor oil

Black Box Warning: Hepatic disease

Precautions: Children, geriatric patients, neutropenia of <1500/mm^3, alcoholism, bone marrow suppression, cardiac dysrhythmias, cardiac/renal disease, diabetes mellitus, peripheral neuropathy, thrombocytopenia, ventricular dysfunction

PHARMACOKINETICS

Metabolized in liver by P45CYP3A4, excreted in feces 65% and urine 21%, terminal half-life 52 hr

INTERACTIONS

Increase: ixabepilone level—CYP3A4 inhibitors (amiodarone, amprenavir, aprepitant, atazanavir, chloramphenicol, clarithromycin, conivaptan, cycloSPORINE, danazol, darunavir, dalforpistin, delavirdine, diltiazem, erythromycin, estradiol, fluconazole, fluvoxamine, fosamprenavir, imatinib, indinavir, isoniazid, itraconazole, ketoconazole, lopinavir, miconazole, nefazodone, nelfinavir, propoxyphene, ritonavir, RU-486, saquinavir, tamoxifen, telithromycin, troleandomycin, verapamil, voriconazole, zafirlukast)

Decrease: ixabepilone levels—CYP3A4 inducers (aminoglutethimide, barbiturates, bexarotene, bosentan, carbamazepine, dexamethasone, efavirenz, griseofulvin, modafinil, nafcillin, nevirapine, oxcarbazepine, phenytoin, rifamycin, topiramate)

Drug/Herb

- Avoid use with St. John's wort

Drug/Food

- Avoid use with grapefruit products

NURSING CONSIDERATIONS

Assess:

- CBC, differential, platelet count prior to and q wk; withhold product if WBC is <1500/mm^3 or platelet count is <100,000/mm^3, notify prescriber
- Monitor temp q4hr (may indicate beginning infection)
- Liver function tests before, during therapy (bilirubin, AST, ALT, LDH) prn or q mo; check for jaundiced skin and sclera, dark urine, clay-colored stool, itchy skin, abdominal pain, fever, diarrhea
- VS during 1st hr of infusion; check IV site for signs of infiltration

⚠ Hypersensitive reactions, anaphylaxis including hypotension, dyspnea, angioedema, generalized urticaria; discontinue infusion immediately; keep emergency equipment available

- Effects of alopecia on body image; discuss feelings about body changes

Administer:

- Antiemetic 30-60 min before giving product and prn

IV route

- Let kit stand at room temperature for 30 min; to reconstitute, withdraw supplied diluent (8 ml for 15-mg vials, 23.5 ml for 45-mg vials); slowly inject solution into vial; gently swirl and invert to mix, final conc 2 mg/ml; further dilute in LR in DEHP-free bags, final conc should be between 0.2 and 0.6 mg/ml; after added, mix by manual rotation
- Diluted sol are stable for 6 hr at room temperature; inf must be completed within 6 hr
- Use in-line filter 0.2-1.2 micron
- Give over 3 hr

Evaluate:
- Therapeutic response: decreased tumor size, spread of malignancy

Teach patient/family:
- To report signs of infection: fever, sore throat, flulike symptoms
- To report signs of anemia: fatigue, headache, faintness, SOB
- To report any complaints or side effects to nurse or prescriber
- That hair may be lost during treatment; a wig or hairpiece may make patient feel better; new hair may be different in color, texture
- That pain in muscles and joints 2-5 days after inf is common
- To use nonhormonal type of contraception
- To avoid receiving vaccinations while on this product

Rarely Used

kanamycin (℞)

(kan-a-mye′sin)
kanamycin sulfate
Func. class.: Antiinfective
Chem. class.: Aminoglycoside

Uses: Severe systemic infections of CNS; respiratory, GI, urinary tract; bone, skin, soft tissues caused by *Escherichia coli, Acinetobacter, Proteus, Klebsiella pneumoniae, Pseudomonas aeruginosa, Serratia marcescens;* also used as adjunct in hepatic coma, peritonitis, preoperatively to sterilize bowel; decreases ammonia-producing bacteria in bowel and intraperitoneally after fecal spill during surgery

DOSAGE AND ROUTES

Severe systemic infections
- *Adult and child:* **IV INF** 15 mg/kg/day in divided doses q8-12hr; diluted 500 mg/200 ml of NS or D_5W given over 30-60 min, not to exceed 1.5 g/day; **IM** 15 mg/kg/day in divided doses q8-12hr, not to exceed 1.5 g/day, irrigation not to exceed 1.5 g/day; **NEB/INH** 250 mg qid

Preoperative bowel sterilization
- *Adult:* **PO** 1 g q hr × 4 doses, then q6hr × 36-72 hr

Renal dose
- *Adult:* **IM/IV** 7.5 mg/kg, may increase or decrease dose based on renal status

Contraindications: Pregnancy (D), bowel obstruction, severe renal disease, hypersensitivity

ketoconazole (℞)

(kee-toe-koe′na-zole)
Func. class.: Antifungal
Chem. class.: Imidazole derivative

Action: Alters cell membrane permeability and inhibits several fungal enzymes leading to cell death

Uses: Systemic candidiasis, chronic mucocandidiasis, oral thrush, candiduria, coccidioidomycosis, histoplasmosis, chromomycosis, para-coccidioidomycosis, blastomycosis; tinea cruris, tinea corporis, tinea versicolor, *Pityrosporum ovale*

Unlabeled uses: Cushing's syndrome, advanced prostatic cancer

DOSAGE AND ROUTES

- *Adult:* **PO** 200-400 mg/day for 1-2 wk (candidiasis), 6 wk (other infections)
- *Child >2 yr:* **PO:** 3.3-6.6 mg/kg/day as single daily dose

Prostate cancer (unlabeled)
- *Adult:* **PO** 400 mg tid

Available forms: Tabs 200 mg; oral susp 100 mg/5 ml ✤

SIDE EFFECTS

CNS: Headache, dizziness, somnolence
GI: Nausea, vomiting, anorexia, diarrhea, abdominal pain, **hepatotoxicity**
GU: Gynecomastia, impotence
HEMA: **Thrombocytopenia, leukopenia, hemolytic anemia**

INTEG: Pruritus, fever, chills, photophobia, rash, dermatitis, purpura, urticaria
SYST: **Anaphylaxis**
Contraindications: Breastfeeding, hypersensitivity, fungal meningitis
Black Box Warning: Coadministration with other products

Precautions: Pregnancy (C), children <2 yr, renal disease, achlorhydria (product-induced)
Black Box Warning: Hepatic disease

PHARMACOKINETICS

PO: Peak 1-2 hr; half-life 2 hr, terminal 8 hr; metabolized in liver; excreted in bile, feces; requires acid pH for absorption; distributed poorly to CSF; highly protein bound

INTERACTIONS

- Ketoconazole may decrease theophylline effect
- Inhibited metabolism: paclitaxel

Increase: hepatotoxicity—other hepatotoxic products, alcohol
Increase: anticoagulant effect—warfarin, anticoagulants
Decrease: CYP 4503A4 pathway, toxicity: alfentanil, alprazolam, amprenavir, atorvastatin, calcium channel blockers, carbamazepine, cerivastatin, clarithromycin, corticosteroids, cyclophosphamide, cycloSPORINE, donepezil, erythromycin, fentanyl, ifosfamide, indinavir, lovastatin, midazolam, nelfinavir, nisoldipine, quinidine, ritonavir, saquinavir, sildenafil, simvastatin, sufentanil, tamoxifen, triazolam, vinBLAStine, vinca alkaloids, vinCRIStine, zolpidem
Decrease: action of ketoconazole—antacids, H_2-receptor antagonists, anticholinergics, phenytoin, isoniazid, rifampin, ddI, gastric acid pump inhibitors
Decrease: effect of oral contraceptives
Drug/Herb
Increase: nephrotoxicity—gossypol
Decrease: ketoconazole action—yew

NURSING CONSIDERATIONS

Assess:

- For infection symptoms before and after treatment
- Hepatic studies (ALT, AST, bilirubin) if on long-term therapy
- For allergic reaction: rash, photosensitivity, urticaria, dermatitis

⚠ For hepatotoxicity: nausea, vomiting, jaundice, clay-colored stools, fatigue

Administer:

- In the presence of acid products only; do not use alkaline products, proton pump inhibitors, H_2-antagonists, antacids within 2 hr of product; may give coffee, tea, acidic fruit juices, cola
- With food to decrease GI symptoms
- With HCl if achlorhydria is present; dissolve tab/4 ml of aqueous sol 0.2 N hydrochloric acid; use straw to avoid contact; rinse with water afterward and swallow

Perform/provide:

- Storage in tight container at room temperature

Evaluate:

- Therapeutic response: decreased fever, malaise, rash, negative C&S for infecting organism, absence of scaling

Teach patient/family:

- That long-term therapy may be needed to clear infection (1 wk-6 mo depending on infection)
- To avoid hazardous activities if dizziness occurs
- To take 2 hr before administration of other products that increase gastric pH (antacids, H_2-blockers, omeprazole, sucralfate, anticholinergics)
- The importance of compliance with product regimen

⚠ To notify prescriber of GI symptoms, signs of hepatic dysfunction (fatigue, nausea, anorexia, vomiting, dark urine, pale stools)

- Use sunglasses to prevent photophobia
- To use alternative method of contraception while taking this product

ketoconazole topical
See Appendix B

ketoprofen (OTC, ℞)
(ke-toe-proe'fen)
Apo-Keto ♣, Apo-Keto-E ♣, ketoprofen, Orudis-E ♣, Orudis-SR ♣, Rhodis ♣
Func. class.: Nonsteroidal antiinflammatory product (NSAID), antirheumatic
Chem. class.: Propionic acid derivative

Action: Inhibits prostaglandin synthesis by decreasing enzyme needed for biosynthesis; analgesic, antiinflammatory, antipyretic
Uses: Mild to moderate pain, osteoarthritis, rheumatoid arthritis, dysmenorrhea; OTC relief of minor aches, pains
Unlabeled uses: Ankylosing spondylitis, bone pain, gouty arthritis

DOSAGE AND ROUTES
Antiinflammatory
- *Adult:* **PO** 150-300 mg in divided doses tid-qid, max 300 mg/day or **EXT REL** 200 mg/day

Analgesic
- *Adult:* **PO** 25-50 mg q6-8hr, max 300 mg/day

Available forms: Caps 50, 75 mg; ext rel cap 200 mg

SIDE EFFECTS
CNS: Dizziness, drowsiness, fatigue, tremors, confusion, insomnia, anxiety, depression, headache
CV: Tachycardia, peripheral edema, palpitations, dysrhythmias, hypertension, **CV thrombotic events, MI, stroke**
EENT: Tinnitus, hearing loss, blurred vision
GI: Nausea, anorexia, vomiting, diarrhea, jaundice, **hepatitis,** constipation, flatulence, cramps, dry mouth, peptic ulcer, **GI bleeding**
GU: **Nephrotoxicity: dysuria, hematuria, oliguria, azotemia**
HEMA: **Blood dyscrasias**
INTEG: Purpura, rash, pruritus, sweating
SYST: **Anaphylaxis**

Contraindications: Pregnancy (D) (2nd/3rd trimester), hypersensitivity to this product, NSAIDs, salicylates, asthma, severe renal/hepatic disease, ulcer disease

Black Box Warning: Perioperative pain in CABG

Precautions: Pregnancy (B) 1st trimester, breastfeeding, children, geriatric patients, bleeding, GI/cardiac disorders, hypersensitivity to other antiinflammatory agents

Black Box Warning: GI bleeding, MI, stroke

K

PHARMACOKINETICS
PO: Peak 1.2 hr; ext rel 6.8 hr, half-life 2-4 hr; 5.4 hr ext rel, metabolized in liver, excreted in urine (metabolites), excreted in breast milk, 99% plasma protein binding

INTERACTIONS
Increase: hypoglycemia—insulin, sulfonylureas
Increase: toxicity—cycloSPORINE, lithium, methotrexate, phenytoin, alcohol
Increase: bleeding risk—anticoagulants, cefamandole, cefoperazone, cefotetan, clopidogrel, eptifibatide, plicamycin, thrombolytics, ticlopidine, tirofiban, valproic acid
Increase: ketoprofen levels—aspirin, probenecid
Increase: adverse GI reactions—aspirin, corticosteroids, NSAIDs, alcohol
Increase: hematologic toxicity—radiation, antineoplastics
Decrease: effect of diuretics, antihypertensives

Drug/Herb

Increase: bleeding risk—anise, arnica, bogbean, chondroitin chamomile, clove, dong quai, feverfew, garlic, ginger, ginkgo, ginseng *(Panax)*

Increase: gastric irritation—arginine, gossypol

Increase: NSAIDs effect—bearberry, bilberry

Drug/Lab Test

Increase: potassium, BUN, alk phos, AST, ALT, LDH, creatinine, bleeding time

Decrease: blood glucose, HCT, Hgb, platelets, CCr, leukocyte

Interference: urine albumin, 17 KS, 17-hydroxycorticosteroid, bilirubin

NURSING CONSIDERATIONS

Assess:

- For pain: type, location, intensity, ROM before and 1-2 hr after treatment
- Renal, hepatic, blood studies: BUN, creatinine, AST, ALT, Hgb, before treatment, periodically thereafter

⚠ For aspirin sensitivity, asthma; these patients may be more likely to develop hypersensitivity to NSAIDs

- Audiometric, ophthalmic exam before, during, after treatment
- For eye, ear problems: blurred vision, tinnitus; may indicate toxicity
- For GI bleeding: blood in sputum, emesis, stools
- For CV thrombotic events: MI, stroke

Administer:

- Do not break, crush, or chew ext rel caps
- With food to decrease GI symptoms; however, taking on empty stomach best facilitates absorption

Perform/provide:

- Storage at room temperature

Evaluate:

- Therapeutic response: decreased pain, stiffness in joints, decreased swelling in joints, ability to move more easily; decreased fever

Teach patient/family:

- To report blurred vision, ringing, roaring in ears; may indicate toxicity
- To avoid driving, other hazardous activities if dizziness, drowsiness occurs, especially geriatric patients
- To report change in urine pattern, increased weight, edema, increased pain in joints, fever, blood in urine; indicate nephrotoxicity; rash, itching, blurred vision, ringing in the ears, flulike symptoms
- That therapeutic effects may take up to 1 mo, to take with 8 oz of water and sit upright for ½ hr after administration to prevent GI irritation
- To avoid aspirin, alcohol, steroids, acetaminophen or other medications, supplements unless approved by prescriber
- To wear sunscreen to prevent photosensitivity
- To report use to all health care providers

ketorolac (℞)

(kee-toe′role-ak)

Func. class.: Nonsteroidal anti-inflammatory/nonopioid analgesic

Chem. class.: Acetic acid

Action: Inhibits prostaglandin synthesis by decreasing an enzyme needed for biosynthesis; analgesic, antiinflammatory, antipyretic effects

Uses: Mild to moderate pain (short term); seasonal allergic conjunctivitis (ophthalmic)

DOSAGE AND ROUTES

- *Adult <65 yr:* **PO** 20 mg then 10 mg q4-6hr prn, max 40 mg/day; **IM** (single dose) 30-60 mg, **IV** 15-30 mg; **IM/IV** (multiple dosing) 15 mg q6hr, max 60 mg/day × 5 day combined either **PO/IM/IV**
- *Adult >65 yr, renal disease, <50 kg:* **PO** 10 mg q4-6hr prn, max 40 mg/day; **IM** (single dose) 30 mg, **IV** 15 mg; **IM/IV**

(multiple dosing) 15 mg q6hr, max 60 mg/day × 5 days combined either **PO/IM/IV**

Available forms: Inj 15, 30 mg/ml (prefilled syringes); tab 10 mg

SIDE EFFECTS

CNS: Dizziness, *drowsiness,* tremors, **seizures**

CV: Hypertension, flushing, syncope, pallor, edema, vasodilation, **CV thrombotic events, MI, stroke**

EENT: Tinnitus, hearing loss, blurred vision

GI: Nausea, anorexia, vomiting, diarrhea, constipation, flatulence, cramps, dry mouth, peptic ulcer, **GI bleeding, perforation,** taste change, **hepatitis, hepatic failure**

GU: **Nephrotoxicity: dysuria, hematuria, oliguria, azotemia**

HEMA: **Blood dyscrasias,** prolonged bleeding

INTEG: Purpura, rash, pruritus, sweating, **angioedema, Stevens-Johnson syndrome, toxic epidermal necrolysis**

Contraindications: Pregnancy (D) 3rd trimester, hypersensitivity, asthma, hepatic disease, peptic ulcer disease, CV bleeding

Black Box Warning: Breastfeeding, severe renal disease, L&D, perioperative pain in CABG, prior to major surgery, epidural/intrathecal administration, GI bleeding, hypovolemia

Precautions: Pregnancy (C), GI/cardiac disorders, hypersensitivity to other antiinflammatory agents, CCr <25 ml/min

Black Box Warning: Children, geriatric patients, bleeding, MI, stroke

PHARMACOKINETICS

Half-life 6 hr, enters breast milk, <50% metabolized by liver, excreted by kidneys

PO: Peak 2-3 hr, duration 4-6 hr

IM: Peak 50 min

INTERACTIONS

Increase: toxicity—methotrexate, lithium, cycloSPORINE, pentoxifylline, probenecid

Increase: bleeding risk—anticoagulants, cefamandole, cefoperazone, cefotetan, clopidogrel, eptifibatide, plicamycin, salicylates, ticlopidine, tirofiban, thrombolytics, valproic acid, SSRIs, SNRIs

Increase: renal impairment—ACE inhibitors

⚠ ***Increase:*** ketorolac levels—aspirin, other NSAIDs, contraindicated

Increase: GI effects—steroids, alcohol, aspirin, NSAIDs, potassium products

Decrease: effects—antihypertensives, diuretics

Drug/Herb

Increase: gastric irritation—arginine, gossypol

Increase: NSAIDs effect—bearberry, bilberry

Increase: bleeding risk—anise, arnica, bogbean, chamomile, chondroitin, clove, dong quai, feverfew, garlic, ginger, ginkgo, ginseng *(Panax)*

Drug/Lab Test

Increase: AST, ALT, LDH, alk phos, bleeding time, BUN, creatinine, potassium

Decrease: blood glucose, Hct/Hgb, platelets

NURSING CONSIDERATIONS

Assess:

- Patients with aspirin sensitivity, asthma; may be more likely to develop hypersensitivity to NSAIDs, monitor for hypersensitivity
- For pain: type, location, intensity, ROM before and 1 hr after treatment
- Renal, hepatic, blood studies: BUN, creatinine, AST, ALT, Hgb before treatment, periodically thereafter; check for dehydration
- Bleeding times; check for bruising, bleeding; test for occult blood in urine
- For eye, ear problems: blurred vision, tinnitus (may indicate toxicity)

⚠ Hepatic dysfunction: jaundice, yellow sclera and skin, clay-colored stools

K

⚠ For CV thrombotic events: MI, stroke

• Audiometric, ophthalmic exam before, during, after treatment

• GI bleeding: blood in sputum, emesis, stools

Administer:

• Not to exceed 5 days

• IM inj deeply in large muscle mass

IV route

• Give undiluted over ≥15 sec

Solution compatibility: D_5W, 0.9% NaCl, LR, D_5, Plasma-Lyte A

Syringe compatibilities: Sufentanil

Y-site compatibilities: Cisatracurium, remifentanil, sufentanil

Perform/provide:

• Storage at room temperature, protect from light

Evaluate:

• Therapeutic response: decreased pain, stiffness, swelling in joints, ability to move more easily

Teach patient/family:

• To report blurred vision or ringing, roaring in ears (may indicate toxicity)

• To avoid driving, other hazardous activities if dizziness or drowsiness occurs

• To report change in urine pattern, weight increase, edema; pain increase in joints, fever, blood in urine (indicates nephrotoxicity); bruising, black tarry stools (indicates bleeding)

• To avoid alcohol, salicylates, other NSAIDs, acetaminophen

• To report use to all health care providers

ketorolac ophthalmic

See Appendix B

ketotifen ophthalmic

See Appendix B

labetalol (℞)

(la-bet′a-lole)

Trandate

Func. class.: Antihypertensive, antianginal

Chem. class.: α/β-Blocker

Do not confuse:

Trandate/Tridrate

Action: Produces decreases in B/P without reflex tachycardia or significant reduction in heart rate through mixture of α-blocking, β-blocking effects; elevated plasma renins are reduced

Uses: Mild to moderate hypertension; treatment of severe hypertension (IV)

Unlabeled uses: Hypertension in patients with pheochromocytoma, hypertension in clonidine withdrawal

DOSAGE AND ROUTES

Hypertension

• *Adult:* **PO** 100 mg bid; may be given with a diuretic; may increase to 200 mg bid after 2 days; may continue to increase q1-3days; max 2400 mg/day in divided doses

Hypertensive crisis

• *Adult:* **IV INF** 200 mg/160 ml D_5W, run at 2 mg/min or 1.6 ml/min; stop inf at desired response, repeat q6-8hr as needed; **IV BOL** 20-80 mg over 2 min, may repeat 20-80 mg q10min, not to exceed 300 mg

Available forms: Tabs 100, 200, 300 mg; inj 5 mg/ml in 20-ml amps

SIDE EFFECTS

CNS: Dizziness, mental changes, drowsiness, fatigue, headache, catatonia, depression, anxiety, nightmares, paresthesias, lethargy

CV: Orthostatic hypotension, bradycardia, **CHF**, chest pain, **ventricular dysrhythmias,** AV block, scalp tingling

EENT: Tinnitus, visual changes; sore throat; double vision; dry, burning eyes

GI: Nausea, vomiting, diarrhea, dyspepsia, taste distortion

GU: Impotence, dysuria, ejaculatory failure

HEMA: **Agranulocytosis, thrombocytopenia, purpura** (rare)

INTEG: Rash, alopecia, urticaria, pruritus, fever

RESP: **Bronchospasm,** dyspnea, wheezing

Contraindications: Hypersensitivity to β-blockers, cardiogenic shock, heart block (2nd or 3rd degree), sinus bradycardia, CHF, bronchial asthma

Precautions: Pregnancy (C), breastfeeding, geriatric patients, major surgery, diabetes mellitus, thyroid/renal/hepatic disease, COPD, well-compensated heart failure, CAD, nonallergic bronchospasm, peripheral vascular disease

Black Box Warning: Abrupt discontinuation

PHARMACOKINETICS

Half-life 2.5-8 hr, metabolized by liver (metabolites inactive), excreted in urine, crosses placenta, excreted in breast milk, protein binding 50%

PO: Onset ½-2 hr, peak 1-4 hr, duration 8-24 hr

IV: Onset 5 min, peak 15 min, duration 2-4 hr

INTERACTIONS

- Do not use within 2 wk of MAOIs

Increase: myocardial depression—hydantoins, general anesthetics, verapamil

Increase: hypotension—diuretics, other antihypertensives, cimetidine, nitroglycerin, alcohol

Decrease: effects—sympathomimetics, lidocaine, indomethacin, theophylline, β-blockers, bronchodilators, xanthines

Decrease: labetolol effect—glutethimide

Decrease: antihypertensive effect—NSAIDs, salicylates

Drug/Herb

Increase: toxicity, death—aconite

Increase: antihypertensive effect—barberry, betony, black catechu, black cohosh, bloodroot, broom, burdock, cat's claw, dandelion, goldenseal, hawthorn, Irish moss, Jamaican dogwood, kelp, khella, mistletoe, parsley

Increase or decrease: antihypertensive effect—astragalus, cola tree

Decrease: antihypertensive effect—coltsfoot, guarana, khat, licorice, yohimbe

Drug/Lab Test

Increase: ANA titer, blood glucose, alk phos, LDH, AST, ALT, BUN, potassium, triglyceride, uric acid

False increase: urinary catecholamines

NURSING CONSIDERATIONS

Assess:

⚠ I&O, weight daily; fluid overload: weight gain, jugular venous distention, edema, crackles in lungs

- B/P during beginning treatment, periodically thereafter, pulse q4hr; note rate, rhythm, quality
- Apical/radial pulse before administration; notify prescriber of any significant changes
- Baselines in renal, hepatic studies before therapy begins
- Edema in feet, legs daily
- Skin turgor, dryness of mucous membranes for hydration status

Administer:

- PO before meals, at bedtime; tab may be crushed or swallowed whole, give with meals to increase absorption
- Reduced dosage in renal dysfunction

IV route

- Undiluted or diluted in LR, D_5W, D_5 in 0.2%, 0.9%, 0.33% NaCl or Ringer's inj, give undiluted 20 mg or less/2 min; inf is titrated to patient response; 200 mg of product/160 ml sol = 1 mg/ml; 300 mg of product/240 ml sol = 1 mg/ml; 200 mg of product/250 ml sol = 2 mg/3 ml; use inf pump
- Keeping patient recumbent during and for 3 hr after administration, monitor VS q5-15min

Solution compatibilities: D_5R, D_5LR, $D_{2½}$/0.45% NaCl, D_5/0.2% NaCl, D_5/0.33% NaCl, D_5/0.9% NaCl, D_5W, Ringer's, LR

Y-site compatibilities: Amikacin, aminophylline, amiodarone, ampicillin, butorphanol, calcium gluconate, cefazolin, ceftazidime, ceftizoxime, chloramphenicol, cimetidine, clindamycin, diltiazem, DOBUTamine, DOPamine, enalaprilat, epinephrine, erythromycin, esmolol, famotidine, fentanyl, gentamicin, hydromorphone, lidocaine, lorazepam, magnesium sulfate, meperidine, metronidazole, midazolam, milrinone, morphine, niCARdipine, nitroglycerin, norepinephrine, nitroprusside, oxacillin, penicillin G potassium, piperacillin, potassium chloride, potassium phosphate, propofol, ranitidine, sodium acetate, tobramycin, trimethoprim-sulfamethoxazole, vancomycin, vecuronium

Perform/provide:
- Storage in dry area at room temperature; do not freeze

Evaluate:
- Therapeutic response: decreased B/P after 1-2 wk

Teach patient/family:
- Not to discontinue product abruptly; taper over 2 wk; may cause precipitate angina
- Not to use OTC products containing α-adrenergic stimulants (nasal decongestants, OTC cold preparations) unless directed by prescriber
- To report bradycardia, dizziness, confusion, depression, fever
- To take pulse at home, advise when to notify prescriber
- To avoid alcohol, smoking, increased sodium intake
- To comply with weight control, dietary adjustments, modified exercise program
- To carry emergency ID to identify product, allergies
- To avoid hazardous activities if dizziness is present
- To report symptoms of CHF: difficulty breathing, especially on exertion or when lying down, night cough, swelling of extremities
- To take medication at bedtime to prevent effect of orthostatic hypotension, to rise slowly
- To wear support hose to minimize effects of orthostatic hypotension

Treatment of overdose: Lavage, IV atropine for bradycardia, IV theophylline for bronchospasm, digoxin, O_2, diuretic for cardiac failure; hemodialysis is useful for removal, hypotension; administer vasopressor (norepinephrine)

lacosamide (℞)

(la-koe'sa-mide)

Vimpat

Func. class.: Anticonvulsant

Chem. class.: Functionalized amino acid

Action: May act through action at sodium channels; exact action is unknown

Uses: Adjunctive therapy of partial seizures

DOSAGE AND ROUTES

- *Adult and child ≥17 yr:* **PO** 50 mg bid, may increase q wk by 100 mg bid to 200-400 mg/day; **IV** 50 mg 2×/day, infuse over 30-60 min, may be increased by 100 mg/day weekly, up to 200-400 mg/day maintenance

Available forms: Film coated tabs 50, 100, 150, 200 mg; IV 20 ml single-use vials (200 mg/20 ml)

SIDE EFFECTS

CNS: Dizziness, syncope, tremor, vertigo, ataxia, drowsiness, fever, hypoesthesia, paresthesias, depression, fatigue, headache, confusion, irritability, psychological dependence, **suicidal ideation**

CV: **Atrial fibrillation/flutter, AV block,** bradycardia, myocarditis, orthostatic hypotension, palpitations, **QT prolongation**

EENT: Diplopia, blurred vision, nystagmus, tinnitus

GI: Nausea, constipation, vomiting, **hepatitis,** diarrhea, dyspepsia

HEMA: **Anemia, neutropenia**

INTEG: Rash, erythema, inj site reaction, pruritus, xerostomia

MS: Asthenia, dysarthria

Contraindications: Hypersensitivity
Precautions: Pregnancy (C), breastfeeding, children <17 yr, geriatric patients, allergies, cardiac/renal/hepatic disease, acute MI, atrial fibrillation/flutter, AV block, bradycardia, CHD, dehydration, depression, dialysis, hazardous activity, electrolyte imbalance, heart failure, labor, QT prolongation, sick sinus syndrome, substance abuse, suicidal ideation, syncope, torsade de pointes

PHARMACOKINETICS

Metabolized by liver; excreted by kidneys, 95% unchanged; protein binding <15%
PO: Peak 1-4 hr; half-life 13 hr

INTERACTIONS

⚠ ***Increase:*** QT prolongation—class 1A/III antidysrhythmics, some phenothiazines, β-agonists, local anesthetics, tricyclics, bepridil, haloperidol, methadone, chloroquine, clarithromycin, droperidol, erythromycin, grepafloxacin, halofantrine, pentamidine, probucol, sparfloxacin
Drug/Lab Test
Increase: LFTs

NURSING CONSIDERATIONS

Assess:
- For seizures: duration, type, intensity precipitating factors
- Renal function: albumin concentration
- CV status: orthostatic hypotension, QT prolongation; monitor cardiac status throughout treatment
- Mental status: mood, sensorium, affect, memory (long, short), depression, suicidal ideation, psychological dependence
- For rash, hypersensitivity reactions

Administer:
PO route
- Give without regard to meals

IV route
- May give undiluted or mixed in 0.9%NaCl, D_5, or LR
- Infuse over 30-60 min
- Do not use if discolored or particulates are present; discard unused portions

Perform/provide:
- Storage of PO products/IV vials at room temperature; solution is stable for 24 hr when mixed with compatible diluents in glass or PVC bags at room temperature

Evaluate:
- Therapeutic response: decrease in severity of seizures

Teach patient/family:
- Not to discontinue product abruptly; seizures may occur
- To avoid hazardous activities until stabilized on product
- To carry emergency ID stating product use
- To notify prescriber of suicidal thoughts or actions, syncope, cardiac changes
- To notify prescriber if pregnancy is planned or suspected
- That interactions with other medications may occur
- Give patient MedGuide for proper use and risks

lactulose (℞)

(lak'tyoo-lose)
Cephulac, Cholac, Chronulac, Constilac, Constulose, Duphalac, Enulose, Evalose, Heptalac, Kristalose, Lactulax ♣, Lactulose PSE, Portalac
Func. class.: Laxative; ammonia detoxicant (hyperosmotic)
Chem. class.: Lactose synthetic derivative

Action: Prevents absorption of ammonia in colon by acidifying stool; increases water in stool
Uses: Chronic constipation, portal-systemic encephalopathy in patients with hepatic disease

DOSAGE AND ROUTES

Constipation

• *Adult:* **PO** 15-30 ml/day (10-20 g) may increase to 60 ml/day prn

• *Child (unlabeled):* **PO** 7.5 ml/day

Encephalopathy

• *Adult:* **PO** 30-45 ml tid or qid until stools are soft; **RETENTION ENEMA** 300 ml diluted

• *Child (unlabeled):* **PO** 40-90 ml/day in divided doses given 2-4×/day

• *Infant (unlabeled):* **PO** 2.5-10 ml/day in divided doses

Available forms: Syr 10 g/15 ml; single-use packets (Kristalose) 10, 20 g

SIDE EFFECTS

GI: Nausea, vomiting, anorexia, abdominal cramps, diarrhea, flatulence, distention, belching

META: Hypernatremia

Contraindications: Hypersensitivity, low-galactose diet

Precautions: Pregnancy (B), breastfeeding, geriatric patients, debilitated patients, diabetes mellitus

PHARMACOKINETICS

Metabolized in colon, excreted by kidneys, onset 1-2 days, peak unknown, duration unknown

INTERACTIONS

• Do not use with other laxatives

Decrease: lactulose effects—neomycin, other oral antiinfectives

Drug/Herb

Increase: laxative action—flax, senna

NURSING CONSIDERATIONS

Assess:

• Stool: amount, color, consistency

• Blood ammonia level (30-70 mg/100 ml); may decrease ammonia level by 25%-50%

• Blood, urine electrolytes if product is used often; may cause diarrhea, hypokalemia, hyponatremia

• I&O ratio to identify fluid loss

• Cause of constipation; determine whether fluids, bulk, or exercise is missing from lifestyle, constipating products

• Cramping, rectal bleeding, nausea, vomiting; if these symptoms occur, product should be discontinued

• Clearing of confusion, lethargy, restlessness, irritability if portal-systemic encephalopathy

Administer:

PO route

• With 8 oz fruit juice, water, milk to increase palatability of oral form

Rectal route

• Retention enema by diluting 300 ml lactose/700 ml of water; administer by rectal balloon catheter

• Increased fluids to 2 L/day; do not give with other laxatives; if diarrhea occurs, reduce dosage

Evaluate:

• Therapeutic response: decreased constipation, decreased blood ammonia level, clearing of mental state

Teach patient/family:

• Not to use laxatives long-term

• To dilute with water or fruit juice to counteract sweet taste

• To store in cool environment; do not freeze

• To take on an empty stomach for rapid action

• To report diarrhea; may indicate overdose

lamivudine (℞)

(lam-i-voo′deen)

Epivir, Epivir-HBV, 3TC

Func. class.: Antiretroviral

Chem. class.: Nucleoside reverse transcriptase inhibitor (NRTI)

Do not confuse:

lamivudine/lamotrigine

Action: Inhibits replication of HIV virus by incorporating into cellular DNA by viral reverse transcriptase, thereby terminating cellular DNA chain

Uses: HIV-1 infection in combination with other antiretrovirals; chronic hepatitis B (Epivir-HBV)

Unlabeled uses: Prophylaxis of HIV—postexposure with indinavir and zidovudine

DOSAGE AND ROUTES

HIV

• *Adult and child >12 yr:* **PO** 150 mg bid or 300 mg/day

• *Child 3 mo-12 yr:* **PO** 4 mg/kg bid, max 150 mg bid

Renal dose

• *Adult:* **PO** CCr 30-49 ml/min 150 mg/day; CCr 15-29 ml/min 150 mg (1st dose), then 100 mg/day; CCr 5-14 ml/min 150 mg/day (1st dose), then 50 mg/day; CCr <5 ml/min, 50 mg (1st dose), then 25 mg/day

Chronic hepatitis B

• *Adult:* **PO** 100 mg/day

• *Child and adolescent 2-17 yr:* **PO** 3 mg/kg/day, max 100 mg

Available forms: (Epivir) oral sol 10 mg/ml; tabs 100, 150, 300 mg; (Epivir-HBV) oral sol 5 mg/ml; tabs 100 mg

SIDE EFFECTS

CNS: Fever, headache, malaise, dizziness, insomnia, depression, fatigue, chills, **seizures**

EENT: Taste change, hearing loss, photophobia

GI: Nausea, vomiting, diarrhea, anorexia, cramps, dyspepsia, **hepatomegaly with steatosis, pancreatitis**

HEMA: **Neutropenia, anemia, thrombocytopenia**

INTEG: Rash

MS: Myalgia, arthralgia, pain

RESP: Cough

SYST: **Lactic acidosis, anaphylaxis, Stevens-Johnson syndrome**

Contraindications: Hypersensitivity

Black Box Warning: Lactic acidosis

Precautions: Pregnancy (C), breastfeeding, children, geriatric patients, granulocyte count <1000/mm^3 or Hgb <9.5 g/dl, renal disease, pancreatitis, peripheral neuropathy

Black Box Warning: Severe hepatic dysfunction

PHARMACOKINETICS

Rapidly absorbed, distributed to extravascular space, excreted unchanged in urine, protein binding <36%, terminal half-life 5-7 hr

INTERACTIONS

• May decrease both products: zalcitabine

Increase: lamivudine level—trimethoprim-sulfamethoxazole

Increase: level—zidovudine

Drug/Lab Test

Increase: ALT, bilirubin

Decrease: Hgb, neutrophil, platelet count

NURSING CONSIDERATIONS

Assess:

• Blood counts q2wk; watch for neutropenia, thrombocytopenia, Hgb, CD4, viral load; if low, therapy may have to be discontinued and restarted after hematologic recovery; blood transfusions may be required

• Hepatic studies: AST, ALT, bilirubin; amylase, lipase, triglycerides, CD4, viral load periodically during treatment

• Children for pancreatitis: abdominal pain, nausea, vomiting

⚠ Lactic acidosis, severe hepatomegaly with steatosis: obtain baseline LFTs, if elevated discontinue treatment; discontinue even if LFTs are normal if lactic acidosis, severe hepatomegaly develop

Administer:

• PO daily or bid, without regard to meals

Perform/provide:

• With other antiretrovirals only

• Storage in cool environment; protect from light

Evaluate:

• Blood dyscrasias: bruising, fatigue, bleeding, poor healing

Teach patient/family:

- That GI complaints, insomnia resolve after 3-4 wk of treatment
- That product is not a cure for HIV, but will control symptoms
- To notify prescriber of sore throat, swollen lymph nodes, malaise, fever; other infections may occur
- That patient is still infective, may pass HIV virus on to others
- That follow-up visits must be continued since serious toxicity may occur; blood counts must be done q2wk
- That product must be taken as prescribed, even if patient feels better
- That other products may be necessary to prevent other infections
- That product may cause fainting or dizziness

lamotrigine (℞)

(la-moe′tri-geen)
Lamictal, Lamictal CD, Lamictal ODT, Lamictal XR, Lamictal Chewable Dispersible

Func. class.: Anticonvulsant—miscellaneous

Chem. class.: Phenyltriazine

Do not confuse:
lamotrigine/lamivudine
Lamictal/Lomotil/Lamisil

Action: Unknown, may inhibit voltage-sensitive sodium channels

Uses: Adjunct in the treatment of partial, tonic-clonic seizures; children with Lennox-Gastaut syndrome, bipolar disorder

Unlabeled uses: Absence, seizures

DOSAGE AND ROUTES

Seizures: monotherapy

- *Adult:* **PO** 50 mg/day for wk 1-2, then increase to 100 mg divided bid for wk 3-4; maintenance 300-500 mg/day; receiving enzyme-inducing AEDs (carbamazepine, phenobarbital, phenytoin, primidone) but not valproic acid EXT REL 50 mg/day × 1-2 wk, then 100 mg/day during wk 3-4, then 200 mg/day during wk 5, then 300 mg/day during wk 6, then 400 mg/day during wk 7, after wk 7 range is 400-600 mg/day
- *Child:* **PO** 0.3 mg/kg/day wk 1 and 2; then 0.6 mg/kg/day wk 3 and 4; depends on use of AED; usual dose 4.5-7.5 mg/kg/day, max 300 mg/day

Seizures: multiple therapy with valproate

- *Adult:* **PO** 25 mg every other day, then 25 mg/day wk 3-4, increase by 25-50 mg q1-2wk, maintenance 100-400 mg/day
- *Child:* **PO** 0.1-0.2 mg/kg/day initially, then increase q2wk as needed to 2 mg/kg/day or 150 mg/day

Bipolar disorder

- *Adult:* **PO** Wk 1-2 25 mg/day; wk 3-4 50 mg/day; wk 5 100 mg/day; wk 6-7 200 mg/day; for patients taking valproic acid: wk 1-2 25 mg every other day, wk 3-4 25 mg/day; wk 5 50 mg/day; wk 6 100 mg/day; wk 7 100 mg/day

Hepatic dose

- *Adult:* **PO** (Child-Pugh B) Reduce by 25%; (Child-Pugh C) reduce by 50%

Absence seizures (unlabeled)

- *Adolescent and child 3-13 yr:* **PO** 0.5 mg/kg/day in 2 divided doses × 2 wk, then 1 mg/kg/day in 2 divided doses × 2 wk, adjusted q5days

Available forms: Tabs 25, 100, 150, 200 mg; PO ext rel 25-50-100, 50-100-200 mg titration kit; PO 25-100 mg starter kit; ext rel 25, 50, 100, 250 mg; chew dispersible tabs 5, 25 mg; oral disintegrating tab 25, 50, 100, 200 mg; oral disintegrating tab 25-50, 50-100 mg, 25-50-100 mg titration kit

SIDE EFFECTS

CNS: Dizziness, ataxia, *headache,* fever, insomnia, tremor, depression, anxiety, **suicidal ideation**

EENT: Nystagmus, *diplopia, blurred vision*

GI: Nausea, vomiting, anorexia, abdominal pain, **hepatotoxicity**

GU: Dysmenorrhea

HEMA: Anemia, **DIC, leukopenia, thrombocytopenia**

INTEG: **Rash (potentially life-threatening),** alopecia, photosensitivity
SYST: **Stevens-Johnson syndrome, angioedema, toxic epidermal necrolysis**

Contraindications: Hypersensitivity
Precautions: Pregnancy (C) (cleft lip/palate in 1st trimester), breastfeeding, geriatric patients, renal/hepatic/cardiac disease, severe depression, suicidal, blood dyscrasias

Black Box Warning: Children <16 yr

PHARMACOKINETICS

Half-life varies depending on dose; terminal half-life 24 hr, 15 hr with enzyme inducers rapidly, completely absorbed; metabolized by glucuronic acid conjunction; protein binding 55%; peak 1.4-2.3 hr; crosses placenta; excreted in breast milk

INTERACTIONS

Decrease: metabolic clearance of lamotrigine—valproic acid, 3A4 inhibitors
Decrease: lamotrigine serum concentration—carbamazepine, rifamycins, oral contraceptives, acetaminophen, phenytoin, primodone, phenobarbital, oxcarbazepine, succinimides, estrogen

Drug/Herb
Increase: anticonvulsant effect—ginkgo
Decrease: anticonvulsant effect—ginseng, santonica

NURSING CONSIDERATIONS

Assess:

- For seizure activity: duration, type, intensity, halo before seizure
- ⚠ For rash (Stevens-Johnson syndrome or toxic epidermal necrolysis) in pediatric patients, product should be discontinued at first sign of rash
- ⚠ Mental status: suicidal thoughts/behaviors

Administer:

- Correct starter kit, errors have occurred
- Chewable dispersible tabs: swallow whole, chew, or dispersed in water or diluted fruit juice; if chewed, drink a small amount of water
- Round to nearest whole tab (adult)

Evaluate:

- Therapeutic response: decrease in severity of seizures

Teach patient/family:

- To take PO doses divided with or after meals to decrease adverse effects, not to discontinue product abruptly; seizures may occur
- To avoid hazardous activities until stabilized on product
- To carry emergency ID, to notify prescriber of skin rash or increased seizure activity, to use sunscreen and protective clothing if photosensitivity occurs
- To notify prescriber if pregnant or intend to become pregnant

lansoprazole (℞, OTC)

(lan-so-prey′zole)
Prevacid, Prevacid 24 HR
Prevacid IV, Prevacid SoluTab
Func. class.: Antiulcer, proton pump inhibitor
Chem. class.: Benzimidazole

Do not confuse:
Prevacid/Pravachol/Prinivil

Action: Suppresses gastric secretion by inhibiting hydrogen/potassium ATPase enzyme system in gastric parietal cell; characterized as gastric acid pump inhibitor, since it blocks final step of acid production

Uses: Gastroesophageal reflux disease (GERD), severe erosive esophagitis, poorly responsive systemic GERD, pathologic hypersecretory conditions (Zollinger-Ellison syndrome, systemic mastocytosis, multiple endocrine adenomas); possibly effective for treatment of duodenal, gastric ulcers, maintenance of healed duodenal ulcers

Unlabeled uses: GERD in pediatrics

DOSAGE AND ROUTES

Frequent heartburn

• *Adult:* **PO** 15 mg daily up to 14 days

NG tube

• *Adult:* Use intact granules mixed in 40 ml of apple juice and injected through **NG** tube, then flush with apple juice

Duodenal ulcer

• *Adult:* **PO** 15 mg/day before eating for 4 wk, then 15 mg/day to maintain healing of ulcers; associated with *Helicobacter pylori*—30 mg lansoprazole, 500 mg clarithromycin, 1 g amoxicillin bid × 14 days or 30 mg lansoprazole, 1 g amoxicillin tid × 14 days

Erosive esophagitis

• *Adult:* **IV** 30 mg over 30 min or for up to 7 days; switch to PO as soon as patient can tolerate, for 6-8 wk

Pathologic hypersecretory conditions

• *Adult:* **PO** 60 mg/day, may give up to 90 mg bid, administer doses of >120 mg/day in divided doses

GERD/esophagitis

• *Adult and adolescent:* **PO** 15-30 mg/day × 8 wk

• *Child 1-11 yr (>30 kg):* **PO** 30 mg/day ≤12 wk

• *Child 1-11 yr (≤30 kg):* **PO** 15 mg/day ≤12 wk

• *Infant (unlabeled):* **PO** 1-1.74 mg/kg/day; limited data are available

• *Neonate (unlabeled):* **PO** 0.5-1 mg/kg/day

Available forms: Del rel caps 15, 30 mg; granules for oral susp 15, 30 mg/packet; orally disintegrating tabs 15, 30 mg; lyophilized powder for IV inj 30 mg/vial

SIDE EFFECTS

CNS: Headache, dizziness, confusion, agitation, amnesia, depression

CV: Chest pain, angina, tachycardia, bradycardia, palpitations, **CVA,** hypo/hypertension, **MI, shock,** vasodilation

EENT: Tinnitus, taste perversion, deafness, eye pain, otitis media

GI: Diarrhea, abdominal pain, vomiting, nausea, constipation, flatulence, acid regurgitation, anorexia, irritable colon, microscopic colitis

GU: **Hematuria,** glycosuria, impotence, kidney calculus, breast enlargement

HEMA: **Hemolysis,** anemia

INTEG: Rash, urticaria, pruritus, alopecia

META: Weight gain/loss, gout

RESP: Upper respiratory infections, cough, epistaxis, asthma, bronchitis, dyspnea, **pneumonia**

Contraindications: Hypersensitivity

Precautions: Pregnancy (B), breastfeeding, children

PHARMACOKINETICS

Absorption after granules leave stomach—>80%; plasma half-life 1½-2 hr; protein binding 97%; extensively metabolized in liver; excreted in urine, feces; clearance decreased in the geriatric patient, renal/hepatic impairment

INTERACTIONS

• Delayed lansoprazole absorption: sucralfate

Decrease: absorption of ketoconazole, itraconazole, iron, indinivir, calcium carbonate

NURSING CONSIDERATIONS

Assess:

• GI system: bowel sounds q8hr, abdomen for pain, swelling, anorexia

• Hepatic studies: AST, ALT, alk phos during treatment

Administer:

• Swallow caps whole before eating; do not crush or chew caps; caps may be opened and contents sprinkled on food

Evaluate:

• Therapeutic response: absence of epigastric pain, swelling, fullness

Teach patient/family:

• To report severe diarrhea; product may have to be discontinued

• That diabetic patient should know that hypoglycemia may occur

• To avoid hazardous activities; dizziness may occur

• To avoid alcohol, salicylates, ibuprofen; may cause GI irritation

Rarely Used

lanthanum (℞)

(lan′-tha-num)

Fosrenol

Func. class.: Phosphate binder

Uses: End-stage renal disease

DOSAGE AND ROUTES

• *Adult:* **PO** 750-1500 mg/day in divided doses with meals; titrate dose q2-3wk until an acceptable phosphate level is reached; tabs should be chewed completely before swallowing; intact tabs should not be swallowed; maintenance dose 1500-3000 mg/day divided with meals

Contraindications: Hypophosphatemia, hypersensitivity

lapatinib (℞)

(la-pa′tin-ib)

Tykerb

Func. class.: Antineoplastic—miscellaneous

Chem. class.: Biologic response modifier, signal transduction inhibitor (STIs)

Action: Reverses tyrosine kinase of both the epidermal growth factor receptor (ERbB1) and human epidermal receptor type 2 (HER2) (ERbB2)

Uses: Advanced metastatic breast cancer patients with tumor that overexpresses HER2 protein and who has received previous chemotherapy

DOSAGE AND ROUTES

• *Adult:* **PO** 1250 mg (5 tabs)/day 1 hr before or after food on days 1-21 plus capecitabine 2000 mg/m^2/day in 2 divided doses on days 1-14 in a repeating 21-day cycle; continue until therapeutic response or toxicity occurs

Hepatic dose

• *Adult:* **PO** (Child-Pugh C) 750 mg/day

Available forms: Tabs 250 mg

SIDE EFFECTS

CNS: Fatigue, insomnia, palmar-plantar erythrodysesthesia (hand/foot syndrome)

CV: **Heart failure,** palpitations, **QT prolongation**

GI: Anorexia, diarrhea, dyspepsia, mouth ulcerations, nausea, vomiting, xerosis

HEMA: **Anemia, neutropenia, thrombocytopenia**

INTEG: Rash

RESP: Dyspnea, pneumonitis

Contraindications: Pregnancy (D), breastfeeding, hypersensitivity, torsade de pointes

Precautions: Geriatric patients, cardiac disease, bradycardia, hypertension, hypokalemia, hypomagnesemia, QT prolongation

Black Box Warning: Hepatic disease

L

PHARMACOKINETICS

Bioavailability incomplete; peak 4 hr; >99% protein bound; extensively metabolized by the liver by P450 enzymes CYP3A4, CYP3A5; elimination half-life 24 hr; steady state 6-7 days; increased half-life in hepatic disease

INTERACTIONS

Increase: effect of lapatinib—CYP3A4 inhibitors (amiodarone, amprenavir, aprepitant, atazanavir, chloramphenicol, clarithromycin, conivaptan, dalfopristin, danazol, darunavir, delavirdine, diltiazem, efavirenz, erythromycin, estradiol, fluconazole, fluvoxamine, imatinib, indinavir, isoniazid, itraconazole, ketoconazole, miconazole, mifepristone, nefazodone, nelfinavir, propoxyphene, quinupristin, ritonavir, RU-486, saquinavir, telithromycin, troleandomycin, verapamil, voriconazole, zafirlukast); avoid concurrent use

Increase: QT prolongation—CYP3A4 inhibitors (amiodarone, clarithromycin, erythromycin, telithromycin, troleandomycin); class IA/III antidysrhythmics, arsenic trioxide, bepridil, chlorpromazine, chloroquine, grepafloxacin, halofantrine, haloperidol, levomethadyl, mesoridazine, pentamine, probucol, sparfloxacin, thioridazine

Increase: effect of these products, QT prolongation: CYP3A4 substrates (methadone, pimozide, quetiapine, quinidine, risperidone, terfenadine, ziprasidone)

NURSING CONSIDERATIONS

Assess:

• Cardiac status: EEG for QT prolongation, ejection fraction; chest pain, palpitations, dyspnea

• Hepatic status: Liver function tests; jaundice of sclera, skin; dose should be reduced in hepatic disease

• For skin toxicities NCI CTC grade 2 or greater; discontinue use in those with decreased left ventricular ejection fraction (LVEF) or for a LVEF that drops below the institution's lower limit of normal; the product may be restarted after 2 wk if the LVEF recovers to normal at 1000 mg/day; restart at 1250 mg/day when toxicity improves to grade 1 or better

Administer:

• Once a day, with water, on an empty stomach, 1 hr before or after food

• Do not use with grapefruit products

Perform/provide:

• Storage at room temperature, away from heat

Evaluate:

• Therapeutic response: decrease in breast cancer progression

Teach patient/family:

• To take with a full glass of water, once a day, 1 hr before or after food; do not take with food or grapefruit products

• To take as directed only; if a dose is missed, take as soon as remembered; if it is close to the next dose, take only that dose; do not double

• To report to prescriber: chest pain, difficulty breathing, fever, chills, sore throat, bleeding, bruising, yellow skin or eyes, severe fatigue, dizziness, palpitations

• The other side effects that may occur, but do not need to be reported: nausea, diarrhea, heartburn, mouth sores, rash, numbness/pain in hands/feet

• To use adequate contraception, as the fetus could be damaged from this product

latanoprost ophthalmic

See Appendix B

leflunomide (℞)

(leh-floo′noh-mide)

Arava

Func. class.: Antirheumatic (DMARDs)

Chem. class.: Immune modulator, pyrimidine synthesis inhibitor

Action: Inhibits an enzyme involved in pyrimidine synthesis and has antiproliferative, antiinflammatory effect

Uses: RA, to reduce disease process and symptoms

Unlabeled uses: Juvenile RA

DOSAGE AND ROUTES

Rheumatoid arthritis

• *Adult:* **PO** Loading dose 100 mg/day × 3 days, maintenance 20 mg/day, may be decreased to 10 mg/day if not well tolerated

Juvenile rheumatoid arthritis (unlabeled)

• *Adolescent and child >40 kg:* **PO** 20 mg

• *Adolescent and child 20-40 kg:* **PO** 15 mg

• *Adolescent and child 10-19.9 kg:* **PO** 10 mg

Available forms: Tabs 10, 20, 100 mg

SIDE EFFECTS

CNS: Headache, dizziness, insomnia, depression, paresthesia, anxiety, migraine, neuralgia

CV: Palpitations, hypertension, chest pain, angina pectoris, peripheral edema

EENT: Pharyngitis, oral candidiasis, stomatitis, dry mouth, blurred vision

GI: Nausea, anorexia, vomiting, constipation, flatulence, diarrhea, elevated LFTs, **hepatotoxicity**

HEMA: Anemia, ecchymosis, hyperlipidemia

INTEG: Rash, pruritus, alopecia, acne, hematoma, herpes infections

RESP: Pharyngitis, rhinitis, bronchitis, cough, respiratory infection, pneumonia, sinusitis

SYST: **Opportunistic/fatal infections**

Contraindications: Breastfeeding, hypersensitivity, jaundice, lactase deficiency, hepatic disease

Black Box Warning: Pregnancy (X)

Precautions: Children, renal disorders, vaccinations, infection, alcoholism, immunosuppression

PHARMACOKINETICS

Metabolized in liver to active metabolite, excreted in urine

INTERACTIONS

Increase: NSAIDs effect—NSAIDs

Increase: leflunomide side effects—hepatotoxic agents, methotrexate

Increase: rifampin levels—rifampin

Decrease: antibody response—live virus vaccines

Decrease: leflunomide effect—activated charcoal, cholestyramine

NURSING CONSIDERATIONS

Assess:

- Screen for latent TB before starting treatment
- Arthritic symptoms: ROM, mobility, swelling of joints baseline and during treatment
- Hepatic studies: if ALT elevations are > twofold ULN, reduce dose to 10 mg/day
- CBC with differential, pregnancy test, serum electrolytes

⚠ For infections; fatal infections can occur

- B/P, weight; edema can occur

Administer:

- With food for GI upset
- To eliminate product: give cholestyramine 8 g tid × 11 days, check levels

Evaluate:

- Therapeutic response: decreased inflammation, pain in joints

Teach patient/family:

- That product must be continued for prescribed time to be effective
- To take with food, milk, or antacids to avoid GI upset
- To use caution when driving; drowsiness, dizziness may occur
- To take with a full glass of water to enhance absorption
- To avoid pregnancy while taking this product; not to breastfeed while taking this product; men should also discontinue product and begin leflunomide removal protocol if a pregnancy is planned
- That hair may be lost, review alternatives
- To avoid vaccinations during treatment (live virus)
- To notify prescriber of weight loss

lenalidomide (℞)

(len-a-lid'o-mide)

Revlimid

Func. class.: Antianemic, biologic response modifier, hormone

Chem. class.: Thalidomide derivative/TNF modifier

Action: Decreases secretion of inflammatory cytokines and increases secretion of antiinflammatory cytokines, also COX-2 inhibition

Uses: Transfusion-dependent anemia due to low- or intermediate-1-risk myelodysplastic syndrome (MDS); multiple myeloma in combination with dexamethasone

DOSAGE AND ROUTES

Transfusion dependent anemia

- *Adult:* **PO** 10 mg/day

Multiple myeloma

• *Adult:* **PO** 25 mg/day on days 1-21 with dexamethasone 40 mg/day on days 1-4, 9-12, 17-20 of each 28-day cycle for first 4 therapy cycles; starting with cycle 5 leave lenalidomide the same, give dexamethasone 40 mg/day on days 1-4 of a 28-day cycle

Treatment of patients with transfusion-dependent anemia due to low- or intermediate-1-risk myelodysplastic syndrome (MDS) associated with a deletion 5q cytogenetic abnormality with or without additional cytogenetic abnormalities

• *Adult:* **PO** 10 mg/day; continue/adjust based on clinical toxicity/laboratory findings

Treatment of multiple myeloma in combination with dexamethasone in patients who have failed to respond to at least one prior therapy

• *Adult:* **PO** 25 mg/day on days 1-21, along with dexamethasone 40 mg/day **PO** on days 1-4, 9-12, and 17-20 of each 28-day cycle for the first 4 therapy cycles; starting with cycle 5, the lenalidomide dose stays the same, but give only dexamethasone 40 mg/day **PO** on days 1-4 q28days; continue/adjust dosing based on clinical and laboratory findings

Dosage adjustments of lenalidomide for hematologic toxicities associated with myelodysplastic syndrome (MDS)

• *Thrombocytopenia or neutropenia that develops within 4 wk of starting at 10 mg/day PO:* Reduce dose from 10 mg/day **PO** to 5 mg/day **PO**; withhold lenalidomide if platelet count <50,000/mm^3 from a baseline of at least 100,000/mm^3, if platelet count falls to 50% of the baseline value if the baseline is <100,000/mm^3, if absolute neutrophil count (ANC) <750/mm^3 from a baseline of at least 1000/mm^3, or if <500/mm^3 from a baseline of <1000/mm^3; the new dose of 5 mg/day **PO** may begin once the platelet count is at least 50,000/mm^3 (30,000/mm^3 if the baseline <60,000/mm^3), and the ANC returns to at least 1000/mm^3 or 500/mm^3 for patients with a baseline <1000/mm^3

• *Thrombocytopenia or neutropenia that develops after 4 wk of starting at 10 mg/day PO:* Reduce dose from 10 mg/day **PO** to 5 mg/day **PO**; withhold lenalidomide if platelet count <30,000/mm^3, if platelet count <50,000/mm^3 and a platelet transfusion, if neutrophils <500/mm^3 for at least 7 days, or if <500/mm^3 and a temperature of at least 38.5° C are present; the new dose of 5 mg/day **PO** may begin once the platelet count is at least 30,000/mm^3 without hemostatic failure and the ANC is at least 500/mm^3

• *Thrombocytopenia or neutropenia that develops while taking 5 mg/day PO:* Reduce dose from 5 mg/day **PO** to 5 mg/day **PO** every other day; withhold lenalidomide if platelet count <30,000/mm^3, platelet count <50,000/mm^3 and a platelet transfusion, neutrophils <500/mm^3 for at least 7 days, or if <500/mm^3 and a temperature of at least 38.5° C are present; the new dose of 5 mg **PO** every other day may begin once the platelet count is at least 30,000/mm^3 without hemostatic failure and the ANC is at least 500/mm^3

Dosage adjustments of lenalidomide for toxicities associated with multiple myeloma

• *Thrombocytopenia:* Reduce dose from 25 mg/day **PO** to 15 mg/day **PO**; withhold lenalidomide if platelet count <30,000/mm^3; check CBC q wk; the new dose of 15 mg/day **PO** may begin once the platelet count is at least 30,000/mm^3; withhold lenalidomide each time the platelet count is <30,000/mm^3; a new dose of 5 mg less than the previous dose should be started once the platelet count is at least 30,000/mm^3; do not dose below 5 mg/day **PO**

• *Neutropenia without other toxicity:* Hold dose; withhold lenalidomide and add G-CSF if neutrophils <1000/mm^3; check CBC weekly; resume lenalidomide at 25 mg/day **PO** once neutrophils are at least 1000/mm^3, and neutropenia is the only toxicity

• *Neutropenia with other toxicity:* Reduce dose from 25 mg/day **PO** to 15 mg/day **PO**; withhold lenalidomide and add G-CSF if neutrophils <1000/mm^3; check CBC q wk; resume lenalidomide at 15 mg/day **PO** once neutrophils are at least 1000/mm^3; withhold lenalidomide and add G-CSF each time the neutrophils are <1000/mm^3; if other toxicity is present, a new dose of 5 mg less than the previous dose should be started once the neutrophils are at least 1000/mm^3; do not dose below 5 mg/day **PO**

• *Other grade 3 or 4 toxicity judged to be related to lenalidomide:* Reduce dose from 25 mg/day **PO** to 15 mg/day **PO**; withhold lenalidomide and resume lenalidomide at 15 mg/day **PO** once the toxicity has resolved to grade 2 or less; withhold lenalidomide each time a grade 3 or 4 toxicity occurs; a new dose of 5 mg less than the previous dose should be started once the toxicity has resolved to grade 2 or less; do not dose below 5 mg/day **PO**

Renal dose

• *Adult:* **PO** CCr 30-59 ml/min 5 mg q24hr (MDS); 10 mg q24hr (multiple myeloma); CCr <30 ml/min (not requiring dialysis) 5 mg q48hr (MDS), 15 mg q48hr (multiple myeloma)

Available forms: Caps 5, 10, 15, 25 mg

SIDE EFFECTS

CNS: Depression, dizziness, fatigue, fever, headache, sweating, peripheral enuropathy

CV: Chest pain, hypotension, palpitations

GI: Abdominal pain, anorexia, constipation, diarrhea, nausea/vomiting, dysgeusia, xerosis

HEMA: **Anemia, leukopenia, neutropenia, pancytopenia, thrombocytopenia**

META: Hypokalemia, hypomagnesemia

MS: Arthralgia, back pain, myalgia

RESP: Cough, dyspnea, **pulmonary embolism,** epistaxis, rhinitis

SYST: **Angioedema**

Contraindications: Breastfeeding, hypersensitivity

Black Box Warning: Pregnancy (X), females

Precautions: Children, geriatric patients, accidental exposure, bone marrow suppression, dental disease, uterine bleeding, fungal/viral infections, smoking

Black Box Warning: Neutropenia/thrombocytopenia, thromboembolic disease

PHARMACOKINETICS

Rapid absorption, elimination half-life 3 hr

INTERACTIONS

Increase: bleeding risk—anticoagulants, salicylates, NSAIDs, thrombolytics, platelet inhibitors

Decrease: immune response—vaccines/toxoids

NURSING CONSIDERATIONS

Assess:

• Blood studies: Hct, Hgb, electrolytes
• B/P for hypotension
• Blood dyscrasias
• For hypersensitivity reactions: skin rashes, urticaria (rare)

Administer:

• PO, with dexamethasone for multiple myeloma
• Do not crush or open caps
• All persons involved must comply with the conditions of rev assist program

Evaluate:

• Therapeutic response: increase in reticulocyte count

Teach patient/family:

• To avoid driving or hazardous activity during beginning of treatment

⚠ High Alert

lepirudin (℞)

(lep-ih-roo′din)

Refludan

Func. class.: Anticoagulant

Chem. class.: Thrombin inhibitor, hirudin

Action: Direct inhibitor of thrombin that is highly specific

Uses: Anticoagulation in those with heparin-induced thrombocytopenia (HIT) and other thromboembolic conditions

Unlabeled uses: Adjunct therapy in unstable angina, acute MI without ST elevation, prevention of DVT, PCI

DOSAGE AND ROUTES

Heparin-induced thrombocytopenia (not receiving thrombolytic therapy concurrently)

• *Adult:* **IV** 0.4 mg/kg over 15-20 sec; then 0.15 mg/kg/hr as a **CONT INF** for 2-10 days or longer

Concomitant use with thrombolytic therapy

• *Adult:* **IV BOL** 0.2 mg/kg initially, then **CONT IV INF** 0.1 mg/kg/hr

Renal dose

• *Adult:* **IV BOL** 0.2 mg/kg over 15-20 sec, then if CCr 45-60 ml/min 0.075 mg/kg/hr; CCr 30-44 ml/min 0.045 mg/kg/hr; CCr 15-29 ml/min 0.0225 mg/kg/hr

Available forms: Powder for inj 50 mg

SIDE EFFECTS

CNS: Fever, **intracranial bleeding**

CV: **Heart failure, pericardial effusion, ventricular fibrillation**

GI: GI bleeding, abnormal LFTs

GU: **Hematuria,** abnormal kidney function, vaginal bleeding

HEMA: **Hemorrhage, thrombocytopenia, anemia**

INTEG: Allergic skin reactions

RESP: Pneumonia, stridor, dyspnea, **bronchospasm**

SYST: **Multiorgan failure, sepsis, anaphylaxis**

Contraindications: Hypersensitivity to hirudins

Precautions: Pregnancy (B), breastfeeding, children, geriatric patients, women, intracranial bleeding, hepatic disease, recent major surgery, hemorrhagic diathesis bacterial endocarditis, severe uncontrolled hypertension, advanced renal disease, recent active peptic ulcer, recent CVA, stroke, intracerebral surgery

PHARMACOKINETICS

May be metabolized by the release of amino acids during catabolism, 50% unchanged in urine, terminal half-life 1.3 hr

INTERACTIONS

Increase: bleeding risk—warfarin derivatives, thrombolytics, NSAIDs, plicamycin, cefamandole, cefotetan, cefoperazone, aspirin, clopidogrel, dipyridamole, eptifibatide, ticlopidine, tirofiban, valproic acid

Drug/Herb

Increase: bleeding risk—agrimony, alfalfa, angelica, anise, basil, bay, bilberry, black haw, bogbean, bromelain, buchu, chondroitin, cinchona bark, dong quai, fenugreek, feverfew, garlic, ginger, ginkgo, ginseng, horse chestnut, Irish moss, kelp, kelpware, khella, lovage, lungwort, meadowsweet, motherwort, mugwort, nettle, papaya, parsley (large amts), pau d'arco, pineapple, poplar, prickly ash, safflower, saw palmetto, tonka bean, turmeric, wintergreen, yarrow

Decrease: anticoagulant effect—chamomile, coenzyme Q10, flax, glucomannan, goldenseal, guar gum

NURSING CONSIDERATIONS

Assess:

• Obtain baseline in aPTT before treatment; do not start treatment if aPTT ratio ≥2.5, then aPTT 4 hr after initiation of treatment and at least daily thereafter; if aPTT above target, stop inf for 2 hr, then restart at 50%, take aPTT in 4 hr; if below target, increase inf rate by 20%, take aPTT in 4 hr, do not exceed inf rate of 0.21 mg/kg/hr without checking for coagulation abnormalities

• aPTT, which should be 1.5-2.5 × control

⚠ Bleeding gums, petechiae, ecchymosis, black tarry stools, hematuria/epistaxis, B/P, vaginal bleeding and possible hemorrhage

• Hct, Hgb, platelets, serum creatinine, urinalysis, stool guaiac

• Fever, skin rash, urticaria

Administer:

• Avoiding all IM inj

• After reconstitution and further dilution under sterile conditions; use water for inj or 0.9% NaCl; for further dilution 0.9% NaCl or D_5; for rapid and complete reconstitution, inject 1 ml of diluent into vial and shake gently; use immediately; warm to room temperature before use

IV, direct route

• Reconstitute each vial with 1 ml sterile water or 0.9% NaCl; shake gently; transfer content of vial into 10-ml syringe and dilute to a volume of 10 ml with sterile water for inj, D_5W, or 0.9% NaCl, final conc 5 mg/ml

CONT IV route

• Reconstitute 2 vials with 1 ml each of sterile water for inj, or 0.9% NaCl; transfer contents into inf bag containing 250 or 500 ml 0.9% NaCl or D_5W for a conc 0.2 mg/ml or 0.4 mg/ml respectively; infuse at 0.15 mg/kg/hr; use inf pump

Evaluate:

• Therapeutic response: anticoagulation

Teach patient/family:

• To use soft-bristle toothbrush to avoid bleeding gums, avoid contact sports, use electric razor, avoid IM inj

• To report any signs of bleeding: gums, under skin, urine, stools

letrozole (℞)

(let′tro-zohl)

Femara

Func. class.: Antineoplastic, nonsteroidal aromatase inhibitor

Action: Binds to the heme group of aromatase; inhibits conversion of androgens to estrogens to reduce plasma estrogen levels

Uses: Early, advanced, or metastatic breast cancer in postmenopausal women

Unlabeled uses: Infertility, idiopathic short stature, constitutional delayed puberty

DOSAGE AND ROUTES

• *Adult:* **PO** 2.5 mg/day

Infertility (unlabeled)

• *Adult:* **PO** 2.5, 5, 7.5 mg/day × 5 days, usually days 3-7 of menstrual cycle

Idiopathic short stature, constitutional delayed puberty (unlabeled)

• *Adolescent and child ≥9 (male):* **PO** 2.5 mg/day; use with testosterone in delayed puberty

Available forms: Tabs 2.5 mg

SIDE EFFECTS

CNS: Headache, lethargy, somnolence, dizziness, depression, anxiety

CV: **Angina, MI, CVA, thromboembolic events,** hypertension, peripheral edema

GI: Nausea, vomiting, anorexia, constipation, heartburn, diarrhea

GU: **Endometrial cancer, vaginal bleeding, endometrial proliferation disorders**

INTEG: Rash, pruritus, alopecia, sweating

MISC: Hot flashes, night sweats, **second malignancies, anaphylaxis, angioedema**

MS: Arthralgia, arthritis, bone fracture, myalgia, osteoporosis

RESP: Dyspnea, cough

Contraindications: Pregnancy (D), premenopausal females, hypersensitivity

Precautions: Respiratory/hepatic disease, osteoporosis

PHARMACOKINETICS

Metabolized in liver, excreted in urine, peak 2-6 wk, terminal half-life 48 hr

INTERACTIONS

Decrease: letrozole effect—estrogens, oral contraceptives

NURSING CONSIDERATIONS

Assess:

- Hepatic studies before, during therapy (bilirubin, AST, ALT, LDH) as needed or monthly

Administer:

- Without regard to meals; use a small glass of water
- May administer biphosphates to increase bone density

Perform/provide:

- Liquid diet, including cola, Jell-O; dry toast or crackers as ordered may be added if patient is not nauseated or vomiting
- Nutritious diet with iron and vitamin supplements as ordered

Evaluate:

- Therapeutic response: decrease in size of tumor

Teach patient/family:

- To report allergic reactions (rash; hives; difficulty breathing; tightness in chest; swelling on mouth, face, lips, tongue)
- To report vaginal bleeding, diarrhea, chest/bone pain
- To use adequate contraception in perimenopausal, recently postmenopausal women

leucovorin (℞)

(loo-koe-vor′in)
citrovorum factor, folinic acid, leucovorin calcium
Func. class.: Vitamin, folic acid/methotrexate antagonist antidote
Chem. class.: Tetrahydrofolic acid derivative

Do not confuse:
leucovorin/Leukeran/leukine
folinic acid/folic acid

Action: Needed for normal growth patterns; prevents toxicity during antineoplastic therapy by protecting normal cells

Uses: Megaloblastic or macrocytic anemia caused by folic acid deficiency, overdose of folic acid antagonist, methotrexate/pyrimethamine/trimetrexate/trimethoprim toxicity, pneumocystosis, toxoplasmosis

DOSAGE AND ROUTES

Megaloblastic anemia caused by enzyme deficiency

- *Adult and child:* **PO/IV/IM** up to 6 mg/day

Megaloblastic anemia caused by deficiency of folate

- *Adult and child:* **IM** 1 mg or less/day until adequate response

Methotrexate toxicity-leucovorin rescue

- *Adult and child:* **PO/IM/IV** Normal elimination given 6 hr after dose of methotrexate (10 mg/m^2) until methotrexate is $<5 \times 10^{-8}$ m, CCr is >50% above prior level, or methotrexate level is 5×10^{-8} m at 24 hr, or at 48-hr level is $>9 \times 10^{-8}$ m; give leucovorin 100 mg/m^2 q3hr until level drops to $<10^{-8}$ m

Pyrimethamine/trimethoprim toxicity

- *Adult and child:* **PO/IM** 5-15 mg/day

Advanced colorectal cancer

- *Adult:* **IV** 200 mg/m^2, then 5-FU 370 mg/m^2; or leucovorin 20 mg/m^2, then 5-FU 425 mg/m^2; give daily × 5 days q4-5wk

Available forms: Tabs 5, 10, 15, 25 mg; inj 3, 5 mg/ml; powder for inj 10 mg/ml

SIDE EFFECTS

HEMA: Thrombocytosis (intraarterial)
INTEG: Rash, pruritus, erythema, urticaria
RESP: Wheezing

Contraindications: Hypersensitivity to this product or folic acid, benzyl alcohol, anemias other than megaloblastic not associated with vit B_{12} deficiency

Precautions: Pregnancy (C), neonates, breastfeeding, geriatric patients, seizures, stomatitis, vomiting

INTERACTIONS

Increase: metabolism of phenobarbital, hydantoins

Increase: toxicity—fluorouracil

Decrease: folate levels—chloramphenicol

NURSING CONSIDERATIONS

Assess:

- CCr, creatinine before leucovorin rescue and daily to detect nephrotoxicity; methotrexate level
- I&O; urine pH q6hr, maintain >7 to prevent neurotoxicity; watch for nausea and vomiting
- Other products taken: alcohol, hydantoins, trimethoprim may cause increased folic acid use by body
- Neurologic status (rescue): weakness, fatigue
- Monitor calcium levels
- Megaloblastic anemia, plasma lactic acid, leticulocyte count, Hct, Hgb

Administer:

- Within 1 hr of folic acid antagonist
- Do not give concurrently with systemic methotrexate

IM route

- No reconstitution needed
- Treatment of megaloblastic anemia uses IM dosing

IV route

- For IV reconstitute 50 mg/5 ml bacteriostatic or sterile H_2O for inj (10 mg/ml) or (100 mg/10 ml); use immediately if sterile H_2O is used
- Give by direct IV over 160 mg/min or less (16 ml of 10 mg/ml sol/min)
- Give by intermittent inf after diluting in 100-500 ml of 0.9% NaCl, D_5W, $D_{10}W$, LR, Ringer's sol

Additive compatibilities: Cisplatin, cisplatin/floxuridine, floxuridine

Syringe compatibilities: Bleomycin, cisplatin, cyclophosphamide, DOXOrubicin, fluorouracil, furosemide, heparin, methotrexate, metoclopramide, mitomycin, vinBLAStine, vinCRIStine

Y-site compatibilities: Amifostine, aztreonam, bleomycin, cefepime, cisplatin, cladribine, cyclophosphamide, DOXOrubicin, DOXOrubicin liposome, filgrastim, fluconazole, fluorouracil, furosemide, granisetron, heparin, methotrexate, metoclopramide, mitomycin, piperacillin/tazobactam, tacrolimus, teniposide, thiotepa, vinBLAStine, vinCRIStine

Perform/provide:

- Increase fluid intake if used to treat folic acid inhibitor overdose
- Protection from light and heat

Evaluate:

- Therapeutic response: increased weight; improved orientation, well-being; absence of fatigue; reversal of toxicity (methotrexate, folic acid antagonist overdose)

Teach patient/family:

- For leucovorin rescue have patient drink 3 L fluid daily of rescue
- For folic acid deficiency eat folic acid rich foods: bran; yeast; dried beans; nuts; fresh, green leafy vegetables
- To take product exactly as prescribed
- To notify prescriber of side effects
- To report signs of hyposensitivity reaction immediately
- To avoid breastfeeding

⚠ High Alert

leuprolide (℞)

(loo-proe′lide)

Eligard, Lupron Depo Ped, Lupron, Lupron Depot, Lupron Depot-3 month, Lupron Depot-4 month, Viadur

Func. class.: Antineoplastic hormone

Chem. class.: Gonadotropin-releasing hormone

Do not confuse:

Lupron/Nuprin/Lopurin

Action: Causes initial increase in circulating levels of LH, FSH; continuous administration results in decreased LH, FSH; in men, testosterone is reduced to castrate levels; in premenopausal women, estrogen is reduced to menopausal levels

Uses: Metastatic prostate cancer (inj implant), management of endometriosis, central precocious puberty, uterine leiomyomata (fibroids)

Unlabeled uses: Breast cancer, recurrent priapism

DOSAGE AND ROUTES

Prostate cancer

- *Adult:* **SUBCUT** 1 mg/day; **IM** 7.5 mg/dose q mo; Viadur implant (72 mg) q yr; or **IM** 22.5 mg q3mo; or **IM** 30 mg q4mo

Endometriosis/fibroids

- *Adult:* **IM** 3.75 mg q mo for 6 mo or 11.25 q3mo for 6 mo or 30 mg q4mo

Central precocious puberty

- *Child:* **SUBCUT** 50 mcg/kg/day; may increase by 10 mcg/kg/day as needed
- *Child >37.5 kg:* **IM** 15 mg q4wk
- *Child 25-37.5 kg:* **IM** 11.25 mg q4wk
- *Child ≤25 kg:* 7.5 mg q4wk

Available forms: Inj 5 mg/ml; powder for inj, lyophilized 7.5 mg; microspheres for inj, lyophilized 3.75, 7.5, 11.25, 15, 22.5, 30 mg; implant 72 mg; depot 7.5, 22.5, 30, 45 mg; depot 3.75, 11.25 mg; intradermal kit 65 mg

SIDE EFFECTS

CNS: Memory impairment, depression, **seizures**

CV: **MI, PE, dysrhythmias**, peripheral edema

GI: Nausea, vomiting, anorexia, diarrhea, **GI bleeding**

GU: Edema, hot flashes, impotence, decreased libido, amenorrhea, vaginal dryness, gynecomastia, **profuse vaginal bleeding**

INTEG: Alopecia

MS: Bone pain

Contraindications: Pregnancy (X), breastfeeding, hypersensitivity to GnRH or analogs, thromboembolic disorders, undiagnosed vaginal bleeding, Viadur implant or Eligard should not be used in women or children

Precautions: Edema, hepatic disease, CVA, MI, seizures, hypertension, diabetes mellitus, CHF, depression, osteoporosis, spinal cord compression, urinary tract obstruction

PHARMACOKINETICS

SUBCUT: Onset 1-2 wk; peak 2-4 wk; absorbed rapidly (SUBCUT), slowly (IM depot); half-life 3 hr

INTERACTIONS

Increase: antineoplastic action—flutamide, megestrol

NURSING CONSIDERATIONS

Assess:

- For symptoms of endometriosis (lower abdominal pain)/fibroids (pelvic pain, excessive vaginal bleeding, bloating) before, during, and after treatment
- For central precocious puberty (CPP) if treatment is for this condition; secondary S_4 characteristics to children <9 yr, estradiol/testosterone levels, GnRH test, tomography of head, adrenal steroids, chorionic gonadotropin, wrist x-ray, height, weight
- Hepatic studies before, during therapy (bilirubin, AST, ALT, LDH) monthly or as

needed; PSA, calcium, testosterone in prostate cancer; bone mineral density
- Pituitary gonadotropic and gonadal function during therapy and 4-8 wk after therapy is decreased
- Worsening of signs and symptoms; normal during beginning therapy
- Fatigue, increased pulse, pallor, lethargy; edema in feet, joints; stomach pain

⚠ Symptoms indicating severe allergic reaction: rash, pruritus, urticaria, purpuric skin lesions, itching, flushing

Administer:
- IM/SUBCUT using syringe and product packaged together; give deep in large muscle mass; rotate sites
- Use depot IM only
- Monthly: reconstitute single-use vial with 1 ml of diluent; if multiple vials used, withdraw 0.5 ml and inject into each vial (1 ml); withdraw all and inject
- 3-month: reconstitute microspheres using 1.5 ml of diluent and inject in vial; shake, withdraw, and inject
- 12-month: insert into upper arm; at the end of 12 months, implant must be removed

Perform/provide:
- Nutritious diet with iron, vitamin supplements as ordered
- Storage in tight container at room temperature

Evaluate:
- Therapeutic response: decreased tumor size and spread of malignancy; decrease in lesions, pain in endometriosis, fibroids, correction of CPP; increased follicle maturation

Teach patient/family:
- To notify prescriber if menstruation continues; menstruation should stop
- To use a nonhormonal method of contraception during therapy
- That bone pain will disappear after 1 wk
- To report any complaints, side effects to nurse or prescriber; hot flashes may occur; record weight, report gain of >2 lb/day
- How to prepare, give; to rotate sites for SUBCUT inj
- To keep accurate records of dose
- That tumor flare may occur: increase in size of tumor, increased bone pain, will subside rapidly; may take analgesics for pain; premenopausal women must use mechanical birth control; ovulation may be induced
- Do not breastfeed while taking this product
- Voiding problems may increase in beginning of therapy, but will decrease in several weeks

levalbuterol (℞)
(lev-al-byoo'ter-ole)
Xopenex, Xopenex HFA
Func. class.: Bronchodilator, adrenergic β_2-agonist

Action: Causes bronchodilation by action on β_2 (pulmonary) receptors by increasing levels of cAMP, which relaxes smooth muscle; produces bronchodilation, CNS, cardiac stimulation, as well as increased diuresis and gastric acid secretion

Uses: Treatment or prevention of bronchospasm (reversible obstructive airway disease)

DOSAGE AND ROUTES
- *Adult and child ≥12 yr:* **INH** 0.63 mg tid, q6-8hr by nebulization, may increase 1.25 mg q8hr
- *Adult/adolescent/child >4 yr:* (HFA, metered dose) 90 mcg (2 **INH**) q4-6hr
- *Child 6-11 yr:* **INH** 0.31 mg tid by nebulization, max 0.63 mg tid

Available forms: Sol, inh 0.63 mg, 1.25 mg/3 ml; 45 mcg per actuation (HFA)

SIDE EFFECTS
CNS: Tremors, anxiety, insomnia, headache, dizziness, stimulation, *restlessness,* hallucinations, flushing, irritability
CV: Palpitations, tachycardia, hypertension, angina, hypotension, dysrhythmias, **QT prolongation**

L

EENT: Dry nose, irritation of nose and throat
GI: Heartburn, nausea, vomiting
INTEG: Rash
META: Hypokalemia, hyperglycemia
MS: Muscle cramps
RESP: Cough
SYST: **Anaphylaxis, angioedema**
Contraindications: Hypersensitivity to sympathomimetics, this product or albuterol, tachydysrhythmias, severe cardiac disease
Precautions: Pregnancy (C), breastfeeding, cardiac disorders, hyperthyroidism, diabetes mellitus, hypertension, prostatic hypertrophy, angle-closure glaucoma, seizures, renal disease, QT prolongation

PHARMACOKINETICS

Metabolized in the liver and tissues; crosses placenta, breast milk, blood-brain barrier; half-life 3.3-4 hr
INH: Onset 5-15 min, peak 1-1½ hr, duration 6-8 hr

INTERACTIONS

Increase: action of aerosol bronchodilators
Increase: levalbuterol action—tricyclics, MAOIs, other adrenergics
Decrease: levalbuterol action—other β-blockers
Drug/Herb
Increase: stimulation—black/green tea, coffee, cola nut, guarana, yerba maté

NURSING CONSIDERATIONS

Assess:
- Respiratory function: vital capacity, forced expiratory volume, ABGs, lung sounds, heart rate and rhythm (baseline); character of sputum: color, consistency, amount
- Cardiac status: palpitations, increase/decrease in B/P, dysrhythmias, QT prolongation

⚠ For evidence of allergic reactions, paradoxical bronchospasm, anaphylaxis, angioedema
- Potassium, blood glucose

Administer:
- By nebulization q6-8hr; wait at least 1 min between inhalation of aerosols

Evaluate:
- Therapeutic response: absence of dyspnea, wheezing after 1 hr, improved airway exchange, improved ABGs

Teach patient/family:
- Not to use OTC medications; excess stimulation may occur
- To avoid getting aerosol in eyes; blurring may result
- To avoid smoking, smoke-filled rooms, persons with respiratory infections

⚠ That paradoxic bronchospasm may occur and to stop product immediately, contact prescriber
- To limit caffeine products such as chocolate, coffee, tea, and colas or herbs such as cola nut, guarana, yerba maté

Treatment of overdose: Administer a β_1-adrenergic blocker

levetiracetam (℞)

(lev-eh-teer-ass′eh-tam)
Keppra, Keppra XR
Func. class.: Anticonvulsant

Do not confuse:
Keppra/Kaletra
Action: Unknown, may inhibit nerve impulses by limiting influx of sodium ions across cell membrane in motor cortex
Uses: Adjunctive therapy in partial-onset seizures, primary generalized tonic-clonic seizures
Unlabeled use: Pediatrics

DOSAGE AND ROUTES

Adjunctive treatment of partial seizures
- *Adult and adolescent ≥16 yr:* **IV** 500 mg bid, may be titrated by 1000 mg/day q2wk, max 3000 mg/day in divided doses; **EXT REL** 1000 mg/day, may increase q2wk, max 3000 mg/day
- *Infant/child/adolescent <16 yr (unlabeled):* **IV** 50.4 mg/kg/day for 4-5 days

Myoclonic seizures/tonic-clonic seizures/partial seizures

- *Adult and adolescent ≥16 yr:* **PO/IV** 500 mg bid, may increase by 1000 mg/day q2wk, max 3000 mg/day

Renal dose

- *Adult:* **PO** CCr 50-80 ml/min 500-1000 mg q12hr; or **EXT REL** 1000-2000 q24hr, max 2000 mg/day; CCr 30-49 ml/min 250-750 mg q12hr or **EXT REL** 500-1500 mg q24hr, max 1500 mg/day; CCr <30 ml/min 250-500 mg q12hr or **EXT REL** 500-1000 q24hr, max 1000 mg/day

Available forms: Tabs 500, 1000 mg; oral sol 100 mg/ml; sol for inj 100 mg/ml; ext rel tab 500 mg

SIDE EFFECTS

CNS: Dizziness, somnolence, asthenia, psychosis, **suicidal ideation**
HEMA: Lowered Hct, Hgb, RBC, infection
MISC: Infection, abdominal pain, pharyngitis

Contraindications: Hypersensitivity, breastfeeding

Precautions: Pregnancy (C), children, geriatric patients, renal/cardiac disease, psychosis

PHARMACOKINETICS

Rapidly absorbed; not protein bound; excreted via kidneys 66% unchanged; half-life 6-8 hr, longer in geriatric/renal disease

INTERACTIONS

- Avoid use with alcohol
- Possible increased carbamazepine toxicity: carbamazepine

Decrease: levetiracetam absorption—sevelamer; separate by 1 hr before, 3 hr after sevelamer

NURSING CONSIDERATIONS

Assess:

- Seizure activity: type, location, duration, and character; provide seizure precautions
- Renal studies: urinalysis, BUN, urine creatinine q3mo
- Blood studies: RBC, Hct, Hgb
- Description of seizures

⚠ Mental status: mood, sensorium, affect, behavioral changes, suicidal thoughts/behaviors; if mental status changes, notify prescriber

Administer:

PO route

- Swallow tab whole; do not break, crush, or chew
- With food, milk to decrease GI symptoms (rare)

IV route

- Single-use vials: dilute in 100 ml of 0.9% NaCl, D_5, LR; give over 15 min

Perform/provide:

- Storage at room temperature (PO)
- Diluted preparation stable for 24 hr at room temperature in polyvinyl bags
- Assistance with ambulation during early part of treatment; dizziness occurs

Evaluate:

- Therapeutic response: decreased seizure activity, document on patient's chart

Teach patient/family:

- To carry emergency ID stating patient's name, products taken, condition, prescriber's name, phone number
- Use oral sol; if swallowing is a problem, measure oral sol in medicine cup or dropper, do not use teaspoon
- To notify prescriber if pregnant or intend to become pregnant
- To avoid driving, other activities that require alertness
- Not to discontinue medication quickly after long-term use, withdrawal seizure may occur
- Not to breastfeed

levobetaxolol ophthalmic

See Appendix B

levobunolol ophthalmic

See Appendix B

L

levocabastine ophthalmic

See Appendix B

levocetirizine (℞)

(lee-voh-she-teer'ah-zeen)

Xyzal

Func. class.: Antihistamine, low sedating

Chem. class.: H_1 histamine blocker, low-sedating

Action: Acts on blood vessels, GI, respiratory system by competing with histamine for H_1-receptor site; decreases allergic response by blocking pharmacologic effects of histamine; minimal anticholinergic action

Uses: Perennial or seasonal rhinitis, allergy symptoms, chronic idiopathic urticaria

DOSAGE AND ROUTES

- *Adult and child ≥12 yr:* **PO** 2.5-5 mg/day in the evening
- *Child 6-11 yr:* **PO** (oral solution) 2.5 mg/day in the evening
- *Child 2-5 yr:* **PO** (oral solution) 1.25 mg/day in the evening
- *Geriatric:* **PO** 2.5-5 mg/day in the evening

Renal dose

- *Adult:* **PO** CCr 50-80 ml/min 2.5 mg/day; CCr 30-50 ml/min 2.5 mg every other day; CCr 10-30 ml/min 2.5 mg 2×/wk; CCr <10 ml/min, do not use

Available forms: Tabs 5 mg; oral sol 2.5 mg/15 ml

SIDE EFFECTS

CNS: Drowsiness, fatigue, asthenia

GI: Dry mouth, increase LFTs

INTEG: Rash, transient

Contraindications: Breastfeeding; children 6-11 yr with renal disease; end-stage renal disease; dialysis; hypersensitivity to this product, cetirizine, hydroxyzine

Precautions: Pregnancy (B)

PHARMACOKINETICS

Absorption rapid; peak 0.9 hr; protein binding 91%-92%; half-life 8 hr; excreted in urine 85.4%, feces 12.9%

INTERACTIONS

Increase: half-life

Increase: CNS depression—alcohol, other CNS depressants

Increase: anticholinergic/sedative effect—MAOIs, phenothiazines, tricyclics

Decrease: clearance of levocetirizine—ritonavir

Drug/Herb

Increase: effect—hops, Jamaican dogwood, kava, senega, valerian

Increase: anticholinergic effect—corkwood

Drug/Lab Test

False negative: Skin allergy tests

NURSING CONSIDERATIONS

Assess:

- Allergy symptoms: pruritus, urticaria, watering eyes, baseline and during treatment
- Respiratory status: rate, rhythm, increase in bronchial secretions, wheezing, chest tightness
- Liver function test, serum creatinine, BUN

Administer:

- Without regard to meals in the evening; tabs are scored and may be broken in half

Perform/provide:

- Storage in tight, light-resistant container

Evaluate:

- Therapeutic response: absence of running or congested nose or rashes

Teach patient/family:

- All aspects of product use; to notify prescriber if confusion, sedation, hypotension occur
- To avoid driving, other hazardous activities if drowsiness occurs
- To avoid alcohol, other CNS depressants
- That product is not recommended during breastfeeding

Treatment of overdose: Administer diazepam, vasopressors, IV phenytoin

Rarely Used

levodopa (℞)

(lee'voe-doe-pa)

Dopar, Larodopa, L-Dopa

Func. class.: Antiparkinson agent

Do not confuse:

L-dopa/levodopa/methyldopa

Uses: Parkinson's disease

DOSAGE AND ROUTES

• *Adult:* **PO** 0.5-1 g daily divided bid-qid with meals; may increase by up to 0.75 g q3-7days not to exceed 8 g/day unless closely supervised

Contraindications: Hypersensitivity, closed-angle glaucoma, undiagnosed skin lesions

levofloxacin (℞)

(lee-voh-floks'a-sin)

Levaquin

Func. class.: Antiinfective

Chem. class.: Fluoroquinolone

Action: Interferes with conversion of intermediate DNA fragments into high-molecular-weight DNA in bacteria; DNA gyrase inhibitor; inhibits topoisomerase IV

Uses: Acute sinusitis, acute chronic bronchitis, community-acquired pneumonia, uncomplicated skin infections, complicated UTI, cellulitis, PID, prostatitis, inhalational anthrax (postexposure), acute pyelonephritis caused by *Streptococcus pneumoniae, Haemophilus influenzae, Haemophilis parainfluenzae, Moraxella catarrhalis, Escherichia coli, Serratia marcescens, Klebsiella pneumoniae, Chlamydia pneumoniae, Legionella pneumophilia, Mycoplasma pneumoniae, Enterococcus faecalis, Staphylococcus epidermidis, Staphylococcus pyogenes,* inhalation anthrax in children

Unlabeled uses: Gonococcal infections, disseminated; otitis media, otitis externa, tonsillitis, pharyngitis, sialadenitis

DOSAGE AND ROUTES

Acute bacterial exacerbation of chronic bronchitis

• *Adult:* **PO/IV** 500 mg q24hr × 7 days

Acute bacterial sinusitis

Adult: **PO** 500 mg q24hr × 10-14 days or 750 mg q24hr × 5 days

Acute pyelonephritis

• *Adult:* **PO** 250 mg q24hr × 10 days or 750 mg q24hr × 5 days

Chronic bacterial prostitis

• *Adult:* **PO** 500 mg q24hr × 28 days

Postexposure inhalational anthrax

• *Adult/adolescent/child >50 kg:* **PO/IV** 500 mg q24hr × 60 days

• *Infant >6 mo and child <50 kg:* **IV** 8 mg/kg q12hr, max 250 mg/dose; × 60 days

Pneumonia, community acquired

• *Adult:* **PO/IV** 500 mg q24hr × 7-14 days or 750 mg q24hr × 5 days

Pneumonia, nosocomial

• *Adult:* **PO/IV** 750 mg q24hr × 7-14 days

SSSI, complicated

• *Adult:* **PO/IV** 750 mg q24hr × 7-14 days

SSSI, uncomplicated

• *Adult:* **PO** 500 mg q24hr × 7-10 days

UTI, complicated

• *Adult:* **PO/IV** 250 mg q24hr × 10 days

UTI, uncomplicated

• *Adult:* **PO** 250 mg q24hr × 3 days

Gonococcal infection, disseminated (unlabeled)

• *Adult:* **IV** 250 mg q24hr × 24-48 hr, then **PO** 500 mg/day × 7 days

PID

• *Adult:* **IV** 500 mg q24hr × 14 days

Otitis media (unlabeled)

• *Adult:* **PO** 100-200 mg bid-tid × 3-14 days

• *Child 6 mo-14 yr:* **PO** 10 mg/kg bid × 10 days or more

Renal disease

• *Adult:* **PO/IV** CCr 20-49 ml/min initial 500 mg, then 250 mg, q24hr; CCr 10-19

L

ml/min 250 or 500 mg, depending on condition; then 250 mg q48hr

Available forms: Single-use vials 500, 750 mg; premixed flexible containers 250 mg/50 ml D_5W, 500 mg/100 ml D_5W, 750 mg/150 ml D_5W; tabs 250, 500, 750 mg

SIDE EFFECTS

CNS: *Headache,* dizziness, *insomnia,* anxiety, **seizures,** encephalopathy, paresthesia

CV: Chest pain, palpitations, vasodilation, QT prolongation

EENT: Dry mouth, visual impairment

GI: *Nausea,* flatulence, *vomiting,* diarrhea, abdominal pain, **pseudomembranous colitis, hepatotoxicity**

GU: Vaginitis, crystalluria

HEMA: Eosinophilia, **hemolytic anemia,** lymphopenia

INTEG: Rash, pruritus, *photosensitivity,* **epidermal necrolysis**

MISC: Hypoglycemia, hypersensitivity, tendinitis, **tendon rupture**

RESP: Pneumonitis

SYST: **Anaphylaxis, multisystem organ failure, Stevens-Johnson syndrome**

Contraindications: Hypersensitivity to quinolones, photosensitivity

Precautions: Pregnancy (C), breastfeeding, children

Black Box Warning: Tendon pain/rupture, tendinitis

PHARMACOKINETICS

Metabolized in liver, excreted in urine unchanged, half-life 6-8 hr, peak 1-2 hr

INTERACTIONS

• Do not use with magnesium in the same IV line

Increase: QT prolongation—other QT prolonging agents

Increase: levofloxacin levels—probenecid

Increase: CNS stimulation, seizures—NSAIDs, foscarnet

Increase: bleeding risk—warfarin

Decrease: levofloxacin absorption—antacids containing aluminum, magnesium; sucralfate, zinc, iron, calcium

Decrease: clearance of theophylline, toxicity may result

Drug/Herb

• Do not use acidophilus with antiinfectives; separate by several hours

Increase: antiinfective effect—cola tree

Drug/Lab Test

Decrease: glucose, lymphocytes

NURSING CONSIDERATIONS

Assess:

• For previous sensitivity reaction

• For signs and symptoms of infection: characteristics of sputum, WBC >10,000/mm^3, fever; obtain baseline information before and during treatment

• C&S before beginning product therapy to identify if correct treatment has been initiated

⚠ For allergic reactions and anaphylaxis: rash, urticaria, pruritus, chills, fever, joint pain; may occur a few days after therapy begins; epinephrine and resuscitation equipment should be available for anaphylactic reaction

• Bowel pattern daily; if severe diarrhea occurs, product should be discontinued

⚠ For overgrowth of infection: perineal itching, fever, malaise, redness, pain, swelling, drainage, rash, diarrhea, change in cough, sputum

• For cardiac function, watch for QT prolongation; for tendon pain, renal function

Administer:

• PO 4 hr before or 2 hr after antacids, iron, calcium, zinc

• Not to use theophylline with this product; toxicity may result

IV route

• Only by slow IV inf over 60-90 min

• Discard any unused sol in the single-dose vial

• Using premix, tear outer wrap at notch and remove sol container; check for leaks; close control clamps; remove cover from port at bottom of container; insert pin into port with a twist; suspend container from hanger; squeeze and release drip chamber to proper fluid level; open flow control to expel air, close clamp; regulate rate with flow control clamps

Solution compatibilities: 0.9% NaCl, D_5W, D_5/0.9% NaCl, D_5LR, D_5/0.45% NaCl, sodium lactate, plasma-lyte 56/D_5W

Perform/provide:

• Increase fluid intake to 2 L/day to prevent crystalluria

Evaluate:

• Therapeutic response: absence of signs/symptoms of infection (WBC <10,000/mm^3, temp WNL)

Teach patient/family:

• To contact prescriber if vaginal itching; loose, foul-smelling stools; furry tongue occur (may indicate superinfection); report itching, rash, pruritus, urticaria

• To notify prescriber of diarrhea with blood or pus

• To take 4 hr before or 2 hr after antacids, iron, calcium, zinc products

• To complete full course of therapy

• To avoid hazardous activities until response is known

• To use frequent rinsing of mouth, sugarless candy or gum for dry mouth

• To avoid other medication unless approved by prescriber

• To prevent sun exposure or use sunscreen to prevent phototoxicity

levofloxacin ophthalmic

See Appendix B

levoleucovorin (℞)

(lee-voe-loo-koe-voe′rin)

Fusilev

Func. class.: Chemotherapy protectant

Chem. class.: Tetrahydrofolic acid derivative

Action: Acts as a replacement to rescue cells from the effects of folate antagonists

Uses: For methotrexate toxicity prophylaxis

Unlabeled uses: Colorectal cancer (to potentiate fluorouracil therapy)

DOSAGE AND ROUTES

For levoleucovorin rescue following high-dose methotrexate treatment for osteosarcoma

• *Adult and child >6 yr:* **IV** 7.5 mg (approximately 5 mg/m^2) q6hr × 10 doses starting 24 hr after the beginning of methotrexate inf; do not give >16 ml (160 mg) of the reconstituted sol/min

For inadvertent overdose of methotrexate

• *Adult and child >6 yr:* **IV** 7.5 mg q6hr until serum methotrexate conc <0.01 micromolar; do not give >16 ml (160 mg) of the reconstituted sol/min

Colorectal cancer (unlabeled)

• *Adult:* **IV** 100-200 mg/m^2 or 175 mg over 2 hr or as a bolus in combination with fluorouracil

Available forms: Powder for inj 50 mg

SIDE EFFECTS

CNS: **Seizures,** syncope

GI: Nausea, vomiting, stomatitis

GU: Abnormal renal function

INTEG: *Rash, pruritus,* anaphylaxis, *urticaria*

RESP: Dyspnea

Contraindications: Hypersensitivity to this agent or folic acid, mannitol; intrathecal administration

Precautions: Pregnancy (C), breastfeeding, children <6 yr, megaloblastic/pernicious anemia, seizure disorder, vitamin B_{12} deficiency

INTERACTIONS

Increase: metabolism of barbiturates, hydantoins

Increase: toxicity—fluorouracil

Decrease: effects of methotrexate, pyrimethamine, trimethoprim, trimetrexate

L

NURSING CONSIDERATIONS

Assess:

- CCr, creatinine before levoleucovorin rescue and daily to detect methotrexate level
- CBC with differential
- Other products taken: hydantoins, trimethoprim may cause increased folic acid use by body
- Neurologic status (rescue): weakness, fatigue

Administer:

- Within 1 hr of folic acid antagonist
- Do not give concurrently with systemic methotrexate

IV route

- For IV reconstitute 50 mg vial/5.3 ml of normal saline (10 mg/ml)

IV, direct route

- Give 160 mg/min or less (16 ml of 10 mg/ml sol/min)

Intermittent IV route

- Further diluting to a final concentration of 0.5 mg/ml-5 mg/ml

Perform/provide:

- Increase fluid intake if used to treat folic acid inhibitor overdose
- Protection from light and heat

Evaluate:

- Therapeutic response: prevention of methotrexate toxicity

Teach patient/family:

- For folic acid deficiency eat folic acid–rich foods: bran; yeast; dried beans; nuts; fresh, green leafy vegetables
- To notify prescriber of side effects
- To report signs of hyposensitivity reaction immediately
- To avoid breastfeeding

levothyroxine (T_4) (℞)

(lee-voe-thye-rox′een)

Eltroxin ✱, Levo-T, Levothroid, levothyroxine sodium, Levoxyl, PMS-Levothyroxine Sodium ✱, Synthroid, T_4, Unithroid

Func. class.: Thyroid hormone

Chem. class.: Levoisomer of thyroxine

Do not confuse:

Synthroid/Symmetrel

Action: Increases metabolic rate, controls protein synthesis, increases cardiac output, renal blood flow, O_2 consumption, body temp, blood volume, growth, development at cellular level, exact mechanism unknown

Uses: Hypothyroidism, myxedema coma, thyroid hormone replacement, thyrotoxicosis, congenital hypothyroidism, some types of thyroid cancer, pituitary TSH suppression

DOSAGE AND ROUTES

Severe hypothyroidism

- *Adult:* **PO** 12.5-25 mcg/day, increase by 25 mcg/day every 2-4 wk, average dose 100-200 mcg/day; max 200 mcg/day **IM/IV** 50-100 mcg/day as a single dose or 50% of usual oral dosage or *(Adult >50 yr without heart disease or <50 yr with heart disease)* **PO** 25-50 mcg/day, titrate q6-8wk or *(Adult >50 yr with heart disease)* **PO** 12.5-25 mcg/day, titrate by 12.5-25 mcg q6-8wk
- *Child >12 yr:* **PO** 2-3 mcg/kg/day as a single dose AM
- *Child 6-12 yr:* **PO** 4-5 mcg/kg/day as a single dose AM
- *Child 1-5 yr:* **PO** 5-6 mcg/kg/day as a single dose AM
- *Child 6-12 mo:* **PO** 6-8 mcg/kg/day as a single dose AM
- *Child to 6 mo:* **PO** 8-10 mcg/kg/day as a single dose AM

Myxedema coma

• *Adult:* **IV** 200-500 mcg, may increase by 100-300 mcg after 24 hr; place on oral medication as soon as possible

Subclinical hypothyroidism

• *Adult:* **PO** 1 mcg/kg/day may be sufficient

Available forms: Powder for inj 200, 500 mcg/vial; tabs 0.025, 0.05, 0.075, 0.088, 0.1, 0.112, 0.125, 0.137, 0.15, 0.175, 0.2, 0.3 mg

SIDE EFFECTS

CNS: Anxiety, insomnia, tremors, headache, **thyroid storm,** excitability

CV: Tachycardia, palpitations, angina, dysrhythmias, hypertension, **cardiac arrest**

GI: Nausea, diarrhea, increased or decreased appetite, cramps

MISC: Menstrual irregularities, weight loss, sweating, heat intolerance, fever, alopecia, decreased bone mineral density

Contraindications: Adrenal insufficiency, recent MI, thyrotoxicosis, hypersensitivity to beef, alcohol intolerance (inj only)

Black Box Warning: Obesity treatment

Precautions: Pregnancy (A), breastfeeding, geriatric patients, angina pectoris, hypertension, ischemia, cardiac disease, diabetes

PHARMACOKINETICS

Half-life euthyroid 6-7 days, hypothyroid 9-10 days, hyperthyroid 3-4 days, distributed throughout body tissues

PO: Onset 3-5 days, peak 6-8 wk, duration 1-3 wk

IV: Onset 6-8 hr, peak 24 hr, duration unknown

INTERACTIONS

Increase: cardiac insufficiency risk—epinephrine products

Increase: effects of anticoagulants, sympathomimetics, tricyclics

Decrease: levothyroxine absorption—cholestyramine, colestipol, ferrous sulfate

Decrease: effects of digoxin, insulin, hypoglycemics

Decrease: levothyroxine effect—estrogens, SSRIs, antacids, sucralfate, aluminum, magnesium, calcium, iron

Drug/Herb

Decrease: thyroid hormone effect—agar, bugleweed carnitine, kelpware, soy, spirulina

Drug/Lab Test

Increase: CPK, LDH, AST, blood glucose

Decrease: thyroid function tests

NURSING CONSIDERATIONS

Assess:

• B/P, pulse periodically during treatment

• Weight daily in same clothing, using same scale, at same time of day

• Height, growth rate of a child

• T_3, T_4, FTIs, which are decreased; radioimmunoassay of TSH, which is increased; radio uptake, which is increased if patient is on too low a dose of medication

• PT may require decreased anticoagulant; check for bleeding, bruising

• Increased nervousness, excitability, irritability, which may indicate too high dose of medication, usually after 1-3 wk of treatment

• Cardiac status: angina, palpitation, chest pain, change in VS

Administer:

PO route

• In AM if possible as a single dose to decrease sleeplessness; at same time each day to maintain product level; take on empty stomach

• Only for hormone imbalances; not to be used for obesity, male infertility, menstrual conditions, lethargy

• Lowest dose that relieves symptoms; lower dose to the geriatric patient and in cardiac diseases

• Crushed and mixed with water; nonsoy formula, or breast milk for infants/children

• Separate antacids, iron, calcium products by 4 hr

IV, direct route

• IV after diluting with provided diluent 0.5 mg/5 ml; shake; give through Y-tube or 3-way stopcock; give 0.1 mg or less over 1 min; do not add to IV inf; 0.1 mg = 1 ml

• Considered to be incompatible in syringe with all other products

Perform/provide:

• Storage in tight, light-resistant container; sol should be discarded if not used immediately

• Withdrawal of medication 4 wk before RAIU test

Evaluate:

• Therapeutic response: absence of depression; increased weight loss, diuresis, pulse, appetite; absence of constipation, peripheral edema, cold intolerance; pale, cool, dry skin; brittle nails, alopecia, coarse hair, menorrhagia, night blindness, paresthesias, syncope, stupor, coma, rosy cheeks

Teach patient/family:

• That hair loss will occur in child, is temporary

• To report excitability, irritability, anxiety, which indicate overdose

• Not to switch brands unless approved by prescriber

• That product may be discontinued after giving birth, thyroid panel evaluated after 1-2 mo

• That hypothyroid child will show almost immediate behavior/personality change

• That product is not to be taken to reduce weight

• To avoid OTC preparations with iodine; read labels; separate antacids, iron, calcium products by 4 hr

• To avoid iodine food, iodized salt, soybeans, tofu, turnips, high-iodine seafood, some bread

• That product is not a cure but controls symptoms and treatment is lifelong

⚠ High Alert

lidocaine (parenteral) (℞)

(lye′doe-kane)

LidoPen Auto-Injector, Xylocaine, Xylocard 🍁, Zingo

Func. class.: Antidysrhythmic (Class Ib)

Chem. class.: Aminoacyl amide

Action: Increases electrical stimulation threshold of ventricle, His-Purkinje system, which stabilizes cardiac membrane, decreases automaticity

Uses: Ventricular tachycardia, ventricular dysrhythmias during cardiac surgery, MI, digoxin toxicity, cardiac catheterization

Unlabeled uses: Attenuation of intracranial pressure increases during intubation/endotracheal tube suctioning

DOSAGE AND ROUTES

• *Adult:* **IV BOL** 50-100 mg (1-1.5 mg/kg) over 2-3 min, repeat q3-5min, not to exceed 300 mg in 1 hr; begin **IV INF; IV INF** 20-50 mcg/kg/min; **IM** 200-300 mg (4.3 mg/kg) in deltoid muscle, may repeat in 1-1½ hr if needed

• *Child:* **ID** (Zingo) 0.5 mg applied 1-3 min prior to needle insertion

CHF, reduced hepatic function

• *Geriatric:* **IV BOL** give ½ adult dose

• *Child:* **IV BOL** 1 mg/kg, then **IV INF** 30 mcg/kg/min

Available forms: IV INF 0.2% (2 mg/ml), 0.4% (4 mg/ml), 0.8% (8 mg/ml); IV ad 4% (40 mg/ml), 10% (100 mg/ml), 20% (200 mg/ml); IV dir 1% (10 mg/ml), 2% (20 mg/ml); IM 10% 300 mg/ml; (Zingo) needle free (powder intradermal)

SIDE EFFECTS

CNS: Headache, dizziness, involuntary movement, confusion, tremor, drowsiness, euphoria, **seizures**

CV: Hypotension, bradycardia, **heart block, CV collapse, arrest**

EENT: Tinnitus, blurred vision
GI: Nausea, vomiting, anorexia
HEMA: **Methemoglobinemia**
INTEG: Rash, urticaria, edema, swelling
MISC: Febrile response, phlebitis at inj site
RESP: Dyspnea, **respiratory depression**

Contraindications: Hypersensitivity to amides, severe heart block, supraventricular dysrhythmias, Adams-Stokes syndrome, Wolff-Parkinson-White syndrome

Precautions: Pregnancy (B), breastfeeding, children, geriatric patients, renal/hepatic disease, CHF, respiratory depression, malignant hyperthermia, myasthenia gravis, weight <50 kg

PHARMACOKINETICS

Half-life 8 min, 1-2 hr (terminal); metabolized in liver; excreted in urine; crosses placenta

IM: Onset 5-15 min, duration 1½ hr

IV: Onset 2 min, duration 20 min

INTERACTIONS

Increase: neuromuscular blockade—neuromuscular blockers, tubocurarine

Increase: lidocaine effects—cimetidine, phenytoin, propranolol, metoprolol

Decrease: lidocaine effects—barbiturates

Drug/Herb

Increase: toxicity, death—aconite

Increase: lidocaine action, effect—aloe, broom, buckthorn (chronic use), cascara sagrada (chronic use), Chinese rhubarb, figwort, fumitory, goldenseal, kudzu, licorice, senna

Increase: serotonin effect—horehound

Decrease: effect—coltsfoot

Drug/Lab Test

Increase: CPK

NURSING CONSIDERATIONS

Assess:

⚠ ECG continuously to determine increased PR or QRS segments; if these develop, discontinue or reduce rate; watch for increased ventricular ectopic beats; may have to rebolus, B/P

- IV inf rate using inf pump; run at <4 mg/min
- Blood levels (therapeutic level: 1.5-5 mcg/ml)
- I&O ratio, electrolytes (K, Na, Cl)

⚠ Malignant hyperthermia: tachypnea, tachycardia, changes in B/P, increased temp

- Respiratory status: rate, rhythm, lung fields for crackles, watch for respiratory depression; lung fields, bilateral crackles may occur in CHF patient; increased respiration, increased pulse; product should be discontinued
- CNS effects: dizziness, confusion, psychosis, paresthesias, convulsions; product should be discontinued

Administer:

- IM inj in deltoid; aspirate to avoid intravascular administration; check site daily for infiltration or extravasation

IV route

- Bolus undiluted (1%, 2% only) give 50 mg or less over 1 min or dilute 1 g/250-500 ml of D_5W; titrate to patient response; use inf pump; pediatric inf is 120 mg of lidocaine/100 ml D_5W; 1-2.5 ml/kg/hr = 20-50 mcg/kg/min; use only 1%, 2% sol for IV bol

Additive compatibilities: Alteplase, aminophylline, amiodarone, atracurium, bretylium, calcium chloride, calcium gluceptate, calcium gluconate, chloramphenicol, chlorothiazide, cimetidine, dexamethasone, digoxin, diphenhydrAMINE, DOBUTamine, DOPamine, ephedrine, erythromycin lactobionate, floxacillin, flumazenil, furosemide, heparin, hydrocortisone, hydrOXYzine, insulin (regular), mephentermine, metaraminol, nafcillin, nitroglycerin, penicillin G potassium, pentobarbital, phenylephrine, potassium chloride, procainamide, prochlorperazine, promazine, ranitidine, sodium bicarbonate, sodium lactate, theophylline, verapamil, vit B/C

Solution compatibilities: D_5W, D_5/0.9% NaCl, D_5/0.45% NaCl, D_5/LR, LR, 0.9% NaCl, 0.45% NaCl

Syringe compatibilities: Cloxacillin, glycopyrrolate, heparin, hydrOXYzine, methicillin, metoclopramide, milrinone, moxalactam, nalbuphine

Y-site compatibilities: Alteplase, amiodarone, amrinone, cefazolin, ciprofloxacin, cisatracurium, diltiazem, DOBUTamine, DOPamine, enalaprilat, etomidate, famotidine, haloperidol, heparin, heparin/hydrocortisone, labetalol, meperidine, morphine, nitroglycerin, nitroprusside, potassium chloride, propofol, remifentanil, streptokinase, theophylline, vit B/C, warfarin

Evaluate:

• Therapeutic response: decreased dysrhythmias

Teach patient/family:

• The use of automatic lidocaine injection device if ordered for personal use

Treatment of overdose: 0_2, artificial ventilation, ECG; administer DOPamine for circulatory depression, diazepam or thiopental for convulsions; decrease product if needed

lidocaine topical

See Appendix B

lindane (℞)

(lin′dane)

GBH, G-Well, Hexit ♣, Kwell, lindane, PMS-Lindane ♣

Func. class.: Scabicide, pediculicide

Chem. class.: Chlorinated hydrocarbon (synthetic)

Action: Stimulates nervous system of arthropods, resulting in seizures, death of organism

Uses: Scabies, lice (head/pubic/body), nits

DOSAGE AND ROUTES

Lice

• *Adult and child:* **CREAM/LOTION** Wash area with soap, water; remove visible crusts; apply to skin surfaces; remove with soap, water in 8-12 hr; may reapply in 1 wk if needed; shampoo using 30 ml: work into lather, rub for 5 min, rinse, dry with towel; comb with fine-toothed comb to remove nits; most require 1 oz, max 2 oz

Scabies

• *Adult and child:* **TOP** Apply 1% cream/lotion to skin, neck to bottom of feet, toes; repeat in 1 wk prn; most require 1 oz, max 2 oz

Available forms: Lotion, shampoo, cream (1%)

SIDE EFFECTS

CNS: Tremors, **seizures, CNS toxicity,** stimulation, dizziness (chronic inhalation of vapors), anxiety, insomnia

CV: **Ventricular fibrillation** (chronic inhalation of vapors)

GI: Nausea, vomiting, diarrhea, liver damage (inhalation of vapors)

GU: **Kidney damage** (chronic inhalation of vapors)

HEMA: **Aplastic anemia** (chronic inhalation of vapors), myelosuppression

INTEG: Pruritus, rash, irritation, contact dermatitis

Contraindications: Hypersensitivity, patients with known seizure disorders, Norwegian (crusted) scabies

Black Box Warning: Premature neonate; inflammation of skin, abrasions, or skin breaks; seizure disorder

Precautions: Pregnancy (C), breastfeeding, infants, children <10 yr, avoid contact with eyes

INTERACTIONS

• Oils may increase absorption; if an oil-based hair dressing is used, shampoo, rinse, dry hair before applying lindane shampoo

NURSING CONSIDERATIONS

Assess:

• Head, hair for lice and nits before and after treatment; if scabies are present check all skin surfaces

• Identify source of infection: school, family, sexual contacts

Administer:

• To body areas, scalp only; do not apply to face, lips, mouth, eyes, any mucous membrane, anus, or meatus
• Topical corticosteroids as ordered to decrease contact dermatitis
• Antihistamines
• Lotions of menthol or phenol to control itching
• Topical antibiotics for infection

Perform/provide:

• Isolation until areas on skin, scalp have cleared and treatment is completed
• Removal of nits by using a fine-toothed comb rinsed in vinegar after treatment; use gloves

Evaluate:

• Therapeutic response: decreased crusts, nits, brownish trails on skin, itching papules in skin folds, decreased itching after several weeks

Teach patient/family:

• To wash all inhabitants' clothing, using insecticide; preventive treatment may be required of all persons living in same house, using lotion or shampoo to decrease spread of infection; use rubber gloves when applying product
• That itching may continue for 4-6 wk
• That product must be reapplied if accidently washed off, or treatment will be ineffective
• Not to apply to face; if accidental contact with eyes occurs, flush with water
• Instruct patient to remove after specified time to prevent toxicity
• To treat sexual contacts simultaneously
• To check for CNS toxicity: dizziness, cramps, anxiety, nausea, vomiting, seizures

linezolid (℞)

(line-zoe'lide)

Zyvox

Func. class.: Broad-spectrum antiinfective

Chem. class.: Oxazolidinone

Action: Inhibits protein synthesis by interfering with translation; binds to bacterial 23S ribosomal RNA of the 50S subunit preventing formation of the bacterial translation process in primarily gram-positive organisms

Uses: Vancomycin-resistant *Enterococcus faecium* infections, nosocomial pneumonia, uncomplicated or complicated skin and skin structure infections, community-acquired pneumonia

DOSAGE AND ROUTES

Vancomycin-resistant* Enterococcus faecium *infections

• *Adult:* **IV/PO** 600 mg q12hr × 14-28 days; max 1200 mg/day

Nosocomial pneumonia/complicated skin infections/community-acquired pneumonia/concurrent bacterial infection

• *Adult:* **IV/PO** 600 mg q12hr × 10-14 days; max 1200 mg/day
• *Child: birth-11 yr:* **PO** 10 mg/kg q8hr × 10-14 days

Uncomplicated skin infections

• *Adult:* **PO** 400 mg q12hr × 10-14 days; max 1200 mg/day
• *Adolescent:* **PO** 600 mg q12hr × 10-14 days; max 1200 mg/day
• *Infant preterm <7 days old:* **PO** 10 mg/kg q12hr × 10-14 days

Available forms: Tabs 600 mg; oral sus 100 mg/5 ml; inj 2 mg/ml

SIDE EFFECTS

CNS: Headache, dizziness, insomnia

GI: Nausea, diarrhea, **pseudomembranous colitis,** increased ALT, AST, *vomiting,* taste change, tongue color change

HEMA: **Myelosuppression**

MISC: Vaginal moniliasis, fungal infection, oral moniliasis, **lactic acidosis**

Contraindications: Hypersensitivity

Precautions: Pregnancy (C), breastfeeding, children, thrombocytopenia, bone marrow suppression

PHARMACOKINETICS

Peak 1-2 hr, terminal half-life 4-5 hr, rapidly and extensively absorbed, protein binding 31%, metabolized by oxidation of the morpholine ring

INTERACTIONS

⚠ Do not use with MAOIs or those that possess MAOI-like action (furazolidone, isoniazid, INH, procarbazine); hypertensive crisis may occur

⚠ ***Increase:*** hypertensive crisis, seizures, coma—amoxapine, maprotiline, mirtazapine, trazodone, cyclobenzaprine, tricyclics

⚠ ***Increase:*** hypertensive crisis—levodopa

Increase: serotonin syndrome—SSRIs

Increase: effects of adrenergic agents, serotonergic agents

Drug/Herb

- Do not use acidophilus with antiinfectives; separate by several hours
- Avoid use with green tea

Drug/Food

- Tyramine foods: avoid, increased pressor response

NURSING CONSIDERATIONS

Assess:

- CBC with differential weekly, assess for myelosuppression (anemias, leukopenia, pancytopenia, thrombocytopenia)
- For serotonin syndrome
- CNS symptoms: headache, dizziness
- Hepatic studies: AST, ALT
- Allergic reactions: fever, flushing, rash, urticaria, pruritus

⚠ For pseudomembranous colitis, product should be discontinued

- For lactic acidosis: nausea, vomiting, low bicarbonate levels

Administer:

PO route

- With or without food
- Store reconstituted oral suspension at room temperature, use within 3 wk

IV route

- 30-120 min; do not use IV inf bag in series connections; do not use with additives in sol; do not use with another product, administer separately

Y-site compatibilities: acyclovir, alfentanil, amikacin, aminophylline, ampicillin, aztreonam, bretylium, buprenorphine, butorphanol, calcium gluconate, carboplatin, cefazolin, cefoperazone, cefotetan, cefoxitin, ceftazidine, ceftizoxime, cefuroxime, cimetidine, ciprofloxacin, cisatracurium, cisplatin, clindamycin, cyclophosphamide, cycloSPORINE, cytarabine, digoxin, furosemide, ganciclovir, gemcitabine, gentamicin, heparin, hydromorphone, ifosfamide, labetalol, leucovorin, levofloxacin, lidocaine, lorazepam, magnesium sulfate, mannitol, meperidine, meropenem, mesna, methotrexate, methylPREDNISolone, metoclopramide, metronidazole, midazolam, minocycline, mitoxantrone, morphine, nalbuphine, naloxone, nitroglycerin, ofloxacin, ondansetron, paclitaxel, pentobarbital, phenobarbital, piperacillin, potassium chloride, prochlorperazine, promethazine, propranolol, ranitidine, remifentanil, sufentanil, theophylline, ticarcillin, tobramycin, vancomycin, vecuronium, verapamil, vinCRIStine, zidovudine

Solution compatibilities: D_5, 0.9% NaCl, LR

Evaluate:

- Therapeutic response: decreased symptoms of infection, blood cultures negative

Teach patient/family:

- If dizziness occurs, to ambulate, perform activities with assistance
- To complete full course of product therapy
- To contact prescriber if adverse reaction occurs
- To inform prescriber if SSRIs or cold products, decongestants are being used
- To inform prescriber if there is a history of hypertension
- To avoid large amounts of high-tyramine foods, drinks (provide list)

liothyronine (T_3) (℞)

(lye-oh-thye′roe-neen)

Cytomel, l-triiodothyronine, T_3, liothyronine sodium, Triostat

Func. class.: Thyroid hormone

Chem. class.: Synthetic T_3

Action: Increases metabolic rates, cardiac output, O_2 consumption, body temp, blood volume, growth, development at cellular level; exact mechanism unknown

Uses: Hypothyroidism, myxedema coma, thyroid hormone replacement, congenital hypothyroidism, nontoxic goiter, T_3 suppression test

DOSAGE AND ROUTES

• *Adult:* **PO** 25 mcg/day, increased by 12.5-25 mcg q1-2wk until desired response, maintenance dose 25-75 mcg/day, max 100 mcg/day

• *Geriatric:* **PO** 5 mcg/day, increase by 5 mcg/day q1-2wk, maintenance 25-75 mcg/day

Congenital hypothyroidism

• *Child >3 yr:* **PO** 50-100 mcg/day

• *Child <3 yr:* **PO** 5 mcg/day, increased by 5 mcg q3-4days titrated to response, maintenance 20 mcg/day

Myxedema, severe hypothyroidism

• *Adult:* **PO** 25-50 mcg then may increase by 5-10 mcg q1-2wk; maintenance dose 50-100 mcg/day

Myxedema coma/precoma

• *Adult:* **IV** 25-50 mcg initially, 5 mcg in geriatric patients, 10-20 mcg in cardiac disease; give doses q4-12hr

Nontoxic goiter

• *Adult:* **PO** 5 mcg/day, increased by 12.5-25 mcg q1-2wk; maintenance dose 75 mcg/day

Suppression test

• *Adult:* **PO** 75-100 mcg/day × 1 wk; radioactive ^{131}I is given before and after 1-wk dose

Available forms: Tabs 5, 25, 50 mcg; inj 10 mcg/ml

SIDE EFFECTS

CNS: Insomnia, tremors, headache, **thyroid storm**

CV: Tachycardia, palpitations, angina, dysrhythmias, hypertension, **cardiac arrest**

GI: Nausea, diarrhea, increased or decreased appetite, cramps

MISC: Menstrual irregularities, weight loss, sweating, heat intolerance, fever, alopecia

Contraindications: Adrenal insufficiency, MI, thyrotoxicosis, untreated hypertension

Black Box Warning: Obesity treatment

Precautions: Pregnancy (A), breastfeeding, geriatric patients, angina pectoris, hypertension, ischemia, cardiac disease, diabetes

PHARMACOKINETICS

PO/IV: Peak 2-3 days, duration 72 hr, half-life 2.5 days

INTERACTIONS

Increase: effects of anticoagulants, sympathomimetics, tricyclics, amphetamines, decongestants, vasopressors

Decrease: absorption of liothyronine—cholestyramine; colestipol; calcium, iron, aluminum, magnesium products

Decrease: effects of digoxin, insulin, hypoglycemics

Decrease: effects of liothyronine—estrogens

Drug/Herb

Decrease: thyroid hormone effect—agar, bugleweed, carnitine, kelpware, soy, spirulina

Drug/Lab Test

Increase: CPK, LDH, AST, PBI, blood glucose

Decrease: thyroid function tests

NURSING CONSIDERATIONS

Assess:

• B/P, pulse, periodically during treatment

- Weight daily in same clothing, using same scale, at same time of day
- Height, growth rate of child
- T_3, T_4, which are decreased; radioimmunoassay of TSH, which is increased; radio uptake, which is increased if patient is on too low a dose of medication
- PT may require decreased anticoagulant; check for bleeding, bruising
- Increased nervousness, excitability, irritability, which may indicate too high dose of medication, usually after 1-3 wk of treatment
- Cardiac status: angina, palpitation, chest pain, change in VS

Administer:

- In AM if possible as a single dose to decrease sleeplessness
- At same time each day to maintain product level
- Only for hormone imbalances; not to be used for obesity, male infertility, menstrual conditions, lethargy
- Lowest dose that relieves symptoms
- Liothyronine after discontinuing other thyroid preparation
- Do not take with calcium, iron, aluminum, magnesium products

Perform/provide:

- Removal of medication 4 wk before RAIU test

Evaluate:

- Therapeutic response: absence of depression; increased weight loss, diuresis, pulse, appetite; absence of constipation, peripheral edema, cold intolerance; pale, cool, dry skin; brittle nails, alopecia, coarse hair, menorrhagia, night blindness, paresthesia, syncope, stupor, coma, rosy cheeks

Teach patient/family:

- That hair loss will occur in child but is temporary
- To report excitability, irritability, anxiety, which indicates overdose
- Not to switch brands unless approved by prescriber
- That hypothyroid child will show almost immediate behavior/personality change
- That product is not to be taken to reduce weight
- To avoid OTC preparations with iodine; read labels; do not take with calcium, iron, aluminum, magnesium products
- To avoid iodine food, iodized salt, soybeans, tofu, turnips, high iodine seafood, some bread
- That product controls symptoms but does not cure; treatment is lifelong

liotrix (℞)

(lye′oh-trix)

Thyrolar, T_3/T_4

Func. class.: Thyroid hormone

Chem. class.: Levothyroxine/liothyronine (synthetic T_4, T_3)

Do not confuse:

Thyrolar/Thyrar

Action: Increases metabolic rates, cardiac output, O_2 consumption, body temp, blood volume, growth, development at cellular level, exact mechanism unknown

Uses: Hypothyroidism, thyroid hormone replacement

DOSAGE AND ROUTES

- *Adult:* **PO** A single dose of Thyrolar ¼ or ½ adult dose, adjust as needed at 2-wk intervals
- *Geriatric:* **PO** ¼ tab, initially, adjust q6-8wk

Available forms: Tabs: Levothyroxine 12.5 mcg/liothyronine 3.1 mcg; levothyroxine 25 mcg/liothyronine 6.25 mcg (Thyrolar-½); levothyroxine 50 mcg/liothyronine 12.5 mcg (Thyrolar-1); levothyroxine 100 mcg/liothyronine 25 mcg (Thyrolar-2); levothyroxine 150 mcg/liothyronine 37.5 mcg (Thyrolar-3)

SIDE EFFECTS

CNS: Insomnia, tremors, headache, **thyroid storm,** nervousness

CV: Tachycardia, palpitations, angina, dysrhythmias, hypertension, **cardiac arrest**

GI: Nausea, vomiting, diarrhea, increased or decreased appetite, cramps

MISC: Menstrual irregularities, weight loss, sweating, heat intolerance, fever

Contraindications: Adrenal insufficiency, MI, thyrotoxicosis

Black Box Warning: Obesity treatment

Precautions: Pregnancy (A), breastfeeding, geriatric patients, angina pectoris, hypertension, ischemia, cardiac disease, diabetes

PHARMACOKINETICS

PO (T_4): Onset unknown, peak 1-3 wk, duration 1-3 wk, terminal half-life 6-7 days

PO (T_3): Onset unknown, peak 24-72 hr, duration 72 hr, terminal half-life 1-2 days

INTERACTIONS

Increase: effects of amphetamines, decongestants, vasopressors, anticoagulants, sympathomimetics, tricyclics, catecholamines

Decrease: absorption of liotrix—cholestyramine, colestipol

Decrease: effects of digoxin, insulin, hypoglycemics, theophylline

Decrease: effects of liotrix—estrogens, phenytoin, carbamazepine, rifampin

Drug/Herb

Decrease: thyroid hormone effect—agar, bugleweed, carnitine, kelpware, soy, spirulina

Drug/Lab Test

Increase: CPK, LDH, AST, PBI, blood glucose

Decrease: thyroid function tests

NURSING CONSIDERATIONS

Assess:

- B/P, pulse periodically during treatment
- Weight daily in same clothing, using same scale, at same time of day
- Height, growth rate of child
- T_3, T_4, FTIs, which are decreased; radioimmunoassay of TSH, which is increased; radio uptake, which is increased if patient is on too low a dose of medication
- PT may require decreased anticoagulant; check for bleeding, bruising
- Increased nervousness, excitability, irritability, which may indicate too high dose of medication, usually after 1-3 wk of treatment
- Cardiac status: angina, palpitation, chest pain, change in VS

Administer:

- Separate products containing calcium, iron by ≥4 hr
- In AM if possible as a single dose to decrease sleeplessness
- At same time each day to maintain product level
- Only for hormone imbalances; not to be used for obesity, male infertility, menstrual conditions, lethargy
- Lowest dose that relieves symptoms

Perform/provide:

- Withdrawal of medication 4 wk before RAIU test
- Storage in airtight, light-resistant container

Evaluate:

- Therapeutic response: absence of depression; increased weight loss, diuresis, pulse, appetite; absence of constipation, peripheral edema, cold intolerance; pale, cool, dry skin; brittle nails, coarse hair, menorrhagia, night blindness, paresthesias, syncope, stupor, coma, rosy cheeks

Teach patient/family:

- That hair loss will occur in child, is temporary
- To report excitability, irritability, chest pain, increased pulse rate, palpitations, excessive sweating, heat intolerance, nervousness, anxiety, which indicate overdose
- Not to switch brands unless approved by prescriber
- That hypothyroid child will show almost immediate behavior/personality change
- That product is not to be taken to reduce weight
- To avoid OTC preparations with iodine; read labels; separate products containing calcium, iron by ≥4 hr

• To avoid iodine food, iodized salt, soybeans, tofu, turnips, high iodine seafood, some bread
• That product does not cure, but controls symptoms; treatment is lifelong

lisdexamfetamine (℞)

(lis-dex'am-fet'a-meen)
Vyvanse
Func. class.: CNS stimulant
Chem. class.: Amphetamine

Controlled Substance Schedule II
Action: Increases release of norepinephrine, DOPamine in cerebral cortex to reticular activating system
Uses: Attention deficit disorder with hyperactivity (ADHD)

DOSAGE AND ROUTES

• *Child 6-12 yr:* **PO** 30 mg/day, may increase by 10-20 mg/day at weekly intervals, max 70 mg/day
Available forms: Caps 30, 50, 70 mg

SIDE EFFECTS

CNS: Hyperactivity, insomnia, restlessness, talkativeness, dizziness, headache, dysphoria, irritability, aggressiveness, CNS tumor, dependence, addiction, mild euphoria, somnolence, lability, psychosis, mania, hallucinations, aggression
CV: Palpitations, tachycardia, hypertension, decrease in heart rate, **dysrhythmias,** MI, **cardiomyopathy**
EENT: Blurred vision, mydriasis, dyplopia
ENDO: Growth inhibition
GI: Anorexia, dry mouth, diarrhea, weight loss
GU: Impotence, change in libido
INTEG: Urticaria, **angioedema, Stevens-Johnson syndrome, toxic epidermal necrolysis**
Contraindications: Breastfeeding, hyperthyroidism, hypertension, glaucoma, severe arteriosclerosis, CV disease, hypersensitivity to sympathomimetic amines
Black Box Warning: Substance abuse
Precautions: Pregnancy (C), children <6 yr, Gilles de la Tourette's disorder, depression, anorexia nervosa, psychosis, seizure disorder, suicidal ideation, MI, heart failure, alcoholism, aortic stenosis, bipolar disorder

PHARMACOKINETICS

Metabolized by liver; urine excretion pH dependent; crosses placenta, breast milk; half-life <1hr

INTERACTIONS

⚠ Hypertensive crisis: MAOIs or within 14 days of MAOIs
Increase: lisdexamfetamine effect—acetaZOLAMIDE, antacids, sodium bicarbonate, urinary alkalinizers
Increase: CNS effect—haloperidol, tricyclics, phenothiazines, modafinil, meperidine, phenobarbital, phenytoin
Increase: CNS stimulation—melatonin
Decrease: absorption of phenytoin
Decrease: lisdexamfetamine effect—ascorbic acid, ammonium chloride, urinary acidifiers
Decrease: effect of adrenergic blockers, antidiabetics
Drug/Herb
• Serotonin syndrome: St. John's wort
Increase: stimulant effect—khat, melatonin, green tea, guarana
Decrease: stimulant effect—eucalyptus
Drug/Food
Increase: amine effect—caffeine

NURSING CONSIDERATIONS

Assess:
• VS, B/P; this product may reverse antihypertensives; check patients with cardiac disease often
• CBC, urinalysis; in diabetes: blood glucose; insulin changes may be required, since eating may decrease
• Height, growth rate in children; growth rate may be decreased
• Mental status: mood, sensorium, affect, stimulation, insomnia, irritability

- Tolerance or dependency: an increased amount may be used to get same effect; will develop after long-term use
- Overdose: pain, fever, dehydration, insomnia, hyperactivity

Administer:

- Give daily in AM
- May give without regard to meals
- Caps: may take whole or opened and contents dissolved in water and taken

Perform/provide:

- Gum, hard candy, frequent sips of water for dry mouth

Evaluate:

- Therapeutic response: increased CNS stimulation, decreased drowsiness

Teach patient/family:

- To decrease caffeine consumption (coffee, tea, cola, chocolate); may increase irritability, stimulation
- To avoid OTC preparations unless approved by prescriber
- To taper product over several weeks; depression, increased sleeping, lethargy may occur
- To avoid alcohol ingestion
- To avoid breastfeeding
- To avoid hazardous activities until stabilized on medication
- To get needed rest; patient will feel more tired at end of day
- To use as part of a comprehensive treatment program

Treatment of overdose: Administer fluids, antihypertensive for increased B/P, ammonium chloride for increased excretion, chlorpromazine for antagonize CNS effect

lisinopril (℞)

(lyse-in'oh-pril)

Prinivil, Zestril

Func. class.: Antihypertensive, angiotensin-converting enzyme (ACE) inhibitor

Chem. class.: Enalaprilat lysine analog

Do not confuse:

lisinopril/Risperdal

Prinivil/Plendil/Proventil/Prilosec

Action: Selectively suppresses renin-angiotensin-aldosterone system; inhibits ACE, preventing conversion of angiotensin I to angiotensin II

Uses: Mild to moderate hypertension, adjunctive therapy of systolic CHF, acute MI

DOSAGE AND ROUTES

Hypertension

- *Adult:* **PO** 10-40 mg/day; may increase to 80 mg/day if required
- *Geriatric:* **PO** 2.5-5 mg/day, increase q7days

CHF

Adult: **PO** 5 mg initially with diuretics/digoxin, range 5-40 mg

Available forms: Tabs 2.5, 5, 10, 20, 30, 40 mg

SIDE EFFECTS

CNS: Vertigo, depression, **stroke,** insomnia, paresthesias, headache, *fatigue,* asthenia, dizziness

CV: Chest pain, hypotension

EENT: Blurred vision, nasal congestion

GI: Nausea, vomiting, anorexia, constipation, flatulence, GI irritation, diarrhea

GU: **Proteinuria, renal insufficiency,** sexual dysfunction, impotence

INTEG: Rash, pruritus

MISC: Muscle cramps, hyperkalemia

RESP: Dry cough, dyspnea

SYST: **Angioedema**

Contraindications: Hypersensitivity, angioedema

Black Box Warning: Pregnancy (D)

Precautions: Breastfeeding, renal disease, hyperkalemia, renal artery stenosis, CHF

PHARMACOKINETICS

Onset 1 hr, peak 6-8 hr, duration 24 hr, excreted unchanged in urine, half-life 12 hr

INTERACTIONS

- Hyperkalemia: potassium salt substitutes, potassium-sparing diuretics, potassium supplements, cycloSPORINE
- Possible toxicity: lithium, digoxin

Increase: hypotensive effect—diuretics, other antihypertensives, probenecid, phenothiazines, nitrates, acute alcohol ingestion

Increase: hypersensitivity—allopurinol

Decrease: lisinopril effects—aspirin, indomethacin, NSAIDs

Drug/Herb

Increase: toxicity, death—aconite

Increase: antihypertensive effect—barberry, betony, black catechu, black cohosh, bloodroot, broom, burdock, cat's claw, dandelion, goldenseal, hawthorn, Irish moss, Jamaican dogwood, kelp, khella, mistletoe, parsley

Increase or decrease: antihypertensive effect—astragalus, cola tree

Decrease: antihypertensive effect—coltsfoot, guarana, khat, licorice, yohimbe

Drug/Food

- High-potassium diet (bananas, orange juice, avocados, nuts, spinach) should be avoided; hyperkalemia may occur

Drug/Lab Test

Interference: glucose/insulin tolerance tests, ANA titer

NURSING CONSIDERATIONS

Assess:

⚠ Blood studies, platelets; WBC with differential baseline and periodically q3mo; if neutrophils <1000/mm^3, discontinue treatment (recommended in collagen-vascular disease)

- B/P, pulse q4hr; note rate, rhythm, quality
- Electrolytes: K, Na, Cl
- Apical/pedal pulse before administration; notify prescriber of any significant changes
- Baselines in renal, hepatic studies before therapy begins and periodically LFTs, uric acid and glucose may be increased
- Edema in feet, legs daily, weight daily in CHF
- Skin turgor, dryness of mucous membranes for hydration status
- Symptoms of CHF: edema, dyspnea, wet crackles

Administer:

- Severe hypotension may occur after 1st dose of this medication; may be prevented by reducing or discontinuing diuretic therapy 3 days before beginning lisinopril therapy

Evaluate:

- Therapeutic response: decreased B/P, CHF symptoms

Teach patient/family:

- Not to discontinue product abruptly
- To rise slowly to sitting or standing position to minimize orthostatic hypotension
- To avoid increasing potassium in the diet

Treatment of overdose: Lavage, IV atropine for bradycardia, IV theophylline for bronchospasm, digoxin, O_2, diuretic for cardiac failure

lithium (℞)

(li'thee-um)

Carbolith ♣, Duralith ♣, Eskalith, Eskalith-CR, lithium carbonate, Lithizine ♣, Lithobid, Lithonate, Lithotabs

Func. class.: Antimanic, antipsychotic

Chem. class.: Alkali metal ion salt

Action: May alter sodium, potassium ion transport across cell membrane in nerve, muscle cells; may balance biogenic amines of norepinephrine, serotonin in CNS areas involved in emotional responses

Uses: Bipolar disorders (manic phase), prevention of bipolar manic-depressive psychosis

DOSAGE AND ROUTES

- *Adult:* **PO** 300-600 mg tid, maintenance 300 mg tid or qid; **SLOW REL TABS** 300 mg bid; dose should be individualized to maintain blood levels at 0.5-1.5 mEq/L
- *Geriatric:* **PO** 300 mg bid, increase q7days by 300 mg to desired dose
- *Child:* **PO** 15-20 mg/kg/day in 2-3 divided doses; increase as needed; do not exceed adult doses; maintain blood levels at 0.4-0.5 mEq/L

Renal dose

- *Adult:* **PO** CCr 10-50 ml/min 50%-75% of dose; CCr <10 ml/min 25%-50% of dose

Available forms: Caps 150, 300, 600 mg; tabs 300 mg; ext rel tabs 300, 450 mg; syr 300 mg/5 ml (8 mEq/5 ml); slow rel caps 150, 300 mg ✤

SIDE EFFECTS

CNS: Headache, drowsiness, dizziness, tremors, twitching, ataxia, **seizure,** slurred speech, restlessness, confusion, stupor, memory loss, clonic movements, fatigue

CV: Hypotension, ECG changes, **dysrhythmias, circulatory collapse,** edema

EENT: Tinnitus, blurred vision

ENDO: Hyponatremia, goiter, hyperglycemia, hypo/hyperthyroidism

GI: Dry mouth, anorexia, nausea, vomiting, diarrhea, incontinence, abdominal pain, metallic taste

GU: **Polyuria, glycosuria, proteinuria, albuminuria,** urinary incontinence, polydipsia

HEMA: **Leukocytosis**

INTEG: Drying of hair, alopecia, rash, pruritus, hyperkeratosis, acneiform lesions, folliculitis

MS: Muscle weakness

Contraindications: Pregnancy (D), breastfeeding, children <12 yr, hepatic disease, brain trauma, organic brain syndrome, schizophrenia, severe cardiac/renal disease, severe dehydration

Precautions: Geriatric patients, thyroid disease, seizure disorders, diabetes mellitus, systemic infection, urinary retention

Black Box Warning: Lithium level >1.5 mmol/L

PHARMACOKINETICS

PO: Onset rapid, peak ½-12 hr, half-life 18-36 hr depending on age, crosses blood-brain barrier, 80% of filtered lithium is reabsorbed by the renal tubules, excreted in urine, crosses placenta, enters breast milk, well absorbed by oral method

L

INTERACTIONS

- Neurotoxicity: haloperidol, thioridazine

Increase: hypothyroid effects—antithyroid agents, calcium iodide, potassium iodide, iodinated glycerol

Increase: effects of neuromuscular blocking agents, phenothiazines

Increase: renal clearance—sodium bicarbonate, acetaZOLAMIDE, mannitol, aminophylline

Increase: toxicity—indomethacin, diuretics, NSAIDs, losartan

Increase: lithium effect/toxicity—carbamazepine, fluoxetine, methyldopa, thiazide diuretics, probenecid

Decrease: lithium effects—theophyllines, urea, urinary alkalinizers

Drug/Herb

Increase: lithium effects, increase toxicity—broom, buchu, dandelion, goldenrod, horsetail, juniper, nettle, parsley

Decrease: lithium levels—black/green tea, coffee, cola nut, guarana, plantain, yerba maté

Drug/Food

- Significant changes in sodium intake will alter lithium excretion

Drug/Lab Test
Increase: potassium excretion, urine glucose, blood glucose, protein, BUN
Decrease: VMA, T_3, T_4, PBI, ^{131}I

NURSING CONSIDERATIONS

Assess:

- Weight daily; check for and report edema in legs, ankles, wrists
- Sodium intake; decreased sodium intake with decreased fluid intake may lead to lithium retention; increased sodium and fluids may decrease lithium retention
- Skin turgor at least daily
- Urine for albuminuria, glycosuria, uric acid during beginning treatment, q2mo thereafter
- Neurologic status: LOC, gait, motor reflexes, hand tremors
- Serum lithium levels q wk initially, then q2mo (therapeutic level: 0.5-1.5 mEq/L); toxic level >1.5 mcg/L

Administer:

- Do not break, crush, or chew caps, ext rel tabs
- Reduced dose to geriatric patients
- With meals to avoid GI upset
- Adequate fluids (2-3 L/day) to prevent dehydration during initial treatment, 1-2 L/day during maintenance

Evaluate:

- Therapeutic response: decrease in excitement, manic phase

Teach patient/family:

- The symptoms of minor toxicity: vomiting, diarrhea, poor coordination, fine motor tremors, weakness, lassitude; major toxicity: coarse tremors, severe thirst, tinnitus, diluted urine
- To monitor urine specific gravity, emphasize need for follow-up care to determine lithium levels; monitor lithium levels to ensure effective levels and treatment
- That contraception is necessary, since lithium may harm fetus
- Not to operate machinery until lithium levels are stable
- That beneficial effects may take 1-3 wk
- About products that interact with lithium (provide list) and discuss need for adequate stable intake of salt and fluids

Treatment of overdose: Induce emesis or lavage, maintain airway, respiratory function; dialysis for severe intoxication

Iodoxamide ophthalmic

See Appendix B

lomustine (℞)

(loe-mus'teen)
CCNU, CeeNU
Func. class.: Antineoplastic alkylating agent
Chem. class.: Nitrosourea

Action: Responsible for crosslinking DNA strands, which leads to cell death; activity is not cell cycle phase specific

Uses: Hodgkin's disease, malignant glioma

Unlabeled uses: Brain, breast, renal, GI tract, bronchogenic carcinoma; melanomas, non-Hodgkin's lymphoma

DOSAGE AND ROUTES

- *Adult:* **PO** 100-130 mg/m^2 as a single dose q6wk or 75-100 mg/m^2 q6wk in combination; titrate dose to WBC; do not give repeat dose unless WBC >4000/mm^3, platelet count >100,000/mm^3

Available forms: Caps 10, 40, 100 mg

SIDE EFFECTS

CNS: Lethargy
GI: Nausea, vomiting, anorexia, stomatitis, **hepatotoxicity**
GU: **Azotemia, renal failure**
HEMA: **Thrombocytopenia, leukopenia, myelosuppression, anemia**
INTEG: Alopecia
RESP: **Fibrosis, pulmonary infiltrate**

Contraindications: Pregnancy (D), breastfeeding, hypersensitivity, "blastic" phase of CML

Black Box Warning: Leukopenia, thrombocytopenia

Precautions: Radiation therapy, pulmonary disease

PHARMACOKINETICS

Metabolized in liver, excreted in urine, half-life 16-48 hr, 50% protein bound, crosses blood-brain barrier, appears in breast milk

INTERACTIONS

• Lomustine potentiation: succinylcholine

Increase: bleeding—aspirin, anticoagulants

Increase: toxicity—barbiturates, cimetidine, phenytoin, chloral hydrate

Increase: lomustine metabolism—phenobarbital

Increase: bone marrow depression—allopurinol

Drug/Lab Test

False positive: cytology tests for breast, bladder, cervix, lung

NURSING CONSIDERATIONS

Assess:

• CBC, differential, platelet count q wk; withhold product if WBC <4000/mm^3 or platelet count <100,000/mm^3; notify prescriber; these may occur after 4-6 wk, and with cumulative doses >600 mg

• Pulmonary function tests, chest x-ray films before, during therapy; chest film should be obtained q2wk during treatment

• Renal studies: BUN, serum uric acid, urine CCr before, during therapy

• I&O ratio; report fall in urine output of 30 ml/hr

• Monitor temp (may indicate beginning infection, usually after 4 wk); no rectal temps

• Hepatic studies before, during therapy (bilirubin, AST, ALT, LDH) as needed or monthly

• Bleeding: hematuria, guaiac, bruising or petechiae, mucosa or orifices

• Dyspnea, crackles, unproductive cough, chest pain, tachypnea

• Jaundiced skin and sclera, dark urine, clay-colored stools, itchy skin, abdominal pain, fever, diarrhea

• Inflammation of mucosa, breaks in skin

• Buccal cavity q8hr for dryness, sores or ulceration, white patches, oral pain, bleeding, dysphagia

• Local irritation, pain, burning, discoloration at inj site

⚠ Symptoms indicating severe allergic reaction: rash, pruritus, urticaria, purpuric skin lesions, itching, flushing

Administer:

• Antiemetic and dexamethasone 30-60 min before giving product to prevent vomiting; no food or drinks for ≥2 hr after administration

Perform/provide:

• Storage in tight container at room temperature

• Strict medical asepsis, protective isolation if WBC levels are low

• Deep-breathing exercises with patient tid-qid; place in semi-Fowler's position

• Rinsing of mouth tid-qid with water, club soda; brushing of teeth bid-tid with soft brush or cotton-tipped applicators for stomatitis; use unwaxed dental floss

Evaluate:

• Therapeutic response: decreased tumor size, spread of malignancy

Teach patient/family:

• About protective isolation

• To report any changes in breathing or coughing

• To avoid foods with citric acid, hot or rough texture if buccal inflammation is present

• To report any bleeding, white spots, or ulcerations in mouth to prescriber; tell patient to examine mouth daily

• To report signs of infection: fever, sore throat

• To use effective contraception, avoid breastfeeding

• To report signs of anemia: fatigue, headache, faintness, shortness of breath, irritability
• To avoid use of razors, commercial mouthwash if thrombocytopenia occurs
• To avoid use of all OTC medications unless approved by prescriber
• To take entire dose at one time

loperamide (OTC, ℞)

(loe-per'a-mide)
loperamide solution, Imodium, Imodium A-D, Imodium A-D Caplet, loperamide, Kaopectate II Caplets, Maalox Antidiarrheal Caplets, Neo-Diaral, Pepto Diarrhea Control

Func. class.: Antidiarrheal
Chem. class.: Piperidine derivative

Do not confuse:
Imodium/Indocin
Loperamide/furosemide

Action: Direct action on intestinal muscles to decrease GI peristalsis; reduces volume, increases bulk, electrolytes not lost

Uses: Diarrhea (cause undetermined), travelers' diarrhea, chronic diarrhea, to decrease amount of ileostomy discharge

Unlabeled uses: Irinotecan-induced diarrhea, irritable bowel syndrome

DOSAGE AND ROUTES

• *Adult:* **PO** 4 mg, then 2 mg after each loose stool, max 16 mg/day
• *Child 9-11 yr:* **PO** 2 mg, then 1 mg after each loose stool, max 6 mg/24 hr
• *Child 2-5 yr:* **PO** 1 mg then 0.1 mg/kg after each loose stool, max 4 mg/24 hr

Irinotecan-induced diarrhea (unlabeled)

• *Adult:* **PO** 4 mg at first sign of late diarrhea (≥24 hr after irinotecan) then 2 mg q2hr × ≥12 hr, at night 4 mg q4hr

Available forms: Caps 2 mg; liq 1 mg/5 ml; tabs 2 mg

SIDE EFFECTS

CNS: Dizziness, drowsiness, fatigue
GI: Nausea, dry mouth, vomiting, constipation, abdominal pain, anorexia, **toxic megacolon,** bacterial enterocolitis, flatulence
INTEG: Rash
MISC: Hyperglycemia
SYST: **Anaphylaxis, angioedema, toxic epidermal necrolysis**

Contraindications: Hypersensitivity, pseudomembranous colitis, constipation, dysentery, GI bleeding/obstruction/perforation, ileus, vomiting

Precautions: Pregnancy (C), breastfeeding, children <2 yr, hepatic disease, dehydration, gastroenteritis, toxic megacolon, geriatric patients, severe ulcerative colitis

PHARMACOKINETICS

PO: Onset 1-3 hr, duration 4-5 hr, half-life 9-14 hr, metabolized in liver, excreted in feces as unchanged product, small amount in urine

INTERACTIONS

Increase: CNS depression—alcohol, antihistamines, analgesics, opioids, sedative/hypnotics

Drug/Herb

Increase: CNS depression—chamomile, hops, kava, skullcap, valerian
Increase: antidiarrheal effect—nutmeg

NURSING CONSIDERATIONS

Assess:

• Stools: volume, color, characteristics
• Electrolytes (K, Na, Cl) if on long-term therapy
• Skin turgor q8hr if dehydration is suspected, fluid replacement
• Bowel pattern before; for rebound constipation
• Response after 48 hr; if no response, product should be discontinued
• Dehydration, CNS problems in children or those with hepatic disease
• Abdominal distention, toxic megacolon; may occur in ulcerative colitis

Administer:

- Do not break, crush, or chew caps
- For 48 hr only
- Do not mix oral sol with other sols

Perform/provide:

- Storage in tight container

Evaluate:

- Therapeutic response: decreased diarrhea

Teach patient/family:

- To avoid OTC products unless directed by prescriber
- That ileostomy patient may take this product for extended time
- That if drowsiness occurs, not to operate machinery
- To use hard candy, sips of water for dry mouth

loracarbef

See cephalosporins—2nd generation

loratadine (OTC, ℞)

(lor-a'ti-deen)

Alavert, Children's Loratadine, Children's ND Non-Drowsy Allergy, Claritin, Claritin Non-Drowsy Allergy, Clear-Atadine, Dimetapp, Tavist ND

Func. class.: Antihistamine, 2nd generation

Chem. class.: Selective histamine (H_1)-receptor antagonist

Do not confuse:

loratadine/lovastatin/lorazepam/losartan

Action: Binds to peripheral histamine receptors, providing antihistamine action without sedation

Uses: Seasonal rhinitis, chronic idiopathic urticaria for those ≥2 yr

DOSAGE AND ROUTES

- *Adult and child ≥6 yr:* **PO** 10 mg/day
- *Child 2-5 yr:* **PO** 5 mg/day

Renal dose

- *Adult:* **PO** CCr <30 ml/min, 10 mg every other day

Hepatic dose

- *Adult:* **PO** 10 mg every other day

Available forms: Tabs 10 mg; rapid-disintegrating tabs 10 mg; orally disintegrating tabs 10 mg; syr 1 mg/ml; susp 5 mg/ml

SIDE EFFECTS

CNS: Sedation (more common with increased doses), headache, fatigue, restlessness

CV: Sinus tachycardia

RESP: Wheezing

Contraindications: Hypersensitivity, acute asthma attacks, lower respiratory tract disease

Precautions: Pregnancy (B), breastfeeding, increased intraocular pressure, bronchial asthma, hepatic/renal disease

PHARMACOKINETICS

Onset 1-3 hr, peak 8-10 hr, duration 24 hr, metabolized in liver to active metabolites, excreted in urine, active metabolite desloratadine half-life 20 hr

INTERACTIONS

Increase: antihistamine effects—MAOIs

Increase: CNS depressant effects—alcohol, antidepressants, other antihistamines, sedative/hypnotics

Increase: loratadine level—cimetidine, ketoconazole, macrolides (clarithromycin, erythromycin)

Drug/Herb

Increase: CNS depression—chamomile, hops, Jamaican dogwood, kava, khat, senega, skullcap, valerian

Increase: anticholinergic effect—corkwood, henbane leaf

Drug/Lab Test

False negative: skin allergy tests (discontinue antihistamine 3 days before testing)

NURSING CONSIDERATIONS

Assess:

- Allergy: hives, rash, rhinitis; monitor respiratory status
- LFTs, serum creatinine/BUN

Administer:

- Rapid-disintegrating tabs by placing on tongue, then swallow after disintegrated with or without water
- Use within 6 mo of opening pouch and immediately after opening blister pack
- On empty stomach daily

Perform/provide:

- Storage in tight container at room temperature
- Increased fluids to 2 L/day to decrease secretions

Evaluate:

- Therapeutic response: absence of running or congested nose, other allergy symptoms

Teach patient/family:

- To avoid driving, other hazardous activities if drowsiness occurs
- To use sunscreen or stay out of the sun to prevent photosensitivity
- To avoid use of other CNS depressants
- To increase fluids to 2 L/day to decrease secretions

lorazepam (℞)

(lor-a'ze-pam)

Apo-Lorazepam ✱, Ativan, lorazepam, Novo-Lorazem ✱, Nu-Loraz ✱

Func. class.: Sedative, hypnotic; antianxiety

Chem. class.: Benzodiazepine, short acting

Controlled Substance Schedule IV

Do not confuse:

lorazepam/alprazolam/clonazepam

Action: Potentiates the actions of GABA, especially in the limbic system and reticular formation

Uses: Anxiety, irritability in psychiatric or organic disorders, preoperatively, insomnia, adjunct in endoscopic procedures

Unlabeled uses: Antiemetic prior to chemotherapy, status epilepticus, rectal use, alcohol withdrawal, seizure prophylaxis

DOSAGE AND ROUTES

Anxiety

- *Adult:* **PO** 2-6 mg/day in divided doses, max 10 mg/day
- *Geriatric:* **PO** 1-2 mg/day in divided doses; or 0.5-1 mg at bedtime
- *Child ≥12 yr:* **PO** 0.05 mg/kg/dose, q4-8hr

Insomnia

- *Adult:* **PO** 2-4 mg at bedtime; only minimally effective after 2 wk continuous therapy
- *Geriatric:* **PO** 0.5-1 mg initially

Preoperatively

- *Adult:* **IM** 50 mcg/kg 2 hr prior to surgery; **IV** 44 mcg/kg 15-20 min prior to surgery, max 2 mg 15-20 min prior to surgery
- *Child ≥12 yr:* **IV** 0.05 mg/kg

Status epilepticus

- *Neonate:* **IV** 0.05 mg/kg
- *Child:* **IV** 0.1 mg/kg up to 4 mg/dose; **RECT** (unlabeled) 0.05-0.1 mg × 2; wait 7 min before giving 2nd dose

Alcohol withdrawal (unlabeled)

- *Adult:* **PO** 2 mg q6hr × 4 doses, then 1 mg q6hr, for 8 doses

Available forms: Tabs 0.5, 1, 2 mg; inj 2, 4 mg/ml; conc oral sol 2 mg/ml

SIDE EFFECTS

CNS: Dizziness, drowsiness, confusion, headache, anxiety, tremors, stimulation, fatigue, depression, insomnia, hallucinations, weakness, unsteadiness

CV: Orthostatic hypotension, **ECG changes, tachycardia,** hypotension; **apnea, cardiac arrest (IV, rapid)**

EENT: Blurred vision, tinnitus, mydriasis

GI: Constipation, dry mouth, nausea, vomiting, anorexia, diarrhea

INTEG: Rash, dermatitis, itching

MISC: Acidosis

Contraindications: Pregnancy (D), breastfeeding, hypersensitivity to benzodiazepines, benzyl alcohol; closed-angle glaucoma, psychosis, history of drug abuse, COPD, sleep apnea
Precautions: Children <12 yr, geriatric patients, debilitated, renal/hepatic disease, addiction, suicidal ideation

PHARMACOKINETICS

Metabolized by liver; excreted by kidneys; crosses placenta, breast milk; half-life 14 hr
PO: Onset ½ hr, peak 1-6 hr, duration 12-24 hr
IM: Onset 15-30 min, peak 1-1½ hr, duration 6-8 hr
IV: Onset 5-15 min, peak unknown, duration 6-8 hr

INTERACTIONS

Increase: lorazepam effects—CNS depressants, alcohol, disulfiram, oral contraceptives
Decrease: lorazepam effects—valproic acid

Drug/Herb
Increase: hypotension—black cohosh
Increase: CNS depression—catnip, chamomile, clary, cowslip, hops, kava, lavender, mistletoe, nettle, pokeweed, poppy, Queen Anne's lace, senega, skullcap, valerian

Drug/Lab Test
Increase: AST, ALT, serum bilirubin
Decrease: RAIU
False increase: 17-OHCS

NURSING CONSIDERATIONS

Assess:
• B/P (lying, standing), pulse; if systolic B/P drops 20 mm Hg, hold product, notify prescriber; respirations q5-15min if given IV
• Blood studies: CBC during long-term therapy; blood dyscrasias have occurred rarely
• Hepatic studies: AST, ALT, bilirubin, creatinine, LDH, alk phos
• Mental status: mood, sensorium, affect, sleeping pattern, drowsiness, dizziness
• Physical dependency, withdrawal symptoms: headache, nausea, vomiting, muscle pain, weakness, tremors, seizures, after long-term, excessive use
⚠ Suicidal tendencies

Administer:
• With food or milk for GI symptoms
• Crushed if patient is unable to swallow medication whole
• Sugarless gum, hard candy, frequent sips of water for dry mouth
• Deep into large muscle mass (IM inj)
• Give largest dose before bedtime, if giving in divided doses
• Concentrate: use calibrated dropper; add to food/drink; consume immediately

IV route
• Prepare immediately before use, short stability time
• IV after diluting in equal vol sterile H_2O, 5% dextrose or 0.9% NaCl for inj; give through Y-tube or 3-way stopcock; give at 2 mg or less over 1 min

Syringe compatibilities: Cimetidine, hydromorphone
Y-site compatibilities: Acyclovir, albumin, allopurinol, amifostine, amikacin, amoxicillin, amoxicillin/clavulanate, amphotericin B cholesteryl, amsacrine, atracurium, bumetanide, cefepime, cefotaxime, ciprofloxacin, cisatracurium, cisplatin, cladribine, clonidine, cyclophosphamide, cytarabine, dexamethasone, diltiazem, DOBUTamine, DOPamine, DOXOrubicin, DOXOrubicin liposome, epinephrine, erythromycin, etomidate, famotidine, fentanyl, filgrastim, fluconazole, fludarabine, furosemide, gentamicin, granisetron, haloperidol, heparin, hydrocortisone, hydromorphone, ketanserin, labetalol, melphalan, methotrexate, metronidazole, midazolam, milrinone, morphine, niCARdipine, nitroglycerin, norepinephrine, paclitaxel, pancuronium, piperacillin, piperacillin/tazobactam, potassium chloride, propofol, ranitidine, remifentanil, tacrolimus, teniposide, thiotepa, trimethoprim-

sulfamethoxazole, vancomycin, vecuronium, vinorelbine, zidovudine

Perform/provide:

- Assistance with ambulation during beginning therapy, since drowsiness/dizziness occurs
- Check to see if PO medication has been swallowed
- Refrigerate parenteral form

Evaluate:

- Therapeutic response: decreased anxiety, restlessness, insomnia

Teach patient/family:

- That product may be taken with food
- Not to use product for everyday stress or longer than 4 mo unless directed by prescriber
- Not to take more than prescribed amount; may be habit forming
- To avoid OTC preparations (cough, cold, hay fever) unless approved by prescriber
- To avoid driving, activities that require alertness, since drowsiness may occur
- To avoid alcohol ingestion, other psychotropic medications, unless directed by prescriber
- Not to discontinue medication abruptly after long-term use
- To rise slowly or fainting may occur, especially geriatric patients
- That drowsiness may worsen at beginning of treatment
- To use birth control if child-bearing age

Treatment of overdose: Lavage, VS, supportive care, flumazenil

losartan (℞)

(lo-zar′tan)

Cozaar

Func. class.: Antihypertensive

Chem. class.: Angiotensin II receptor (type AT_1) antagonist

Do not confuse:

losartan/valsartan

Cozaar/Zocor

Action: Blocks the vasoconstrictor and aldosterone-secreting effects of angiotensin II; selectively blocks the binding of angiotensin II to the AT_1 receptor found in tissues

Uses: Hypertension, alone or in combination, nephropathy in type 2 diabetes, hypertension with left ventricular hypertrophy

DOSAGE AND ROUTES

Hypertension

- *Adult:* **PO** 50 mg/day alone or 25 mg/day when used in combination with diuretic; maintenance 25-100 mg/day

Hepatic dose

- *Adult:* **PO** 25 mg/day as starting dose

Hypertension with left ventricular hypertrophy

- *Adult:* **PO** 50 mg/day, add hydrochlorothiazide 12.5 mg/day and/or increase losartan to 100 mg/day, then increase hydrochlorothiazide to 25 mg/day

Nephropathy in type 2 diabetic patients

- *Adult:* **PO** 50 mg/day, may increase to 100 mg/day

Available forms: Tabs 25, 50, 100 mg

SIDE EFFECTS

CNS: Dizziness, insomnia, anxiety, confusion, abnormal dreams, migraine, tremor, vertigo, headache, malaise

CV: Angina pectoris, 2nd-degree AV block, **cerebrovascular accident,** hypotension, **MI,** *dysrhythmias*

EENT: Blurred vision, burning eyes, conjunctivitis

GI: Diarrhea, dyspepsia, anorexia, constipation, dry mouth, flatulence, gastritis, vomiting

GU: Impotence, nocturia, urinary frequency, UTI, **renal failure**

HEMA: Anemia, **thrombocytopenia**

INTEG: Alopecia, dermatitis, dry skin, flushing, photosensitivity, rash, pruritus, sweating, **angioedema**

META: Gout

MS: Cramps, myalgia, pain, stiffness

RESP: Cough, upper respiratory infection, congestion, dyspnea, bronchitis

Contraindications: Hypersensitivity

Black Box Warning: Pregnancy (D) 2nd/3rd trimesters

Precautions: Pregnancy (C) 1st trimester, breastfeeding, children, geriatric patients; hypersensitivity to ACE inhibitors; hepatic disease, angioedema, renal artery stenosis

PHARMACOKINETICS

Peak 1-4 hr, extensively metabolized, half-life 2 hr, metabolite 6-9 hr, excreted in urine and feces, protein binding 98.7%

INTERACTIONS

Increase: lithium toxicity—lithium
Increase: antihypertensive effect—fluconazole
Increase: hyperkalemia—potassium sparing diuretics, potassium supplements, ACE inhibitors
Decrease: antihypertensive effect—NSAIDs, phenobarbital, rifamycin, salicylates

Drug/Herb

Increase: toxicity, death—aconite
Increase: antihypertensive effect—barberry, betony, black catechu, black cohosh, bloodroot, broom, burdock, cat's claw, dandelion, goldenseal, hawthorn, Irish moss, Jamaican dogwood, kelp, khella, mistletoe, parsley
Increase or decrease: antihypertensive effect—astragalus, cola tree
Decrease: antihypertensive effect—coltsfoot, guarana, khat, licorice, yohimbe

NURSING CONSIDERATIONS

Assess:

- B/P with position changes, pulse q4hr; note rate, rhythm, quality
- Electrolytes: K, Na, Cl
- Baselines in renal, hepatic studies before therapy begins
- Edema in feet, legs daily
- Skin turgor, dryness of mucous membranes for hydration status

Administer:

- Without regard to meals

Evaluate:

- Therapeutic response: decreased B/P

Teach patient/family:

- To avoid sunlight or wear sunscreen if in sunlight; photosensitivity may occur
- To comply with dosage schedule, even if feeling better; do not discontinue abruptly
- To notify prescriber of mouth sores, fever, swelling of hands or feet, irregular heartbeat, chest pain
- That excessive perspiration, dehydration, vomiting, diarrhea may lead to fall in B/P; consult prescriber if these occur
- That product may cause dizziness, fainting; light-headedness may occur
- To rise slowly to sitting or standing position to minimize orthostatic hypotension
- To use contraception while taking this product
- To avoid salt substitutes, alcohol, grapefruit juice, OTC products unless approved by prescriber

loteprednol ophthalmic

See Appendix B

lovastatin (℞)

(loh-vah-stat′in)

Altocor, Altoprev, Mevacor

Func. class.: Antilipemic

Chem. class.: HMG-CoA reductase inhibitor

Do not confuse:
lovastatin/Lotensin

Action: Inhibits HMG-CoA reductase enzyme, which reduces cholesterol synthesis

Uses: As an adjunct in primary hypercholesterolemia (types IIa, IIb), atherosclerosis, primary and secondary prevention of coronary events

DOSAGE AND ROUTES

- *Adult:* **PO** 20 mg/day with evening meal; may increase to 20-80 mg/day in

single or divided doses, not to exceed 80 mg/day; dosage adjustments should be made q mo, reduce dose in renal disease; **EXT REL** 20-60 mg/day at bedtime
Available forms: Tabs 10, 20, 40 mg; ext rel tab (Altocor) 10, 20, 40, 60 mg

SIDE EFFECTS

CNS: Dizziness, headache, tremor, insomnia, paresthesia, **Lou Gehrig's disease (ALS)**
EENT: Blurred vision, lens opacities
GI: Flatus, nausea, constipation, diarrhea, dyspepsia, abdominal pain, heartburn, **hepatic dysfunction,** vomiting, acid regurgitation, dry mouth, dysgeusia
HEMA: **Thrombocytopenia, hemolytic anemia, leukopenia**
INTEG: Rash, pruritus, photosensitivity
MS: Muscle cramps, myalgia, **myositis, rhabdomyolysis,** leg, shoulder or localized pain
Contraindications: Pregnancy (X), breastfeeding, hypersensitivity, active hepatic disease
Precautions: Children, past hepatic disease, alcoholism, severe acute infections, trauma, hypotension, uncontrolled seizure disorders, severe metabolic disorders, electrolyte imbalances, visual disorder

PHARMACOKINETICS

PO: Peak 2-4 hr; peak response 4-6 wk; metabolized in liver (metabolites); highly protein bound; excreted in urine 10%, feces 83%; crosses placenta; excreted in breast milk; half-life 3-4 hr

INTERACTIONS

Increase: myalgia, myositis—azole antifungals, clarithromycin, clofibrate, cycloSPORINE, dalfopristin, danazol, diltiazem, erythromycin, gemfibrozil, niacin, protease inhibitors, quinupristin, telithromycin, verapamil
Increase: bleeding—warfarin
Increase: effects of digoxin
Decrease: effects of lovastatin—bile acid sequestrants, exonatide, bosentan

Drug/Herb
Increase: effect—glucomannan
Decrease: effect—gotu kola, St. John's wort

Drug/Food
- Possible toxicity: grapefruit juice

Increase: levels of lovastatin with food, must be taken with food
Decrease: absorption—oat bran

Drug/Lab Test
Increase: CPK, LFTs

NURSING CONSIDERATIONS

Assess:
- Diet, obtain diet history including fat, cholesterol in diet
- Fasting cholesterol, LDL, HDL, triglycerides periodically during treatment
- Hepatic studies q1-2mo during the first 1½ yr of treatment; AST, ALT, LFTs may increase
- Renal function in patients with compromised renal system: BUN, creatinine, I&O ratio

⚠ For muscle pain, tenderness, obtain CPK baseline and if these occur, product may need to be discontinued

Administer:
- In evening with meal; if dose is increased, take with breakfast and evening meal

Perform/provide:
- Storage in cool environment in airtight, light-resistant container

Evaluate:
- Therapeutic response: cholesterol at desired level after 8 wk

Teach patient/family:
- To report suspected pregnancy, pregnancy category (X)
- That blood work and ophthalmic exam will be necessary during treatment
- To report blurred vision, severe GI symptoms, dizziness, headache, muscle pain, weakness
- To use sunscreen or stay out of the sun to prevent photosensitivity
- That previously prescribed regimen will continue: low-cholesterol diet, exercise program, smoking cessation
- That product should be taken with food

loxapine (℞)

(lox'a-peen)

Loxapac ✦, loxapine succinate ✦, Loxitane, Loxitane IM

Func. class.: Antipsychotic, neuroleptic

Chem. class.: Dibenzoxazepine

Do not confuse:

Loxitane/Soriatane

Action: Depresses cerebral cortex, hypothalamus, limbic system, which control activity and aggression; blocks neurotransmission produced by DOPamine at synapse; exhibits strong α-adrenergic, anticholinergic blocking action; mechanism for antipsychotic effects is unclear

Uses: Psychotic disorders, nonpsychotic symptoms associated with dementia

Unlabeled uses: Depression, anxiety

DOSAGE AND ROUTES

- *Adult:* **PO** 10 mg bid-qid initially, may be rapidly increased depending on severity of condition, maintenance 60-100 mg/day; **IM** 12.5-50 mg q4-6hr or more until desired response, then start **PO** form, max 250 mg/day
- *Geriatric:* **PO** 5-10 mg daily-bid, increase q4-7days by 5-10 mg, max 250 mg/day

Available forms: Caps 5, 10, 25, 50 mg; tabs 5, 10, 25, 50 mg; conc 25 mg/ml; inj 50 mg/ml

SIDE EFFECTS

CNS: EPS: pseudoparkinsonism, akathisia, dystonia, tardive dyskinesia, drowsiness, headache, **seizures,** confusion, **neuroleptic malignant syndrome**

CV: Orthostatic hypotension, **cardiac arrest,** ECG changes, tachycardia

EENT: Blurred vision, glaucoma

GI: Dry mouth, nausea, vomiting, anorexia, constipation, diarrhea, jaundice, weight gain

GU: Urinary retention, urinary frequency, enuresis, impotence, amenorrhea, gynecomastia

HEMA: **Anemia, leukopenia, leukocytosis, agranulocytosis**

INTEG: Rash, photosensitivity, dermatitis

RESP: **Laryngospasm,** dyspnea, **respiratory depression**

Contraindications: Hypersensitivity, blood dyscrasias, coma, brain damage, bone marrow depression, alcohol and barbiturate withdrawal states, severe CNS depression, closed-angle glaucoma

Precautions: Pregnancy (C), breastfeeding, children <16 yr, geriatric patients, seizure disorders, cardiac/renal/hepatic disease, prostatic hypertrophy, cardiac conditions

Black Box Warning: Dementia

PHARMACOKINETICS

Metabolized by liver, excreted in urine, crosses placenta, enters breast milk, initial half-life 5 hr, terminal half-life 19 hr

PO: Onset 20-30 min, peak 2-4 hr, duration 12 hr

IM: Onset 15-30 min, peak 15-20 min, duration 12 hr

INTERACTIONS

Increase: toxicity—epinephrine

Increase: EPS—other antipsychotics

Increase: CNS depression—MAOIs, antidepressants, alcohol

Decrease: effects—guanadrel, guanethidine, levodopa

Drug/Herb

Increase: CNS depression—chamomile, cola tree, hops, kava, nettle, nutmeg, skullcap, valerian

Increase: EPS—betel palm, kava

NURSING CONSIDERATIONS

Assess:

- Mental status before initial administration
- Swallowing of PO medication; check for hoarding or giving of medication to other patients

L

• I&O ratio; palpate bladder if low urinary output occurs, urinary retention may be the cause
• Bilirubin, CBC, LFTs q mo
• Urinalysis is recommended before and during prolonged therapy
• Affect, orientation, LOC, reflexes, gait, coordination, sleep pattern disturbances
• B/P standing and lying; take pulse and respirations q4hr during initial treatment; establish baseline before starting treatment; report drops of 30 mm Hg
• Dizziness, faintness, palpitations, tachycardia on rising
• EPS including akathisia (inability to sit still, no pattern to movements), tardive dyskinesia (bizarre movements of the jaw, mouth, tongue, extremities), pseudoparkinsonism (rigidity, tremors, pill rolling, shuffling gait)

⚠ For neuroleptic malignant syndrome: muscle rigidity, increased CPK, altered mental status, hyperthermia
• Constipation, urinary retention daily; if these occur, increase bulk, water in diet

Administer:
• Reduced dose to geriatric patients
• Anticholinergic agent if EPS symptoms occur

PO route
• Concentrate mixed in orange or grapefruit juice

IM route
• IM inj into large muscle mass

Perform/provide:
• Decreased sensory input by dimming lights, avoiding loud noises
• Supervised ambulation until stabilized on medication; do not involve in strenuous exercise program because fainting is possible; patient should not stand still for long periods
• Increased fluids to prevent constipation
• Sips of water, candy, gum for dry mouth
• Storage in airtight, light-resistant container

Evaluate:
• Therapeutic response: decrease in emotional excitement, hallucinations, delusions, paranoia; reorganization of patterns of thought, speech

Teach patient/family:
• That orthostatic hypotension may occur and to rise from sitting or lying position gradually
• To remain lying down after IM injection for at least 30 min
• To avoid hot tubs, hot showers, tub baths, as hypotension may occur; that in hot weather heat stroke may occur; take extra precautions to stay cool
• To avoid abrupt withdrawal of this product, or EPS may result; product should be withdrawn slowly
• To avoid OTC preparations (cough, hay fever, cold) unless approved by prescriber; serious product interactions may occur; avoid use with alcohol, CNS depressants; increased drowsiness may occur
• To avoid hazardous activities until stabilized on medication
• To use sunscreen during sun exposure to prevent burns
• About necessity for meticulous oral hygiene, since oral candidiasis may occur
• To report impaired vision, jaundice, tremors, muscle twitching

Treatment of overdose: Lavage if orally ingested; provide an airway

lubiprostone (℞)

(loo bee-pros′-tone)
Amitiza
Func. class.: Gastrointestinal agent—miscellaneous

Action: Locally acting chloride channel activator, enhances a chloride-rich intestinal fluid secretion without altering other electrolytes; increases motility in the intestine, increasing softening and passage of stool

Uses: Chronic idiopathic constipation, constipation predominant irritable bowel syndrome in women >18 yr

DOSAGE AND ROUTES

Chronic idiopathic constipation

• *Adult:* **PO** 24 mcg bid with food/water

IBS with constipation (females)

• *Adult and adolescent ≥18 yr:* **PO** 8 mcg bid with food and water

Available forms: Caps 8, 24 mcg

SIDE EFFECTS

CNS: Headache, dizziness, depression, fatigue, insomnia

CV: Hypertension, chest pain

GI: Nausea, abdominal pain, eructation, abdominal distention, constipation, diarrhea, dry mouth, dyspepsia, flatulence, gastroenteritis viral, gastroesophageal reflux disease, vomiting, fecal incontinence, fecal urgency

GU: UTI

MISC: Chest pain, peripheral edema, influenza, pyrexia, viral infection

MS: Back pain, arthralgia, muscle cramps, pain in extremities

RESP: Bronchitis, cough, dyspnea, nasopharyngitis, sinusitis, upper respiratory tract infection

Contraindications: Hypersensitivity, GI obstruction

Precautions: Pregnancy (C), breastfeeding, children, diarrhea, inflammatory bowel disease

PHARMACOKINETICS

Peak 1.14 hr; 94% protein binding; half-life 0.9-1.4 hr; metabolism rapid, extensively in stomach, jejunum

INTERACTIONS

Decrease: effect by antidiarrheals and anticholinergics

NURSING CONSIDERATIONS

Assess:

• GI symptoms: nausea, abdominal pain

• Periodically need for continued treatment

Administer:

• With foods, bid

Perform/provide:

• Store at room temperature

Evaluate:

• Therapeutic response: decreased constipation

Teach patient/family:

• To notify prescriber of GI symptoms, diarrhea, hypersensitivity reactions

lymphocyte immune globulin (antithymocyte) (℞)

Atgam, Thymoglobulin

Func. class.: Immune globulins—immunosuppressant

Action: Produces immunosuppression by inhibiting the function of lymphocytes (T)

Uses: Organ transplants to prevent rejection, aplastic anemia

Unlabeled uses: MS; myasthenia gravis; immunosuppressant in liver, bone marrow, heart, and other organ transplants; pure red-cell aplasia; scleroderma

DOSAGE AND ROUTES

Renal allograft

• *Adult:* **IV** 10-30 mg/kg/day

• *Child:* **IV** 5-25 mg/kg/day

Delay of renal allograft rejection

• *Adult:* **IV** 15 mg/kg/day × 7-14 days, then every other day × 14 days for a total of 21 doses in 28 days

Aplastic anemia

• *Adult:* **IV** 10-20 mg/kg/day × 8-14 days, then every other day for up to 21 total doses

Available forms: Inj 50 mg horse gamma globulin/ml

SIDE EFFECTS

Renal transplant

CNS: Fever, chills, headache, dizziness, weakness, faintness, **seizures**

CV: Chest pain, hyper/hypotension, tachycardia

GI: Diarrhea, nausea, vomiting, epigastric pain, **GI bleeding**

INTEG: Rash, pruritus, urticaria, wheal

SYST: **Anaphylaxis**

Aplastic anemia
CNS: Fever, chills, headache, **seizures,** light-headedness, encephalitis, postviral encephalopathy
CV: Bradycardia, myocarditis, irregularity
GI: Nausea, LFTs abnormality
HEMA: **Thrombocytopenia**
Contraindications: Hypersensitivity to this product or equine/leporine protein, acute viral illness
Precautions: Pregnancy (C), breastfeeding, children, severe renal/hepatic disease, leukopenia, thrombocytopenia
Black Box Warning: Infection, neoplastic disease

PHARMACOKINETICS

Onset rapid, half-life 5-7 days

NURSING CONSIDERATIONS

Assess:
- For infection; if infection occurs, evaluation will be needed to continue therapy
- Renal studies: BUN, creatinine at least monthly during treatment, 3 mo after treatment
- Hepatic studies: alk phos, AST, ALT, bilirubin
- CBC with differential

Administer:
- Do not infuse <4 hr; usually given over 4-8 hr

Aplastic anemia
- Skin testing must be completed prior to treatment; use intradermal inj of 0.1 ml of a 1:1000 dilution (5 mcg horse IgG) in 0.9% NaCl, if a wheal or rash >10 mm or both, use caution during inf
- Dilute in saline sol before inf; invert IV bag so undiluted product does not contact the air inside; concentration should not be >1 mg/ml; do not shake
- Keep emergency equipment nearby for severe allergic reaction

Evaluate:
- Therapeutic response: absence of rejection; hematologic recovery (aplastic anemia)

Teach patient/family:
- To report fever, chills, sore throat, fatigue, since serious infections may occur
- To use contraceptive measures during treatment, for 12 wk after ending therapy

mafenide topical

See Appendix B

magaldrate (OTC)

(mag′al-drate)
Riopan
Func. class.: Antacid
Chem. class.: Aluminum/magnesium hydroxide

Action: Neutralizes gastric acidity; product is dissolved in gastric contents; combination of aluminum, magnesium
Uses: Antacid, hyperacidity, indigestion, heartburn, hiatal hernia
Unlabeled uses: Gastritis prophylaxis, peptic ulcer disease (adjunct), duodenal, gastric ulcers, reflux esophagitis

DOSAGE AND ROUTES

- *Adult/child/geriatric:* **SUSP** 5-10 ml (480-1080 mg) with water between meals, at bedtime

Available forms: Susp 540 mg/5 ml

SIDE EFFECTS

GI: Constipation, diarrhea, anorexia
META: Hypermagnesemia, hypophosphatemia
Contraindications: Hypersensitivity to this product or benzyl alcohol
Precautions: Pregnancy (C), geriatric patients, fluid restriction, decreased GI motility, GI obstruction, dehydration, renal disease, sodium-restricted diets, bone disease, hypertension, appendicitis, diverticulitis, ulcerative colitis, neonates/infants, hypermagnesemia, hypophosphatemia

PHARMACOKINETICS

PO: Onset 10-20 min, duration 60 min

INTERACTIONS

Increase: action when taken in large amounts—quinidine, flecainide, amphetamines

Decrease: absorption of chlordiazepoxide, cimetidine, corticosteroids, fluoroquinolones, iron salts, isoniazid, ketoconazole, phenothiazines, phenytoin, salicylates, tetracyclines, itraconazole, biphosphonates, gabapentin, thyroid hormones, cephalosporins, protease inhibitors

Decrease: action when taken in large amounts—salicylates

NURSING CONSIDERATIONS

Assess:

• GI status: location of pain, intensity, characteristics, heartburn, hematemesis

• Serum magnesium levels with impaired renal function; calcium, phosphate, potassium if using long term; may increase calcium, decrease phosphate

• Constipation: increase bulk in diet if needed

Administer:

• Laxatives or stool softeners if constipation occurs

• After shaking; give between meals and bedtime

Evaluate:

• Therapeutic response: absence of pain, decreased acidity

Teach patient/family:

• To separate enteric-coated products and antacid by 2 hr

• To notify prescriber immediately of coffee-ground emesis, emesis with frank blood, black tarry stools

magnesium salts (OTC)
(mag-nee'zee-um)

magnesium chloride (℞)
Chloromag, Slo-Mag

magnesium citrate (OTC)
Citrate of Magnesia, Citroma, CitroMag ♣

magnesium gluconate (OTC)
Almoate, Magonate, Magtrate OTC

magnesium oxide (OTC)
Mag-Ox 400, Maox, Uro-Mag

magnesium hydroxide (OTC)
Phillips' Magnesia Tablets, Phillips' Milk of Magnesia, MOM

magnesium sulfate (OTC, ℞)
epsom salts; magnesium sulfate (IV)—**HIGH ALERT**

Func. class.: Electrolyte; anticonvulsant; saline laxative, antacid

Action: Increases osmotic pressure, draws fluid into colon, neutralizes HCl

Uses: Constipation, bowel preparation before surgery or exam, anticonvulsant in preeclampsia, eclampsia (magnesium sulfate), electrolyte

Unlabeled uses: *Magnesium sulfate:* persistent pulmonary hypertension of the newborn (PPHN), cardiac arrest, CPR, digitoxin/digoxin toxicity, premature labor, seizure prophylaxis, status asthmaticus, torsade de pointes, ventricular fibrillation/tachycardia

DOSAGE AND ROUTES

Laxative

• *Adult:* **PO** (Milk of Magnesia) 15-60 ml at bedtime

• *Adult and child >12 yr:* **PO** (magnesium sulfate) 15 g in 8 oz H_2O; **PO** (Concentrated Milk of Magnesia) 10-20 ml; **PO** (magnesium citrate) 5-10 oz at bedtime
• *Child 2-5 yr:* **PO** (Milk of Magnesia) 5-15 ml/day

Prevention of magnesium deficiency
• *Adult and child ≥10 yr:* **PO** (male) 350-400 mg/day; (female) 280-300 mg/day; (breastfeeding) 335-350 mg/day; (pregnancy) 320 mg/day
• *Child 8-10 yr:* **PO** 170 mg/day
• *Child 4-7 yr:* **PO** 120 mg/day

Magnesium sulfate deficiency
• *Adult:* **PO** 200-400 mg in divided doses tid-qid; **IM** 1 g q6hr × 4 doses; **IV** 5 g (severe)
• *Child 6-12 yr:* **PO** 3-6 mg/kg/day in divided doses tid-qid

Pre-eclampsia/eclampsia magnesium sulfate
• *Adult:* **IM/IV** 4-5 g IV inf; with 5 g **IM** in each gluteus, then 5 g q4hr or 4 g **IV INF**, then 1-2 g/hr **CONT INF**, max 40 g/day or 20 g/48 hr in severe renal disease

Persistent pulmonary hypertension of the newborn (PPHN) in mechanically ventilated neonates (unlabeled)
• *Premature infants >33 wk and term neonates:* **IV** (magnesium sulfate) 200 mg/kg over 20-30 min, then **CONT IV INF** 20-150 mg/kg/hr to maintain blood magnesium levels at 3.5-5.5 mmol/L

Status asthmaticus (unlabeled)
• *Adult:* **IV** (magnesium sulfate) 2 g
• *Child:* **IV INF** (PALS) (magnesium sulfate) 25-50 mg/kg diluted in D_5W and given over 10-20 min, max 2 g/dose

Premature labor (unlabeled)
• *Adult:* **IV INF** (magnesium sulfate) 4-6 g given as a loading dose over 20-30 min, then 2-4 g/hr **CONT INF;** use infusion pump until contractions cease; continue inf at lowest dose over 12-24 hr; **PO** (magnesium chloride/gluconate/oxide) 648-1200 mg/day elemental magnesium in divided dose

Torsade de pointes/cardiac dysrhythmias with hypomagnesemia (unlabeled)
• *Adult:* **IV** (magnesium sulfate) use ACLS guidelines or 1-2 g in 50-100 ml D_5W given over 5-20 min in emergent cases or over 5-60 min

Available forms: *Chloride:* sus rel tabs 535 mg (64 mg Mg) enteric tabs 833 mg (100 mg Mg); *citrate:* oral sol 240, 296, 300 ml bottles (77 mEq/100 ml); *oxide:* tabs 400 mg; caps 140 mg; *hydroxide:* liq 400 mg/5 ml; conc liq 800 mg/5 ml; chew tabs 300, 600 mg; *sulfate:* powder for oral; bulk packages; epsom salts, bulk packages; inj 10%, 12.5%, 25%, 50%

SIDE EFFECTS

CNS: Muscle weakness, flushing, sweating, confusion, sedation, depressed reflexes, **flaccid paralysis,** hypothermia
CV: Hypotension, heart block, **circulatory collapse,** vasodilation
GI: Nausea, vomiting, anorexia, cramps, diarrhea
HEMA: Prolonged bleeding time
META: Electrolyte, fluid imbalances
RESP: Respiratory depression/paralysis

Contraindications: Hypersensitivity, abdominal pain, nausea/vomiting, obstruction, acute surgical abdomen, rectal bleeding, heart block, myocardial damage

Precautions: Pregnancy (A); (B) (magnesium sulfate), renal/cardiac disease

PHARMACOKINETICS

PO: Onset 1-2 hr
IM: Onset 1 hr, duration 4 hr
IV: Duration ½ hr
Excreted by kidney, effective anticonvulsant serum levels 2.5-7.5 mEq/L

INTERACTIONS

Increase: effect of neuromuscular blockers
Increase: hypotension—antihypertensives
Decrease: absorption of tetracyclines, fluoroquinolones, nitrofurantoin
Decrease: effect of digoxin

NURSING CONSIDERATIONS

Assess:

• I&O ratio; check for decrease in urinary output
• Cause of constipation; lack of fluids, bulk, exercise
• Cramping, rectal bleeding, nausea, vomiting; product should be discontinued
⚠ Magnesium toxicity: thirst, confusion, decrease in reflexes

Administer:

PO route

• With 8 oz H_2O
• Refrigerate magnesium citrate before giving
• Shake susp before using as antacid at least 2 hr after meals

IM route (magnesium sulfate)

• Give deeply in gluteal site

IV route (magnesium sulfate)

• Only when calcium gluconate available for magnesium toxicity

IV, direct route

• IV undiluted 1.5 ml of 10% sol over 1 min

Intermittent IV INF route

• May dilute to 20% sol, infuse over 3 hr
• IV at less than 150 mg/min; circulatory collapse may occur
• Use inf pump

Additive compatibilities: Cephalothin, chloramphenicol, cisplatin, heparin, hydrocortisone, isoproterenol, meropenem, methyldopate, norepinephrine, penicillin G potassium, potassium phosphate, verapamil

Y-site compatibilities: Acyclovir, aldesleukin, amifostine, amikacin, ampicillin, aztreonam, cefazolin, cefoperazone, cefotaxime, cefoxitin, cephalothin, cephapirin, chloramphenicol, cisatracurium, DOBUTamine, doxycycline, DOXOrubicin liposome, enalaprilat, erythromycin, esmolol, famotidine, fludarabine, gallium, gentamicin, granisetron, heparin, hydromorphone, idarubicin, insulin, kanamycin, labetalol, meperidine, metronidazole, minocycline, morphine, moxalactam, nafcillin, ondansetron, oxacillin, paclitaxel, penicillin G potassium, piperacillin, piperacillin/tazobactam, potassium chloride, propofol, remifentanil, sargramostim, thiotepa, ticarcillin, tobramycin, trimethoprim-sulfamethoxazole, vancomycin, vit B complex/C

Evaluate:

• Therapeutic response: decreased constipation

Teach patient/family:

• Not to use laxatives for long-term therapy; bowel tone will be lost
• That chilling helps the taste of magnesium citrate
• To shake suspension well
• To not give at bedtime as a laxative; may interfere with sleep
• To give citrus fruit after administering to counteract unpleasant taste

mannitol (℞)

(man′i-tole)
mannitol, Osmitrol, Resectisol
Func. class.: Diuretic, osmotic
Chem. class.: Hexahydric alcohol

M

Action: Acts by increasing osmolarity of glomerular filtrate, which inhibits reabsorption of water and electrolytes and increases urinary output

Uses: Edema, promote systemic diuresis in cerebral edema, decrease intraocular pressure, improve renal function in acute renal failure, chemical poisoning

DOSAGE AND ROUTES

Oliguria, prevention

• *Adult:* **IV** 50-100 g of a 5%-25% sol, may use test dose 0.2 g/kg over 3-5 min

Oliguria, treatment

• *Adult:* **IV** 300-400 mg/kg of a 20%-25% sol up to 100 g of a 15%-20% sol over 30-60 min
• *Child (unlabeled):* **IV** 0.25-2 g/kg as a 15%-20% sol, run over 2-6 hr (maintenance)

Intraocular pressure/ICP

• *Adult:* **IV** 1.5-2 g/kg of a 15%-25% sol over 30-60 min
• *Child:* **IV** 1-2 g/kg (30-60 g/m^2) as a 15%-20% sol run over 2-6 hr

Renal failure

• *Adult:* **IV** 50-200 g/24 hr, adjusting to maintain output of 30-50 mg/hr

Diuresis in drug intoxication

• *Adult and child >12 yr:* 5%-10% sol continuously up to 200 g **IV,** while maintaining 100-500 ml urine output/hr

Available forms: Inj 5%, 10%, 15%, 20%, 25%; GU irrigation: 5%

SIDE EFFECTS

CNS: Dizziness, headache, **seizures, rebound increased ICP,** confusion

CV: Edema, thrombophlebitis, hypo/hypertension, **tachycardia,** angina-like chest pains, fever, chills, **CHF, circulatory overload**

EENT: Loss of hearing, blurred vision, nasal congestion, decreased intraocular pressure

ELECT: Fluid, electrolyte imbalances, *acidosis,* electrolyte loss, dehydration, hypo/hyperkalemia

GI: Nausea, vomiting, dry mouth, diarrhea

GU: Marked diuresis, urinary retention, thirst

RESP: Pulmonary congestion

Contraindications: Active intracranial bleeding, hypersensitivity, anuria, severe pulmonary congestion, edema, severe dehydration, progressive heart, renal failure

Precautions: Pregnancy (C), breastfeeding, geriatric patients, dehydration, severe renal disease, CHF, electrolyte imbalances

PHARMACOKINETICS

IV: Onset 30-60 min for diuresis, ½-1 hr for intraocular pressure, 25 min for cerebrospinal fluid; duration 4-6 hr for intraocular pressure, 3-8 hr for cerebrospinal fluid; excreted in urine, half-life 100 min

INTERACTIONS

Increase: elimination of mannitol—lithium

Drug/Food

• Potassium foods: increased hyperkalemia

Drug/Lab Test

Interference: inorganic phosphorus, ethylene glycol

NURSING CONSIDERATIONS

Assess:

• Weight, I&O daily to determine fluid loss; effect of product may be decreased if used daily; output q hr prn

• Rate, depth, rhythm of respiration, effect of exertion

• B/P lying, standing; postural hypotension may occur

• Electrolytes: K, Na, Cl; include BUN, CBC, serum creatinine, blood pH, ABGs, CVP, PAP

• Signs of metabolic acidosis: drowsiness, restlessness

• Signs of hypokalemia: postural hypotension, malaise, fatigue, tachycardia, leg cramps, weakness, or hyperkalemia

• Rashes, temp daily

• Confusion, especially in geriatric patients; take safety precautions if needed

• Hydration including skin turgor, thirst, dry mucous membranes

• For blurred vision, pain in eyes, before and during treatment (increased intraocular pressure); neurologic checks, intracranial pressure during treatment (increased intracranial pressure)

Administer:

IV route

• In 15%-25% sol with filter; give over ½-1½ hr; rapid inf may worsen CHF; warm in hot water and shake to dissolve crystals

• Test dose in severe oliguria, 0.2 g/kg over 3-5 min; if no urine increase, give second test dose; if no response, reassess patient

Irrigation

• 100 ml of 25%/900 ml of sterile water for inj (2.5% sol)

Additive compatibilities: Amikacin, bretylium, cefamandole, cefoxitin, cimetidine, cisplatin, DOPamine, fosphenytoin, furosemide, gentamicin, metoclopramide, nizatidine, ofloxacin, ondansetron, sodium bicarbonate, tobramycin, verapamil

Y-site compatibilities: Allopurinol, amifostine, amphotericin B cholesteryl, aztreonam, cisatracurium, cladribine, docetaxel, etoposide, fludarabine, fluorouracil, gatifloxacin, gemcitabine, idarubicin, linezolid, melphalan, ondansetron, paclitaxel, piperacillin, propofol, remifentanil, sargramostim, teniposide, thiotepa, vinorelbine

Evaluate:
- Therapeutic response: improvement in edema of feet, legs, sacral area daily if medication is being used in CHF; decreased intraocular pressure, prevention of hypokalemia, increased excretion of toxic substances; decreased ICP

Teach patient/family:
- To rise slowly from lying or sitting position
- The reason for and method of treatment
- To report signs of electrolyte imbalance; confusion

Treatment of overdose: Discontinue inf; correct fluid, electrolyte imbalances; hemodialysis; monitor hydration, CV status, renal function

maraviroc (℞)

(mah-rav′er-rock)

Selzentry

Func. class.: Antiretroviral

Chem. class.: Fusion inhibitor

Action: Interferes with entry into HIV-1 by inhibiting the fusion of the virus and cell membrane

Uses: CCR5-tropic HIV in combination with other antiretroviral agents in treating experienced patients

DOSAGE AND ROUTES

Those not taking any CYP3A inducers/inhibitors
- *Adult:* **PO** 300 mg bid

Those taking CYP3A4 inhibitors with/without a CYP3A inducer
- *Adult:* **PO** 150 mg bid

Those taking CYP3A4 inducers without a strong CYP3A inhibitor
- *Adult:* **PO** 600 mg bid

Available forms: Tabs 150, 300 mg

SIDE EFFECTS

CV: **MI, cardiac ischemia, orthostatic hypotension**

CNS: Dizziness, depression, **viral meningitis,** disturbances in consciousness, peripheral neuropathy, paresthesia, dysesthesia, fever

EENT: Gingival hyperplasia

GI: Diarrhea, constipation, dyspepsia, **pseudomembranous colitis, hepatotoxicity**

INTEG: Rash, urticaria, pruritus, folliculitis

MS: Joint pain, leg pain, muscle cramps

RESP: Cough, upper respiratory tract infection, sinusitis, bronchitis, pneumonia, **bronchospasm, obstruction**

SYST: Herpes virus

Contraindications: Hypersensitivity

Precautions: Pregnancy (B), Asian patients, breastfeeding, renal/hepatic/cardiac disease, electrolyte imbalance, dehydration, immune reconstitution syndrome, infection, MI, orthostatic hypotension, children, geriatric patients

Black Box Warning: Hepatitis

PHARMACOKINETICS

Metabolized by P450 system; CYP3A metabolism; excreted 20% urine, 76% feces, protein binding 76%, terminal half-life 14-18 hr

INTERACTIONS

Increase: maraviroc levels—CYP3A inhibitors (amiodarone, aprepitant, chloramphenicol, clarithromycin, conivaptan, cycloSPORINE, dalfopristin, danazol, diltiazem, erythromycin, estradiol, fluconazole, fluvoxamine, imatinib, isoniazid, itraconazole, ketoconazole, miconazole, nefazodone, niCARdipine, propoxyphene, RU-486, tamoxifen, telithromycin, troleandomycin, verapamil, voriconazole, zafirlukast)

M

Decrease: maraviroc levels—CYP3A4 inducers (efavirenz, aminoglutethimide, barbiturates, bexaroten, bosentan, carbamazepine, dexamethasone, griseofulvin, modafinil, nafcillin, oxcarbazepine, phenytoin, fosphenytoin, rifabutin, rifampin, rifapentine, topiramate, tipranavir)

Drug/Food

- High fat meal decreases absorption 33%

NURSING CONSIDERATIONS

Assess:

- Signs of infection
- Blood studies: CD_4, T-cell count, plasma HIV RNA
- Renal studies: serum creatinine
- C&S before product therapy; product may be taken as soon as culture is taken; repeat C&S after treatment; determine the presence of other infections
- Bowel pattern before, during treatment
- Skin eruptions: rash, urticaria, itching
- Allergies before treatment, reaction of each medication

Administer:

- May give without regard to meals, with 8 oz of water

Perform/provide:

- Storage at room temperature

Evaluate:

- Therapeutic response: improvement in CD4, viral load, T-cell count

Teach patient/family:

- To take as prescribed; if dose is missed, take as soon as remembered up to 1 hr before next dose; do not double dose; that product does not cure the condition
- That product does not cure infection, just controls symptoms and does not prevent infecting others

⚠ To report sore throat, fever, fatigue (may indicate superinfection)

- That product must be taken in equal intervals around the clock to maintain blood levels for duration of therapy
- To notify prescriber of side effects

mebendazole (℞)

(me-ben′da-zole)

Func. class.: Anthelmintic

Chem. class.: Carbamate

Action: Inhibits glucose uptake, degeneration of cytoplasmic microtubules in the cell; interferes with absorption, secretory function

Uses: Pinworms, roundworms, hookworms, whipworms, thread-worms, pork tapeworms, dwarf tapeworms, beef tapeworms, hydatid cyst

DOSAGE AND ROUTES

- *Adult and child >2 yr:* **PO** 100 mg as a single dose (pinworms) or bid × 3 days (whipworms, roundworms, or hookworms); course may be repeated in 3 wk if needed, max 200 mg/day

Available forms: Chew tabs 100 mg

SIDE EFFECTS

CNS: Dizziness, fever, headache, **seizures (rare)**

GI: Transient diarrhea, abdominal pain, nausea, vomiting, constipation, **hepatitis**

INTEG: Rash

Contraindications: Hypersensitivity

Precautions: Pregnancy (C) (1st trimester), breastfeeding, children <2 yr, Crohn's disease, hepatic disease, inflammatory bowel disease, ulcerative colitis

PHARMACOKINETICS

PO: Peak ½-7 hr; excreted in feces primarily (metabolites), small amount in urine (unchanged); highly bound to plasma proteins 95%

INTERACTIONS

Decrease: mebendazole effect—carbamazepine, hydantoins

Drug/Food

Increase: absorption—high-fat meal

NURSING CONSIDERATIONS

Assess:

- Stools during entire treatment; specimens must be sent to lab while still warm, also 1-3 wk after treatment is completed
- For allergic reaction: rash (rare)
- For diarrhea during expulsion of worms; avoid self-contamination with patient's feces
- For infection in other family members, since infection from person to person is common
- Blood studies: AST, ALT, alk phos, BUN, CBC during treatment

Administer:

- May be crushed, chewed, swallowed whole, mixed with food
- PO after meals to avoid GI symptoms
- Second course after 3 wk if needed; usually recommended

Perform/provide:

- Storage in tight container

Evaluate:

- Therapeutic response: expulsion of worms and 3 negative stool cultures after completion of treatment

Teach patient/family:

- Proper hygiene after BM, including hand-washing technique; tell patient to avoid putting fingers in mouth; clean fingernails
- That infected person should sleep alone; do not shake bed linen, change bed linen daily, wash in hot water, change and wash undergarments daily
- To clean toilet daily with disinfectant (green soap solution)
- The need for compliance with dosage schedule, duration of treatment
- To wear shoes, wash all fruits and vegetables well before eating; use commercial fruit/vegetable cleaner
- That all members of the family should be treated (pinworms)
- To report jaundice, liver pain

mecasermin (℞)

(mec-a'sir-men)

Increlex

Func. class.: Biologic response modifier; insulin-like growth factor

Action: Stimulates growth; IGF-1 is the principal hormonal mediator of statural growth; GH binds to its receptor in the liver and other tissues

Uses: Growth failure in children with severe primary insulin-like growth factor-1 (IGF-1) deficiency (primary IGFD) or with growth hormone (GH) gene deletion who have developed neutralizing antibodies to GH

Unlabeled uses: ALS

DOSAGE AND ROUTES

- *Child:* **SUBCUT** 0.04-0.08 mg/kg (40-80 mcg/kg) bid; if well tolerated for 1 wk, may increase by 0.04 mg/kg/dose, max 0.12 mg/kg bid

Available forms: Inj 10 mg/ml

M

SIDE EFFECTS

CNS: Headache, **seizures,** dizziness, cardiac valvulopathy, increased intracranial pressure

CV: Cardiac murmur

EENT: Ear pain, otitis media, abnormal tympanometry, papilledema, visual impairment, tonsillar hypertrophy

ENDO: **Hypoglycemia, ketosis, hypothyroidism**

GI: Vomiting

HEMA: Thymus hypertrophy

MISC: Bruising, lipohypertrophy, hypersensitivity reactions, inj site reaction

MS: Arthralgia, joint pain, slipped upper femoral epiphysis

RESP: Snoring, **apnea**

SYST: **Antibodies to growth hormone**

Contraindications: Hypersensitivity, benzyl alcohol, closed epiphyses, active/suspected neoplasia, IV use

Precautions: Pregnancy (C), breastfeeding, children <2 yr, diabetes mellitus, hypothyroidism, lymphoid tissue hypertrophy, increased intracranial pressure, malnutrition, scoliosis, sleep apnea

PHARMACOKINETICS

Bioavailability almost 100%, metabolized in liver/kidney, half-life 5.8 hr

INTERACTIONS

Increase: hypoglycemia—antidiabetics, corticosteroids

NURSING CONSIDERATIONS

Assess:

- Monitor preprandial glucose at beginning of treatment and until well tolerated
- By funduscopic exam at beginning and periodically during treatment
- For allergic reactions; if present, interrupt treatment and notify prescriber
- Growth rate of child at intervals during treatment

Administer:

SUBCUT route

- Give within 20 min of meal or snack
- Rotate inj site; use sterile, disposable syringe/needles; use small-volume syringe for accurate measurement

Perform/provide:

- Storage in refrigerator before opening, avoid freezing; after opening, stable for 30 days after initial vial entry, store in refrigerator, do not use if particulate matter is present, avoid direct light, do not use after expiration date

Evaluate:

- Therapeutic response: growth in children

Teach patient/family:

- That treatment may continue for years; regular assessments are required
- To avoid hazardous activities, driving within 2-3 hr of dosing
- Correct administration and needle disposal

mechlorethamine (℞)

(me-klor-eth′a-meen)

Mustargen, nitrogen mustard

Func. class.: Antineoplastic alkylating agent

Chem. class.: Nitrogen mustard

Action: Responsible for cross-linking DNA strands leading to cell death; rapidly degraded, a vesicant; activity is not cell cycle phase specific

Uses: Hodgkin's disease, leukemias, lymphomas, lymphosarcoma; ovarian, breast, lung carcinoma; neoplastic effusions, pericardial/peritoneal/pleural effusion, polycythemia vera

DOSAGE AND ROUTES

- *Adult:* **IV** 0.4 mg/kg or 6 mg/m^2 as a single dose or 2-4 divided doses over 2-4 days; second course after 3 wk depending on blood cell count

Neoplastic effusions

- *Adult:* **Intracavity** 0.2-0.4 mg/kg

Polycythemia vera

- *Adult:* **IV** 0.4 mg/kg or 6 mg/m^2 as a single dose q mo or as needed

Available forms: Inj 10 mg

SIDE EFFECTS

CNS: Headache, dizziness, drowsiness, paresthesia, peripheral neuropathy, **coma**

EENT: Tinnitus, hearing loss

GI: Nausea, vomiting, diarrhea, stomatitis, weight loss, colitis, **hepatotoxicity**

HEMA: **Thrombocytopenia, leukopenia, agranulocytosis,** anemia

INTEG: Alopecia, pruritus, herpes zoster, extravasation

Contraindications: Breastfeeding, acute herpes zoster, infection

Black Box Warning: Pregnancy (D), myelosuppression

Precautions: Radiation therapy, chronic lymphocytic leukopenia

Black Box Warning: Accidental exposure, extravasation

PHARMACOKINETICS

Metabolized in liver, excreted in urine

INTERACTIONS

Increase: blood dyscrasias—amphotericin B

Increase: bleeding—aspirin, anticoagulants, NSAIDs

Increase: toxicity—antineoplastics, radiation

Decrease: antibody reaction—live virus vaccines

NURSING CONSIDERATIONS

Assess:

- CBC, differential, platelet count q wk; withhold product if WBC is <1000/mm^3 or platelet count is <75,000/mm^3; notify prescriber, recovery of WBCs, platelets within 20 days
- Renal function tests: BUN, serum uric acid, urine CCr before, during therapy
- I&O ratio; report fall in urine output of 30 ml/hr
- Monitor temp (may indicate beginning infection); no rectal temps
- Hepatic studies before, during therapy (bilirubin, AST, ALT, LDH) as needed or monthly
- Bleeding: hematuria, guaiac, bruising or petechiae, mucosa or orifices
- Jaundiced skin and sclera, dark urine, clay-colored stools, itchy skin, abdominal pain, fever, diarrhea
- Effects of alopecia on body image; discuss feelings about body changes
- Buccal cavity for dryness, sores, ulceration, white patches, oral pain, bleeding, dysphagia
- Local irritation, pain, burning, discoloration at inj site, a vesicant, watch for extravasation

⚠ Symptoms indicating severe allergic reaction: rash, pruritus, urticaria, purpuric skin lesions, itching, flushing

Administer:

- After using guidelines for preparation of cytotoxic products
- Antiemetic and dexamethasone 30-60 min before giving product and prn
- IV after diluting 10 mg/10 ml sterile H_2O or NaCl; leave needle in vial, shake, withdraw dose, give through Y-tube or 3-way stopcock or directly over 3-5 min
- Watch for infiltration; infiltrate area with isotonic sodium thiosulfate; apply ice for 6-12 hr
- Topical or systemic analgesics for pain
- Local or systemic products for infection

Y-site compatibilities: Amifostine, aztreonam, filgrastim, fludarabine, granisetron, melphalan, ondansetron, sargramostim, teniposide, vinorelbine

Perform/provide:

- Storage at room temperature in dry form
- Increase fluid intake to 2-3 L/day to prevent urate deposits, calculi formation
- Diet low in purines: organ meats (kidney, liver), dried beans, peas to maintain alkaline urine
- Preparation under hood using gloves and mask
- Rinsing of mouth tid-qid with water, club soda; brushing of teeth bid-tid with soft brush or cotton-tipped applicators for stomatitis; use unwaxed dental floss
- Warm compresses at inj site for inflammation if no extravasation

Evaluate:

- Therapeutic response: decreased tumor size, spread of malignancy

Teach patient/family:

- The rationale for and techniques of protective isolation
- That sterility, amenorrhea can occur; reversible after discontinuing treatment
- That hair may be lost during treatment; a wig or hairpiece may make patient feel better; new hair may be different in color, texture
- To avoid foods with citric acid, hot or rough texture

• To report any bleeding, white spots, or ulcerations in mouth to prescriber; tell patient to examine mouth daily
• To report signs of infection: fever, sore throat, flulike symptoms
• To report signs of anemia: fatigue, headache, faintness, shortness of breath, irritability
• To avoid use of razors, commercial mouthwash
• To avoid use of aspirin products, NSAIDs
• To notify prescriber if pregnancy is suspected; to use contraception during treatment

meclizine (OTC, ℞)

(mek′li-zeen)

Antivert, Bonamine ♣, Bonine, Dramamine Less Drowsy Formula, meclizine HCl, Medivert, Travel Sickness, Wal-Dram II

Func. class.: Antiemetic, antihistamine, anticholinergic

Chem. class.: H_1-Receptor antagonist, piperazine derivative

Action: Acts centrally by blocking chemoreceptor trigger zone, which in turn acts on vomiting center

Uses: Vertigo, motion sickness

DOSAGE AND ROUTES

Vertigo

• *Adult/adolescent:* **PO** 25-100 mg/day in divided doses

Motion sickness

• *Adult/adolescent:* **PO** 25-50 mg 1 hr before traveling, repeat dose q24hr prn

Available forms: Tabs 12.5, 25, 50 mg; chew tabs 25 mg; caps 25, 30 mg

SIDE EFFECTS

CNS: ***Drowsiness,*** fatigue, restlessness, headache, insomnia

CV: Hypotension

EENT: Dry mouth, blurred vision

GI: Nausea, anorexia, constipation, increased appetite

GU: Urinary retention

Contraindications: Hypersensitivity to cyclizines, shock

Precautions: Pregnancy (B), breastfeeding, children, geriatric patients, closed-angle glaucoma, urinary retention, prostatic hypertrophy, CV disease, hypertension, seizure disorder

PHARMACOKINETICS

PO: Onset 1 hr, duration 8-24 hr, half-life 6 hr

INTERACTIONS

Increase: effect of alcohol, opioids, other CNS depressants

Drug/Herb

Increase: anticholinergic effect—corkwood, henbane leaf

Increase: sedative effect—hops, Jamaican dogwood, khat, senega

Drug/Lab Test

False negative: allergy skin testing

NURSING CONSIDERATIONS

Assess:

• VS, B/P

⚠ Signs of toxicity of other products or masking of symptoms of disease: brain tumor, intestinal obstruction

• Observe for drowsiness, dizziness, level of consciousness

• For nausea/vomiting after 1 hr

Administer:

PO route

• Tablets may be swallowed whole, chewed, or allowed to dissolve; give with food to decrease GI upset

• Lowest possible dose in geriatric patients, anticholinergic effects

Evaluate:

• Therapeutic response: absence of dizziness, vomiting

Teach patient/family:

• That a false-negative result may occur with skin testing for allergies; these procedures should not be scheduled for 4 days after discontinuing use

• To avoid hazardous activities, activities requiring alertness; dizziness may occur; instruct patient to request assistance with ambulation
• To avoid alcohol, other depressants; breastfeeding

* medroxyPROGESTERone (℞)

(me-drox'ee-proe-jess'te-rone)
Amen, Depo-Provera, medroxyPROGESTERone, Provera
Func. class.: Antineoplastic, hormone, contraceptive
Chem. class.: Progesterone derivative

Do not confuse:
medroxyPROGESTERone/methylPREDNISolone
Amen/Ambien
Provera/Premarin/Covera

Action: Inhibits secretion of pituitary gonadotropins, which prevents follicular maturation and ovulation; stimulates growth of mammary tissue; antineoplastic action against endometrial cancer

Uses: Uterine bleeding (abnormal), secondary amenorrhea, prevent endometrial changes associated with estrogen replacement therapy (ERT), contraceptive

Unlabeled uses: Hot flashes, symptoms of menopause; paraphilia (men), hot flashes (men) in prostate cancer

DOSAGE AND ROUTES

Secondary amenorrhea
• *Adult:* **PO** 5-10 mg/day × 5-10 days

Uterine bleeding
• *Adult:* **PO** 5-10 mg/day × 5-10 days starting on 16th or 21st day of menstrual cycle

With ERT
• *Adult:* **PO** 5-10 mg daily × 10-14 or more days/mo (sequential estrogen); 2.5-5 mg daily (continuous estrogen)

Contraceptive
• *Adult:* **IM** 150 mg q12wk

Hot flashes/symptoms of menopause (unlabeled)
• *Adult (female):* **PO** 20 mg/day; **IM** 150 mg q mo

Hot flashes (men) in prostate cancer (unlabeled)
• *Adult (male):* **IM** Depot 150 or 400 mg

Available forms: Tabs 2.5, 5, 10 mg; inj susp 50, 150, 400 mg/ml; 104 mg/0.65 ml

SIDE EFFECTS

CNS: Dizziness, headache, migraines, depression, fatigue, nervousness
CV: Hypotension, thrombophlebitis, edema, **thromboembolism, stroke, PE, MI**
EENT: Diplopia
GI: Nausea, vomiting, anorexia, cramps, increased weight, **cholestatic jaundice,** abdominal pain
GU: Amenorrhea, cervical erosion, breakthrough bleeding, dysmenorrhea, vaginal candidiasis, breast changes, *gynecomastia, testicular atrophy, impotence,* endometriosis, **spontaneous abortion**
INTEG: Rash, urticaria, acne, hirsutism, alopecia, oily skin, seborrhea, purpura, melasma, photosensitivity
META: Hyperglycemia
MS: Decreased bone density
SYST: **Angioedema, anaphylaxis**

Contraindications: Pregnancy (X), breast cancer, hypersensitivity, thromboembolic disorders, reproductive cancer, genital bleeding (abnormal, undiagnosed), missed abortion

Precautions: Breastfeeding, hypertension, asthma, blood dyscrasias, gallbladder disease, CHF, diabetes mellitus, bone disease, depression, migraine headache, seizure disorders, renal/hepatic disease, family history of cancer of breast or reproductive tract, bone mineral density loss, ocular disorders

Black Box Warning: Cardiac disease, dementia, osteoporosis

M

PHARMACOKINETICS

PO: Duration 24 hr, excreted in urine and feces, metabolized in liver

INTERACTIONS

Decrease: medroxyPROGESTERone action—aminoglutethimide

Drug/Lab Test

Increase: alk phos, sodium (urine), pregnanediol, amino acids

Decrease: GTT, HDL

NURSING CONSIDERATIONS

Assess:

⚠ Symptoms indicating severe allergic reaction, angioedema, have epinephrine and rescusitative equipment available

- Weight daily; notify prescriber of weekly weight gain >5 lb; bone mineral density
- B/P at beginning of treatment and periodically
- I&O ratio; be alert for decreasing urinary output, increasing edema
- Hepatic studies: ALT, AST, bilirubin, periodically during long-term therapy
- Edema, hypertension, cardiac symptoms, jaundice
- Mental status: affect, mood, behavioral changes, depression

Administer:

- Titrated dose; use lowest effective dose
- Oil solution deep in large muscle mass (IM); rotate sites
- With food or milk to decrease GI symptoms (PO)

Perform/provide:

- Storage in dark area

Evaluate:

- Therapeutic response: decreased abnormal uterine bleeding, absence of amenorrhea

Teach patient/family:

- To avoid sunlight or use sunscreen; photosensitivity can occur
- Cushingoid symptoms: weight gain, moon face, buffalo hump, acne

⚠ To report breast lumps, vaginal bleeding, edema, jaundice, dark urine, clay-colored stools, dyspnea, headache, blurred vision, abdominal pain, sudden change in speech/coordination, numbness or stiffness in legs, chest pain; male to report impotence or gynecomastia

- To report suspected pregnancy; fertility returns in 6-12 mo after discontinuing
- Long-term use decreases bone density; exercise and calcium supplements can help lessen this

medrysone ophthalmic

See Appendix B

megestrol (℞)

(me-jess'trole)

Megace, Megace ES, megestrol

Func. class.: Antineoplastic hormone

Chem. class.: Progestin

Do not confuse:

Megace/Reglan

Action: Affects endometrium by antiluteinizing effect; this is thought to bring about cell death

Uses: Breast, endometrial cancer, renal cell cancer; cachexia anorexia weight loss in AIDs

Unlabeled uses: Hot flashes in women (menopause) or men (prostate cancer), unexplained weight loss in geriatric patients, endometriosis, renal cell cancer (palliative), endometrial cancer, breast cancer (metastatic)

DOSAGE AND ROUTES

Endometrial/ovarian carcinoma

- *Adult:* **PO** 40-320 mg/day in divided doses

Breast carcinoma

- *Adult:* **PO** 40 mg qid or 160 mg/day

Anorexia (AIDS)

- *Adult:* **PO** 800 mg/day (oral susp) or 625 mg/day (ES)

Hot flashes (unlabeled)
• *Adult:* **PO** 20 mg/bid
Metastatic breast/prostate/renal cell cancer (unlabeled)
• *Adult:* **PO** 40 mg qid × ≥2 mo
Metastatic endometrial cancer (unlabeled)
• *Adult:* **PO** 40-320 mg/day in divided doses × ≥2 mo
Prostate cancer (unlabeled)
• *Adult:* **PO** 120 mg as a single daily dose in combination with diethylstilbesterol 0.1 mg

Available forms: Tabs 20, 40 mg; oral susp 40, 125 mg/ml

SIDE EFFECTS

CNS: Mood swings, insomnia
CV: **Thrombophlebitis, thromboembolism,** hypertension
ENDO: Adrenal insufficiency
GI: Nausea, vomiting, diarrhea, abdominal cramps, weight gain, flatus, indigestion
GU: Gynecomastia, fluid retention, hypercalcemia, vaginal bleeding, discharge, impotence, decreased libido
INTEG: Alopecia, rash, pruritus, purpura, itching, sweating
META: Hyperglycemia

Contraindications: Pregnancy (D), (tabs), (X) (susp) hypersensitivity
Precautions: Diabetes, thrombosis, adrenal insufficiency

PHARMACOKINETICS

PO: Duration 1-3 days; half-life 60 min; metabolized in liver; excreted in feces, breast milk; food increases bioavailability of oral sol

INTERACTIONS

• Do not use with dofetilide

Drug/Lab Test
Increase: alk phos, urinary sodium, urinary pregnanediol, plasma amino acids
Decrease: HDL, glucose tolerance test
False positive: urine glucose

NURSING CONSIDERATIONS

Assess:
• PSA levels in men (prostate cancer)
• I&O ratio; weights
• Effects of alopecia on body image; discuss feelings about body changes
⚠ Symptoms indicating severe allergic reaction: rash, pruritus, urticaria, purpuric skin lesions, itching, flushing
• Frequency of stools, characteristics: cramping, acidosis, signs of dehydration (rapid respirations, poor skin turgor, decreased urine output, dry skin, restlessness, weakness)
• Anorexia, nausea, vomiting, constipation, weakness, loss of muscle tone
⚠ Thrombophlebitis: Homans' sign, edema, pain in calf, thigh, notify prescriber immediately

Administer:
• Oral susp for AIDS patients; shake well
• Tablets for carcinoma

Perform/provide:
• Nutritious diet with iron, vitamin supplements as ordered
• Storage in tight container at room temperature

Evaluate:
• Therapeutic response: decreased tumor size, spread of malignancy; weight gain in AIDS patients; resolved dysfunctional uterine bleeding

Teach patient/family:
• To report vaginal bleeding
• That nonhormonal contraception should be used during and 4 mo after treatment
• That gynecomastia alopecia can occur; reversible after discontinuing treatment
⚠ To recognize signs of fluid retention, thromboemboli and to report immediately
• To monitor blood glucose if diabetic

M

meloxicam (℞)

(mel-ox'i-kam)

Mobic

Func. class.: Nonsteroidal anti-inflammatory drugs/nonopioid analgesic (NSAIDs)

Chem. class.: Oxicam

Action: Inhibits prostaglandin synthesis by decreasing an enzyme needed for biosynthesis; analgesic, antiinflammatory, antipyretic effects

Uses: Osteoarthritis, RA, juvenile arthritis

DOSAGE AND ROUTES

• *Adult:* **PO** 7.5 mg/day, may increase to 15 mg/day; max 15 mg/day

Available forms: Tabs 7.5, 15 mg; susp 7.5 mg/5 ml

SIDE EFFECTS

CNS: Dizziness, drowsiness, tremors, headache, nervousness, malaise, fatigue, insomnia, depression, **seizures**

CV: Hypertension, angina, **cardiac failure, MI,** hypotension, palpitations, **dysrhythmias,** tachycardia, stroke

EENT: Tinnitus, hearing loss, blurred vision

GI: Pancreatitis, nausea, colitis, GERD, vomiting, diarrhea, constipation, flatulence, cramps, dry mouth, peptic ulcer, **GI bleeding, perforation,** jaundice

GU: **Nephrotoxicity: dysuria, hematuria, oliguria, azotemia**

HEMA: **Blood dyscrasias,** anemia, prolonged bleeding

INTEG: Rash, urticaria, photosensitivity

SYST: **Angioedema, anaphylaxis, Stevens-Johnson syndrome, toxic epidermal necrolysis**

Contraindications: Pregnancy (D) 2nd/3rd trimester, breastfeeding; hypersensitivity, asthma, severe renal/hepatic disease, peptic ulcer disease, L&D, CV bleeding

Black Box Warning: Perioperative pain in CABG surgery

Precautions: Pregnancy (C), children, geriatric patients, bleeding disorders, GI disorders, cardiac disorders, hypersensitivity to other antiinflammatory agents, CCr <25 ml/min

Black Box Warning: GI bleeding, MI, stroke

PHARMACOKINETICS

PO: Peak 4-5 hr

IM: Peak 50 min

Half-life 15-20 hr, enters breast milk, <50% metabolized by liver, excreted by kidneys/feces, protein binding 99.4%

INTERACTIONS

Increase: nephrotoxicity—cycloSPORINE, tacrolimus

Increase: meloxicam action—phenytoin, sulfonamides, salicylates

Increase: action of aminoglycosides, hydantoins, diuretics, anticoagulants, lithium, methotrexate

Decrease: meloxicam action—cholestyramine

Decrease: action of β-blockers, ACE inhibitors, thiazides, other antihypertensives

Drug/Herb

Increase: gastric irritation—arginine, gossypol

Increase: NSAIDs effect—bearberry, bilberry

Increase: bleeding risk—bogbean, chondroitin

NURSING CONSIDERATIONS

Assess:

• Renal, hepatic, blood studies: BUN, creatinine, AST, ALT, Hgb before treatment, periodically thereafter

• Bleeding times; check for bruising, bleeding; test for occult blood in urine

⚠ For anaphylaxis and angioedema; emergency equipment should be nearby

⚠ Hepatic dysfunction: jaundice, yellow sclera and skin, clay-colored stools

• Audiometric, ophthalmic exam before, during, after treatment

• GI condition, hypertension, cardiac conditions

Administer:
- May take without regard to meals, to take with food for GI upset
- Take with full glass of water and sit upright for ½ hr

Perform/provide:
- Storage at room temperature

Evaluate:
- Therapeutic response: decreased pain, stiffness, swelling in joints, ability to move more easily

Teach patient/family:
- To report blurred vision or ringing, roaring in ears (may indicate toxicity)
- To avoid driving, other hazardous activities if dizziness or drowsiness occurs
- To report change in urine pattern, weight increase, edema, pain increase in joints, fever, blood in urine (indicates nephrotoxicity); to report rash, black stools, or continuing headache
- To avoid alcohol, aspirin, acetaminophen, NSAIDs without consulting prescriber
- To report use to all health care providers

⚠ High Alert

melphalan (℞)

(mel'fa-lan)

Alkeran

Func. class.: Antineoplastic, alkylating agent

Chem. class.: Nitrogen mustard

Do not confuse:
melphalan/Myleran

Action: Responsible for cross-linking DNA strands leading to cell death; activity is not cell cycle phase specific

Uses: Multiple myeloma, malignant melanoma, advanced ovarian cancer

Unlabeled uses: Breast, testicular, prostate carcinoma; osteogenic sarcoma, chronic myelogenous leukemia, non-Hodgkin's lymphoma, pediatric rhabdomyosarcoma, stem cell transplant, bone marrow ablation, AML, myelodysplastic syndrome

DOSAGE AND ROUTES

Multiple myeloma
- *Adult:* **PO** 6 mg daily × 2-3 wk, adjust dose based on blood counts or 10 mg daily × 7-10 day and 2 mg daily once WBC >4000 cells/mm^3, platelets >100,000 cells/mm^3, then 2-4 mg/day or 7 mg/m^2 × 5 day q5-6wk
- *Adult:* **IV INF** 16 mg/m^2, reduce in renal insufficiency, give over 15-20 min, give at 2-wk intervals × 4 doses, then at 4-wk intervals

Ovarian carcinoma
- *Adult:* **PO** 200 mcg/kg/day for 5 days q4-5wk

Testicular cancer/breast cancer/ non-Hodgkin's lymphoma/ osteogenic sarcoma (unlabeled)
- *Adult:* **PO** 150 mcg/kg/day × 7 days q4wk; when leukocytes are normal give 50 mcg/kg/day maintenance

Pediatric rhabdomyosarcoma (unlabeled)
- *Child:* **IV** 10-35 mg/m^2 q21-28days

Stem cell transplant/bone marrow ablation/acute myelogenous leukemia/myelodysplastic syndrome (unlabeled)
- *Adult and child:* **IV** 140 mg/m^2 on day 1 or divided over 2 days prior to SCT

Available forms: Tabs 2 mg, powder for inj 50 mg

SIDE EFFECTS

GI: Nausea, vomiting, stomatitis, diarrhea, **hepatitis**

GU: Amenorrhea, hyperuricemia, gonadal suppression

HEMA: **Thrombocytopenia, neutropenia, leukopenia,** anemia

INTEG: Rash, urticaria, alopecia, pruritus

RESP: **Fibrosis, dysplasia,** dyspnea, pneumonitis

SYST: **Anaphylaxis,** allergic reactions, **secondary malignancies,** edema

M

Contraindications: Pregnancy (D), breastfeeding, other nitrogen mustards

Black Box Warning: Hypersensitivity to this product

Precautions: Children, radiation therapy, infections, renal disease

Black Box Warning: Bone marrow depression, secondary malignancy

PHARMACOKINETICS

Metabolized in liver, excreted in urine, half-life 1½ hr, protein binding 80%-90%

INTERACTIONS

Increase: toxicity—antineoplastics, radiation

Increase: pulmonary toxicity—carmustine

Increase: renal failure risk—cycloSPORINE

Increase: enterocolitis risk—nalidixic acid

Increase: bleeding risk—NSAIDs, anticoagulants

Decrease: antibody response—live virus vaccines

NURSING CONSIDERATIONS

Assess:

- CBC, differential, platelet count q wk; withhold product if WBC is <3000/mm^3 or platelet count is <100,000/mm^3; notify prescriber; recovery usually occurs in 6 wk
- Renal studies: BUN, serum uric acid, before, during therapy
- I&O ratio; report fall in urine output to 30 ml/hr
- For infection: fever, cough, temp, sore throat, notify prescriber
- For bleeding: bruising, blood in urine, stools, emesis
- Hepatic studies before, during therapy (bilirubin, AST, ALT, LDH) as needed
- Bleeding: hematuria, guaiac, bruising or petechiae, mucosa or orifices q8hr
- Jaundiced skin and sclera, dark urine, clay-colored stools, itchy skin, abdominal pain, fever, diarrhea
- Buccal cavity q8hr for dryness, sores, ulceration, white patches, oral pain, bleeding, dysphagia
- Local irritation, pain, burning, discoloration at inj site

⚠ Symptoms indicating severe allergic reaction: rash, pruritus, urticaria, purpuric skin lesions, itching, flushing; assess allergy to chlorambucil, cross-sensitivity may occur

Administer:

- Antiemetic 30-60 min before giving product to prevent vomiting

PO route

- Give on empty stomach

IV route

- Use gloves during administration; if skin exposure occurs, wash immediately with soap and water
- Give by intermittent inf after reconstituting with 10 ml diluent provided (5 mg/ml), shake, dilute dose with 0.9% NaCl (≤0.45 mg/ml), give within 1 hr, run over ≥15 min

Y-site compatibilities: Acyclovir, amikacin, aminophylline, ampicillin, aztreonam, bleomycin, bumetanide, buprenorphine, butorphanol, calcium gluconate, carboplatin, carmustine, cefazolin, cefepime, cefoperazone, cefotaxime, cefotetan, ceftazidime, ceftizoxime, ceftriaxone, cefuroxime, cimetidine, cisplatin, clindamycin, cyclophosphamide, cytarabine, dacarbazine, dactinomycin, DAUNOrubicin, dexamethasone, diphenhydrAMINE, DOXOrubicin, doxycycline, droperidol, enalaprilat, etoposide, famotidine, floxuridine, fluconazole, fludarabine, fluorouracil, furosemide, gallium, ganciclovir, gentamicin, granisetron, haloperidol, heparin, hydrocortisone, hydrocortisone sodium phosphate, hydromorphone, hydrOXYzine, idarubicin, ifosfamide, imipenem-cilastatin, lorazepam, mannitol, mechlorethamine, meperidine, mesna, methotrexate, methylPREDNISolone, metoclopramide, metronidazole, miconazole, minocycline, mitomycin, mitoxantrone, morphine, nalbuphine, netilmicin, ondansetron, pentostatin, piperacillin, plicamycin, potassium chloride, prochlorperazine, promethazine, ranitidine, sodium bicarbonate, streptozocin, teniposide, thiotepa, ticarcillin, ticarcillin/clavulanate, tobramycin, trimethoprim-sulfamethoxazole, vancomycin, vinBLAStine, vinCRIStine, vinorelbine, zidovudine

Perform/provide:

- Storage in airtight, light-resistant container
- Strict medical asepsis, protective isolation if WBC levels are low
- Increase fluid intake to 2-3 L/day to prevent urate deposits, calculi formation
- Diet low in purines: organ meats (kidney, liver), dried beans, peas to maintain alkaline urine
- Rinsing of mouth tid-qid with water, club soda; brushing of teeth bid-tid with soft brush or cotton-tipped applicators for stomatitis; use unwaxed dental floss
- Warm compresses at inj site for inflammation

Evaluate:

- Therapeutic response: decreased tumor size, spread of malignancy

Teach patient/family:

- That usually sterility, amenorrhea can occur; reversible after discontinuing treatment
- To avoid foods with citric acid, hot or rough texture
- To report any bleeding, white spots, or ulcerations in mouth to prescriber; tell patient to examine mouth daily
- To report signs of infection: fever, sore throat, flulike symptoms
- To report suspected pregnancy; to use contraception during treatment
- To report signs of anemia: fatigue, headache, faintness, shortness of breath, irritability
- To avoid use of razors, commercial mouthwash
- To avoid use of aspirin products, NSAIDs, alcohol

memantine (℞)

(me-man′teen)

Namenda

Func. class.: Anti-Alzheimer agent

Chem. class.: NMDA receptor antagonist

Action: Antagonist action of CNS NMDA receptors that may contribute to the symptoms of Alzheimer's disease

Uses: Treatment of moderate to severe dementia in Alzheimer's disease

Unlabeled uses: Vascular dementia, acquired pendular nystagmus

DOSAGE AND ROUTES

- *Adult:* **PO** 5 mg/day, may increase dose in 5-mg increments ≥1 wk intervals; recommended target dose 20 mg/day as 10 mg bid

Available forms: Tabs 5, 10 mg; tab titration pak 5, 10 mg; oral sol 2 mg/ml (10 mg/5 ml)

M

SIDE EFFECTS

CNS: *Dizziness, confusion,* somnolence, headache, hallucinations

CV: Hypertension

GI: Vomiting, constipation

INTEG: Rash

MISC: Back pain, fatigue, pain

RESP: Coughing, dyspnea

Contraindications: Breastfeeding, children, hypersensitivity, renal failure

Precautions: Pregnancy (B), renal disease, GU conditions that raise urine pH, seizures, severe hepatic disease

PHARMACOKINETICS

Rapidly absorbed PO, 44% protein binding, very little metabolism, 57%-82% excreted unchanged in urine, terminal elimination half-life 60-80 hr

INTERACTIONS

- May alter levels of both products: hydrochlorothiazide, triamterene, cimetidine, quinidine, ranitidine, nicotine

Increase: effect—levodopa, some ergots

Decrease: clearance of memantine—products which make the urine alkaline (sodium bicarbonate, carbonic anhydrase inhibitors)

NURSING CONSIDERATIONS

Assess:

- B/P: hypertension
- Mental status: affect, mood, behavioral changes; hallucinations, confusion
- GI status: vomiting, constipation, add bulk, increase fluids for constipation
- GU status: urinary frequency
- Respiratory status: dyspnea

Administer:

- Can be taken without regard to meals
- Twice a day if dose >5 mg
- Dosage adjusted to response no more than q1wk
- Oral sol using device provided; remove dosing syringe, green cap, and plastic tube from plastic; attach tube to green cap; open cap by pushing down on cap and turning counterclockwise; remove unscrewed cap; carefully remove seal from bottle and discard; insert plastic tube fully into bottle and screw green cap tightly onto bottle by turning cap clockwise; keeping bottle upright on table, remove the lid; with plunger fully depressed, insert tip of syringe into cap; while holding syringe, gently pull up on plunger; remove syringe; invert syringe and slowly press plunger to a level that removes large air bubbles; keep plunger in inverted position; a few small air bubbles may be present

Perform/provide:

- Assistance with ambulation during beginning therapy; dizziness may occur

Evaluate:

- Therapeutic response: decrease in confusion, improved mood

Teach patient/family:

- To report side effects: restlessness, psychosis, visual hallucinations, stupor, LOC; indicate overdose
- To use product exactly as prescribed; product is not a cure
- To use oral solution dispenser

menotropins (℞)

(men-oh-troe′pins)

Menopur, Pergonal, Repronex

Func. class.: Gonadotropin

Chem. class.: Exogenous gonadotropin

Action: In women, increases follicular growth, maturation; in men, when given with hCG, stimulates spermatogenesis

Uses: Infertility, anovulation in women, stimulates spermatogenesis in men

DOSAGE AND ROUTES

Infertility

- *Men:* **IM** 1 ampule 3 × wk with hCG 2000 units 2 × wk × 4 mo
- *Women:* **IM** 75 international units FSH, LH daily × 9-12 days, then 10,000 units hCG 1 day after these products; repeat × 2 menstrual cycles, then increase to 150 international units FSH, LH daily × 9-12 days, then 10,000 units hCG 1 day after these products × 2 menstrual cycles

Anovulation

- *Women:* **IM** (Humegon, Pergonal) 75 international units FSH, LH daily × 7-12 days, then 10,000 units hCG 1 day after last dose of these products; repeat × 1-3 menstrual cycles; **IM/SUBCUT** (Repronex only) 75 international units FSH/LH activity daily × 5 days, adjust dose by no more than 75-150 international units/day q2days

Available forms: Powder for inj lyophilized 75 international units FSH, LH activity 150 international units FSH, LH activity

SIDE EFFECTS

CNS: Fever, hot flashes, dizziness

CV: **Hypovolemia,** tachycardia

GI: Nausea, vomiting, diarrhea, anorexia

GU: **Ovarian hyperstimulation syndrome (OHSS),** *abdominal distention/pain,* multiple births, sudden ovarian enlargement, ascites with or without pain, ectopic pregnancy, gynecomastia in men

HEMA: **Hemoperitoneum, arterial thromboembolism**
INTEG: Rash, swelling of inj site
RESP: **ARDS, PE, pulmonary infarction, pleural effusion,** atelectasis, dyspnea, tachypnea
SYST: **Anaphylaxis**

Contraindications: Pregnancy (X), primary ovarian failure, abnormal bleeding, thyroid/adrenal dysfunction, organic intracranial lesion, ovarian cysts, primary testicular failure, high FSH, neoplastic disease

Precautions: Ascites, children, geriatric patients, endometriosis, polycystic ovary syndrome, thromboembolic disease, uterine leiomyomata, smoking

NURSING CONSIDERATIONS

Assess:

- Weight daily; notify prescriber if weight increases rapidly
- Estrogen excretion level; if >100 mcg/24 hr, product is withheld; serum progesterone, LH, estradiol level, pelvic exam, ovarian ultrasound
- I&O ratio; be alert for decreasing urinary output
- Ovarian enlargement, abdominal distention/pain

Administer:

IM route

- After reconstituting with 1-2 ml sterile saline inj; use immediately

Evaluate:

- Therapeutic response: ovulation, pregnancy

Teach patient/family:

- To report abdominal pain/distention
- That multiple births are possible; if pregnancy occurs, usually 4-6 wk after start of treatment
- To keep appointment during treatment daily × 2 wk

⚠ High Alert

meperidine (℞)

(me-per′i-deen)

Demerol, meperidine, Meperitab

Func. class.: Opioid analgesic
Chem. class.: Phenylpiperidine derivative

Controlled Substance Schedule II

Do not confuse:
meperidine/hydromorphone/meprobamate/morphine
Demerol/Dilaudid

Action: Depresses pain impulse transmission at the spinal cord level by interacting with opioid receptors

Uses: Moderate to severe pain, preoperatively, postoperatively

Unlabeled uses: Obstetric/regional analgesic, acute severe headache/migraine, shaking chills induced by IV amphotericin B or postoperative shivering

M

DOSAGE AND ROUTES

Pain

- *Adult:* **PO/SUBCUT/IM** 50-150 mg q3-4hr prn; **IV** 15-35 mg/hr as a **CONT INF;** PCA 10 mg, then 1-5 mg incremental dose; lockout interval 6-10 min
- *Geriatric:* **PO/SUBCUT/IM** start with 50 mg, increase as needed q3-4hr
- *Child:* **PO/SUBCUT/IM** 1-1.8 mg/kg q3-4hr prn, not to exceed 100 mg q4hr

Labor analgesia

- *Adult:* **SUBCUT/IM** 50-100 mg given when contractions are regularly spaced, repeat q1-3hr prn

Preoperatively

- *Adult:* **IM/SUBCUT** 50-100 mg 30-90 min before surgery; dose should be reduced if given **IV**
- *Child:* **IM/SUBCUT** 1-2.2 mg/kg 30-90 min before surgery

Shaking, chills induced by amphotericin B or postoperative shivering (unlabeled)

- *Adult:* **IV** 25-50 mg as a single dose

• *Child and adolescent:* **IV** 0.35-1 mg/kg, max 50 mg, use lowest effective dose
Available forms: Inj 10, 25, 50, 75, 100 mg/ml; tabs 50, 100 mg; syr 50 mg/5 ml

SIDE EFFECTS

CNS: Drowsiness, dizziness, confusion, headache, sedation, euphoria, **increased intracranial pressure**, **seizures,** serotonin syndrome
CV: Palpitations, bradycardia, hypotension, change in B/P, tachycardia (IV)
EENT: Tinnitus, blurred vision, miosis, diplopia, depressed corneal reflex
GI: Nausea, vomiting, anorexia, constipation, cramps, biliary spasm, paralytic ileus
GU: Urinary retention, dysuria
INTEG: Rash, urticaria, bruising, flushing, diaphoresis, pruritus
RESP: **Respiratory depression**
SYST: **Anaphylaxis**
Contraindications: Hypersensitivity
Precautions: Pregnancy (B), breastfeeding, children <18 yr, geriatric patients, addictive personality, increased intracranial pressure, MI (acute), severe heart disease, respiratory depression, renal/hepatic disease, seizure disorder, abrupt discontinuation

PHARMACOKINETICS

Metabolized by liver (to active/inactive metabolites), excreted by kidneys; crosses placenta, excreted in breast milk; half-life 3-4 hr; toxic by-product accumulation can result from regular use or in renal disease, protein binding 65%-75%
PO: Onset 15 min, peak ½-1 hr, duration 2-4 hr, absorption 50%
SUBCUT/IM: Onset 10 min, peak ½-1 hr, duration 2-4 hr, well absorbed
IV: Onset 5 min, duration 2 hr

INTERACTIONS

⚠ May cause fatal reaction: MAOIs, procarbazine
Increase: effects with other CNS depressants, alcohol, opioids, sedative/hypnotics, antipsychotics, skeletal muscle relaxants
Increase: adverse reactions—protease inhibitor antiretrovirals
Decrease: meperidine effect—phenytoin

Drug/Herb
Increase: CNS depression—chamomile, hops, gotu kola, Jamaican dogwood, kava, lavender, mistletoe, nettle, pokeweed, poppy, senega, skullcap, St. John's wort, valerian
Increase: Parsley may promote serotonin syndrome; avoid concurrent medicinal use

Drug/Lab Test
Increase: amylase, lipase

NURSING CONSIDERATIONS

Assess:
• Pain: location, type, character; give before pain becomes extreme; reassess after 60 min (IM, SUBCUT, PO) and 5-10 min (IV)
• Renal function prior to initiating therapy; poor renal function can lead to accumulation of toxic metabolite and seizures
• I&O ratio; check for decreasing output; may indicate urinary retention
• For constipation; increase fluids, bulk in diet; give stimulant laxatives if needed
• CNS changes: dizziness, drowsiness, hallucinations, euphoria, LOC, pupil reactions; at chronic or high-dose use
• Allergic reactions: rash, urticaria
• Respiratory dysfunction: depression, character, rate, rhythm; notify prescriber if respirations are <12/min
• CNS stimulation: occurs with chronic or high doses

Administer:
• Patient should remain recumbent for 1 hr after IM/SUBCUT route
• With antiemetic for nausea, vomiting
• When pain is beginning to return; determine dosage interval by patient response
• In gradually decreasing dose after long-term use; withdrawal symptoms may occur

IV route

- After diluting with 5 ml or more sterile H_2O or NS; give directly over 4-5 min; may be further diluted in sol to 1 mg/ml during anesthesia in D_5W or NS; if diluted in NS, may be given through patient-controlled inf device

Additive compatibilities: Cefazolin, clonidine, DOBUTamine, metoclopramide, ondansetron, parecoxib, scopolamine, succinylcholine, triflupromazine, verapamil

Syringe compatibilities: Butorphanol, chlorproMAZINE, cimetidine, dimenhyDRINATE, diphenhydrAMINE, droperidol, fentanyl, glycopyrrolate, hydrOXYzine, ketamine, metoclopramide, midazolam, pentazocine, perphenazine, prochlorperazine, promazine, promethazine, ranitidine, scopolamine

Y-site compatibilities: Amifostine, amikacin, ampicillin, atenolol, aztreonam, bumetanide, cefazolin, cefotaxime, cefotetan, cefoxitin, ceftazidime, ceftizoxime, ceftriaxone, cefuroxime, cephalothin, cephapirin, chloramphenicol, cisatracurium, cladribine, clindamycin, dexamethasone, diltiazem, diphenhydrAMINE, DOBUTamine, DOPamine, DOXOrubicin liposome, doxycycline, droperidol, erythromycin, famotidine, filgrastim, fluconazole, fludarabine, gallium, gentamicin, granisetron, heparin, hydrocortisone, insulin (regular), kanamycin, labetalol, lidocaine, methyldopate, magnesium sulfate, melphalan, methylPREDNISolone, metoclopramide, metoprolol, metronidazole, moxalactam, ondansetron, oxacillin, oxytocin, paclitaxel, penicillin G potassium, piperacillin, potassium chloride, propofol, propranolol, ranitidine, remifentanil, sargramostim, teniposide, thiotepa, ticarcillin, ticarcillin/clavulanate, tobramycin, trimethoprim-sulfamethoxazole, vancomycin, verapamil, vinorelbine

Perform/provide:

- Storage in light-resistant container at room temperature
- Assistance with ambulation
- Safety measures: night-light, call bell within easy reach

Evaluate:

- Therapeutic response: decrease in pain

Teach patient/family:

- To report any symptoms of CNS changes, allergic reactions
- That physical dependency may result from extended use
- That drowsiness, dizziness may occur; to call for assistance
- That withdrawal symptoms may occur: nausea, vomiting, cramps, fever, faintness, anorexia
- To make position changes slowly; orthostatic hypotension can occur
- To avoid OTC medications, alcohol unless directed by prescriber

Treatment of overdose: Naloxone (Narcan) 0.2-0.8 mg IV, O_2, IV fluids, vasopressors

mercaptopurine (℞)

(mer-kap-toe-pyoor′een)

Purinethol, 6-MP

Func. class.: Antineoplastic-antimetabolite

Chem. class.: Purine analog

Action: Inhibits purine metabolism at multiple sites, which inhibits DNA and RNA synthesis, S phase of cell cycle specific

Uses: Chronic myelocytic or acute lymphoblastic leukemia in children

Unlabeled uses: Polycythemia vera, psoriatic arthritis, ulcerative colitis, Crohn's disease, AML, CML, lymphoma

DOSAGE AND ROUTES

Acute lymphocytic leukemia

- *Adult:* **PO** 2.5-5 mg/kg/day or 80-100 mg/m^2/day, maintenance 1.5-2.5 mg/kg/day
- *Child:* **PO** 2.5-5 mg/kg/day, maintenance 1.5-2.5 mg/kg/day or 70-100 mg/m^2/day

Acute myelogenous leukemia (unlabeled)
- *Adult and child:* **PO** 2.5 mg/kg/day

Chronic myelogenous leukemia (unlabeled)
- *Adult:* **PO** Chronic phase 60-75 mg/m^2/day; blast crisis 100 mg/m^2 q12hr × 5-7 days

Crohn's disease/ulcerative colitis (unlabeled)
- *Adult:* **PO** 1.5-2 mg/kg/day

Available forms: Tabs 50 mg

SIDE EFFECTS

CNS: Weakness
GI: Nausea, vomiting, anorexia, diarrhea, stomatitis, **hepatotoxicity** (high doses), jaundice, gastritis, **pancreatitis**
GU: **Renal failure,** hyperuricemia, **oliguria,** crystalluria, **hematuria**
HEMA: **Thrombocytopenia, leukopenia, myelosuppression, anemia**
INTEG: Rash, dry skin, urticaria, alopecia
Contraindications: Pregnancy (D), breastfeeding, patients with prior product resistance, leukopenia, thrombocytopenia, anemia
Precautions: Renal/hepatic disease

PHARMACOKINETICS

Incompletely absorbed when taken orally, metabolized in liver, excreted in urine, peak 1-2 hr, terminal half-life 1-1.5 hr

INTERACTIONS

Increase: effects—radiation or other antineoplastics, immunosuppressants
Increase: bone marrow depression—allopurinol, co-trimoxazole
Increase: anticoagulant action—anticoagulants, NSAIDs, thrombolytics, platelet inhibitors
Decrease: antibodies—live virus vaccines

NURSING CONSIDERATIONS

Assess:
- CBC, differential, platelet count q wk; withhold product if WBC is <3500 or platelet count is <100,000; notify prescriber; product should be discontinued
- Renal studies: BUN, serum uric acid, urine CCr, electrolytes before, during therapy
- I&O ratio; report fall in urine output to <30 ml/hr
- Monitor temp; fever may indicate beginning infection; no rectal temps
- Hepatic studies before, during therapy: bilirubin, alk phos, AST, ALT, q wk during beginning therapy
- Bleeding: hematuria, guaiac, bruising, petechiae; mucosa or orifices
- Buccal cavity for dryness, sores, ulceration, white patches, oral pain, bleeding, dysphagia

⚠ Symptoms indicating severe allergic reaction: rash, urticaria, itching, flushing

Administer:
- Give product after evening meal before bedtime on an empty stomach
- Allopurinol or sodium bicarbonate to maintain uric acid levels, alkalinization of urine

Perform/provide:
- Strict medical asepsis, protective isolation if WBC levels are low
- Increase fluid intake to 2-3 L/day to prevent urate deposits, calculi formation, unless contraindicated
- Diet low in purines: absence of organ meats (kidney, liver), dried beans, peas to maintain alkaline urine
- Rinsing of mouth tid-qid with water, club soda; brushing of teeth bid-tid with soft brush or cotton-tipped applicators for stomatitis; use unwaxed dental floss
- Storage in tightly closed container in cool environment

Evaluate:
- Therapeutic response: decreased size of tumor, spread of malignancy

Teach patient/family:
- To avoid foods with citric acid, hot or rough texture for stomatitis
- To report stomatitis: any bleeding, white spots, ulcerations in mouth; tell patient to examine mouth daily, report symptoms

- That contraceptive measures are recommended during therapy; to avoid breastfeeding
- To drink 10-12 (8 oz) glasses of fluid/day
- To notify prescriber of fever, chills, sore throat, nausea, vomiting, anorexia, diarrhea, bleeding, bruising, which may indicate blood dyscrasias
- To report signs of infection: fever, sore throat, flulike symptoms
- To report signs of anemia: fatigue, headache, faintness, shortness of breath, irritability
- To report bleeding: avoid use of razors, commercial mouthwash
- To avoid use of aspirin products, NSAIDs
- To take entire dose at one time

meropenem (℞)

(mer-oh-pen′em)

Merrem IV

Func. class.: Antiinfective—miscellaneous

Chem. class.: Carbapenem

Action: Bactericidal, interferes with cell wall replication of susceptible organisms; osmotically unstable cell wall swells, bursts from osmotic pressure

Uses: Serious infections caused by gram-positive bacteria: *Streptococcus pneumoniae,* group A β-hemolytic streptococci, enterococcus; gram-negative: *Klebsiella, Proteus, Escherichia coli, Pseudomonas aeruginosa;* appendicitis, peritonitis caused by *viridans* group streptococci; *Bacteroides fragilis, Bacteroides thetaiotaomicron,* bacterial meningitis (≥3 mo)

Unlabeled uses: Febrile neutropenic, community-acquired pneumonia

DOSAGE AND ROUTES

- *Adult:* **IV** 1 g q8hr, given over 15-30 min or as an **IV BOL** 5-20 ml given over 3-5 min
- *Child ≥3 mo:* **IV** 20-40 mg/kg q8hr (max 2 g q8hr meningitis)
- *Child >50 kg:* **IV** 1 g q8hr (intraabdominal infection) or 2 g q8hr (meningitis) given over 15-30 min or as an **IV BOL** 5-20 ml over 3-5 min; max 2 g q8hr

Renal disease

- *Adult:* **IV** CCr 26-50 ml/min 1 g q12hr; CCr 10-25 ml/min 500 mg q12hr; CCr <10 ml/min 500 mg q24hr

Febrile neutropenia (unlabeled)

- *Adult:* **IV** 1 g q8hr

Community-acquired pneumonia (CAP) (unlabeled)

- *Adult:* **IV** 500 mg q8hr with ciprofloxacin or with an aminoglycoside plus fluoroquinolone

Available forms: Powder for inj 500 mg, 1 g

SIDE EFFECTS

CNS: Fever, somnolence, **seizures,** dizziness, weakness, myoclonia, *headache,* confusion

CV: Hypotension, palpitations, tachycardia

GI: Diarrhea, nausea, vomiting, **pseudomembranous colitis, hepatitis,** glossitis

HEMA: **Eosinophilia, neutropenia,** decreased Hgb, Hct, **agranulocytosis**

INTEG: *Rash,* urticaria, *pruritus,* pain at inj site, phlebitis, erythema at inj site

RESP: Chest discomfort, dyspnea, hyperventilation, **PE**

SYST: **Anaphylaxis, Stevens-Johnson syndrome, angioedema**

Contraindications: Hypersensitivity to this product, carbapenems, cephalosporins, penicillins

Precautions: Pregnancy (B), breastfeeding, geriatric patients, renal disease, seizure disorder

PHARMACOKINETICS

IV: Onset immediate, peak dose dependent, half-life 1 hr, excreted unchanged in urine (70%)

INTERACTIONS

Increase: meropenem plasma levels—probenecid

Decrease: effect of valproic acid

Drug/Herb
• Do not use acidophilus with antiinfectives; separate by several hours
Drug/Lab Test
Increase: AST, ALT, LDH, BUN, alk phos, bilirubin, creatinine
False positive: direct Coombs' test

NURSING CONSIDERATIONS

Assess:
• Sensitivity to carbapenem antibiotics, penicillins
• Renal disease: lower dose may be required
• Bowel pattern daily; if severe diarrhea occurs, product should be discontinued; may indicate pseudomembranous colitis
• For infection: temp, sputum, characteristics of wound, before, during, and after treatment
⚠ Allergic reactions, anaphylaxis: rash, urticaria, pruritus; may occur few days after therapy begins
• Overgrowth of infection: perineal itching, fever, malaise, redness, pain, swelling, drainage, rash, diarrhea, change in cough, sputum
Administer:
• By IV inf or IV bol
• After C&S is taken
• Reconstitute with 0.9% NaCl, D_5W, LR; dilute in 5-20 ml comp sol; give by direct IV over 3-5 min; give by intermittent inf, dilute in 5-20 ml of comp sol; give over 15-30 min
Additive compatibilities: Aminophylline, atropine, cimetidine, dexamethasone, DOBUTamine, DOPamine, enalaprilat, fluconazole, furosemide, gentamicin, heparin, insulin (regular), magnesium sulfate, metoclopramide, morphine, norepinephrine, phenobarbital, ranitidine, vancomycin
Y-site compatibilities: Aminophylline, atenolol, atropine, cimetidine, dexamethasone, digoxin, diphenhydrAMINE, enalaprilat, fluconazole, furosemide, gentamicin, heparin, insulin (regular), metoclopramide, morphine, norepinephrine, phenobarbital, vancomycin

Evaluate:
• Therapeutic response: negative C&S; absence of symptoms and signs of infection
Teach patient/family:
• To report severe diarrhea; may indicate pseudomembranous colitis
• To report sore throat, bruising, bleeding, joint pain; may indicate blood dyscrasias (rare)
• To report overgrowth of infection: black, furry tongue; vaginal itching; foul-smelling stools
• To avoid breastfeeding; product is excreted in breast milk
• Treatment of anaphylaxis: Epinephrine, antihistamines; resuscitate if needed

mesalamine, 5-ASA (℞)

(mez-al'a-meen)
Apriso, Asacol, Canasa, Lialda, Pentasa, Rowasa
Salofalk ♣
Func. class.: GI antiinflammatory
Chem. class.: 5-Aminosalicylic acid

Do not confuse:
Asacol/Ansaid/Os-Cal
Action: May diminish inflammation by blocking cyclooxygenase, inhibiting prostaglandin production in colon; local action only
Uses: Mild to moderate active distal ulcerative colitis, proctosigmoiditis, proctitis
Unlabeled uses: Crohn's disease

DOSAGE AND ROUTES

• *Adult:* **RECT** 60 ml (4 g) at bedtime, retained for 8 hr × 3-6 wk; **PO** 1000 mg qid for up to 8 wk; del rel tab 1.2 g/day; **DEL REL TAB** (Lialda) 2.4 g/day; **DEL REL TAB** (Asacol) 800 mg tid × 6 wk; **CONTROLLED REL CAP** (Pentasa) 1 g qid up to 8 wk; **EXT REL** cap (Apriso) 1500 mg (4 caps) qAM daily up to 6 mo, **RECT SUPP** 500 mg bid retained for 1-3 hr × 3-6 wk until remission, may increase tid if needed

Available forms: Enema 4 g/60 ml; ext rel tab 500 mg; ext rel cap 250, 500 mg; 0.375 g (Apriso); del rel tab 400 mg; del rel tab (Lialda) 1.2 g; rectal supp 1000 mg

SIDE EFFECTS

CNS: Headache, fever, dizziness, insomnia, asthenia, weakness, fatigue
CV: Pericarditis, myocarditis, chest pain, palpitations
EENT: Sore throat, cough, pharyngitis, rhinitis
GI: Cramps, gas, nausea, diarrhea, rectal pain, constipation
INTEG: Rash, itching, acne
SYST: Flulike symptoms, malaise, back pain, peripheral edema, leg and joint pain, arthralgia, dysmenorrhea, **anaphylaxis,** acute intolerance syndrome

Contraindications: Hypersensitivity to this product or salicylates, 5-aminosalicylates

Precautions: Pregnancy (B), breastfeeding, children, geriatric patients, renal disease, sulfite sensitivity, pyloric stenosis

PHARMACOKINETICS

RECT: Primarily excreted in feces but some in urine as metabolite; half-life 1 hr, metabolite half-life 5-10 hr

INTERACTIONS

Increase: mesalamine absorption—omeprazole
Increase: action of azathioprine
Decrease: digoxin level—digoxin
Decrease: mesalamine absorption—lactulose

Drug/Lab Test

Increase: AST, ALT, alk phos, LDH, GGTP, amylase, lipase

NURSING CONSIDERATIONS

Assess:

- For allergy to salicylates, sulfonamides, if allergic reactions occur, discontinue product
- Renal studies: BUN, creatinine before and during treatment; renal toxicity may occur
- GI symptoms: cramps, gas, nausea, diarrhea, rectal pain; if severe, product should be discontinued
- I&O ratios, increase fluids to 1500 ml daily to prevent crystalluria

Administer:

PO route

- Swallow tabs whole; do not break, crush, or chew tabs

Rectal route

- Product should be given at bedtime, retained until morning; empty bowel before insertion

Perform/provide:

- Storage at room temperature

Evaluate:

- Therapeutic response: absence of pain, bleeding from GI tract, decrease in number of diarrhea stools

Teach patient/family:

- That usual course of therapy is 3-6 wk
- To shake bottle well (rectal susp)
- Method of rectal administration
- To inform prescriber of GI symptoms
- To report abdominal cramping, pain, diarrhea with blood, headache, fever, rash, chest pain; product should be discontinued

M

metaproterenol (℞)

(met-a-proe-ter′e-nole)
Func. class.: Bronchodilator-selective β_2-agonist

Action: Relaxes bronchial smooth muscle by direct action on β_2-adrenergic receptors with increased levels of cAMP with increased bronchodilation, diuresis, cardiac CNS stimulation

Uses: Bronchial asthma, bronchospasm

DOSAGE AND ROUTES

- *Adult and child >12 yr:* **INH** 2-3 inhalations; may repeat q3-4hr, not to exceed 12 inhalations/day; **IPPB** or **NEB** 0.2-0.3

ml of 5% sol diluted in 2.5 ml of ½ NS or NS; or 2.5 ml of 0.4, 0.6% sol q4hr prn
- *Adult:* **PO** 20 mg q6-8hr
- *Geriatric:* **PO** 10 mg tid-qid, initially
- *Child 6-12 yr:* **IPPB/NEB** 0.1-0.2 ml of a 5% sol diluted in NS to a final volume of 3 ml q4hr prn
- *Child >9 yr or >27 kg:* **PO** 20 mg q6-8hr or 0.4-0.9 mg/kg tid
- *Child 6-9 yr or <27 kg:* **PO** 10 mg q6-8hr or 0.4-0.9 mg/kg tid
- *Child 2-6 yr:* **PO** 1.3-2.6 mg/kg divided q6-8hr
- *Child 1-2 yr:* **PO** 0.4 mg/kg q6-8hr

Available forms: Tabs 10, 20 mg; aerosol inhaler 0.65 mg/dose; syr 10 mg/5 ml; neb inhaler 0.4%, 0.6%, 5%

SIDE EFFECTS

CNS: *Tremors,* anxiety, insomnia, headache, dizziness, stimulation
CV: Palpitations, tachycardia, hypertension, dysrhythmias, **cardiac arrest** (high dose)
GI: Nausea, vomiting, dry mouth
MISC: Hypokalemia, pyrosis
RESP: **Paradoxical bronchospasm**

Contraindications: Hypersensitivity to sympathomimetics, closed-angle glaucoma, cardiac dysrhythmias with tachycardia

Precautions: Pregnancy (C), children <6 yr (NEB), children <12 yr (INH), geriatric patients, cardiac disorders, hyperthyroidism, diabetes mellitus, prostatic hypertrophy, seizure disorder

PHARMACOKINETICS

PO: Onset 15-30 min, peak 1 hr, duration 1-4 hr, excreted in urine as metabolites

INH: Onset 1 min, peak 1 hr, duration 1-2½ hr

NEB: Onset 5-30 min, peak 1 hr, duration 1-2½ hr

INTERACTIONS

⚠ Hypertensive crisis: MAOIs, tricyclics
Increase: effects of both products—other sympathomimetics, bronchodilators
Decrease: β-blockers action

Drug/Herb
Increase: effect—black/green tea, coffee, cola nut, guarana, yerba maté

Drug/Lab Test
Decrease: potassium

NURSING CONSIDERATIONS

Assess:
- Respiratory function: vital capacity, forced expiratory volume, ABGs; also B/P; lung sounds, secretions before and after treatment
- Cardiac status: hypertension, dysrhythmias, palpitations, tachycardia; cardiac arrest can occur at high doses
- Tolerance over long-term therapy; dose may have to be changed; check for rebound bronchospasm

Administer:
- 2 hr before bedtime to avoid sleeplessness
- PO with food for GI upset

Perform/provide:
- Storage at room temperature; do not use discolored sol
- Spacer device for geriatric patients

Evaluate:
- Therapeutic response: absence of dyspnea, wheezing; improved ABGs

Teach patient/family:
- To increase fluid intake (2-3 L/day) to liquefy secretions unless contraindicated
- Not to use OTC medications; excess stimulation may occur
- To notify prescriber of headaches, chest pain, weakness, dizziness, anxiety
- Use of inhaler; review package insert with patient
- To avoid getting aerosol in eyes
- To wash inhaler in warm water and dry daily
- All aspects of product; avoid smoking, smoke-filled rooms, persons with respiratory infections

metformin (℞)

(met-for′min)

Fortamet, Glucophage, Glucophage XR, Glumetza, Novo-Metformin ✤, Riomet

Func. class.: Antidiabetic, oral

Chem. class.: Biguanide

Action: Inhibits hepatic glucose production and increases sensitivity of peripheral tissue to insulin

Uses: Type 2 diabetes mellitus

Unlabeled uses: Precocious puberty or early-normal onset of puberty to delay menarche, polycystic ovary syndrome, infertility

DOSAGE AND ROUTES

Diabetes mellitus

• *Adult:* **PO** 500 mg bid initially, then increase to desired response 1-2 g; dosage adjustment q2-3wk or 850 mg/day with morning meal with dosage increased every other wk, max 2550 mg/day, **EXT REL** (Glucophage XR) 500 mg daily with evening meal, may increase by 500 mg q wk, max 2000 mg/day; (Glumetza) 1000 mg daily with food, preferably with the PM meal, may increase by 500 mg q wk max 2000 mg daily; (Fortamet) 500-1000 mg daily with PM meal, may increase by 500 mg q wk, max 2550 mg daily

• *Geriatric:* **PO** Use lowest effective dose

To delay early menarche and to prolong pubertal growth with early onset of puberty (unlabeled)

• *Child 8-9 yr:* **PO** 825 mg/day with dinner

To delay clinical puberty and early menarche in precocious puberty (unlabeled)

• *Child >6 yr:* **PO** 425 mg/day with dinner

Polycystic ovary syndrome/infertility related to hyperinsulinemia secondary to polycystic ovary syndrome (unlabeled)

• *Adult (female):* **PO** 500 mg tid

Available forms: Tabs 500, 850, 1000 mg; ext rel tab 500, 1000 mg

SIDE EFFECTS

CNS: Headache, weakness, dizziness, drowsiness, tinnitus, fatigue, vertigo, *agitation*

CV: **Heart failure**

ENDO: **Lactic acidosis,** hypoglycemia

GI: Nausea, vomiting, diarrhea, heartburn, anorexia, metallic taste

HEMA: **Thrombocytopenia,** decreased vit B_{12} levels

INTEG: Rash

Contraindications: Hypersensitivity; hepatic disease; creatinine >1.5 mg/ml (males), ≥1.4 (females); alcoholism; cardiopulmonary disease; acidemia; acute MI; cardiogenic shock; diabetic ketoacidosis; metabolic acidosis

Black Box Warning: History of lactic acidosis

Precautions: Pregnancy (B), geriatric patients, previous hypersensitivity, thyroid disease, CHF

M

PHARMACOKINETICS

Excreted by the kidneys unchanged 35%-50%, half-life 1½-5 hr, terminal 6-20 hr, peak 1-3 hr

INTERACTIONS

• Do not give with radiologic contrast media; may cause renal failure

Increase: metformin level—cimetidine, digoxin, morphine, procainamide, quinidine, ranitidine, triamterene, vancomycin

Increase: hypoglycemia—cimetidine, calcium channel blockers, corticosteroids, estrogens, oral contraceptives, phenothiazines, sympathomimetics, diuretics, phenytoin

Drug/Herb

Increase: hyperglycemia—glucosamine

Increase: hypoglycemia—chromium, coenzyme Q-10, fenugreek

Increase: metformin level—quinine

Increase: antidiabetic effect—alfalfa, aloe, basil, bay, bilberry, bitter melon,

black catechu, buchu, burdock, coriander, dandelion, eyebright (po), fenugreek, garlic, ginseng, glucomannan, glucosamine, goat's rue, gymnema, horehound, horse chestnut, jambul, myrrh, myrtle
Decrease: antidiabetic effect—bee pollen, blue cohosh, broom, chromium, elecampane, eucalyptus, gotu kola

NURSING CONSIDERATIONS

Assess:

- For hypoglycemic reactions (sweating, weakness, dizziness, anxiety, tremors, hunger), hyperglycemic reactions soon after meals; these occur rarely with this product
- CBC (baseline, q3mo) during treatment; check LFTs periodically AST, LDH, renal studies: BUN, creatinine during treatment; glucose, A1c

⚠ For lactic acidosis: malaise, myalgia, abdominal distress; risk increases with age, poor renal function; monitor electrolytes, lactate, pyruvate, blood pH, ketones, glucose

Administer:

PO route

- Do not break, crush, chew ext rel tab
- Twice a day given with meals to decrease GI upset and provide best absorption; may also be taken as a single dose; titrate slowly to therapeutic response, side effect tolerance
- Immediate release tabs crushed and mixed with meal or fluids for patients with difficulty swallowing

Perform/provide:

- Conversion from other oral hypoglycemic agents; change may be made without gradual dosage change; monitor serum glucose and urine ketones tid during conversion
- Storage in tight container in cool environment

Evaluate:

- Therapeutic response: decrease in polyuria, polydipsia, polyphagia; clear sensorium; absence of dizziness; stable gait; blood glucose, A1c at normal level

Teach patient/family:

⚠ Lactic acidosis symptoms: hyperventilation, fatigue, malaise, chills, myalgia, somnolence; to notify prescriber immediately

- To use regular self-monitoring of blood glucose using blood glucose meter
- The symptoms of hypo/hyperglycemia, what to do about each (rare)
- That product must be continued on daily basis; explain consequence of discontinuing product abruptly
- To avoid OTC medications, alcohol unless approved by prescriber
- That diabetes is a lifelong illness; that this product is not a cure; only controls symptoms
- To carry emergency ID and glucagon emergency kit for emergencies
- That Glucophage XR tab may appear in stool
- To take with first meal of the day

⚠ High Alert

methadone (℞)

(meth'a-done)

Dolophine, methadone, Methadose

Func. class.: Opioid analgesic
Chem. class.: Synthetic diphenylheptane derivative

Controlled Substance Schedule II

Do not confuse:
methadone/methylphenidate

Action: Depresses pain impulse transmission at the spinal cord level by interacting with opioid receptors, produce CNS depression

Uses: Severe pain, opioid withdrawal

DOSAGE AND ROUTES

Severe pain

- *Adult:* **PO/SUBCUT/IM** 2.5-10 mg q8-12hr prn

Opioid withdrawal

- *Adult:* **PO** 15-40 mg/day individualized initially, then 20-120 mg/day titrated to patient response

Renal disease

• *Adult:* May need to be modified, no quantitative recommendations

Available forms: Inj 10 mg/ml; tabs 5, 10 mg; oral sol 5, 10 mg/5 ml, 10 mg/ml

SIDE EFFECTS

CNS: Drowsiness, dizziness, confusion, headache, sedation, euphoria, **seizures**

CV: Palpitations, bradycardia, change in B/P, **cardiac arrest, shock,** hypotension, **torsade de pointes, QT prolongation**

EENT: Tinnitus, blurred vision, miosis, diplopia

GI: Nausea, vomiting, anorexia, constipation, cramps, biliary tract spasm

GU: Increased urinary output, dysuria, urinary retention, impotence

INTEG: Rash, urticaria, bruising, flushing, diaphoresis, pruritus

RESP: **Respiratory depression, respiratory arrest**

Contraindications: Hypersensitivity to this product or chlorobutanol (inj), asthma, ileus

Black Box Warning: Respiratory depression

Precautions: Pregnancy (C), breastfeeding, children <18 yr, geriatric patients, addictive personality, increased intracranial pressure, MI (acute), severe heart disease, respiratory depression, pulmonary/renal/hepatic disease, respiratory insufficiency, torsade de pointes, COPD

Black Box Warning: QT prolongation, pain

PHARMACOKINETICS

Metabolized by liver; excreted by kidneys; crosses placenta; excreted in breast milk; half-life 8-59 hr, extended interval with continued dosing; 90% bound to plasma proteins

PO: Onset 30-60 min, peak 1-1.5 hr, duration 6-8 hr, cumulative 22-48 hr; PO half as active as INJ

SUBCUT/IM: Onset 10-20 min, peak 1½-2 hr, duration 4-6 hr, cumulative 22-48 hr

INTERACTIONS

⚠ Unpredictable reactions: MAOIs, do not use together

Increase: effects with other CNS depressants—alcohol, opiates, sedative/hypnotics, antipsychotics, skeletal muscle relaxants

Increase: toxicity—CYP3A4 inhibitors (aprepitant, antiretroviral protease inhibitors, clarithromycin, danazol, delavirdine, diltiazem, erythromycin, fluconazole, fluoxetine, fluroxamine, imatinib, ketoconazole, mibefradil, nefazodone, telithromycin, voriconazole)

Increase: QT prolongation—class IA antiarrhythmics (disopyramide, procainamide, quinidine), class III antiarrhythmics (amiodarone, bretylium, dofetilide, ibutilide, sotalol), astemizole, arsenic trioxide, bepridil, cisapride, chloroquine, clarithromycin, levomethadye, pentamidine, some phenothiazines, pimozide, probucol, sparfloxacin, terfenadine

Decrease: analgesia—rifampin, phenytoin, nalbuphine, pentazine

Decrease: methadone effect—CYP3A4 inducers (barbiturates, bosentan, carbamazepine, efavirenz, phenytoins, nevirapine, rifabutin, rifampin)

Drug/Herb

• Avoid use with St. John's wort

Increase: CNS depression—chamomile, hops, Jamaican dogwood, kava, lavender, mistletoe, nettle, pokeweed, poppy, senega, skullcap, valerian

Increase: anticholinergic effect—corkwood

Drug/Lab Test

Increase: amylase, lipase

NURSING CONSIDERATIONS

Assess:

• For pain: type, location, intensity, grimacing before and 1½-2 hr after administration; use pain scoring

• I&O ratio; check for decreasing output; may indicate urinary retention
• CNS changes: dizziness, drowsiness, hallucinations, euphoria, LOC, pupil reaction
• Allergic reactions: rash, urticaria
• Respiratory dysfunction: respiratory depression, character, rate, rhythm; notify prescriber if respirations are <10/min
• For opioid detoxification: no analgesia occurs, only prevention of withdrawal symptoms
• B/P, pulse, ECG; QT prolongation, hypotension, palpitations may occur
• Bowel changes, bulk, fluids, laxatives should be used for constipation

Administer:

• With antiemetic if nausea/vomiting occurs
• When pain is beginning to return; determine dosage interval by patient response
• Rotating inj sites, give deep in large muscle mass (IM)

Perform/provide:

• Storage in light-resistant container at room temperature
• Assistance with ambulation
• Safety measures: night-light, call bell within easy reach

Evaluate:

• Therapeutic response: decrease in pain, successful opioid withdrawal

Teach patient/family:

• To report any symptoms of CNS changes, allergic reactions
• That physical dependency may result from extended use

⚠ Withdrawal symptoms may occur: nausea, vomiting, cramps, fever, faintness, anorexia

Treatment of overdose: Naloxone (Narcan) 0.2-0.8 mg IV, O_2, IV fluids, vasopressors

methimazole (℞)

(meth-im'a-zole)
Tapazole
Func. class.: Thyroid hormone antagonist (antithyroid)
Chem. class.: Thioamide

Do not confuse:
methimazole/metoprolol/minoxidil

Action: Inhibits synthesis of thyroid hormones by decreasing iodine use in manufacture of thyroglobin and iodothyronine; does not affect circulatory T_4, T_3

Uses: Hyperthyroidism, preparation for thyroidectomy, thyrotoxic crisis, thyroid storm

DOSAGE AND ROUTES

Hyperthyroidism

• *Adult:* **PO** 15 mg/day (mild hyperthyroidism); 30-40 mg/day (moderate-severe); 60 mg/day (severe); maintenance 5-15 mg/day; may be divided
• *Child:* **PO** 0.4 mg/kg/day in divided doses q8hr; continue until euthyroid; maintenance dose 0.2 mg/kg/day in divided doses q8hr, max 30 mg/24 hr; may be divided

Preparation for thyroidectomy

• *Adult and child:* **PO** Same as above; iodine may be added × 10 days before surgery

Thyrotoxic crisis

• *Adult and child:* **PO** Same as hyperthyroidism with iodine and propranolol

Available forms: Tabs 5, 10, 15, 20 mg

SIDE EFFECTS

CNS: Drowsiness, headache, vertigo, fever, paresthesias, neuritis
ENDO: Enlarged thyroid
GI: Nausea, diarrhea, vomiting, **jaundice, hepatitis,** loss of taste
GU: **Nephritis**
HEMA: **Agranulocytosis, leukopenia, thrombocytopenia, hypothrombinemia, lymphadenopathy,** bleeding, vasculitis

INTEG: ***Rash, urticaria, pruritus, alopecia, hyperpigmentation,*** lupus-like syndrome
MS: Myalgia, arthralgia, nocturnal muscle cramps
Contraindications: Pregnancy (D), breastfeeding, hypersensitivity
Precautions: Infection, bone marrow depression, hepatic disease, bleeding disorders

PHARMACOKINETICS

Onset 12-18 hr; duration 36-72 hr; half-life 4-12 hr; excreted in urine, breast milk; crosses placenta

INTERACTIONS

- Agranulocytosis: phenothiazines

Increase: bone marrow depression—radiation, antineoplastic agents
Increase: response to digoxin
Decrease: effectiveness—amiodarone, potassium iodide
Decrease: Anticoagulant effect—warfarin
Drug/Lab Test
Increase: PT, AST, ALT, alk phos

NURSING CONSIDERATIONS

Assess:

- Pulse, B/P, temp
- I&O ratio; check for edema: puffy hands, feet, periorbits; indicate hypothyroidism
- Weight daily; same clothing, scale, time of day
- T_3, T_4, which are increased; serum TSH, which is decreased; free thyroxine index, which is increased if dosage is too low; discontinue product 3-4 wk before RAIU

⚠ Blood work: CBC for blood dyscrasias: leukopenia, thrombocytopenia, agranulocytosis; if these occur, product should be discontinued and other treatment initiated; LFTs

- Hypersensitivity: rash, enlarged cervical lymph nodes; product may have to be discontinued
- Hypoprothrombinemia: bleeding, petechiae, ecchymosis
- Clinical response: after 3 wk should include increased weight, pulse; decreased T_4

⚠ Bone marrow depression: sore throat, fever, fatigue

Administer:

- With meals to decrease GI upset
- At same time each day to maintain product level
- Lowest dose that relieves symptoms; discontinue before RAIU

Perform/provide:

- Storage in light-resistant container
- Fluids to 3-4 L/day, unless contraindicated

Evaluate:

- Therapeutic response: weight gain, decreased pulse, decreased T_4, B/P

Teach patient/family:

- Not to breastfeed
- To take pulse daily
- To report redness, swelling, sore throat, mouth lesions, fever, which indicate blood dyscrasias
- To keep graph of weight, pulse, mood
- To avoid OTC products that contain iodine
- That seafood, other iodine products may be restricted
- Not to discontinue this medication abruptly; thyroid crisis may occur; stress patient response
- That response may take several mo if thyroid is large
- The symptoms and signs of overdose: periorbital edema, cold intolerance, mental depression
- The symptoms of inadequate dose: tachycardia, diarrhea, fever, irritability
- To take medication as prescribed; do not skip or double dose

M

methocarbamol (℞)

(meth-oh-kar′ba-mole)
methocarbamol, Relaxin, Robaxin
Func. class.: Skeletal muscle relaxant, central acting
Chem. class.: Carbamate derivative

Do not confuse:
Relaxin/Reglan/Relafen/Rolephin
Action: Depresses multisynaptic pathways in the spinal cord, causing skeletal muscle relaxation
Uses: Adjunct for relief of spasm and pain in musculoskeletal conditions, tetanus

DOSAGE AND ROUTES

Musculoskeletal pain

- *Adult:* **PO** 1.5 g qid × 2-3 days, then 1 g qid; **IM** 500 mg in each gluteal region, may repeat q8hr; **IV BOL** 1-3 g/day, max 3 ml/min; **IV INF** 1 g/250 ml D_5W or NS, max 3 g/day
- *Geriatric:* **PO** 500 mg qid, titrate to needed dose

Tetanus management

- *Adult:* **IV direct** 1-2 g or **IV INF** 1-3 g q6hr, max 3 g
- *Child:* **IV** 15 mg/kg q6hr prn, max 1.8 g/m^2/day for 3 consecutive days, max 3 ml/min IV

Available forms: Tabs 500, 750 mg; inj 100 mg/ml

SIDE EFFECTS

CNS: Dizziness, weakness, drowsiness, headache, tremor, depression, confusion, insomnia; **seizures (IV, IM use)**
CV: Postural hypotension, **bradycardia**
EENT: Diplopia, temporary loss of vision, blurred vision, nystagmus, syncope, flushing, conjunctivitis, nasal congestion
GI: Nausea, vomiting, hiccups, anorexia, metallic taste, dyspepsia, jaundice
GU: Brown, black, green urine
HEMA: Hemolysis, increased hemoglobin, **leukopenia (IV only)**
INTEG: Rash, pruritus, fever, facial flushing, urticaria, phlebitis, extravasation
SYST: **Anaphylaxis, angioneurotic edema (IM, IV)**
Contraindications: Hypersensitivity to this product or PEG 300 (inj); children <12 yr, intermittent porphyria, renal disease (IM/IV)
Precautions: Pregnancy (C), breastfeeding, renal/hepatic disease, addictive personalities, myasthenia gravis, epilepsy

PHARMACOKINETICS

Metabolized in liver, excreted in urine unchanged, crosses placenta
PO: Onset ½ hr, peak 1-2 hr, half-life 1-2 hr
IM/IV: Onset rapid

INTERACTIONS

Increase: CNS depression—alcohol, tricyclics, opioids, barbiturates, sedatives, hypnotics
Drug/Herb
Increase: CNS depression—chamomile, hops, kava, skullcap, St. John's wort, valerian
Drug/Lab Test
False increase: VMA, urinary 5-HIAA

NURSING CONSIDERATIONS

Assess:

- Blood studies: CBC, WBC, differential; blood dyscrasias may occur
- During and after inj: CNS effects, rash, conjunctivitis, nasal congestion may occur
- Hepatic studies: AST, ALT, alk phos; hepatitis may occur; renal studies: BUN, creatinine with IV use
- EEG in epileptic patients; poor seizure control has occurred
- Allergic reactions: rash, fever, respiratory distress
- Severe weakness, numbness in extremities
- Tolerance: increased need for medication, more frequent requests for medication, increased pain

• CNS depression: dizziness, drowsiness, psychiatric symptoms

Administer:

PO route

• With meals for GI symptoms

IM route

• IM deep in large muscle mass; rotate sites

• Do not give SUBCUT

• Considered incompatible with any product in sol or syringe

IV route

• IV undiluted over 1 min or more; give 300 mg or less/1 min or longer; may be diluted in 250 ml or less D_5 or isotonic NaCl sol for slow IV inf

• By slow IV to prevent phlebitis; keep recumbent for 15 min to prevent orthostatic hypotension; check for extravasation

• Considered incompatible with any product in sol or syringe

Perform/provide:

• Storage in tight container at room temperature

• Assistance with ambulation if dizziness/drowsiness occurs

• Recumbent position during and 10-15 min after IV administration

Evaluate:

• Therapeutic response: decreased pain, spasticity

Teach patient/family:

• Not to discontinue medication quickly; insomnia, nausea, headache, spasticity, tachycardia will occur; product should be tapered off over 1-2 wk

• That urine may turn green, black, or brown

• Not to take with alcohol, other CNS depressants

• To avoid altering activities while taking this product

• To avoid hazardous activities if drowsiness, dizziness occurs

• To avoid using OTC medication: cough preparations, antihistamines, unless directed by prescriber

Treatment of overdose: Activated charcoal, dialysis; have epinephrine, antihistamines, and corticosteroids available, enhance elimination with osmotic diuresis, IV fluids for hypotension

⚠ High Alert

methotrexate (amethopterin, MTX) (℞)

(meth-oh-trex′ate)

methotrexate, Rheumatrex Dose Pack, Trexall

Func. class.: Antineoplastic-antimetabolite

Chem. class.: Folic acid antagonist

Do not confuse:

methotrexate/metolazone/mitoxantrone

Action: Inhibits an enzyme that reduces folic acid, which is needed for nucleic acid synthesis in all cells; S phase of cell cycle specific; immunosuppressive

Uses: Acute lymphocytic leukemia, in combination for breast, lung, head, neck carcinoma; lymphosarcoma, gestational choriocarcinoma, hydatidiform mole, psoriasis, RA, mycosis fungoides, osteosarcoma

Unlabeled uses: Burkitt's lymphoma, bladder/ovarian cancer, carcinomatous meningitis, desmoid tumor, fibromatosis, asthma, active Crohn's disease, ulcerative colitis, GVHD prophylaxis, ectopic pregnancy, pregnancy termination, psoriatic arthritis, pruritus due to cholestasis/primary biliary cirrhosis, SLE, sarcoidosis

DOSAGE AND ROUTES

Acute lymphocytic leukemia

• *Adult and child:* **PO/IM/IV** 3.3 mg/m^2/day × 4-6 wk until remission, then 20-30 mg/m^2 **PO/IM** q wk in 2 divided doses or 2.5 mg/kg **IV** × 2 wk

Choriocarcinoma

• *Adult and child:* **PO/IM** 15-30 mg/day × 5 days, then off 1 wk; may repeat

Meningeal leukemia

• *Adult and child:* 12 mg/m^2 **INTRATHECALLY** q2-5days until CSF is normal, then 1 additional dose, max 15 mg

M

Lymphosarcoma (stage III)
• *Adult:* **PO/IM/IV** 0.625-2.5 mg/kg/day
Osteosarcoma
• *Adult and child:* **IV** 12 g/m^2 given over 4 hr, then leucovorin rescue
Mycosis fungoides
• *Adult:* **PO** 2.5-10 mg/day until cleared (may be many months); **IM** 50 mg q wk or 25 mg 2×/wk
Psoriasis
• *Adult:* **PO/IM/IV** 10-25 mg q wk or 2.5 mg **PO** q12hr × 3 doses qwk, may increase to 25 mg q wk
Breast cancer
• *Adult:* **IV** 40-60 mg/m^2 on day 1 of every 21-28 days with other antineoplastics
Rheumatoid arthritis
• *Adult:* **PO** 7.5 mg/wk or divided doses of 2.5 mg q12hr × 3 given q wk; max 20 mg/wk
Polyarticular-course juvenile RA
• *Child:* **PO/IM** 10 mg/m^2 q wk
Burkitt's lymphoma (stages I, II, III) (unlabeled)
• *Adult:* **PO** 10-25 mg/day × 4-8 days with 7-day rest period
Bladder cancer (unlabeled)
• *Adult:* **IV** 30 mg/m^2 on days 1, 15, 22 q28days in combination with vinBLAStine, DOXOrubicin, cisplatin (MVAC) regimen
Desmoid tumor/fibromatosis (unlabeled)
• *Adult and child:* **IV** 20-30 mg/m^2 q wk in combination with vinBLAStine
Ovarian cancer (unlabeled)
• *Adult:* **IV** 40 mg/m^2 on days 1, 8 q28 days with hexamethylmelamine, cyclophosphamide, fluorouracil
Active Crohn's disease/ulcerative colitis (unlabeled)
• *Adult:* **IM** 25 mg q wk; **SUBCUT** 15 mg/kg q wk × 16 wk
GVHD prophylaxis (unlabeled)
• *Adult and child:* **IV** 15 mg/m^2 on day 1 after transplant, then 10 mg/m^2 on days 3, 6, 11
Ectopic pregnancy (unlabeled)
• *Adult:* **IM** 50 mg/m^2, may be used in combination with mifepristone
Pregnancy termination prior to 63rd day of pregnancy (unlabeled)
• *Adult:* **IM** 50 mg/m^2, then intravaginal misoprostol 5-7 days later
Psoriatic arthritis (unlabeled)
• *Adult:* **PO** 5-7.5 mg q wk

Available forms: Tabs 2.5, 5, 7.5, 10, 15 mg; inj 25 mg/ml; powder for inj 20 mg, 1 g

SIDE EFFECTS

CNS: Dizziness, **seizures, leukoencephalopathy,** headache, confusion, hemiparesis, malaise, fatigue, chills, fever; **arachnoiditis** (intrathecal)
EENT: Blurred vision, optic neuropathy
GI: Nausea, vomiting, anorexia, diarrhea, ulcerative stomatitis, **hepatotoxicity,** cramps, ulcer, gastritis, **GI hemorrhage,** abdominal pain, hematemesis, **hepatic fibrosis, acute toxicity**
GU: Urinary retention, **renal failure,** menstrual irregularities, defective spermatogenesis, **hematuria, azotemia, uric acid nephropathy**
HEMA: **Leukopenia, thrombocytopenia, myelosuppression, anemia**
INTEG: Rash, alopecia, dry skin, urticaria, photosensitivity, folliculitis, vasculitis, petechiae, ecchymosis, acne, alopecia, **severe fatal skin reaction**
RESP: **Methotrexate-induced lung disease**
SYST: **Sudden death,** *Pneumocystis jiroveci*

Contraindications: Hypersensitivity, leukopenia (<3500/mm^3), thrombocytopenia (<100,000/mm^3), anemia, psoriatic patients with severe renal disease, alcoholism, HIV

Black Box Warning: Pregnancy (X), hepatic disease

Precautions: Breastfeeding, children

Black Box Warning: Renal disease, ascites, diarrhea, exfoliative dermatitis, infection, intrathecal administration, lymphoma, pleural effusion, pulmonary disease, radiation therapy, stomatitis, tumor lysis syndrome

PHARMACOKINETICS

Not metabolized; excreted in urine (unchanged); crosses placenta, blood-brain barrier; 50% plasma protein bound; terminal half-life 10-12 hr

PO: Readily absorbed

PO/IM/IV: Onset, duration unknown

IT: Onset, peak, duration unknown

INTERACTIONS

Increase: toxicity—salicylates, sulfa products, other antineoplastics, radiation, alcohol, probenecid, NSAIDs, phenylbutazone, theophylline, penicillins

Increase: hypoprothrombinemia—oral anticoagulants

Decrease: effect of oral digoxin, vaccines, phenytoin, fosphenytoin

Decrease: effect of methotrexate—folic acid supplements

NURSING CONSIDERATIONS

Assess:

- Make sure that product is taken weekly in RA, JRA

⚠ CBC, differential, platelet count weekly; withhold product if WBC is <3500/mm^3 or platelet count is <100,000/mm^3; notify prescriber; WBC, platelet nadirs occur on day 7

- Renal studies: BUN, serum uric acid, urine CCr, electrolytes before, during therapy, I&O ratio; report fall in urine output to <30 ml/hr
- Monitor temp; fever may indicate beginning infection; no rectal temps
- Hepatic studies before and during therapy: bilirubin, alk phos, AST, ALT; liver biopsy should be done before start of therapy (psoriasis patients)
- Bleeding time, coagulation time during treatment; bleeding: hematuria, guaiac, bruising or petechiae, mucosa or orifices
- Effects of alopecia on body image; discuss feelings about body changes

⚠ Hepatotoxicity: jaundiced skin and sclera, dark urine, clay-colored stools, pruritus, abdominal pain, fever, diarrhea

- Monitor methotrexate levels, adjust leucovorin dose based on the level
- Buccal cavity for dryness, sores, ulceration, white patches, oral pain, bleeding, dysphagia

⚠ Symptoms indicating severe allergic reaction: rash, urticaria, itching, flushing

Administer:

- Chemotherapeutic handling
- Antiemetic 30-60 min before giving product
- Allopurinol or sodium bicarbonate to maintain uric acid levels, alkalinization of urine (pH >6.5), adequate fluids

IV route

- After diluting 5 mg/2 ml of sterile H_2O for inj; give through Y-tube or 3-way stopcock

⚠ Leucovorin calcium within 24 hr of this product to prevent tissue damage; check agency policy, continue until methotrexate level <10^{-8}m

⚠ Give sodium bicarbonate tabs or IV fluids to prevent precipitation of product at high doses; urine pH should be >7; may need to reduce dosage if BUN 20-30 mg/dl or creatinine is 1.2-2 mg/dl; stop product if BUN >30 mg/dl or creatinine is >2 mg/dl

Additive compatibilities: Cephalothin, cyclophosphamide, cytarabine, fluorouracil, hydrOXYzine, mercaptopurine, ondansetron, sodium bicarbonate, vinCRIStine

Solution compatibilities: Amino acids, 4.25%/D_{25}, D_5W, sodium bicarbonate 0.05 mol/L, sodium chloride 0.9%

Syringe compatibilities: Bleomycin, cisplatin, cyclophosphamide, doxapram, DOXOrubicin, fluorouracil, furosemide, heparin, leucovorin, mitomycin, vinBLAStine, vinCRIStine

Y-site compatibilities: Allopurinol, amifostine, amphotericin B cholesteryl, asparaginase, aztreonam, bleomycin, cefepime, ceftriaxone, cimetidine, cisplatin, cyclophosphamide, cytarabine, DAUNOrubicin, dexchlorpheniramine, diphenhydrAMINE, DOXOrubicin, DOXOrubicin liposome, etoposide, famotidine, filgrastim, fludarabine, fluorouracil, furo-

M

semide, gallium, ganciclovir, granisetron, heparin, hydromorphone, imipenem/cilastatin, leucovorin, lorazepam, melphalan, mesna, methylPREDNISolone, metoclopramide, mitomycin, morphine, ondansetron, oxacillin, paclitaxel, piperacillin/tazobactam, prochlorperazine, ranitidine, sargramostim, teniposide, thiotepa, vinBLAStine, vinCRIStine, vinorelbine

Perform/provide:

- Strict medical asepsis and protective isolation if WBC levels are low
- Liquid diet: carbonated beverage, Jell-O; dry toast, crackers may be added when patient is not nauseated or vomiting
- Increased fluid intake to 2-3 L/day to prevent urate deposits, calculi formation, unless contraindicated
- Diet low in purines: absence of organ meats (kidney, liver), dried beans, peas to maintain alkaline urine
- Rinsing of mouth tid-qid with water, club soda; brushing of teeth bid-tid with soft brush or cotton-tipped applicators for stomatitis; use unwaxed dental floss
- Nutritious diet with iron, vitamin supplements, no folic acid
- Storage in tightly closed container in cool environment; store injection, powder for inj in dark, dry area

Evaluate:

- Therapeutic response: decreased tumor size, spread of malignancy; decreased joint inflammation, pain in RA

Teach patient/family:

- To report any complaints, side effects to nurse or prescriber: black tarry stools, chills, fever, sore throat, bleeding, bruising, cough, SOB, dark or bloody urine, seizures
- That hair may be lost during treatment; wig or hairpiece may make patient feel better; tell patient that new hair may be different in color, texture (alopecia is rare)
- To avoid foods with citric acid, hot or rough texture if stomatitis is present
- To report stomatitis: any bleeding, white spots, ulcerations in mouth to prescriber; tell patient to examine mouth daily, report symptoms to nurse, use good oral hygiene
- That contraceptive measures are recommended during therapy and for at least 8 wk following cessation of therapy, to discontinue breastfeeding; toxicity to infant may occur
- To drink 10-12 glasses of fluid/day
- To avoid alcohol, salicylates, live vaccines
- To avoid use of razors, commercial mouthwash
- To use sunblock to prevent burns

methoxy polyethylene glycol-epoetin beta (℞)

(meth-ox′ee pol′ee-eth′i-leen glye′kol-e-poe′e-tin bay′ta)

Mircera

Func. class.: Antianemic, biologic modifier, hormone

Chem. class.: Amino acid polypeptide

Action: Erythropoietin is one factor controlling rate of red cell production; product is developed by recombinant DNA technology

Uses: Anemia caused by reduced endogenous erythropoietin production, primarily end-stage renal disease; to correct hemostatic defect in uremia on all dosages

DOSAGE AND ROUTES

For all dosages

- *Adult and geriatric:* Reduce by 25% if Hgb >1 g/dl in any 2 wk period or if Hgb is close to 12 g/dl; if Hgb continues to rise after decrease, hold until Hgb starts to decrease

Treatment of anemia in chronic renal failure (dialysis dependant/independent)—not currently using ESA

- *Adult and geriatric:* **IV/SUBCUT** 0.6 mcg q2wk

Using >80 mcg/wk darbepoetin or >16,000 units/wk epoetin

- *Adult and geriatric:* **IV/SUBCUT** 180 mcg q2wk or 360 mcg q4wk

Using 40-80 mcg/wk darbepoetin or 8000-16,000 units/wk epoetin

- *Adult and geriatric:* **IV/SUBCUT** 100 mcg q2wk

Using <40 mcg/wk darbepoetin or <8000 units/wk epoetin

- *Adult and geriatric:* **IV/SUBCUT** 60 mcg q2wk or 120 mcg q4wk

SIDE EFFECTS

CNS: **Seizures, encephalopathy,** headache

CV: *Hypertension,* edema, **heart failure,** hypotension, **sinus tachycardia, stroke, MI**

GI: Diarrhea

HEMA: **Anemia, red cell aplasia, thrombocytopenia, thromboembolism, thrombosis**

INTEG: Pruritus, rash, erythema, inj site reaction

MS: Muscle spasms, back pain

SYST: Antibody formation

Contraindications: Red cell aplasia, neoplastic disease, hypersensitivity to mannitol

Black Box Warning: Hgb >12 g/dl

Precautions: Pregnancy (C), breastfeeding, children <1 mo, multidose preserved formulation contains benzyl alcohol and should not be used in premature infants, seizure disorder, porphyria, CV disease, hemodialysis, latex allergy, surgery, hypertension, history of CABG

Black Box Warning: Neoplastic disease

PHARMACOKINETICS

SUBCUT: Half-life 139 ± 67 hr rise in reticulocytes on day 7, rise in Hgb in 7-14 days

IV: Half-life 134 ± 65 hr

INTERACTIONS

- Adverse reactions: other erythropoiesis stimulating agents (ESA) (epoetin, darbepoetin); do not give concurrently

Increase: action of methoxy polyethylene glycol-epoetin—androgens

NURSING CONSIDERATIONS

Assess:

- Renal studies: urinalysis, protein, blood, BUN, creatinine; I&O, report drop in output <50 ml/hr
- ⚠ CBC, blood studies: ferritin, transferrin monthly; transferrin ≥20%, ferritin ≥100 ng/ml; Hct 2×/wk until stabilized in target range (30%-36%) then at regular intervals; those with endogenous erythropoietin levels of <500 units/L respond to this agent; monitor Hct 2×/wk in chronic renal failure; patients treated with zidovudine or patients with cancer should be monitored weekly, then periodically after stabilization; death may occur in Hgb >12 g/dl
- B/P; check for rising B/P as Hct rises, antihypertensives may be needed; hypertension may occur rapidly leading to hypertensive encephalopathy
- CNS symptoms: for seizures if Hct is increased within 2 wk by 4 pts
- For hypersensitivity reactions: skin rashes, urticaria (rare), antibody development
- ⚠ For pure cell aplasia in absence of other causes, evaluate by testing sera for recombinant erythropoetin antibodies; any loss of response to epoetin should be evaluated
- Dialysis patients: thrill, bruit of shunts, monitor for circulation impairment

Administer:

- Do not shake vial
- Iron supplements as needed; adequate iron stores are needed for this agent to work properly

SUBCUT route

- Inject into outer aspect of upper arms, abdomen (except for 2 inches around navel) or front aspect of middle thigh; do

M

not inject in areas that have stretch marks, or are scarred or bruised

- Rotate inj sites

IV route

- Additional heparin to lower chance of clots
- By direct inj or bolus into venous line at end of dialysis

Solution compatibilities: Do not dilute or administer with other solutions

Evaluate:

- Therapeutic response: increase in reticulocyte count in 2-6 wk, Hgb/Hct; increased appetite, enhanced sense of well-being

Teach patient/family:

- To avoid driving or hazardous activity during beginning of treatment
- To monitor B/P
- To take iron supplements, vit B_{12}, folic acid as directed

methylcellulose (OTC)

(meth-ill-sell′yoo-lose)

Citrucel

Func. class.: Laxative, bulk forming

Chem. class.: Hydrophilic semisynthetic cellulose derivative

Do not confuse:

Citrucel/Citracal

Action: Attracts water, expands in intestine to increase peristalsis; also absorbs excess water in stool; decreases diarrhea

Uses: Chronic constipation

DOSAGE AND ROUTES

- *Adult:* **PO** up to 6 g/day in divided doses
- *Child 6-12 yr:* **PO** 3 g/day in divided doses

Available forms: Powder 105 mg/g, 196 mg/g

SIDE EFFECTS

GI: **Obstruction,** abdominal distention

Contraindications: Hypersensitivity, GI obstruction, hepatitis

PHARMACOKINETICS

PO: Onset 12-24 hr, peak 1-3 days

INTERACTIONS

Decrease: absorption—digoxin, nitrofurantoin, salicylates, tetracyclines, oral anticoagulants

Drug/Herb

Increase: laxative action—flax senna

NURSING CONSIDERATIONS

Assess:

- Blood, urine electrolytes if used often
- I&O ratio to identify fluid loss
- Cause of constipation; lack of fluids, bulk, exercise, constipating products
- Cramping, rectal bleeding, nausea, vomiting; product should be discontinued

Administer:

PO route

- Alone for better absorption; do not take within 1 hr of other products
- In morning or evening (oral dose)

Evaluate:

- Therapeutic response: decrease in constipation

Teach patient/family:

- To mix powder in water
- To increase fluid intake
- That normal bowel movements do not always occur daily
- Not to use in presence of abdominal pain, nausea, vomiting
- To notify prescriber if constipation unrelieved or if symptoms of electrolyte imbalance occur: muscle cramps, pain, weakness, dizziness, excessive thirst

methyldopa/methyldopate (℞)

(meth-ill-doe′pa)

Apo-Methyldopa ♣, Dopamet ♣, methyldopa/methyldopate, Novo-medopa ♣, Nu-Medopa ♣

Func. class.: Antihypertensive

Chem. class.: Centrally acting α-adrenergic inhibitor

Do not confuse:
methyldopa/L-dopa/levodopa

Action: Stimulates central inhibitory α-adrenergic receptors or acts as false transmitter, resulting in reduction of arterial pressure

Uses: Hypertension, hypertensive crisis

DOSAGE AND ROUTES

- *Adult:* **PO** 250-500 mg bid or tid, then adjusted q2days as needed, 0.5-2 g/day in 2-4 divided doses (maintenance), max 3 g/day; **IV** 250-500 mg in 100 ml D_5W q6hr, run over 30-60 min, max 1 g q6hr, switch to oral as soon as possible
- *Geriatric:* **PO** 125 mg bid-tid, increase q2days as needed, max 3 g/day
- *Child:* **PO** 10 mg/kg/day in 2-4 divided doses, max 65 mg/kg or 3 g/day, whichever is less; **IV** 20-40 mg/kg/day in 4 divided doses, max 65 mg/kg or 3 g, whichever is less

Available forms: *Methyldopa:* tabs 125, 250, 500 mg; oral susp 50 mg/ml; *methyldopate:* inj 50 mg/ml

SIDE EFFECTS

CNS: Drowsiness, weakness, dizziness, sedation, headache, depression, psychosis paresthesias, parkinsonism, Bell's palsy, nightmares

CV: Bradycardia, **myocarditis,** orthostatic hypotension, angina, edema, weight gain, **CHF,** paradoxical pressor response (IV use)

EENT: Nasal congestion

ENDO: Breast enlargement, gynecomastia, breastfeeding, amenorrhea

GI: Nausea, vomiting, diarrhea, constipation, **hepatic dysfunction,** sore or "black" tongue, **pancreatitis,** colitis, flatulence

GU: Impotence, failure to ejaculate

HEMA: **Leukopenia, thrombocytopenia, hemolytic anemia, granulocytopenia,** positive Coombs' test

INTEG: Rash, **toxic epidermal necrolysis,** lupuslike syndrome

Contraindications: Active hepatic disease, hypersensitivity

Precautions: Pregnancy (B), geriatric patients, cardiac disease, autoimmune disease, depression, dialysis, hemolytic anemia, Parkinson's disease, pheochromocytoma, sulfite hypersensitivity

PHARMACOKINETICS

PO: Peak 2-4 hr, duration 12-24 hr
IV: Peak 2 hr, duration 10-16 hr
Metabolized by liver, excreted in urine, half-life 2 hr

M

INTERACTIONS

- Lithium toxicity: lithium

Increase: pressor effect—sympathomimetic amines, MAOIs

Increase: hypotension, CNS toxicity—levodopa

Increase: hypotension—diuretics, other antihypertensives

Increase: psychosis—haloperidol

Increase: CNS depression—alcohol, antihistamines, antidepressants, analgesics, sedative/hypnotics

Increase: B/P—phenothiazines, β-blockers, amphetamines, NSAIDs, tricyclics, barbiturates

Increase: hypoglycemia—TOLBUTamide

Decrease: methyldopa absorption—iron

Drug/Herb

Increase: toxicity, death—aconite

Increase: antihypertensive effect—barberry, betony, black catechu, black cohosh, bloodroot, broom, burdock, cat's claw, dandelion, goldenseal, hawthorn, Irish moss, Jamaican dogwood, kelp, khella, mistletoe, parsley

Increase or decrease: antihypertensive effect—astragalus, cola tree
Decrease: effect—capsicum, Indian snakeroot
Decrease: antihypertensive effect—coltsfoot, guarana, khat, licorice, yohimbe
Drug/Lab Test
Interference: urinary uric acid, serum creatinine, AST
False increase: urinary catecholamines

NURSING CONSIDERATIONS

Assess:
- Blood studies: neutrophils, decreased platelets
- Direct Coombs' test before/after 6, 12 mo of therapy
- Baselines in renal, hepatic studies, before therapy begins
- B/P when beginning treatment, periodically thereafter, report significant changes
- Allergic reaction: rash, fever, pruritus, urticaria; product should be discontinued if antihistamines fail to help
- CNS symptoms, especially in the geriatric patient, depression, change in mental status
- Symptoms of CHF: edema, dyspnea, wet crackles, B/P
- Renal symptoms: polyuria, oliguria, urinary frequency; I&O ratio, weight, report weight gain >5 lb

Administer:
PO route
- Shake susp before use

IV route
- After diluting with 100 ml D_5W; run over ½-1 hr

Additive compatibilities: Aminophylline, ascorbic acid, chloramphenicol, diphenhydrAMINE, heparin, magnesium sulfate, multivitamins, netilmicin, potassium chloride, promazine, sodium bicarbonate, succinylcholine, verapamil, vit B/C

Solution compatibilities: D_5W, D_5/0.9% NaCl, Ringer's, sodium bicarbonate 5%, 0.9% NaCl, amino acids 4.25%/D_{25}, $Dextran_6$/0.9% NaCl, Normosol R, Normosol M/D_5W

Y-site compatibilities: Esmolol, heparin, meperidine, morphine, theophylline

Perform/provide:
- Storage of tabs in tight container

Evaluate:
- Therapeutic response: decrease in B/P in hypertension

Teach patient/family:
- To avoid hazardous activities
- Not to discontinue product abruptly, or withdrawal symptoms may occur: anxiety, increased B/P, headache, insomnia, increased pulse, tremors, nausea, sweating
- Not to use OTC (cough, cold, allergy) products unless directed by prescriber
- To comply with dosage schedule even if feeling better
- To rise slowly to sitting or standing position to minimize orthostatic hypotension
- To notify prescriber of mouth sores, sore throat, fever, swelling of hands or feet, irregular heartbeat, chest pain, signs of angioedema
- That excessive perspiration, dehydration, vomiting, diarrhea may lead to fall in B/P; consult prescriber
- That dizziness, fainting, light-headedness may occur during first few days of therapy
- That compliance is necessary; not to skip or stop product unless directed by prescriber
- That product may cause skin rash or impaired perspiration

Treatment of overdose: Gastric evacuation, sympathomimetics may be indicated; if severe, hemodialysis

methylergonovine (℞)

(meth-ill-er-goe-noe'veen)
Methergine, methylergonovine
Func. class.: Oxytocic
Chem. class.: Ergot alkaloid

Action: Stimulates uterine, vascular, smooth muscle, causing contractions; decreases bleeding; arterial vasoconstriction

Uses: Treatment of hemorrhage postpartum or postabortion, uterine contractions

DOSAGE AND ROUTES

• *Adult:* **PO** 200 tid-qid up to 7 days; **IM/IV** 200 mcg q2-4hr for 1-5 doses

Available forms: Inj 200 mcg/ml; tabs 200 mcg

SIDE EFFECTS

CNS: Headache, dizziness, **seizures**
CV: **Hypotension,** chest pain, palpitation, **hypertension, dysrhythmias, CVA (IV)**
EENT: Tinnitus
GI: Nausea, vomiting
GU: Cramping
INTEG: Sweating, rash, allergic reactions
RESP: Dyspnea

Contraindications: Pregnancy, hypertension, PID, respiratory/cardiac disease, peripheral vascular disease, angina, arteriosclerosis, CAD, dysfunctional uterine bleeding, eclampsia, MI, neonates, Raynaud's disease, sepsis, stroke, Buerger's disease, thrombophlebitis, hypersensitivity to ergot preparations

Precautions: Pregnancy (C), severe renal/hepatic disease, jaundice, diabetes mellitus, seizure disorders, sepsis, CAD

PHARMACOKINETICS

Metabolized in liver, excreted in urine
PO: Onset 5-25 min, duration 3 hr
IM: Onset 2-5 min, duration 3 hr
IV: Onset immediate, duration 45 min

INTERACTIONS

Increase: vasoconstriction—vasopressors, nicotine

NURSING CONSIDERATIONS

Assess:

• B/P, pulse, character and amount of vaginal bleeding; watch for indications of hemorrhage
• Respiratory rate, rhythm, depth; notify prescriber of abnormalities
• For uterine relaxation; observe for severe cramping
• Ergot toxicity: tinnitus, hypertension, palpitations, chest pain, nausea, vomiting, weakness; cold, numb extremities

Administer:

• Only during fourth stage of labor; not to be used to augment labor
• IM in deep muscle mass; rotate inj sites of additional doses

IV route

• Undiluted through Y-tube or 3-way stopcock; give 0.2 mg or less/min or diluted in 5 ml 0.9% NaCl given through Y-site
• With crash cart available on unit; IV route used only in emergencies

Y-site compatibilities: Heparin, hydrocortisone sodium succinate, potassium chloride, vit B/C

Evaluate:

• Therapeutic response: absence of hemorrhage

Teach patient/family:

• To report increased blood loss, severe abdominal cramps, fever or foul-smelling lochia
• To avoid smoking
• Not to breastfeed while taking this product

M

methylnaltrexone (℞)

(meth-il-nal-trex′one)
Relistor
Func. class.: Opioid antagonist

Action: Peripheral mu-opioid receptor antagonist that reduces constipation associated with opiate agonists

Uses: Treatment of opioid-induced constipation in patients with advanced illness who are receiving palliative care when response to laxative therapy has been insufficient

Unlabeled uses: Pruritus, nausea/vomiting related to morphine, urinary retention from opioids

DOSAGE AND ROUTES

Opiate-agonist induced constipation

• *Adult >114 kg:* **SUBCUT** 0.15 mg/kg every other day prn

• *Adult 62-114 kg:* **SUBCUT** 12 mg every other day prn
• *Adult 38-<62 kg:* **SUBCUT** 8 mg every other day prn
• *Adult <38 kg:* **SUBCUT** 0.15 mg/kg every other day prn

Renal dose

• *Adult:* **SUBCUT** CCr <30 ml/min, reduce normal adult dose by 50%

Pruritus, nausea/vomiting related to morphine (unlabeled) (oral dose investigational)

• *Adult:* **PO** 19.2 mg/kg 20 min prior to morphine

Available forms: Solution for inj 12 mg/0.6 ml

SIDE EFFECTS

CNS: Dizziness, migraines, obsessive-compulsive disorder
GI: Nausea, vomiting, diarrhea, flatulence, abdominal pain

Contraindications: Hypersensitivity, GI obstruction, IV route

Precautions: Pregnancy (B), breastfeeding, children, geriatric patients, renal disease, diarrhea, driving, operating machinery

PHARMACOKINETICS

Terminal half-life 8 hr, protein binding 11%-15.3%; renal impairment has a marked effect on the renal excretion of methylnaltrexone, dose adjustment is required for patients with CCr <30 ml/min, renal clearance decreased and total systemic exposure increase in patients with severe renal impairment who received a single SUBCUT dose of 0.3 mg/kg

SUBCUT: Peak 30 min

NURSING CONSIDERATIONS

Assess:

• Serum creatinine
• For stool characteristics

Administer:

• SUBCUT only; oral dose is investigational and not currently available
• Do not give IV; IV dosing for urinary retention is investigational

SUBCUT route

• Inspect the solution before use; it should be a clear, colorless to pale yellow aqueous solution; do not use if particulate matter or discoloration are present
• Withdraw the needed amount of solution into a sterile syringe; if immediate administration is impossible, the syringe may be kept at room temperature for up to 24 hr; the syringe does not need to be kept away from light during the 24-hr period; immediately discard any unused portion in the vile; no preservatives are present
• Administer into the upper arm, abdomen, or thigh no more than 1×/24 hr; rotate inj sites; do not inject the same spot each time; do not inject into areas where skin is tender, bruised, red, or hard; avoid areas with scars or stretch marks
• If using with retractable needle, slowly push down on the plunger past the resistance point until the syringe is empty and a click is heard

Perform/provide:

• Storage at 15°-30° C (59°-86° F); do not freeze
• Storage away from light

Evaluate:

• Therapeutic response: decreasing constipation

Teach patient/family:

• Not to drive or operate machinery until effect is known

methylphenidate (℞)

(meth-ill-fen′i-date)
Concerta, Daytrana, Metadate CD, Methylin, Methylin ER, Methidate, PMS-Methylphenidate ✱, Riphenidate ✱, Ritalin, Ritalin LA, Ritalin SR

Func. class.: Cerebral stimulant
Chem. class.: Piperidine derivative

Controlled Substance Schedule II

Do not confuse:
methylphenidate/methadone

Action: Increases release of norepinephrine, DOPamine in cerebral cortex to reticular activating system; exact action not known

Uses: Attention deficit disorder (ADD), attention deficit hyperactivity disorder (ADHD); narcolepsy (except Concerta, Metadate CD, Ritalin LA)

DOSAGE AND ROUTES

Attention deficit hyperactivity disorder

- *Adult:* **PO** 20-30 mg/day; **EXT REL** (Concerta) 18-36 mg/day
- *Child >6 yr:* **PO** (immediate release tabs, chew tabs, oral sol) 5 mg before breakfast and lunch, increasing by 5-10 mg/wk, max 60 mg/day; **EXT REL** 20 mg daily-tid, max 60 mg/day

Attention deficit hyperactivity disorder, conversion from PO to transdermal

- *Child 6-12 yr:* Week 1, 12.5 cm^2 (10 mg); week 2, 18.75 cm^2 (15 mg); week 3, 25 cm^2 (20 mg); week 4, 37.5 cm^2 (30 mg)

Narcolepsy

- *Adult:* **PO** 10 mg bid-tid, 30-45 min before meals, may increase up to 60 mg/day

Major depression/post-stroke depression

- *Adult and geriatric:* **PO** 2.5 mg QAM, increase q3days by 2.5 mg to desired dose, max 20 mg/day

Available forms: Tabs 5, 10, 20 mg; ext rel tabs 10, 20, mg; ext rel tabs (Concerta) 18, 27, 36, 54 mg; ext rel caps 10, 20, 30, 40 mg; oral sol 5 mg, 10 mg/ml; chew tabs (Methylin) 2.5, 5, 10 mg; transdermal patch 12.5 cm^2 (10 mg), 18.75 cm^2 (15 mg), 25 cm^2 (20 mg), 37.5 cm^2 (30 mg)

SIDE EFFECTS

CNS: Hyperactivity, insomnia, restlessness, talkativeness, dizziness, drowsiness, toxic psychosis, headache, akathisia, dyskinesia, masking or worsening of Gilles de la Tourette's syndrome, **seizures,** hallucinations, **malignant neuroleptic syndrome**

CV: Palpitations, tachycardia, B/P changes, angina, **dysrhythmias**

ENDO: Growth retardation

GI: Nausea, anorexia, dry mouth, weight loss, abdominal pain

HEMA: **Leukopenia, anemia, thrombocytopenic purpura**

INTEG: **Exfoliative dermatitis,** urticaria, rash, erythema multiforme, **hypersensitivity reactions**

MISC: Fever, arthralgia, scalp hair loss

Contraindications: Children <6 yr, hypersensitivity, anxiety, history of Gilles de la Tourette's syndrome; glaucoma, anorexia nervosa, tartrazine dye hypersensitivity

Precautions: Pregnancy (C), breastfeeding, hypertension, depression, seizures

Black Box Warning: Substance abuse

PHARMACOKINETICS

PO: Onset ½-1 hr, duration 4-6 hr, metabolized by liver, excreted by kidneys, half-life 3-4 hr

INTERACTIONS

- Hypertensive crisis: MAOIs or within 14 days of MAOIs, vasopressors

Increase: effects of tricyclics, SSRIs, anticonvulsants

Decrease: effect of guanethidine

M

Drug/Herb

• Synergistic effect: melatonin

Increase: CNS stimulation—cola nut, guarana, horsetail, yerba maté, yohimbe

Drug/Food

Increase: stimulation—caffeine

NURSING CONSIDERATIONS

Assess:

• VS, B/P; may reverse antihypertensives; check patients with cardiac disease more often for increased B/P

• CBC, urinalysis, in diabetes: blood glucose, urine glucose; insulin changes may have to be made, since eating will decrease

• Height, growth rate q3mo in children; growth rate may be decreased

• Mental status: mood, sensorium, affect, stimulation, insomnia, aggressiveness

⚠ Withdrawal symptoms: headache, nausea, vomiting, muscle pain, weakness

• Appetite, sleep, speech patterns

• For attention span, decreased hyperactivity in ADHD persons

Administer:

PO route

• Do not crush or chew ext rel medication; caps may be opened and beads sprinkled over spoonful of applesauce

• Gum, hard candy, frequent sips of water for dry mouth

• Give immediate rel dose 30-45 min prior to meals

• Chew tab with adequate water to prevent choking; contains phenylalanine

• Avoid metadate CD on day of surgery

Transdermal route

• Place on clean, dry area of the hip; avoid waist; removal is 9 hr after application; fold after removal and flush down toilet

• If patch falls off, apply a new patch to a different site; total wear time should be 9 hr

Evaluate:

• Therapeutic response: decreased hyperactivity (ADHD) or ability to stay awake (narcolepsy)

Teach patient/family:

• To decrease caffeine consumption (coffee, tea, cola, chocolate); may increase irritability, stimulation; not to use guarana, yerba maté, cola nut

• To avoid OTC preparations unless approved by prescriber

• To taper off product over several weeks, or depression, increased sleeping, lethargy will occur

• To avoid driving, hazardous activities if dizziness, blurred vision occur

• To avoid alcohol ingestion

• To avoid hazardous activities until stabilized on medication

• To get needed rest; patients will feel more tired at end of day

• That shell of Concerta tab may appear in stools

• To take regular tab at least 6 hr prior to sleep; 10 hr for ext rel

• That for transdermal patch, once tray is opened, use within 2 mo; do not store patches without protective patch

Treatment of overdose: Administer fluids; hemodialysis or peritoneal dialysis; antihypertensive for increased B/P; administer short-acting barbiturate before lavage

*methylPREDNISolone (℞)

(meth-il-pred-niss′oh-lone)

A-Methapred, depMedalone, Depoject, Depo-Medrol, Depopred, Depo-Predate, Medrol, Duralone, Medralone, Rep-Pred, Solu-Medrol

Func. class.: Corticosteroid, synthetic

Chem. class.: Glucocorticoid, immediate acting

Do not confuse:

methylPREDNISolone/predniSONE/ medroxyPROGESTERone/ methylTESTOSTERone

Action: Decreases inflammation by suppression of migration of polymorphonuclear leukocytes, fibroblasts; reversal of increased capillary permeability and lysosomal stabilization

Uses: Severe inflammation, shock, adrenal insufficiency, collagen disorders, management of acute spinal cord injury, multiple sclerosis

Unlabeled uses: Multiple myeloma, bronchospasm prophylaxis, airway-obstructing hemangioma, noncardiogenic pulmonary edema, idiopathic pulmonary fibrosis, carpal tunnel syndrome, temporal arteritis, Churg-Strauss syndrome, mixed connective tissue disease, polyarteritis nodosa, relapsing polychondritis, polymyalgia rheumatica, vasculitis, Wegener's granulomatosis, *Pneumocystis jiroveci* pneumonia in AIDS patients, acute spinal cord injury, severe acute respiratory syndrome (SARS), acute interstitial nephritis

DOSAGE AND ROUTES

Adrenal insufficiency/inflammation

- *Adult:* **PO** 2-60 mg in 4 divided doses; **IM** 10-80 mg (acetate); **IM/IV** 10-250 mg (succinate); **INTRAARTICULAR** 4-30 mg (acetate); **RECT** 40 mg 3-7 × wk for ≥2 wk
- *Child:* **IV** 0.5-1.7 mg/kg in 3-4 divided doses (succinate); **RECT** 0.5-1 mg/kg (15-30 mg/m^2) daily or every other day × 1 wk or more

Shock

- *Adult:* **IV** 100-250 mg q2-6hr or 30 mg/kg, then q4-6hr prn, for 2-3 days (succinate)

Multiple sclerosis

- *Adult:* **PO** 160 mg/day × 1 wk, then 64 mg every other day × 30 days

Multiple myeloma/temporal arteritis/Churg-Strauss syndrome/ mixed connective tissue disease/ polyarteritis nodosa/relapsing polychondritis/polymyalgia rheumatica/vasculitis/Wegener's granulomatosis (unlabeled)

- *Adult:* **PO** 4-48 mg/day in 4 divided doses; **IM** 10-120 mg (acetate); **IV** 10-40 mg over several min (sodium succinate)
- *Child:* **PO/IM** 0.5-1.7 mg/kg or 5-25 mg/m^2/day in divided doses q6-12hr

Bronchospasm prophylaxis (unlabeled)

- *Adult and adolescent:* **PO/IV** 40-80 mg/day in 1-2 divided doses
- *Child:* **PO/IV** 1 mg/kg in 2 divided doses (max 60 mg)

Airway-obstructing hemangioma (unlabeled)

- *Child:* **PO** 0.5-1.7 mg/kg or 5-25 mg/m^2/day in divided doses q6-12hr

Idiopathic pulmonary fibrosis (unlabeled)

- *Adult:* **IV** 1-2 g q wk or every other week

Carpal tunnel syndrome (unlabeled)

- *Adult:* **INJ** (local) 40-80 mg as a single inj

Available forms: Tabs 2, 4, 6, 8, 16, 24, 32 mg; inj 20, 40, 80 mg/ml acetate; inj 40, 125, 500, 1000, 2000 mg/vial succinate; susp for inj 20, 40, 80 mg/ml; dose pack 4 mg tabs; enema 40 mg

SIDE EFFECTS

CNS: Depression, flushing, sweating, headache, mood changes

CV: Hypertension, **circulatory collapse, thrombophlebitis, embolism,** tachycardia

EENT: Fungal infections, increased intraocular pressure, blurred vision, cataracts

GI: Diarrhea, nausea, abdominal distention, **GI hemorrhage,** increased appetite, pancreatitis

HEMA: **Thrombocytopenia**

INTEG: Acne, poor wound healing, ecchymosis, petechiae

MS: Fractures, osteoporosis, weakness

Contraindications: Hypersensitivity, Cushing's syndrome, measles, varicella, fungal infections

Precautions: Pregnancy (C), breastfeeding, diabetes mellitus, glaucoma, osteoporosis, seizure disorders, ulcerative colitis, CHF, myasthenia gravis, renal disease, esophagitis, peptic ulcer, tartrazine, benzyl alcohol, corticosteroid hypersensitivity, viral infection, TB, traumatic brain injury

PHARMACOKINETICS

Half-life >3½ hr (plasma), 18-36 hr (tissue); crosses placenta, enters breast milk in small amounts; metabolized in liver; excreted by kidneys (unchanged)

PO: Peak 1-2 hr, duration 1½ days, well absorbed

IM: Peak 4-8 days, duration 1-4 wk, well absorbed

Intraarticular: Peak 1 wk

INTERACTIONS

Increase: side effects—amphotericin B, diuretics

Increase: methylPREDNISolone action—oral contraceptives

Increase: adrenal suppression—CYP3A4 inhibitors (aprepitant, antiretroviral protease inhibitors, clarithromycin, danazol, delavirdine, diltiazem, erythromycin, fluconazole, fluoxetine, fluvoxamine, imatinib, ketoconazole, mibefradil, nefazodone, telithromycin, voriconazole)

Decrease: methylPREDNISolone effect—CYP3A4 inducers (barbiturates, bosentan, carbamazepine, efavirenz, phenytoins, nevirapine, rifabutin, rifampin)

Decrease: effects of antidiabetics, vaccines, somatrem

Drug/Herb

- Avoid use with St. John's wort

Increase: hypokalemia—aloe, buckthorn, cascara sagrada, Chinese rhubarb, senna

Increase: corticosteroid effect—aloe, licorice, perilla

Drug/Food

- Do not use with grapefruit juice; level of methylPREDNISolone will be increased

Drug/Lab Test

Increase: cholesterol, sodium, blood glucose, uric acid, calcium, urine glucose

Decrease: Ca, K, T_4, T_3, thyroid ^{131}I uptake test, urine 17-OHCS, 17-KS

False negative: skin allergy tests

NURSING CONSIDERATIONS

Assess:

- Potassium depletion: parethesias, fatigue, nausea, vomiting, depression, polyuria, dysrhythmias, weakness
- Edema, hypertension, cardiac symptoms
- Mental status: affect, mood, behavioral changes, aggression
- Potassium, blood glucose, urine glucose while on long-term therapy; hypokalemia and hyperglycemia
- Joint mobility, pain, edema if given intraarticularly
- B/P q4hr, pulse; notify prescriber of chest pain, crackles
- I&O ratio; be alert for decreasing urinary output, increasing edema; weight daily; notify prescriber of weekly gain >5 lb
- Adrenal insufficiency: weight loss, nausea, vomiting, confusion, anxiety, hypotension, weakness
- Plasma cortisol levels during long-term therapy (normal level: 138-635 nmol/L SI units when drawn at 8 AM)
- Growth in children on long-term treatment

Administer:

- Titrated dose; use lowest effective dose
- IM inj deep in large muscle mass; rotate sites; avoid deltoid; use 21G needle; after shaking suspension (parenteral)
- In one dose in AM to prevent adrenal suppression; avoid SUBCUT administration; may damage tissue
- With food or milk to decrease GI symptoms (PO)

⚠ Do not give Solu-Medrol intrathecally

IV route

- After diluting with diluent provided; agitate slowly; give 500 mg or less/1 min or longer; may be given as IV inf in its own diluent over 10-20 min

Additive compatibilities: Chloramphenicol, cimetidine, clindamycin, DOPamine, granisetron, heparin, norepinephrine, penicillin G potassium, ranitidine, theophylline, verapamil

Syringe compatibilities: Granisetron, metoclopramide

Y-site compatibilities: Acyclovir, amifostine, amphotericin B cholesteryl, amrinone, aztreonam, cefepime, cisplatin, cladribine, cyclophosphamide, cytarabine, DOPamine, DOXOrubicin, enalaprilat, famotidine, fludarabine, granisetron, heparin, melphalan, meperidine, methotrexate, metronidazole, midazolam, morphine, piperacillin/tazobactam, remifentanil, sodium bicarbonate, tacrolimus, teniposide, theophylline, thiotepa

Perform/provide:

- Assistance with ambulation in patient with bone tissue disease to prevent fractures

Evaluate:

- Therapeutic response: ease of respirations, decreased inflammation; decreased symptoms of adrenal insufficiency
- Infection: increased temp, WBC, even after withdrawal of medication; product masks infection

Teach patient/family:

- To increase intake of potassium, calcium, protein
- To carry emergency ID (corticosteroid user)
- To notify prescriber if therapeutic response decreases; dosage adjustment may be needed

⚠ Not to discontinue abruptly, or adrenal crisis can result

- To avoid OTC products: salicylates, alcohol in cough products, cold preparations unless directed by prescriber; to avoid vaccinations, since immunosuppression occurs
- About cushingoid symptoms
- To recognize the symptoms of adrenal insufficiency: nausea, anorexia, fatigue, dizziness, dyspnea, weakness, joint pain

metipranolol ophthalmic

See Appendix B

metoclopramide (℞)

(met-oh-kloe-pra'mide)

Apo-Metoclop ♣, Emex ♣, Maxeran ♣, metoclopramide, Octamide, Reglan, Sensamide IV

Func. class.: Cholinergic, antiemetic

Chem. class.: Central DOPamine receptor antagonist

Do not confuse:

metoclopramide/metolazone

Reglan/Megace/Renagel

Action: Enhances response to acetylcholine of tissue in upper GI tract, which causes contraction of gastric muscle; relaxes pyloric, duodenal segments; increases peristalsis without stimulating secretions, blocks DOPamine in chemoreceptor trigger zone of CNS

Uses: Prevention of nausea, vomiting induced by chemotherapy, radiation, delayed gastric emptying, gastroesophageal reflux

M

Unlabeled uses: Hiccups, migraines, breastfeeding induction, lung cancer

DOSAGE AND ROUTES

Renal dose

- *Adult:* CCr <40 ml/min 50% of dose

Nausea/vomiting (chemotherapy)

- *Adult:* **IV** 1-2 mg/kg 30 min before administration of chemotherapy, then q2hr × 2 doses, then q3hr × 3 doses
- *Child (unlabeled):* **IV** 1-2 mg/kg/dose

Facilitate small bowel intubation, in radiologic exams

- *Adult and child >14 yr:* **IV** 10 mg over 1-2 min
- *Child <6 yr:* **IV** 0.1 mg/kg
- *Child 6-14 yr:* **IV** 2.5-5 mg

Diabetic gastroparesis

- *Adult:* **PO** 10 mg 30 min before meals, at bedtime × 2-8 wk
- *Geriatric:* **PO** 5 mg ½ hr before meals, at bedtime, increase to 10 mg if needed

Gastroesophageal reflux

- *Adult:* **PO** 10-15 mg qid 30 min before meals and at bedtime

• *Child:* **PO** 0.4-0.8 mg/kg/day in 4 divided doses

Lactation induction (unlabeled)

• *Adult:* **PO** 10 mg bid-tid, may increase to 20-45 mg/day in divided doses

Non–small cell lung cancer (NSCLC) radiation sensitizer (unlabeled)

• *Adult:* **IV** (Sensamide IV) 2 mg/kg given 1 hr prior to radiation therapy 3×/wk

Hiccups (unlabeled)

• *Adult:* **PO/IM/IV** 10 mg q6hr

Available forms: Tabs 5, 10 mg; syr 5 mg/5 ml; inj 5 mg/ml; conc sol 10 mg/ml

SIDE EFFECTS

CNS: ***Sedation, fatigue, restlessness, headache, sleeplessness, dystonia,*** dizziness, drowsiness, **suicide ideation, seizures,** EPS, **neuroleptic malignant syndrome; tardive dyskinesia (>3 mo, high doses)**

CV: Hypotension, supraventricular tachycardia

GI: Dry mouth, constipation, nausea, anorexia, vomiting, diarrhea

GU: Decreased libido, prolactin secretion, amenorrhea, galactorrhea

HEMA: **Neutropenia, leukopenia, agranulocytosis**

INTEG: Urticaria, rash

Contraindications: Hypersensitivity to this product or procaine or procainamide, seizure disorder, pheochromocytoma, breast cancer (prolactin dependent), GI obstruction

Precautions: Pregnancy (B), breastfeeding, GI hemorrhage, CHF, Parkinson's disease

Black Box Warning: Tardive dyskinesia

PHARMACOKINETICS

Metabolized by liver, excreted in urine, half-life 4 hr

PO: Onset ½-1 hr, duration 1-2 hr

IM: Onset 10-15 min, duration 1-2 hr

IV: Onset 1-3 min, duration 1-2 hr

INTERACTIONS

• Avoid use with MAOIs

Increase: sedation—alcohol, other CNS depressants

Increase: risk for EPS—haloperidol, phenothiazines

Decrease: action of metoclopramide—anticholinergics, opiates

Drug/Lab Test

Increase: prolactin, aldosterone, thyrotropin

NURSING CONSIDERATIONS

Assess:

• For EPS and tardive dyskinesia, more likely to occur in geriatric patients

• Mental status: depression, anxiety, irritability

• GI complaints: nausea, vomiting, anorexia, constipation

Administer:

PO route

• ½-1 hr before meals for better absorption

• Gum, hard candy, frequent rinsing of mouth for dry oral cavity

IV route

• DiphenhydrAMINE IV for EPS

• Undiluted if dose is ≤10 mg; give over 2 min; more than 10 mg may be diluted in 50 ml or more D_5W, NaCl, Ringer's, LR and given over 15 min or more

Syringe compatibilities: Aminophylline, ascorbic acid, atropine, benztropine, bleomycin, butorphanol, chlorproMAZINE, cisplatin, cyclophosphamide, cytarabine, dexamethasone, dimenhyDRINATE, diphenhydrAMINE, DOXOrubicin, droperidol, fentanyl, fluorouracil, heparin, hydrocortisone, hydrOXYzine, insulin (regular), leucovorin, lidocaine, magnesium sulfate, meperidine, methotrimeprazine, methylPREDNISolone, midazolam, mitomycin, morphine, pentazocine, perphenazine, prochlorperazine, promazine, promethazine, ranitidine, scopolamine, sufentanil, vinBLAStine, vinCRIStine, vit B/C

Y-site compatibilities: Acyclovir, aldesleukin, amifostine, aztreonam, bleomycin, ciprofloxacin, cisatracurium, cisplatin, cladribine, cyclophosphamide, cytarabine, diltiazem, DOXOrubicin, droperidol, famotidine, filgrastim, fluconazole, fludarabine, fluorouracil, foscarnet, gallium, granisetron, heparin, idarubicin, leucovorin, melphalan, meperidine, meropenem, methotrexate, mitomycin, morphine, ondansetron, paclitaxel, piperacillin/tazobactam, propofol, remifentanil, sargramostim, sufentanil, tacrolimus, teniposide, thiotepa, vinBLAStine, vinCRIStine, vinorelbine, zidovudine

Perform/provide:

- Protect from light with aluminum foil during inf
- Discard open ampules

Evaluate:

- Therapeutic response: absence of nausea, vomiting, anorexia, fullness

Teach patient/family:

- To avoid driving, other hazardous activities until patient is stabilized on this medication
- To avoid alcohol, other CNS depressants that will enhance sedating properties of this product

metolazone (℞)

(me-tole'a-zone)

Zaroxolyn

Func. class.: Diuretic, antihypertensive

Chem. class.: Thiazide-like quinazoline derivative

Do not confuse:
metolazone/methotrexate/metoclopramide

Action: Acts on distal tubule by increasing excretion of water, sodium, chloride, potassium, magnesium, bicarbonate

Uses: Edema, hypertension, CHF, nephrotic syndrome

DOSAGE AND ROUTES

Edema

- *Adult:* **PO** 2.5-20 mg/day; max 20 mg/day

Hypertension

- *Adult:* **PO** 2.5-5 mg/day

Available forms: Tabs 2.5, 5, 10 mg

SIDE EFFECTS

CNS: Anxiety, depression, ***headache, dizziness, fatigue, weakness***

CV: Orthostatic hypotension, palpitations, volume depletion, hypotension, chest pain

EENT: Blurred vision

ELECT: ***Hypokalemia,*** hypercalcemia, hyponatremia

GI: ***Nausea, vomiting, anorexia,*** constipation, diarrhea, cramps, pancreatitis, GI irritation, dry mouth, jaundice

GU: ***Urinary frequency,*** polyuria, **uremia, glucosuria,** nocturia, impotence

HEMA: **Aplastic anemia, hemolytic anemia, leukopenia, agranulocytosis, neutropenia**

INTEG: ***Rash,*** urticaria, purpura, photosensitivity, fever, dry skin

META: ***Hyperglycemia,*** increased creatinine, BUN

MS: Muscle cramps, joint pain, swelling

Contraindications: Hypersensitivity to thiazides or sulfonamides, anuria

Black Box Warning: Hepatic encephalopathy

Precautions: Pregnancy (B), breastfeeding, geriatric patients, hypokalemia, renal/hepatic disease, gout, COPD, lupus erythematosus, diabetes mellitus, hypotension, history of pancreatitis, hypersensitivity to sulfonamides, thiazides

PHARMACOKINETICS

Onset 1 hr, peak 2 hr, duration 12-24 hr, excreted unchanged by kidneys, crosses placenta, enters breast milk, half-life 8-14 hr

INTERACTIONS

Increase: hypokalemia—mezlocillin, piperacillin, amphotericin B, glucocorticoids, digoxin, stimulant laxatives

Increase: hypotension—alcohol (large amounts), nitrates, antihypertensives, barbiturates, opioids

Increase: toxicity—lithium

M

Increase: metolazone effects—loop diuretics
Decrease: action of metolazone—NSAIDs, salicylates

Drug/Herb

Increase: hypokalemia—aloe, buckthorn, cascara sagrada, rhubarb, senna
Increase: toxicity, death—aconite
Increase: antihypertensive effect—barberry, betony, black catechu, black cohosh, bloodroot, broom, burdock, cat's claw, dandelion, goldenseal, Irish moss, Jamaican dogwood, kelp, khella, mistletoe, parsley
Increase or decrease: antihypertensive effect—astragalus, cola tree
Decrease: antihypertensive effect—coltsfoot, guarana, khat, licorice

NURSING CONSIDERATIONS

Assess:

- Weight, I&O daily to determine fluid loss; effect of product may be decreased if used daily
- Rate, depth, rhythm of respiration, effect of exertion
- B/P lying, standing; postural hypotension may occur
- Electrolytes: K, Mg, Na, Cl; include BUN, blood glucose, CBC, serum creatinine, blood pH, ABGs, uric acid, calcium
- Improvement in edema of feet, legs, sacral area daily if medication is being used in CHF
- Improvement in CVP q8hr
- Signs of metabolic alkalosis: drowsiness, restlessness
- Signs of hypokalemia: postural hypotension, malaise, fatigue, tachycardia, leg cramps, weakness
- Rashes, fever daily
- Confusion, especially in geriatric patients; take safety precautions if needed

Administer:

- In AM to avoid interference with sleep if using product as a diuretic
- Potassium replacement if potassium <3 mg/dl
- With food, if nausea occurs; absorption may be decreased slightly
- Extended product is Zaroxolyn, prompt product is Mykrox; they are not interchangeable

Evaluate:

- Therapeutic response: decreased edema, B/P

Teach patient/family:

- To increase fluid intake to 2-3 L/day unless contraindicated, to rise slowly from lying or sitting position
- To notify prescriber of muscle weakness, cramps, nausea, dizziness
- That product may be taken with food or milk
- To use sunscreen for photosensitivity
- That blood glucose may be increased in diabetics
- To take early in day to avoid nocturia
- To avoid alcohol
- To avoid sodium food, increase potassium foods in diet

Treatment of overdose: Lavage if taken orally; monitor electrolytes; administer dextrose in saline; monitor hydration, CV, renal status

metoprolol (℞)

(meh-toe'proe-lole)
Betaloc ♣, Betaloc Durules ♣, Lopresor ♣, Lopressor, Lopressor SR ♣, Nu-Metop ♣, Novometoprol ♣, Toprol-XL
Func. class.: Antihypertensive, antianginal
Chem. class.: β_1-Blocker

Do not confuse:
metoprolol/misoprostol

Action: Lowers B/P by β-blocking effects; reduces elevated renin plasma levels; blocks β_2-adrenergic receptors in bronchial, vascular smooth muscle only at high doses, negative chronotropic effect

Uses: Mild to moderate hypertension, acute MI to reduce cardiovascular mortality, angina pectoris, NYHA class II, III heart failure

Unlabeled uses: Migraine prevention, heart rate control in atrial fibrillation/flutter without accessory pathway, essential tremor, unstable angina

DOSAGE AND ROUTES

Hypertension

• *Adult:* **PO** 50 mg bid, or 100 mg/day; may give up to 200-450 mg in divided doses; **EXT REL** 25-100 mg daily, titrate at weekly intervals; max 400 mg/day

• *Geriatric:* **PO** 25 mg/day initially, increase weekly as needed

• *Child and adolescent 6-16 yr:* **PO ER** 1 mg/kg up to 50 mg daily

Myocardial infarction

• *Adult:* **IV BOL** (early treatment) 5 mg q2min × 3, then 50 mg **PO** 15 min after last dose and q6hr × 48 hr; (late treatment) **PO** maintenance 100 mg bid for ≥3 mo

Heart failure (NYHA class II/III)

• *Adult:* **PO EXT REL** 25 mg daily × 2 wk (class II); 12.5 mg daily (class III); **PO** (unlabeled) 5 mg bid, titrate to 100-150 mg/day in 2-3 divided doses

Angina

• *Adult:* **PO** 100 mg/day as a single dose or in two divided doses, increase q wk prn or 100 mg **EXT REL** daily

Migraine prevention (unlabeled)

• *Adult:* **PO** 50-100 mg bid-qid; 50-200 mg daily (XL)

Heart rate control in atrial fibrillation/flutter without accessory pathway (unlabeled)

• *Adult:* **IV BOL** (acute setting) 2.5-5 mg over 2 min, may repeat dose × 3; **PO** (nonacute setting) 25-100 mg bid

Essential tremor (unlabeled)

• *Adult:* **PO** 50 mg/day, may increase, max 300 mg/day in divided doses; **EXT REL** 100 mg/day

Available forms: Tabs 50, 100 mg; inj 1 mg/ml; ext rel tab (succinate) (XL) 25, 50, 100, 200 mg; ext rel tabs, tartrate: 100 mg

SIDE EFFECTS

CNS: *Insomnia, dizziness,* mental changes, hallucinations, depression, anxiety, headaches, nightmares, confusion, fatigue

CV: Hypotension, **bradycardia,** CHF, *palpitations,* dysrhythmias, **cardiac arrest, AV block, pulmonary/peripheral edema, chest pain**

EENT: Sore throat; dry, burning eyes

GI: *Nausea, vomiting,* colitis, cramps, *diarrhea,* constipation, flatulence, dry mouth, *hiccups*

GU: Impotence

HEMA: **Agranulocytosis, eosinophilia, thrombocytopenia, purpura**

INTEG: Rash, purpura, alopecia, dry skin, urticaria, pruritus

RESP: **Bronchospasm,** dyspnea, wheezing

Contraindications: Hypersensitivity to β-blockers, cardiogenic shock, heart block (2nd, 3rd degree), sinus bradycardia, pheochromocytoma, sick sinus syndrome

Precautions: Pregnancy (C), breastfeeding, geriatric patients, major surgery, diabetes mellitus, thyroid/renal/hepatic disease, COPD, CAD, nonallergic bronchospasm, CHF, bronchial asthma, CVA, children, depression, vasospastic angina

Black Box Warning: Abrupt discontinuation

PHARMACOKINETICS

Half-life 3-4 hr, metabolized in liver (metabolites), excreted in urine, crosses placenta, enters breast milk

PO: Peak 2-4 hr, duration 13-19 hr

PO-ER: Peak 6-12 hr, duration 24 hr

IV: Onset immediate, peak 20 min, duration 6-8 hr

INTERACTIONS

• Do not use with MAOIs

Increase: hypotension, bradycardia—reserpine, hydrALAZINE, methyldopa, prazosin, amphetamines, epinephrine, H_2-antagonists, calcium channel blockers

Increase: hypoglycemic effects—insulin, oral antidiabetics

Increase: metoprolol effect—cimetidine

Increase: effects of benzodiazepines

Decrease: antihypertensive effect—salicylates, NSAIDs

Decrease: metoprolol level—barbiturates

Decrease: effects of DOPamine, DOBUTamine, xanthines

Drug/Herb

Increase: toxicity, death—aconite

Increase: antihypertensive effect—barberry, betony, black catechu, black cohosh, bloodroot, broom, burdock, cat's claw, dandelion, goldenseal, Irish moss, Jamaican dogwood, kelp, khella, mistletoe, parsley

Increase or decrease: antihypertensive effect—astragalus, cola tree

Decrease: antihypertensive effect—coltsfoot, guarana, khat, licorice

Drug/Food

Increase: absorption with food

Drug/Lab Test

Increase: BUN, potassium, ANA titer, serum lipoprotein, triglycerides, uric acid, alk phos, LDH, AST, ALT

NURSING CONSIDERATIONS

Assess:

- ECG directly when giving IV during initial treatment
- I&O, weight daily
- B/P during initial treatment, periodically thereafter; pulse q4hr; note rate, rhythm, quality
- Apical/radial pulse before administration; notify prescriber of any significant changes or pulse <50 bpm
- Baselines in renal, hepatic studies before therapy begins
- Edema in feet, legs daily
- Skin turgor, dryness of mucous membranes for hydration status

Administer:

PO route

- Do not break, crush, or chew ext rel tabs
- Regular release tab after meals, at bedtime; tab may be crushed or swallowed whole; take at same time each day

IV route

- IV, undiluted, give over 1 min, × 3 doses at 2-5 min intervals; start **PO** 15 min after last IV dose

Y-site compatibilities: Alteplase, meperidine, morphine

Perform/provide:

- Storage in dry area at room temperature, do not freeze

Evaluate:

- Therapeutic response: decreased B/P after 1-2 wk, decreased anginal pain

Teach patient/family:

- To take immediately after meals
- Not to discontinue product abruptly; taper over 2 wk; may cause precipitate angina
- Not to use OTC products containing α-adrenergic stimulants (nasal decongestants, OTC cold preparations) unless directed by prescriber
- To report bradycardia, dizziness, confusion, depression, fever, sore throat, SOB, decreased vision to prescriber
- To take pulse, B/P at home; advise when to notify prescriber
- To avoid alcohol, smoking, sodium intake
- To comply with weight control, dietary adjustments, modified exercise program
- To carry emergency ID to identify product, allergies
- To monitor blood glucose closely, if diabetic
- To avoid hazardous activities if dizziness is present
- To report symptoms of CHF: difficult breathing, especially on exertion or when lying down, night cough, swelling of extremities
- To take medication at bedtime to prevent effect of orthostatic hypotension
- To wear support hose to minimize effects of orthostatic hypotension
- To report Raynaud's symptoms

Treatment of overdose: Lavage, IV atropine for bradycardia, IV theophylline for bronchospasm, digoxin, O_2, diuretic for cardiac failure, hemodialysis, hypotension administer vasopressor (norepinephrine)

metronidazole (℞)

(me-troe-ni′da-zole)
Apo-Metronidazole ♣, Flagyl, Flagyl ER, Flagyl IV, Flagyl IV RTU, metronidazole, Novonidazole ♣, Trikacide ♣
Func. class.: Antiinfective—miscellaneous
Chem. class.: Nitroimidazole derivative

Action: Direct-acting amebicide/trichomonacide binds, disrupts DNA structure inhibiting bacterial nucleic acid synthesis

Uses: Intestinal amebiasis, amebic abscess, trichomoniasis, refractory trichomoniasis, bacterial anaerobic infections, giardiasis, septicemia, endocarditis, bone, joint infections, lower respiratory tract infections, rosacea

Unlabeled uses: Crohn's disease, urethritis, amebiasis due to *Dientamoeba fragilis, Entamoeba polecki,* giardiasis, pruritus; gastric ulcer, dyspepsia *(H. pylori),* pseudomembranous colitis, guinea worm disease, periodontitis

DOSAGE AND ROUTES

Trichomoniasis

- *Adult:* **PO** 250 mg tid × 7 days or 2 g in single dose; do not repeat treatment for 4-6 wk
- *Child (unlabeled):* **PO** 15 mg/kg/day divided in 3 doses × 7-10 days

Refractory trichomoniasis

- *Adult:* **PO** 250 mg bid × 10 days

Amebic hepatic abscess

- *Adult:* **PO** 500-750 mg tid × 5-10 days
- *Child:* **PO** 35-50 mg/kg/day in 3 divided doses × 10 days

Intestinal amebiasis

- *Adult:* **PO** 750 mg tid × 5-10 days
- *Child:* **PO** 35-50 mg/kg/day in 3 divided doses × 10 days; then oral iodoquinol

Anaerobic bacterial infections

- *Adult:* **IV INF** 15 mg/kg over 1 hr, then 7.5 mg/kg **IV** or **PO** q6hr, not to exceed 4 g/day; first maintenance dose should be administered 6 hr following loading dose

Bacterial vaginosis

- *Adult:* **PO** ext rel 750 mg/day × 7 days

Persistent urethritis (unlabeled)

- *Adult and adolescent:* **PO** 2 g as a single dose with azithromycin

Dientamoeba fragilis *(unlabeled)*

- *Child:* **PO** 250 mg tid × 7 days

Entamoeba polecki *(unlabeled)*

- *Adult:* **PO** 750 mg tid × 10 days
- *Child:* **PO** 30-50 mg/kg/day in 3 divided doses × 5-10 days

Guinea worm disease (unlabeled)

- *Adult:* **PO** 250 mg tid × 10 days
- *Child:* **PO** 25 mg/kg/day in 3 divided doses × 10 days

Crohn's disease (unlabeled)

- *Adult:* **PO** 250 mg tid-qid

Giardiasis (unlabeled)

- *Adult:* **PO** 250 mg tid × 5 days
- *Child:* **PO** 5 mg/kg tid × 5 days

Antibiotic-associated pseudomembranous colitis (unlabeled)

- *Adult:* **PO** 250-500 mg 3-4 ×/day × 7-14 days
- *Child:* **PO** 20 mg/kg/day (max 2 g) divided q6hr

Available forms: Tabs 250, 500 mg; ext rel tab (ER) 750 mg; caps 375, 500 mg; inj 500 mg/100 ml; powder for inj 500-mg single dose

SIDE EFFECTS

CNS: Headache, dizziness, confusion, irritability, restlessness, ataxia, depression, fatigue, drowsiness, insomnia, paresthesia, peripheral neuropathy, **seizures,** incoordination, depression, encephalopathy

CV: Flattening of T waves

EENT: Blurred vision, sore throat, retinal edema, dry mouth, metallic taste, furry

M

tongue, glossitis, stomatitis, photophobia
GI: *Nausea, vomiting, diarrhea,* epigastric distress, *anorexia,* constipation, *abdominal cramps,* **pseudomembranous colitis**
GU: Darkened urine, vaginal dryness, polyuria, **albuminuria,** dysuria, cystitis, decreased libido, **neurotoxicity,** incontinence, dyspareunia, candidiasis
HEMA: **Leukopenia, bone marrow, depression, aplasia**
INTEG: Rash, pruritus, urticaria, flushing
Contraindications: Pregnancy 1st trimester, breastfeeding, hypersensitivity to this product, GI/renal/hepatic disease, contracted visual or color fields, blood dyscrasias, CNS disorders
Precautions: Pregnancy (B) 2nd/3rd trimesters, geriatric patients, *Candida* infections, heart failure, fungal infection, dental disease, bone marrow suppression, hematologic disease

Black Box Warning: Secondary malignancy

PHARMACOKINETICS

Crosses placenta, enters breast milk, metabolized by liver 30%-60%, excreted in urine (60%-80%)
PO: Peak 1-2 hr, half-life 6-11 hr, absorbed 80%-85%
IV: Onset immediate, peak end of inf

INTERACTIONS

- Disulfiram reaction: alcohol

Increase: metronidazole level—cimetidine
Increase: lithium, CYP3A4 substrates
Increase: action of warfarin
Increase: leukopenia—azathioprine, fluorouracil
Decrease: metronidazole action—phenobarbital, phenytoin, cimetidine

Drug/Herb

- Do not use acidphilus with antiinfectives; separate by several hours

Drug/Lab Test

Altered: AST, ALT, LDH

NURSING CONSIDERATIONS

Assess:

- For infection: WBC, wound symptoms, fever, skin or vaginal secretions; start treatment after C&S
- For opportunistic fungal infections
- Stools during entire treatment; should be clear at end of therapy; stools should be free of parasites for 1 yr before patient is considered cured (amebiasis)
- Vision by ophthalmic exam during, after therapy; vision problems often occur
- I&O; weight daily; stools for number, frequency, character

⚠ Neurotoxicity: peripheral neuropathy, seizures, dizziness, uncoordination, pruritus, joint pains; product may be discontinued

- Allergic reaction: fever, rash, itching, chills; product should be discontinued if these symptoms occur
- Superinfection: fever, monilial growth, fatigue, malaise
- Renal and reproductive dysfunction: dysuria, polyuria, impotence, dyspareunia, decreased libido

Administer:

PO route

- Do not break, crush, or chew ER products
- PO with or after meals to avoid GI symptoms, metallic taste; crush tabs if needed

IV route

- Prediluted; metronidazole IV, dilute with 4.4 ml sterile H_2O or 0.9% NaCl; must be diluted further with 8 mg/ml or more 0.9% NaCl, D_5W, or LR; must neutralize with 5 mEq $NaCO_3$/500 mg; CO_2 gas will be generated and may require venting; run over 1 hr or more; primary IV must be discontinued; may be given as cont inf; do not use aluminum products; IV may require venting

Additive compatibilities: Amikacin, aminophylline, cefazolin, cefotaxime, ceftazidime, ceftizoxime, ceftriaxone, cefuroxime, chloramphenicol, ciprofloxacin, clindamycin, disopyramide, floxacillin, fluconazole, gentamicin, heparin, moxalactam, multielectrolyte concentrate, multivitamins, netilmicin, penicillin G potassium, tobramycin

Y-site compatibilities: Acyclovir, allopurinol, amifostine, amiodarone, cefepime, cisatracurium, cyclophosphamide, diltiazem, DOPamine, DOXOrubicin liposome, enalaprilat, esmolol, fluconazole, foscarnet, granisetron, heparin, hydromorphone, labetalol, lorazepam, magnesium sulfate, melphalan, meperidine, methylPREDNISolone, midazolam, morphine, perphenazine, piperacillin/tazobactam, remifentanil, sargramostim, tacrolimus, teniposide, theophylline, thiotepa, vinorelbine

Perform/provide:

• Storage in light-resistant container; do not refrigerate

Evaluate:

• Therapeutic response: decreased symptoms of infection

Teach patient/family:

• That urine may turn dark-reddish brown, product may cause metallic taste
• Proper hygiene after BM; hand-washing technique
• To notify physician for numbness or tingling of extremities
• To avoid hazardous activities, since dizziness can occur
• Need for compliance with dosage schedule, duration of treatment
• To use condoms if treatment for trichomoniasis, or cross-contamination may occur; notify prescriber if pregnant or plan to become pregnant
• To use frequent sips of water, sugarless gum, candy for dry mouth
• That treatment of both partners is necessary in trichomoniasis
• Not to drink alcohol or use preparations containing alcohol during use or for 48 hr after use of product; disulfiram-like reaction can occur

metronidazole topical

See Appendix B

mexiletine (℞)

(mex-il'e-teen)

Func. class.: Antidysrhythmic (Class IB)

Chem. class.: Lidocaine analog

Action: Increases electrical stimulation threshold of ventricle, His-Purkinje system, which stabilizes cardiac membrane

Uses: Life-threatening ventricular tachycardia; because of proarrhythmic effects, use with lesser dysrhythmias not recommended

Unlabeled uses: Neuropathic pain

DOSAGE AND ROUTES

• *Adult:* **PO** 200-400 mg (loading dose), then 200 mg q8hr, then 200-400 mg q8hr

Neuropathic pain (unlabeled)

• *Adult:* **PO** 450-600 mg/day

Available forms: Caps 150, 200, 250 mg

SIDE EFFECTS

CNS: Headache, dizziness, confusion, **seizures,** tremors, psychosis, nervousness, paresthesias, weakness, fatigue, coordination difficulties, change in sleep habits

CV: Hypotension, bradycardia, angina, PVCs, **heart block, CV collapse or arrest,** sinus node slowing, **left ventricular failure,** syncope, **cardiogenic shock, AV conduction disturbances, CHF, atrial dysrhythmias, palpitations, ventricular dysrhythmias, ventricular tachycardia, other ventricular arrhythmias in acute phase of MI**

EENT: Blurred vision, tinnitus

GI: Nausea, vomiting, anorexia, diarrhea, abdominal pain, **hepatitis,** dry mouth, peptic ulcer, altered taste, **GI bleeding,** constipation

GU: Urinary hesitancy, decreased libido

HEMA: **Thrombocytopenia, leukopenia, agranulocytosis**

INTEG: Rash, alopecia, dry skin

MISC: Edema, arthralgia, fever, SLE syndrome
RESP: Dyspnea

Contraindications: Hypersensitivity, cardiogenic shock, severe heart block (if no pacemaker)

Precautions: Pregnancy (C), breastfeeding, children, renal/hepatic disease, CHF, seizure disorder, hypotension, blood dyscrasias, electrolyte imbalances, Parkinson's disease

Black Box Warning: MI, cardiac arrhythmias

PHARMACOKINETICS

PO: Peak 2-3 hr; half-life 12 hr, metabolized by liver, excreted unchanged by kidneys (10%), excreted in breast milk

INTERACTIONS

Increase: mexiletine effects—metoclopramide, urinary alkalinizers
Increase: levels of caffeine, theophylline
Decrease or increase: mexiletine effects—cimetidine
Decrease: mexiletine levels—phenytoin, phenobarbital, rifampin, urinary acidifiers, aluminum/magnesium hydroxide, atropine, opiates
Decrease: product effect—smoking

Drug/Herb

Increase: hypokalemia, increase antidysrhythmic action—aloe, buckthorn, cascara sagrada, rhubarb, senna
Increase: toxicity, death—aconite
Increase: effect—aloe, broom, chronic buckthorn use, cascara sagrada (chronic use), Chinese rhubarb, figwort, fumitory, goldenseal, kudzu, licorice
Increase: serotonin effect—horehound
Decrease: effect—coltsfoot

Drug/Lab Test

Increase: CPK, LFTs

NURSING CONSIDERATIONS

Assess:

- ECG continuously for increased PR or QRS segments; discontinue or reduce rate; watch for increased ventricular ectopic beats; may have to rebolus
- Blood levels (therapeutic level 0.5-2 mcg/ml)
- B/P continuously for fluctuations in cardiac rate
- I&O ratio, electrolytes (K, Na, Cl), liver enzymes

⚠ Malignant hyperthermia: tachypnea, tachycardia, changes in B/P, fever

- Respiratory status: rate, rhythm, lung fields for crackles, watch for respiratory depression
- CNS effects: dizziness, confusion, psychosis, paresthesias, seizures; product should be discontinued
- Lung fields, bilateral crackles may occur in CHF patient
- Increased respiration, increased pulse; product should be discontinued

Administer:

- With food for GI upset

Evaluate:

- Therapeutic response: decreased dysrhythmias

Teach patient/family:

- To take with food or antacid; to take as directed; do not skip doses
- Avoid changes in diet that could drastically acidify or alkalinize urine
- Notify prescriber of side effects
- Not to stop abruptly

Treatment of overdose: O_2, artificial ventilation, ECG; administer DOPamine for circulatory depression, diazepam or thiopental for seizures, to acidify urine

micafungin (℞)

(my-ca-fun'gin)
Mycamine
Func. class.: Antifungal, systemic
Chem. class.: Echinocandin

Action: Inhibits an essential component in fungal cell walls; causes direct damage to fungal cell wall

Uses: Treatment of esophageal candidiasis; prophylaxis of candida infections in patients undergoing hematopoietic stem cell transplantation (HSCT); susceptible

candida species: *C. albicans, C. glabrata, C. krusei, C. parapsilosis, C. tropicalis*
Unlabeled uses: *Aspergillus* sp., pediatrics to prevent Candidiasis

DOSAGE AND ROUTES

Esophageal candidiasis

- *Adult:* **IV INF** 150 mg/day, given over 1 hr

Prophylaxis of candida infections

- *Adult:* **IV INF** 50 mg/day, given over 1 hr
- *Adolescent/child/infant ≥6 mo (unlabeled):* **IV INF** 1 mg/kg/day, max 50 mg/day

Aspergillus *sp. (unlabeled)*

- *Adult:* **IV INF** 25-150 mg/day × ≥30 days

Available forms: Powder for inj 50 mg, in single-dose vials 50, 100 mg vial

SIDE EFFECTS

CNS: **Seizures,** dizziness, *headache, somnolence*
CV: Flushing, hypertension, phlebitis
GI: Abdominal pain, *nausea, anorexia, vomiting, diarrhea, increased AST, ALT, alk phos, blood dehydrogenase, hyperbilirubinemia*
HEMA: **Neutropenia, thrombocytopenia, leukopenia, coagulopathy, anemia, hemolytic anemia**
INTEG: Rash, pruritus, inj site pain
META: Hypokalemia, hypocalcemia, hypomagnesemia
MS: Rigors
Contraindications: Hypersensitivity to this product or other echinocandins
Precautions: Pregnancy (C), breastfeeding, children, geriatric patients, severe hepatic disease

PHARMACOKINETICS

Metabolized in liver; excretion feces, urine; terminal half-life 14-20 hr; protein binding 99%

INTERACTIONS

Increase: plasma concentrations—sirolimus, NIFEdipine; may need dosage reduction

NURSING CONSIDERATIONS

Assess:

- For signs and symptoms of infection, clearing of cultures during treatment; obtain culture baseline and throughout; product may be started as soon as culture is taken (esophageal candidiasis); monitor cultures during HSCT for prevention of candida infections
- CBC (RBC, Hct, Hgb), differential, platelet count periodically; notify prescriber of results
- Renal studies: BUN, urine CCr, electrolytes before and during therapy
- Hepatic studies before and during treatment: bilirubin, AST, ALT, alk phos, as needed
- Bleeding: hematuria, heme-positive stools, bruising or petechiae, mucosa or orifices; blood dyscrasias can occur
- For hypersensitivity: rash, pruritus, facial swelling; also for phelibits
- For hemolytic anemia
- GI symptoms: frequency of stools, cramping, if severe diarrhea occurs, electrolytes may need to be given

Administer:

- Do not use if cloudy or precipitated; do not admix
- Flush line before and after administration with 0.9% NaCl

IV route

- For candida prevention, reconstitute with provided dilutent 0.9% NaCl without bacteriostatic product; 50-mg vial/5 ml (10 mg/ml), swirl to dissolve, do not shake; further dilute with 100 ml 0.9% NaCl, only; run over 1 hr
- For candida infection, reconstitute with provided diluent 50 mg/5 ml (10 mg/ml); further dilute 3 reconstituted vials in 100 ml of 0.9% NaCl, run over 1 hr

Perform/provide:

• Storage at room temperature, away from light, do not freeze; discard unused solution

Evaluate:

• Therapeutic response: prevention of candida infection in HSCT; or decreased symptoms of candida infection, negative culture

Teach patient/family:

• To notify prescriber if pregnancy is suspected or planned; use nonhormonal form of contraception while taking this product

• To avoid breastfeeding while taking this product

• To inform prescriber of kidney or liver disease

• To report bleeding, facial swelling, wheezing, difficulty breathing, itching, rash, hives, increasing warmth, flushing

• To report signs of infection: increased temp, sore throat, flulike symptoms

• To notify prescriber of nausea, vomiting, diarrhea, jaundice, anorexia, clay-colored stools, dark urine; heptatotoxicity may occur

miconazole topical

See Appendix B

miconazole vaginal antifungal

See Appendix B

midazolam (℞)

(mid'ay-zoe-lam)

Func. class.: Sedative, hypnotic, antianxiety

Chem. class.: Benzodiazepine, short-acting

Controlled Substance Schedule IV

Action: Depresses subcortical levels in CNS; may act on limbic system, reticular formation; may potentiate γ-aminobutyric acid (GABA) by binding to specific benzodiazepine receptors

Uses: Preoperative sedation, general anesthesia induction, sedation for diagnostic endoscopic procedures, intubation, anxiety

Unlabeled uses: Refractory status epilepticus

DOSAGE AND ROUTES

Preoperative sedation

• *Adult and child ≥12 yr:* **IM** 0.07-0.08 mg/kg ½-1 hr before general anesthesia

• *Child 1-6 mo:* **IM** 0.1-0.15 mg/kg, may give up to 0.5 mg/kg if needed, max 10 mg

• *Child 6 mo-5 yr:* **IV** 0.05-0.1 mg/kg, a total dose of 0.6 mg/kg may be necessary

• *Child 6 yr-11 yr:* **IV** 0.025-0.05 mg/kg, a total dose of 0.4 mg/kg may be necessary

Induction of general anesthesia

• *Adult >55 yr:* (ASA I/II) **IV** 150-300 mcg/kg over 30 sec; (ASA III/IV) limit dose to 250 mcg/kg (nonpremedicated) or 150 mcg/kg (premedicated)

• *Adult <55 yr:* **IV** 200-350 mcg/kg over 20-30 sec; if patient has not received premedication, may repeat by giving 20% of original dose; if patient has received premedication reduce dose by 50 mcg/kg

• *Child:* No safe and effective dose established; however doses of 50-200 mcg/kg **IV** have been used

Continuous infusion for intubation (critical care)

• *Adult:* **IV** 0.01-0.05 mg/kg over several min; repeat at 10-15 min intervals, until adequate sedation; then 0.02-0.10 mg/kg/hr maintenance, adjust as needed

• *Child:* **IV** 0.05-0.2 mg/kg over 2-3 min, then 0.06-0.12 mg/kg/hr by cont inf; adjust as needed

• *Neonate:* **IV** 0.03-0.06 mg/kg/hr, titrate using lowest dose

Status epilepticus (unlabeled)

• *Child and infant >2 mo:* **IV** 0.15 mg/kg, then **CONT IV** 1 mcg/kg/min, titrate upward q5min until seizures controlled

Available forms: Inj 1, 5 mg/ml, syr 2 mg/ml

SIDE EFFECTS

CNS: Retrograde amnesia, euphoria, confusion, headache, anxiety, insomnia, slurred speech, paresthesia, tremors, weakness, chills, agitation, paradoxical reactions

CV: Hypotension, PVCs, tachycardia, bigeminy, nodal rhythm, **cardiac arrest**

EENT: Blurred vision, nystagmus, diplopia, loss of balance

GI: Nausea, vomiting, increased salivation, hiccups

INTEG: Urticaria, pain at inj site, swelling at inj site, rash, pruritus at inj site

RESP: Coughing, **apnea, bronchospasm, laryngospasm,** dyspnea, **respiratory depression**

Contraindications: Pregnancy (D), hypersensitivity to benzodiazepines, acute closed-angle glaucoma, status asthmaticus

Precautions: Breastfeeding, children, geriatric patients, COPD, CHF, chronic renal failure, chills, debilitated, hepatic disease, shock, coma, alcohol intoxication

Black Box Warning: Neonates (contains benzyl alcohol), IV administration, respiratory depression/insufficiency

PHARMACOKINETICS

Protein binding 97%; half-life 1.8-6.4 hr, metabolized in liver; metabolites excreted in urine; crosses placenta, blood-brain barrier

PO: Onset 20-30 min

IM: Onset 15 min, peak ½-1 hr, duration 2-3 hr

IV: Onset 3-5 min, onset of anesthesia 1½-2½ min, duration 2 hr

INTERACTIONS

Increase: extended half-life—CYP3A4 inhibitors (cimetidine, erythromycin, ranitidine)

Increase: respiratory depression—other CNS depressants, alcohol, barbiturates, opiate analgesics, verapamil, ritonavir, indinavir, fluvoxamine

Decrease: midazolam metabolism—CYP3A4 inducers (azole antifungals, theophylline)

Drug/Herb

Increase: hypotension—black cohosh

Increase: CNS depression—catnip, chamomile, clary, cowslip, hops, kava, lavender, mistletoe, nettle, pokeweed, poppy, Queen Anne's lace, senega, skullcap, valerian, tan-shen, St. John's wort

Drug/Food

Increase: (PO) midazolam effect—grapefruit juice

NURSING CONSIDERATIONS

Assess:

- Inj site for redness, pain, swelling
- Degree of amnesia in geriatric patients; may be increased
- Anterograde amnesia
- Vital signs for recovery period in obese patient, since half-life may be extended
- Apnea, respiratory depression that may be increased in geriatric patients

Administer:

PO route

- Remove cap of press-in bottle adaptor and push adaptor into neck of bottle; close with cap; remove cap and insert tip of dispenser and insert into adaptor; turn upside-down and withdraw correct dose; place in mouth

IM route

- IM deep into large muscle mass

IV route

- May be given diluted or undiluted
- After diluting with D_5W or 0.9% NaCl to 0.25 mg/ml; give over 2 min (conscious sedation) or over 30 sec (anesthesia induction)

Additive compatibility: Hydromorphone

Syringe compatibilities: Alfentanil, atracurium, atropine, benzquinamide, buprenorphine, butorphanol, chlorproMAZINE, cimetidine, cisatracurium, diphenhydrAMINE, droperidol, fentanyl, glycopyrrolate, hydromorphone, hydrOXYzine, ketamine, meperidine, metoclopramide, morphine, nalbuphine, promazine,

M

promethazine, remifentanil, scopolamine, sufentanil, thiethylperazine, trimethobenzamide

Y-site compatibilities: Abciximab, alfentamil, amikacin, amiodarone, argatroban, atracurium, atropine, aztreonam, benzotropine, calcium gluconate, cefazolin, cefotaxime, cefoxitine, ceftriaxone, cimetidine, ciprofloxacin, cisplatin, clindamycin, clonidine, cyanocobalamin, cyclosporine, dactinomycin, digoxin, diltiazem, diphenhydramine, docetaxal, DOPamine, doxycyclin, enalaprilat, epinephrine, erythromycin, esmolol, etomidate, etoposide, famotidine, fentanyl, fluconazole, folic acid, gatifloxacin, gemcitabine, gentamicin, glycopyrrolate, granisetron, heparin, hetastarch, hydromorphone, hydroxyzine, inamrinone, isoproterenol, labetalol, lactated Ringer's, levofloxacin, lidocaine, linezolid, lorazepam, magnesium, mannitol, meperdine, methadone, methyldopa, methylPREDNISolone, metoclopromide, metomolol, metronidazole, milrinone, morphine, nalbuphine, naloxone, niCARdipine, nitroglycerin, nitroprusside, norepinephrine, ondansetron, oxacillin, oxytocin, paclitaxel, palonasetron, pancuronium, papaverin, phentolamine, phytonadione, piperacillin, potassium chloride, propanolol, protamine, pyridoxine, ranitidine, remifentanil, sodium nitroprusside, streptokinase, succinylcholine, sufentanil, teniposide, theophylline, thiotepa, ticarcillin, tobramycin, vancomycin, vasopressin, vecuronium, verapamil, voriconazole

Perform/provide:

- Assistance with ambulation until drowsy period relieved
- Storage at room temperature, protect from light
- Immediate availability of resuscitation equipment, O_2 to support airway; do not give by rapid bolus

Evaluate:

- Therapeutic response: induction of sedation, general anesthesia

Teach patient/family:

- That amnesia occurs; events may not be remembered

Treatment of overdose: Flumazenil, O_2

midodrine (℞)

(mye′doh-dreen)

ProAmatine

Func. class.: Vasopressor

Chem. class.: α_1 agonist

Do not confuse:

ProAmatine/Protamine

Action: Activates α-adrenergic receptors of arteriolar, venous vasculature by increasing vascular tone

Uses: Orthostatic hypotension

Unlabeled uses: Urinary incontinence

DOSAGE AND ROUTES

- *Adult:* **PO** 10 mg tid, max 40 mg/day

Urinary incontinence (unlabeled)

- *Adult:* **PO** 2.5-5 mg bid-tid

Renal dose

- *Adult:* **PO** 2.5 mg tid

Available forms: Tabs 2.5, 5, 10 mg

SIDE EFFECTS

CNS: Drowsiness, restlessness, headache, *paresthesia, pain,* chills, confusion

CV: **Supine hypertension,** vasodilation, flushing face

EENT: Dry mouth, blurred vision

GI: Nausea, anorexia

GU: Dysuria

INTEG: Pruritus, piloerection, rash

Contraindications: Hypersensitivity, acute renal disease, pheochromocytoma, thyrotoxicosis, urinary retention

Black Box Warning: Severe organic heart disease, persistent/excessive supine hypertension

Precautions: Pregnancy (C), breastfeeding, children, hepatic impairment, diabetes, heart failure, renal disease, visual disturbance, dialysis, thyroid disease

PHARMACOKINETICS

Peak 1-2 hr, half-life 3-4 hr, bioavailability 90%, excreted in urine 80% active metabolite

INTERACTIONS

• Do not give concurrently with MAOIs or any products with MAOI-type activity
Increase: bradycardia—β-blockers, psychotropics, cardiac glycosides, tricyclics
Increase: pressor effects—α-agonist
Increase: supine hypertension—fludrocortisone
Increase: lactic acidosis—metformin

NURSING CONSIDERATIONS

Assess:

• VS, B/P (standing, supine); notify prescriber if B/P supine is increased
• Observe for drowsiness, dizziness, LOC

Administer:

• Tablets may be swallowed whole, chewed, or allowed to dissolve
• Upon arising, midday, and late afternoon (no later than 6 PM)
• Avoid administering if patient is to be supine during day

Evaluate:

• Therapeutic response: decreased orthostatic hypotension

Teach patient/family:

• To avoid hazardous activities, activities requiring alertness; dizziness may occur; instruct patient to request assistance with ambulation
• To avoid alcohol, other depressants, OTC products; multiple drug–drug interactions

mifepristone, RU-486 (℞)

(mif-ee-press'tone)
Mifeprex
Func. class.: Abortifacient
Chem. class.: Antiprogestational

Action: Stimulates uterine contractions, causing complete abortion

Uses: Abortion through 49 days' gestation

Unlabeled uses: Postcoital contraception/contragestation, intrauterine fetal death, endometriosis, Cushing's syndrome, unresectable meningioma

DOSAGE AND ROUTES

• *Adult:* **PO** 600 mg day 1, 400 mcg misoprostol day 3 if needed

Cushing's syndrome (unlabeled)

• *Adult:* **PO** (Corlux) 5-20 mg/kg/day during a 9-wk period

Advanced breast cancer/ unresectable or malignant meningioma (unlabeled)

• *Adult:* **PO** 200-400 mg/day

Uterine leiomyomata (unlabeled)

• *Adult:* **PO** 25-50 mg/day

Endometriosis (unlabeled)

• *Adult:* **PO** 50 mg/day

Available forms: Tabs 200 mg

SIDE EFFECTS

CNS: Dizziness, insomnia, anxiety, syncope, fainting, headache
GI: Nausea, vomiting, diarrhea, dyspepsia
GU: Uterine cramping, uterine hemorrhage, vaginitis, pelvic pain
MISC: Fatigue, back pain, fever, viral infections, chills, sinusitis

Contraindications: Severe respiratory/cardiac/renal/hepatic disease, IUD, ectopic pregnancy, chronic adrenal failure, bleeding disorder, inherited porphyrias, PID, hypersensitivity to this product, misoprostol, or prostaglandins

Precautions: Pregnancy (C), asthma, anemia, jaundice, diabetes mellitus, convulsive disorders, women >35 yr/smoke ≥10 cigarettes/day, past uterine surgery

Black Box Warning: Infection, sepsis, vaginal bleeding

PHARMACOKINETICS

Rapidly absorbed, peak 90 min, 98% bound to plasma proteins, albumin, glycoprotein, excretion via feces, urine

M

INTERACTIONS

• Do not use with anticoagulants, long-term corticosteroids

Decrease: metabolism of erythromycin, ketoconazole, itraconazole

Drug/Herb

Decrease: by St. John's wort

Drug/Food

Decrease: metabolism of mifepristone—grapefruit juice

NURSING CONSIDERATIONS

Assess:

• B/P, pulse; watch for change that may indicate hemorrhage

• Respiratory rate, rhythm, depth; notify prescriber of abnormalities

• For length, duration of contraction; notify prescriber of contractions lasting over 1 min or absence of contractions

• For incomplete abortion, pregnancy must be terminated by another method; product is teratogenic

Perform/provide:

• Emotional support before and after abortion

Evaluate:

• Therapeutic response: expulsion of fetus

Teach patient/family:

• To report increased blood loss, abdominal cramps, increased temp, foul-smelling lochia

• Some methods of comfort control and pain control

• Must continue with follow-up

• That cramping and vaginal bleeding will occur

miglitol (℞)

(mig′lih-tol)

Glyset

Func. class.: Oral hypoglycemic

Chem. class.: α-Glucosidase inhibitor

Action: Delays digestion and absorption of ingested carbohydrates, results in smaller rise in blood glucose after meals; does not increase insulin production

Uses: Type 2 diabetes mellitus

DOSAGE AND ROUTES

• *Adult:* **PO** 25 mg tid initially, with first bite of meal; maintenance dose may be increased to 50 mg tid; may be increased to 100 mg tid if needed with dosage adjustment at 4-8 wk intervals

Available forms: Tabs 25, 50, 100 mg

SIDE EFFECTS

GI: Abdominal pain, diarrhea, flatulence, **hepatotoxicity**

HEMA: Low iron

INTEG: Rash

Contraindications: Hypersensitivity, diabetic ketoacidosis, cirrhosis, inflammatory bowel disease, colonic ulceration, partial intestinal obstruction, chronic intestinal disease, ileus

Precautions: Pregnancy (B), breastfeeding, children, renal/hepatic disease

PHARMACOKINETICS

Peak 2-3 hr, not metabolized, excreted in urine as unchanged product, half-life 2 hr

INTERACTIONS

Decrease: levels of digoxin, propranolol, ranitidine

Decrease: miglitol levels—digestive enzymes, intestinal adsorbents; do not use together

Drug/Herb

• Improved glucose tolerance: karela

Decrease: hypoglycemic effect—broom, buchu, dandelion, juniper

Increase or decrease: hypoglycemic effect—chromium, fenugreek, ginseng

Drug/Food

Increase: diarrhea—carbohydrates

NURSING CONSIDERATIONS

Assess:

• Hypoglycemia, hyperglycemia; even though product does not cause hypoglycemia, if patient is on sulfonylureas or insulin, hypoglycemia may be additive (rare)

- Blood glucose levels, hemoglobin, A1c LFTs; if hypoglycemia occurs with monotherapy, treat with glucose

Administer:

- Tid with first bite of each meal

Perform/provide:

- Storage in tight container at room temperature

Evaluate:

- Therapeutic response: decreased signs/symptoms of diabetes mellitus (polyuria, polydipsia, polyphagia; clear sensorium, absence of dizziness; stable gait); improved blood glucose, A1c

Teach patient/family:

- The symptoms of hypo/hyperglycemia, what to do about each, that during periods of stress, infection, surgery, insulin may be required
- That medication must be taken as prescribed; explain consequences of discontinuing medication abruptly
- To avoid OTC medications unless approved by health care provider
- That diabetes is lifelong illness; that this product is not a cure
- To carry ID for emergency purposes
- That diet and exercise regimen must be followed
- Regarding GI side effects

Rarely Used

miglustat (℞)

(mih'glue-stat)

Zavesca

Func. class.: Miscellaneous agent

Uses: Adults with mild to moderate type 1 Gaucher disease

DOSAGE AND ROUTES

- *Adult:* **PO** 100 mg tid, without regard to food

Contraindications: Pregnancy (X), hypersensitivity

⚠ High Alert

milrinone (℞)

(mill'rih-nohn)

Func. class.: Inotropic/vasodilator agent with phosphodiesterase activity

Chem. class.: Bipyridine derivative

Action: Positive inotropic agent, increases contractility of cardiac muscle with vasodilator properties; reduces preload and afterload by direct relaxation on vascular smooth muscle

Uses: Short-term management of advanced heart failure that has not responded to other medication; can be used with digoxin

Unlabeled uses: Adolescents, children, infants

DOSAGE AND ROUTES

- *Adult:* **IV BOL** 50 mcg/kg given over 10 min; start inf of 0.375-0.75 mcg/kg/min; reduce dose in renal impairment
- *Adolescent/child/infant (unlabeled):* **IV** 50-75 mcg/kg over 10-60 min, then 0.5-0.75 mcg/kg/min

Available forms: Inj 1 mg/ml; premixed inj 200 mcg/ml in D_5W

SIDE EFFECTS

CV: **Dysrhythmias,** hypotension, chest pain

GI: Nausea, vomiting, anorexia, abdominal pain, **hepatotoxicity, jaundice**

HEMA: **Thrombocytopenia**

MISC: Headache, hypokalemia, tremor, inj site reactions

Contraindications: Hypersensitivity to this product, severe aortic disease, severe pulmonic valvular disease, acute MI

Precautions: Pregnancy (C), breastfeeding, children, geriatric patients, renal/hepatic disease, atrial flutter/fibrillation

PHARMACOKINETICS

IV: Onset 2-5 min, peak 10 min, duration variable; half-life 2.4 hr; metabolized in liver; excreted in urine as product (83%) and metabolites (12%)

M

INTERACTIONS

Increase: effects of antihypertensives, diuretics

NURSING CONSIDERATIONS

Assess:

⚠ ECG continuously during IV, ventricular dysrhythmia can occur
- B/P and pulse q5min during inf; if B/P drops 30 mm Hg, stop inf and call prescriber
- Electrolytes: K, Na, Cl, Ca; renal studies: BUN, creatinine; blood studies: platelet count
- ALT, AST, bilirubin daily
- I&O ratio and weight daily; diuresis should increase with continuing therapy
- If platelets are <150,000/mm^3, product is usually discontinued and another product started
- Extravasation; change site q48hr

Administer:
- Potassium supplements if ordered for potassium levels <3 mg/dl

IV route
- Give IV loading dose undiluted over 10 min
- Into running dextrose inf through Y-connector or directly into tubing; dilute with 0.9% NaCl to 1-3 mg/ml; do not mix with glucose for long-term inf
- By inf pump for doses other than bolus

Additive compatibilities: Quinidine

Syringe compatibilities: Atropine, calcium chloride, digoxin, epinephrine, lidocaine, morphine, propranolol, sodium bicarbonate, verapamil

Y-site compatibilities: Digoxin, diltiazem, DOBUTamine, DOPamine, epinephrine, fentanyl, heparin, hydromorphone, labetalol, lorazepam, midazolam, morphine, niCARdipine, nitroglycerin, norepinephrine, propranolol, quinidine, ranitidine, thiopental, vecuronium

Evaluate:
- Therapeutic response: increased cardiac output, decreased PCWP, adequate CVP, decreased dyspnea, fatigue, edema, ECG

Teach patient/family:
- To report angina immediately during infusion
- To report headache, which can be treated with analgesics

Treatment of overdose: Discontinue product, support circulation

minocycline (℞)

(min-oh-sye'kleen)

Arestin, Dynacin, Minocin, Myrac, Soledyn

Func. class.: Broad-spectrum antiinfective

Chem. class.: Tetracycline

Action: Inhibits protein synthesis, phosphorylation in microorganisms by binding to 30S ribosomal subunits, reversibly binding to 50S ribosomal subunits; bacteriostatic

Uses: Syphilis, *Chlamydia trachomatis,* gonorrhea, lymphogranuloma venereum, rickettsial infections, inflammatory acne, *Neisseria meningitidis, Neisseria gonorrhoeae, Treponema pallidum, Chlamydia trachomatis, Ureaplasma urealyticum, Mycoplasma pneumoniae, Nocardia,* periodontitis, methicillin-resistant *S. aureus* (MRSA) infection

Unlabeled uses: Rheumatoid arthritis, bullous pemphigoid, dental infection

DOSAGE AND ROUTES

- *Adult:* **PO/IV** 200 mg, then 100 mg q12hr or 50 mg q6hr, max 400 mg/24 hr **IV; SUBGINGIVAL** inserted into periodontal pocket
- *Child >8 yr:* **PO/IV** 4 mg/kg then 4 mg/kg/day **PO** in divided doses q12hr

Gonorrhea
- *Adult:* **PO** 200 mg, then 100 mg q12hr × 4 days or more

Chlamydia trachomatis
- *Adult:* **PO** 100 mg bid × 7 days

Syphilis
- *Adult:* **PO** 200 mg, then 100 mg q12hr × 10-15 days

Uncomplicated gonococcal urethritis in men

• *Adult:* **PO** 100 mg q12hr × 5 days

Rheumatoid arthritis (unlabeled)

• *Adult:* **PO** 100 mg bid for ≤48 wk

Bullous pemphigus (unlabeled)

• *Adult:* **PO** 50 mg/day may increase to 100 mg/day after 1-2 wk

Available forms: Caps 50, 75, 100 mg; oral susp 50 mg/5 ml; powder for inj 100 mg; caps, pellet filled 50, 100 mg; tabs 50, 75, 100 mg; ext rel tabs 45, 90, 135 mg

SIDE EFFECTS

CNS: Dizziness, fever, light-headedness, vertigo, **seizures, increased intracranial pressure**

CV: Pericarditis

EENT: Dysphagia, glossitis, decreased calcification of deciduous teeth, permanent discoloration of teeth, oral candidiasis

GI: Nausea, abdominal pain, *vomiting, diarrhea,* anorexia, enterocolitis, **hepatotoxicity,** flatulence, abdominal cramps, epigastric burning, stomatitis

GU: Increased BUN, polyuria, polydipsia, **renal failure, nephrotoxicity**

HEMA: **Eosinophilia, neutropenia, thrombocytopenia, hemolytic anemia, pancytopenia**

INTEG: Rash, urticaria, photosensitivity, increased pigmentation, **exfoliative dermatitis,** pruritus, blue-gray color of skin, mucous membranes

MS: Myalgia, arthritis, bone discoloration, joint stiffness

SYST: **Angioedema, Stevens-Johnson syndrome**

Contraindications: Pregnancy (D), children <8 yr, hypersensitivity to tetracyclines

Precautions: Hepatic disease, breastfeeding

PHARMACOKINETICS

PO: Peak 2-3 hr, half-life 11-17 hr; excreted in urine, feces, breast milk; crosses placenta; 70%-75% protein bound

INTERACTIONS

Increase: effect of warfarin, digoxin, insulin, oral anticoagulants, theophylline

Decrease: effect of minocycline—antacids, sodium bicarbonate, alkali products, iron, kaolin/pectin, cimetidine

Decrease: effect of barbiturates, carbamazepine, phenytoin, penicillins, oral contraceptives, calcium

Drug/Herb

• Do not use acidophilus with antiinfectives; separate by several hours

Drug/Lab Test

False negative: urine glucose with Clinistix or Tes-Tape

NURSING CONSIDERATIONS

Assess:

• I&O ratio

• Age and tooth development

• Blood tests: PT, CBC, AST, ALT, BUN, creatinine

• Signs of anemia: Hct, Hgb, fatigue

• Allergic reactions: rash, itching, pruritus, angioedema

• Nausea, vomiting, diarrhea; administer antiemetic, antacids as ordered

• Overgrowth of infection: fever, malaise, redness, pain, swelling, drainage, perineal itching, diarrhea, changes in cough or sputum, black, furry tongue

Administer:

• After C&S obtained

• With a full glass of water; with food for GI symptoms

PO route

• 2 hr before or after laxative or ferrous products; 3 hr after antacid

IV route

• After diluting 100 mg/5 ml sterile H_2O for inj; further dilute in 500-1000 ml of NaCl, dextrose sol, LR, Ringer's sol; run 100 mg/6 hr

Y-site compatibilities: Alfentanil, amikacin, atracurium, benztropine, bretylium, buprenorphine, butorphanol, calcium chloride, carboplatin, caspofungin, cefonicid, chlorpromazine, cimetidine, cisatracurium, codeine, cyclophosphamide, cycloSPORINE, cytarabine, dactinomycin, dexmedetomidine, diltiazem, diphenhydrAMINE, DOBUTamine, docetaxel, doxacurium, doxycycline, enalaprilat, ephedrine, epinephrine, eptifibatide, etoposide, fenoldopam, fentanyl, filgrastim, fludarabine, gatafloxacin, gemcitabine, gentamicin, glycopyrrolate, granisetron, heparin, hetastarch, idarubicin, ifosfamide, inamrinone, isoproterenol, labetalol, levofloxacin, lidocaine, linezolid, lorazepam, magnesium sulfate, mannitol, melphalan, metaraminol, methotrexate, methyldopa, metoclopramide, metoprolol, midazolam, mitoxantrone, nalbuphine, naloxone, perphenazine, potassium chloride, remifentanil, sargramostim, teniposide, vinorelbine, vit B/C

Perform/provide:

- Storage in airtight, light-resistant container at room temperature

Evaluate:

- Therapeutic response: decreased temp, absence of lesions, negative C&S

Teach patient/family:

- To avoid sunlight; sunscreen does not seem to decrease photosensitivity
- That all prescribed medication must be taken to prevent superinfection; not to use outdated product, Fanconi's syndrome may occur
- To avoid taking with antacids, iron, cimetidine; absorption may be decreased
- That teeth discoloration, joint/muscle pain may occur

minoxidil (℞, OTC)

(mi-nox′i-dill)

minoxidil, Rogaine (topical)

Func. class.: Antihypertensive

Chem. class.: Vasodilator, peripheral

Do not confuse:

minoxidil/Monopril

Action: Directly relaxes arteriolar smooth muscle, causing vasodilation

Uses: Severe hypertension unresponsive to other therapy (use with diuretic); topically to treat alopecia

Unlabeled uses: Scleroderma renal crisis (SRC) to control hypertension

DOSAGE AND ROUTES

Severe hypertension

- *Adult:* **PO** 2.5-5 mg/day in 1-2 divided doses; max 100 mg/day; usual range 10-40 mg/day in single doses
- *Geriatric:* **PO** 2.5 mg/day, may be increased gradually
- *Child <12 yr:* **PO** (initial) 0.1-0.2 mg/kg/day; (effective range) 0.25-1 mg/kg/day; (max) 50 mg/day

Alopecia

- *Adult:* **TOP** 1 ml bid, rub into scalp daily, max 2 ml/day

Scleroderma renal crisis (unlabeled)

- *Adult:* **PO** 5 mg/day in 1-2 divided doses, increase after 3 days by 10-20 mg/day to reach desired B/P, max 100 mg/day

Available forms: Tabs 2.5, 10 mg; topical 2% sol

SIDE EFFECTS

Systemic

CNS: Headache, fatigue

CV: *Severe rebound hypertension on withdrawal in children,* tachycardia, angina, increased T wave, **CHF, pulmonary edema, pericardial effusion,** edema, sodium, water retention

GI: Nausea, vomiting

GU: Breast tenderness

HEMA: Hct, Hgb, erythrocyte count may decrease initially

INTEG: Pruritus, **Stevens-Johnson syndrome,** rash, hirsutism

Contraindications: Dissecting aortic aneurysm, hypersensitivity, pheochromocytoma

Black Box Warning: Acute MI

Precautions: Pregnancy (C), breastfeeding, children, geriatric patients, renal disease, CVD

Black Box Warning: CAD, CHF, cardiac disease, cardiac tamponade, edema, hypotension, orthostatic hypotension, pericardial effusion

PHARMACOKINETICS

PO: Onset 30 min, peak 2-3 hr, duration 48-120 hr; half-life 4.2 hr; metabolized in liver; metabolites excreted in urine, feces

INTERACTIONS

Increase: orthostatic hypotension—antihypertensives

Decrease: antihypertensive effect—NSAIDs, salicylates

Drug/Herb

Increase: antihypertensive effect—hawthorn

Decrease: antihypertensive effect—yohimbe

Drug/Lab Test

Increase: renal studies

Decrease: Hgb/Hct/RBC

NURSING CONSIDERATIONS

Assess:

⚠ Monitor closely, usually given with β-blocker to prevent tachycardia and increased myocardial workload, usually given with diuretic to prevent serious fluid accumulation, patient should be hospitalized during beginning treatment

- Nausea, edema in feet, legs daily
- Skin turgor, dryness of mucous membranes for hydration status
- Crackles, dyspnea, orthopnea
- Electrolytes: K, Na, Cl, CO_2
- Renal studies: catecholamines, BUN, creatinine
- Hepatic studies: AST, ALT, alk phos
- B/P, pulse
- Weight daily, I&O

Administer:

PO route

- With meals for better absorption, to decrease GI symptoms
- With β-blocker and/or diuretic for hypertension

Topical route

- 1 ml no matter how much balding has occurred; increasing dosage does not speed growth

Perform/provide:

- Storage protected from light and heat

Evaluate:

- Therapeutic response: decreased B/P or increased hair growth

Teach patient/family:

- That body hair will increase but is reversible after discontinuing treatment
- Not to discontinue product abruptly
- To report pitting edema, dizziness, weight gain >5 lb, SOB, bruising or bleeding, heart rate >20 beats/min over normal, severe indigestion, dizziness, lightheadedness, panting, new or aggravated symptoms of angina
- To take product exactly as prescribed, or serious side effects may occur

Topical

- That for topical use, treatment must continue long-term or new hair will be lost
- Not to use except on scalp

Treatment of overdose: Administer normal saline IV, vasopressors

M

mirtazapine (℞)

(mer-ta'za-peen)

Remeron, Remeron Soltab

Func. class.: Antidepressant

Chem. class.: Tetracyclic

Action: Blocks reuptake of norepinephrine, serotonin into nerve endings, increasing action of norepinephrine, serotonin in nerve cells, antagonist of central α_2-receptors, blocks histamine receptors

Uses: Depression, dysthymic disorder, bipolar disorder—depressed, agitated depression

Unlabeled uses: Resting tremor, benign familial tremor, levodopa-induced dyskinesias, pruritus

DOSAGE AND ROUTES

- *Adult:* **PO** 15 mg/day at bedtime, maintenance to continue for 6 mo, titrate up to 45 mg/day; **ORALLY DISINTEGRATING** tabs open blister pack, place tab on tongue, allow to disintegrate, swallow

• *Geriatric:* **PO** 7.5 mg at bedtime, increase by 7.5 mg q1-2wk to desired dose, max 45 mg/day

Resting tremor/benign familial tremor/levodopa-induced dyskinesias (unlabeled)

• *Adult:* **PO** Titrate, then 30 mg at bedtime

Pruritus (unlabeled)

• *Adult:* **PO** 15-30 mg/day

Available forms: Tabs 15, 30, 45 mg; orally disintegrating tab (soltab) 15, 30, 45 mg

SIDE EFFECTS

CNS: Dizziness, drowsiness, confusion, headache, anxiety, tremors, stimulation, weakness, nightmares, EPS (geriatric patients), increased psychiatric symptoms, **seizures**

CV: Orthostatic hypotension, ECG changes, tachycardia, **hypertension,** palpitations

EENT: Blurred vision, tinnitus, mydriasis

GI: Diarrhea, dry mouth, nausea, vomiting, **paralytic ileus,** increased appetite, cramps, epigastric distress, constipation, **jaundice, hepatitis,** stomatitis

GU: Urinary retention, **acute renal failure**

HEMA: **Agranulocytosis, thrombocytopenia, eosinophilia, leukopenia**

INTEG: Rash, urticaria, sweating, pruritus, photosensitivity

SYST: Flulike symptoms, increased cholesterol levels

Contraindications: Hypersensitivity to tricyclics, recovery phase of MI, agranulocytosis, jaundice

Precautions: Pregnancy (C), geriatric patients, suicidal patients, severe depression, increased intraocular pressure, closed-angle glaucoma, urinary retention, cardiac/renal/hepatic disease, hypo/hyperthyroidism, electroshock therapy, elective surgery, seizure disorder, bone marrow suppression, thrombocytopenia

Black Box Warning: Suicidal ideation, children

PHARMACOKINETICS

PO: Peak 12 hr, metabolized by liver; excreted in urine, feces; crosses placenta; half-life 20-40 hr

INTERACTIONS

⚠ Hyperpyretic crisis, seizures, hypertensive episode: MAOIs

Increase: CNS depression—alcohol, barbiturates, benzodiazepines, other CNS depressants

Decrease: effects of clonidine, indirect-acting sympathomimetics (ephedrine)

Drug/Herb

• Serotonin syndrome: SAM-e, St. John's wort

Increase: anticholinergic effect—belladonna, henbane

Increase: antidepressant action—scopolia

Increase: CNS depression—chamomile, hops, kava, skullcap, valerian

Drug/Lab Test

Increase: serum bilirubin, blood glucose, alk phos

Decrease: VMA, 5-HIAA

False increase: urinary catecholamines

NURSING CONSIDERATIONS

Assess:

• B/P (lying, standing), pulse q4hr; if systolic B/P drops 20 mm Hg, hold product, notify prescriber; vital signs q4hr in patients with CV disease

• Blood studies: CBC, leukocytes, differential, cardiac enzymes if patient is receiving long-term therapy

• Hepatic studies: AST, ALT, bilirubin, creatinine

• Weight q wk; appetite may increase with product

• ECG for flattening of T wave, bundle branch block, AV block, dysrhythmias in cardiac patients

• EPS primarily in geriatric patients: rigidity, dystonia, akathisia

• Mental status: mood, sensorium, affect, suicidal tendencies, increase in psychiatric symptoms: depression, panic

• Alcohol consumption; if alcohol is consumed, hold dose until morning

Administer:

• Increased fluids, bulk in diet for constipation, especially geriatric patients

• With food, milk for GI symptoms

• Dosage at bedtime if oversedation occurs during day; may take entire dose at bedtime; geriatric patients may not tolerate once/day dosing

• Gum, hard candy, or frequent sips of water for dry mouth

• Orally disintegrating tab: no water needed; allow to dissolve on tongue, do not split

Perform/provide:

• Storage in tight container at room temperature; do not freeze

• Assistance with ambulation during beginning therapy, since drowsiness/dizziness occurs

• Safety measures, including side rails, primarily in geriatric patients

• Checking to see PO medication swallowed

Evaluate:

• Therapeutic response: decreased depression

Teach patient/family:

• That therapeutic effects may take 2-3 wk; take at bedtime

• To use caution in driving, other activities requiring alertness, because of drowsiness, dizziness, blurred vision

• To report immediately urinary retention, worsening of depression, suicidal thoughts/behavior

• To avoid alcohol ingestion, other CNS depressants

• How to take orally disintegrating tabs; dissolve on tongue, swallow

• Not to use within 14 days of MAOIs

Treatment of overdose: ECG monitoring, lavage, activated charcoal; administer anticonvulsant

misoprostol (℞)

(mye-soe-prost′ole)

Cytotec

Func. class.: Gastric mucosa protectant, antiulcer

Chem. class.: Prostaglandin E_1-analog

Do not confuse:

misoprostol/metoprolol

Cytotec/Cytoxan

Action: Inhibits gastric acid secretion; may protect gastric mucosa; can increase bicarbonate, mucus production

Uses: Prevention of NSAID-induced gastric ulcers

Unlabeled uses: Pregnancy termination, postpartum hemorrhage, cervical ripening/labor induction (vaginal), active duodenal/gastric ulcer, kidney transplant rejection prophylaxis

DOSAGE AND ROUTES

• *Adult:* **PO** 200 mcg qid with food for duration of NSAID therapy with last dose at bedtime; if 200 mcg is not tolerated, 100 mcg may be given

Active duodenal/gastric ulcer (unlabeled)

• *Adult:* **PO** 100-200 mcg qid with meals at bedtime × 4-8 wk

Pregnancy termination prior to 63rd day (unlabeled)

• *Adult:* **INTRAVAGINALLY** 800 mcg 5-7 days after methotrexate IM

Cervical ripening induction for term pregnancy (unlabeled)

• *Adult:* **INTRAVAGINALLY** 25 mcg q3-6hr

Available forms: Tabs 100, 200 mcg

SIDE EFFECTS

GI: Diarrhea, nausea, vomiting, flatulence, constipation, dyspepsia, abdominal pain

GU: Spotting, cramps, hypermenorrhea, menstrual disorders

M

Contraindications: Hypersensitivity to this product or prostaglandins

Black Box Warning: Pregnancy (X), females

Precautions: Breastfeeding, children, geriatric patients, renal disease, CV disease

PHARMACOKINETICS

PO: Peak 12 min, plasma steady state achieved within 2 days, excreted in urine

INTERACTIONS

Drug/Food

Decrease: maximum concentrations when taken with food

NURSING CONSIDERATIONS

Assess:

- GI symptoms: hematemesis, occult or frank blood in stools, gastric aspirate, cramping, severe diarrhea
- Obtain a negative pregnancy test; miscarriages are common
- Gastric pH (>5 should be maintained)

Administer:

- PO with meals for prolonged product effect; avoid use of magnesium antacids

Perform/provide:

- Storage at room temperature

Evaluate:

- Therapeutic response: absence of pain or GI complaints; prevention of ulcers

Teach patient/family:

- To take only as directed, read patient information leaflet
- Not to take if pregnant (can cause miscarriage) and not to become pregnant while taking this medication; if pregnancy occurs during therapy, discontinue product, notify prescriber; not to administer to nursing mothers
- Not to give product to anyone else or take for more than 4 wk unless directed by prescriber
- To avoid OTC preparations: aspirin, cough, cold products; condition may worsen

⚠ High Alert

mitomycin (℞)

(mye-toe-mye'sin)

mitomycin

Func. class.: Antineoplastic, antibiotic

Do not confuse:

mitomycin/mithramycin/mitotane/mitoxantrone

Action: Inhibits DNA synthesis, primarily; derived from *Streptomyces caespitosus;* appears to cause cross-linking of DNA, a vesicant

Uses: Pancreatic, stomach, colorectal, bladder cancer

Unlabeled uses: Palliative treatment of anal, bladder, head, neck, colon, breast, biliary, cervical, lung malignancies; bone marrow ablation, desmoid tumor, mesothelioma, stem cell transplant preparation

DOSAGE AND ROUTES

- *Adult:* **IV** 10-20 mg/m^2 q6-8wk

Available forms: Inj 5, 20, 40 mg/vial

SIDE EFFECTS

CNS: Fever, headache, confusion, drowsiness, syncope, fatigue

EENT: Blurred vision

GI: Nausea, vomiting, anorexia, stomatitis, **hepatotoxicity**, diarrhea

GU: Urinary retention, **renal failure,** edema

HEMA: **Thrombocytopenia, leukopenia, anemia**

INTEG: Rash, alopecia, **extravasation,** nail discoloration

MISC: **Hemolytic uremic syndrome, CHF**

RESP: **Fibrosis, pulmonary infiltrate,** dyspnea

Contraindications: Pregnancy (D) 1st trimester, breastfeeding, hypersensitivity, as a single agent, coagulation disorders

Black Box Warning: Thrombocytopenia

Precautions: Accidental exposure, acute bronchospasm, anemia, children, dental disease/work, extravasation, females, infection, radiation therapy, surgery, vaccines, renal/respiratory disease

Black Box Warning: Bone marrow suppression, hemolytic-uremic syndrome

PHARMACOKINETICS

Half-life 1 hr, metabolized in liver, 10% excreted in urine (unchanged)

INTERACTIONS

Increase: toxicity—other antineoplastics, radiation

Increase: bleeding risk—NSAIDs, anticoagulants

Drug/Herb

- Avoid use with black cohosh

NURSING CONSIDERATIONS

Assess:

- CBC, differential, platelet count weekly; withhold product if WBC is <2000/mm^3, granulocyte count <1000/mm^3, or platelet count is <100,000/mm^3; notify prescriber
- Pulmonary function tests, chest x-ray before, during therapy; chest x-ray should be obtained q2wk during treatment

⚠ Fatal hemolytic uremic syndrome: hypertension, thrombocytopenia, microangiopathic hemolytic anemia, occurs in those on long-term therapy

- Renal studies: BUN, serum uric acid, urine CCr, electrolytes before, during therapy, adjust dose based on renal function
- I&O ratio; report fall in urine output to <30 ml/hr
- Monitor temp q4hr; fever may indicate beginning infection
- Hepatic studies before, during therapy: bilirubin, AST, ALT, alk phos as needed or monthly; check for jaundiced skin and sclera, dark urine, clay-colored stools, itchy skin, abdominal pain, fever, diarrhea
- Bleeding: hematuria, guaiac, bruising, petechiae, mucosa, or orifices q8hr

⚠ Pulmonary fibrosis: bronchospasm

- Dyspnea, crackles, unproductive cough; chest pain, tachypnea, fatigue, increased pulse, pallor, lethargy
- Effects of alopecia on body image; discuss feelings about body changes
- Inflammation of mucosa, breaks in skin
- Buccal cavity q8hr for dryness, sores, ulceration, white patches, oral pain, bleeding, dysphagia
- Local irritation, pain, burning at inj site
- GI symptoms: frequency of stools, cramping
- Acidosis, signs of dehydration: rapid respirations, poor skin turgor, decreased urine output, dry skin, restlessness, weakness

Administer:

IV route

- Apply ice compress for extravasation; stop inf
- Antiemetic 30-60 min before giving product to prevent vomiting
- IV after diluting 5 mg/10 ml or 10 mg/40 ml sterile H_2O for inj; shake, allow to stand, give through Y-tube or 3-way stopcock; give slow IV push or infuse over 15-30 min; color of reconstituted sol is gray

Additive compatibilities: Dexamethasone, hydrocortisone

Solution compatibilities: LR, 0.3% NaCl, 0.5% NaCl

Syringe compatibilities: Bleomycin, cisplatin, cyclophosphamide, DOXOrubicin, droperidol, fluorouracil, furosemide, heparin, leucovorin, methotrexate, metoclopramide, vinBLAStine, vinCRIStine

Y-site compatibilities: Allopurinol, amifostine, bleomycin, cisplatin, cyclophosphamide, DOXOrubicin, droperidol, fluorouracil, furosemide, granisetron, heparin, leucovorin, melphalan, methotrexate, metoclopramide, ondansetron, teniposide, thiotepa, vinBLAStine, vinCRIStine

Perform/provide:

- Adequate fluids 2-3 L/day unless contraindicated

M

• Rinsing of mouth tid-qid with water; brushing of teeth with baking soda bid-tid with soft brush or cotton-tipped applicators for stomatitis; use unwaxed dental floss
• Storage at room temperature 1 wk after reconstituting or 2 wk refrigerated

Evaluate:
• Therapeutic response: decreased tumor size, spread of malignancy

Teach patient/family:
• To report any complaints, side effects to nurse or prescriber
• That hair may be lost during treatment and wig or hairpiece may make the patient feel better; tell patient that new hair may be different in color, texture
• To avoid foods with citric acid, hot or rough texture
• To report any bleeding, white spots, ulcerations in mouth; tell patient to examine mouth daily
• To avoid crowds, persons with infections if granulocyte count is low
• To report immediately urine retention, absence of urine, dyspnea, bleeding, jaundice

Rarely Used

mitotane (℞)

(mye'toe-tane)
Lysodren
Func. class.: Antineoplastic

Do not confuse:
mitotane/mitomycin/mithramycin/mitoxantrone

Uses: Adrenocortical carcinoma

DOSAGE AND ROUTES

• *Adult:* **PO** 1-6 g/day in 3-4 divided doses then 9-10 g/day in divided doses tid or qid; may have to decrease dose for severe reaction, start with reduced dose and gradually increase, 1-6 g/day in 3-4 divided doses

Contraindications: Hypersensitivity

Black Box Warning: Adrenal insufficiency

⚠ High Alert

mitoxantrone (℞)

(mye-toe-zan'trone)
Novantrone
Func. class.: Antineoplastic, antiinfective, immunomodulator
Chem. class.: Synthetic anthraquinone

Do not confuse:
mitoxantrone/mitomycin/mithramycin/mitotane

Action: DNA reactive agent, cytocidal effect on both proliferating and nonproliferating cells, topoisomerase II inhibitor (vesicant)

Uses: Acute myelogenous leukemia (adult), relapsed leukemia, breast cancer; used with steroids to treat bone pain (advanced prostate cancer), multiple sclerosis (MS)

Unlabeled uses: Liver malignancies, non-Hodgkin's lymphoma, breast cancer, ALL

DOSAGE AND ROUTES

Acute nonlymphatic leukemia/induction
• *Adult:* **IV INF** 12 mg/m^2/day on days 1-3, and 100 mg/m^2 cytosine arabinoside × 7 days as a continuous 24-hr inf

Consolidation
• *Adult:* **IV** 12 mg/m^2 given as a short 5-15 min inf

Advanced prostate cancer
• *Adult:* **IV** 12-14 mg/m^2 as a single dose or short inf q21days

Multiple sclerosis
• *Adult:* **IV INF** 12 mg/m^2 as a 5-15 min inf q3mo

Available forms: Inj 2, 10, 12.5, 15 mg/ml

SIDE EFFECTS

CNS: Headache, **seizures,** fatigue
CV: **CHF, cardiopathy, dysrhythmias**
EENT: Conjunctivitis, blue/green sclera, blurred vision

GI: Nausea, vomiting, diarrhea, anorexia, mucositis, **hepatotoxicity**
GU: Amenorrhea, menstrual disorders
HEMA: **Thrombocytopenia, leukopenia, myelosuppression, anemia, secondary leukemia**
INTEG: Rash, necrosis at inj site, dermatitis, thrombophlebitis at inj site, alopecia
MISC: Fever
RESP: Cough, dyspnea

Contraindications: Pregnancy (D), hypersensitivity

Precautions: Breastfeeding, children; myelosuppression, renal/cardiac/hepatic disease; gout

Black Box Warning: Secondary malignancy, neutropenia, intrathecal administration, extravasation, heart failure

PHARMACOKINETICS

Protein binding 78%; metabolized in liver; excreted via renal, hepatobiliary systems; half-life 23-215 hr

INTERACTIONS

- Do not mix with heparin; precipitate will form
- Do not mix with any other product

Increase: bone marrow depression toxicity—radiation, other antineoplastics
Increase: adverse reactions—live virus vaccines
Increase: bleeding risk—NSAIDs, anticoagulants

Drug/Herb

- Avoid use with black cohosh, dong quai

NURSING CONSIDERATIONS

Assess:

- CBC, differential, platelet count q wk; withhold product if WBC is <4000/mm^3 or platelet count is <75,000/mm^3; neutrophil count or ANC; notify prescriber of these results
- Hepatic studies before, during therapy: bilirubin, AST, ALT, alk phos prn or q mo; dose reduction needed in hepatic disease
- Renal studies: BUN, serum uric acid, urine CCr, electrolytes before, during therapy
- Bleeding, hematuria, guaiac, bruising or petechiae, mucosa or orifices q8hr
- Jaundiced skin and sclera, dark urine, clay-colored stools, itchy skin, abdominal pain, fever, diarrhea

⚠ ECG, ECHO, chest x-ray, MUGA, RAI angiography; assess ejection fraction before and during treatment; cardiotoxic may develop during treatment or months to years after treatment; use vigilant cardiac monitoring in MS

- Acidosis, signs of dehydration: rapid respirations, poor skin turgor, decreased urine output, dry skin, restlessness, weakness

⚠ For secondary acute myelogenous leukemia (AML) that can develop after taking this product

⚠ For MS: obtain MUGA, LVEF baselines; repeat LVEF if symptoms of CHF occur or if cumulative dose is >100 mg/m^2; do not administer to patients who have received a lifetime dose of ≥140 mg/m^2 or if LVEF <50% or significant LVEF

- Do not administer to patients with MS if neutrophils <1500 cells/mm^3, except in AML
- Obtain pregnancy test in all women of childbearing age, even if birth control is used

Administer:

- Medications by oral route if possible; avoid IM, SUBCUT, IV routes
- Antiemetic 30-60 min before giving product to prevent vomiting

IV route

- IV after diluting with 50 ml or more NS or D_5W; give over 3-5 min, running IV of D_5W or NS; may be diluted further in D_5W, NS and run over 15-30 min; check for extravasation; give into freely flowing IV inf; do not give IM, SUBCUT, or intraarterially

Additive compatibilities: Cyclophosphamide, cytarabine, fluorouracil, hydrocortisone, potassium chloride

Solution compatibilities: D_5/0.9 NaCl, D_5W, 0.9% NaCl

M

Y-site compatibilities: Allopurinol, amifostine, cladribine, filgrastim, fludarabine, granisetron, melphalan, ondansetron, sargramostim, teniposide, thiotepa, vinorelbine

Perform/provide:

- Liquid diet: carbonated beverages, Jell-O; dry toast, crackers may be added if patient is not nauseated or vomiting
- Rinsing of mouth tid-qid with water, club soda; brushing of teeth bid-qid with soft brush or cotton-tipped applicators for stomatitis; use unwaxed dental floss
- Increase fluids to 2-3 L/day unless contraindicated

Evaluate:

- Therapeutic response: decreased tumor size, spread of malignancy

Teach patient/family:

- To immediately report bleeding, dyspnea, possible infections, seizure, jaundice
- To avoid foods with citric acid, rough texture, or hot
- To report any bleeding, white spots, ulcerations in mouth; tell patient to examine mouth daily
- To avoid crowds, persons with infections
- That sclera, urine may turn blue or green, hair loss may occur
- To notify prescriber if pregnancy is suspected or planned, use effective contraception

modafinil (℞)

(mo-daf′i-nil)

Alertec ♣, Provigil

Func. class.: CNS stimulant

Chem. class.: Racemic compound

Controlled substance IV

Action: Similar action as sympathomimetics, doesn't alter release of DOPamine, norepinephrine

Uses: Narcolepsy, shift work sleep disturbance, obstructive sleep apnea

DOSAGE AND ROUTES

- *Adult:* **PO** 200 mg daily

Hepatic dose (severe hepatic disease)

- *Adult:* **PO** 100 mg daily

Available forms: Tabs 100, 200 mg

SIDE EFFECTS

*CNS: **Headache***, anxiety, cataplexy, depression, dizziness, insomnia, amnesia, confusion, ataxia, tremors, paresthesia, dyskinesia, **suicidal ideation**

CV: Dysrhythmias, hyper/hypotension, chest pain, vasodilation

EENT: Change in vision, ***rhinitis,*** pharyngitis, epistaxis

GI: Nausea, vomiting, changes in LFTs, anorexia, diarrhea, thirst, mouth ulcers, thirst

GU: Ejaculation disorder, urinary retention, albuminuria

HEMA: Eosinophilia

INTEG: Rash, dry skin, herpes simplex, **Stevens-Johnson syndrome**

MISC: Infection, hyperglycemia, neck pain

*RESP: **Dyspnea***, lung changes

Contraindications: Hypersensitivity, ischemic heart disease, left ventricular hypertrophy, chest pain, dysrhythmias

Precautions: Pregnancy (C), breastfeeding, child <16 yr, geriatric patients, unstable angina, history of MI, severe hepatic disease

PHARMACOKINETICS

Absorbed rapidly, 60% protein binding, metabolized by the liver (90%), half-life 15 hr, peak 2-4 hr

INTERACTIONS

Increase: effects of—diazepam, tricylic antidepressants, phenytoin, propranolol, warfarin

Decrease: effects of—cyclosporine, hormonal contraceptives, theophylline

Drug/Herb

Increase: stimulation—cola nut, guarana, mate, coffee, tea

Drug/Lab Test

Increase: LFTs, glucose, eosinophils

NURSING CONSIDERATIONS

Assess:

- For narcolepsy, shift work, history of sleep apnea
- For depression, suicidal ideation
- Monitor B/P in those with hypertension

Administer:

- Give 1 hr before start of shift work, or in the AM for those with narcolepsy or sleep apnea

Perform/provide:

- Storage at room temperature

Evaluate:

- Ability to stay awake

Teach patient/family:

- To take only as directed, may be taken with or without food
- To use other form of contraception during and at least 30 days after discontinuing medication, if using hormonal birth control
- To notify prescriber if pregnancy is planned or suspected, or if breastfeeding
- To notify prescribed of allergic reaction, tremors, confusion
- To avoid all OTC medications unless approved by prescriber
- To avoid hazardous activities until drug effect is known

moexipril (℞)

(moe-ex′ih-prill)

Univasc

Func. class.: Antihypertensive

Chem. class.: Angiotensin-converting enzyme inhibitor

Action: Selectively suppresses renin-angiotensin-aldosterone system; inhibits ACE; prevents conversion of angiotensin I to angiotensin II; results in dilation of arterial, venous vessels

Uses: Hypertension, alone or in combination with thiazide diuretics

DOSAGE AND ROUTES

- *Adult:* **PO** 7.5 mg 1 hr before meals initially, may be increased or divided depending on B/P response; maintenance dosage 7.5-30 mg/day in 1-2 divided doses 1 hr before meals

Renal dose

- *Adult:* **PO** CCr <40 ml/min 3.75 mg/day titrate to desired dose; max 15 mg/day

Available forms: Tabs 7.5, 15 mg

SIDE EFFECTS

CNS: Fever, chills

CV: Hypotension, postural hypotension

GI: Loss of taste

GU: Impotence, dysuria, nocturia, proteinuria, nephrotic syndrome, acute reversible renal failure, polyuria, oliguria, frequency

HEMA: **Neutropenia**

INTEG: Rash

META: Hypokalemia

RESP: **Bronchospasm**, dyspnea, dry cough

SYST: **Angioedema, anaphylaxis**

Contraindications: Breastfeeding, children, hypersensitivity, heart block, bilateral renal stenosis, history of angioedema

Black Box Warning: Pregnancy (D)

Precautions: Dialysis patients, hypovolemia, leukemia, scleroderma, lupus erythematosus, blood dyscrasias, CHF, diabetes mellitus, thyroid/renal disease, COPD, asthma, potassium-sparing diuretics

PHARMACOKINETICS

Peak 1.5 hr, metabolized by liver (metabolites); excreted in urine, crosses placenta, excreted in breast milk, protein binding 50%-70%, half-life 2-10 hr

INTERACTIONS

- Do not use with potassium-sparing diuretics, sympathomimetics, potassium supplements

Increase: hypotension—diuretics, other antihypertensives, ganglionic blockers, adrenergic blockers, phenothiazines

Increase: toxicity—digoxin, lithium

Increase: hyperkalemia—cycloSPORINE, potassium-sparing diuretics

Increase: myelosuppression—azathioprine
Decrease: antihypertensive effect—NSAIDs
Drug/Herb
Increase: antihypertensive effect—hawthorn
Decrease: antihypertensive effect—yohimbe
Drug/Lab Test
False positive: urine acetone

NURSING CONSIDERATIONS

Assess:

- Blood tests: neutrophils, decreased platelets
- B/P
- Renal studies: protein, BUN, creatinine; watch for increased levels that may indicate nephrotic syndrome
- Baselines in renal, hepatic studies before therapy begins
- Potassium levels, although hyperkalemia rarely occurs
- Edema in feet, legs daily
- Allergic reaction: rash, fever, pruritus, urticaria; product should be discontinued if antihistamines fail to help
- Symptoms of CHF; edema, dyspnea, wet crackles, B/P
- Renal symptoms: polyuria, oliguria, frequency

Administer:

- 1 hr before meals
- Do not use with potassium-sparing diuretics, sympathomimetics, potassium supplements

Perform/provide:

- Storage in tight container at 86° F (30° C) or less

Evaluate:

- Therapeutic response: decrease in B/P in hypertension

Teach patient/family:

- To take 1 hr before meals
- Not to discontinue product abruptly
- Not to use OTC (cough, cold, or allergy) products unless directed by prescriber
- To comply with dosage schedule, even if feeling better
- To rise slowly to sitting or standing position to minimize orthostatic hypotension
- To notify prescriber of mouth sores, sore throat, fever, swelling of hands or feet, irregular heartbeat, chest pain, signs of angioedema
- That excessive perspiration, dehydration, vomiting, diarrhea may lead to fall in blood pressure; consult prescriber if these occur
- That dizziness, fainting, lightheadedness may occur during first few days of therapy
- That skin rash or impaired perspiration may occur
- How to take B/P

Treatment of overdose: 0.9% NaCl IV inf, hemodialysis

montelukast (℞)

(mon-teh-loo'kast)
Singulair
Func. class.: Bronchodilator
Chem. class.: Leukotriene antagonist, cysteinyl

Action: Inhibits leukotriene (LTD_4) formation; leukotrienes exert their effects by increasing neutrophil, eosinophil migration; aggregation of neutrophils, monocytes; smooth muscle contraction, capillary permeability; these actions further lead to bronchoconstriction, inflammation, edema

Uses: Chronic asthma in adults and children, seasonal allergic rhinitis

Unlabeled uses: Chronic urticaria

DOSAGE AND ROUTES

- *Adult and child ≥15 yr:* **PO** 10 mg/day PM
- *Child 6-14 yr:* **PO** 5 mg chew tab/day PM
- *Child 2-5 yr:* **PO** chew tab 4 mg/day

Asthma

- *Child 12-23 mo:* **PO** 1 packet (4 mg) of granules taken PM

Exercise-induced bronchoconstriction

• *Adult and adolescent ≥15 yr:* **PO** 10 mg 2 hr prior to exercise; do not take another dose within 24 hr

Available forms: Tabs 10 mg; chew tabs 4, 5 mg; oral granules 4 mg/packet

SIDE EFFECTS

CNS: Dizziness, fatigue, headache, behavior changes, **suicidal ideation, suicide,** hallucinations, **seizures,** agitation, anxiety, depression, fever

GI: Abdominal pain, dyspepsia, nausea, vomiting, diarrhea

INTEG: Rash

MS: Asthenia

RESP: Influenza, cough, nasal congestion

SYST: **Anaphylaxis, angioedema**

Contraindications: Hypersensitivity

Precautions: Pregnancy (B), breastfeeding, children <6 yr, acute attacks of asthma, alcohol consumption, aspirin sensitivity, severe hepatic disease

PHARMACOKINETICS

Rapidly absorbed, peak 3-4 hr, half-life 2.7-5.5 hr; protein binding 99%; metabolized by liver, excreted via bile

INTERACTIONS

Decrease: montelukast levels—phenobarbital, rifampin

Drug/Herb

Increase: stimulation—black, green tea, guarana

Drug/Lab Test

Increase: ALT, AST

NURSING CONSIDERATIONS

Assess:

⚠ Adult patients carefully for symptoms of Churg-Strauss syndrome (rare), including eosinophilia, vasculitic rash, worsening pulmonary symptoms, cardiac complications, and/or neuropathy

• CBC, blood chemistry, during treatment

• Respiratory rate, rhythm, depth; auscultate lung fields bilaterally; notify prescriber of abnormalities

• Allergic reactions: rash, urticaria; product should be discontinued

⚠ For behavior changes and suicidal ideation

Administer:

PO route

• In PM daily for all uses except exercise-induced bronchoconstriction; then take 2 hr prior to exercise

• Granules directly in the mouth or mixed with a spoonful of soft food (carrots, applesauce, ice cream, rice)

• Do not open granules packet until ready to use; mix whole dose; give within 15 min

Evaluate:

• Therapeutic response: ability to breathe more easily

Teach patient/family:

• To check OTC medications, current prescription medications for ephedrine, which will increase stimulation; to avoid alcohol

• To avoid hazardous activities; dizziness may occur

• That product is not to be used for acute asthma attacks

• If aspirin sensitivity is known, do not take NSAIDs while taking this product

• To continue to use inhaled β-agonists if exercise-induced asthma occurs

M

⚠ High Alert

morphine (℞)

(mor′feen)

Astramorph, Astramorph PF, Avinza, Duramorph, Epimorph ✦, Infumorph, Kadian, morphine sulfate, Morphitec ✦, M.O.S. ✦, M.O.S.-S.R. ✦, MS Contin, MSIR, OMS Concentrate, Oramorph SR, RMS, Roxanol, Roxanol Rescudose, Roxanol-T, Statex

Func. class.: Opioid analgesic
Chem. class.: Alkaloid

Controlled Substance Schedule II

Do not confuse:

morphine/hydromorphone

Roxanol/Roxicet

Action: Depresses pain impulse transmission at the spinal cord level by interacting with opioid receptors

Uses: Moderate to severe pain

DOSAGE AND ROUTES

• *Adult:* **SUBCUT/IM** 5-20 mg q4hr prn; **PO** 10-30 mg q4hr prn; **EXT REL** 15-30 mg q8-12hr; **RECT** 10-20 mg q4hr prn; **IV** 2.5-15 mg diluted in 4-5 ml H_2O for inj, over 5 min; **SUS REL** caps (Kadian), **EXT REL** caps (Avinza) give total daily dose q24hr; for those with no tolerance to opioids, 30 mg/day; may adjust by no more than 30 mg q4days

• *Child:* **SUBCUT/IV** 0.05-0.2 mg/kg, max 15 mg; **PO** 0.2-0.5 mg/kg q4-6hr (reg rel), q12hr (sus rel)

Available forms: Inj 0.5, 1, 2, 3, 4, 5, 8, 10, 15, 25, 50 mg/ml; sol tabs 10, 15, 30 mg; oral sol 10, 20 mg/5 ml, 20 mg/10 ml, 20 mg/ml; oral tabs 15, 30 mg; rect supp 5, 10, 20, 30 mg; ext rel tabs 15, 30, 60, 100, 200 mg; caps 15, 30 mg; syr 1, 5 mg/ml; cont rel cap pellets (Kadian) 20, 30, 50, 60, 100 mg; ext rel caps (Avinza) 30, 60, 90, 120 mg

SIDE EFFECTS

CNS: Drowsiness, dizziness, confusion, headache, sedation, euphoria, insomnia, **seizures**

CV: Palpitations, **bradycardia,** change in B/P, **shock, cardiac arrest,** chest pain, hypo/hypertension, edema, **tachycardia**

EENT: Tinnitus, blurred vision, miosis, diplopia

GI: Nausea, vomiting, anorexia, constipation, cramps, biliary tract pressure

GU: Urinary retention

HEMA: **Thrombocytopenia**

INTEG: Rash, urticaria, bruising, flushing, diaphoresis, pruritus

RESP: **Respiratory depression, respiratory arrest, apnea**

Contraindications: Hypersensitivity, addiction (opioid), hemorrhage, bronchial asthma, increased intracranial pressure

Black Box Warning: Respiratory depression

Precautions: Pregnancy (C), breastfeeding, children <18 yr, geriatric patients, addictive personality, acute MI, severe heart disease, renal/hepatic disease, bowel impaction

Black Box Warning: Abrupt discontinuation, accidental exposure, epidural/intrathecal administration, opioid-naive patients, substance abuse

PHARMACOKINETICS

PO: Onset variable, peak variable, duration variable

IM: Onset ½ hr, peak ½-1 hr, duration 3-7 hr

SUBCUT: Onset 15-20 min, peak 50-90 min, duration 3-5 hr

IV: Peak 20 min

RECT: Peak ½-1 hr, duration 4-5 hr

Intrathecal: Onset rapid, duration up to 24 hr

Metabolized by liver, crosses placenta; excreted in urine, breast milk; half-life 1½-2 hr

INTERACTIONS

• Unpredictable reaction, avoid use: MAOIs

Increase: effects with other CNS depressants—alcohol, opiates, sedative/hypnotics, antipsychotics, skeletal muscle relaxants

Decrease: morphine action—rifampin

Drug/Herb

Increase: anticholinergic effect—corkwood

Increase: CNS depression—chamomile, hops, Jamaican dogwood, kava, lavender, mistletoe, nettle, pokeweed, poppy, senega, skullcap, St. John's wort, valerian

Drug/Food

Decrease: morphine effect—cranberry juice (excessive amounts), oats

Drug/Lab Test

Increase: amylase

NURSING CONSIDERATIONS

Assess:

• Pain: location, type, character; give dose before pain becomes severe

• Bowel status; constipation common, use stimulant laxative if needed

• I&O ratio; check for decreasing output; may indicate urinary retention

• B/P, pulse, respirations (character, depth, rate)

• CNS changes: dizziness, drowsiness, hallucinations, euphoria, LOC, pupil reaction

• Allergic reactions: rash, urticaria

• Respiratory dysfunction: depression, character, rate, rhythm; notify prescriber if respirations are <12/min

Administer:

• May be given by patient: controlled analgesia

• Epidural cautiously in the geriatric patients

• Kadian is not bioequivalent to other controlled release forms

• Kadian caps may be opened and sprinkled on applesauce immediately before use; pellets in the cap should not be chewed, crushed, or dissolved, which may lead to overdose; adjustments may need to be made when converting from another form of morphine

PO route

• Do not break, crush, or chew controlled or sus rel products

• With antiemetic for nausea, vomiting

• When pain is beginning to return; determine dosage interval by response; continuous dosing is more effective than prn

IV route

• After diluting with 5 ml or more sterile H_2O or NS; give 15 mg or less over 4-5 min; give through Y- tube or 3-way stopcock; may be added to IV sol, each 0.1-1 mg diluted in 1 ml D_5W, $D_{10}W$, 0.9% NaCl, 0.45% NaCl, Ringer's sol, LR, given with inf pump titrated to patient response

Additive compatibilities: Alteplase, atracurium, baclofen, bupivacaine, DOBUTamine, fluconazole, furosemide, meropenem, metoclopramide, ondansetron, succinylcholine, verapamil

Syringe compatibilities: Atropine, benzquinamide, bupivacaine, butorphanol, cimetidine, dimenhyDRINATE, diphenhydrAMINE, droperidol, fentanyl, glycopyrrolate, hydrOXYzine, ketamine, metoclopramide, midazolam, milrinone, pentazocine, perphenazine, promazine, ranitidine, scopolamine

Y-site compatibilities: Allopurinol, amifostine, amikacin, aminophylline, amiodarone, ampicillin, ampicillin/sulbactam, amsacrine, atenolol, atracurium, aztreonam, bumetanide, calcium chloride, cefamandole, cefazolin, cefmetazole, cefoperazone, cefotaxime, cefotetan, cefoxitin, ceftazidime, ceftizoxime, ceftriaxone, cefuroxime, cephalothin, cephapirin, chloramphenicol, cisatracurium, cisplatin, cladribine, clindamycin, cyclophosphamide, cytarabine, dexamethasone, digoxin, diltiazem, DOBUTamine, DOPamine, doxycycline, enalaprilat, epinephrine, erythromycin, esmolol, etomidate, famotidine, fentanyl, filgrastim, fluconazole, fludarabine, foscarnet, gentamicin, granisetron, heparin, hydrocortisone, hydromorphone, IL-2, insulin (regular), kanamycin, labetalol, lidocaine, loraz-

M

epam, magnesium sulfate, melphalan, meropenem, methotrexate, methyldopate, methylPREDNISolone, metoclopramide, metoprolol, metronidazole, mezlocillin, midazolam, milrinone, moxalactam, nafcillin, niCARdipine, nitroglycerin, norepinephrine, ondansetron, oxacillin, oxytocin, paclitaxel, pancuronium, penicillin G potassium, piperacillin, piperacillin/tazobactam, potassium chloride, propofol, propranolol, ranitidine, remifentanil, sodium bicarbonate, sodium nitroprusside, teniposide, thiotepa, ticarcillin, ticarcillin/clavulanate, tobramycin, trimethoprim-sulfamethoxazole, vancomycin, vecuronium, vinorelbine, vit B/C, warfarin, zidovudine

Perform/provide:

- Storage in light-resistant container at room temperature
- Assistance with ambulation
- Safety measures: side rails, night-light, call bell within easy reach
- Gradual withdrawal after long-term use

Evaluate:

- Therapeutic response; decrease in pain intensity

Teach patient/family:

- To change position slowly; orthostatic hypotension may occur
- To report any symptoms of CNS changes, allergic reactions
- That physical dependency may result from long-term use
- To avoid use of alcohol, CNS depressants
- That withdrawal symptoms may occur: nausea, vomiting, cramps, fever, faintness, anorexia

Treatment of overdose: Naloxone (Narcan) 0.2-0.8 mg IV, O_2, IV fluids, vasopressors

moxifloxacin (℞)

Avelox, Avelox IV

Func. class.: Antiinfective

Chem. class.: Fluoroquinolone

Action: Interferes with conversion of intermediate DNA fragments into high-molecular-weight DNA in bacteria; DNA gyrase inhibitor

Uses: Acute bacterial sinusitis: *Streptococcus pneumoniae, Haemophilus influenzae, Moraxella catarrhalis;* acute bacterial exacerbation of chronic bronchitis: *S. pneumoniae, H. influenzae, Haemophilus parainfluenzae, Klebsiella pneumoniae, Staphylococcus aureus, M. catarrhalis;* community-acquired pneumonia: *S. pneumoniae, H. influenzae, Mycoplasma pneumoniae, Chlamydia pneumoniae, M. catarrhalis;* uncomplicated skin/skin structure infections: *S. aureus, Streptococcus pyogenes;* complicated intraabdominal infections including polymicrobial infections: *E. coli, Bacterioides fragilis, S. anginosus, S. constellatus, Enterococcus faecalis, Proteus mirabilis, Clostridium perfringens, Bacteroides thetaiotaomicron, Peptostreptococcus* sp; complicated skin, skin structure infections caused by methicillin-susceptible: *S. aureus, E. coli, K. pneumoniae, Enterobacter cloacae*

DOSAGE AND ROUTES

Acute bacterial sinusitis

- *Adult:* **PO/IV** 400 mg q24hr × 10 days

Acute bacterial exacerbation of chronic bronchitis

- *Adult:* **PO/IV** 400 mg q24hr × 5 days

Community-acquired pneumonia

- *Adult:* **PO/IV** 400 mg q24hr × 7-14 days

Uncomplicated skin/skin structure infections

- *Adult:* **PO/IV** 400 mg q24hr × 7 days

Complicated intraabdominal infections

- *Adult:* **IV** 400 mg/day × 5-14 days

Complicated skin, skin structure infections

- *Adult:* **PO/IV** 400 mg/day × 7-21 days

Available forms: Tabs 400 mg; inj premix 400 mg/250 ml

SIDE EFFECTS

CNS: Headache, dizziness, fatigue, insomnia, depression, *restlessness,* **seizures,**

confusion, **increased intracranial pressure,** peripheral neuropathy
CV: **Prolonged QT interval, dysrhythmias, torsade de pointes,** tachycardia
EENT: Blurred vision, tinnitus, taste changes
GI: Nausea, diarrhea, increased ALT, AST, flatulence, heartburn, *vomiting,* oral candidiasis, dysphagia, **pseudomembranous colitis**
INTEG: Rash, pruritus, urticaria, photosensitivity, flushing, fever, chills
MS: Tremor, arthralgia, tendinitis, **tendon rupture,** myalgia
SYST: **Anaphylaxis, Stevens-Johnson syndrome**
Contraindications: Hypersensitivity to quinolones
Precautions: Pregnancy (C), breastfeeding, children, hepatic/cardiac/renal/GI disease, epilepsy, uncorrected hypokalemia, prolonged QT interval, patients receiving class IA, III antidysrhythmics, seizure disorder

Black Box Warning: Tendon pain/rupture, tendinitis

PHARMACOKINETICS

Excreted in urine as active product, metabolites; parent product excreted in urine and feces; terminal half-life PO 12 hr, IV 15 hr

INTERACTIONS

• Prolonged QT: antidysrhythmics class IA/III, other drugs that increase QT prolongation
Increase: moxifloxacin serum levels—probenecid
Increase: warfarin, cycloSPORINE effect
Increase: seizure risk—NSAIDs
Decrease: moxifloxacin absorption—magnesium antacids, aluminum hydroxide, zinc, iron, sucralfate, calcium, enteral feeding, didanosine

Drug/Herb

• Do not use acidophilus with antiinfectives; separate by several hours
Increase: antiinfective effect—cola tree

NURSING CONSIDERATIONS

Assess:

• CNS symptoms: headache, dizziness, fatigue, insomnia, depression, seizures
• Renal, hepatic studies: BUN, creatinine, AST, ALT
• I&O ratio, urine pH <5.5 is ideal
⚠ Allergic reactions, Stevens-Johnson syndrome, toxic epidermal necrolysis, and anaphylaxis: fever, flushing, rash, urticaria, pruritus; keep epinephrine, emergency equipment nearby for anaphylaxis
⚠ For tendon pain, rupture, tendinitis, if tendon becomes inflamed, drug should be discontinued
⚠ Cardiac status: prolonged QT, or use of drugs that increase QT prolongation
⚠ GI status: watch for pseudomembranous colitis

Administer:

PO route
• 4 hr before or 8 hr after antacids, zinc, iron, calcium

IV route
• Discontinue primary IV while administering moxifloxacin
• Do not give SUBCUT, IM

Solution compatibilities: 0.9% NaCl, D_5, D_{10}, LR, sterile water for inj

Perform/provide:

• Limited intake of alkaline foods, products: milk, dairy products, alkaline antacids, sodium bicarbonate
• That fluids must be increased to 3 L/day to avoid crystallization in kidneys

Evaluate:

• Therapeutic response: decreased pain, C&S; absence of infection

Teach patient/family:

• Not to take any products containing magnesium or calcium (such as antacids), iron, or aluminum with this product or within 8 hr of product
• That photosensitivity may occur; patient should avoid sunlight or use sunscreen to prevent burns
• To use frequent rinsing of mouth, sugarless candy or gum for dry mouth
• To take as prescribed, not to double or miss doses

M

• If dizziness occurs, to ambulate, perform activities with assistance
• To complete full course of product therapy
• To contact prescriber if abnormal heart rhythm or seizures occur or if inflammation or pain in tendon occurs

moxifloxacin ophthalmic

See Appendix B

multivitamins (OTC, ℞)

Adavite, Dayalets, LKV Drops, Multi-75, Multiday, One-A-Day, Optilets, Poly-Vi-sol, Quin tabs, Ru-Lets, Sesame Street Vitamins, Tab-A-Vite, Therabid, Theragran, Unicaps, Vita-Bob, Vita-Kid, many other brands

Func. class.: Vitamins, multiple

Do not confuse:
Theragran/Phenergan

Action: Needed for adequate metabolism

Uses: Prevention and treatment of vitamin deficiencies

DOSAGE AND ROUTES

• *Adult and child:* **PO/IV** Depends on brand

Available forms: Many

SIDE EFFECTS

None known at recommended dosage

Precautions: Pregnancy (A)

NURSING CONSIDERATIONS

Assess:
• Vitamin deficiency: usually more than one vitamin is deficient

Administer:
• Liquid multivitamins diluted or dropped into patient's mouth using dropper provided with some brands
• Chew tabs should be chewed, not swallowed whole
• Give by cont IV inf only after diluting 5-10 ml multivitamins/500-1000 ml of D_5W, $D_{10}W$, $D_{20}W$, LR, D_5/LR, D_5/0.9% NaCl, 0.9% NaCl, 3% NaCl
• Do not use sol with crystals, precipitate, or color other than bright yellow

Additive compatibilities: Cefoxitin, isoproterenol, methyldopate, metoclopramide, metronidazole, netilmicin, norepinephrine, sodium bicarbonate, verapamil

Y-site compatibilities: Acyclovir, ampicillin, cefazolin, cephalothin, cephapirin, diltiazem, erythromycin, fludarabine, gentamicin, tacrolimus

Evaluate:
• Therapeutic response: check each individual vitamin for guidelines

Teach patient/family:
• That adequate nutrition must be maintained to prevent further deficiencies
• To comply with regimen
• To avoid presenting flavored multivitamins as candy; child may overdose
• To store out of children's reach

mupirocin topical

See Appendix B

muromonab-CD3 (℞)

(mur-oo-mone'ab)

Orthoclone OKT3

Func. class.: Immunosuppressant
Chem. class.: Murine monoclonal antibody

Action: Reverses graft rejection by blocking T-cell function

Uses: Acute allograft rejection in renal, cardiac/hepatic transplant patients

DOSAGE AND ROUTES

• *Adult:* **IV BOL** 5 mg/day × 10-14 days
• *Child ≤30 kg:* **IV** 2.5 mg daily × 10-14 days

Cardiac/hepatic allograft rejection, steroid resistant

• *Adult:* **IV BOL** 5 mg/day × 10-14 days; begin when it is known that rejection has not been reversed by steroids

Available forms: Inj 5 mg/5 ml

SIDE EFFECTS

CNS: Pyrexia, chills, tremors, **aseptic meningitis,** *fever,* headache

CV: Chest pain

EENT: Vision impairment

GI: Vomiting, nausea, diarrhea

MISC: **Infection, cytokine release syndrome, anaphylaxis,** malaise

MS: Myalgia, arthralgia

RESP: Dyspnea, wheezing, **pulmonary edema**

Contraindications: CHF, uncontrolled hypertension, hypersensitivity to murine origin

Black Box Warning: Fluid overload, seizures

Precautions: Pregnancy (C), children <2 yr, fever, cerebral edema, thrombus, CV/vascular disease

Black Box Warning: Angioedema, immunosuppression

PHARMACOKINETICS

Trough level steady state 3-14 days

INTERACTIONS

Increase: immunosuppression—immunosuppressants

Increase: infection risk—cycloSPORINE, corticosteroids, azathioprine

Increase: CNS symptoms—indomethacin

Decrease: immune response—vaccines

Drug/Herb

• Interference with immunosuppression: astragalus, echinacea, melatonin

Decrease: effect—ginseng, maitake, mistletoe, schisandra, St. John's wort, turmeric

NURSING CONSIDERATIONS

Assess:

▲ For cytokine release syndrome (CRS): nausea, vomiting, chills, fever, joint pain, weakness, dizziness, diarrhea, tremors, abdominal pain; usually occurs within 30-48 hr and may last 6 hr; treat with antihistamines, acetaminophen

▲ For hypersensitivity, anaphylaxis: dyspnea, bronchospasm, urticaria, tachycardia, angioedema; emergency equipment must be available

• Blood studies: Hgb, WBC, platelets during treatment q mo; if leukocytes are <3000/mm^3, product should be discontinued; CD3, CD4, CD8, CD3 ≤25 cells/mm^3

• Hepatic studies: alk phos, AST, ALT, bilirubin

▲ Hepatotoxicity: dark urine, jaundice, itching, light-colored stools; product should be discontinued

• For infection: sore throat, fever, chills, temp, notify prescriber immediately

▲ For aseptic meningitis: fever, headache, photophobia

▲ For fluid overload: increased weight, I&O, edema, crackles, B/P

Administer:

• Pretreat with corticosteroids, acetaminophen, or antihistamines

• For several days before transplant surgery

• All medications PO if possible; avoid IM inj, since infection may occur

IV route

• IV undiluted; withdraw with a 0.2-0.22 low protein-binding μm filter, discard and use new needle for administration; give over 1 min

• Incompatible with any product in syringe or sol; do not admix

Evaluate:

• Therapeutic response: absence of graft rejection

Teach patient/family:

• To report fever, chills, sore throat, fatigue, since serious infection may occur; rash, dyspnea, fast heartbeat; change in mental status

• To use contraceptive measures during treatment

• To report cytokine release syndrome, give symptoms

M

- To avoid vaccinations during treatment
- To avoid persons with infections, crowds; infections may occur

mycophenolate (℞)

(mye-koe-phen′oh-late)

CellCept, Myfortic

Func. class.: Immunosuppressant

Action: Inhibits inflammatory responses that are mediated by the immune system; prolongs the survival of allogenic transplants

Uses: Organ transplants (to prevent rejection); prophylaxis of organ rejection in allogenic cardiac, hepatic, renal transplants

Unlabeled uses: Refractory uveitis, second-line therapy for Churg-Strauss syndrome, diffuse proliferative lupus nephritis (in combination), rheumatoid arthritis, psoriasis, GVHD, kidney disease, myasthenia gravis, atopic dermatitis

DOSAGE AND ROUTES

Renal transplant

- *Adult:* **PO/IV** Give initial dose 72 hr prior to transplantation; 1 g bid given to renal transplant patients in combination with corticosteroids, cycloSPORINE; **TAB ER** 720 mg bid on empty stomach
- *Child:* **PO-ER** 400 mg/m^2 bid, max 720 mg bid

Renal dose

- *Adult:* **PO/IV** GFR <25 ml/min, max 2 g/day

Cardiac transplant

- *Adult:* **PO/IV** 1.5 g bid, **IV** can be started ≤24 hr after transplant, switch to **PO** when able

Hepatic transplant

- *Adult:* **PO** 1.5 g bid; **IV** 1 g over ≥2 hr

Refractory acute kidney transplant rejection (unlabeled)

- *Adult:* **PO** 1.5 g bid

Rheumatoid arthritis (unlabeled)

- *Adult:* **PO** 250 mg-2 g/day

GVHD (unlabeled)

- *Adult:* **PO** 2 g/day with cycloSPORINE and prednisoLONE

Diffuse proliferative lupus nephritis (unlabeled)

- *Adult:* **PO** 1 g/day

Uveitis (unlabeled)

- *Adult:* **PO** 1 g bid × 6-41 mo

Atopic dermatitis (unlabeled)

- *Adult:* **PO** 1 g bid × 4 wk
- *Child ≥2 yr/adolescent:* **PO** 30-50 mg/kg/day in 2 divided doses

Available forms: Caps 250 mg; tabs 500 mg; inj (powder) 500 mg/20-ml vial; powder for oral susp 200 mg/ml; ext rel tab (Myfortic) 180, 360 mg

SIDE EFFECTS

CNS: Tremor, dizziness, insomnia, headache, fever, **progressive multifocal leukoencephalopathy**

CV: Hypertension, chest pain

GI: Diarrhea, constipation, nausea, vomiting, stomatitis, **GI bleeding**

GU: UTI, hematuria, **renal tubular necrosis**

HEMA: **Leukopenia, thrombocytopenia, anemia, pancytopenia, pure red cell aplasia**

INTEG: Rash

META: Peripheral edema, hypercholesterolemia, hypophosphatemia, edema, hyperkalemia, hypokalemia, hyperglycemia, hypocalcemia, hypomagnesemia

MS: Arthralgia, muscle wasting

RESP: Dyspnea, respiratory infection, increased cough, pharyngitis, bronchitis, pneumonia

SYST: **Lymphoma,** *nonmelanoma skin carcinoma,* **sepsis**

Contraindications: Hypersensitivity to this product or mycophenolic acid

Black Box Warning: Pregnancy (D)

Precautions: Breastfeeding, lymphomas, neutropenia, renal disease

Black Box Warning: Infection, neoplastic disease

PHARMACOKINETICS

Rapidly and completely absorbed, metabolized to active metabolite (MPA), excreted in urine, feces, protein binding (MPA) 97%, half-life (MPA) 17.9 hr

INTERACTIONS

• Avoid administration with azathioprine
Increase: effects of phenytoin, theophylline
Increase: concentration of both products—acyclovir, ganciclovir
Increase: mycophenolate levels—probenecid, salicylates
Decrease: mycophenolate levels—antacids, cholestyramine
Decrease: protein binding of phenytoin, theophylline
Decrease: effect of live attenuated vaccines, oral contraceptives

Drug/Herb

Interference with immunosuppression: astragalus, echinacea, melatonin

Drug/Food

Decrease: absorption if taken with food

NURSING CONSIDERATIONS

Assess:

⚠ For progressive multifocal leukoencephalopathy, may be fatal; ataxia, confusion, apathy, hemiparesis, visual problems, weakness; side effects should be reported to the FDA
• Blood studies: CBC during treatment monthly
• Hepatic studies: alk phos, AST, ALT, bilirubin
• Renal studies and electrolytes

Administer:

• 72 hr prior to transplantation; may be given in combination with corticosteroids, cycloSPORINE

PO route

• Do not break, crush, or chew tabs; do not open caps
• At same time each day
• Avoid inhalation or direct contact with skin, mucous membranes, teratogenic in animals
• Oral susp: tap the closed bottle several times to loosen powder, use 94 ml of water in graduated cylinder, add ½ the total amount of water for constitution and shake the closed bottle, add remaining water and shake, again remove child resistant cap and push adapter into neck of the bottle, close tightly
• Give alone for better absorption

IV route

• Do not give by rapid or bolus inj; reconstitute and dilute to 6 mg/ml with D_5W, give over ≥2 hr
• Do not admix with mycophenolate IV in inf catheter or with other IV products or inf admixtures

Evaluate:

• Therapeutic response: absence of graft rejection

Teach patient/family:

• To report fever, rash, severe diarrhea, chills, sore throat, fatigue, since serious infections may occur
• To reduce risk of infection by avoiding crowds
• The need for repeated lab tests
• To limit exposure to sunlight/UV light
• To use contraception before, during, and 6 wk after therapy
• To take at same time each day

nabilone (℞)

(nab′ih-lohn)

Cesamet

Func. class.: Antiemetic

Chem. class.: Cannabinoid—miscellaneous

Action: Orally, active cannabinoid, chemically related to marijuana; may decrease nausea by action on cannabinoid receptors in the CNS

Uses: Prevention of nausea, vomiting associated with cancer chemotherapy, in those who have not responded to other treatment; not to be used on an as-needed basis

DOSAGE AND ROUTES

• *Adult:* **PO** 1-2 mg bid; give initial dose 1-3 hr prior to chemotherapy; start with lower dose and increase as needed; may give dose of 1-2 mg the night before chemotherapy; may give 2-3 ×/day during chemotherapy cycle

Available forms: Caps 1 mg

SIDE EFFECTS

CNS: Headache, ataxia, drowsiness, dysphoria, euphoria, sleep disturbance, vertigo, asthenia, concentration difficulties, depression, syncope, hallucinations

CV: Chest discomfort, **tachycardia,** orthostatic hypotension

GI: Dry mouth, nausea, *anorexia*, increased appetite

INTEG: Allergic reactions, rash, photosensitivity, pruritus

MS: Back, joint, muscle, neck pain

Contraindications: Hypersensitivity to this product or cannabinoids

Precautions: Pregnancy (C), breastfeeding, depression, mental disorders, severe renal/hepatic disease, hypertension, tachycardia, CV disorders

PHARMACOKINETICS

Absorption rapid, 10%-20% absorbed, duration is unpredictable, psychiatric symptoms may occur for up to 72 hr after treatment is concluded, terminal half-life 2 hr, metabolized by the liver, excreted via biliary system in feces

INTERACTIONS

• Hypomanic reaction: disulfiram and possibly fluoxetine

Increase: hypertension, tachycardia, and possibly cardiotoxicity—sympathomimetics (amphetamines, cocaine)

Increase: tachycardia, drowsiness—anticholinergics (antihistamines, atropine, scopolamine)

Increase: drowsiness, CNS depression—CNS depressants (alcohol, barbiturates, benzodiazepines, busPIRone, lithium, muscle relaxants, opioids)

Increase: action or nabilone—naltrexone

Increase: action of both—opioids

Increase: tachycardia, hypertension, drowsiness—tricyclics

Decrease: metabolism of theophylline

NURSING CONSIDERATIONS

Assess:

• For absence of nausea and vomiting during chemotherapy

• CNS symptoms: headache, depression, ataxia, drowsiness, dysphoria, euphoria, sleep disturbances, concentration difficulties

• CV symptoms, cardiac status: tachycardia, orthostatic hypo/hypertension

• Psychiatric symptoms: euphoria, depression, sleep disturbance

Administer:

• PO, not to be used on an as-needed basis

Perform/provide:

• Storage of capsules at room temperature, away from light and moisture

Evaluate:

• Therapeutic response: decreased nausea and vomiting associated with chemotherapy

Teach patient/family:

• That mood, behavioral changes may occur while taking this product

• To notify prescriber if pregnancy is suspected

• To avoid breastfeeding while taking this product

• Not to use alcohol or other CNS depressants unless approved by prescriber

• Not to operate machinery or perform other hazardous activities while taking this product

nabumetone (℞)

(na-byoo′me-tone)

Func. class.: Nonsteroidal antiinflammatory

Chem. class.: Acetic acid derivative

Action: Metabolite inhibits COX-1, COX-2 by blocking arachidonate; analgesic, antiinflammatory, antipyretic

Uses: Osteoarthritis, rheumatoid arthritis, acute or chronic treatment

DOSAGE AND ROUTES

• *Adult:* **PO** 1 g as a single dose or divided bid; may increase to 2 g/day if needed; may give daily or bid as a divided dose

Available forms: Tabs 500, 750 mg

SIDE EFFECTS

CNS: Dizziness, headache, drowsiness, fatigue, tremors, confusion, insomnia, anxiety, depression, nervousness

EENT: Tinnitus

CV: Tachycardia, peripheral edema, palpitations, dysrhythmias, **CHF, MI, stroke**

GI: Nausea, anorexia, vomiting, diarrhea, jaundice, **cholestatic hepatitis,** constipation, flatulence, cramps, dry mouth, peptic ulcer, gastritis, **ulceration, perforation, bleeding**

GU: **Nephrotoxicity, dysuria, hematuria, oliguria, azotemia,** cystitis

HEMA: **Blood dyscrasias**

INTEG: Purpura, rash, pruritus, sweating, photosensitivity

RESP: Dyspnea, pharyngitis, **bronchospasm**

SYST: **Anaphylaxis, angioneurotic edema**

Contraindications: Pregnancy (D) 3rd trimester, hypersensitivity to this product or aspirin, iodides, NSAIDs

Black Box Warning: Perioperative pain in CABG surgery

Precautions: Pregnancy (C), breastfeeding, children, geriatric patients, bleeding/GI/cardiac/renal disorders, hepatic dysfunction, asthma, bone marrow suppression, lupus (SLE), ulcerative colitis, blood dyscrasias

Black Box Warning: MI, stroke, GI bleeding

PHARMACOKINETICS

PO: Peak 2½-4 hr, plasma protein binding >90%, half-life 22-30 hr; metabolized in liver to active metabolite; excreted in urine (metabolites), breast milk

INTERACTIONS

Increase: bleeding risk—anticoagulants, thrombolytics, valproic acid, cefamandole, cefotetan, cefoperazone, plicamycin, clopidogrel, eptifibatide, ticlopidine

Increase: hematologic toxicity—antineoplastics, radiation

Increase: GI reactions—salicylates, NSAIDs, alcohol, potassium, corticosteroids

Increase: effect of—lithium, methotrexate

Decrease: effect of diuretics, antihypertensives

Drug/Herb

Increase: gastric irritation—arginine, gossypol

Increase: NSAIDs effect—bearberry, bilberry

Increase: bleeding risk—garlic, ginger, ginkgo

Drug/Lab Test

Increase: bleeding time, K, BUN, AST, ALT, LDH, alk phos, creatinine

Decrease: CCr, blood glucose, Hct, Hgb

NURSING CONSIDERATIONS

Assess:

⚠ Cardiac status: CV thrombotic events, MI, stroke; may be fatal

⚠ GI status: ulceration, bleeding, perforation; may be fatal

• Pain: frequency, intensity, characteristics; relief of pain after med

• Asthma, aspirin sensitivity, or nasal polyps; increased hypersensitivity reactions

N

• Renal, hepatic studies: BUN, creatinine, AST, ALT, Hgb, LDH, blood glucose, WBC, platelets, CCr before treatment, periodically thereafter
• Audiometric, ophthalmic exam before, during, after treatment
• For eye, ear problems: blurred vision, tinnitus; may indicate toxicity

Administer:
• With food for GI symptoms

Perform/provide:
• Storage at room temperature

Evaluate:
• Therapeutic response: decreased pain and stiffness in joints

Teach patient/family:
• To avoid alcoholic beverages and aspirin
• To report blurred vision, ringing, roaring in ears; may indicate toxicity
• To avoid driving, other hazardous activities if dizziness, drowsiness occur
• To report change in urine pattern, increased weight, edema, increased pain in joints, fever, blood in urine; indicates nephrotoxicity
• That therapeutic effects may take up to 1 mo
• To take with a full glass of water to enhance absorption and sit upright for 30 min
• To report dark stools; may indicate GI bleeding
• To use sunscreen, protective clothing if in the sun
• To report use to all health care providers

nadolol (℞)

(nay-doe'lole)
Corgard, Syn-Nadolol ♣
Func. class.: Antihypertensive, antianginal
Chem. class.: β-Adrenergic receptor blocker

Do not confuse:
Corgard/Cognex

Action: Long-acting, nonselective β-adrenergic receptor blocking agent, blocks β_1 in the heart and β_2 in the lungs, uterus, and circulatory system; mechanism is similar to that of propranolol

Uses: Chronic stable angina pectoris, mild to moderate hypertension

Unlabeled uses: Tachydysrhythmias, aggression, anxiety, tremors, esophageal varices (rebleeding only), hyperthyroidism adjunctive therapy, prophylaxis of migraine headaches

DOSAGE AND ROUTES

• *Adult:* **PO** 40 mg/day, increase by 40-80 mg q3-7days; maintenance 40-240 mg/day for angina, 40-320 mg/day for hypertension
• *Geriatric:* **PO** 20 mg/day, may increase by 20 mg until desired dose

Renal dose
• *Adult:* **PO** CCr 31-50 ml/min give q24-36hr; CCr 10-30 ml/min give q24-48hr; CCr <10 ml/min give q40-60hr

Available forms: Tabs 20, 40, 80, 120, 160 mg

SIDE EFFECTS

CNS: Depression, dizziness, *fatigue,* lethargy, paresthesias, headache, *weakness,* insomnia, memory loss, nightmares
CV: **Bradycardia,** *hypotension,* **CHF,** palpitations, **AV block,** chest pain, peripheral ischemia, flushing, edema, vasodilation, conduction disturbances
EENT: Blurred vision, dry eyes, nasal congestion
ENDO: Hyperglycemia, hypoglycemia
GI: Nausea, vomiting, diarrhea, colitis, constipation, cramps, dry mouth, flatulence, hepatomegaly, **pancreatitis,** taste distortion
GU: *Impotence,* decreased libido
HEMA: **Agranulocytosis, thrombocytopenia**
INTEG: Rash, pruritus, fever, alopecia
RESP: Dyspnea, respiratory dysfunction, **bronchospasm,** cough, wheezing, **pulmonary edema,** pharyngitis, **laryngospasm**

Contraindications: Hypersensitivity to this product, cardiac failure, cardiogenic shock, 2nd/3rd degree heart block, bronchospastic disease, sinus bradycardia, CHF, COPD

Precautions: Pregnancy (C), breastfeeding, diabetes mellitus, renal disease, hyperthyroidism, peripheral vascular disease, myasthenia gravis, major surgery, nonallergic bronchospasm

Black Box Warning: Abrupt discontinuation

PHARMACOKINETICS

PO: Onset variable, peak 3-4 hr, duration 17-24 hr; half-life 20-24 hr; not metabolized; excreted in urine (unchanged), bile, breast milk; protein binding 30%

INTERACTIONS

- Do not use with MAOIs; bradycardia may occur
- Peripheral ischemia: ergots

Increase: bradycardia—digoxin

Increase: hypotension, bradycardia—clonidine, epinephrine

Increase: hypotensive effects—other hypotensive agents, phenothiazines

Decrease: β-blocking effect—thyroid hormones

Decrease: antihypertensive effect—NSAIDs

Drug/Herb

Increase: toxicity, death—aconite

Increase: antihypertensive effect—barberry, betony, black catechu, black cohosh, bloodroot, broom, burdock, cat's claw, dandelion, goldenseal, Irish moss, Jamaican dogwood, kelp, khella, mistletoe, parsley

Increase or decrease: antihypertensive effect—astragalus, cola tree

Decrease: antihypertensive effect—coltsfoot, guarana, khat, licorice

Drug/Lab Test

Increase: serum potassium, serum uric acid, ALT, AST, alk phos, LDH, blood glucose, cholesterol, ANA, triglycerides

NURSING CONSIDERATIONS

Assess:

- B/P, pulse, respirations during beginning therapy, orthostatic hypotension may occur
- Weight daily; report gain of 5 lb
- I&O ratio, CCr if kidney damage is diagnosed; crackles, jugular vein distention, fatigue, dyspnea
- Pain: duration, time started, activity being performed, character
- Headache, light-headedness, decreased B/P; may indicate a need for decreased dosage

Administer:

- With 8 oz water

Evaluate:

- Therapeutic response: decreased B/P, heart rate, symptoms of angina

Teach patient/family:

- That product may mask signs of hypoglycemia or alter blood glucose in diabetics

⚠ Not to discontinue abruptly, serious dysrhythmias may occur

- To avoid OTC products unless prescriber approves
- To avoid hazardous activities if dizziness occurs
- To comply with complete medical regimen, to report weight gain >5 lb, swelling, unusual bruising, bleeding
- To rise slowly to prevent orthostatic hypotension
- How and when to check B/P and pulse; to hold dose and contact prescriber if pulse ≤50 bpm, systolic B/P <90 mm Hg

nafarelin (℞)

(naf-ah-rell′in)

Synarel

Func. class.: Gonadotropin

Chem. class.: Analog of gonadotropin-releasing hormone

Action: Stimulates the release of LH and FSH, which increases ovarian steroid production; repeated dosing prevents stimulation of the pituitary gland

N

Uses: Endometriosis, gonadotropin-central precocious puberty

DOSAGE AND ROUTES

• *Adult:* **NASAL** 400 mcg/day as one spray (200 mcg) into one nostril in morning and one spray into other nostril in evening; start treatment between days 2 and 4 of menstrual cycle; may increase to 800 mcg/day (one spray into each nostril twice a day); recommended duration of treatment is 6 mo

• *Child:* **NASAL** 2 sprays in each nostril AM and PM, may increase to 3 sprays alternating nostril tid

Available forms: Nasal spray 2 mg/ml (200 mcg/spray)

SIDE EFFECTS

CNS: Headache, flushing, depression, insomnia, *emotional lability,* hot flashes

GU: Decreased libido, vaginal dryness, breast tenderness, increased pubic hair, *impaired fertility, reduction in breast size, absence of menses,* impotence, irregular periods

INTEG: Acne

META: Decreased bone density, increased cholesterol, triglycerides

MISC: Body odor, seborrhea, rhinitis, *nasal irritation*

SENSITIVITY: Shortness of breath, chest pain, urticaria, pruritus

Contraindications: Pregnancy (X), breastfeeding, hypersensitivity to this product, GnRH, sorbitol; undiagnosed abnormal vaginal bleeding

Precautions: Children, females, menstruation, osteoporosis, pituitary insufficiency

PHARMACOKINETICS

Rapidly absorbed, peak 10-40 min, half-life 3 hr; 80% bound to plasma proteins

INTERACTIONS

Decrease: nafarelin absorption—nasal decongestants (nasal sprays)

NURSING CONSIDERATIONS

Assess:

• Abdominal pain (endometriosis) during treatment

• Central precocious puberty: endocrine studies, bone age, sex steroids, RHCg, GnRH, baseline q8wk

• For precocious puberty including secondary sex characteristics

• Test results: pituitary/hypothalamus dysfunction (decreased LH); postmenopausal (increased LH)

Administer:

• Repeated doses may be necessary to elevate pituitary gonadotropin reserve; in endometriosis treatment continues for up to 6 mo

• Tilting head back slightly; wait 30 sec between sprays; do not use decongestant until 12 hr later

Perform/provide:

• Storage at room temperature; protect from light

Evaluate:

• Therapeutic response: decreased symptoms of endometriosis; adequate resolution of central precocious puberty

Teach patient/family:

• To use nonhormonal contraception

• About correct nasal use; one spray in right nostril AM, one in left nostril PM for endometriosis; 2 sprays in each nostril in AM and PM for central precocious puberty

• That medication may cause hot flashes, decreased libido, vaginal dryness

• To avoid use of nasal decongestants or separate by 12 hr

• That growth of facial hair, increased body odor and vaginal discharge may occur in females

nafcillin (℞)

(naf-sill'in)

nafcillin sodium, Unipen

Func. class.: Antiinfective, broad-spectrum

Chem. class.: Penicillinase-resistant penicillin

Action: Interferes with cell wall replication of susceptible organisms; cell lysis mediated by cell wall autolytic enzymes

Uses: Effective for gram-positive cocci *(Staphylococcus aureus, Streptococcus viridans, Streptococcus pneumoniae)*, infections caused by penicillinase-producing *Staphylococcus*

DOSAGE AND ROUTES

- *Adult:* **IV** 500-2000 mg q4hr
- *Child and infant >1 mo:* **IV** 50-200 mg/kg/day in divided doses q4-6hr
- *Neonates >7 days (weight >2 kg):* **IV** 25 mg/kg q8hr
- *Neonates ≤7 days (weight <2 kg):* **IV** 25 mg/kg q12hr

Meningitis

- *Adult:* **IV** 100-200 mg/kg/day divided q4-6hr, max 12 g/day
- *Neonates >7 days (weight >2 kg):* **IV** 50 mg/kg q6hr
- *Neonates ≤7 days (weight <2 kg):* **IV** 50 mg/kg q12hr

Available forms: Powder for inj 1, 2, 10 g

SIDE EFFECTS

CNS: Lethargy, hallucinations, anxiety, depression, twitching, **coma, seizures**

GI: Nausea, vomiting, diarrhea, increased AST, ALT, abdominal pain, glossitis, **pseudomembranous colitis**

GU: Oliguria, **proteinuria, hematuria,** vaginitis, moniliasis, **glomerulonephritis,** interstitial nephritis

HEMA: Anemia, increased bleeding time, **bone marrow depression, granulocytopenia**

SYST: **Anaphylaxis, serum sickness, Stevens-Johnson syndrome**

Contraindications: Hypersensitivity to penicillins or corn

Precautions: Pregnancy (B), breastfeeding, neonates, hypersensitivity to cephalosporins or carbapenems, GI disease, asthma

PHARMACOKINETICS

Half-life 1 hr, metabolized by liver, excreted in bile, urine

INTERACTIONS

- Avoid use with tetracyclines

Increase: nafcillin concentrations—probenecid

Decrease: effect of cycloSPORINE

Drug/Herb

- Do not use acidophilus with antiinfectives; separate by several hours

Decrease: absorption—khat

Drug/Food

Decrease: absorption—food, carbonated drinks, citrus fruit juices

Drug/Lab Test

False positive: urine glucose, urine protein

N

NURSING CONSIDERATIONS

Assess:

- I&O ratio; report hematuria, oliguria, since penicillin in high doses is nephrotoxic

⚠ Any patient with compromised renal system, since product is excreted slowly in poor renal system function; toxicity may occur rapidly

- Hepatic studies: AST, ALT
- Blood studies: WBC, RBC, Hct, Hgb, bleeding time
- Renal studies: urinalysis, protein, blood, BUN, creatinine
- C&S before product therapy; product may be given as soon as culture is taken
- Bowel pattern before and during treatment
- Respiratory status: rate, character, wheezing, and tightness in chest

⚠ Allergies before initiation of treatment; monitor for anaphylaxis, dyspnea, rash, laryngeal edema; stop product; keep emergency equipment nearby; skin eruptions after administration of penicillin to 1 wk after discontinuing product

• Differential WBC in patients on long-term therapy

Administer:

• Product after C&S has been completed

IV route

• After diluting 1 g/3.4 ml or 2 g/6.8 ml to 250 mg/ml sterile H_2O for inj; further dilute 15-30 ml sterile H_2O or NS sol; give through Y-tube or 3-way stopcock; 500 mg or less/5-10 min; may be further diluted and run over 24 hr

Additive compatibilities: Chloramphenicol, chlorothiazide, dexamethasone, diphenhydrAMINE, ephedrine, heparin, hydrOXYzine, lidocaine, potassium chloride, prochlorperazine, sodium bicarbonate, sodium lactate

Syringe compatibilities: Cimetidine, heparin

Y-site compatibilities: Acyclovir, atropine, cyclophosphamide, diazepam, enalaprilat, esmolol, famotidine, fentanyl, fluconazole, foscarnet, hydromorphone, magnesium sulfate, morphine, perphenazine, propofol, theophylline, zidovudine

Perform/provide:

• Adrenalin, suction, tracheostomy set, endotracheal intubation equipment

• Adequate fluid intake (2 L) during diarrhea episodes

• Scratch test to assess allergy after securing order from prescriber; usually done when penicillin is only product of choice

• Storage in tight container; refrigerate reconstituted sol

Evaluate:

• Therapeutic response: absence of fever, draining wounds

Teach patient/family:

• To report sore throat, fever, fatigue (may indicate superinfection); CNS reactions, pseudomembraneous colitis

• To wear or carry emergency ID if allergic to penicillins

• To notify prescriber of diarrhea

Treatment of anaphylaxis: Withdraw product; maintain airway; administer epinephrine, aminophylline, O_2, IV corticosteroids

⚠ High Alert

nalbuphine (℞)

(nal′byoo-feen)

nalbuphine HCl

Func. class.: Opioid analgesic

Chem. class.: Synthetic opioid agonist, antagonist

Action: Depresses pain impulse transmission at the spinal cord level by interacting with opioid receptors

Uses: Moderate to severe pain

DOSAGE AND ROUTES

Analgesic

• *Adult:* **SUBCUT/IM/IV** 10 mg q3-6hr prn, not to exceed 160 mg/day

Balanced anesthesia supplement

• *Adult:* **IV** 0.3-3 mg/kg given over 10-15 min, may give 0.25-0.5 mg/kg as needed for maintenance

Available forms: Inj 10, 20 mg/ml

SIDE EFFECTS

CNS: Drowsiness, dizziness, confusion, headache, sedation, euphoria, dysphoria (high doses), hallucinations, dreaming, tolerance, physical, psychological dependency

CV: Palpitations, bradycardia, change in B/P, orthostatic hypotension, **cardiac arrest**

EENT: Tinnitus, blurred vision, miosis, diplopia

GI: Nausea, vomiting, anorexia, constipation, cramps, abdominal pain, dyspepsia, xerostomia, bitter taste

GU: Increased urinary output, dysuria, urinary retention, urgency

INTEG: Rash, urticaria, bruising, flushing, diaphoresis, pruritus

RESP: **Respiratory depression,** pulmonary edema

Contraindications: Hypersensitivity, addiction (opiate)

Precautions: Pregnancy (C), breastfeeding, addictive personality, increased intracranial pressure, MI (acute), severe heart disease, respiratory depression, renal/hepatic disease, bowel impaction

PHARMACOKINETICS

SUBCUT/IM/IV: Peak 30 min, onset 2-15 min, duration 3-6 hr, metabolized by liver, excreted by kidneys, half-life 3-6 hr

INTERACTIONS

⚠ Avoid use with MAOIs, unpredictable reactions may occur

Increase: effects with other CNS depressants—alcohol, opiates, sedative/hypnotics, antipsychotics, skeletal muscle relaxants

Drug/Herb

Increase: CNS depression—chamomile, hops, Jamaican dogwood, kava, lavender, mistletoe, nettle, pokeweed, poppy, senega, skullcap, valerian, St. John's wort, gotu kola

Increase: anticholinergic effect—corkwood

Drug/Lab Test

Increase: amylase, lipase

NURSING CONSIDERATIONS

Assess:

- I&O ratio; check for decreasing output; may indicate urinary retention
- Bowel status; constipation is common

⚠ For withdrawal reactions in opiate-dependent individuals: PE, vascular occlusion; abscesses, ulcerations, nausea, vomiting, seizures; however, there is a low potential for dependence

- CNS changes: dizziness, drowsiness, hallucinations, euphoria, LOC, pupil reaction
- Allergic reactions: rash, urticaria
- Respiratory dysfunction: respiratory depression, character, rate, rhythm; notify prescriber if respirations are <10/min
- Need for pain medication by pain sedation scoring, physical dependency

Administer:

- With antiemetic if nausea, vomiting occur
- When pain is beginning to return; determine dosage interval by response

IM route

- IM deep in large muscle mass, rotate inj sites

IV route

- Undiluted 10 mg or less over 3-5 min

Syringe compatibilities: Atropine, cimetidine, diphenhydrAMINE, droperidol, glycopyrrolate, hydrOXYzine, lidocaine, midazolam, prochlorperazine, ranitidine, scopolamine, trimethobenzamide

Y-site compatibilities: Amifostine, aztreonam, cefmetazole, cisatracurium, cladribine, filgrastim, fludarabine, granisetron, melphalan, paclitaxel, propofol, remifentanil, teniposide, thiotepa, vinorelbine

Perform/provide:

- Storage in light-resistant area at room temperature
- Assistance with ambulation
- Safety measures: night-light, call bell within easy reach

Evaluate:

- Therapeutic response: decrease in pain

Teach patient/family:

- To report any symptoms of CNS changes, allergic reactions
- That physical dependency may result from long-term use
- That withdrawal symptoms may occur: nausea, vomiting, cramps, fever, faintness, anorexia
- Avoid CNS depressants, alcohol
- Avoid driving, operating machinery if drowsiness occurs

Treatment of overdose: Naloxone (Narcan) 0.2-0.8 mg IV, O_2, IV fluids, vasopressors

N

naloxone (℞)

(nal-oks'one)

naloxone HCl

Func. class.: Opioid antagonist, antidote

Chem. class.: Thebaine derivative

Action: Competes with opioids at opiate receptor sites

Uses: Respiratory depression induced by opioids, pentazocine, propoxyphene; refractory circulatory shock, asphyxia neonatorum, coma, hypotension

Unlabeled uses: IBS, opiate agonist dependence, opiate agonist-induced constipation, pruritus, urinary retention

DOSAGE AND ROUTES

Opioid-induced respiratory depression

• *Adult:* **IV/SUBCUT/IM** 0.4-2 mg, repeat q2-3min if needed, max 10 mg

• *Child <5 yr or ≤20 kg:* **IV/SUBCUT/IM** 0.01 mg/kg slowly followed by 0.1 mg/kg if needed or as **INF** titrated to response

Postoperative opioid-induced respiratory depression

• *Adult:* **IV** 0.1-0.2 mg q2-3min prn

• *Child:* **IV/SUBCUT/IM** 0.005-0.01 mg/kg q2-3min prn

Opioid overdose

• *Adult:* **IV/SUBCUT/IM** 0.4 mg (10 mcg/kg) (not opioid dependent) may repeat q2-3min; 0.1-0.2 mg q2-3min (opioid dependent)

Diagnosis of opiate agonist dependence (unlabeled)

• *Adult:* **IM** 0.16 mg; if no withdrawal symptoms in 20-30 min, give 0.24 mg **IV**

Available forms: Inj 0.02, 0.4 mg/ml

SIDE EFFECTS

CNS: Drowsiness, nervousness, **seizures**, tremor

CV: Rapid pulse, increased systolic B/P (high doses), **ventricular tachycardia, fibrillation,** hypo/hypertension, **cardiac arrest, sinus tachycardia**

GI: Nausea, vomiting, **hepatotoxicity**

RESP: Hyperpnea, **pulmonary edema**

Contraindications: Hypersensitivity

Precautions: Pregnancy (C), breastfeeding, children, neonates, CV disease, opioid dependency, seizure disorder, drug dependency

PHARMACOKINETICS

Well absorbed IM, SUBCUT; metabolized by liver, crosses placenta; excreted in urine, breast milk; half-life 1 hr

IM/SUBCUT: Onset 2-5 min, duration 45-60 min

IV: Onset 1 min, duration 45 min

INTERACTIONS

Decrease: effect of opioid analgesics

Drug/Lab Test

Interference: urine VMA, 5-HIAA, urine glucose

NURSING CONSIDERATIONS

Assess:

• Withdrawal: cramping, hypertension, anxiety, vomiting, signs of withdrawal in drug-dependent individuals may occur up to 2 hr after administration

• VS q3-5min

• ABGs including Po_2, Pco_2

• Cardiac status: tachycardia, hypertension; monitor ECG

• Respiratory dysfunction: respiratory depression, character, rate, rhythm; if respirations are <10/min, administer naloxone; probably due to opioid overdose; monitor LOC

• For pain: duration, intensity, location, before and after administration; may be used for respiratory depression

Administer:

• Only with resuscitative equipment, O_2 nearby

• Only sol prepared within 24 hr

IV route

- Undiluted with sterile H_2O for inj; may be further diluted with NS or D_5 and given as an inf; give 0.4 mg or less over 15 sec or titrate inf to response

Additive compatibilities: Verapamil

Syringe compatibilities: Benzquinamide, heparin, ondansetron

Y-site compatibilities: Gatifloxacin, linezolid, propofol

Perform/provide:

- Dark storage at room temperature

Evaluate:

- Therapeutic response: reversal of respiratory depression; LOC—alert

naltrexone (℞)

(nal-trex′one)

ReVia, Vivitrol

Func. class.: Opioid antagonist

Chem. class.: Thebaine derivative

Action: Competes with opioids at opioid receptor sites

Uses: Blockage of opioid analgesics, used in treatment of opiate addiction, alcoholism

Unlabeled uses: Nicotine withdrawal, opiate agonist withdrawal, pruritus

DOSAGE AND ROUTES

Adjunct in opiate agonist dependence

- *Adult:* **PO** 25 mg; if no withdrawal symptoms in 1 hr, then 25 mg additionally; if no withdrawal symptoms, then 50-150 mg/day or in divided doses

Adjunct in alcoholism treatment

- *Adult:* **PO** 50 mg/day with food × 12 wk; **IM** (Vivitrol) 380 mg q4wk

Pruritus (unlabeled)

- *Adult:* **PO** 50 mg/day × 7 days to 4 wk

Nicotine withdrawal (unlabeled)

- *Adult:* **PO** 50 mg/day

Ultrarapid opiate detoxification (unlabeled)

- *Adult:* **PO** 50 mg prior to sedation with midazolam

Available forms: Tabs 25, 50, 100 mg; susp for inj 380 mg

SIDE EFFECTS

CNS: Stimulation, drowsiness, dizziness, confusion, **seizures,** headache, flushing, hallucinations, nervousness, irritability, **suicidal ideation,** syncope, anxiety

CV: Rapid pulse, **pulmonary edema,** hypertension, DVT

EENT: Tinnitus, hearing loss, blurred vision

GI: Nausea, vomiting, diarrhea, heartburn, anorexia, **hepatitis,** constipation, abdominal pain

GU: Delayed ejaculation, decreased potency

INTEG: Rash, urticaria, bruising, oily skin, acne, pruritus, inj site reactions

MISC: Increased thirst, chills, fever

MS: Joint and muscle pain

RESP: Wheezing, hyperpnea, nasal congestion, rhinorrhea, sneezing, sore throat, pneumonia

Contraindications: Hypersensitivity, opioid dependence

Black Box Warning: Hepatic failure, hepatitis

Precautions: Pregnancy (C), breastfeeding, children, renal disease, depression, suicidal ideation

Black Box Warning: Hepatic disease

PHARMACOKINETICS

Metabolized by liver, excreted by kidneys; crosses placenta, excreted in breast milk; half-life 4 hr; extensive first-pass metabolism; protein binding 21%-28%

PO: Onset 15-30 min, peak 1-2 hr, duration is dose dependent

IM: Peak 2 hr

INTERACTIONS

Increase: lethargy—phenothiazines

Increase: hepatotoxicity—disulfiram

Decrease: effect of analgesics, antidiarrheals, cough preparations

NURSING CONSIDERATIONS

Assess:

- ABGs including Po_2, Pco_2, LFTs, VS q3-5min

N

• Signs of withdrawal in drug-dependent individuals
• Cardiac status: tachycardia, hypertension
• Respiratory dysfunction: respiratory depression, character, rate, rhythm; if respirations are <10/min, respiratory stimulant should be administered
• Mental status: depression, suicidal ideation

Administer:

PO route

• Give with food, antacid to prevent nausea/vomiting

IM route

• IM deep in gluteal, alternate inj sites, use supplied needle to prevent inj site reaction, aspirate before injecting
• Only if resuscitative equipment is nearby

Perform/provide:

• Storage in tight container

Evaluate:

• Therapeutic response: blocking opiate ingestion; successful nicotine, alcohol withdrawal

Teach patient/family:

• That they must be drug-free to start treatment
• That using opioid while taking this product could prove fatal because high dose is needed to overcome this antagonist; do not self-dose with OTC products unless approved by prescriber
• To carry emergency ID stating med used
• If surgery is needed, all involved should be aware of this product
• To use caution while driving or performing other hazardous tasks until effect is known
• That suicidal thoughts/behavior may occur, report immediately

nandrolone (℞)

(nan'droe-lone)
Deca-Durabolin, Hybolin Decanoate, Kabolin
Func. class.: Androgenic anabolic steroid, antianemic
Chem. class.: Halogenated testosterone derivative

Controlled Substance Schedule III

Action: May stimulate bone marrow development, stimulates erythropoietin production, increases Hgb and RBCs

Uses: Anemia associated with renal disease

DOSAGE AND ROUTES

• *Adult and child ≥14 yr:* **IM** (women) 50-100 mg q1-4wk; (men) 100-200 mg q1-4wk
• *Child 2-13 yr:* **IM** 25-50 mg q3-4wk

Available forms: Inj 50, 100, 200 mg/ml

SIDE EFFECTS

CNS: Dizziness, headache, fatigue, tremors, paresthesias, flushing, sweating, anxiety, lability, insomnia, carpal tunnel syndrome, chills, depression
CV: Increased B/P, edema
EENT: Conjunctival edema, nasal congestion
ENDO: Abnormal GTT, *virilism (women, prepubescent boys)*
GI: Nausea, vomiting, constipation, weight gain, **cholestatic jaundice**, diarrhea, **hepatic necrosis/failure, peliosis, hepatitis**
GU: **Hematuria,** amenorrhea, vaginitis, decreased libido, decreased breast size, clitoral hypertrophy, testicular atrophy, priapism, voiding change, impotence
INTEG: Rash, acneiform lesions, oily hair/skin, flushing, sweating, acne vulgaris, alopecia, hirsutism
MISC: Hypercalcemia, chills, blood coagulation disorder, electrolyte imbalance
MS: Cramps, spasms

Contraindications: Pregnancy (X), breastfeeding, severe cardiac disease, hypersensitivity to this product or benzyl alcohol, abnormal genital bleeding, males with cancer of breast, prostate, females

Black Box Warning: Hepatic disease, hypercholesterolemia

Precautions: Diabetes mellitus, CV disease, MI, prostatic hypertrophy, renal disease, hypercalcemia

Black Box Warning: Hepatocellular cancer

PHARMACOKINETICS

Well absorbed, peak up to 6 days

INTERACTIONS

Increase: bleeding—anticoagulants, NSAIDs, salicylates

Increase: hepatotoxicity—hepatotoxics

Drug/Lab Test

Increase: serum cholesterol, blood glucose, urine glucose, LDL

Decrease: serum calcium, serum potassium, T_4, T_3, thyroid ^{131}I uptake test, urine 17-OHCS, 17-KS, PBI, HDL

NURSING CONSIDERATIONS

Assess:

- Anemia symptoms: dyspnea, fatigue, weakness, pallor
- Weight daily; notify prescriber if weekly weight gain is >5 lb
- B/P q4hr
- I&O ratio; be alert for decreasing urinary output, increasing edema
- Growth rate in children, since growth rate may be uneven (linear/bone growth) with extended use
- Electrolytes: K, Na, Cl, Ca; cholesterol
- Hepatic studies: ALT, AST, bilirubin
- Blood studies: CBC, Hct, Hgb, lipid panel
- Edema, hypertension, cardiac symptoms, jaundice
- Mental status: affect, mood, behavioral changes, aggression
- Signs of masculinization in female: increased libido, deepening of voice, decreased breast tissue, enlarged clitoris, menstrual irregularities; male: gynecomastia, impotence, testicular atrophy
- Hypercalcemia: lethargy, polyuria, polydipsia, nausea, vomiting, constipation, product may have to be decreased
- Hypoglycemia in diabetics, since oral antidiabetic action is increased

Administer:

- Titrated dose; use lowest effective dose
- Inject deeply, use large muscle mass

Perform/provide:

- Diet with increased calories, protein; decrease sodium if edema occurs

Evaluate:

- Therapeutic response: increased appetite, increased stamina

Teach patient/family:

- Not to discontinue abruptly
- About changes in sex characteristics

naphazoline nasal agent

See Appendix B

naphazoline ophthalmic

See Appendix B

naproxen (℞, OTC)

(na-prox'en)

Apo-Naproxen ♣, EC-Naprosyn, Naprosyn-E ♣, Naprosyn-SR ♣, Naxen ♣, Novo-Naprox ♣, Nu-Naprox ♣

naproxen sodium (℞, OTC)

Aleve, Anaprox, Anaprox DS, Apo-Napro-Na ♣, Midol Extended Relief, Novo-Naprox Sodium ♣, Novo-Naprox Sodium DS ♣, Synflex ♣, Synflex DS ♣

Func. class.: Nonsteroidal antiinflammatory, nonopioid analgesic

Chem. class.: Propionic acid derivative

Do not confuse:
Naprosyn/natacyn/naprelan

Action: Completely inhibits COX-1, COX-2 by blocking arachidonate; analgesic, antiinflammatory, antipyretic

Uses: Osteoarthritis; rheumatoid, gouty arthritis; primary dysmenorrhea; ankylosing spondylitis, bursitis, tendinitis

Unlabeled uses: Juvenile RA, bone pain, migraine/migraine prophylaxis, heterotropic ossification, bone pain

DOSAGE AND ROUTES

Antiinflammatory/analgesic/antidysmenorrheal

- *Adult:* **PO** 250-500 mg bid, max 1250 mg/day; **DEL REL** 375-500 mg bid
- *Child ≥2 yr:* **PO** 5-7 mg/kg q8-12hr

Antigout

- *Adult:* **PO** 750 mg, then 250 mg q8hr

OTC use

- *Adult:* **PO** 200 mg q8-12hr or 400 mg, then 200 mg q12hr; max 600 mg/24hr, taken no longer than 10 days
- *Geriatric >65 yr:* **PO** Max 200 mg q12hr

Available forms: *Naproxen:* tabs 250, 375, 500 mg; del rel tabs (EC-Naprosyn, Naprosyn-E) 250 ♣, 375, 500 mg; oral susp 125 mg/5 ml; ext rel tabs (SR) 375, 500, 750 mg ♣; *naproxen sodium:* tabs 220, 275, 550 mg tab, ext rel 220 mg

SIDE EFFECTS

CNS: Dizziness, drowsiness, fatigue, tremors, confusion, insomnia, anxiety, depression

CV: Tachycardia, peripheral edema, palpitations, dysrhythmias, **MI, stroke**

EENT: Tinnitus, hearing loss, blurred vision

GI: Nausea, anorexia, vomiting, diarrhea, jaundice, **hepatitis,** constipation, flatulence, cramps, peptic ulcer, **GI ulceration, bleeding, perforation**

GU: **Nephrotoxicity: dysuria, hematuria, oliguria, azotemia**

HEMA: **Blood dyscrasias**

INTEG: Purpura, rash, pruritus, sweating

SYST: **Anaphylaxis**

Contraindications: Pregnancy (D) 2nd/3rd trimester, hypersensitivity to NSAIDs, salicylates; asthma, severe renal/hepatic disease, ulcer disease

Black Box Warning: Perioperative pain in CABG surgery

Precautions: Pregnancy (B) 1st trimester, breastfeeding, children <2 yr, geriatric patients, bleeding disorders, GI disorders, cardiac disorders, hypersensitivity to other antiinflammatory agents, CCr <30 ml/min

Black Box Warning: MI, GI bleeding, stroke

PHARMACOKINETICS

PO: Peak 2-4 hr, half-life 12-17 hr; metabolized in liver; excreted in urine (metabolites), breast milk; 99% protein binding

INTERACTIONS

- Possible renal impairment: ACE inhibitors
- Toxicity risk: methotrexate, lithium, antineoplastics, probenecid, radiation treatment

Increase: bleeding risk—oral anticoagulants, thrombolytic agents, eptifibatide, tirofiban, cefamandole, cefotetan, cefo-

perazone, clopidogrel, ticlopidine, plicamycin, SSRIs, tricyclics, valproic acid
Increase: GI side effects risk—aspirin, corticosteroids, alcohol, NSAIDs
Decrease: effect of antihypertensives, diuretics
Decreased: absorption of naproxen—antacids, sucralfate, antilipidemics
Drug/Herb
• Bleeding risk: anise, arnica, bogbean, chamomile, chondroitin, clove, dong quai, fenugreek, feverfew, garlic, ginger, ginkgo, ginseng *(Panax),* horse chestnut, licorice, red clover
Increase: gastric irritation—arginine, gossypol
Increase: NSAIDs effect—bearberry, bilberry
Drug/Lab Test
Increase: BUN, alk phos
False increase: 5-HIAA, 17KS

NURSING CONSIDERATIONS

Assess:
⚠ Cardiac status: CV thrombotic events, MI, stroke; may be fatal
⚠ GI status: ulceration, bleeding, perforation; may be fatal
• Pain: frequency, characteristics, intensity; relief prior to and 1-2 hr after med
⚠ Asthma, aspirin hypersensitivity or nasal polyps, increased risk of hypersensitivity
• Renal, hepatic, blood studies: BUN, creatinine, AST, ALT, Hgb, LDH, blood glucose, Hct, WBC, platelets CCr before treatment, periodically thereafter
• Audiometric, ophthalmic exam before, during, after treatment
• For eye, ear problems: blurred vision, tinnitus (may indicate toxicity)
Administer:
• With food to decrease GI symptoms; take on empty stomach to facilitate absorption
• Do not crush, break, or chew delayed release tabs
• OTC for ≤10 days, unless approved by prescriber
Perform/provide:
• Storage at room temperature
Evaluate:
• Therapeutic response: decreased pain, stiffness, swelling in joints, ability to move more easily
Teach patient/family:
• To use sunscreen to prevent photosensitivity
• To report blurred vision, ringing, roaring in ears (may indicate toxicity)
• To avoid driving, other hazardous activities if dizziness or drowsiness occurs
• To report change in urine pattern, weight increase, edema (face, lower extremities), pain increase in joints, fever, blood in urine (indicates nephrotoxicity); black stools, flulike symptoms
• That therapeutic effects may take up to 1 mo
• To avoid ASA, alcohol, steroids or other OTC medications without prescriber approval
• To report use to all health care providers

N

naratriptan (℞)

(nair′ah-trip-tan)
Amerge
Func. class.: Antimigraine agent, abortive
Chem. class.: 5-HT_1 receptor agonist, triptan

Action: Binds selectively to the vascular 5-HT_1 receptor subtype, exerts antimigraine effect; causes vasoconstriction in cranial arteries
Uses: Acute treatment of migraine with or without aura

DOSAGE AND ROUTES

• *Adult:* **PO** 1 or 2.5 mg with fluids; if headache returns, repeat once after 4 hr; max 5 mg/24 hr
Hepatic/renal dose
• *Adult:* **PO** Max 2.5 mg/24 hr
Available forms: Tabs 1, 2.5 mg

SIDE EFFECTS

CNS: Dizziness, sedation, fatigue

CV: Increased B/P, palpitations, **tachydysrhythmias, PR, QTc prolongation, ST/T wave changes, PVCs, atrial flutter/fibrillation, coronary vasospasm**

EENT: EENT infections, photophobia

GI: Nausea, vomiting

MISC: Temperature change sensations; tightness, pressure sensations

MS: Weakness, neck stiffness, myalgia

Contraindications: Hypersensitivity, angina pectoris, history of MI, documented silent ischemia, ischemic heart disease, concurrent ergotamine-containing preparations, uncontrolled hypertension, CV syndromes, hemiplegic or basilar migraines, severe renal disease (CCr <15 ml/min); severe hepatic disease (Child-Pugh grade C)

Precautions: Pregnancy (C), breastfeeding, children, geriatric patients, postmenopausal women, men >40 yr, risk factors for CAD, hypercholesterolemia, obesity, diabetes, impaired renal/hepatic function, peripheral vascular disease

PHARMACOKINETICS

Onset 2-3 hr; peak 2-3 hr; 28%-31% protein binding; half-life 6 hr; metabolized in the liver (metabolite); excreted in urine, feces; may be excreted in breast milk

INTERACTIONS

Increase: weakness, hyperreflexia, incoordination—SSRIs (fluoxetine, fluvoxamine, paroxetine, sertraline)

Increase: vasospastic effects—ergot, ergot derivatives, other 5-HT_1 agonists

Increase: adverse reactions risk—MAOIs, do not use together

Increase: naratriptan effect—sibutramine

Drug/Herb

- Serotonin syndrome: SAM-e, St. John's wort

Increase: effect—butterbur

NURSING CONSIDERATIONS

Assess:

- Migraine symptoms: aura, duration, effect on lifestyle, aggravating/alleviating factors
- For stress level, activity, recreation, coping mechanisms
- Neurologic status: LOC blurred vision, nausea, vomiting, tingling in extremities preceding headache

Administer:

- With fluids as soon as symptoms appear, may take another dose after 4 hr; do not take >5 mg in any 24-hr period

Perform/provide:

- Quiet, calm environment with decreased stimulation for noise, bright light, excessive talking

Evaluate:

- Therapeutic response: decrease in frequency, severity of headache

Teach patient/family:

- To report pain, tightness in chest, neck, throat, or jaw; notify prescriber immediately if sudden, severe abdominal pain occurs
- Not to use if another 5-HT_1 agonist or an ergot preparation has been used in the past 24 hr; avoid using >2 days/wk, rebound headache may occur
- Advise patient to notify prescriber if pregnancy is planned or suspected, avoid breastfeeding

natalizumab (℞)

(na-ta-liz'u-mab)

Tysabri

Func. class.: Biologic response modifier, immunoglobulins, monoclonal antibody

Action: Action not clearly understood; biologic response modifying properties mediated through specific receptors on cells, may be secondary of blockade of the interaction by inflammatory cells on vascular endothelial cells

Uses: Ambulatory patients with relapsing-remitting MS who have not responded to other treatment, moderate-severe Crohn's disease

DOSAGE AND ROUTES

• *Adult:* **IV INF** 300 mg q4wk; give over 1 hr; observe during and for 1 hr after infusion

Available forms: Single-use vial, 300 mg/100 ml 0.9% NaCl

SIDE EFFECTS

CNS: Headache, fatigue, rigors, syncope, tremors, *depression,* **progressive multifocal leukoencephalopathy (PML), suicidal ideation,** anxiety

CV: Chest discomfort, hypo/hypertension, tachycardia

GI: Abdominal discomfort, abnormal LFT, gastroentritis, **severe hepatic injury**

GU: Amenorrhea, *UTI, irregular menses,* vaginitis, urinary frequency

INTEG: Rash, dermatitis, pruritus, **skin melanoma,** inf-related reactions

MS: Arthralgia, myalgia

RESP: Lower respiratory tract infection, dyspnea

SYST: **Anaphylaxis, angioedema**

Contraindications: Hypersensitivity, immunocompromised individuals (HIV, AIDS, leukemia, lymphoma, transplants), PML, murine (mouse) protein allergy

Black Box Warning: Progressive multifocal leukoencephalopathy

Precautions: Pregnancy (C), breast-feeding, geriatric patients, chronic progressive MS, depression, mental disorders, diabetes, TB, active infections, hepatotoxicity

PHARMACOKINETICS

Half-life approximately 11 days

INTERACTIONS

• Do not use with vaccines

Increase: infection—immunosuppressants, antineoplastics, immunomodulators

NURSING CONSIDERATIONS

Assess:

• Blood, renal, hepatic studies: CBC, differential, platelet counts, BUN, creatinine, ALT, urinalysis, for hypersensitivity reactions

• CNS symptoms: headache, fatigue, depression, rigors, tremors

• GI status: abdominal discomfort, gastroenteritis, severe hepatic injury, abnormal LFTs

• Mental status: depression, depersonalization, suicidal thoughts, insomnia

• For MS symptoms; this product should only be used in patients who have not responded to other treatments

⚠ Anaphylaxis: shortness of breath, hives; swelling, tightness in throat, chest pain; usually within 2 hr of inf

• PML using gadolinium-enhanced MRI scan of the brain, possibly cerebrospinal fluid for JC viral DNA; signs/symptoms of PML (decreased cognition, vision; ataxia, dysphagia)

Administer:

• Acetaminophen for fever, headache

• Only after being enrolled in the TOUCH Prescribing Program

Intermittent IV INF route

• Use only clear, colorless solution, without particulates

• Withdraw 15 ml from the vial using aseptic technique: inj concentration into 100 ml 0.9% NaCl; do not use other diluents; mix completely; do not shake; infuse immediately or refrigerate for up to 8 hr; warm to room temperature before using; flush with 0.9% NaCl before and after inf; do not admix or use in same line with other agents

• Withhold product at first sign of PML

Perform/provide:

• Storage of solution in refrigerator; do not freeze or shake; protect from light; use within 8 hr of preparation

Evaluate:

• Therapeutic response: decreased symptoms of MS

Teach patient/family:
- To provide patient or family member with written, detailed information about the product
- That female patients may experience irregular menses, amenorrhea
- To use sunscreen to prevent photosensitivity
- To notify prescriber if pregnancy is suspected
- To avoid breastfeeding while taking this product
- To notify prescriber of possible infection: sore throat, cough, increased temp

natamycin ophthalmic
See Appendix B

nebivolol (℞)
(ne-biv′oh-lol)
Bystolic
Func. class.: Antihypertensive
Chem. class.: β_1-blocker

Action: Competitively blocks stimulation of β-adrenergic receptors within vascular smooth muscle; decreases rate of SA node discharge, increases recovery time, slows conduction of AV node resulting in decreased heart rate (negative chronotropic effect), which decreases O_2 consumption in myocardium due to β_1-receptor antagonism; also decreases renin-aldosterone-angiotensin system at high doses, inhibits β_2-receptors in bronchial system (high doses)
Uses: Hypertension alone or in combination
Unlabeled uses: Heart failure

DOSAGE AND ROUTES
Hypertension
- *Adult:* **PO** 5 mg/day, may be increased to desired response q2wk; max 40 mg/day
- *Geriatric:* **PO** Not to exceed 40 mg/day

Renal dose
- *Adult:* **PO** CCr <30 ml/min, 2.5 mg/day; may increase cautiously

Hepatic dose
- *Adult:* **PO** (Child-Pugh class B) 2.5 mg daily, use dose escalation cautiously

Heart failure (unlabeled)
- *Adult:* **PO** 1.25 mg titrated to max 10 mg/day

Available forms: Tabs 2.5, 5, 10, 20 mg

SIDE EFFECTS
CNS: Insomnia, fatigue, dizziness, mental changes, drowsiness, headache
CV: **Bradycardia, MI**, AV heart block, edema
GI: Nausea, diarrhea, vomiting, abdominal pain
GU: Impotence
HEMA: **Thrombocytopenia**
INTEG: Rash, pruritus, vasculitis, urticaria, psoriasis, **angioedema**
MISC: **Renal failure, pulmonary edema,** hyperuricemia, hypercholesterolemia
RESP: **Bronchospasm,** dyspnea
Contraindications: Cardiogenic shock, heart failure, severe hepatic disease, severe bradycardia, sick sinus syndrome, AV heart block, hypersensitivity to this agent or β-blockers
Precautions: Pregnancy (C), breastfeeding, children, major surgery, peripheral vascular disease, diabetes mellitus, thyrotoxicosis disease, COPD, asthma, well-compensated heart failure, renal/hepatic disease, abrupt discontinuation, acute bronchospasm

PHARMACOKINETICS
Peak 1.5-4 hr; half-life 12 hr; metabolized in liver by CYP2D6; 38% excreted in urine, 44% in feces

INTERACTIONS
- Do not give with other β-blockers, mefloquine

Increase: nebivolol action—CYP2D6 inhibitors (amiodarone, buPROPion, chloroquine, chlorpheniramine, chlorproM-

AZINE, cinacalcet, diphenhydrAMINE, duloxetine, fluoxetine, haloperidol, imatinib, paroxetine, promethazine, propoxyphene, quinidine, quinine, ritonavir, terbinafine, thioridazine), cimetidine, calcium channel blockers (nondihydropyridine)
Decrease: nebivolol action—CYP2D6 inducers (rifampin), sildenafil

Drug/Herb

• May increase nebivolol effect—hawthorn

Drug/Lab Test

Increase: serum lipoprotein levels, BUN, potassium, triglycerides, uric acid, LDH, AST, ALT, blood glucose, alk phos
Positive: ANA titer

NURSING CONSIDERATIONS

Assess:

• B/P during beginning treatment, periodically thereafter; pulse q4hr; note rate, rhythm, quality
• Apical/radial pulse before administration; notify prescriber of any significant changes (pulse <50 bpm); signs of CHF (dyspnea, crackles, weight gain, jugular vein distention)
• Baselines in renal, hepatic function tests before therapy begins and periodically
• Edema in feet, legs daily: monitor I&O
• Skin turgor, dryness of mucous membranes for hydration status, especially geriatric patients

Administer:

PO route

• Without regard to meals; tab may be crushed or swallowed whole; give with food to prevent GI upset

Perform/provide:

• Storage protected from light, moisture; place in cool environment

Evaluate:

• Therapeutic response: decreased B/P after 1-2 wk; decreased dysrhythmias

Teach patient/family:

⚠ Not to discontinue product abruptly, severe cardiac reactions may occur, taper over 2 wk; do not double dose; if a dose is missed, take as soon as remembered up to 4 hr before next dose
• Product may mask signs of hypoglycemia or alter blood glucose levels
• Not to use OTC products containing α-adrenergic stimulants (such as nasal decongestants, OTC cold preparations) unless directed by prescriber
• To report low pulse, dizziness, confusion, depression, fever
• To take pulse, B/P at home; advise when to notify prescriber
• To comply with weight control, dietary adjustments, modified exercise program
• To carry emergency ID to identify product, allergies
• To avoid hazardous activities if dizziness, drowsiness is present
• To report symptoms of CHF: difficulty breathing, especially on exertion or when lying down, night cough, swelling of extremities
• To continue with required lifestyle changes (exercise, diet, weight loss, stress reduction)

Treatment of overdose: Lavage, IV atropine for bradycardia, IV theophylline for bronchospasm, digoxin, O_2, diuretic for cardiac failure, IV glucose for hypoglycemia, IV diazepam (or phenytoin) for seizures, IV fluids, IV pressors

N

nelarabine (℞)

(nella-ra′ben)

Arranon

Func. class.: Antineoplastic
Chem. class.: Purine analog

Action: Leukemic blasts allow for incorporation into DNA, thus interfering with cell replication lending to cell death

Uses: T-cell lymphoblastic leukemia, T-cell lymphoblastic lymphoma post relapse or treatment failure with at least two chemotherapeutic agents

DOSAGE AND ROUTES

• *Adult:* **IV** 1500 mg/m^2 over 2 hr on days 1, 3, 5, repeated q21days
• *Child:* **IV** 650 mg/m^2 over 1 hr/day × 5 days, repeated q21days

Available forms: Sol for inj 5 mg/ml (50 ml)

SIDE EFFECTS

CNS: Dizziness, *fatigue,* insomnia, rigors, **seizures,** peripheral neuropathy, **paralysis,** confusion, headache, **Guillain-Barré syndrome,** depression, drowsiness, encephalopathy
CV: Edema
GI: Nausea, vomiting, anorexia, diarrhea, stomatitis, constipation
HEMA: **Neutropenia,** leukopenia, **thrombocytopenia,** anemia
META: Decreased potassium, calcium, magnesium, albumin, bilirubin, AST, ALT, hyperuricemia; increased glucose
MS: Myalgia, arthralgia, back pain, weakness
RESP: **Pleural effusion,** cough, dyspnea, wheezing, epistaxis
SYST: Tumor lysis syndrome (TLS)
Contraindications: Pregnancy (D), hypersensitivity

Black Box Warning: Severe neurotoxicity

Precautions: Breastfeeding, children, geriatric patients, renal/hepatic disease

Black Box Warning: Seizure disorder, IM administration, neurologic disease, peripheral neuropathy

PHARMACOKINETICS

Metabolized in the liver, excreted kidneys, half-life 30 min-3 hr

INTERACTIONS

• Do not use with live virus vaccinations/toxoids
Increase: bleeding risk—NSAIDs, anticoagulants, platelet inhibitors, salicylates

NURSING CONSIDERATIONS

Assess:
• CBC (RBC, Hct, Hgb), differential platelet count weekly; withhold product if WBC is <4000/mm^3, platelet count is <75,000/mm^3, or RBC, Hct, Hgb low; notify prescriber of these results
• Renal studies: BUN, serum uric acid, urine CCr, electrolytes before and during therapy
• Monitor temp; fever may indicate beginning infection; no rectal temps
• Hepatic studies before and during therapy: bilirubin, ALT, AST, alk phos as needed or monthly
• Bleeding: hematuria, heme-positive stools, bruising or petechiae, mucosa or orifices q8hr
• Neurotoxicity: somnolence, confusion, seizures, ataxia, paresthesias, hypoesthesia, coma, status epilepticus, craniospinal demyelination; contact prescriber immediately
• Dyspnea, crackles, unproductive cough, chest pain, tachypnea, fatigue, increased pulse, pallor, lethargy, personality changes
• Buccal cavity for dryness, sores or ulceration, white patches, oral pain, bleeding, dysphagia
• GI symptoms: frequency of stools, cramping; if severe diarrhea occurs, fluid and electrolytes may need to be given

Administer:
• IV hydration, and allopurinol in risk of hyperuricemia
• Use procedures for proper handling/disposal of anticancer products

Perform/provide:
• Rinsing of mouth tid-qid with water, club soda; brushing of teeth bid-tid with soft brush or cotton-tipped applicators for stomatitis; use unwaxed dental floss
• Storage at room temperature

Evaluate:
• Therapeutic response: decreased spread of malignancy

Teach patient/family:
• To avoid foods with citric acid, hot or rough texture if stomatitis is present; OTC products
• Use contraception while taking this product
• To avoid using while lactating
• To report signs of infection: increased temp, sore throat, flulike symptoms

• To report signs of anemia: fatigue, headache, faintness, shortness of breath, irritability
• To report bleeding; to avoid use of razors, commercial mouthwash
• To report numbness, paresthesias, weakness
• That seizures may occur, do not operate machinery or drive until effects are known
• Not to receive vaccinations while taking this product

nelfinavir (℞)

(nell-fin'a-ver)

Viracept

Func. class.: Antiretroviral

Chem. class.: HIV protease inhibitor

Action: Inhibits human immunodeficiency virus (HIV-1) protease, which prevents maturation of the infectious virus

Uses: HIV-1 in combination with other antiretrovirals

DOSAGE AND ROUTES

HIV infection

• *Adult and child >13 yr:* **PO** 750 mg tid or 1250 mg bid
• *Child 2-13 yr:* **PO** 20-30 mg/kg tid, max 2500 mg/day

Prevention of HIV infection after exposure

• *Adult:* **PO** 1250 mg bid with two other antiretroviral agents × 4 wk

Available forms: Tabs 250, 625 mg; powder, oral 50 mg/g/scoop

SIDE EFFECTS

CNS: Headache, asthenia, poor concentration, **seizures, suicidal ideation**

CV: Bleeding

ENDO: Hyperglycemia, hyperlipidemia

GI: *Diarrhea,* anorexia, dyspepsia, *nausea, flatulence,* **hepatitis, pancreatitis**

HEMA: **Anemia, leukopenia, thrombocytopenia,** Hgb abnormalities

INTEG: *Rash,* dermatitis

MS: Pain, arthralgia, myalgia, myopathy

OTHER: **Hypoglycemia,** redistribution/accumulation of body fat

Contraindications: Hypersensitivity to protease inhibitors

Precautions: Pregnancy (B), breastfeeding, renal/hepatic disease, hemophilia, PKU, pancreatitis, diabetes, infection

PHARMACOKINETICS

Half-life 3½-5 hr, excreted urine/feces, peak 2-4 hr, 98% protein binding, metabolized by CYP3A4 enzyme system, a potent inhibitor of CYP3A4

INTERACTIONS

Drug/Herb

⚠ Serious dysrhythmias: amiodarone, ergots, lovastatin, midazolam, pimozide, quinidine, simvastatin, triazolam

Increase: effect—atorvastatin, azithromycin, rifabutin, indinavir, saquinavir, cycloSPORINE, tacrolimus, sirolimus, sildenafil, alfentanil, alosetron, buprenorphine, busPIRone, bortezomib, calcium channel blockers, cilostazol, disopyramide, dofetilide, docetaxel, donepezil, ethosuximide, fentanyl, galantamine, gefitinib, halofantrine, levomethadyl, systemic lidocaine, paclitaxel, sibutramine, sufentanil, vinca alkaloids, ziprasidone, zonisamide

Increase: nelfinavir levels—ketoconazole, indinavir, ritonavir

Increase: protease inhibitor levels—delavirdine, HIV protease inhibitors

Decrease: nelfinavir levels—rifamycins, nevirapine, phenobarbital, phenytoin, carbamazepine

Decrease: effect of didanosine, methadone, oral contraceptives, phenytoin

Drug/Herb

Decrease: antiretroviral effect—St. John's wort

Drug/Food

Increase: absorption with food

Drug/Lab Test

Increase: AST, ALT, alk phos, total bilirubin, CPK, LDH

N

NURSING CONSIDERATIONS

Assess:

- Resistance testing at initiation and failure of treatment
- Signs of infection, anemia
- Hepatic studies: ALT, AST
- C&S before drug therapy; product may be taken as soon as culture is taken; repeat C&S after treatment; determine the presence of other sexually transmitted diseases
- Bowel pattern before, during treatment; if severe abdominal pain with bleeding occurs, product should be discontinued; monitor hydration
- Skin eruptions, rash, urticaria, itching
- Allergies before treatment, reaction of each medication; place allergies on chart
- Blood studies: Serum lipid profile, plasma HIV RNA, blood glucose, viral load, CD4 cell counts baseline and throughout treatment

Administer:

- Oral powder mixed with fluids if desired; do not mix with juice or acidic fluids; stable mixed for 6 hr

Teach patient/family:

- To avoid taking with other medications unless directed by prescriber
- That product does not cure, but does manage symptoms; does not prevent transmission of HIV to others
- To use a nonhormonal form of birth control while taking this product
- If dose is missed, to take as soon as remembered up to 1 hr before next dose; do not double dose
- To take with food
- To report symptoms of hyperglycemia

Rarely Used

neomycin (℞)

(nee-oh-mye′sin)

Myciguent, Neo-Fradin, Neo-Rx

Func. class.: Antiinfective

Uses: Severe systemic infections of CNS, respiratory, GI, urinary tract, eye, bone, skin, soft tissues caused by *Pseudomonas aeruginosa, Escherichia coli, Enterobacter, Klebsiella pneumoniae, Proteus vulgaris;* also used for hepatic coma, preoperatively to sterilize bowel, infectious diarrhea caused by enteropathogenic *E. coli*

DOSAGE AND ROUTES

Hepatic encephalopathy

- *Adult:* **PO** 4-12 g/day in divided doses × 5-6 days
- *Child:* **PO** 50-100 mg/kg/day in divided doses q6hr × 5-6 days

Preoperative intestinal antisepsis

- *Adult:* **PO** 1 g qhr × 4hr, then 1 g q4hr for remaining 24 hr

Contraindications: Infants, children, bowel obstruction (oral use), severe renal disease, hypersensitivity, GI disease

neomycin topical

See Appendix B

neostigmine (℞)

(nee-oh-stig′meen)

neostigmine, Prostigmin

Func. class.: Cholinergic stimulant; anticholinesterase

Chem. class.: Quaternary compound

Action: Inhibits destruction of acetylcholine, which increases concentration at sites where acetylcholine is released; this facilitates transmission of impulses across myoneural junction

Uses: Diagnosis/treatment of myasthenia gravis, nondepolarizing neuromuscular blocker antagonist, postoperative ileus, urinary retention

DOSAGE AND ROUTES

Myasthenia gravis diagnosis

- *Adult:* **IM** 0.02 mg/kg as a single dose
- *Child:* **IM** 0.04 mg/kg as a single dose

Myasthenia gravis treatment

- *Adult:* **PO** 15 mg tid, may increase to 375 mg/day; **IM/IV** 0.5-2.5 mg q1-3hr up to 10 mg/day

• *Child:* **PO** 2 mg/kg/day q3-4hr; **IM/IV/SUBCUT** 0.01-0.04 mg/kg q2-4hr
Nondepolarizing neuromuscular blocker antagonist
• *Adult:* **IV** 0.5-2.5 mg slowly, may repeat if needed, max 5 mg (give 0.6-1.2 mg atropine several min before this product)
• *Infant and child:* **IV** 0.025-0.08 mg/kg/dose (give atropine several min before this product)
Postoperative abdominal distention/ileus
• *Adult:* **IM/SUBCUT** 0.25-1 mg (1:4000) q4-6hr depending on condition × 2-3 days
Urinary retention treatment
• *Adult:* **IM/SUBCUT** 0.5-1 mg q3hr × 5 doses after bladder is emptied
Renal dose
• CCr 10-50 ml/min 50% of dose; CCr <10 ml/min 25% of dose
Available forms: Tabs 15 mg; inj 1:1000, 1:2000, 1:4000

SIDE EFFECTS

CNS: Dizziness, headache, sweating, weakness, **seizures,** incoordination, **paralysis,** drowsiness, loss of consciousness
CV: Tachycardia, dysrhythmias, bradycardia, hypotension, AV block, ECG changes, **cardiac arrest,** syncope
EENT: Miosis, blurred vision, lacrimation, visual changes
GI: Nausea, diarrhea, vomiting, cramps, increased peristalsis, salivary and gastric secretions
GU: Urinary frequency, incontinence, urgency
INTEG: Rash, urticaria, flushing
RESP: **Respiratory depression, bronchospasm, constriction, laryngospasm, respiratory arrest,** dyspnea
SYST: **Anaphylaxis**
Contraindications: Obstruction of intestine, renal system, bromide sensitivity, peritonitis, urinary tract obstruction, ileus
Precautions: Pregnancy (C), breastfeeding, children, bradycardia, hypotension, seizure disorders, bronchial asthma, coronary occlusion, hyperthyroidism, dysrhythmias, peptic ulcer, megacolon, poor GI motility

PHARMACOKINETICS

Metabolized in liver, excreted in urine
PO: Onset 45-75 min, peak 1-2 hr, duration 2½-4 hr
IM/SUBCUT: Onset 20-30 min, duration 2½-4 hr
IV: Onset 1-2 min, duration 1-2 hr

INTERACTIONS

Increase: action of decamethonium, succinylcholine
Increase: bradycardia—β-blockers, calcium channel blockers, digoxin
Decrease: neostigmine action—aminoglycosides, antihistamines, antidepressants, atropine, anticholinergics, local/general anesthetics, corticosteroids, haloperidol, phenothiazines, quinidine, disopyramide
Drug/Herb
Increase: effect: pill-bearing spurge

NURSING CONSIDERATIONS

Assess:
• VS, respiration q8hr
• I&O ratio; check for urinary retention or incontinence
⚠ For bradycardia, hypotension, bronchospasm, headache, dizziness, seizures, respiratory depression; product should be discontinued if toxicity occurs
Administer:
• Only with atropine sulfate available for cholinergic crisis
• Only after all other cholinergics have been discontinued
• Increased doses, as ordered if tolerance occurs
• Larger doses after exercise or fatigue, as ordered
PO route
• On empty stomach for better absorption
IV route
• Undiluted, give through Y-tube or 3-way stopcock; give 0.5 mg or less over 1 min
Additive compatibilities: Netilmicin

Syringe compatibilities: Glycopyrrolate, heparin, ondansetron, pentobarbital, thiopental

Y-site compatibilities: Heparin, hydrocortisone, potassium chloride, vit B/C

Perform/provide:

- Storage at room temperature

Evaluate:

- Therapeutic response: increased muscle strength, hand grasp, improved gait, absence of labored breathing (if severe)

Teach patient/family:

- That product is not a cure; it only relieves symptoms
- To wear emergency ID specifying myasthenia gravis, products taken
- To avoid driving, other hazardous activities until effect is known
- To report respiratory distress, cardiac dysrhythmias

Treatment of overdose: Respiratory support, atropine 1-4 mg (IV), aggressive hydration

nepafenac ophthalmic

See Appendix B

⚠ High Alert

nesiritide (℞)

(neh-seer′ih-tide)

Natrecor

Func. class.: Vasodilator

Chem. class.: Human B-type natriuretic peptide

Action: Uses DNA technology; human B-type natriuretic peptide binds to the receptor in vascular smooth muscle and endothelial cells, leading to smooth muscle relaxation

Uses: Acutely decompensated CHF

DOSAGE AND ROUTES

- *Adult:* **IV BOL** 2 mcg/kg, then **CONT IV INF** 0.01 mcg/kg/min

Available forms: Powder for inj, 1.5-mg single-use vial

SIDE EFFECTS

CNS: Headache, insomnia, dizziness, anxiety, confusion, paresthesia, tremor

CV: Hypotension, **tachycardia,** dysrhythmias, bradycardia, ventricular tachycardia, ventricular extrasystoles, atrial fibrillation

GI: Vomiting, nausea

INTEG: Rash, sweating, pruritus, inj site reaction

MISC: Abdominal pain, back pain

RESP: Increased cough, hemoptysis, **apnea**

Contraindications: Hypersensitivity to this product or *Escherichia coli* protein, cardiogenic shock or B/P <90 mm Hg as primary therapy

Precautions: Pregnancy (C); breastfeeding; children; mitral stenosis; significant valvular stenosis, restriction, or obstructive cardiomyopathy, or any condition that is dependent on venous return; renal disease; constrictive pericarditis

PHARMACOKINETICS

Half-life 18 min

INTERACTIONS

Increase: symptomatic hypotension with ACE inhibitors

NURSING CONSIDERATIONS

Assess:

- PCWP, RAP, cardiac index, MPAP
- B/P, pulse during treatment until stable
- I&O, daily weight, serum creatinine, BUN
- For CHF: weight gain, dyspnea, crackles, edema

Administer:

IV route

- Do not administer nesiritide through a central catheter containing other products; administer other products through a separate catheter or a central line heparin-coated catheter as nesiritide binds to heparin

Prime IV fluid with inf of 25 ml before connecting to patient's vascular access port and before bolus dose or IV inf

Reconstitute one 1.5-mg vial/5 ml of diluent from prefilled 250-ml plastic IV bag with diluent of choice (D_5, 0.9% NaCl, D_5/½ NaCl, D_5/0.2% NaCl); do not shake vial, roll gently; use only clear sol

Withdraw all contents of reconstituted vial and add to the 250-ml plastic IV bag (6 mcg/ml), invert bag several times

Use within 24 hr of reconstituting

IV, direct route

- Withdraw prescribed bolus dose (volume) from prepared inf bag; give over 1 min through IV port

Intermittent IV INF route

- After bolus dose, use inf, give at 0.1 ml/kg/hr (0.01 mcg/kg/min)

Y-site compatibilities: Bumetanide, enalaprilat, furosemide, heparin, hydrALAZINE, regular insulin

Evaluate:

- Therapeutic response: improvement in CHF with improved PCWP, RAP, MPAP

Teach patient/family:

- To explain purpose of medication and expected results
- To report dizziness, blurred vision, light-headedness, sweating

nevirapine (℞)

(ne-veer′a-peen)

Viramune

Func. class.: Antiretroviral

Chem. class.: Nonnucleoside reverse transcriptase inhibitor (NNRTI)

Do not confuse

nevirapine/nelfinavir

Viramune/Viracept

Action: Binds directly to reverse transcriptase and blocks RNA, DNA, causing a disruption of the enzyme's site

Uses: HIV-1 in combination with other highly active antiretroviral therapy (HAART)

DOSAGE AND ROUTES

Treatment of HIV infection in combination with other antiretroviral agents

- *Adult and adolescent:* **PO** 200 mg/day × 2 wk, then 200 mg bid in combination
- *Neonate ≥15 days old/infant/child:* **PO** 150 mg/m²/day × 14 days, then 150 mg/m² bid, max 400 mg/day

Perinatal transmission prophylaxis (unlabeled)

- *Females with no previous antiretroviral therapy:* **PO** 200 mg as a single dose at onset of labor with zidovudine 2 mg/kg over 1 hr followed by zidovudine 1 mg/kg/hr until delivery
- *Neonate ≥34 wk gestation:* **PO** Nevirapine 2 mg/kg as single dose at age 48-72 hr and **PO** zidovudine 2 mg/kg q12hr for 6 wk

Available forms: Tabs 200 mg; oral susp 50 mg/5 ml

SIDE EFFECTS

CNS: Paresthesia, headache, fever, peripheral neuropathy

GI: Diarrhea, abdominal pain, *nausea, stomatitis,* **hepatotoxicity, hepatic failure**

HEMA: **Neutropenia, anemia, thrombocytopenia**

INTEG: Rash, **toxic epidermal necrolysis**

MISC: **Stevens-Johnson syndrome, anaphylaxis**

MS: Pain, myalgia, **rhabdomyolysis**

Contraindications:

Black Box Warning: Hypersensitivity, hepatic disease

Precautions: Pregnancy (B), breastfeeding, children, renal disease

Black Box Warning: Females, hepatitis

PHARMACOKINETICS

Rapidly absorbed, peak 4 hr, 60% bound to plasma proteins, metabolized by liver; metabolized by hepatic P450 enzyme system, excreted 91% in urine, terminal half-life 25-30 hr, 50% removed by peritoneal dialysis, in hepatic disease, Hispanics, African Americans there is slower rate of clearance

INTERACTIONS

Increase: nevirapine levels—cimetidine, macrolide antiinfectives

Decrease: effects of protease inhibitors, oral contraceptives, ketoconazole, methadone, itraconazole

Decrease: nevirapine levels—rifamycins, anticonvulsants, clonazepam, diazepam, warfarin

Drug/Herb

Decrease: action of antiretroviral—St. John's wort, do not use concurrently

Drug/Lab Test

Increase: ALT, AST, GGT, bilirubin, Hgb

Decrease: neutrophil count

NURSING CONSIDERATIONS

Assess:

• Resistance testing prior to starting and when therapy fails

⚠ Signs of infection, anemia, hepatotoxicity, immune reconstitution syndrome

• Hepatic, blood studies during treatment: ALT, AST, viral load, CD4, plasma HIV RNA, renal studies; if LFTs are elevated significantly, product should be withheld; glucose levels in diabetic patients

• C&S before product therapy; product may be taken as soon as culture is taken; repeat C&S after treatment; determine the presence of other sexually transmitted disease

• Bowel pattern before, during treatment; if severe abdominal pain with bleeding occurs, product should be discontinued; monitor hydration

⚠ Allergies before treatment, reaction to each medication; skin eruptions; rash, urticaria, itching; if rash is severe or systemic symptoms occur, discontinue immediately

Administer:

• Do not initiate treatment in females when CD4 counts >250 cells/mm^3, or in males when >400 cells/mm^3 unless benefit outweighs risks

• Without regard to meals

• Oral susp should be shaken prior to giving

Evaluate:

• Therapeutic response: absence of AIDS defining symptoms, improvement in quality of life

Teach patient/family:

⚠ To report any right quadrant pain, jaundice, rash immediately

• That product may be taken with food, antacids, didanosine

• To take as prescribed; if dose is missed, take as soon as remembered up to 1 hr before next dose; do not double dose

• That product is not a cure, does not prevent transmission, controls symptoms of HIV

• To avoid OTC agents unless approved by prescriber

• To use a nonhormonal form of contraception during treatment

• That product must be taken in equal intervals around the clock to maintain blood levels for duration of therapy

niacin (OTC, ℞)

(nye'a-sin)

Edur-Acin, Nia-Bid, Niac, Niacels, Niacor, Niaspan, Nicobid, Nico-400, Nicolar, Nicotinex

nicotinic acid (OTC, ℞)

Novo-Niacin ♣, Slo-Niacin, vitamin B

niacinamide (OTC, ℞)

nicotinamide (OTC, ℞)

Func. class.: Vit B_3, antihyperlipidemic

Chem. class.: Water-soluble vitamin

Do not confuse:

Nicobid/Nitro-Bid

Action: Needed for conversion of fats, protein, carbohydrates, by oxidation reduction; acts directly on vascular smooth muscle, causing vasodilation; reduces total cholesterol, LDL, VLDL, triglycerides; increases HDL

Uses: Pellagra, hyperlipidemias (types 4, 5), peripheral vascular disease that presents a risk for pancreatitis

DOSAGE AND ROUTES

Niacin deficiency

• *Adult:* **PO** 100-500 mg/day in divided doses; **IM/SUBCUT** 5-100 mg 5 or more ×/day; **IV** 25-100 mg bid or tid

• *Child*: **PO** Up to 300 mg/day in divided doses

Adjunct in hyperlipidemia

• *Adult:* **PO** 250 mg after evening meal; may increase dose at 1-4 wk intervals to 1-2 g tid, max 6 g/day; **EXT REL** 500 mg at bedtime × 4 wk, then 1000 mg at bedtime for wk 5-8; do not increase by more than 500 mg q4wk, max 2000 mg/day

Pellagra

• *Adult:* **PO** 300-500 mg/day in divided doses

• *Child:* **PO** 100-300 mg/day in divided doses

Peripheral vascular disease

• *Adult:* **PO** 250-800 mg/day in 3-5 divided doses

Available forms: *Niacin:* tabs 25, 50, 100, 250, 500, 1000 mg; time rel caps 250, 500 mg; ext rel caps 250, 400 mg; sus rel tabs 500 mg; cont rel tabs 250, 500, 750 mg; sus rel cap 125, 500 mg; elix 50 mg/5 ml; *nicotinamide:* tabs 100, 250, 500 mg

SIDE EFFECTS

CNS: Paresthesias, headache, dizziness, anxiety

CV: Postural hypotension, vasovagal attacks, dysrhythmias, vasodilation

EENT: Blurred vision, ptosis

GI: Nausea, vomiting, anorexia, **jaundice, hepatotoxicity**, diarrhea, peptic ulcer, dyspepsia, **hepatitis**

GU: Hyperuricemia, **glycosuria, hypoalbuminemia**

INTEG: Flushing, dry skin, rash, pruritus, itching, tingling

Contraindications: Breastfeeding, hypersensitivity, peptic ulcer, hepatic disease, hemorrhage, severe hypotension

Precautions: Pregnancy (C), breastfeeding, glaucoma, cardiovascular disease, CAD, diabetes mellitus, gout, schizophrenia

PHARMACOKINETICS

PO: Peak 30-70 min (depends on formulation) half-life 45 min; metabolized in liver; 30% excreted unchanged in urine

INTERACTIONS

• Postural hypotension: ganglionic blockers

Increase: myopathy, rhabdomyolysis—HMG-CoA reductase inhibitors

Increase: flushing, pruritus—alcohol, avoid use

Drug/Herb

Increase: myopathy, rhabdomyolysis—red yeast rice

Drug/Lab Test

Increase: bilirubin, alk phos, hepatic enzymes, LDH, uric acid, glucose

Decrease: cholesterol

False increase: urinary catecholamines

False positive: urine glucose

NURSING CONSIDERATIONS

Assess:

• Hepatic studies: AST, ALT, bilirubin, uric acid, alk phos; blood glucose before and during treatment

• Cardiac status: rate, rhythm, quality; postural hypotension, dysrhythmias

• Nutritional status: liver, yeast, legumes, organ meat, lean poultry; fat in diet

• Hepatic dysfunction: clay-colored stools, itching, dark urine, jaundice

• CNS symptoms: headache, paresthesias, blurred vision

• For symptoms of niacin deficiency: nausea, vomiting, anemia, poor memory, confusion, dermatitis

• For lipid, triglyceride, cholesterol level, if using for hyperlipidemia

Administer:
• Do not break, crush, or chew ext rel tabs, caps
• With meals for GI symptoms, and 81-325 mg aspirin or NSAIDs ½ hr before dose to decrease flushing

Evaluate:
• Therapeutic response: decreased lipids, warm extremities, absence of numbness in extremities

Teach patient/family:
• That flushing and increase in feelings of warmth will occur several hr after taking product (PO); after 2 wk of therapy, these side effects diminish
• To remain recumbent if postural hypotension occurs; to rise slowly to prevent orthostatic hypotension
• To abstain from alcohol if product is prescribed for hyperlipidemia
• To avoid sunlight if skin lesions are present
⚠ To report clay-colored stools, anorexia, jaundiced sclera, skin; dark urine, hepatotoxicity may occur

*niCARdipine (℞)

(nye-card'i-peen)
Cardene IV, Cardene SR
Func. class.: Calcium channel blocker, antianginal, antihypertensive
Chem. class.: Dihydropyridine

Do not confuse:
niCARdipine/NIFEdipine
Cardene/Cardizem
Cardene SR/Cardizem SR

Action: Inhibits calcium ion influx across cell membrane during cardiac depolarization; produces relaxation of coronary vascular smooth muscle, peripheral vascular smooth muscle; dilates coronary vascular arteries; increases myocardial oxygen delivery in patients with vasospastic angina

Uses: Chronic stable angina pectoris, hypertension

DOSAGE AND ROUTES

Hypertension
• *Adult:* **PO** 20 mg tid initially; may increase after 3 days (range 20-40 mg tid) or 30 mg bid **SUS REL;** may increase to 60 mg bid or **IV** 5 mg/hr; may increase by 2.5 mg/hr q15min; max 15 mg/hr

Angina
• *Adult:* **PO** 20 mg tid; may be adjusted q3days; may use 20-40 mg tid

Renal dose
• *Adult:* **PO** 20 mg tid or **SUS REL** 30 mg bid

Hepatic dose
• *Adult:* **PO** 20 mg bid

Available forms: Caps 20, 30 mg; sus rel caps 30, 45, 60 mg; inj 2.5 mg/ml

SIDE EFFECTS

CNS: Headache, dizziness, anxiety, depression, confusion, paresthesia, somnolence, *flushing*
CV: Edema, bradycardia, hypotension, palpitations, **pulmonary edema,** chest pain, tachycardia, increased angina, **arrhythmias, CHF**
GI: Nausea, vomiting, gastric upset, constipation, **hepatitis,** abdominal cramps, dry mouth, sore throat
GU: Nocturia, polyuria
INTEG: Rash, inf site discomfort, **Stevens-Johnson syndrome**
OTHER: Blurred vision, flushing, sweating, SOB, impotence

Contraindications: Sick sinus syndrome, 2nd-/3rd-degree heart block, hypersensitivity, advanced aortic stenosis

Precautions: Pregnancy (C), breastfeeding, children, geriatric patients, CHF, hypotension, hepatic injury, renal disease

PHARMACOKINETICS

Metabolized by liver, excreted in urine 60%, 35% feces
PO: Onset 30 min, peak 1-2 hr, duration 8 hr
PO-SR: Onset unknown, peak 2-6 hr, duration 10-12 hr, half-life 2-5 hr

INTERACTIONS

Increase: effects of digoxin, neuromuscular blocking agents, theophylline, other antihypertensives, nitrates, alcohol, quinidine

Increase: niCARdipine effects—cimetidine

Increase: toxicity risk—cycloSPORINE, prazosin, carbamazepine, quinidine, propranolol

Decrease: antihypertensive effect—NSAIDs, rifampin

Drug/Herb

Increase: effect—barberry, betel palm, burdock, goldenseal, khat, khella, lily of the valley, plantain

Decrease: effect—yohimbe

Drug/Food

Increase: hypotensive effect—grapefruit juice

NURSING CONSIDERATIONS

Assess:

⚠ Cardiac status: B/P, pulse, respiration, ECG during long-term treatment

- Anginal pain: intensity, location, duration, alleviating factors
- Potassium, renal, hepatic studies, periodically

⚠ CHF: weight gain, crackles, jugular venous distention, dyspnea, I&O

Administer:

PO route

- Do not break, crush, chew, or open sus rel cap
- Without regard to meals

IV route

- Dilute each 25 mg/240 ml of compatible sol (0.1 mg/ml), give slowly
- Stable at room temperature 24 hr

Solution compatibilities: D_5W, D_5/0.45% NaCl, D_5/0.9% NaCl

Y-site compatibilities: Diltiazem, DOBUTamine, DOPamine, epinephrine, fentanyl, hydromorphone, labetalol, lorazepam, midazolam, milrinone, morphine, nitroglycerin, norepinephrine, ranitidine, vecuronium

Evaluate:

- Therapeutic response: decreased anginal pain, decreased B/P

Teach patient/family:

- To avoid hazardous activities until stabilized on product, dizziness is no longer a problem
- To limit caffeine consumption, take no alcohol products
- To avoid OTC products unless directed by prescriber
- To comply in all areas of medical regimen: diet, exercise, stress reduction, product therapy

⚠ To notify prescriber of irregular heartbeat, SOB, swelling of feet and hands, pronounced dizziness, constipation, nausea, hypotension, change in severity/pattern/incidence of angina

Treatment of overdose: Defibrillation, β-agonists, IV calcium, diuretics, atropine for AV block, vasopressor for hypotension

nicotine (OTC, ℞)
(nik′o-teen)

nicotine chewing gum (OTC, ℞)
Nicorette

nicotine inhaler (OTC, ℞)
Nicotrol Inhaler

nicotine lozenge (OTC)
Commit

nicotine nasal spray (℞)
Nicotrol NS

nicotine transdermal (OTC, ℞)
Clear Nicoderm CQ, Habitrol, Nicoderm CQ, Nicotrol, Nicotrol TD

Func. class.: Smoking deterrent
Chem. class.: Ganglionic cholinergic agonist

Action: Agonist at nicotinic receptors in peripheral, central nervous systems; acts at sympathetic ganglia, on chemorecep-

tors of aorta, carotid bodies; also affects adrenalin-releasing catecholamines
Uses: Deter cigarette smoking
Unlabeled uses: Gilles de la Tourette's syndrome

DOSAGE AND ROUTES

Nicotine chewing gum

• *Adult:* If patient smokes <25 cigarettes/day, start with 2 mg gum; if >25 cigarettes/day, start with 4 mg gum; then 1 piece of gum q1-2hr × 6 wk; then 1 piece of gum q2-4hr × 2 wk, then 1 piece of gum q4-8hr × 2 wk, then discontinue; not to exceed 24/day

Nicotine inhaler

• *Adult:* **INH** 6 cartridges/day for first 3-6 wk, max 16/day × 12 wk

Nicotine lozenge

• *Adult:* If cigarette is desired >30 min after awakening, start with 1 2-mg lozenge; if <30 min after awakening, start with 4-mg lozenge; then 1 q1-2hr, max 20 lozenges/day or 5 lozenges/6 hr × 6 wk, then 1 lozenge q2-4hr × 2 wk, then 1 lozenge q4-8hr × 2 wk, then discontinue

Nicotine nasal spray

• *Adult:* 1 spray in each nostril 1-2×/hr, max 5×/hr or 40×/day, max 3 mo

Nicotine transdermal/inhaler system

• *Habitrol, Nicoderm:* 21 mg/day × 4-8 wk; 14 mg/day × 2-4 wk; 7 mg/day × 2-4 wk

• *Nicotrol:* 15 mg/day × 12 wk; 10 mg/day × 2 wk; 5 mg/day × 2 wk

• *Nicotrol Inhaler:* Delivers 30% of what a smoker receives from an actual cigarette

Gilles de la Tourette's syndrome (unlabeled)

• *Adult and child:* **Chewing gum** 2 mg chewed × ½ hr bid for 1-6 mo; **TRANSDERMAL** 7- or 10-mg patch daily × 2 days

Available forms: Transdermal patch (Habitrol, Nicoderm, nicotine transdermal system) delivering 7, 14, 21 mg/day; (Nicoderm) 5, 10, 15 mg/day; nicotine inhaler 4 mg delivered; nasal spray 0.5 mg nicotine/actuation; gum 2 mg/piece; lozenge 2 mg, 4 mg

SIDE EFFECTS

CNS: Dizziness, vertigo, insomnia, headache, confusion, seizures, depression, euphoria, numbness, tinnitus, strange dreams

CV: Dysrhythmias, tachycardia, palpitations, edema, flushing, hypertension

EENT: Jaw ache, irritation in buccal cavity

GI: Nausea, vomiting, anorexia, indigestion, diarrhea, abdominal pain, constipation, eructation, irritation

RESP: Breathing difficulty, cough, hoarseness, sneezing, wheezing, bronchial spasm

Contraindications: Pregnancy (X), gum; (D), transdermal; hypersensitivity, immediate post MI recovery period, severe angina pectoris

Precautions: Breastfeeding, vasospastic disease, dysrhythmias, diabetes mellitus, hyperthyroidism, pheochromocytoma, esophagitis, peptic ulcer, coronary/renal/hepatic disease; MRI (patch)

PHARMACOKINETICS

Onset 15-30 min, metabolized in liver, excreted in urine, half-life 2-3 hr, 30-120 hr (terminal)

INTERACTIONS

• Smoking cessation increases diuretic effects of furosemide

Increase: absorption—SUBCUT insulin

Increase: blood levels with cessation of smoking—caffeine, theophylline, pentazocine, imipramine, oxazepam, propranolol, acetaminophen

Decrease: absorption—glutethimide

Decrease: metabolism of propoxyphene

Drug/Herb

Increase: effect—blue cohosh, lobelia

Decrease: effect—oats

NURSING CONSIDERATIONS

Assess:

• Adverse reaction: irritation of buccal cavity, dislike of taste, jaw ache

Administer:

Gum

- Chew gum slowly for 30 min to promote buccal absorption of the product; do not chew over 45 min
- Begin product withdrawal after 3 mo use; do not exceed 6 mo

Transdermal patch

- Once a day to a nonhairy, clean, dry area of skin on upper body or upper outer arm; rotate sites to prevent skin irritation

Inhaler

- Puffing on mouthpiece delivers nicotine through the mouth

Evaluate:

- Therapeutic response: decrease in urge to smoke, decreased need for gum after 3-6 mo

Teach patient/family:

Gum

- All aspects of product use; give package insert to patient and explain
- That gum will not stick to dentures, dental appliances
- That gum is as toxic as cigarettes; to be used only to deter smoking
- Not to use during pregnancy; birth defects may occur

Transdermal patch

- That patch is as toxic as cigarettes; to be used only to deter smoking
- Not to use during pregnancy; birth defects may occur
- To keep used and unused system out of reach of children and pets
- To stop smoking immediately when beginning patch treatment
- To apply promptly after removing from protective patch; system may lose strength

*NIFEdipine (℞)

(nye-fed'i-peen)

Adalat, Adalat CC, Apo-Nifed PA ♣, Nifediac CC, Nifedical XL, Novo-Nifedin ♣, Nu-Nifedin ♣, Procardia, Procardia XL

Func. class.: Calcium-channel blocker, antianginal, antihypertensive

Chem. class.: Dihydropyridine

Do not confuse:

NIFEdipine/niCARdipine/nimodipine

Action: Inhibits calcium ion influx across cell membrane during cardiac depolarization; relaxes coronary vascular smooth muscle; dilates coronary arteries; increases myocardial oxygen delivery in patients with vasospastic angina; dilates peripheral arteries

Uses: Chronic stable angina pectoris, vasospastic angina, hypertension

Unlabeled uses: Migraines, preterm labor, chronic/acute hypertension (pediatrics), diabetic nephropathy, proteinuria, hiccups

N

DOSAGE AND ROUTES

- *Adult:* **PO** Immediate release 10 mg tid, increase in 10-mg increments q7-14days, max 180 mg/24 hr or single dose of 30 mg; **SUS REL** 30-60 mg/day, may increase q7-14days, doses >120 mg not recommended

Hypertension

- *Adult:* **PO EXT REL** 30-60 mg daily titrate upward as needed, max 90 mg/day (Adalat CC), 120 mg/day (Procardia XL)
- *Child/adolescent (unlabeled):* **PO EXT REL** 0.25-0.5 mg/kg/day, max 3 mg/kg/day

Acute hypertensive episodes in pediatric patients (unlabeled)

- *Infant/child/adolescent:* **PO** 0.2-0.5 mg/kg/dose up to 10 mg (total dose)

Migraine prophylaxis (unlabeled)

- *Adult:* **PO** 30-180 mg/day

Preterm labor (unlabeled)

• *Pregnant female:* **PO** Immediate release (Procardia, Adalat) 30 mg loading dose, then 10-20 mg q4-6hr; use in monitored settings

Available forms: Caps 5 ✱, 10, 20 mg; ext rel tabs (CC, XL) 10 ✱, 20 ✱, 30, 60, 90 mg; tabs 10 mg ✱

SIDE EFFECTS

CNS: Headache, fatigue, drowsiness, *dizziness,* anxiety, depression, weakness, insomnia, light-headedness, paresthesia, tinnitus, blurred vision, nervousness, tremor, *flushing*

CV: **Dysrhythmias,** edema, hypotension, palpitations, tachycardia

GI: Nausea, vomiting, diarrhea, gastric upset, constipation, increased LFTs, dry mouth, flatulence, gingival hyperplasia, **hepatotoxicity**

GU: Nocturia, polyuria

HEMA: Bruising, bleeding, petechiae

INTEG: Rash, pruritus, flushing, hair loss

MISC: Sexual difficulties, cough, fever, chills

SYST: **Stevens-Johnson syndrome**

Contraindications: Hypersensitivity to this product or dihydropyridine

Precautions: Pregnancy (C), breastfeeding, children, CHF, hypotension, sick sinus syndrome, 2nd-/3rd-degree heart block, hypotension <90 mm Hg systolic, hepatic injury, renal disease, acute MI, aortic stenosis, cardiogenic shock, GERD, heart failure

PHARMACOKINETICS

Metabolized by liver; excreted in urine 60%-80% (metabolites), feces 15%; protein binding 90%-98%

PO: Onset 20 min, peak 0.5-6 hr, duration 6-8 hr, half-life 2-5 hr, well absorbed

PO-ER: Duration 24 hr

INTERACTIONS

Increase: level of digoxin, phenytoin, cycloSPORINE, prazosin, carbamazepine

Increase: NIFEdipine, toxicity—cimetidine, ranitidine

Increase: effects of β-blockers, antihypertensives

Decrease: antihypertensive effect—NSAIDs

Decrease: effects of quinidine

Decrease: NIFEdipine level—smoking

Drug/Herb

Increase: effect—barberry, betel palm, burdock, goldenseal, khat, khella, lily of the valley, plantain

Decrease: effect—yohimbe

Drug/Food

Increase: NIFEdipine level—grapefruit juice

Drug/Lab Test

Increase: CPK, LDH, AST

Positive: ANA, direct Coombs' test

NURSING CONSIDERATIONS

Assess:

• Anginal pain: location, intensity, duration, character, alleviating, aggravating factors

• Cardiac status: B/P, pulse, respiration, ECG

• Potassium, renal, hepatic studies periodically during treatment

• For bruising, petechiae, bleeding

Administer:

• Do not break, crush, or chew ext rel tabs

• Without regard to meals

Evaluate:

• Therapeutic response: decreased anginal pain, B/P, activity tolerance

Teach patient/family:

• To avoid hazardous activities until stabilized on product, dizziness is no longer a problem

• To limit caffeine consumption; take no alcohol products

• To avoid OTC products unless directed by a prescriber

• That ext rel nonabsorbable shell may appear in stools

• To comply with all areas of medical regimen: diet, exercise, stress reduction, product therapy

• To change position slowly; orthostatic hypotension is common

⚠ To notify prescriber of dyspnea, edema of extremities, nausea, vomiting, severe ataxia, severe rash; changes in pattern/frequency/severity of angina

• To increase fluid intake to prevent constipation

• To check for gingival hyperplasia and report promptly

• Not to discontinue abruptly, gradually taper

Treatment of overdose: Defibrillation, atropine for AV block, vasopressor for hypotension

nilotinib (℞)

(nye-loe'ti-nib)

Tasigna

Func. class.: Antineoplastic—miscellaneous

Chem. class.: Protein-tyrosine kinase inhibitor

Action: Inhibits BCR-ABL tyrosine kinase created in chronic myeloid leukemia (CML)

Uses: Chronic phase/accelerated phase Philadelphia chromosome–positive CML that is resistant/intolerant to imatinib

DOSAGE AND ROUTES

• *Adult:* **PO** 400 mg q12hr, continue until disease progression or unacceptable toxicity

Escalation regimen for those taking a strong CYP3A4 inducer

• *Adult:* **PO** Increase dose as required

Adjustment following discontinuation of a strong CYP3A4 inducer

• *Adult:* **PO** Reduce to 400 mg/bid

For those taking a strong CYP3A4 inhibitor

• *Adult:* **PO** Reduce dose to 400 mg/day

QT prolongation

• *QTc >480 msec*: Withhold dose

Myelosuppression

• *ANC 1 × 10^9/L or platelets <50 × 10^9/L*: Withhold dose

Available forms: Caps 200 mg

SIDE EFFECTS

CNS: Headache, dizziness, fatigue, fever, flushing, paresthesia

CV: **QT prolongation,** palpitations, **torsade de pointes**

GI: Nausea, **hepatotoxicity, vomiting, dyspepsia,** *anorexia, abdominal pain,* constipation, **pancreatitis,** diarrhea

HEMA: **Neutropenia, thrombocytopenia, anemia, pancytopenia**

INTEG: Rash, alopecia, erythema

META: Hyperamylasemia, hyperbilirubinemia, hyperglycemia, hyperkalemia, hypocalcemia, hyponatremia, hypomagnesemia

MISC: Diaphoresis

MS: Arthralgia, myalgia, back/bone pain, muscle cramps

RESP: Cough, dyspnea

SYST: **Bleeding**

Contraindications: Pregnancy (D), breastfeeding, hypersensitivity

Black Box Warning: Hypokalemia, hypomagnesemia, QT prolongation

Precautions: Children, females, geriatric patients, active infections, anemia, cardiac disease, bone marrow suppression, cholestasis, diabetes, gelatin hypersensitivity, infertility, galactose-free diet, lactase deficiency, neutropenia, pancreatitis, thrombocytopenia

Black Box Warning: Hepatic disease

PHARMACOKINETICS

Protein binding 98%, metabolized by CYP3A4, plasma levels 3 hr, elimination half-life 17 hr

INTERACTIONS

• Product interactions are numerous

• Do not use with phenothiazines, pimozide, ziprasidone

Increase: hepatotoxicity—acetaminophen

Increase: concentrations—ketoconazole, itraconazole, erythromycin, clarithromycin

Increase: plasma concentrations of simvastatin, calcium channel blockers

N

Increase: plasma concentration of warfarin; avoid use with warfarin, use low-molecular-weight anticoagulants instead
Decrease: concentrations—dexamethasone, phenytoin, carbamazepine, rifampin, phenobarbital
Drug/Herb
Decrease: concentration—St. John's wort
Drug/Food
Increase: plasma concentrations—grapefruit juice

NURSING CONSIDERATIONS

Assess:
- ANC and platelets; if ANC <1 $\times 10^9$/L and/or platelets <50 $\times 10^9$/L, stop until ANC >1.5 $\times 10^9$/L and platelets >75 $\times 10^9$/L
- CV status: hypertension, QT prolongation can occur; monitor left ventricular ejection fraction (LVEF) baseline periodically
- For renal toxicity: if bilirubin >3 × IULN, withhold until bilirubin levels return to <1.5 × IULN
- For hepatotoxicity: monitor LFTs, before treatment and q mo; if liver transaminases >5 × IULN, withhold until transaminase levels return to <2.5 × IULN
- CBC, differential, platelet count weekly; withhold product if WBC is <3500/mm^3 or platelet count <100,000/mm^3; notify prescriber of these results; product should be discontinued
- For bleeding: epistaxis rectal, gingival, upper GI, genital and wound bleeding; tumor-related hemorrhage may occur rapidly
- Electrolytes: calcium, potassium, magnesium, sodium; lipase, phosphate; hypokalemia, hypomagnesemia should be corrected prior to use

Administer:
- Do not break, crush, or chew caps
- On an empty stomach; separate doses by 12 hr; a make-up dose should not be taken if a dose is missed

Perform/provide:
- Storage at 15° C-30° C (59° F- 86° F)

Evaluate:
- Therapeutic response: decrease in progression of disease

Teach patient/family:
- To report adverse reactions immediately: SOB, bleeding
- Reason for treatment, expected result
- That many adverse reactions may occur
- To avoid persons with known upper respiratory tract infections; immunosuppression is common
- To watch for signs/symptoms of low potassium or magnesium

nilutamide (℞)

(nye-loo'ta-mide)
Anandron ✱, Nilandron
Func. class.: Antineoplastic-hormone
Chem. class.: Antiandrogen

Action: Interferes with testosterone uptake in the nucleus or testosterone activity in target tissues; arrests tumor growth in androgen-sensitive tissue (e.g., prostate gland); prostatic carcinoma is androgen-sensitive, so tumor growth is arrested

Uses: Metastatic prostatic carcinoma, stage D2 in combination with surgical castration (only to be used by men)

DOSAGE AND ROUTES

- *Adult:* **PO** 300 mg/day × 30 days, then 150 mg/day

Available forms: Tabs 50, 100 ✱, 150 mg

SIDE EFFECTS

CNS: Hot flashes, drowsiness, insomnia, dizziness, hyperthesia, depression
CV: **Heart failure,** hypertension
EENT: Delay in adaptation to dark
GI: Diarrhea, nausea, vomiting, increased LFTs, constipation, dyspepsia, **hepatotoxicity**

GU: Decreased libido, impotence, testicular atrophy, UTI, hematuria, nocturia, gynecomastia
HEMA: Anemia
INTEG: Rash, sweating, alopecia, dry skin
MISC: Edema
RESP: Dyspnea, URI, pneumonia, **interstitial pneumonitis**

Contraindications: Women, hypersensitivity, severe hepatic impairment

Black Box Warning: Severe respiratory disease

Precautions: Pregnancy (C)

PHARMACOKINETICS

Rapidly and completely absorbed; excreted in urine and feces as metabolites

INTERACTIONS

Increase: toxicity of vit K, phenytoin, theophylline

NURSING CONSIDERATIONS

Assess:

⚠ Hepatic studies: AST, ALT, alk phos, which may be elevated; if elevated 3× normal, discontinue product
- For CNS symptoms: drowsiness, insomnia, dizziness
- Chest x-rays, routinely, baseline pulmonary function studies; dyspnea, cough, which may indicate interstitial pneumonitis; discontinue treatment if this condition is suspected
- PSA, improvement in bone pain
- For hyperglycemia, increased BUN, creatinine, alk phos, leukopenia

Administer:
- Without regard to meals
- Start therapy on day of or after surgery

Perform/provide:
- Storage at room temperature

Evaluate:
- Therapeutic response: decrease in prostatic tumor size, decrease in spread of cancer

Teach patient/family:

⚠ To report side effects: decreased libido, impotence, breast enlargement, hot flashes, diarrhea, dyspnea, cough, SOB; if SOB occurs, notify prescriber immediately

⚠ To report signs of hepatotoxicity: dark urine, abdominal pain, clay-colored stools, jaundice eyes, skin
- To wear tinted lens to alleviate delay in adapting to the dark
- That product is started on day of or day after surgical removal of testes
- To avoid alcohol consumption

Treatment of overdose: Induce vomiting, provide supportive care

nisoldipine (℞)
(nye-sole′dih-peen)
Sular
Func. class.: Calcium channel blocker, antihypertensive
Chem. class.: Dihydropyridine

Action: Inhibits calcium ion influx across cell membrane, resulting in dilation of peripheral arteries

Uses: Essential hypertension, alone or with other antihypertensives

Unlabeled uses: Variant (Prinzmetal's) angina, stable angina pectoris

N

DOSAGE AND ROUTES

Hypertension
- *Adult:* **PO** 17 mg/day initially, may increase by 8.5 mg/wk, usual dose 17-34 mg/day, max 34 mg/day
- *Geriatric/hepatic dose:* **PO** 8.5 mg/day, increase based on response

Variant (Prinzmetal's) angina/stable angina pectoris (unlabeled)
- *Adult:* **PO** 17-34 mg/day, max 34 mg/day

Available forms: Ext rel tabs 8.5, 17, 20, 25.5, 30, 34, 40 mg

SIDE EFFECTS

CNS: Headache, fatigue, drowsiness, dizziness, anxiety, depression, nervousness, insomnia, light-headedness, paresthesia, tinnitus, psychosis, somnolence, ataxia, confusion, malaise, migraine

CV: Dysrhythmia, edema, **CHF**, hypotension, palpitations, **MI, pulmonary edema,** tachycardia, syncope, AV block, angina, chest pain, ECG abnormalities

GI: Nausea, vomiting, diarrhea, gastric upset, constipation, increased LFTs, dry mouth, dyspepsia, dysphagia, flatulence

GU: Nocturia, hematuria, dysuria

HEMA: **Anemia, leukopenia,** petechiae

INTEG: Rash, pruritus

MISC: Sexual difficulties, cough, nasal congestion, SOB, wheezing, epistaxis, dyspnea, gingival hyperplasia, chills, fever, gout, sweating

Contraindications: Hypersensitivity; sick sinus syndrome; 2nd-/3rd-degree heart block; aortic stenosis

Precautions: Pregnancy (C), breastfeeding, children, geriatric patients, CHF, hypotension <90 mm Hg systolic, hepatic injury, renal disease, acute MI, unstable angina, CAD, cardiogenic shock

PHARMACOKINETICS

Metabolized by liver, excreted in urine, peak 6-12 hr, protein binding 99%, half-life 7-12 hr

INTERACTIONS

Increase: effects of β-blockers, antihypertensives, digoxin

Increase: nisoldipine level—CYP3A4 inhibitors, cimetidine, ranitidine, azole antifungals

Decrease: nisoldipine effect—CYP3A4 inducers, hydantoins

Drug/Herb

Increase: effect—barberry, betel palm, burdock, goldenseal, hawthorn, khat, khella, lily of the valley, plantain

Decrease: effect—St. John's wort, yohimbe

Drug/Food

Increase: nisoldipine level—high-fat foods

Increase: hypotensive effect—grapefruit juice

NURSING CONSIDERATIONS

Assess:

- Cardiac status: B/P, pulse, respiration, ECG
- I&O ratios, weight daily
- For CHF: weight gain, jugular vein distention, edema, crackles

Administer:

- Swallow whole; do not break, crush, or chew
- Once daily as whole tablet; avoid high-fat foods, grapefruit juice

Evaluate:

- Therapeutic response: decreased B/P

Teach patient/family:

- To avoid hazardous activities until stabilized on product, dizziness is no longer a problem
- To report nausea, dizziness, edema, SOB, palpitations
- To limit caffeine consumption
- To avoid OTC products unless directed by a prescriber
- The importance of complying with all areas of medical regimen: diet, exercise, stress reduction, product therapy
- To rise slowly to prevent orthostatic hypotension

Treatment of overdose: Defibrillation, atropine for AV block, vasopressor for hypotension

nitazoxanide (℞)

(nye-taz-ox'a-nide)

Alinia

Func. class.: Antiprotozoal

Action: Interferes with DNA/RNA synthesis in protozoa

Uses: Diarrhea caused by *Cryptosporidium parvum* or *Giardia lamblia*

DOSAGE AND ROUTES

- *Adult:* **PO** 500 mg q12hr × 3 days
- *Child 4-11 yr:* **PO** 10 ml (200 mg) q12hr × 3 days
- *Child 12-47 mo:* **PO** 5 ml (100 mg) q12hr × 3 days

Available forms: Powder for oral susp 100 mg/5 ml; tab 500 mg

SIDE EFFECTS

CNS: Dizziness, fever, headache
CV: Hypotension
GI: Nausea, anorexia, flatulence, increased appetite, enlarged salivary glands, abdominal pain, diarrhea, vomiting
HEMA: Anemia, **leukopenia,** neutropenia
INTEG: Pruritus, sweating
MISC: Increased creatinine, pale yellow eye discoloration, rhinitis, discolored urine, infection, malaise
Contraindications: Hypersensitivity
Precautions: Pregnancy (B), breastfeeding, children <1 yr or >11 yr, renal/hepatic disease, diabetes mellitus (contains sucrose), HIV, immunocompromised patients

PHARMACOKINETICS

Excreted in urine, bile, feces; hydrolyzed to active metabolite, which undergoes conjugation; metabolite protein binding >99%

INTERACTIONS

• Competes for binding sites: other highly protein-bound products; phenytoin, salicylates

NURSING CONSIDERATIONS

Assess:
• Signs of infection
• Bowel pattern before, during treatment

Administer:

PO route
• With food
• Shake oral suspension before giving

Evaluate:
• Therapeutic response: C&S negative for organism, decreased diarrhea

Teach patient/family:
• To take with food; shake susp well before each dose

Rarely Used

nitisinone (℞)

(ni-tiz'i-none)
Orfadin
Func. class.: Orphan drug

Uses: Hereditary tyrosinemia type I

DOSAGE AND ROUTES

• *Adult/adolescent/child/infant:* **PO** 1 mg/kg/day divided in AM and PM
Contraindications: Hypersensitivity, tyrosine/phenylalanine intake

nitrofurantoin (℞)

(nye-troe-fyoor'an-toyn)
Apo-Nitrofurantoin ♣, Furadantin, Macrobid, Macrodantin, nitrofurantoin
Func. class.: Urinary tract antiinfective
Chem. class.: Synthetic nitrofuran derivative

Action: Inhibits bacterial acetyl-CoA intefering with carbohydrate metabolism
Uses: Urinary tract infections caused by *Escherichia coli, Klebsiella, Pseudomonas, Proteus vulgaris, Proteus morganii, Serratia, Citrobacter, Staphylococcus aureus, Staphylococcus epidermidis, Enterococcus, Salmonella, Shigella*

DOSAGE AND ROUTES

Active infections
• *Adult:* **PO** 50-100 mg qid after meals or 50-100 mg at bedtime for long-term treatment
• *Child:* **PO** 5-7 mg/kg/day in 4 divided doses; 1-2 mg/kg/day for long-term treatment, max 7 mg/kg/day

Chronic suppression
• *Adult:* **PO** 50-100 mg q PM
• *Child:* **PO** 1-2 mg/kg/day q PM or 0.5-1 mg/kg q12hr if dose is not well tolerated
Available forms: Caps 25, 50, 100 mg; tabs 50, 100 mg; susp 25 mg/5 ml; macrocrystal caps (Macrodantin) 25, 50,

100 mg; Macrobid cap 100 mg (25 macrocrystals, 75 monohydrate)

SIDE EFFECTS

CNS: *Dizziness, headache,* drowsiness, peripheral neuropathy, chills, confusion, vertigo
CV: **Bundle branch block,** chest pain
GI: *Nausea, vomiting, abdominal pain, diarrhea,* **cholestatic jaundice,** loss of appetite, **pseudomembranous colitis, hepatitis, pancreatitis**
HEMA: **Anemia, agranulocytosis, hemolytic anemia, leukopenia, thrombocytopenia**
INTEG: Pruritus, rash, urticaria, angioedema, alopecia, tooth staining, **exfoliative dermatitis**
MS: Arthralgia, myalgia, numbness, peripheral neuropathy
RESP: Cough, dyspnea, pneumonitis, pulmonary fibrosis/infiltrate
SYST: **Stevens-Johnson syndrome, superinfection,** SLE-like syndrome
Contraindications: Infants <1 mo, hypersensitivity, anuria, severe renal disease, CCr <60 ml/min
Precautions: Pregnancy (B), breastfeeding, geriatric patients, G6PD deficiency, GI disease, diabetes, cholestatic jaundice due to nitrofurantoin therapy

PHARMACOKINETICS

PO: Half-life 20-60 min; crosses blood-brain barrier, placenta; enters breast milk; excreted as inactive metabolites in liver, unchanged in urine; protein binding 60%-90%

INTERACTIONS

Increase: antagonistic effect—norfloxacin
Increase: levels of nitrofurantoin—probenecid
Decrease: absorption of magnesium trisilicate antacid

Drug/Herb

- Do not use acidophilus with antiinfectives; separate by several hours

Drug/Lab Test

Increase: BUN, alk phos, bilirubin, creatinine, blood glucose

NURSING CONSIDERATIONS

Assess:

- Blood count during chronic therapy
- Urinary tract infection: burning, pain on urination, fever, cloudy, foul-smelling urine; I&O ratio: C&S before treatment, after completion
- CNS symptoms: insomnia, vertigo, headache, drowsiness, seizures
- Allergy: fever, flushing, rash, urticaria, pruritus

Administer:

PO route

- Do not break, crush, chew, or open tabs, caps
- Two daily doses if urine output is high or if patient has diabetes
- Use calibrated device to measure liquid product; may mix water, fruit juice; rinse mouth after liquid product; staining of teeth may occur

Evaluate:

- Therapeutic response: decreased dysuria, fever; negative C&S

Teach patient/family:

- To notify prescriber of diarrhea containing mucus or if pus occurs; pseudomembranous colitis may occur
- To take with food or milk; avoid alcohol
- To protect susp from freezing and shake well before taking
- That product may cause drowsiness; instruct client to seek aid in walking and other activities; advise client not to drive or operate machinery while on medication
- That diabetics should monitor blood glucose level
- That product may turn urine rust-yellow to brown

⚠ To notify prescriber of symptoms of pseudomembranous colitis: fever, diarrhea with mucus, pus, or blood; MS reactions: myalgia, arthralgia

nitrofurazone topical
See Appendix B

nitroglycerin (℞)
(nye-troe-gli'ser-in)

transmucosal tablets (℞)
Nitrogard, Nitrogard SR ♣

extended release caps (℞)
Nitrocot, Nitroglyn E-R, Nitropar, Nitro-Time, Nitrong

extended release buccal tabs (℞)
Nitrogard, Nitrogard SR ♣

IV (℞)
Nitro-Bid I.V., Tridil

ointment (℞)
Nitro-Bid, Nitrol

SL (℞)
Nitrostat, NitroQuick

translingual spray (℞)
Nitrolingual Translingual Spray

transdermal (℞)
Deponit, Minitran, Nitrek, Nitrocine, Nitrodisc, Nitro-Dur, Transderm-Nitro

Func. class.: Coronary vasodilator, antianginal
Chem. class.: Nitrate

Do not confuse:
Nitro-Bid/Nicobid

Action: Decreases preload, afterload, which is responsible for decreasing left ventricular end-diastolic pressure, systemic vascular resistance; dilates coronary arteries, improves blood flow through coronary vasculature, dilates arterial, venous beds systemically

Uses: Chronic stable angina pectoris, prophylaxis of angina pain, CHF associated with acute MI, controlled hypotension in surgical procedures

DOSAGE AND ROUTES

• *Adult:* **SL** Dissolve tab under tongue when pain begins; may repeat q5min until relief occurs; take no more than 3 tabs/15 min; use 1 tab prophylactically 5-10 min before activities; **SUS CAP** q6-12hr on empty stomach; **TOP** 1-2 in q8hr, increase to 4 in q4hr as needed; **IV** 5 mcg/min, then increase by 5 mcg/min q3-5min; if no response after 20 mcg/min, increase by 10-20 mcg/min until desired response; **TRANS PATCH** apply a pad daily to a site free of hair; remove patch at bedtime to provide 10-12 hr nitrate-free interval to avoid tolerance; **BUCCAL** 1 mg q5hr

• *Child:* **IV** Initially 0.25-0.5 mcg/kg/min, titrate to patient response, usual dose 1-3 mcg/kg/min transmucosal

Available forms: Buccal tabs 1, 2, 3 mg; translingual aero 0.4 mg/metered spray; sus rel caps 2.5, 6.5, 9, 13 mg; sus rel tabs 2.6, 6.5, 9 mg; SL tabs 0.3, 0.4, 0.6 mg; oint 2%; trans syst 0.1, 0.2, 0.3, 0.4, 0.6, 0.8 mg/hr; inj sol 25 mg/250 ml, 50 mg/250 ml, 50 mg/500 ml, 100 mg/250 ml, 200 mg/500 ml

SIDE EFFECTS

CNS: Headache, flushing, dizziness
CV: Postural hypotension, tachycardia, **collapse,** syncope, palpitations
GI: Nausea, vomiting
INTEG: Pallor, sweating, rash

Contraindications: Hypersensitivity to this product or nitrites, severe anemia, increased intracranial pressure, cerebral hemorrhage, closed-angle glaucoma, cardiac tamponade, cardiomyopathy, constrictive pericarditis

Precautions: Pregnancy (C), breastfeeding, children, postural hypotension, severe renal/hepatic disease, acute MI, abrupt discontinuation, hyperthyroidism

PHARMACOKINETICS

Metabolized by liver, excreted in urine, half-life 1-4 min

SUS REL: Onset 20-45 min, duration 3-8 hr

N

SL: Onset 1-3 min, duration 30 min
TRANSDERMAL: Onset ½-1 hr, duration 12-24 hr
TRANSMUCOSAL: Onset 1-2 min, duration 3-5 hr
AEROSOL: Onset 2 min, duration 30-60 min
TOPICAL OINT: Onset 30-60 min, duration 2-12 hr
IV: Onset 1-2 min, duration 3-5 min

INTERACTIONS

- Severe hypotension, CV collapse: alcohol

Increase: effects of β-blockers, diuretics, antihypertensives, calcium channel blockers
Increase: hypotension—sildenafil, tadalafil, vardenafil
Increase: nitrate level—aspirin
Decrease: heparin—IV nitroglycerin

Drug/Lab Test

Increase: urine catecholamine, urine VMA
False increase: cholesterol

NURSING CONSIDERATIONS

Assess:

- Pain: duration, time started, activity being performed, character
- Orthostatic B/P, pulse prior to and after administration
- Tolerance if taken over long period
- Headache, light-headedness, decreased B/P; may indicate a need for decreased dosage

Administer:

PO route

- Swallow sus rel products whole; do not break, crush, or chew
- With 8 oz H_2O on empty stomach (oral tablet) 1 hr before or
- 2 hr after meals
- SL should be dissolved under tongue, not swallowed
- Aerosol sprayed under tongue, not inhaled

Transdermal route

- Transmucosal tab should be placed between cheek and gum line
- Topical ointment should be measured on papers supplied
- Apply a new TD patch daily and remove after 12-14 hr to prevent tolerance

IV route

- Diluted in amount specified D_5, D_5W, 0.9% NaCl for inf; use glass inf bottles, non–polyvinyl chloride inf tubing; titrate to patient response; do not use filters

Y-site compatibilities: Amiodarone, amphotericin B cholesteryl, amrinone, atracurium, cefmetazole, cisatracurium, diltiazem, DOBUTamine, DOPamine, epinephrine, esmolol, famotidine, fentanyl, fluconazole, furosemide, haloperidol, heparin, hydromorphone, insulin (regular), labetalol, lidocaine, lorazepam, midazolam, milrinone, morphine, niCARdipine, norepinephrine, pancuronium, propofol, ranitidine, remifentanil, sodium nitroprusside, streptokinase, tacrolimus, theophylline, thiopental, vecuronium, warfarin

Evaluate:

- Therapeutic response: decrease, prevention of anginal pain

Teach patient/family:

- To place buccal tab between lip and gum above incisors or between cheek and gum
- To keep tabs in original container; to replace q6mo, as effectiveness is lost; keep away from heat, moisture, light
- If 3 SL tabs in 15 min do not relieve pain, to seek immediate medical attention
- To avoid alcohol
- That product may cause headache; tolerance usually develops; use nonopioid analgesic
- That product may be taken before stressful activity: exercise, sexual activity
- That SL may sting when product comes in contact with mucous membranes
- To avoid hazardous activities if dizziness occurs
- To comply with complete medical regimen
- To make position changes slowly to prevent fainting

⚠ To never use erectile dysfunction products (sildenafil, tadalafil, vardenafil); may cause severe hypotension, death

⚠ High Alert

nitroprusside (℞)

(nye-troe-pruss′ide)

Nitropress, sodium nitroprusside

Func. class.: Antihypertensive, vasodilator

Action: Directly relaxes arteriolar, venous smooth muscle, resulting in reduction in cardiac preload, afterload

Uses: Hypertensive crisis, to decrease bleeding by creating hypotension during surgery, acute CHF

DOSAGE AND ROUTES

- *Adult and child:* **IV INF** 0.25-10 mcg/kg/min; max 10 mcg/kg/min

Available forms: Inj 50 mg

SIDE EFFECTS

CNS: *Dizziness, headache,* agitation, twitching, decreased reflexes, restlessness

CV: Bradycardia, ECG changes, tachycardia, hypotension

GI: Nausea, vomiting, abdominal pain

INTEG: Pain, irritation at inj site, sweating

MISC: **Cyanide, thiocyanate toxicity,** flushing, hypothyroidism

Contraindications: Hypersensitivity, hypertension (compensatory) due to aortic coarctation or AV shunting, acute CHF associated with reduced peripheral vascular resistance, AV shunt, Leber's disease, toxic amblyopia

Black Box Warning: Cyanide toxicity

Precautions: Pregnancy (C), breastfeeding, children, geriatric patients, fluid, electrolyte imbalances, renal/hepatic disease, hypothyroidism

Black Box Warning: Hypotension

PHARMACOKINETICS

IV: Onset 1-2 min, duration 1-10 min, half-life 3 days in patients with abnormal renal function, circulating half-life 2 min; metabolized in liver, excreted in urine

INTERACTIONS

- Severe hypotension: ganglionic blockers, volatile liquid anesthetics, halothane, enflurane, circulatory depressants

Drug/Herb

Increase: toxicity, death—aconite

Increase: antihypertensive effect—barberry, betony, black catechu, black cohosh, bloodroot, broom, burdock, cat's claw, dandelion, goldenseal, Irish moss, Jamaican dogwood, kelp, khella, mistletoe, parsley

Increase or decrease: antihypertensive effect—astragalus, cola tree

Decrease: antihypertensive effect—coltsfoot, guarana, khat, licorice

NURSING CONSIDERATIONS

Assess:

- Electrolytes: K, Na, Cl, CO_2, CBC, serum glucose, serum methemoglobin if pulmonary O_2 levels are decreased; use IV 1-2 mg/kg methylene blue given over several min for methemoglobinemia
- Renal studies: catecholamines, BUN, creatinine
- Hepatic studies: AST, ALT, alk phos
- B/P by direct means if possible; check ECG continuously; pulse, jugular vein distention; PCWP; rebound hypertension may occur after nitroprusside is discontinued
- Weight daily, I&O

⚠ Thiocyanate, lactate, cyanide levels daily in inf >3 mcg/kg/min; thiocyanate level should be ≤1 mmol/L; thiocyanate toxicity includes confusion, weakness, seizures, hyperreflexia, psychosis, tinnitus, coma

- Nausea, vomiting, diarrhea
- Edema in feet, legs daily; skin turgor, dryness of mucous membranes for hydration status

N

- Crackles, dyspnea, orthopnea q30min
- For decrease in bicarbonate, Pco_2 blood pH, acidosis

Administer:

- Antidote is sodium thiosulfate

IV route

- Depending on B/P reading q15min
- IV after diluting 50 mg/2-3 ml of D_5W, further dilute in 250 ml of D_5W; use an infusion pump only; wrap bottle with aluminum foil to protect from light; observe for color change in the inf; discard if highly discolored (blue, green, dark red); titrate to patient response

Syringe compatibilities: Heparin

Y-site compatibilities: Amrinone, atracurium, diltiazem, DOBUTamine, DOPamine, enalaprilat, famotidine, lidocaine, nitroglycerin, pancuronium, tacrolimus, theophylline, vecuronium

Evaluate:

- Therapeutic response: decreased B/P, absence of bleeding

Teach patient/family:

- To report headache, dizziness, loss of hearing, blurred vision, dyspnea, faintness
- The reason for giving product and expected results

nizatidine (OTC, ℞)

(ni-za'ti-deen)

Axid, Axid AR

Func. class.: H_2-receptor antagonist

Chem. class.: Substituted thiazole

Action: Blocks H_2-receptors, thereby reducing gastric acid output

Uses: Benign gastric and duodenal ulceration, prevention of duodenal ulcer recurrence, symptomatic relief of gastroesophageal reflux, heartburn prevention

DOSAGE AND ROUTES

Gastric and duodenal ulcer

- *Adult:* **PO** 300 mg at night or 150 mg bid for 4-8 wk; maintenance 150 mg at night

Prophylaxis of duodenal ulcer

- *Adult:* **PO** 150 mg/day at bedtime

Gastroesophageal reflux

- *Adult and child ≥12 yr:* **PO** 150 mg bid, up to 12 wk, max 300 mg/day

Heartburn prevention

- *Adult:* **PO** 75 mg before eating bid

Renal dose

- *Adult:* **PO** CCr 20-50 ml/min give 150 mg every other day; CCr <20 ml/min give 150 mg q72hr

Available forms: Caps 150, 300 mg; tabs 75 mg

SIDE EFFECTS

CNS: Headache, somnolence, confusion, abnormal dreams, dizziness

CV: **Cardiac dysrhythmias, cardiac arrest**

ENDO: Gynecomastia

GI: Elevated hepatic enzymes, **hepatitis,** jaundice, nausea

HEMA: **Thrombocytopenia, agranulocytosis, aplastic anemia**

INTEG: Pruritus, sweating, urticaria, **exfoliative dermatitis**

METAB: Hyperuricemia

MS: Myalgia

RESP: **Bronchospasm, laryngeal edema, pneumonia**

Contraindications: Hypersensitivity

Precautions: Pregnancy (B), breastfeeding, renal/hepatic impairment (reduce dose in renal impairment)

PHARMACOKINETICS

Partially metabolized by liver, excreted by kidneys, plasma half-life 1-2.8 hr, 70% absorbed orally, small amount (0.1% of plasma concentration) enters breast milk, 35% bound to plasma proteins

INTERACTIONS

Decrease: effect of—ketoconazole, itraconazole

NURSING CONSIDERATIONS

Assess:

⚠ CBC with differential if on long-term therapy, agranulocytosis may occur

- Gastric pH (>5 should be maintained)
- Fluid balance, I&O

Administer:
- With meals for prolonged product effect; antacids 1 hr before or 1 hr after product; at bedtime if taken daily

Evaluate:
- Mental status, confusion, dizziness, depression, anxiety, weakness, tremors, psychosis, diarrhea, jaundice, report immediately
- For GI symptoms: nausea, vomiting, diarrhea, cramps

Teach patient/family:
- That gynecomastia, impotence may occur, are reversible
- To avoid driving or other hazardous activities until patient is stabilized on this medication; dizziness may occur
- To avoid black pepper, caffeine, alcohol, harsh spices, extremes in temperature of food
- To avoid OTC preparations: aspirin, cough, cold preparations

Treatment of overdose: Symptomatic and supportive therapy is recommended; activated charcoal, emesis, or lavage may reduce absorption

⚠ High Alert

norepinephrine (℞)

(nor-ep-i-nef′rin)

Levophed

Func. class.: Adrenergic

Chem. class.: Catecholamine

Do not confuse:
norepinephrine/epinephrine

Action: Causes increased contractility and heart rate by acting on β-receptors in heart; also acts on α-receptors, causing vasoconstriction in blood vessels; B/P is elevated, coronary blood flow improves, cardiac output increases

Uses: Acute hypotension, shock

DOSAGE AND ROUTES

- *Adult:* **IV INF** 0.5-1 mcg/min titrated to B/P maintenance 2-4 mcg/min; max 30 mcg/min
- *Child:* **IV INF** 0.1-0.2 mcg/kg/min titrated to B/P; max 2 mcg/kg/min

Available forms: Inj 1 mg/ml

SIDE EFFECTS

CNS: Headache, anxiety, dizziness, insomnia, restlessness, tremor, **cerebral hemorrhage**

CV: Palpitations, tachycardia, hypertension, ectopic beats, angina

GI: Nausea, vomiting

GU: Decreased urine output

INTEG: Necrosis, tissue sloughing with extravasation, **gangrene**

RESP: Dyspnea

SYST: **Anaphylaxis**

Contraindications: Hypersensitivity to this product or cyclopropane/halothane anesthesia, ventricular fibrillation, tachydysrhythmias, pheochromocytoma, hypotension, hypovolemia

Precautions: Pregnancy (C), breastfeeding, geriatric patients, arterial embolism, peripheral vascular disease, hypertension, hyperthyroidism, cardiac disease

Black Box Warning: Extravasation

PHARMACOKINETICS

IV: Onset 1-2 min; metabolized in liver; excreted in urine (inactive metabolites); crosses placenta

INTERACTIONS

- Dysrhythmias: general anesthetics, bretylium
- Incompatible with alkaline solutions: sodium, HCO_3^-
- Severe hypertension: guanethidine

⚠ Do not use within 2 wk of MAOIs, antihistamines, ergots, methyldopa, oxytocics, tricyclics, guanethidine, or hypertensive crisis may result

Increase: B/P—oxytocics

Increase: pressor effect—tricyclics, MAOIs

Decrease: norepinephrine action—α-blockers

NURSING CONSIDERATIONS

Assess:
- I&O ratio; notify prescriber if output <30 ml/hr

N

• ECG during administration continuously; if B/P increases, product is decreased
• B/P and pulse q2-3min after parenteral route
• CVP or PWP during inf if possible
• For paresthesias and coldness of extremities; peripheral blood flow may decrease
• Inj site: tissue sloughing; administer phentolamine mixed with 0.9% NaCl
• Sulfite sensitivity, which may be life-threatening

Administer:
• Plasma expanders for hypovolemia
• IV after diluting with 500-1000 ml D_5W or D_5/0.9% NaCl; average dilution is 4 mg/1000 ml diluent (4 mcg base/ml); give as inf 2-3 ml/min; titrate to response
• Using 2-bottle setup so product may be discontinued while IV is still running; use inf pump

Additive compatibilities: Amikacin, calcium chloride, calcium gluconate, cimetidine, corticotropin, dimenhyDRINATE, DOBUTamine, heparin, hydrocortisone, magnesium sulfate, meropenem, methylPREDNISolone, multivitamins, netilmicin, potassium chloride, succinylcholine, verapamil, vit B/C
Syringe compatibilities: Heparin
Y-site compatibilities: Amiodarone, amrinone, cisatracurium, diltiazem, DOBUTamine, DOPamine, epinephrine, esmolol, famotidine, fentanyl, furosemide, haloperidol, heparin, hydrocortisone, hydromorphone, labetalol, lorazepam, meropenem, midazolam, milrinone, morphine, niCARdipine, nitroglycerin, potassium chloride, propofol, ranitidine, remifentanil, vecuronium, vit B/C

Perform/provide:
• Storage of reconstituted sol in refrigerator no longer than 24 hr
• Do not use discolored sol

Evaluate:
• Therapeutic response: increased B/P with stabilization

Teach patient/family:
• The reason for product administration and to report dyspnea, dizziness, chest pain

Treatment of overdose: Administer fluids, electrolyte replacement

norethindrone (℞)

(nor-eth-in′drone)
Aygestin, Camila, Errin, Jolivette, Micronor, Nora-BE, Nor-QD, Ortho Micronor
Func. class.: Progestogen
Chem. class.: Progesterone derivative

Action: Inhibits secretion of pituitary gonadotropins, which prevents follicular maturation, ovulation; stimulates growth of mammary tissue; antineoplastic action against endometrial cancer
Uses: Uterine bleeding (abnormal), amenorrhea, endometriosis, contraception

DOSAGE AND ROUTES

Amenorrhea, abnormal uterine bleeding (Aygestin)
• *Adult:* **PO** 2.5-10 mg/day on days 5-25 of menstrual cycle

Endometriosis (Aygestin)
• *Adult:* **PO** 5 mg/day × 2 wk, then increased by 2.5 mg/day × 2 wk, up to 15 mg/day, may continue for 6-9 mo

Contraception
• *Adult:* **PO** 0.35 mg on 1st day of menses, then 0.35 mg/day

Available forms: Tabs (Aygestin) 5 mg; tabs 0.35 mg

SIDE EFFECTS

CNS: Dizziness, headache, migraines, depression, fatigue
CV: Hypotension, **thrombophlebitis,** edema, **thromboembolism, CVA, stroke, PE, MI**
EENT: Diplopia
GI: Nausea, vomiting, anorexia, cramps, increased weight, **cholestatic jaundice**
GU: Amenorrhea, cervical erosion, breakthrough bleeding, dysmenorrhea, vaginal

candidiasis, breast changes, (gynecomastia, testicular atrophy, impotence), endometriosis, **spontaneous abortion,** breast tenderness
INTEG: Rash, urticaria, acne, hirsutism, alopecia, oily skin, seborrhea, purpura, melasma
META: Hyperglycemia
Contraindications: Pregnancy (X), breast cancer, hypersensitivity, thromboembolic disorders, reproductive cancer, genital bleeding (abnormal, undiagnosed), liver tumors
Precautions: Breastfeeding, hypertension, asthma, blood dyscrasias, CHF, diabetes mellitus, depression, migraine headache, seizure disorders, bone/gallbladder/renal/hepatic disease, family history of breast or reproductive tract cancer, smoking

PHARMACOKINETICS

Duration 24 hr, excreted in urine, feces, metabolized in liver

INTERACTIONS

Decrease: progestin effect—barbiturates, carbamazepine, fosphenytoin, phenytoin, rifampin
Drug/Herb
Increase: stimulation—black/green tea, coffee, cola nut, guarana, yerba maté
Decrease: contraception—St. John's wort
Drug/Food
Increase: caffeine level—caffeine
Drug/Lab Test
Increase: alk phos, nitrogen (urine), pregnanediol, amino acids, factors VII, VIII, IX, X
Decrease: GTT, HDL

NURSING CONSIDERATIONS

Assess:
- Weight daily: notify prescriber of weekly weight gain >5 lb
- B/P at beginning of treatment and periodically
- I&O ratio; be alert for decreasing urinary output, increasing edema
- Hepatic studies: ALT, AST, bilirubin, periodically during long-term therapy
- Edema, hypertension, cardiac symptoms, jaundice, thromboembolism
- Mental status: affect, mood, behavioral changes, depression
- Hypercalcemia

Administer:
- Titrated dose; use lowest effective dose
- One dose in AM; do not interrupt between pill packs
- With food or milk to decrease GI symptoms

Perform/provide:
- Storage in dark area

Evaluate:
- Therapeutic response: decreased abnormal uterine bleeding, absence of amenorrhea

Teach patient/family:
- About cushingoid symptoms
- To report breast lumps, vaginal bleeding, amenorrhea, edema, jaundice, dark urine, clay-colored stools, dyspnea, headache, blurred vision, abdominal pain, numbness or stiffness in legs, chest pain; men to report impotence or gynecomastia
- To take at same time of day; do not interrupt between pill packs
- To report suspected pregnancy immediately, to wait ≥3 mo after stopping medication to become pregnant
- To avoid smoking; CV reactions may occur
- Does not protect against HIV, STDs
- May mask onset of menopause

norfloxacin (℞)

(nor-flox′-a-sin)
Noroxin
Func. class.: Urinary antiinfective
Chem. class.: Fluoroquinolone

Action: Interferes with conversion of intermediate DNA fragments into high-molecular-weight DNA in bacteria, inhibits DNA gyrase
Uses: Adult urinary tract infections (including complicated) caused by *Esche-*

richia coli, Enterobacter cloacae, Proteus mirabilis, Klebsiella pneumoniae, group D strep, indole-positive *Proteus, Citrobacter freundii, Staphylococcus aureus;* uncomplicated gonorrhea; prostatitis; cystitis

DOSAGE AND ROUTES

Uncomplicated infections

• *Adult:* **PO** 400 mg bid × 3-10 days 1 hr before or 2 hr after meals

Complicated infections

• *Adult:* **PO** 400 mg bid × 10-21 days; 400 mg/day × 7-10 days in impaired renal function

Uncomplicated gonorrhea

• *Adult:* **PO** 800 mg as a single dose

Prostatitis

• *Adult:* **PO** 400 mg bid × 28 days

Renal dose

• *Adult:* **PO** CCr ≤30 ml/min 400 mg/day

Available forms: Tabs 400 mg

SIDE EFFECTS

CNS: Headache, dizziness, fatigue, somnolence, depression, insomnia

CV: **QT prolongation, torsade de pointes, dysrhythmias**

EENT: Visual disturbances

GI: Nausea, constipation, **hepatic necrosis,** increased ALT, AST, flatulence, heartburn, vomiting, diarrhea, dry mouth, **pseudomembranous colitis**

HEMA: **Agranulocytosis, hemolytic anemia**

INTEG: Rash, photosensitivity

MS: Tendinitis, **tendon rupture**

SYST: **Stevens-Johnson syndrome, angioedema**

Contraindications: Hypersensitivity to quinolones

Black Box Warning: Tendon pain/rupture, tendinitis

Precautions: Pregnancy (C), breastfeeding, children, renal disease, seizure disorders, acute MI, atrial fibrillation, dehydration, females, QT prolongation, pseudomembranous colitis, torsade de pointes

PHARMACOKINETICS

Peak 1 hr; half-life 3-4 hr; steady state 2 days; metabolized via liver; excreted in urine as active product, metabolites

INTERACTIONS

Increase: levels, toxicity—theophylline, caffeine; do not use together

⚠ ***Increase:*** QT prolongation—class IA/III antidysrhythmics, some phenothiazines, β-agonists, local anesthetics, tricyclics, bepridil, haloperidol, methadone, chloroquine, clarithromycin, droperidol, erythromycin, grepafloxacin, halofantrine, pentamidine, probucol, sparfloxacin

Increase: serum concentrations of cycloSPORINE

Increase: norfloxacin level—probenecid

Increase: anticoagulation—warfarin

Increase: toxicity risk—products metabolized by CYP1A2

Decrease: effects of norfloxacin—nitrofurantoin; monitor closely

Decrease: norfloxacin effect—antacids, iron products, sucralfate; give 2 hr apart

Drug/Herb

• Do not use acidophilus with antiinfectives; separate by several hours

Drug/Lab Test

Increase: AST, ALT, BUN, creatinine, alk phos

NURSING CONSIDERATIONS

Assess:

• Renal, hepatic studies: BUN, creatinine, AST, ALT

• I&O ratio

• For tendon pain

• CNS symptoms: insomnia, vertigo, headache, agitation, confusion

• Allergic reactions: fever, flushing, rash, urticaria, pruritus

Administer:

• After clean-catch urine for C&S

• Two daily doses if urine output is high or if patient has diabetes

Evaluate:

• Therapeutic response: decreased pain, frequency, urgency, C&S, absence of infection

Teach patient/family:

- That if dizziness occurs, to walk, perform activities with assistance
- To complete full course of product therapy, to take at same time of day
- To contact prescriber if adverse reaction occurs
- To take 1 hr before or 2 hr after meals; not to take antacids with or within 2 hr of this product; to sip water or use hard candy for dry mouth

norfloxacin ophthalmic

See Appendix B

norgestrel (℞)

(nor-jess'trel)

Ovrette

Func. class.: Progestogen

Chem. class.: Progesterone derivative

Action: Inhibits secretion of pituitary gonadotropins, which prevents follicular maturation, ovulation, stimulates growth of mammary tissue, antineoplastic action against endometrial cancer

Uses: Female contraception

DOSAGE AND ROUTES

- *Adult:* **PO** 1 tab/day

Available forms: Tabs 0.075 mg

SIDE EFFECTS

CNS: Dizziness, headache, migraines, depression, fatigue

CV: Hypotension, **thrombophlebitis,** edema, **thromboembolism, stroke, PE, MI**

EENT: Diplopia

GI: Nausea, vomiting, anorexia, cramps, increased weight, **cholestatic jaundice**

GU: Amenorrhea, cervical erosion, breakthrough bleeding, dysmenorrhea, vaginal candidiasis, breast changes, *gynecomastia, testicular atrophy, impotence,* endometriosis, **spontaneous abortion**

INTEG: Rash, urticaria, acne, hirsutism, alopecia, oily skin, seborrhea, purpura, melasma

META: Hyperglycemia

Contraindications: Pregnancy (X), breastfeeding, breast cancer, hypersensitivity, thromboembolic disorders, reproductive cancer, genital bleeding (abnormal, undiagnosed), cerebral hemorrhage

Precautions: Hypertension, asthma, blood dyscrasias, CHF, diabetes mellitus, depression, migraine headache, seizure disorders, bone/gallbladder/renal/hepatic disease, family history of breast or reproductive tract cancer

PHARMACOKINETICS

Duration 24 hr; excreted in urine, feces; metabolized in liver

INTERACTIONS

Decrease: norgestrel effect—barbiturates, carbamazepine, oxcarbazepine, phenytoin, rifampin

Drug/Lab Test

Increase: alk phos, nitrogen (urine), pregnanediol, amino acids, factors VII, VIII, IX, X

Decrease: GTT, HDL

NURSING CONSIDERATIONS

Assess:

- Weight daily; notify prescriber of weekly weight gain >5 lb
- B/P at beginning of treatment and periodically
- I&O ratio; be alert for decreasing urinary output, increasing edema
- Hepatic studies: ALT, AST, bilirubin, periodically during long-term therapy
- Edema, hypertension, cardiac symptoms, jaundice
- Mental status: affect, mood, behavioral changes, depression

Administer:

- In one dose in AM
- With food or milk to decrease GI symptoms

Perform/provide:

- Storage in dark area

Evaluate:

- Therapeutic response: absence of pregnancy

Teach patient/family:

- Avoid smoking
- About cushingoid symptoms
- To report breast lumps, vaginal bleeding, edema, jaundice, dark urine, clay-colored stools, dyspnea, headache, blurred vision, abdominal pain, numbness or stiffness in legs, chest pain
- To report suspected pregnancy, to wait ≥3 mo after stopping medication to get pregnant, use another form of birth control if a pill is missed
- To monitor blood glucose if diabetic
- That product does not protect against HIV or STDs
- To take at same time of day

nortriptyline (℞)

(nor-trip′ti-leen)

Pamelor

Func. class.: Antidepressant, tricyclic

Chem. class.: Dibenzocycloheptene—secondary amine

Do not confuse:
nortriptyline/amitriptyline

Action: Blocks reuptake of norepinephrine, serotonin into nerve endings, increasing action of norepinephrine, serotonin in nerve cells

Uses: Major depression

Unlabeled uses: Chronic pain management, PMDD, social phobia, neuropathy, panic disorder enuresis, migraine prophylaxis

DOSAGE AND ROUTES

- *Adult:* **PO** 25 mg tid or qid; may increase to 150 mg/day; may give daily dose at bedtime
- *Adolescent:* **PO** 1-3 mg/kg/day in 3-4 divided doses or daily at bedtime, max 150 mg/day
- *Child 6-12 yr (unlabeled):* **PO** 1-3 mg/kg/day in 3-4 divided doses, max 150 mg/day
- *Geriatric:* **PO** 10-25 mg at bedtime, increase by 10-25 mg at weekly intervals to desired dose; usual maintenance 75 mg/day

Available forms: Caps 10, 25, 50, 75 mg; sol 10 mg/5 ml

SIDE EFFECTS

CNS: Dizziness, drowsiness, confusion, headache, anxiety, tremors, stimulation, weakness, insomnia, nightmares, EPS (geriatric patients), increased psychiatric symptoms, **seizures**

CV: Orthostatic hypotension, ECG changes, tachycardia, **hypertension,** palpitations, **dysrhythmias**

EENT: Blurred vision, tinnitus, mydriasis

GI: Constipation, dry mouth, nausea, vomiting, **paralytic ileus,** increased appetite, cramps, epigastric distress, jaundice, **hepatitis,** stomatitis

GU: Urinary retention, **acute renal failure**

HEMA: **Agranulocytosis, thrombocytopenia, eosinophilia, leukopenia**

INTEG: Rash, urticaria, sweating, pruritus, photosensitivity

Contraindications: Pregnancy (D), hypersensitivity to tricyclics, recovery phase of MI, seizure disorders, prostatic hypertrophy

Precautions: Breastfeeding, suicidal patients, severe depression, increased intraocular pressure, closed-angle glaucoma, urinary retention, cardiac/hepatic disease, hyperthyroidism, electroshock therapy, elective surgery

Black Box Warning: Children, suicidal ideation

PHARMACOKINETICS

PO: Steady state 4-19 days; metabolized by liver; excreted by kidneys; crosses placenta; excreted in breast milk; half-life 18-28 hr

INTERACTIONS

- Heavy smoking: decreased product effect

⚠ Hyperpyretic crisis, seizures, hypertensive episode: MAOI

Increase: effects of direct-acting sympathomimetics (epinephrine), alcohol, barbiturates, benzodiazepines, CNS depressants, products increasing QT interval

Decrease: effects of guanethidine, clonidine, indirect-acting sympathomimetics (ephedrine)

Drug/Herb

• Serotonin syndrome: SAM-e, St. John's wort

Increase: anticholinergic effect—belladonna, corkwood, henbane, jimsonweed

Increase: antidepressant action—scopolia

Increase: CNS effect—hops, lavender

Drug/Lab Test

Increase: serum bilirubin, blood glucose, alk phos

Decrease: VMA, 5-HIAA

False increase: urinary catecholamines

NURSING CONSIDERATIONS

Assess:

• B/P (lying, standing), pulse q4hr; if systolic B/P drops 20 mm Hg, hold product, notify prescriber; VS q4hr in patients with CV disease

• Blood studies: CBC, leukocytes, differential, cardiac enzymes if patient is receiving long-term therapy

• Hepatic studies: AST, ALT, bilirubin

• Weight q wk; appetite may increase with product

• ECG for flattening of T wave, bundle branch block, AV block, dysrhythmias in cardiac patients

• EPS primarily in geriatric patients: rigidity, dystonia, akathisia

• Mental status changes: mood, sensorium, affect, suicidal tendencies, increase in psychiatric symptoms, depression, panic

• Urinary retention, constipation; constipation is more likely to occur in children

⚠ Withdrawal symptoms: headache, nausea, vomiting, muscle pain, weakness; do not usually occur unless product was discontinued abruptly

• Alcohol intake; if alcohol is consumed, hold dose until AM

Administer:

• Increased fluids, bulk in diet if constipation occurs

• With food, milk for GI symptoms

• Dosage at bedtime for oversedation during day; may take entire dose at bedtime; geriatric patients may not tolerate once/day dosing

• Gum, hard candy, frequent sips of water for dry mouth

• Concentrate with fruit juice, water, or milk to disguise taste

Perform/provide:

• Storage in tight, light-resistant container at room temperature

• Assistance with ambulation during beginning therapy, since drowsiness/dizziness occurs

• Safety measures including side rails, primarily for geriatric patients

• Checking to see if PO medication swallowed

Evaluate:

• Therapeutic response: decreased depression

Teach patient/family:

• That therapeutic effects may take 2-3 wk

• To use caution in driving, other activities requiring alertness because of drowsiness, dizziness, blurred vision

• To avoid alcohol ingestion, other CNS depressants; MAOIs within 14 days

• Not to discontinue medication quickly after long-term use; may cause nausea, headache, malaise

• To wear sunscreen or large hat, since photosensitivity occurs

• To report immediately urinary retention, worsening depression, suicidal thoughts/behavior

Treatment of overdose: ECG monitoring; lavage, activated charcoal; administer anticonvulsant

N

nystatin (℞)

(nye-stat'in)

Bio-Statin, Mycostatin, Nadostine ✦, Nilstat, Nystex, PMS-Nystatin ✦, Pastilles, nystatin

Func. class.: Antifungal

Chem. class.: Amphoteric polyene

Action: Interferes with fungal DNA replication; binds sterols in fungal cell membrane, which increases permeability, leaking of cell nutrients

Uses: Lozenges, oral: *Candida* species causing oral, intestinal infections

DOSAGE AND ROUTES

Oral infection

- *Adult:* **SUSP** 400,000-600,000 units qid, use ½ dose in each side of mouth, swish and swallow
- *Infant:* **SUSP** 200,000 units qid (100,000 units in each side of mouth)
- *Newborn and premature infant:* **SUSP** 100,000 units qid
- *Adult and child:* **TROCHES** 200,000-400,000 units qid × up to 2 wk

GI infection

- *Adult:* **PO** 500,000-1,000,000 units tid

Available forms: Tabs 500,000 units; powder for oral susp 50 million, 150 million, 500 million, 1 billion, 2 billion, 5 billion units; susp 100,000 units per ml; troches 200,000 units; oral caps 500,000, 1,000,000 units

Side effects/adverse reactions:

GI: Nausea, vomiting, anorexia, diarrhea, cramps

INTEG: Rash, urticaria (rare)

Contraindications: Hypersensitivity

Precautions: Pregnancy (B)

PHARMACOKINETICS

PO: Little absorption, excreted in feces

NURSING CONSIDERATIONS

Assess:

- For allergic reaction: rash, urticaria; product may have to be discontinued
- For predisposing factors: antibiotic therapy, pregnancy, diabetes mellitus, sexual partner infection (vaginal infections)

Administer:

- Oral susp dose by placing ½ in each cheek, then swallow
- Topical dose after cleansing area; mouth may be swabbed

Perform/provide:

- Storage in refrigerator for oral susp; tabs in tight, light-resistant containers at room temperature

Evaluate:

- Therapeutic response: culture negative for *Candida*

Teach patient/family:

- That long-term therapy may be needed to clear infection; to complete entire course of medication
- Using no commercial mouthwashes for mouth infection
- Shake susp before measuring each dose
- To notify prescriber of irritation; product may have to be discontinued

nystatin topical

See Appendix B

nystatin vaginal antifungal

See Appendix B

octreotide (℞)

(ok-tree'oh-tide)

Sandostatin, Sandostatin LAR Depot

Func. class.: Hormone, antidiarrheal

Chem. class.: Octapeptide

Action: A potent growth hormone similar to somatostatin

Uses: Sandostatin: acromegaly, improves symptoms in carcinoid tumors, vasoactive intestinal peptide tumors (VIPomas); LAR Depot: long-term maintenance of acromegaly, carcinoid tumors, VIPomas

Unlabeled uses: GI fistula, variceal bleeding, diarrheal conditions, pancreatic fistula, irritable bowel syndrome, dumping syndrome

DOSAGE AND ROUTES

Acromegaly

• *Adult:* **SUBCUT/IV** (Sandostatin) 50-100 mcg bid-tid, adjust q2wk based on growth hormone levels, or **IM** (Sandostatin LAR) 20 mg q4wk × 3 mo, adjust by growth hormone levels

VIPomas

• *Adult:* **SUBCUT/IV** (Sandostatin) 200-300 mcg/day in 2-4 doses for 2 wk, max 450 mcg/day, or **IM** (Sandostatin LAR) 20 mg q2wk × 2 mo, adjust dose

Carcinoid tumors

• *Adult:* **SUBCUT/IV** (Sandostatin) 100-600 mcg/day in 2-4 doses for 2 wk, titrated to patient response, or **IM** (Sandostatin LAR) 20 mg q4wk × 2 mo, adjust dose

GI fistula

• *Adult:* **SUBCUT** (Sandostatin) 50-200 mcg q8hr

Antidiarrheal in AIDS patients (unlabeled)

• *Adult:* **SUBCUT** (Sandostatin) 50 mcg q8hr prn, increase to 500 mcg q8hr

Irritable bowel syndrome (unlabeled)

• *Adult:* **SUBCUT** (Sandostatin) 100 mcg single dose to 125 mcg bid

Dumping syndrome (unlabeled)

• *Adult:* **SUBCUT** (Sandostatin) 50-150 mcg/day

Variceal bleeding (unlabeled)

• *Adult:* **IV** (Sandostatin) 25-50 mcg/hr **CONT IV INF** for 18 hr-5 days

Available forms: Inj (Sandostatin) 0.05, 0.1, 0.2, 0.5, 1 mg/ml; inj (LAR depot) 10, 20, 30 mg/5 ml

SIDE EFFECTS

CNS: Headache, dizziness, fatigue, weakness, depression, anxiety, tremors, **seizure,** paranoia

CV: Sinus bradycardia, conduction abnormalities, **dysrhythmias,** chest pain, shortness of breath, thrombophlebitis, ischemia, **CHF,** hypertension, palpitations, **QT prolongation, ST-T wave changes**

ENDO: Hypo/hyperglycemia, ketosis, hypothyroidism, galactorrhea, diabetes insipidus

GI: Diarrhea, nausea, abdominal pain, vomiting, flatulence, distention, constipation, **hepatitis,** increased LFTs, **GI bleeding, pancreatitis,** cholelithiasis, ileus

GU: UTI

HEMA: Hematoma of inj site, bruise

INTEG: Rash, urticaria, pain; inflammation at inj site

MS: Joint and muscle pain

Contraindications: Hypersensitivity

Precautions: Pregnancy (B), breastfeeding, children, geriatric patients, diabetes mellitus, hypothyroidism, renal disease

PHARMACOKINETICS

Absorbed rapidly, completely, peak ½ hr, half-life 1.7 hr, duration 12 hr, excreted unchanged in urine

INTERACTIONS

Increase: QT prolongation—other products that prolong QT

Decrease: effect of—cycloSPORINE

Drug/Food

Decrease: absorption of dietary fat, vit B_{12} levels

Drug/Lab Test

Decrease: T_4

NURSING CONSIDERATIONS

Assess:

• Growth hormone antibodies, IGF-1, 1-4 hr intervals for 8-12 hr post dose in acromegaly; 5-HIAA, plasma serotonin; blood glucose, serotonin levels (carcinoid tumors), plasma substance P, plasma vasoactive intestinal peptide (VIP) (VIPoma)

• Thyroid function tests: T_3, T_4, T_7, TSH to identify hypothyroidism

• Fecal fat, serum carotene

• Allergic reaction: rash, itching, fever, nausea, wheezing

• For cardiac status: bradycardia, conduction abnormalities, dysrhythmias;

O

monitor ECG for QT prolongation, low voltage, axis shifts, early repolarization, R/S transition, early wave progression

Administer:

IM route

- Reconstitute with diluent provided; give into gluteal

SUBCUT route

- Rotate inj site; use hip, thigh, abdomen
- Avoid using medication that is cold; allow to reach room temperature

IV route

- May use IV bolus if required; give over 3 min
- To use by intermittent inf, dilute in 50-200 ml D_5W, 0.9% NaCl; give 15-30 min
- In an emergency carcinoid crisis, give rapid bolus

Perform/provide:

- Storage in refrigerator for unopened amps, vials; or room temperature for 2 wk, protect from light; do not use discolored or cloudy sol

Evaluate:

- Therapeutic response: relief of diarrhea in AIDS, improves symptoms in carcinoid or VIP tumors, data is insufficient if products decrease size/rate of tumor growth, decreasing symptoms of acromegaly

Teach patient/family:

- Regular assessments are required
- Regarding SUBCUT inj if patient or other persons will be giving inj
- To change position slowly to prevent orthostatic hypotension

ofloxacin (℞)

(o-flox′a-sin)

Func. class.: Antiinfective

Chem. class.: Fluoroquinolone

Action: Interferes with conversion of intermediate DNA fragments into high-molecular-weight DNA in bacteria, inhibits DNA gyrase

Uses: Treatment of lower respiratory tract infections (pneumonia, bronchitis), genitourinary infections (prostatitis, UTIs) caused by *Escherichia coli, Klebsiella pneumoniae, Chlamydia trachomatis,* skin and skin structure infections; conjunctivitis (ophthalmic) (refer to Appendix B)

Unlabeled uses: Leprosy

DOSAGE AND ROUTES

Lower respiratory tract infections/ skin and skin structure infections

- *Adult:* **PO/IV** 400 mg q12hr × 10 days

Cervicitis, urethritis

- *Adult:* **PO/IV** 300 mg q12hr × 7 days

Prostatitis

- *Adult:* **PO/IV** 300 mg q12hr × 6 wk

Urinary tract infection

- *Adult:* **PO/IV** 200 mg q12hr × 3-10 days

Pelvic inflammatory disease

- *Adult:* **PO** 400 mg q12hr × 10-14 days

Renal dose

- *Adult:* **PO** CCr 20-50 ml/min give q24hr; CCr <20 ml/min give ½ of dose q24hr

Available forms: Tabs 200, 300, 400 mg; inj 20, 40 mg/ml; 200 mg/50 ml; 400 mg/100 ml

SIDE EFFECTS

CNS: Dizziness, headache, fatigue, somnolence, depression, insomnia, lethargy, malaise, **seizures,** vertigo

CV: **QT prolongation, dysrhythmias,** chest pain

EENT: Visual disturbances

GI: Diarrhea, nausea, vomiting, anorexia, flatulence, heartburn, dry mouth, increased AST, ALT, abdominal pain, constipation, **pseudomembranous colitis,** abnormal taste

HEMA: **Blood dyscrasias**

INTEG: Rash, pruritus, photosensitivity

MS: Tendinitis, **tendon rupture, rhabdomyolysis**

SYST: **Anaphylaxis, Stevens-Johnson syndrome, toxic epidermal necrolysis**

Contraindications: QT prolongation, hypersensitivity to quinolones

Precautions: Pregnancy (C), breastfeeding, children, geriatric patients, renal disease, seizure disorders, excessive sunlight, hypokalemia

Black Box Warning: Tendon pain/rupture, tendinitis

PHARMACOKINETICS

PO: Peak 1-2 hr; half-life 4-8 hr; steady state 2 days; excreted in urine as active product, metabolites; 90%-95% bioavailability

INTERACTIONS

• May alter blood glucose levels: antidiabetics

• Possible theophylline toxicity: theophylline, do not use together

⚠ ***Increase:*** QT prolongation—class IA/III antidysrhythmics, some phenothiazines, β-agonists, local anesthetics, tricyclics, bepridil, haloperidol, methadone, chloroquine, clarithromycin, droperidol, erythromycin, grepafloxacin, halofantrine, pentamidine, probucol, sparfloxacin

Increase: CNS stimulation, seizures—NSAIDs

Increase: anticoagulation—warfarin

Decrease: absorption—antacids with aluminum, magnesium, iron products, sucralfate, zinc products; separate by 2 hr

Drug/Herb

• Do not use acidophilus with antiinfectives; separate by several hours

Increase: effect—cola nut

NURSING CONSIDERATIONS

Assess:

• Renal, hepatic studies: BUN, creatinine, AST, ALT

• Cardiac status: QT prolongation

• CNS symptoms: insomnia, vertigo, headache, agitation, confusion

• Allergic reactions: rash, flushing, urticaria, pruritus

Administer:

PO route

• 2 hr before or 2 hr after antacids, calcium, iron, zinc products

• After clean-catch urine for C&S

IV route

• Dilute to 4 mg/ml with 0.9% NaCl, D_5W, D_5/LR, D_5/0.9% NaCl, 5% $NaCO_3$, D_5 plasmalyte 56, sodium lactate; give over 1 hr or more

Y-site compatibilities: Ampicillin, bivalrudin, cefotaxime, ceftazidime, cisatracurium, clindamycin, docetaxel, etoposide, gemcitabine, gentamicin, granisetron, linezolid, piperacillin, propofol, remifentanil, thiotepa, tobramycin, vancomycin

Perform/provide:

• Storage for 2 wk refrigerated or 6 mo frozen after reconstitution

Evaluate:

• Therapeutic response: urine culture, absence of symptoms of infection

Teach patient/family:

• That if dizziness or light-headedness occurs, ambulate, perform activities with assistance

• To complete full course of therapy

• To avoid iron- or mineral-containing supplements within 2 hr before or after dose

• To avoid sun exposure, photosensitivity can occur

O

ofloxacin ophthalmic

See Appendix B

olanzapine (℞)

(oh-lanz'a-peen)

Zyprexa Zydis, Zyprexa, Zyprexa IntraMuscular

Func. class.: Antipsychotic, neuroleptic

Chem. class.: Thienbenzodiazepine

Do not confuse:

olanzapine/osalazine

Zyprexa/Celexa/Zyrtec

Action: Unknown; may mediate antipsychotic activity by both DOPamine and serotonin type 2 (5-HT2) antagonist; also, may antagonize muscarinic receptors, histaminic (H_1)- and α-adrenergic receptors

Uses: Schizophrenia, acute manic episodes in bipolar disorder
Unlabeled uses: Dementia related to Alzheimer's disease, OCD

DOSAGE AND ROUTES

Schizophrenia
• *Adult:* **PO** 5-10 mg/day initially, may increase dosage by 5 mg at 1 wk or more intervals; **ORALLY DISINTEGRATING** tabs open blister pack, place tab on tongue, let disintegrate, swallow, max 20 mg/day
• *Geriatric:* **PO** 5 mg, may increase cautiously at 1-wk intervals, max 20 mg/day

Bipolar mania
• *Adult:* **PO** 10-15 mg/day, may increase dose >24 hr by 5 mg

Agitation associated with schizophrenia, bipolar I mania
• *Adult:* **IM** 10 mg

Dementia in geriatric patients (unlabeled)
• *Adult:* **PO** 2.5-5 mg/day

Available forms: Tab 2.5, 5, 7.5, 10, 15, 20 mg; orally disintegrating tabs 5, 10, 15, 20 mg; powder for inj 10 mg

SIDE EFFECTS

CNS: EPS: (pseudoparkinsonism, akathisia, dystonia, tardive dyskinesia), **seizures,** headache, **neuroleptic malignant syndrome (rare),** agitation, nervousness, hostility, *dizziness,* hypertonia, *tremor,* euphoria, confusion, *drowsiness,* fatigue, *abnormal gait, insomnia, fever*
CV: Hypotension, tachycardia, chest pain, **heart failure, sudden death (geriatric patients, IM),** orthostatic hypotension
ENDO: Increased prolactin levels, hypoglycemia
GI: Dry mouth, nausea, vomiting, appetite, dyspepsia, anorexia, *constipation,* abdominal pain, *weight gain,* jaundice, **hepatitis**
GU: Urinary retention, urinary frequency, enuresis, impotence, amenorrhea, gynecomastia, breast engorgement, premenstrual syndrome
HEMA: **Neutropenia**
INTEG: Rash
MISC: Peripheral edema, accidental injury, hypertonia, hyperlipidemia
MS: Joint pain, twitching
RESP: Cough, pharyngitis; **fatal pneumonia (geriatric patients, IM)**
Contraindications: Hypersensitivity
Precautions: Pregnancy (C), breastfeeding, geriatric patients, hypertension, cardiac/renal/hepatic disease, diabetes, agranulocytosis, abrupt discontinuation, Asian patients, closed-angle glaucoma, coma, leukopenia, QT prolongation, tardive dyskinesia, torsade de pointes
Black Box Warning: Dementia

PHARMACOKINETICS

Well absorbed (60%), peak 6 hr, metabolized by liver, glucuronidation/oxidation by CYP1A2 and CYP2D6, excreted in urine (57%), feces (30%), 93% bound to plasma proteins, half-life 21-54 hr, extended in geriatric patients; clearance decreased in women, increased in smokers

INTERACTIONS

Increase: sedation—other CNS depressants, alcohol, barbiturate anesthetics, antihistamines, sedatives/hypnotics, antidepressants
Increase: olanzapine levels—CYP1A2 inhibitors (fluvoxamine)
Increase: hypotension—antihypertensives, alcohol, diazepam
Increase: anticholinergic effects—anticholinergics
Decrease: olanzapine levels—CYP1A2 inducers: carbamazepine, omeprazole, rifampin
Decrease: antiparkinson activity—levodopa, bromocriptine, other DOPamine agonists

Drug/Herb
Increase: EPS—betel palm, kava
Increase: effect—cola tree, hops, nettle, nutmeg

Drug/Lab Test
Increase: LFTs, prolactin, CPK

NURSING CONSIDERATIONS

Assess:

- Mental status: orientation, mood, behavior, presence of hallucinations and type before initial administration and monthly
- Swallowing of PO medication: check for hoarding or giving of medication to other patients
- I&O ratio; palpate bladder if low urinary output occurs, urinary retention may be the cause especially in geriatric patients
- Bilirubin, CBC
- Urinalysis recommended before, during prolonged therapy
- Affect, orientation, LOC, reflexes, gait, coordination, sleep pattern disturbances
- B/P sitting, standing, lying: take pulse and respirations q4hr during initial treatment; establish baseline before starting treatment; report drops of 30 mm Hg; obtain baseline ECG
- Dizziness, faintness, palpitations, tachycardia on rising

⚠ Geriatric patients for serious reactions: fatal pneumonia, heart failure, stroke leading to death (IM)

⚠ For neuroleptic malignant syndrome: hyperpyrexia, muscle rigidity, increased CPK, altered mental status, for acute dystonia (check chewing, swallowing, eyes, pill rolling)

- EPS, including akathisia (inability to sit still, no pattern to movements), tardive dyskinesia (bizarre movements of the jaw, mouth, tongue, extremities), pseudoparkinsonism (rigidity, tremors, pill rolling, shuffling gait)
- Skin turgor daily
- Constipation, urinary retention daily; increase bulk, H_2O in diet
- Weight gain, hyperglycemia, metabolic changes in diabetes

Administer:

- Anticholinergic agent for EPS
- Decreased dose in geriatric patients

PO route

- With full glass of water, milk; or with food to decrease GI upset
- Orally disintegrating tabs: open blister pack; place tab on tongue until dissolved; swallow; no water needed

IM route

- Dissolve contents of vials with 2.1 ml sterile water for injection (5 mg/ml), use immediately
- Do not use IV or SUBCUT
- Inject slowly, deep into muscle mass

Perform/provide:

- Decreased stimuli by dimming light, avoiding loud noises
- Supervised ambulation until stabilized on medication; do not involve in strenuous exercise program because fainting is possible; patient should not stand still for long periods
- Increased fluids, bulk in diet to prevent constipation
- Sips of water, candy, gum for dry mouth
- Storage in tight, light-resistant container

Evaluate:

- Therapeutic response: decrease in emotional excitement, hallucinations, delusion, paranoia, reorganization of patterns of thought, speech

Teach patient/family:

- To use good oral hygiene; frequent rinsing of mouth, sugarless gum, candy, ice chips for dry mouth
- To avoid hazardous activities until product response is determined
- That orthostatic hypotension occurs often and to rise from sitting or lying position gradually
- To avoid hot tubs, hot showers, tub baths, since hypotension may occur
- To avoid abrupt withdrawal of this product, or EPS may result; product should be withdrawn slowly
- To avoid OTC preparations (cough, hay fever, cold) unless approved by prescriber, since serious product interactions may occur; avoid use with alcohol, CNS depressants; increased drowsiness may occur
- That in hot weather, heat stroke may occur; take extra precautions to stay cool

Treatment of overdose: Lavage if orally ingested; provide airway; do not induce vomiting or use epinephrine

olmesartan (℞)

(ol-meh-sar'tan)
Benicar
Func. class.: Antihypertensive
Chem. class.: Angiotensin II receptor (type AT_1) antagonist

Action: Blocks the vasoconstrictor and aldosterone-secreting effects of angiotensin II; selectively blocks the binding of angiotensin II to the AT_1 receptor found in tissues

Uses: Hypertension, alone or in combination with other antihypertensives

DOSAGE AND ROUTES

- *Adult:* **PO** Single agent 20 mg/day initially in patients who are not volume depleted, may be increased to 40 mg/day if needed after 2 wk

Available forms: Tabs 5, 20, 40 mg

SIDE EFFECTS

CNS: Dizziness, fatigue, headache, insomnia

CV: Chest pain, peripheral edema, tachycardia

EENT: Sinusitis, rhinitis, pharyngitis

GI: Diarrhea, abdominal pain

MS: Arthralgia, pain

RESP: Upper respiratory infection, bronchitis

SYST: **Angioedema**

Contraindications: Hypersensitivity

Black Box Warning: Pregnancy (D) 2nd/3rd trimesters

Precautions: Pregnancy (C) 1st trimester, breastfeeding, children, geriatric patients, hepatic disease, CHF

PHARMACOKINETICS

Peak 12 hr, excreted in urine and feces, half-life 13 hr, protein binding 99%

INTERACTIONS

Increase: antihypertensive effects—other antihypertensives, diuretics

Increase: hyperkalemia—potassium supplements, potassium-sparing diuretics

Increase: effect of lithium

Decrease: antihypertensive effect—NSAIDs, salicylates

Drug/Herb

Increase: toxicity, death—aconite

Increase: antihypertensive effect—barberry, betony, black catechu, black cohosh, bloodroot, broom, burdock, cat's claw, dandelion, goldenseal, hawthorn, Irish moss, Jamaican dogwood, kelp, khella, mistletoe, parsley

Increase or decrease: antihypertensive effect—astragalus, cola tree

Decrease: antihypertensive effect—coltsfoot, guarana, khat, licorice, yohimbe

NURSING CONSIDERATIONS

Assess:

⚠ For pregnancy; this product can cause fetal death when given in pregnancy

- Response and adverse reactions especially in renal disease
- B/P, pulse q4hr; note rate, rhythm, quality; electrolytes: K, Na, Cl; baselines in renal, hepatic studies before therapy begins
- Skin turgor, dryness of mucous membranes for hydration status; for angioedema: facial swelling, dyspnea

Administer:

- Without regard to meals

Evaluate:

- Therapeutic response: decreased B/P

Teach patient/family:

- To comply with dosage schedule, even if feeling better
- To notify prescriber of mouth sores, fever, swelling of hands or feet, irregular heartbeat, chest pain
- That excessive perspiration, dehydration, vomiting, diarrhea may lead to fall in B/P; to consult prescriber if these occur
- That product may cause dizziness, fainting; light-headedness may occur
- To rise slowly to sitting or standing position to minimize orthostatic hypotension
- To notify prescriber immediately if pregnant; not to use during breastfeeding

• To avoid all OTC medications, unless approved by prescriber
• To inform all health care providers of medication use
• To use proper technique for obtaining B/P and acceptable parameters

olopatadine nasal agent
See Appendix B

olopatadine ophthalmic
See Appendix B

olsalazine (℞)
(ohl-sal'ah-zeen)
Dipentum
Func. class.: Antiinflammatory
Chem. class.: Salicylate derivative

Action: Bioconverted to 5-aminosalicylic acid, which decreases inflammation
Uses: Maintenance of remission of ulcerative colitis in patients intolerant to sulfasalazine

DOSAGE AND ROUTES
• *Adult:* **PO** 500 mg bid
Available forms: Caps 250 mg

SIDE EFFECTS
CNS: Headache, hallucinations, depression, vertigo, fatigue, dizziness
GI: Nausea, vomiting, abdominal pain, **hepatitis,** diarrhea, bloating, pancreatitis
HEMA: **Leukopenia, neutropenia, thrombocytopenia, agranulocytosis, anemia**
INTEG: Rash, dermatitis, urticaria
Contraindications: Hypersensitivity to salicylates
Precautions: Pregnancy (C), breastfeeding, children <14 yr; impaired renal/hepatic function; severe allergy; bronchial asthma

PHARMACOKINETICS
Partially absorbed, peak 1½ hr, half-life 5-10 hr, excreted in urine as 5-aminosalicylic acid and metabolites, crosses placenta

INTERACTIONS
Drug/Lab Test
Increase: AST, ALT

NURSING CONSIDERATIONS
Assess:
⚠ Blood dyscrasias: skin rash, fever, sore throat, bruising, bleeding, fatigue, joint pain (rare)
• Allergic reaction: rash, dermatitis, urticaria, pruritus, dyspnea, bronchospasm
Administer:
• Medication after C&S; repeat C&S after full course of medication
• Total daily dose evenly spaced to minimize GI intolerance, with food
Perform/provide:
• Storage in tight, light-resistant container at room temperature
Evaluate:
• Therapeutic response: absence of fever, mucus in stools
Teach patient/family:
• To report diarrhea
• To take even if feeling better

omalizumab (℞)
(oh-mah-lye-zoo'mab)
Xolair
Func. class.: Antiasthmatic
Chem. class.: Monoclonal antibody

Action: Recombinant DNA-derived humanized IgG murine monoclonal antibody that selectively binds to IgE to limit the release of mediators in the allergic response
Uses: Moderate to severe persistent asthma

Unlabeled uses: Seasonal allergic rhinitis, food allergy

DOSAGE AND ROUTES

• *Adult/adolescent/child ≥12 yr:* **SUBCUT** 150-375 mg × 2-4 wk, divide inj into 2 sites if dose is >150 mg; dose is adjusted based on IgE levels and significant changes in body weight

Available forms: Powder for inj, lyophilized 202.5 mg (150 mg/1.2 ml after reconstitution)

SIDE EFFECTS

CV: **Heart failure,** cardiomyopathy, hypotension

HEMA: **Serious systemic eosinophilia**

INTEG: Pruritus, dermatitis, inj site reactions, rash

MISC: Earache, dizziness, fatigue, pain, **malignancies**, viral infections, **anaphylaxis, thrombocytopenia,** headache

MS: Arthralgia, fracture, leg, arm pain

RESP: Sinusitis, upper respiratory infections, pharyngitis, pulmonary hypertension, **bronchospasm**

Contraindications: Hypersensitivity to hamster protein

Black Box Warning: Hypersensitivity to this product

Precautions: Pregnancy (B), breastfeeding, children <12 yr, acute attacks of asthma, lymphoma, nephrotic disease, bronchospasm, neoplastic disease, status asthmatics

PHARMACOKINETICS

Slowly absorbed, peak 7-8 days, half-life 26 days, degradation by liver, excretion in bile

INTERACTIONS

• Use cautiously with live virus vaccines

NURSING CONSIDERATIONS

Assess:

• Respiratory rate, rhythm, depth; auscultate lung fields bilaterally; notify prescriber of abnormalities; monitor pulmonary function tests; serum IgE

• ⚠ Anaphylaxis, allergic reactions: rash, urticaria, inability to breathe, edema of throat; product should be discontinued; have emergency equipment available, observe for 2 hr, reaction can occur up to 24 hr

Administer:

SUBCUT route

• Reconstitute using 1.4 ml sterile water for inj; gently swirl to dissolve; invert vial to allow to drain; use large-bore needle to withdraw medication; replace needle with small-bore needle

• Given q2-4wk, product is viscous; if >150 mg is given divide into two sites; the inj may take 5-10 seconds to administer

Evaluate:

• Therapeutic response: ability to breathe more easily

Teach patient/family:

• That improvement will not be immediate

• Not to stop taking or decrease current asthma medications unless instructed by prescriber

• Avoid live virus vaccines while taking this product

• To report signs of allergic reaction

omeprazole (OTC, ℞)

(oh-mep′ray-zole)

Losec ✦, Prilosec, Prilosec OTC

Func. class.: Antiulcer, proton pump inhibitor

Chem. class.: Benzimidazole

Do not confuse:

Prilosec/Prinivil/Prozac/predniSONE

Action: Suppresses gastric secretion by inhibiting hydrogen/potassium ATPase enzyme system in gastric parietal cell; characterized as gastric acid pump inhibitor, since it blocks final step of acid production

Uses: Gastroesophageal reflux disease (GERD), severe erosive esophagitis, poorly responsive systemic GERD, pathologic hypersecretory conditions (Zollinger-Ellison

syndrome, systemic mastocytosis, multiple endocrine adenomas); treatment of active duodenal ulcers with or without anti-infectives for *Helicobacter pylori*
Unlabeled uses: GERD-related laryngitis, enhancing pancreatin

DOSAGE AND ROUTES

Active duodenal ulcers
- *Adult:* **PO** 20 mg/day × 4-8 wk; associated with *H. pylori* 40 mg QAM and clarithromycin 500 mg tid on days 1-14, then 20 mg/day on days 15-28

Severe erosive esophagitis/poorly responsive GERD
- *Adult:* **PO** (del rel cap/del rel susp) 20 mg/day × 4-8 wk

Pathologic hypersecretory conditions
- *Adult:* **PO** 60 mg/day; may increase to 120 mg tid; daily doses >80 mg should be divided

Gastric ulcer
- *Adult:* **PO** 40 mg/day 4-8 wk
- *Geriatric:* **PO** ≤20 mg/day

Heartburn (OTC)
- *Adult:* **PO** 1 delayed rel tab (20 mg)/day before AM meal with glass of water

Laryngitis (unlabeled)
- *Adult:* **PO** 20-40 mg at bedtime × 6-24 wk or 20 mg bid × 4-12 wk

Available forms: Del rel caps 10, 20, 40 mg; del rel tabs (Prilosec OTC) 20 mg; granules for oral susp 2.5, 10 mg (del rel)

SIDE EFFECTS

CNS: Headache, dizziness, asthenia
CV: Chest pain, angina, tachycardia, bradycardia, palpitations, peripheral edema, **heart failure**
EENT: Tinnitus, taste perversion
GI: Diarrhea, abdominal pain, vomiting, nausea, constipation, flatulence, acid regurgitation, abdominal swelling, anorexia, irritable colon, esophageal candidiasis, dry mouth, **hepatic failure**
GU: UTI, urinary frequency, increased creatinine, **proteinuria, hematuria,** testicular pain, glycosuria
HEMA: **Pancytopenia, thrombocytopenia, neutropenia, leukocytosis,** anemia
INTEG: Rash, dry skin, urticaria, pruritus, alopecia
META: Hypoglycemia, increased hepatic enzymes, weight gain
MISC: Back pain, fever, fatigue, malaise
RESP: Upper respiratory infections, cough, epistaxis, **pneumonia**
SYST: **Angioedema, exfoliative dermatitis, Stevens-Johnson syndrome, toxic epidermal necrolysis**

Contraindications: Hypersensitivity
Precautions: Pregnancy (C), breastfeeding, children

PHARMACOKINETICS

Bioavailabity 30%-40%; peak ½-3½ hr; half-life ½-1 hr; protein binding 95%; eliminated in urine as metabolites and in feces; in geriatric patients elimination rate decreased, bioavailability increased; metabolized by CYP450 enzyme system

INTERACTIONS

Increase: bleeding—warfarin
Increase: serum levels of diazepam, phenytoin, flurazepam, triazolam, cycloSPORINE, disulfiram, digoxin
Decrease: effect of iron salts, ketoconazole, cyanocobalamin, calcium carbonate, ampicillin, indinavir, gefitinib

Drug/Lab Test
Increase: alk phos, AST, ALT, bilirubin, gastrin

NURSING CONSIDERATIONS

Assess:
- GI system: bowel sounds q8hr, abdomen for pain, swelling, anorexia
- Hepatic enzymes: AST, ALT, alk phos during treatment; blood studies: CBC, differential during treatment

Administer:
- Swallow caps whole; do not crush or chew

- Caps may be opened and sprinkled over applesauce
- Before eating, usually in the AM

Evaluate:

- Therapeutic response: absence of epigastric pain, swelling, fullness

Teach patient/family:

- To report severe diarrhea; product may have to be discontinued
- That diabetic patient should know hypoglycemia may occur
- To avoid hazardous activities; dizziness may occur
- To avoid alcohol, salicylates, ibuprofen; may cause GI irritation

ondansetron (℞)

(on-dan-seh'tron)

Zofran, Zofran ODT

Func. class.: Antiemetic

Chem. class.: 5-HT_3 receptor antagonist

Do not confuse:

Zofran/Zantac

Action: Prevents nausea, vomiting by blocking serotonin peripherally, centrally, and in the small intestine

Uses: Prevention of nausea, vomiting associated with cancer chemotherapy, radiotherapy, and prevention of postoperative nausea, vomiting

Unlabeled uses: Pruritus (rectal use), alcoholism, hyperemesis gravidarum

DOSAGE AND ROUTES

Prevention of nausea/vomiting of cancer chemotherapy

- *Adult and child 4-18 yr:* **IV** 0.15 mg/kg infused over 15 min, 30 min before start of cancer chemotherapy; 0.15 mg/kg given 4 hr and 8 hr after first dose or 32 mg as a single dose; dilute in 50 ml of D_5 or 0.9% NaCl before giving; **RECT** (unlabeled) 16 mg/day 2 hr prior to chemotherapy; **PO** 8 mg ½ hr prior to chemotherapy, repeat 4, 8 hr after 1st dose
- *Child ≥4 yr:* **PO** 4 mg ½ hr prior to chemotherapy

Prevention of nausea/vomiting of radiotherapy

- *Adult:* **PO** 8 mg tid, may repeat q8hr

Prevention of postoperative nausea/vomiting

- *Adult:* **IV/IM** 4 mg undiluted over >30 sec prior to induction of anesthesia
- *Child 2-12 yr:* **IV** 0.1 mg/kg (≤40 kg); **IV** 4 mg (≥40 kg) give ≥30 sec

Hepatic dose

- *Adult:* **PO/IM/IV** Max dose 8 mg/day

Hyperemesis gravidarum (unlabeled)

- *Adult:* **PO/IV** 4-8 mg bid-tid

Pruritus (unlabeled)

- *Adult:* **PO** 4 mg bid

Alcoholism (unlabeled)

- *Adult:* **PO** 4 mcg/kg bid

Available forms: Inj 2 mg/ml, 32 mg/50 ml (premixed); tabs 4, 8 mg; oral sol 4 mg/5 ml; oral disintegrating tabs 4, 8 mg

SIDE EFFECTS

CNS: Headache, dizziness, drowsiness, fatigue, EPS

GI: Diarrhea, constipation, abdominal pain, dry mouth

MISC: Rash, **bronchospasm** (rare), *musculoskeletal pain, wound problems, shivering, fever, hypoxia, urinary retention*

Contraindications: Hypersensitivity; phenylketonuric hypersensitivity (oral disintegrating tab), torsade de pointes

Precautions: Pregnancy (B), breastfeeding, children, geriatric patients, granisetron hypersensitivity

PHARMACOKINETICS

IV: Mean elimination half-life 3.5-4.7 hr, plasma protein binding 70%-76%, extensively metabolized in the liver, excreted 45%-60% in urine

INTERACTIONS

Decrease: ondansetron effect—rifampin, carbamazepine, phenytoin

NURSING CONSIDERATIONS

Assess:

- For absence of nausea, vomiting during chemotherapy
- Hypersensitivity reaction: rash, bronchospasm
- For EPS: shuffling gait, tremors, grimacing, rigidity

Administer:

PO route

- Oral disintegrating tab: do not push through foil; gently remove and immediately place on tongue to dissolve; swallow with saliva

IV route

- After diluting a single dose in 50 ml NS or D_5W, 0.45% NaCl or NS; give over 15 min

Additive compatibilities: Cisplatin, cyclophosphamide, cytarabine, dacarbazine, dexamethasone, DOXOrubicin, etoposide, fluconazole, hydromorphone, meperidine, methotrexate, morphine

Solution compatibilities: May also be diluted with D_5W, lactated Ringer's, D_5/0.9% NaCl, D_5/0.45% NaCl

Y-site compatibilities: Aldesleukin, amifostine, amikacin, aztreonam, bleomycin, carboplatin, carmustine, cefazolin, cefmetazole, cefotaxime, cefoxitin, ceftazidime, ceftizoxime, cefuroxime, chlorproMAZINE, cimetidine, cisatracurium, cisplatin, cladribine, clindamycin, cyclophosphamide, cytarabine, dacarbazine, dactinomycin, DAUNOrubicin, dexamethasone, diphenhydrAMINE, DOPamine, DOXOrubicin, DOXOrubicin liposome, doxycycline, droperidol, etoposide, famotidine, filgrastim, floxuridine, fluconazole, fludarabine, gallium, gentamicin, haloperidol, heparin, hydrocortisone, hydromorphone, hydrOXYzine, ifosfamide, imipenem/cilastatin, magnesium sulfate, mannitol, mechlorethamine, melphalan, meperidine, mesna, methotrexate, metoclopramide, miconazole, mitomycin, mitoxantrone, morphine, paclitaxel, pentostatin, piperacillin/tazobactam, potassium chloride, prochlorperazine, promethazine, ranitidine, remifentanil, streptozocin, teniposide, thiotepa, ticarcillin, ticarcillin/clavulanate, vancomycin, vinBLAStine, vinCRIStine, vinorelbine, zidovudine

Perform/provide:

- Storage at room temperature 48 hr after dilution

Evaluate:

- Therapeutic response: absence of nausea, vomiting during cancer chemotherapy

Teach patient/family:

- To report diarrhea, constipation, rash, or changes in respirations or discomfort at insertion site
- Headache requiring analgesic is common

orlistat (℞, OTC)

(or′lih-stat)

Alli, Xenical

Func. class.: Weight control agent

Chem. class.: Lipase inhibitor

Action: Inhibits the absorption of dietary fats

Uses: Obesity management

DOSAGE AND ROUTES

- *Adult:* **PO** (Alli) 60 mg, (Xenical) 120 mg tid with each main meal containing fat, max 360 mg/day

Available forms: Caps (Alli) 60 mg, (Xenical) 120 mg

SIDE EFFECTS

CNS: Insomnia, depression, anxiety, dizziness, headache, fatigue

GI: Oily spotting, flatus with discharge, fecal urgency, fatty/oily stool, oily evacuation, fecal incontinence, frequent defecation, nausea, vomiting, abdominal pain, infectious diarrhea, rectal pain, tooth disorder, hypovitaminosis, **hepatic failure, hepatitis, pancreatitis**

GU: UTI, vaginitis, menstrual irregularity

INTEG: Dry skin, rash

MS: Back pain, arthritis, myalgia, tendinitis

RESP: Influenza, URI, LRI, EENT symptoms

Contraindications: Breastfeeding, hypersensitivity, chronic malabsorption syndrome, cholestasis

Precautions: Pregnancy (B), children, hypothyroidism, other organic causes of obesity, anorexia nervosa, bulimia, nephrolithiasis, GI disease, diabetes, fat-soluble vitamin deficiency

PHARMACOKINETICS

Minimal absorption, peak 8 hr, 99% protein binding, excretion in feces, half-life 1-2 hr

INTERACTIONS

Increase: lipid-lowering effect—pravastatin

Increase: effects of warfarin

Decrease: absorption—fat-soluble vitamins (A, D, E, K), cycloSPORINE

NURSING CONSIDERATIONS

Assess:

- Weight weekly, diabetic patients may need reduction in oral hypoglycemics
- For misuse in certain populations (anorexia nervosa, bulimia)
- For liver injury: jaundice, weakness, abdominal pain

Administer:

- For obesity only if patient is on weight-reduction program that includes dietary changes, exercise; patient should be on a diet with 30% of calories from fat, omit dose of orlistat if a meal contains no fat

Evaluate:

- Therapeutic response: decrease in weight

Teach patient/family:

- That the 60 mg cap can be obtained OTC; 60 mg tid is the highest OTC dose
- Safety and effectiveness beyond 2 yr have not been determined
- By instructing patient to read patient's information sheet, discuss unpleasant GI side effects
- To take a multivitamin containing fat-soluble vitamins 2 hr before or after orlistat; phyllium taken with each dose or at bedtime may decrease GI symptoms
- To avoid hazardous activities until stabilized on medication, discuss unpleasant side effects
- To notify prescriber if pregnancy is planned or suspected

oseltamivir (℞)

(oss-el-tam′ih-veer)

Tamiflu

Func. class.: Antiviral

Chem. class.: Neuramidase inhibitor

Action: Inhibits influenza virus neuraminidase with possible alteration of virus particle aggregation and release

Uses: Prevention/treatment of influenza type A or B

Unlabeled uses: Avian flu (H5N1), avian influenzae A (H5N1), swine flu (H1N1), encephalitis

DOSAGE AND ROUTES

Treatment of influenza

- *Adult and child >40 kg:* **PO** 75 mg bid × 5 days, begin treatment within 2 days of onset of symptoms
- *Child 23-40 kg and ≥1 yr:* **PO** 60 mg bid
- *Child 15-23 kg and ≥1 yr:* **PO** 45 mg bid
- *Child ≤15 kg and ≥1 yr:* **PO** 30 mg bid

Prevention of influenza

- *Adult and child ≥13 yr:* **PO** 75 mg/day × ≥7 days; begin treatment within 2 days of contact, max use 6 wk

Renal dose

- *Adult:* **PO** CCr 10-30 ml/min 75 mg/day × 5 days (treatment); 75 mg every other day or 30 mg/day (prophylaxis)

H1N1 influenzae A virus (swine flu) (unlabeled)

- *Adult/adolescent/child >40 kg:* **PO** 75 mg bid × 5 days
- *Adolescent/child 24-40 kg:* **PO** 60 mg bid × 5 days
- *Child >1 yr and 15-23 kg:* **PO** 45 mg bid × 5 days

• *Child >1 yr and ≤15 kg:* **PO** 30 mg bid × 5 days

Available forms: Caps 30, 45, 75 mg; powder for oral susp 12 mg/ml after reconstitution

SIDE EFFECTS

CNS: *Headache, dizziness,* fatigue, *insomnia,* delirium, **self-injury (children)**

ENDO: Hyperglycemia

GI: *Nausea, vomiting,* diarrhea, abdominal pain

INTEG: **Toxic epidermal necrolysis, Stevens-Johnson syndrome, erythema multiforme**

RESP: Cough

Contraindications: Hypersensitivity

Precautions: Pregnancy (C), neonates, breastfeeding, infants, children, geriatric patients, renal/hepatic/pulmonary/cardiac disease, psychosis, viral infection

PHARMACOKINETICS

Rapidly absorbed, protein binding 40%-45%, converted to oseltamivir carboxylate, half-life 1-3 hr, metabolite 6-10 hr, excreted in urine (99%), protein binding 3%

INTERACTIONS

• Avoid use with H1N1 virus vaccine, intranasal influenzae vaccine

NURSING CONSIDERATIONS

Assess:

• Bowel pattern before, during treatment

• Signs of infection: fever, fatigue, sore throat, headache, muscle soreness, aches

Administer:

• Within 2 days of symptoms of influenza; continue for 5 days

• At least 4 hr before bedtime to prevent insomnia

Perform/provide:

• Storage in tight, dry container

Evaluate:

• Therapeutic response: absence of fever, malaise, cough, dyspnea in infection

Teach patient/family:

• About aspects of product therapy

• To avoid hazardous activities if dizziness occurs

• To take missed dose as soon as remembered within 2 hr of next dose

⚠ To stop immediately; report to prescriber skin rash, delirium (child)

oxacillin (℞)

(ox-a-sill'in)

oxacillin sodium

Func. class.: Broad-spectrum antiinfective

Chem. class.: Penicillinase-resistant penicillin

Action: Interferes with cell wall replication of susceptible organisms; osmotically unstable cell wall swells, bursts from osmotic pressure

Uses: Effective for gram-positive cocci *(Staphylococcus aureus, Streptococcus pneumoniae),* infections caused by penicillinase-producing *Staphylococcus*

Unlabeled uses: *Corynebacterium diphtheriae,* erysipelothrix rhusiopathiae

O

DOSAGE AND ROUTES

• *Adult:* **IM/IV** 2-12 g/day in divided doses q4-6hr

• *Child:* **IM/IV** 50-200 mg/kg/day in divided doses q4-6hr, max 4 g/day

Available forms: Powder for inj 250, 500 mg, 1, 2, 4, 10 g

SIDE EFFECTS

CNS: Lethargy, hallucinations, anxiety, depression, twitching, **coma, seizures**

GI: *Nausea, vomiting, diarrhea,* increased AST, ALT, abdominal pain, glossitis, colitis, **pseudomembranous colitis, hepatotoxicity**

GU: **Oliguria, proteinuria, hematuria,** *vaginitis, moniliasis,* **glomerulonephritis, acute interstitial nephritis**

HEMA: Anemia, increased bleeding time, **bone marrow depression, granulocytopenia,** eosinophilia
INTEG: **Exfoliative dermatitis,** rash
SYST: **Anaphylaxis, serum sickness, Stevens-Johnson syndrome**
Contraindications: Hypersensitivity to penicillins or corn
Precautions: Pregnancy (B), breastfeeding, neonates, hypersensitivity to cephalosporins, GI/renal/hepatic disease, hypersensitivity to cephalosporins/carbapenem

PHARMACOKINETICS

Metabolized in the liver; excreted in urine, bile, breast milk; crosses placenta
IM: Peak 30-60 min, duration 4-6 hr
IV: Peak 5 min, duration 4-6 hr, half-life 30-60 min

INTERACTIONS

- Do not mix or give together with aminoglycosides

Increase: oxacillin concentrations—probenecid
Decrease: oxacillin antimicrobial effectiveness—tetracyclines, rifampin, erythromycins, chloramphenicol, cholestyramine, colestipol, sulfonamides
Drug/Herb
Decrease: absorption—acidophilus, khat, separate by ≥2 hr
Drug/Lab Test
False positive: urine glucose, urine protein

NURSING CONSIDERATIONS

Assess:

- I&O ratio; report hematuria, oliguria, since penicillin in high doses is nephrotoxic
- ⚠ Any patient with compromised renal system, since product is excreted slowly in poor renal system function; toxicity may occur rapidly
- Hepatic studies: AST, ALT
- Blood studies: WBC, RBC, Hct, Hgb, bleeding time
- Renal studies: urinalysis, protein
- C&S before therapy; product may be given as soon as culture is taken
- Bowel pattern before and during treatment
- Skin eruptions after administration of penicillin to 1 wk after discontinuing product
- Respiratory status: rate, character, wheezing, tightness in chest
- Allergies before initiation of treatment, and reaction of each medication

Administer:

- Product after C&S completed
- IM inj deep in gluteal muscle

IV route

- After diluting 500 mg or less/5 ml sterile H_2O or NaCl for inj; may dilute further in D_5W, NS, LR and give 1 g over 10 min; may be given as inf over 6 hr

Additive compatibilities: Cephapirin, chloramphenicol, DOPamine, potassium chloride, sodium bicarbonate
Y-site compatibilities: Acyclovir, cyclophosphamide, diltiazem, famotidine, fluconazole, foscarnet, heparin, hydrocortisone, hydromorphone, labetalol, magnesium sulfate, meperidine, methotrexate, morphine, perphenazine, potassium chloride, tacrolimus, vit B/C, zidovudine
Perform/provide:

- Adrenalin, suction, tracheostomy set, endotracheal intubation equipment
- Scratch test to assess allergy, after securing order from prescriber; usually done when penicillin is only product of choice

Evaluate:

- Therapeutic response: absence of fever, draining wounds

Teach patient/family:

- All aspects of product therapy, including need to complete course of medication to ensure organism death (10-14 days); culture may be taken after completed course
- To report sore throat, fever, fatigue (may indicate superinfection); persistent

diarrhea (pseudomembranous colitis); CNS toxicity

• To wear or carry emergency ID if allergic to penicillins

Treatment of anaphylaxis: Withdraw product, maintain airway, administer epinephrine, aminophylline, O_2, IV corticosteroids

oxaliplatin (℞)

(ox-al-i'plat-in)

Eloxatin

Func. class.: Antineoplastic

Chem. class.: 3rd generation platinum analog

Action: Forms crosslinks, inhibiting DNA replication and transcription, cell cycle nonspecific

Uses: Metastatic carcinoma of the colon or rectum in combination with 5-FU/leucovorin

Unlabeled uses: Relapsed or refractory non-Hodgkin lymphoma; advanced ovarian cancer; breast, head/neck, testicular, pancreatic, gastric cancer; mesothelioma

DOSAGE AND ROUTES

Dosage protocols may vary

Colorectal cancer

• *Adult:* **IV INF** *Day 1:* oxaliplatin 85 mg/m^2 in 250-500 ml D_5W and leucovorin 200 mg/m^2 in D_5W, give both over 2 hr at the same time in separate bags using a Y-line, followed by 5-FU 400 mg/m^2 **IV BOL** over 2-4 min, then 5-FU 600 mg/m^2 **IV INF** in 500 ml D_5W as a 22-hr **CONT INF;** *Day 2:* leucovorin 200 mg/m^2 **IV INF** over 2 hr, then 5-FU 400 mg/m^2 **IV BOL** over 2-4 min, then 5-FU 600 mg/m^2 **IV INF** in 500 ml D_5W as a 22-hr **CONT INF;** repeat cycle q2wk

Advanced ovarian cancer (unlabeled)

• *Adult:* **IV** 130 mg/m^2 q3wk as a single agent in those previously treated

Advanced breast cancer (unlabeled)

• *Adult:* **IV** 130 mg/m^2 on day 1 plus 5-fluorouracil (1000 mg/m^2 **CONT IV INF** days 1-4) q3wk

Pancreatic cancer (unlabeled)

• *Adult:* **IV** 100 mg/m^2 on day 2, with gemcitabine 1000 mg/m^2 on day 1, repeat q2wk; 625 mg/m^2 bid throughout treatment or fluorouracil 200 mg/m^2/day throughout treatment

Gastric cancer (unlabeled)

• *Adult:* **IV** 130 mg/m^2 over 2 hr on day 1 with epirubic 50 mg/m^2 and capecitabine

Available forms: Powder for inj 50, 100-mg single-use vials

SIDE EFFECTS

CNS: Peripheral neuropathy, fatigue, headache, dizziness, insomnia

CV: Cardiac abnormalities, **thromboembolism**

EENT: Decreased visual acuity, tinnitus, hearing loss

GI: Severe nausea, vomiting, diarrhea, weight loss, stomatitis, anorexia, gastroesophageal reflux, constipation, dyspepsia, mucositis, flatulence

GU: Hematuria, dysuria, creatinine

HEMA: **Thrombocytopenia, leukopenia, pancytopenia, neutropenia, anemia, hemolytic uremic syndrome**

INTEG: Alopecia, rash, flushing, extravasation, redness, swelling, pain at inj site

META: Hypokalemia

RESP: **Fibrosis,** dyspnea, cough, rhinitis, URI, pharyngitis

SYST: **Anaphylaxis, angioedema**

Contraindications: Pregnancy (D), breastfeeding, radiation therapy or chemotherapy within 1 mo, thrombocytopenia, smallpox vaccination

Black Box Warning: Hypersensitivity to this product or other platinum products

Precautions: Children, geriatric patients, pneumococcus vaccination, renal disease

O

PHARMACOKINETICS

Metabolized in liver, excreted in urine; after administration, 15% of platinum is in systemic circulation, 85% is either in tissues or being eliminated in urine; half-life 390 hr; protein binding >90%

INTERACTIONS

Increase: bleeding risk—aspirin, NSAIDs, alcohol, anticoagulants
Increase: oxaliplatin toxicity—tannins
Increase: myelosuppression—myelosuppressive agents, radiation
Increase: nephrotoxicity—aminoglycosides, loop diuretics
Decrease: antibody response—live virus vaccines

Drug/Lab Test

Increase: ALT, AST, bilirubin, creatinine
Decrease: potassium, neutrophils, WBC, platelets

NURSING CONSIDERATIONS

Assess:

For bone marrow depression

- CBC, differential, platelet count each cycle; withhold product if WBC is <4000 or platelet count is <100,000; notify prescriber of results
- Renal studies: BUN, creatinine, serum uric acid, urine CCr before, electrolytes during therapy; dose should not be given if BUN >19 mg/dl; creatinine <1.5 mg/dl; I&O ratio; report fall in urine output of <30 ml/hr

⚠ For anaphylaxis: wheezing, tachycardia, facial swelling, fainting; discontinue product and report to prescriber; resuscitation equipment should be nearby

⚠ For pulmonary fibrosis: cough, crackles, dyspnea, pulmonary infiltrate; discontinue immediately, death may occur

- Monitor temp (may indicate beginning infection)
- Hepatic studies before each cycle (bilirubin, AST, ALT, LDH) as needed or monthly
- Bleeding: hematuria, guaiac, bruising or petechiae, mucosa or orifices; obtain prescription for viscous lidocaine (Xylocaine)
- Effects of alopecia on body image; discuss feelings about body changes
- Jaundice of skin, sclera; dark urine; clay-colored stools; itchy skin; abdominal pain; fever; diarrhea
- Edema in feet, joint pain, stomach pain, shaking

Administer:

IV route

- Do not reconstitute or dilute with sodium chloride or any chloride-containing solutions
- Do not use aluminum equipment during any preparation or administration, will degrade platinum; do not refrigerate unopened powder or solution; do not freeze; protect from light
- Use cytotoxic handling procedures; prepare in biologic cabinet using gown, gloves, mask; do not allow product to come in contact with skin; use soap and water if contact occurs
- Hydrate patient with 0.9% NaCl over 8-12 hr before treatment
- Epinephrine, antihistamines, corticosteroids for hypersensitivity reaction
- Antiemetic 30-60 min before giving product and prn
- Diuretic (furosemide 40 mg IV) or mannitol after inf

Perform/provide:

- Comprehensive oral hygiene
- All medications PO, if possible, avoid IM inj when platelets <100,000/mm^3
- Increase fluid intake to 2-3 L/day to prevent urate deposits, calculi formation; elimination of product
- Blankets, hat, gloves for cold prevention

Evaluate:

- Therapeutic response: decreased tumor size, spread of malignancy

Teach patient/family:

- To report signs of infection: increased temp, sore throat, flulike symptoms
- To report signs of anemia: fatigue, headache, faintness, shortness of breath, irritability

- To report bleeding: avoid use of razors, commercial mouthwash
- To avoid aspirin, ibuprofen, NSAIDs, alcohol; may cause GI bleeding
- To report any complaints or side effects to nurse or prescriber
- To report any changes in breathing, coughing
- That hair may be lost during treatment; a wig or hairpiece may make patient feel better; new hair may be different in color, texture
- To report numbness, tingling in face or extremities, poor hearing or joint pain, swelling
- Not to receive vaccines during treatment
- To use contraception during treatment and 4 mo after; this product may cause infertility
- To avoid contact with cold (air, ice, liquid) causes acute dysesthesias

oxaprozin (℞)

(ox-a-proe′zin)

Daypro

Func. class.: Nonsteroidal antiinflammatory, antirheumatics

Chem. class.: Propionic acid derivative

Do not confuse:
Daypro/Diupres

Action: Completely inhibits COX-1, COX-2 by blocking arachidonate; analgesic, antiinflammatory, antipyretic

Uses: Acute and long-term management of osteoarthritis, RA, juvenile RA

DOSAGE AND ROUTES

- *Adult:* **PO** 600-1200 mg/day; max 1800 mg/day or 26 mg/kg, whichever is lower
- *Adult <50 kg:* **PO** 600 mg/day

Juvenile rheumatoid arthritis

- *Child 6-16 yr:* **PO** (22-31 kg) 600 mg/dose; (32-54 kg) 900 mg/dose; (≥55 kg) 1200 mg/dose

Available forms: Tabs 600 mg; tabs oxaprozin potassium 678 mg (equal to 600 mg oxaprozin); caps 600 mg

SIDE EFFECTS

CNS: Dizziness, headache, drowsiness, fatigue, tremors, confusion, insomnia, anxiety, depression

CV: Tachycardia, peripheral edema, palpitations, dysrhythmias, **MI, stroke**

EENT: Tinnitus, hearing loss, blurred vision

GI: Nausea, anorexia, vomiting, diarrhea, jaundice, **cholestatic hepatitis,** constipation, flatulence, cramps, dry mouth, peptic ulcer, **GI bleeding, perforation, ulceration,** dyspepsia

GU: **Nephrotoxicity: dysuria, hematuria, oliguria, azotemia**

HEMA: **Increased bleeding time, pancytopenia**

INTEG: Purpura, rash, pruritus, sweating, photosensitivity

MISC: **Anaphylaxis, angioneurotic edema, toxic epidermal necrolysis, Stevens-Johnson syndrome**

Contraindications: Pregnancy (D), 3rd trimester, hypersensitivity, asthma, patients in whom aspirin and iodides have induced symptoms of allergic reactions or asthma

Black Box Warning: Perioperative pain in CABG surgery

Precautions: Pregnancy (C), breastfeeding, children, geriatric patients, bleeding/GI/cardiac disorders, hypersensitivity to other antiinflammatory agents, severe renal/hepatic disease, CHF

Black Box Warning: GI bleeding, MI, stroke

PHARMACOKINETICS

PO: Onset 1 wk, peak 1.5-3.5 hr, duration unknown, half-life 40-50 hr; metabolized in liver; excreted in urine/feces (metabolites), breast milk; 99% protein binding

INTERACTIONS

Increase: toxicity—aspirin, cycloSPORINE, methotrexate, probenecid

Increase: bleeding risk—oral anticoagulants, thrombolytics, cefamandole, ce-

fotetan, cefoperazone, clopidogrel, eptifibatide, plicamycin, ticlopidine, tirofiban
Increase: levels of phenytoin, lithium, avoid concomitant use
Increase: GI side effects—aspirin, corticosteroids, NSAIDs, alcohol, potassium supplements
Decrease: effect—antihypertensives, diuretics

Drug/Herb

• Increase NSAIDs effect: bearberry, bilberry
Increase: bleeding risk—anise, arnica, chamomile, clove, dong quai, fenugreek, feverfew, garlic, ginger, ginkgo, ginseng *(Panax)*, licorice, bogbean, chondroitin
Increase: gastric irritation—arginine, gossypol

Drug/Lab Test

Increase: BUN, alkaline phosphatase
False positive: increased 5-HIAA
False increase: 17-KS

NURSING CONSIDERATIONS

Assess:

• Pain: frequency, intensity, characteristics; relief of pain after med
⚠ Cardiac status: CV thrombotic events, MI, stroke; may be fatal
⚠ GI status: ulceration, bleeding, perforation; may be fatal
⚠ For Stevens-Johnson syndrome, anaphylaxis, toxic epidermal necrolysis, angioneurotic edema
⚠ Asthma, aspirin hypersensitivity, oronasal polyps; increased hypersensitivity reactions
• Renal, hepatic, blood studies: BUN, creatinine, AST, ALT, Hgb, before treatment, periodically thereafter
• Audiometric, ophthalmic exam before, during, after treatment
• For eye, ear problems: blurred vision, tinnitus; may indicate toxicity

Administer:

• With food, antacids to decrease GI symptoms

Perform/provide:

• Storage at room temperature

Evaluate:

• Therapeutic response: decreased pain, stiffness in joints, decreased swelling in joints, ability to move more easily

Teach patient/family:

⚠ To report blurred vision, ringing, roaring in ears; may indicate toxicity
• To avoid driving, other hazardous activities if dizziness/drowsiness occurs
⚠ To report change in urine pattern, increased weight, edema, increased pain in joints, fever, blood in urine; indicates nephrotoxicity
• That therapeutic effects may take up to 1 mo
• To take with a full glass of water to enhance absorption, sit upright for ½ hr after dose
• To avoid prolonged sun exposure, use sunscreen, protective clothing
• To avoid ASA, alcohol or other OTC medications without prescriber approval
• To inform all health care providers that product is being used

oxazepam (℞)

(ox-ay′ze-pam)
Apo-Oxazepam ✦, Novoxapam ✦, oxazepam
Func. class.: Sedative/hypnotic; antianxiety
Chem. class.: Benzodiazepine, short acting

Controlled Substance Schedule IV

Action: Potentiates the actions of GABA, especially in limbic system and reticular formation

Uses: Anxiety, alcohol withdrawal, insomnia

DOSAGE AND ROUTES

Anxiety

• *Adult:* **PO** 10-30 mg tid-qid, max 120 mg/day
• *Geriatric:* **PO** 5 mg daily-bid initially, may increase, max 15 mg qid

Alcohol withdrawal

• *Adult:* **PO** 15-30 mg tid-qid

Available forms: Caps 10, 15, 30 mg; tab 15 mg

SIDE EFFECTS

CNS: Dizziness, drowsiness, confusion, headache, anxiety, tremors, fatigue, depression, insomnia, hallucinations, paradoxical excitement, transient amnesia
CV: Orthostatic hypotension, **ECG changes, tachycardia,** hypotension
EENT: Blurred vision, tinnitus, mydriasis
GI: Nausea, vomiting, anorexia
HEMA: Leukopenia
INTEG: Rash, dermatitis, itching
SYST: Dependence
Contraindications: Pregnancy (D), breastfeeding, children <12 yr, hypersensitivity to benzodiazepines, closed-angle glaucoma, psychosis
Precautions: Geriatric patients, debilitated, renal/hepatic disease, depression, suicidal ideation, dementia, sleep apnea, seizure disorder

PHARMACOKINETICS

Peak 2-4 hr; metabolized by liver; excreted by kidneys; half-life 5-15 hr; crosses placenta, breast milk; protein binding 97%

INTERACTIONS

Increase: oxazepam effects—CNS depressants, alcohol, disulfiram, oral contraceptives
Decrease: oxazepam effects—oral contraceptives, phenytoin, theophylline, valproic acid
Decrease: effects of levodopa
Drug/Herb
Increase: CNS depression—catnip, chamomile, clary, cowslip, hops, kava, lavender, mistletoe, nettle, pokeweed, poppy, Queen Anne's lace, senega, skullcap, valerian
Increase: hypotension—black cohosh
Drug/Lab Test
Increase: AST, ALT, serum bilirubin
Decrease: RAIU
False increase: 17-OHCS

NURSING CONSIDERATIONS

Assess:

- B/P (lying, standing), pulse; if systolic B/P drops 20 mm Hg, hold product, notify prescriber
- Blood studies: CBC during long-term therapy; blood dyscrasias have occurred rarely
- Hepatic studies: AST, ALT, bilirubin, creatinine, LDH, alk phos if taking long term
- Mental status: mood, sensorium, affect, sleeping pattern, drowsiness, dizziness

⚠ Physical dependency, withdrawal symptoms: headache, nausea, vomiting, muscle pain, weakness, tremors, seizures (long-term use)

- Suicidal tendencies

Administer:

- With food, milk for GI symptoms
- Sugarless gum, hard candy, frequent sips of water for dry mouth

Perform/provide:

- Assistance with ambulation during beginning therapy; drowsiness/dizziness occurs
- Safety measures, including side rails
- Check to see if PO medication has been swallowed

Evaluate:

- Therapeutic response: decreased anxiety, restlessness, insomnia

Teach patient/family:

- That product may be taken with food
- That medication is not to be used for everyday stress or used longer than 4 mo unless directed by prescriber; not to take more than prescribed dose; may be habit forming
- To avoid OTC preparations (cough, cold, hay fever) unless approved by prescriber
- To avoid driving, activities that require alertness, since drowsiness may occur
- To avoid alcohol ingestion, other psychotropic medications unless directed by prescriber
- Not to discontinue medication abruptly after long-term use

• To rise slowly, or fainting may occur, especially geriatric patients
• That drowsiness may worsen at beginning of treatment

Treatment of overdose: Lavage, VS, supportive care, flumazenil

oxcarbazepine (℞)

(ox′kar-baz′uh-peen)
Trileptal
Func. class.: Anticonvulsant
Chem. class.: Carbamazepine analog

Action: May inhibit nerve impulses by limiting influx of sodium ions across cell membrane in motor cortex

Uses: Partial seizures

Unlabeled uses: Trigeminal neuralgia, atypical panic disorder, bipolar disorder

DOSAGE AND ROUTES

Seizures, adjunctive therapy

• *Adult:* **PO** 300 mg bid, may be increased by 600 mg/day in divided doses bid at weekly intervals; maintenance 1200 mg/day
• *Child 4-16 yr:* **PO** 8-10 mg/kg/day divided bid; dose is determined by weight, increase by 5 mg/kg/day q3days, max doses are weight dependent

Conversion to monotherapy in partial seizures

• *Adult:* **PO** 300 mg bid with reduction in other anticonvulsants; increase oxcarbazepine by 600 mg/day q1wk over 2-4 wk; withdraw other anticonvulsants over 3-6 wk; max 2400 mg/day

Initiation of monotherapy in partial seizures

• *Adult:* **PO** 300 mg bid, increase by 300 mg/day q3days to 1200 mg divided bid

Renal dose

• *Adult:* **PO** CCr <30 ml/min 150 mg bid and increase slowly

Bipolar disorder/trigeminal neuralgia (unlabeled)

• *Adult:* **PO** 300 mg bid, may increase by ≤600 mg/day

Available forms: Film-coated tabs 150, 300, 600 mg; oral susp 300 mg/5 ml

SIDE EFFECTS

CNS: Headache, dizziness, confusion, fatigue, feeling abnormal, ataxia, abnormal gait, tremors, anxiety, agitation, **worsening of seizures, suicidal ideation/behavior**

CV: Hypotension, chest pain, edema

EENT: Blurred vision, diplopia, nystagmus, rhinitis, sinusitis

GI: Nausea, constipation, diarrhea, anorexia, vomiting, abdominal pain, gastritis, dry mouth, thirst, **rectal hemorrhage**

GU: Frequency, UTI, vaginitis

INTEG: Purpura, rash, acne

RESP: Rhinitis, URI

SYST: **Angioedema, anaphylaxis, Stevens-Johnson syndrome, toxic epidermal necrolysis**

Contraindications: Hypersensitivity

Precautions: Pregnancy (C), breastfeeding, children <4 yr, hypersensitivity to carbamazepine, renal disease, fluid restriction, hyponatremia

PHARMACOKINETICS

PO: Onset unknown; peak 4-6 hr; metabolized by liver to active metabolite; terminal half-life 7-9 hr metabolite; inhibits P450 CYP2C19, induces CYP3A4/5

INTERACTIONS

• Contraindicated: MAOIs, ranolazine, nisoldipine

Increase: CNS depression—alcohol

Decrease: effects—felodipine, oral contraceptive, carbamazepine

Decrease: oxcarbazepine levels—carbamazepine, phenobarbital, phenytoin, valproic acid, verapamil

Drug/Herb

Increase: anticonvulsant effect—ginkgo

Decrease: anticonvulsant effect—ginseng, santonica

NURSING CONSIDERATIONS

Assess:

- Description of seizures: frequency, duration, aura
- For hyponatremia: headache, nausea, confusion
- Electrolyte: sodium; T_4; phenytoin (when given together)

⚠ For serious reactions: angioedema, anaphylaxis, Stevens-Johnson syndrome

- CNS/mental status: mood, sensorium, affect, behavioral changes, confusion; if mental status changes, notify prescriber
- Eye problems: need for ophthalmic exams before, during, after treatment (slit lamp, funduscopy, tonometry)

Administer:

PO route

- With food, milk to decrease GI symptoms

Perform/provide:

- Storage at room temperature
- Hard candy, gum, frequent rinsing for dry mouth
- Assistance with ambulation during early part of treatment; dizziness occurs

Evaluate:

- Therapeutic response: decreased seizure activity

Teach patient/family:

- To carry emergency ID stating patient's name, products taken, condition, prescriber's name and phone number
- To avoid driving, other activities that require alertness
- Not to discontinue medication quickly after long-term use
- To inform prescriber if hypersensitive to carbamazepine
- To avoid use of alcohol while taking this medication
- To use alternative contraception if using hormonal method

Treatment of overdose: Activated charcoal, give 0.9% NaCl (hypotensive state), atropine (bradycardia), use benzodiazepines, barbiturates for seizures

oxybutynin (℞)

(ox-i-byoo′ti-nin)
Ditropan, Ditropan XL, oxybutynin, Gelnique, Oxytrol Transdermal
Func. class.: Anticholinergic
Chem. class.: Synthetic tertiary amine

Do not confuse:
Ditropan/diazepam

Action: Relaxes smooth muscles in urinary tract by inhibiting acetylcholine at postganglionic sites

Uses: Antispasmodic for neurogenic bladder, overactive bladder

DOSAGE AND ROUTES

- *Adult:* **PO** 5 mg bid-tid, max 5 mg qid; **ER** 5-10 mg/day, may increase by 5 mg, max 30 mg/day; **TD** apply one patch to abdomen, hip, buttock 2×/wk (q3-4 days); **GEL** apply contents of 1 packet to abdomen, upper arms, shoulders, thighs
- *Geriatric:* **PO** 2.5-5 mg bid-tid, increase by 2.5 mg q several days
- *Child >6 yr:* **PO** 5 mg bid, max 5 mg tid; **ER** 5 mg/day, max 20 mg/day
- *Child 1-5 yr:* **PO** 0.2 mg/kg/dose 2-4×/day

Available forms: Syr 5 mg/5 ml; tabs 5 mg; ext rel tabs 5, 10, 15 mg; TD 3.9 mg/day; top gel 10% (Gelnique)

SIDE EFFECTS

CNS: Anxiety, restlessness, dizziness, somnolence, insomnia, nervousness, **seizures,** headache, drowsiness, confusion

CV: Palpitations, sinus tachycardia, hypertension, peripheral edema

EENT: Blurred vision, dry eyes, increased intraocular tension, *dry mouth,* throat

GI: Nausea, vomiting, anorexia, abdominal pain, *constipation, dyspepsia,* diarrhea, taste perversion, GERD

GU: Dysuria, impotence, urinary retention, hesitancy

O

Contraindications: Hypersensitivity, GI obstruction, GU obstruction, glaucoma, severe colitis, myasthenia gravis, unstable CV disease, dementia, infants

Precautions: Pregnancy (B), breastfeeding, children <12 yr, geriatric patients, suspected glaucoma, cardiac disease, dementia

PHARMACOKINETICS

Onset ½-1 hr, peak 3-6 hr, duration 6-10 hr; metabolized by liver, excreted in urine

INTERACTIONS

- Altered pharmacokinetic parameters: CYP3A4 inhibitors

Increase: CNS depression—benzodiazepines, sedatives, hypnotics, opioids

Increase: levels of atenolol, digoxin, nitrofurantoin

Increase: anticholinergic effects—antihistamines, amantidine, other anticholinergics

Increase or decrease: levels of phenothiazines

Decrease: levels of acetaminophen, haloperidol, levodopa

Decrease: effects of oxybutynin—CYP3A4 inducers

Drug/Herb

Increase: constipation—black catechu

Increase: anticholinergic action—butterbur, jimsonweed, scopolia

Decrease: anticholinergic effect—jaborandi tree, pill-bearing spurge

NURSING CONSIDERATIONS

Assess:

- Urinary patterns: distention, nocturia, frequency, urgency, incontinence
- Allergic reactions: rash, urticaria; if these occur, product should be discontinued
- CNS effects: confusion, anxiety; anticholinergic effects in the geriatric patients

Administer:

PO route

- Do not crush, break, or chew ext rel tabs
- Without regard to meals

Topical route

- Rotate sites
- Delivers 100 mg

Transdermal route

- Delivers 3.9 mg/day

Evaluate:

- Urinary status: dysuria, frequency, nocturia, incontinence

Teach patient/family:

- To avoid hazardous activities; dizziness, blurred vision may occur
- To avoid OTC medications with alcohol, other CNS depressants
- To prevent photophobia by wearing sunglasses
- Avoid hot weather, strenuous activity, product decreases perspiration
- Rotate site of patch with each application

⚠ High Alert

oxycodone (℞)

(ox-i-koe'done)

Endocodone, M-Oxy, Oxy-Contin, OxyFAST, OxyLR, Roxicodone, Roxicodone SR, Supeudol ✦

oxycodone/aspirin (℞)

Endodan ✦, Oxycodan ✦, Percodan, Percodan-Demi, Roxiprin

oxycodone/acetaminophen (℞)

Endocet ✦, Oxycocet ✦, Percocet, Roxicet, Roxilox, Tylox

oxycodone/ibuprofen (℞)

Combunox

Func. class.: Opiate analgesic

Chem. class.: Semisynthetic derivative

Controlled Substance Schedule II

Do not confuse:

Percodan/Decadron

Roxicet/Roxanol

Tylox/Xanax/Trimox/Wymox

Action: Inhibits ascending pain pathways in CNS, increases pain threshold, alters pain perception

Uses: Moderate to severe pain

Unlabeled uses: Postherpetic neuralgic (cont rel)

DOSAGE AND ROUTES

• *Adult:* **PO** 10-30 mg q4hr (5 mg q6hr for OxyLR, OxyFAST) **OxyFAST Conc Sol is extremely concentrated; do not use interchangeably CONT REL** 10 mg q12hr in opiate-naive patients

Available forms: *Oxycodone:* cont rel tabs (Oxy Contin) 10, 20, 40, 80, 160 mg; immediate rel tabs 15, 30 mg; tabs 5 mg; immediate rel caps 5 mg; oral sol 5 mg/5 ml, 20 mg/ml; *oxycodone with acetaminophen:* tabs 5 mg/325 mg; caps 5 mg/500 mg; oral sol 5 mg/325 mg/5 ml; *oxycodone with aspirin:* 2.44 mg/325 mg, 4.88/325 mg

SIDE EFFECTS

CNS: *Drowsiness, dizziness, confusion, headache, sedation, euphoria,* fatigue, abnormal dreams/thoughts, hallucinations

CV: Palpitations, bradycardia, change in B/P

EENT: Tinnitus, blurred vision, miosis, diplopia

GI: *Nausea, vomiting, anorexia, constipation, cramps,* gastritis, dyspepsia, biliary spasms

GU: Increased urinary output, dysuria, urinary retention

INTEG: *Rash,* urticaria, bruising, flushing, diaphoresis, pruritus

RESP: **Respiratory depression**

Contraindications: Hypersensitivity, addiction (opiate), asthma, ileus

Black Box Warning: Respiratory depression

Precautions: Pregnancy (B), breastfeeding, children <18 yr, addictive personality, increased intracranial pressure, MI (acute), severe heart disease, renal/hepatic disease, bowel impaction

Black Box Warning: Opioid-naive patients, substance abuse

PHARMACOKINETICS

PO: Onset 15-30 min, peak 1 hr, duration 3-4 hr, metabolized by liver, excreted in urine, crosses placenta, excreted in breast milk, half-life 3-5 hr, protein binding 45%

INTERACTIONS

Increase: effects with other CNS depressants—alcohol, opioids, sedative/hypnotics, antipsychotics, skeletal muscle relaxants

Increase: toxicity—cimetidine, MAOIs

Drug/Herb

Increase: anticholinergic effect—corkwood

Increase: sedative effect—gotu kola, Jamaican dogwood, kava, lavender, mistletoe, nettle, pokeweed, poppy, senega, St. John's wort, valerian

Drug/Lab Test

Increase: amylase, lipase

NURSING CONSIDERATIONS

Assess:

• I&O ratio; check for decreasing output; may indicate urinary retention

• CNS changes: dizziness, drowsiness, hallucinations, euphoria, LOC, pupil reaction

• Allergic reactions: rash, urticaria

• Respiratory dysfunction: respiratory depression, character, rate, rhythm; notify prescriber if respirations are <10/min; also B/P, pulse

• For pain: intensity, location, type, characteristics; need for pain medication by pain/sedation scoring; physical dependence

• Bowel status: constipation; stimulate laxative may be needed

Administer:

• Do not break, crush, or chew controlled rel tabs; give q12hr, no more frequently

O

• 80, 160 mg cont rel tabs (OxyContin) only in opioid-tolerant patients
• With antiemetic if nausea, vomiting occur
• When pain is beginning to return; determine dosage interval by response

Perform/provide:
• Storage in light-resistant area at room temperature
• Assistance with ambulation
• Safety measures: night-light, call bell within easy reach

Evaluate:
• Therapeutic response: decrease in pain

Teach patient/family:
• To report any symptoms of CNS changes, allergic reactions
• That physical dependency may result from extended use
• That withdrawal symptoms may occur: nausea, vomiting, cramps, fever, faintness, anorexia
• Avoid CNS depressants, alcohol
• Avoid driving, operating machinery if drowsiness occurs

Treatment of overdose: Naloxone (Narcan) 0.2-0.8 mg IV, O_2, IV fluids, vasopressors

oxymetazoline nasal agent
See Appendix B

oxymetazoline ophthalmic
See Appendix B

⚠ High Alert

oxymorphone (℞)
(ox-i-mor′fone)
Numorphan, Opana, Opana ER

Func. class.: Opiate analgesic
Chem. class.: Semisynthetic phenanthrene derivative

Controlled Substance Schedule II

Action: Inhibits ascending pain pathways in CNS, increases pain threshold, alters pain perception

Uses: Moderate to severe pain

DOSAGE AND ROUTES
• *Adult:* **IM/SUBCUT** 1-1.5 mg q4-6hr prn; **IV** 0.5 mg q4-6hr prn; **RECT** 5 mg q4-6hr prn; **PO** (immediate release only) 5-20 mg q4-6hr prn; **PO-ER** 5 mg q12hr in those requiring around the clock dosing

Labor analgesia
• *Adult:* **IM** 0.5-1 mg

Available forms: Inj 1, 1.5 mg/ml; supp 5 mg; ER tab 5, 10, 20, 40 mg; tabs 5, 10 mg

SIDE EFFECTS
CNS: Drowsiness, dizziness, confusion, headache, hallucinations, **increased intracranial pressure,** *sedation,* **seizures,** *euphoria (geriatric patients)*
CV: Palpitations, **bradycardia,** change in B/P, hypotension
EENT: Tinnitus, blurred vision, miosis, diplopia
GI: Nausea, vomiting, anorexia, constipation, cramps
GU: Dysuria, urinary retention
INTEG: Rash, urticaria, bruising, flushing, diaphoresis, pruritus
RESP: **Respiratory depression**

Contraindications: Hypersensitivity, addiction (opiate), asthma, hepatic disease, ileus, intrathecal use, surgery

Black Box Warning: Respiratory depression

Precautions: Pregnancy (B) (short-term), breastfeeding, children <18 yr, addictive personality, increased intracranial pressure, MI (acute), severe heart disease, respiratory depression, renal/hepatic disease, bowel impaction

Black Box Warning: Alcoholism, opioid-naive patients, substance abuse

PHARMACOKINETICS

Metabolized by liver, excreted in urine, crosses placenta, half-life 2.5-4 hr
PO: Peak 1 hr (fasting)
SUBCUT/IM: Onset 10-15 min, peak 1½ hr, duration, 3-6 hr
RECT: Onset 15-30 min, duration 3-6 hr
IV: Onset 5-10 min, peak 15-30 min, duration 3-6 hr

INTERACTIONS

Increase: effects with other CNS depressants—alcohol, opiates, sedative/hypnotics, antipsychotics, skeletal muscle relaxants

⚠ ***Increase:*** unpredictable effects/reactions—MAOIs

Drug/Herb

Increase: anticholinergic effect—corkwood

Increase: sedative effect—gotu kola, Jamaican dogwood, kava, lavender, mistletoe, nettle, pokeweed, poppy, senega, St. John's wort, valerian

Drug/Lab Test

Increase: amylase

NURSING CONSIDERATIONS

Assess:

- For pain: location, intensity, type, other characteristics, before and 1 hr after (IM) IV 30 min; need for pain medication, physical dependence
- I&O ratio for decreasing output; may indicate urinary retention
- Bowel status: Constipation; may need stimulative laxative
- CNS changes: dizziness, drowsiness, hallucinations, euphoria, LOC, pupil reaction
- Allergic reactions: rash, urticaria
- Respiratory dysfunction: respiratory depression, character, rate, rhythm; notify prescriber if respirations are <10/min

Administer:

- 1 hr before or 2 hr after food (PO)
- With antiemetic for nausea, vomiting
- Do not break, crush, chew ER product
- When pain is beginning to return; determine interval by response

IV route

- After diluting with 5 ml sterile H_2O or NS for inj; give over 2-5 min through Y-tube or 3-way stopcock

Syringe compatibilities: Glycopyrrolate, hydrOXYzine, ranitidine

Perform/provide:

- Storage in light-resistant area at room temperature
- Assistance with ambulation
- Safety measures: night-light, call bell within easy reach

Evaluate:

- Therapeutic response: decrease in pain

Teach patient/family:

- To report any symptoms of CNS changes, allergic reactions
- That physical dependency may result from extended use
- That withdrawal symptoms may occur: nausea, vomiting, cramps, fever, faintness, anorexia
- Not to drive or operate machinery if drowsiness occurs
- To avoid CNS depressants, alcohol

Treatment of overdose: Naloxone (Narcan) 0.2-0.8 mg IV, O_2, IV fluids, vasopressors

⚠ **High Alert**

oxytocin (℞)
(ox-i-toe'sin)
Pitocin
Func. class.: Hormone
Chem. class.: Oxytocic, uterine-active agent

Action: Acts directly on myofibrils, producing uterine contraction; stimulates milk ejection by the breast; vasoactive antidiuretic effect

Uses: Stimulation, induction of labor; missed or incomplete abortion; postpartum bleeding

DOSAGE AND ROUTES

Postpartum hemorrhage

• *Adult:* **IV** 10-40 units in 1000 ml nonhydrating diluent infused at 20-40 mU/min

• *Adult:* **IM** 10 units after delivery of placenta

Contraction stress test (CST)

• *Adult:* **IV** 0.5 mU/min, increase q20min until 3 contractions within 10 min

Stimulation of labor

• *Adult:* **IV** 1-2 mU/min, increase by 1-2 mU q15-60min until contractions occur; then decrease dose

Incomplete abortion

• *Adult:* **IV INF** 10 units/500 ml D_5W or 0.9% NaCl at 10-20 mU/min, max 30 units/12 hr

Available forms: Inj 10 units/ml

SIDE EFFECTS

CNS: **Seizures, tetanic contractions**

CV: Hypo/hypertension, dysrhythmias, increased pulse, bradycardia, tachycardia, PVC

FETUS: Dysrhythmias, jaundice, hypoxia, **intracranial hemorrhage**

GI: Anorexia, nausea, vomiting, constipation

GU: **Abruptio placentae, decreased uterine blood flow**

HEMA: Increased hyperbilirubinemia

INTEG: Rash

RESP: **Asphyxia**

SYST: Water intoxication of mother

Contraindications: Hypersensitivity, serum toxemia, cephalopelvic disproportion, fetal distress, hypertonic uterus, prolapsed umbilical cord, active genital herpes

Precautions: Cervical/uterine surgery, uterine sepsis, primipara >35 yr, 1st/2nd stage of labor

Black Box Warning: Elective induction of labor

PHARMACOKINETICS

IM: Onset 3-7 min, duration 1 hr, half-life 12-17 min

IV: Onset 1 min, duration 30 min, half-life 12-17 min

INTERACTIONS

• Hypertension: vasopressors

Drug/Herb

• Hypertension: ephedra

NURSING CONSIDERATIONS

Assess:

• I&O ratio

• Respiration

• B/P, pulse; watch for changes that may indicate hemorrhage

• Respiratory rate, rhythm, depth; notify prescriber of abnormalities

• Length, intensity, duration of contraction; notify prescriber of contractions lasting over 1 min or absence of contractions; turn patient on her side; discontinue oxytocin

• FHTs, fetal distress; watch for acceleration, deceleration; notify prescriber if problems occur; fetal presentation, pelvic dimensions; turn patient on left side if FHT change in rate, give O_2

⚠ For signs and symptoms of water intoxication; confusion, anuria, drowsiness, headache

Administer:

Labor induction

• After diluting 10 units/L of 0.9% NS or D_5 NS run at 1-2 mU/min at 15-30 min intervals to begin normal labor; dilute 10-40 mU/min; titrate to control postpartum bleeding; dilute 10 units/500 ml sol; run 10 units-20 mU/ml; administer by only 1 route at a time; use inf pump; rotate inf to provide mixing; do not shake

Control of postpartum bleeding

• Dilute 10-40 units/1 L of sol; run at 10-20 mU/min; adjust rate as needed

• With crash cart available on unit (magnesium sulfate at bedside)

Additive compatibilities: Chloramphenicol, metaraminol, netilmicin, sodium bicarbonate, thiopental, verapamil

Y-site compatibilities: Heparin, hydrocortisone, insulin (regular), meperidine, morphine, potassium chloride, vit B/C, warfarin

Evaluate:

- Therapeutic response: stimulation of labor, control of postpartum bleeding

Teach patient/family:

- To report increased blood loss, abdominal cramps, fever, foul-smelling lochia
- That contractions will be similar to menstrual cramps, gradually increasing in intensity

paclitaxel (℞)

(pa-kli-tax′el)

Onxol, Taxol

paclitaxel nanoparticle albumin-bound (℞)

Abraxane

Func. class.: Antineoplastic—miscellaneous

Chem. class.: Toxoid

Do not confuse:

paclitaxel/paroxetine/Paxil

Taxol/Paxil/Taxotere

Action: Inhibits reorganization of microtubule network needed for interphase and mitotic cellular functions; also causes abnormal bundles of microtubules during cell cycle and multiple esters of microtubules during mitosis

Uses: Taxol: metastatic carcinoma of the ovary, breast; AIDS-related Kaposi's sarcoma (2nd-line), non–small cell lung cancer (1st-line), adjuvant treatment for node-positive breast cancer; Onxol: failure of other treatment in breast cancer, advanced carcinoma in ovarian cancer

Unlabeled uses: Advanced head, neck, small cell lung cancer; non-Hodgkin's lymphoma, adenocarcinoma of the upper GI tract, hormone-refractory prostate cancer, bladder cancer

DOSAGE AND ROUTES

Paclitaxel

Ovarian carcinoma

- *Adult:* **IV INF** 135 mg/m^2 given over 24 hr q3wk then cisplatin 75 mg/m^2; or 175 mg/m^2 over 3 hr q3wk; or 175 mg/m^2 over 3 hr

Advanced ovarian carcinoma

- *Adult:* **IV/INF** 175 mg/m^2 with cisplatin 75 mg/m^2 using a 3-hr regimen q3wk

Breast carcinoma

- *Adult:* **IV INF** 175 mg/m^2 over 3 hr q3wk × 4 courses

AIDS-related Kaposi's sarcoma

- *Adult:* **IV INF** 135 mg/m^2 over 3 hr q3wk or 100 mg/m^2 over 3 hr q2wk

1st-line non–small cell lung cancer

- *Adult:* **IV INF** 135 mg/m^2/24 hr inf with cisplatin 75 mg/m^2 × 3 wk

Bladder cancer (unlabeled)

- *Adult:* **IV** 175 mg/m^2 over 3 hr and carboplatin

Head/neck cancer (unlabeled)

- *Adult:* **IV** 250 mg/m^2 over 24 hr or 175-300 mg/m^2 over 3 hr

Stem cell transplant/bone marrow ablation (unlabeled)

- *Adult:* **IV** 250-775 mg/m^2 over 24 hr in combination with other chemotherapy

Paclitaxel protein-bound particles

- *Adult:* **IV** 260 mg/m^2 q3wk

Available forms: Inj 30 mg/5-ml vial, 100 mg/16.7-ml vial, 150 mg/24-ml vial, 300 mg/5-ml vial; powder for inj, lyophilized 100 mg in single-use vials (Abraxane)

SIDE EFFECTS

CNS: Peripheral neuropathy

CV: Bradycardia, *hypotension,* abnormal ECG, **supraventricular tachycardia (SVT)**

GI: Nausea, vomiting, diarrhea, mucositis, increased bilirubin, alk phos, AST

HEMA: **Neutropenia, leukopenia, thrombocytopenia, anemia,** bleeding, infections

INTEG: Alopecia, **tissue necrosis,** generalized urticaria

P

MS: Arthralgia, myalgia

RESP: **Pulmonary embolism,** dyspnea

SYST: Hypersensitivity reactions, **anaphylaxis, Stevens-Johnson syndrome, toxic epidermal necrolysis, angioedema**

Contraindications: Pregnancy (D), hypersensitivity to paclitaxel or other products with polyoxyethylated castor oil, albumin

Black Box Warning: Neutropenia of <1500/mm³

Precautions: Breastfeeding, children, cardiovascular/hepatic/renal disease, CNS disorder, bone marrow suppression, dental disease/work, extravasation, females, geriatric patients, herpes, infection, infertility, jaundice, ocular exposure, radiation therapy, thrombocytopenia, vaccination

Black Box Warning: Taxane hypersensitivity

PHARMACOKINETICS

89%-98% of product is serum protein bound, metabolized in liver, excreted in bile and urine; terminal half-life 5.3-17.4 hr

INTERACTIONS

Increase: myelosuppression—other antineoplastics, radiation

Increase: DOXOrubicin levels—DOXOrubicin

⚠ ***Increase:*** toxicity, decrease metabolism—ketoconazole; avoid concurrent use

Increase: bleeding risk—NSAIDs, anticoagulants

Decrease: paclitaxel metabolism—verapamil, diazepam, cycloSPORINE, teniposide, etoposide, quinidine, dexamethasone, vinCRIStine, testosterone

Decrease: paclitaxel levels—CYP2C8, CYP2C9 inducers

Decrease: immune response—live virus vaccines

NURSING CONSIDERATIONS

Assess:

- CBC, differential, platelet count prior to and q wk; withhold product if WBC is <1500/mm³ or platelet count is <100,000/mm³, notify prescriber
- Monitor temp q4hr (may indicate beginning infection)
- Hepatic studies before, during therapy (bilirubin, AST, ALT, LDH) prn or q mo, check for jaundiced skin and sclera, dark urine, clay-colored stool, itchy skin, abdominal pain, fever, diarrhea
- VS during 1st hr of infusion, check IV site for signs of infiltration

⚠ Hypersensitive reactions, anaphylaxis including hypotension, dyspnea, angioedema, generalized urticaria; discontinue inf immediately; keep emergency equipment available

- Bleeding: hematuria, guaiac, bruising or petechiae, mucosa or orifices q8hr; obtain prescription for viscous lidocaine (Xylocaine)
- Effects of alopecia on body image; discuss feelings about body changes

Administer:

- Antiemetic 30-60 min before giving product and prn

IV route

- For extravasation if given by regular IV, not port
- After diluting in 0.9% NaCl, D_5, D_5 and 0.9% NaCl, D_5LR to a concentration of 0.3-1.2 mg/ml
- Using an in-line filter ≤0.22 μm
- After premedicating with dexamethasone 20 mg PO 12 hr and 6 hr before paclitaxel, diphenhydrAMINE 50 mg IV ½-1 hr before paclitaxel and cimetidine 300 mg or ranitidine 50 mg IV ½-1 hr before paclitaxel
- Using only glass bottles, polypropylene, polyolefin bags and administration sets; do not use PVC inf bags or sets
- Using gloves and cytotoxic handling precautions

Abraxane

- Reconstitute vial by injecting 20 ml of 0.9% NaCl

- Slowly inject the 20 ml of 0.9% NaCl over at least 1 min to direct the sol flow on wall of vial
- Do not inject 0.9% NaCl directly onto lyophilized cake (foaming will occur)
- Allow vial to sit for at least 5 min to ensure proper wetting of lyophilized cake
- Gently swirl or invert vial slowly for at least 2 min until completely dissolved
- Calculate dosing by dosing vol/ml = total dose (mg) ÷ 5 (mg/ml)

Y-site compatibilities: Acyclovir, amikacin, aminophylline, ampicillin/sulbactam, bleomycin, butorphanol, calcium chloride, carboplatin, cefepime, cefotetan, ceftazidime, ceftriaxone, cimetidine, cisplatin, cladribine, cyclophosphamide, cytarabine, dacarbazine, dexamethasone, diphenhydrAMINE, DOXOrubicin, droperidol, etoposide, famotidine, floxuridine, fluconazole, fluorouracil, furosemide, ganciclovir, gentamicin, granisetron, haloperidol, heparin, hydrocortisone, hydromorphone, ifosfamide, lorazepam, magnesium sulfate, mannitol, meperidine, mesna, methotrexate, metoclopramide, morphine, nalbuphine, ondansetron, pentostatin, potassium chloride, prochlorperazine, propofol, ranitidine, sodium bicarbonate, thiotepa, vancomycin, vinBLAStine, vinCRIStine, zidovudine

Perform/provide:
- Confirmation that dexamethasone was given 12 hr and 6 hr before inf begins
- Storage of prepared sol up to 27 hr in refrigerator

Evaluate:
- Therapeutic response: decreased tumor size, spread of malignancy

Teach patient/family:
- To report signs of infection: fever, sore throat, flulike symptoms
- To report signs of anemia: fatigue, headache, faintness, SOB, irritability
- To report bleeding; avoid use of razors, commercial mouthwash
- To avoid use of aspirin, ibuprofen
- To report any complaints or side effects to nurse or prescriber
- That hair may be lost during treatment; a wig or hairpiece may make patient feel better; new hair may be different in color, texture
- That pain in muscles and joints 2-5 days after inf is common
- To use nonhormonal type of contraception
- To avoid receiving vaccinations while on this product

paliperidone (℞)

(pal-ee-per'i-done)
Invega, Invega Sustenna
Func. class.: Antipsychotic
Chem. class.: Benzisoxazole derivative

Do not confuse:
Invega/Iveegam
paliperidone/risperidone

Action: Mediated through both DOPamine type 2 (D_2) and serotonin type 2 ($5\text{-}HT_2$) antagonism

Uses: Schizophrenia

DOSAGE AND ROUTES

- *Adult:* **PO** 6 mg/day, max 12 mg/day; **IM** 234 mg on day 1, then 156 mg 1 wk later, after 2nd dose, give q mo 117 mg, range 39-234 mg

Renal dose
- *Adult:* **PO** CCr 50-79 ml/min, max 6 mg/day; CCr 10-49 ml/min, max 3 mg/day

Available forms: Ext rel tabs 3, 6, 9 mg; ext rel susp for inj 39 mg/0.25 ml, 78 mg/0.5 ml, 117 mg/0.75 ml, 156 mg/1 ml, 234 mg/1.5 ml

SIDE EFFECTS

CNS: EPS, pseudoparkinsonism, akathisia, dystonia, tardive dyskinesia; drowsiness, insomnia, agitation, anxiety, headache, **seizures, neuroleptic malignant syndrome,** dizziness
CV: Orthostatic hypotension, **tachycardia; heart failure, QT prolongation,** heart block, dysrhythmias
EENT: Blurred vision

P

ENDO: Insulin increase

GI: Nausea, vomiting, *anorexia, constipation,* weight gain, xerostomia

Contraindications: Breastfeeding, geriatric patients, seizure disorders, AV block, QT prolongation, torsade de pointes, hypersensitivity to this product or risperidone

Precautions: Pregnancy (C), children, renal/hepatic disease, obesity, Parkinson's disease

Black Box Warning: Dementia

PHARMACOKINETICS

Peak 24 hr; elimination half-life 23 hr; excreted 80% urine, 11% feces

INTERACTIONS

Increase: sedation—other CNS depressants, alcohol, sedative/hypnotics, opiates

Increase: EPS—other antipsychotics

Increase: QT prolongation—class IA, III antidysrhythmics, azole antifungals, tricyclics (high doses), some phenothiazines, β-blockers, chloroquine, pimozide, droperidol, probucol, some antipsychotics, abarelix, alfuzosin, amoxapine, apomorphine, dasatinib, dolasetron, flecainide, halogenated anesthetics

Decrease: effect of paliperidone—carbamazepine

Decrease: levodopa effect—levodopa

Drug/Herb

Increase: CNS depression—kava

Increase: action—cola tree, hops, nettle, nutmeg

Increase: EPS—betel palm, kava

Drug/Lab Test

Increase: prolactin levels

NURSING CONSIDERATIONS

Assess:

- Mental status before initial administration
- Swallowing of PO medication; check for hoarding or giving of medication to other patients
- I&O ratio; palpate bladder if urinary output is low
- Affect, orientation, LOC, reflexes, gait, coordination, sleep pattern disturbances
- B/P standing and lying; also pulse, respirations; take these q4hr during initial treatment; establish baseline before starting treatment; report drops of 30 mm Hg; watch for ECG changes
- Dizziness, faintness, palpitations, tachycardia on rising
- EPS, including akathisia, tardive dyskinesia (bizarre movements of the jaw, mouth, tongue, extremities), pseudoparkinsonism (rigidity, tremors, pill rolling, shuffling gait)

⚠ For serious reactions in the geriatric patient

⚠ For neuroleptic malignant syndrome: hyperthermia, increased CPK, altered mental status, muscle rigidity

- Skin turgor daily
- Constipation, urinary retention daily; if these occur, increase bulk and water in diet

Administer:

- Do not break, crush, or chew ext rel tabs
- Without regard for food
- Reduced dose in geriatric patients
- Antiparkinsonian agent on order from prescriber, to be used for EPS
- Avoid use with CNS depressants

Perform/provide:

- Supervised ambulation until patient is stabilized on medication; do not involve in strenuous exercise program because fainting is possible; patient should not stand still for a long time
- Decrease stimuli by dimming lights, avoiding loud noise
- Increased fluids to prevent constipation
- Sips of water, candy, gum for dry mouth
- Storage in tight, light-resistant container

Evaluate:

- Therapeutic response: decrease in emotional excitement, hallucinations, delusions, paranoia; reorganization of patterns of thought, speech

Teach patient/family:

- That orthostatic hypotension may occur and to rise from sitting or lying position gradually
- To avoid hot tubs, hot showers, tub baths; hypotension may occur
- To avoid abrupt withdrawal of this product; EPS may result; product should be withdrawn slowly
- To avoid OTC preparations (cough, hay fever, cold) unless approved by prescriber; serious product interactions may occur; avoid use of alcohol; increased drowsiness may occur
- To avoid hazardous activities if drowsy or dizzy
- Compliance with product regimen; nonabsorbable tab shell is expelled in stool
- To report impaired vision, tremors, muscle twitching
- That heat stroke may occur in hot weather; take extra precautions to stay cool
- To use contraception, inform prescriber if pregnancy is planned or suspected

Treatment of overdose: Lavage if orally ingested; provide airway; *do not induce vomiting*

palivizumab (℞)

(pal-ih-viz'uh-mab)

Synagis

Func. class.: Monoclonal antibody

Action: A humanized monoclonal antibody that exhibits neutralizing and fusion-inhibitory activity against respiratory syncytial virus (RSV)

Uses: Prevention of serious lower respiratory tract disease caused by RSV in pediatric patients

Unlabeled uses: IV use

DOSAGE AND ROUTES

- *Infant and child:* **IM** 15 mg/kg monthly, those patients who develop RSV should continue to receive monthly doses during RSV season (November-April); **IV** (unlabeled) 15 mg/kg q mo, must be diluted

Available forms: Powder for reconstitution 50, 100 mg; solution 50 mg/0.5 ml, 100 mg/1 ml

SIDE EFFECTS

CNS: Fever

EENT: Otitis media, rhinitis, pharyngitis

GI: Nausea, vomiting, diarrhea, increased AST

INTEG: Rash, inj site reaction

RESP: Upper respiratory tract infection, **apnea,** cough

SYST: **Anaphylaxis, angioedema**

Contraindications: Hypersensitivity, adults, cyanotic congenital heart disease

Precautions: Pregnancy (C), thrombocytopenia, coagulation disorders, established RSV, congenital heart disease, chronic lung disease, systemic allergic reactions

PHARMACOKINETICS

Mean half-life 20 days

NURSING CONSIDERATIONS

Assess:

- For presence of RSV infection, product is given to prevent infection. For side effects; report if allergic reaction is evident

⚠ For anaphylaxis: difficulty breathing; product should be discontinued and have emergency equipment nearby

Administer:

IM route

- Do not dilute prior to IM administration
- Dosage >1 ml should be divided and injected in different sites
- Do not shake

IV route (unlabeled)

- Dilute liquid sol for inj with 5 ml of sterile water, D_5W to 100 mg vial or 2.5 ml to 50 mg vial to conc (20 mg/ml)
- A filter is not necessary
- Give at 1-2 ml/min (20-40 mg/min)
- Flush line with small amount of D_5W before and after administration

Teach patient/family:

• To report upper respiratory infections, earaches, rash, sore throat

palonosetron (℞)

(pa-lone-o′se-tron)

Aloxi

Func. class.: Antiemetic

Chem. class.: 5-HT_3 receptor antagonist

Action: Prevents nausea, vomiting by blocking serotonin peripherally, centrally, and in the small intestine at the 5-HT_3 receptor

Uses: Prevention of nausea, vomiting associated with cancer chemotherapy, postoperative nausea/vomiting

DOSAGE AND ROUTES

• *Adult:* **PO** 0.5 mg as a single dose 1 hr prior to chemotherapy; **IV** 0.25 mg as a single dose over 30 sec, ½ hr prior to chemotherapy, max 25 mg **IV** over q7days

Postoperative nausea/vomiting prophylaxis for up to 24 hr after surgery

• *Adult:* **IV** 0.075 mg given over 10 sec immediately before induction

Available forms: Inj 0.25/5 ml, 0.075/1.5 ml; caps 0.5 mg

SIDE EFFECTS

CNS: Headache, dizziness, drowsiness, fatigue, insomnia

GI: Diarrhea, constipation, abdominal pain

MISC: Weakness, hyperkalemia, anxiety, rash, **bronchospasm** (rare), arthralgia, *fever, urinary retention*

Contraindications: Hypersensitivity

Precautions: Pregnancy (B), breastfeeding, children, geriatric patients, hypokalemia, hypomagnesium, patients taking diuretics

PHARMACOKINETICS

62% protein bound; metabolized by liver; unchanged product and metabolites excreted by kidney; terminal elimination half-life: 40 hr

INTERACTIONS

• Possible QT prolongation: class 1A antidysrhythmics (disopyramide, procainamide, quinidine), class III antidysrhythmics (amiodarone, bretylium, dofetilide, ibutilide, sotalol), bepridil, chloroquine, clarithromycin, droperidol, erythromycin, grepafloxacin, halofantrine, haloperidol, levomethadyl, methadone, pentamidine, some phenothiazines, diuretics (except potassium sparing)

NURSING CONSIDERATIONS

Assess:

• For agents causing QT prolongation, even though manufacturer has removed QT prolongation from the warnings

• For absence of nausea, vomiting during chemotherapy

• Hypersensitivity reaction: rash, bronchospasm

Administer:

PO route

• Give 1 hr prior to chemotherapy

• May be taken without regard to food

IV route

• Give as a single dose over 30 sec

• Do not mix with other products, flush IV line before and after administration with 0.9% NaCl

Perform/provide:

• Storage at room temperature

Evaluate:

• Therapeutic response: absence of nausea, vomiting during cancer chemotherapy

Teach patient/family:

• To report diarrhea, constipation, rash, or changes in respirations or discomfort at insertion site

• To avoid alcohol, barbiturates

pamidronate (℞)

(pam-i-drone′ate)

Aredia

Func. class.: Bone-resorption inhibitor, electrolyte modifier

Chem. class.: Bisphosphonate

Do not confuse:

Aredia/Adriamycin

Action: Inhibits bone resorption, apparently without inhibiting bone formation and mineralization; adsorbs calcium phosphate crystals in bone and may directly block dissolution of hydroxyapatite crystals of bone

Uses: Moderate to severe Paget's disease, hypercalcemia, osteolytic bone metastases in breast cancer, multiple myeloma patients

Unlabeled uses: Postmenopausal osteoporosis and prevention, osteoporosis prophylaxis, ankylosing spondylitis, osteogenesis imperfecta, hyperparathyroidism

DOSAGE AND ROUTES

Hypercalcemia of malignancy

• *Adult:* **IV INF** 60-90 mg as a single dose in moderate hypercalcemia, 90 mg in severe hypercalcemia over 2-24 hr; dose should be diluted in 1000 ml 0.45% NaCl, 0.9% NaCl or D_5W, wait 7 days before 2nd course

Osteolytic lesions

• *Adult:* **IV** 90 mg/500 ml of D_5W, 0.45% NaCl, or 0.9% NaCl given over 4 hr q mo (multiple myeloma) or over 2 hr q3-4wk (breast carcinoma)

Paget's disease

• *Adult:* **IV INF** 30 mg/day given over 4 hr × 3 days

Severe osteogenesis imperfecta (unlabeled)

• *Child:* **IV** 1.5-3 mg/kg/cycle, cycle dose is divided in 3, administered over slow IV over 4 hr/day × 3 days

Hypercalcemia (hyperparathyroidism) (unlabeled)

• *Adult:* **IV** 15-60 mg as a single dose

Corticosteroid-induced osteoporosis (unlabeled)

• *Adult:* **IV** 30 mg q3mo × 1 yr

Ankylosing spondylitis (unlabeled)

• *Adult:* **IV INF** 60 mg over 4 hr; 6 hr INF for first dose

Osteoporosis prophylaxis in Crohn's disease (unlabeled)

• *Adult:* **IV INF** 30 mg over 1 hr q3mo × 1 yr

Available forms: Powder for inj 30, 90 mg/vial; inj 3, 6, 9 mg/ml

SIDE EFFECTS

CNS: Fever, fatigue

CV: Hypertension, **atrial fibrillation**

EENT: Ocular pain, inflammation, vision impairment

GI: Abdominal pain, anorexia, constipation, nausea, vomiting, dyspepsia

GU: **Renal failure**

INTEG: Redness, swelling, induration, pain on palpation at site of catheter insertion

META: Anemia, *hypokalemia, hypomagnesemia, hypophosphatemia, hypocalcemia,* hypothyroidism

MS: Severe bone pain, myalgia, osteonecrosis of the jaw

RESP: Coughing, dyspnea, upper respiratory tract infection

SYST: **Angioedema, anaphylaxis**

Contraindications: Pregnancy (D), hypersensitivity to bisphosphonates

Precautions: Children, nursing mothers, renal dysfunction, poor dentition

PHARMACOKINETICS

Rapidly cleared from circulation and taken up mainly by bones, primarily in areas of high bone turnover, eliminated primarily by kidneys, half-life 21-35 hr, terminal half-life in bone is 300 days

INTERACTIONS

Increase: hypokalemia—loop diuretics

Increase: nephrotoxicity—aminoglycosides, NSAIDs, vancomycin, radiopaque contrast agents, cycloSPORINE, tacrolimus

Increase: effect of entecavir
Decrease: pamidronate effect—calcium, vit D

NURSING CONSIDERATIONS

Assess:

- Dental health; cover with antiinfectives for dental extractions
- For atrial fibrillation
- Electrolytes, Ca, PO_4, Mg, K
- For hypocalcemia: nausea, vomiting, constipation, thirst, dysrhythmias, hypocalcemia, paresthesia, twitching, laryngospasm, Chvostek's, Trousseau's signs
- For bone pain; use analgesics
- I&O, check for fluid overload edema, crackles, increased B/P; BUN, creatinine

Administer:

IV route

- After reconstituting by adding 10 ml of sterile water for inj to each vial (30 mg/10 ml or 90 mg/10 ml depending on vial used); add to 1000 ml of sterile 0.45%, 0.9% NaCl, D_5W, run over 2-24 hr (hypercalcemia); dilute reconstituted sol in 500 ml of 0.9% NaCl, 0.45% NaCl, or D_5W, give over 4 hr (multiple myeloma, Paget's disease); dilute reconstituted sol in 250 ml of 0.9% NaCl, 0.45% NaCl or D_5W, give over 2 hr (osteolytic bone metastases of breast cancer)
- Do not mix with calcium-containing infusion sol such as Ringer's sol

Perform/provide:

- Storage of inf sol up to 24 hr at room temperature
- Reconstituted sol with sterile water may be stored under refrigeration for up to 24 hr

Evaluate:

- Therapeutic response: decreased calcium levels

Teach patient/family

- To report hypercalcemic relapse: nausea, vomiting, bone pain, thirst; unusual muscle twitching, muscle spasms, severe diarrhea, constipation
- To continue with dietary recommendations including calcium and vit D
- To obtain an analgesic from provider for bone pain
- That if nausea/vomiting occur, small, frequent meals may help
- To report ocular symptoms: blurred vision, edema, inflammation; report to prescriber

pancreatin (℞)

(pan'kree-a-tin)
Creon, Creon Delayed Release, Donnazyne, Encron, Hi-Vegi-Lip, 4× Pancreatin 600 mg, 8× Pancreatin 900 mg, Pancrezyme 4×
Func. class.: Digestant
Chem. class.: Pancreatic enzyme concentrate—bovine/porcine

Action: Pancreatic enzyme needed for breakdown of substances released from the pancreas

Uses: Exocrine pancreatic secretion insufficiency, cystic fibrosis (digestive aid)

DOSAGE AND ROUTES:

- *Adult:* **PO** 2000 units of lipase activity up to 36,000 units/day before or with each meal or snack

Available forms: Tabs 325, 500, 650, 900, 1200, 1500, 2000, 12,000 units, others in combination; caps; Creon Delayed Release

SIDE EFFECTS

EENT: Buccal soreness, cavities
GI: Anorexia, nausea, vomiting, diarrhea, glossitis, anal soreness, abdominal discomfort
GU: Hyperuricuria, hyperuricemia, perianal pain
INTEG: Rash, hypersensitivity

Contraindications: Hypersensitivity to pork, chronic pancreatic disease

Precautions: Pregnancy (C), breastfeeding, ileus, esophageal stricture, Crohn's disease

INTERACTIONS

Decrease: absorption—cimetidine, antacids, oral iron

Decrease: effect of acarbose, miglitol

NURSING CONSIDERATIONS

Assess:

- I&O ratio; watch for increasing urinary output; urinalysis, blood chemistries
- Fecal fat, nitrogen, PT, calcium during treatment
- For polyuria, polydipsia, polyphagia (may indicate diabetes mellitus)
- For allergy to pork

Administer:

PO route

- Swallow tabs whole quickly; do not break, crush, or chew enteric-coated tabs; take with meals
- Caps may be opened and mixed with soft foods or fluids; take immediately; do not chew
- After antacid or H_2-blockers
- Low-fat diet for GI symptoms

Perform/provide:

- Adequate hydration
- Storage in tight container at room temperature

Evaluate:

- Therapeutic response: relief of GI symptoms

pancrelipase (℞)

(pan-kre-li'pase)

Cotazym, Cotazym-65B ✤, Cotazym E.C.S. 8, Cotazym E.C.S. 20, Cotazym Capsules, Cotazym-S, Creon, Ilozyme, Ku-Zyme HP, Lipram-PN16, Lipram-CR20, Lipram-UL12, Lipram-PN10, Pancrease Capsules, Pancrease MT 4, Pancrease MT 10, Pancrease MT 16, Protilase, Ultrase MT 12, Ultrase MT 20, Viokase, Zenpep, Zymase

Func. class.: Digestant

Chem. class.: Pancreatic enzyme—bovine/porcine

Action: Pancreatic enzyme needed for breakdown of substances released from the pancreas

Uses: Exocrine pancreatic secretion insufficiency, cystic fibrosis (digestive aid), steatorrhea, pancreatic enzyme deficiency

DOSAGE AND ROUTES

Many products listed above are not interchangeable

- *Adult and child:* **PO** 1-3 caps/tabs before meals or with meals, or 1 cap/tab with snack or 1-2 powder pkt before meals

Available forms: Powder 16,800 units lipase/70,000 units protease and amylase; caps 8000 units lipase/30,000 units protease and amylase; delayed rel cap 4000 units lipase/12,000 units protease and amylase, 4000 units lipase/25,000 units protease/20,000 units amylase, 5000 units lipase/20,000 units protease and amylase, 10,000 units lipase/30,000 units protease and amylase, 12,000 units lipase/24,000 units protease and amylase, 12,000 units lipase/39,000 units protease and amylase, 16,000 units lipase/48,000 units protease and amylase, 20,000 units lipase/65,000 units protease and amylase, 24,000 units lipase/78,000 units protease and amylase; del rel cap 5000, 15,000 units

SIDE EFFECTS

GI: Anorexia, nausea, vomiting, diarrhea, cramping, bloating
GU: Hyperuricuria, hyperuricemia
Contraindications: Allergy to pork
Precautions: Pregnancy (B), ileus, pancreatitis, Crohn's disease

INTERACTIONS

Decrease: absorption—cimetidine, antacids, oral iron
Decrease: effect of acarbose, miglitol

NURSING CONSIDERATIONS

Assess:

- For appropriate height, weight development; may be delayed
- I&O ratio; watch for increasing urinary output
- Fecal fat, nitrogen, PT during treatment
- For polyuria, polydipsia, polyphagia (may indicate diabetes mellitus)
- For pork sensitivity, cross-sensitivity may occur

Administer:

- Avoid inhaling powder
- After antacid or cimetidine; decreased pH inactivates product
- Powder mixed in prepared fruit juice for infants, children
- Low-fat diet for GI symptoms
- With 8 oz water or more; do not allow to sit in mouth; have patient sit up during administration; give with meals

Perform/provide:

- Adequate hydration
- Storage in tight container at room temperature

Evaluate:

- Therapeutic response: improved digestion of carbohydrates, protein, fat; absence of steatorrhea

Teach patient/family:

- Not to inhale powder; may be very irritating to mucous membranes; some powder may irritate skin
- To notify prescriber of allergic reactions, abdominal pain, cramping, or blood in the urine

⚠ High Alert

pancuronium (℞)

(pan-kyoo-roe'nee-um)
pancuronium bromide
Func. class.: Neuromuscular blocker (nondepolarizing)
Chem. class.: Synthetic curariform

Action: Inhibits transmission of nerve impulses by binding with cholinergic receptor sites, antagonizing action of acetylcholine
Uses: Facilitation of endotracheal intubation, skeletal muscle relaxation during mechanical ventilation, surgery, or general anesthesia

DOSAGE AND ROUTES

- *Adult/child/infant >1 mo:* **IV** 0.06-0.1 mg/kg initially or 0.05 mg/kg after initial dose of succinylcholine; maintenance 0.01 mg/kg 60-100 min after initial dose, then 0.01 mg/kg q25-60min as needed; in obese patients, use ideal body weight
- *Neonate <1 mo:* **IV** Test dose 0.02 mg/kg, then 0.03 mg/kg/dose initially, repeat 2× as needed at 5-10 min intervals; maintenance 0.03-0.09 mg/kg/dose q30min-4 hr as needed

Available forms: Inj 1, 2 mg/ml

SIDE EFFECTS

CV: Bradycardia; tachycardia; increased, decreased B/P; ventricular extrasystoles, edema, hypertension
EENT: Increased secretions
INTEG: Rash, flushing, pruritus, urticaria, sweating, salivation
MS: Weakness to prolonged skeletal muscle relaxation

RESP: **Prolonged apnea, bronchospasm, cyanosis, respiratory depression,** dyspnea
SYST: **Anaphylaxis**
Contraindications: Hypersensitivity to bromide ion
Precautions: Pregnancy (C), breastfeeding, children <2 yr, neuromuscular/cardiac/renal/hepatic disease, electrolyte imbalances, dehydration, previous anaphylactic reactions (other neuromuscular blockers)

Black Box Warning: Respiratory insufficiency

PHARMACOKINETICS

IV: Onset 3-5 min, dose dependent, peak 3-5 min; metabolized (small amounts), excreted in urine (unchanged), crosses placenta

INTERACTIONS

• Dysrhythmias: theophylline
Increase: neuromuscular blockade—aminoglycosides, clindamycin, enflurane, isoflurane, lincomycin, lithium, local anesthetics, opioid analgesics, polymyxin antiinfectives, quinidine, thiazides
Drug/Lab Test
Decrease: cholinesterase

NURSING CONSIDERATIONS

Assess:
• For electrolyte imbalances (K, Mg); may lead to increased action of this product
• VS (B/P, pulse, respirations, airway) until fully recovered; rate, depth, pattern of respirations, strength of hand grip
• I&O ratio; check for urinary retention, frequency, hesitancy
• Recovery: decreased paralysis of face, diaphragm, leg, arm, rest of body; allow to recover fully before neurologic assessment
⚠ Allergic reactions, anaphylaxis: rash, fever, respiratory distress, pruritus; product should be discontinued

Administer:
IV, direct route
• May be given undiluted via rapid IV inj
Additive compatibilities: Verapamil, ciprofloxacin
Syringe compatibilities: Heparin
Y-site compatibilities: Aminophylline, cefazolin, cefuroxime, cimetidine, DOBUTamine, DOPamine, epinephrine, esmolol, fenoldopam, fentanyl, fluconazole, gentamicin, heparin, hydrocortisone, isoproterenol, levofloxacin, lorazepam, midazolam, morphine, nitroglycerin, ranitidine, trimethoprim-sulfamethoxazole, vancomycin
Perform/provide:
• Storage in refrigerator; do not store in plastic; use only fresh sol
• Reassurance if communication is difficult during recovery from neuromuscular blockade
• Frequent (q2hr) instillation of artificial tears and covering eyes to prevent drying of cornea
Evaluate:
• Therapeutic response: paralysis of jaw, eyelid, head, neck, rest of body
Treatment of overdose: Edrophonium or neostigmine, atropine, monitor VS; may require mechanical ventilation

P

panitumumab (℞)

(pan-i-tue′moo-mab)
Vectibix
Func. class.: Antineoplastic—miscellaneous
Chem. class.: Multikinase inhibitor, signal transduction inhibitor

Action: Decreases growth and survival of cancer cells by competitive inhibition of EGF receptor
Uses: EGFR expressing metastatic colorectal cancer, not beneficial in KRAS mutations in codon 12 or 13

DOSAGE AND ROUTES

• *Adult:* **IV INF** 6 mg/kg over 60 min every 2 wk
Available forms: Sol for inj 20 mg/ml

SIDE EFFECTS

CNS: Fatigue
CV: Peripheral edema
EENT: Ocular irritation, ocular hyperemia
GI: Nausea, diarrhea, vomiting, anorexia, mouth ulceration, abdominal pain, constipation
HEMA: Thrombophlebitis
INTEG: Rash, pruritus, **exfoliative dermatitis,** skin fissure, **angioedema, severe/fatal INF reactions**
META: Hypocalcemia, hypomagnesemia, antibody formation
RESP: **Bronchospasm, cough,** dyspnea, **hypoxia, pulmonary fibrosis/embolism,** pneumonitis, wheezing

Contraindications: Hypersensitivity

Precautions: Pregnancy (C), breastfeeding, children, hepatic disease, acute bronchospasm, diarrhea, hamster protein allergy, hypomagnesemia, hypotension, pulmonary fibrosis, sepsis, KRAS mutations

Black Box Warning: Exfoliative dermatitis, infusion-related reactions

PHARMACOKINETICS

Bioavailability 38%-49%; elimination half-life 7.5 days; peak 3 hr; high-fat meal decreases bioavailability; plasma protein binding 99.5%; metabolized in the liver; oxidative metabolism by CYP3A4, glucuronidation by UGT1A9; 77% excreted in feces

INTERACTIONS

- Do not use in combination with other antineoplastics

NURSING CONSIDERATIONS

Assess:

- Serum electrolytes periodically (calcium, magnesium)
- Signs of infection: increased temp
- Signs of infusion reactions: bronchospasm, fever, chills, hypotension
- Signs of ocular toxicity: ocular irritation, hyperemia

Administer:

- Give in hospital or clinic setting with full resuscitation equipment
- Only as IV inf using controlled IV inf pump; do not give IV push or bolus; use low-protein binding 0.2 or 0.22 micron in-line filter; flush line with 0.9% NaCl before and after administration
- Give over 60 min through a peripheral line or indwelling catheter; infuse doses of >1000 mg over 90 min
- Dilute in 100 ml of 0.9% NaCl; dilute doses >1000 mg in 150 ml of 0.9% NaCl; mix by inverting; do not exceed 10 mg/ml; use within 6 hr if stored at room temperature; can be stored between 2° C and 8° C for up to 24 hr

Perform/provide:

- Storage of unopened vials in refrigerator; do not shake; protect from direct sunlight; do not freeze

Evaluate:

- Therapeutic response: decrease in colon carcinoma progression

Teach patient/family:

- ⚠ To report adverse reactions immediately: difficulty breathing, mouth sores, skin rash, ocular toxicity
- Reason for treatment, expected results, adverse reactions
- To have males and females use contraception while taking this product and for 6 months after treatment; do not breastfeed for at least 2 mo after stopping treatment
- To avoid the sun and use sunscreen while taking this product

pantoprazole (℞)

(pan-toe-pray′zole)
Protonix, Prontonix IV
Func. class.: Proton pump inhibitor
Chem. class.: Benzimidazole

Action: Suppresses gastric secretion by inhibiting hydrogen/potassium ATPase enzyme system in gastric parietal cell; characterized as gastric acid pump inhibitor, since it blocks final step of acid production

Uses: Gastroesophageal reflux disease (GERD), severe erosive esophagitis, maintenance, long-term pathologic hypersecretory conditions including Zollinger-Ellison syndrome

Unlabeled uses: Duodenal/gastric ulcer, NSAID ulcer prophylaxis, *Helicobacter pylori*–associated ulcer, dyspepsia

DOSAGE AND ROUTES

GERD

• *Adult:* **PO** 40 mg/day × 8 wk, may repeat course

Erosive esophagitis

• *Adult:* **IV** 40 mg/day × 7-10 day; **PO** 40 mg/day × 8 wk; may repeat **PO** course

Pathologic hypersecretory conditions

• *Adult:* **PO** 40 mg bid; **IV** 80 mg q12hr, max 240 mg/day

Duodenal ulcer/gastric ulcer/ NSAID ulcer prophylaxis (unlabeled)

• *Adult:* **PO** 40 mg/day

H. pylori*–associated ulcers (unlabeled)*

• *Adult:* **PO** 40 mg bid; may be used with other products

Available forms: Delayed rel tabs 20, 40 mg; powder for inj, freeze-dried 40 mg/vial

SIDE EFFECTS

CNS: Headache, insomnia

GI: Diarrhea, abdominal pain, flatulence

INTEG: Rash

META: Hyperglycemia

RESP: **Pneumonia**

Contraindications: Hypersensitivity

Precautions: Pregnancy (C), breastfeeding, children, proton pump hypersensitivity

PHARMACOKINETICS

Peak 2.4 hr, duration >24 hr, half-life 1.5 hr, protein binding 97%, eliminated in urine as metabolites and in feces; in geriatric patients elimination rate decreased

INTERACTIONS

Increase: pantoprazole serum levels—diazepam, phenytoin, flurazepam, triazolam, clarithromycin

Increase: bleeding—warfarin

Decrease: absorption—sucralfate, calcium carbonate, vit B_{12}

NURSING CONSIDERATIONS

Assess:

• GI system: bowel sounds q8hr, abdomen for pain, swelling, anorexia

• Hepatic studies: AST, ALT, alk phos during treatment

• For vit B_{12} deficiency in those on long-term therapy

Administer:

PO route

• Swallow del rel tabs whole; do not break, crush, or chew

• Take del rel tabs at same time of day

• May take with or without food

IV route

• Reconstitute with 10 ml 0.9% NaCl, further dilute with 80 ml LR, D_5, 0.9% NaCl (0.8 mg/ml), give over 15 min (≤6 mg/min) or as IV push over 2 min

Evaluate:

• Therapeutic response: absence of epigastric pain, swelling, fullness

Teach patient/family:

• To report severe diarrhea; product may have to be discontinued

• That diabetic patient should know hyperglycemia may occur

• To avoid hazardous activities; dizziness may occur

• To avoid alcohol, salicylates, ibuprofen; may cause GI irritation

• To notify prescriber if pregnant or plan to become pregnant, do not breastfeed

• To continue taking even if feeling better

P

paricalcitol (℞)

(par-ih-cal′sih-tol)

Zemplar

Func. class.: Vit D analog

Chem. class.: Fat-soluble vitamin

Action: Reduces parathyroid hormone (PTH) levels; suppresses PTH levels in patients with chronic renal failure with absence of hypercalcemia/hyperphosphatemia; serum PO_4, calcium, CaXP may increase

Uses: Hyperparathyroidism in chronic renal failure

Unlabeled uses: Renal osteodystrophy

DOSAGE AND ROUTES

• *Adult:* **IV BOL** 0.04-0.1 mcg/kg (2.8-7 mcg) no more than every other day during dialysis; may increase by 2-4 mcg q2-4wk until target serum intact PTH (1.5 – 3 × nonuremic upper limit of normal) is achieved; **PO** 1 mcg/day or 2 mcg 3×/wk

Available forms: Inj 5 mcg/ml; caps 1, 2, 4 mcg

SIDE EFFECTS

CNS: Light-headedness

CV: Palpitations

GI: Nausea, vomiting, anorexia, dry mouth

OTHER: Pneumonia, edema, chills, fever, flu, **sepsis**

Contraindications: Hypersensitivity, hypercalcemia

Precautions: Pregnancy (C), breastfeeding, children, geriatric patients, CV disease, renal calculi

PHARMACOKINETICS

Crosses placenta, enters breast milk

INTERACTIONS

• Digoxin toxicity: digoxin

NURSING CONSIDERATIONS

Assess:

• Ca, PO_4 2×/wk during initial therapy; after dose is established take calcium and phosphorus q mo

Administer:

IV route

• By IV bolus only

Evaluate:

• Decreased hypoparathyroidism in chronic renal disease

Teach patient/family:

• To report weakness, lethargy, headache, anorexia, loss of weight

• To report nausea, vomiting, palpitations

• To adhere to dietary regimen of calcium supplementation/phosphorus restriction

• Avoid excessive use of aluminum compounds/antacids

• Not to breastfeed

• Not to take mineral oil while taking vit D

• To report signs of digoxin toxicity, if on digoxin

paroxetine (℞)

(par-ox′e-teen)

Paxeva, Paxil, Paxil CR

Func. class.: Antidepressant, SSRI

Chem. class.: Phenylpiperidine derivative

Do not confuse:

paroxetine/paclitaxel

Paxil/paclitaxel/Taxol

Action: Inhibits CNS neuron uptake of serotonin but not of norepinephrine or DOPamine

Uses: Major depressive disorder, obsessive-compulsive disorder, panic disorder, generalized anxiety disorder, posttraumatic stress disorder, premenstrual disorders, social anxiety disorder

Unlabeled uses: Premature ejaculation, hot flashes, menopause

DOSAGE AND ROUTES

Generalized anxiety disorder

• *Adult:* **PO** 20 mg/day AM range 20-50 mg/day

Posttraumatic stress disorder

• *Adult:* **PO** 20 mg/day range 20-60 mg/day

Depression

• *Adult:* **PO** 20 mg/day in AM; after 4 wk if no clinical improvement is noted, dose may be increased by 10 mg/day q wk to desired response, max 50 mg/day or **CONT REL** 25 mg/day, may increase by 12.5 mg/day/wk up to 62.5 mg/day

• *Geriatric:* **PO** 10 mg/day, increase by 10 mg to desired dose, max 40 mg/day

Obsessive-compulsive disorder

• *Adult:* **PO** 40 mg/day in AM, start with 20 mg/day, increase 10 mg/day increments, max 60 mg/day

Panic disorder

• *Adult:* **PO** Start with 10 mg/day and increase in 10 mg/day increments to 40 mg/day, max 60 mg/day or **CONT REL** 12.5 mg/day, max 75 mg/day

Premenstrual disorders

• *Adult:* **CONT REL** 12.5 mg/day in AM

Renal dose

• *Adult:* **PO** CCr <30 ml/min 10 mg/day in AM, may increase by 10 mg/day q wk, max 40 mg/day or **CONT REL** 12.5 mg/day, max 50 mg/day

Menopause symptoms/hot flashes (unlabeled)

• *Adult:* **PO (CONT REL)** 12.5 mg/day, may increase to 25 mg/day after 1 wk

Premature ejaculation (unlabeled)

• *Adult:* **PO** 20 mg/day

Available forms: Tabs 10, 20, 30, 40 mg; oral susp 10 mg/5 ml; cont rel tab 12.5, 25, 37.5 mg

SIDE EFFECTS

CNS: *Headache,* nervousness, insomnia, *drowsiness, anxiety, tremor, dizziness,* fatigue, *sedation,* abnormal dreams, agitation, apathy, euphoria, hallucinations, delusions, psychosis, **seizures, neuroleptic malignant syndrome–like reactions**

CV: Vasodilation, postural hypotension, palpitations

EENT: Visual changes

GI: *Nausea, diarrhea, dry mouth,* anorexia, dyspepsia, *constipation,* cramps, vomiting, taste changes, flatulence, decreased appetite

GU: Dysmenorrhea, decreased libido, urinary frequency, UTI, amenorrhea, cystitis, impotence, *abnormal ejaculation (male)*

INTEG: *Sweating,* rash

MS: Pain, arthritis, myalgia, myopathy, myosthenia

RESP: Infection, pharyngitis, nasal congestion, sinus headache, sinusitis, cough, dyspnea, yawning

SYST: Asthenia, fever, abrupt withdrawal syndrome

Contraindications: Pregnancy (D), hypersensitivity, MAOI use, alcohol use

Precautions: Breastfeeding, geriatric patients, seizure history, patients with history of mania, renal/hepatic disease

Black Box Warning: Children, suicidal ideation

PHARMACOKINETICS

PO: Peak 5.2 hr; metabolized in liver by CYP2D6 enzyme system, unchanged products and metabolites excreted in feces and urine; half-life 21 hr (reg rel); 15-20 hr (cont rel); protein binding 95%

INTERACTIONS

• Paroxetine may decrease digoxin levels

⚠ Do not use with MAOIs, pimozide, thioridazine; potentially fatal reactions can occur

Increase: bleeding—warfarin

Increase: paroxetine plasma levels—cimetidine

Increase: agitation—L-tryptophan

Increase: side effects—highly protein-bound products

Increase: theophylline levels—theophylline

P

Increase: toxicity—CYP2D6 inhibitors (aprepitant, delavirdine, imatinib, nefazodone)
Decrease: paroxetine levels—phenobarbital and phenytoin

Drug/Herb

- Avoid use with St. John's wort, kava
- Possible serotonin syndrome: SAM-e, St. John's wort
- Hypertensive crisis: ephedra

Increase: anticholinergic effect—corkwood, jimsonweed
Increase: sedative—hops, lavender
Increase: CNS stimulation—yohimbe

Drug/Lab Test

Increase: serum bilirubin, blood glucose, alk phos
Decrease: VMA, 5-HIAA
False increase: urinary catecholamines

NURSING CONSIDERATIONS

Assess:

- Mental status: mood, sensorium, affect, suicidal tendencies, increase in psychiatric symptoms, depression, panic; OCD: decreasing obsessive thoughts, compulsive behaviors
- B/P (lying/standing), pulse q4hr; if systolic B/P drops 20 mm Hg, hold product, notify prescriber; take vital signs q4hr in patients with CV disease
- Blood studies: CBC, leukocytes, differential, cardiac enzymes if patient is receiving long-term therapy
- Hepatic studies: AST, ALT, bilirubin, creatinine
- Weight q wk; appetite may decrease with product
- ECG for flattening of T wave, bundle branch, AV block, dysrhythmias in cardiac patients
- EPS primarily in geriatric patients: rigidity, dystonia, akathisia
- Urinary retention, constipation
- Withdrawal symptoms: headache, nausea, vomiting, muscle pain, weakness; not usual unless product discontinued abruptly
- Alcohol intake; if alcohol is consumed, hold dose until morning

Administer:

- Increased fluids, bulk in diet for constipation, urinary retention
- With food, milk for GI symptoms
- Crushed if patient is unable to swallow medication whole (regular release only)
- Dosage at bedtime for oversedation during day; may take entire dose at bedtime; geriatric patients may not tolerate once/day dosing
- Gum, hard candy, frequent sips of water for dry mouth
- Avoid use with other CNS depressants

Perform/provide:

- Storage at room temperature; do not freeze
- Assistance with ambulation during therapy, since drowsiness, dizziness occur
- Safety measures primarily in geriatric patients
- Checking to see if PO medication swallowed

Evaluate:

- Therapeutic response: decreased depression

Teach patient/family:

- That therapeutic effect may take 1-4 wk
- To use caution in driving, other activities requiring alertness because of drowsiness, dizziness, blurred vision
- Not to discontinue medication quickly after long-term use; may cause nausea, headache, malaise (abrupt withdrawal syndrome)
- That depression may worsen, suicidal thoughts/behavior occur
- To avoid alcohol ingestion

Treatment of overdose: Activated charcoal, gastric lavage, airway; for seizures give diazepam, symptomatic treatment

pegaptanib (℞)

(peg-ap′ta-nib)

Macugen

Func. class.: Ophthalmic agent—miscellaneous

Action: Binds to vascular endothelial growth factor (VEGF), thereby inhibiting angiogenesis

Uses: Treatment of neovascular (wet) age-related macular degeneration; may be used alone or with photodynamic therapy

Unlabeled uses: Use in diabetic macular edema

DOSAGE AND ROUTES

• *Adult:* **INTRAVITREAL INJ** 0.3 mg injected q6wk

Available forms: Inj 0.3 mg, single glass syringes

SIDE EFFECTS

EENT: Anterior chamber inflammation, blurred vision, conjunctival hemorrhage, corneal edema, cataract, eye discharge, eye pain, increased intraocular pressure, punctuate keratitis, reduced visual acuity, vitreous floaters, vitreous opacities, blepharitis, conjunctivitis, photophobia, retinal detachment, iatrogenic traumatic cataract

Contraindications: Hypersensitivity, ocular or periocular infections

Precautions: Pregnancy (B), inflammatory eye disease, ocular hypertension

PHARMACOKINETICS:

Half-life 87-100 hr in vitreous humor of the monkey, may remain fully active in the eye for 7-28 days

NURSING CONSIDERATIONS

Assess:

• Visual acuity periodically

• Treated eye for increased intraocular pressure, infection, endophthalmitis

• Perfusion of the optic nerve head immediately after inj, tonometry ½ hr after inj, biomicroscopy 2-7 days after inj

Administer:

• Anesthesia and a broad-spectrum anti-infective agent before inj

• The inj should be done under aseptic conditions

• Remove all air bubbles prior to use

Perform/provide:

• Storage at 36° F-46° F, do not freeze or shake vigorously

Evaluate:

• Therapeutic response: macular degeneration stabilized

Teach patient/family:

• To report any inflammation, bleeding, eye discharge, opacities to prescriber

• To continue with follow-up care during treatment

⚠ High Alert

pegaspargase (℞)

(peg-as′per-gase)

Oncaspar, PEG-L-asparaginase

Func. class.: Antineoplastic

Chem. class.: Escherichia coli enzyme

Action: Indirectly inhibits protein synthesis in tumor cells; without amino acid, DNA, RNA synthesis is halted; asparagine, protein synthesis is halted; G_1 phase; cell-cycle specific; a nonvesicant; a modified version of L-asparaginase

Uses: Acute lymphocytic leukemia in combination with other antineoplastics

DOSAGE AND ROUTES

In combination

• *Adult and child:* **IV/IM** 2500 international units/m^2 q14days, run **IV** over 1-2 hr in 100 ml of NaCl or D_5 through a running **IV**; **IM** should be no more than 2 ml in one inj site used in combination with other chemotherapeutics

P

Available forms: Inj 750 international units/ml in a phosphate buffered saline sol

SIDE EFFECTS

CNS: Neuritis, dizziness, headache, **coma,** depression, fatigue, confusion, hallucinations, **seizures, intracranial bleeding**
CV: Chest pain, **hypotension**
ENDO: Hyperglycemia
GI: Nausea, vomiting, anorexia, cramps, stomatitis, **hepatotoxicity, pancreatitis,** *diarrhea*
GU: Urinary retention, **renal failure,** glycosuria, polyuria, azotemia, uric acid neuropathy
HEMA: **Thrombocytopenia, leukopenia, myelosuppression, anemia, decreased clotting factors, pancytopenia, DIC**
INTEG: Rash, urticaria, chills, fever
RESP: **Fibrosis, pulmonary infiltrate, severe bronchospasm**
SYST: **Anaphylaxis, hypersensitivity, angioedema**

Contraindications: Breastfeeding, infant, hypersensitivity, pancreatitis, acute bronchospasm, bleeding, coagulopathy, coronary thrombosis, DIC, hypotension

Precautions: Pregnancy (C), CNS/renal/hepatic disease, *Escherichia coli* protein hypersensitivity, hemophilia, tumor lysis syndrome, infection

PHARMACOKINETICS

Half-life 5½ days, onset rapid, duration 2 wk, metabolized in reticuloendothelial system

INTERACTIONS

- Do not use with radiation
- Coagulation factor imbalances: heparin, warfarin, aspirin, NSAIDs

Decrease: action of methotrexate

NURSING CONSIDERATIONS

Assess:

⚠ For signs and symptoms of pancreatitis (nausea, vomiting, severe abdominal pain), anaphylaxis (bronchospasm, dyspnea), cyanosis

- CBC, differential, platelet count q wk; withhold product if WBC count is <4000 or platelet count is <75,000; notify prescriber of results
- Pulmonary function tests, chest x-ray studies before and during therapy; chest x-ray film should be obtained q2wk during treatment, watch for severe bronchospasm, fibrosis, pulmonary infiltrate
- Renal studies: BUN, serum uric acid, ammonia, urine CCr, electrolytes before and during therapy
- I&O ratio; report fall in urine output to ≤30 ml/hr, may indicate renal failure
- Temp q4hr (may indicate beginning infection)
- Hepatic studies before and during therapy (bilirubin, AST, ALT, LDH) as needed or monthly, hepatotoxicity can occur; check for jaundiced skin, sclera; dark urine, clay-colored stools, itchy skin, abdominal pain, fever, diarrhea
- RBC, Hct, Hgb; may be decreased
- Serum, urine glucose levels, glycosuria can occur
- Bleeding: hematuria, stool guaiac, bruising or petechiae, mucosa or orifices q8hr
- Dyspnea, crackles, nonproductive cough, chest pain, tachypnea, fatigue, increased pulse, pallor, lethargy, swelling around eyes or lips; anaphylaxis may occur
- B/P, since hypertension can occur
- Local irritation, pain, burning, discoloration at inj site

⚠ Symptoms of severe allergic reaction: rash, pruritus, urticaria, purpuric skin lesions, itching, flushing, dyspnea

- Frequency of stools, characteristics; cramping, acidosis; signs of dehydration: rapid respirations, poor skin turgor, decreased urine output, dry skin, restlessness, weakness

Administer:

- Antispasmodic if GI symptoms occur
- Allopurinol or sodium bicarbonate to reduce uric acid levels, alkalinization of urine

Intermittent IV INF route

- Using 21, 23, 25G needle; administer by slow IV infusion via Y-tube or 3-way stopcock of flowing D_5W or NS inf over 2 hr after diluting
- Considered incompatible with other products in syringe or sol

Perform/provide:

- Deep-breathing exercises with patient tid-qid; place in semi-Fowler's position
- Increase fluid intake to 2-3 L/day to prevent urate deposits, calculi formation
- Diet low in purines: no organ meats (kidney, liver); dried beans, peas to maintain alkaline urine
- Rinsing of mouth tid-qid with water, club soda; brushing of teeth bid-tid with soft brush or cotton-tipped applicator for stomatitis; use unwaxed dental floss
- Warm compresses at inj site for inflammation

Evaluate:

- Therapeutic response: decreased exacerbations in acute lymphocytic leukemia

Teach patient/family:

- To report nausea, vomiting, bruising, bleeding, stomatitis, severe diarrhea, jaundice, chest pain, abdominal pain, trouble breathing, rash
- To avoid vaccinations without advice of prescriber
- Not to use hard-bristled toothbrush, razors
- To avoid OTC medications, alcohol

Treatment of anaphylaxis: Administer epinephrine, diphenhydrAMINE, IV corticosteroids

pegfilgrastim (℞)

(peg-fill-grass'stim)

Neulasta

Func. class.: Hematopoietic agent

Chem. class.: Granulocyte colony-stimulating factor

Action: Stimulates proliferation and differentiation of neutrophils

Uses: To decrease infection in patients receiving antineoplastics that are myelosuppressive; to increase WBC in patients with product-induced neutropenia

DOSAGE AND ROUTES

- *Adult:* **SUBCUT** 6 mg give once per chemotherapy cycle

Available forms: Sol for inj 6 mg/0.6 ml

SIDE EFFECTS

CNS: Fever, fatigue, headache, dizziness, insomnia, peripheral edema

GI: *Nausea,* vomiting, diarrhea, mucositis, anorexia, constipation, dyspepsia, abdominal pain, stomatitis, **splenic rupture**

HEMA: **Leukocytosis, granulocytopenia, sickle cell crisis, hemoglobin S disease with crisis**

INTEG: Alopecia

MISC: Chest pain, hyperuricemia, **anaphylaxis, influenza-like illness**

MS: Skeletal pain

RESP: **Respiratory distress syndrome**

Contraindications: Hypersensitivity to proteins of *Escherichia coli,* filgrastim

Precautions: Pregnancy (C), breastfeeding, children <45 kg, adolescents, myeloid malignancies, sickle cell disease, leukocytosis, splenic rupture, ARDs, allergic-type reactions, peripheral blood stem cell mobilization (PBSC)

PHARMACOKINETICS

Half-life: 15-80 hr; 20-38 hr (children)

INTERACTIONS

- Do not use this product concomitantly or 2 wk before or 24 hr after administration of cytotoxic chemotherapy

Increase: release of neutrophils—lithium

Drug/Lab Test

Increase: uric acid, LDH, alk phos

NURSING CONSIDERATIONS

Assess:

⚠ Allergic reactions, anaphylaxis: rash, urticaria; discontinue this product, have emergency equipment nearby

• Blood studies: CBC, platelet count before treatment and twice weekly; neutrophil counts may be increased for 2 days after therapy
• B/P, respirations, pulse before and during therapy
• Bone pain, give mild analgesics

Administer:
• Using single-use vials; after dose is withdrawn, do not reenter vial
• Do not use 6-mg fixed dose in infants, children, or others <45 kg
• Inspect sol for discoloration, particulates; if present, do not use
• Do not administer in the period 14 days before and 24 hr after cytotoxic chemotherapy

Perform/provide:
• Storage in refrigerator; do not freeze; may store at room temperature up to 6 hr, avoid shaking, protect from light

Evaluate:
• Therapeutic response: absence of infection

Teach patient/family:
• The technique for self-administration: dose, side effects, disposal of containers and needles; provide instruction sheet

peginterferon alfa-2a (℞)
(peg-in-ter-feer′on)
Pegasys

peginterferon alfa-2b (℞)
PegIntron

Func. class.: Immunomodulator

Action: Stimulates genes to modulate many biologic effects, including inhibition of viral replication; inhibits ion cell proliferation, immunomodulation, stimulates effector proteins, decreases leukocyte, platelet counts

Uses: Chronic hepatitis C infections in adults with compensated liver disease; chronic hepatitis B in adults with HBe AG-positive, HBe AG-negative; HCV patients coinfected with HIV, nonresponders or relapsers with chronic hepatitis C

Unlabeled uses: Adenovirus, coronavirus, encephalomyocarditis virus, herpes simplex types 1 and 2, hepatitis D, acute hepatitis C, HIV, HPV, polio virus, rhinovirus, varicella-zoster, variola, vesicular-stomatitis

DOSAGE AND ROUTES

Pegasys
• *Adult:* **SUBCUT** 180 mcg q wk × 48 wk; if poorly tolerated, reduce dose to 135 mcg q wk; in some cases reduction to 90 mcg may be needed

PegIntron
Each dose × 1 yr
• *Adult 137-160 kg:* **SUBCUT** 1 mcg/kg/wk (0.5 ml of 150 mcg vial or Redipen); 107-136 kg 1 mcg/kg/wk (0.5 ml of 120 mcg vial or Redipen); 89-106 kg 1 mcg/kg/wk (0.4 ml of 120 vial or Redipen); 73-88 kg 1 mcg/kg/wk (0.5 ml of 80 mcg vial or Redipen)

Available forms: Inj 180 mcg/0.5 ml

SIDE EFFECTS

CNS: Headache, insomnia, dizziness, anxiety, hostility, lability, nervousness, depression, fatigue, poor concentration, pyrexia, **suicidal ideation, homicidal ideation,** relapse of drug addiction
CV: **Ischemic CV events**
ENDO: Hypothyroidism, diabetes
GI: Abdominal pain, nausea, diarrhea, anorexia, vomiting, dry mouth, **fatal colitis, fatal pancreatitis**
HEMA: **Thrombocytopenia,** neutropenia, anemia, lymphopenia
INTEG: Alopecia, pruritus, rash, dermatitis
MISC: Blurred vision, inj site reaction, rigors
MS: Back pain, myalgia, arthralgia
RESP: Cough, dyspnea

Contraindications: Neonates, infants, sepsis; hypersensitivity to interferons, benzyl alcohol, *Escherichia coli* protein

Precautions: Pregnancy (C), breastfeeding, children <18 yr, geriatric patients, thyroid disorders, myelosuppression, renal/hepatic disease, suicidal/homicidal ideation, preexisting ophthalmologic disorders, pancreatitis, hemodialysis

Black Box Warning: Cardiac disease, depression, autoimmune disease, infection, use with ribavirin

PHARMACOKINETICS

Half-life 15-80 hr, large variability in other pharmacokinetics

INTERACTIONS

• Use caution when giving with theophylline, myelosuppressive agents

Drug/Lab Test

Increase: triglycerides, ALT, neutrophils, platelets

Abnormal: thyroid function test

NURSING CONSIDERATIONS

Assess:

• B/P, blood glucose, ophthalmic exam, pulmonary function

• ALT, HCV viral load; patients who show no reduction in ALT, HCV are unlikely to show benefit of treatment after 6 mo

• Platelet counts, heme concentration, ANC, serum creatinine concentration, albumin, bilirubin, TSH, T_4, AFP

• For myelosuppression, hold dose if neutrophil count is $<500 \times 10^6$/L or if platelets are $<50 \times 10^9$/L

• For hypersensitivity: discontinue immediately if hypersensitivity occurs

Administer:

• In evening to reduce discomfort, sleep through some side effects

• Continue pediatric dose in those who turn 18 yr

Evaluate:

• Therapeutic response: decreased chronic hepatitis C signs/symptoms, undetectable viral load

Teach patient/family:

• Provide patient or family member with written, detailed information about product

• Instructions for home use if appropriate

• Use 2 forms of effective contraception throughout treatment and for 6 mo after treatment (men and women) (combination therapy with ribavirin)

• To avoid driving or other hazardous activity if dizziness, confusion, fatigue, somnolence occur

• To use puncture-resistant container for disposal of needles/syringes if using at home

• To report suicidal/homicidal ideation, visual changes, bleeding/bruising, pulmonary symptoms

⚠ High Alert

pemetrexed (℞)

(pem-ah-trex'ed)

Alimta

Func. class.: Antineoplastic-antimetabolite

Chem. class.: Folic acid antagonist

Action: Inhibits multiple enzymes that reduces folic acid, which is needed for cell replication

Uses: Malignant pleural mesothelioma in combination with cisplatin; non–small cell lung cancer as a single agent; nonsquamous non–small cell lung cancer (first-line treatment)

Unlabeled uses: Bladder, breast, colorectal, gastric, head/neck, pancreatic, renal cell cancers

DOSAGE AND ROUTES

• *Adult:* **IV INF** 500-600 mg/m^2 given over 10 min on day 1 of a 21-day cycle with cisplatin 75 mg/m^2 infused over 2 hr, beginning ½ hr after end of pemetrexed inf

• ANC <500/mm^3 and platelets ≥50,000/mm^3, 75% of previous dose

Available forms: Inj, single-use vials, 500 mg

SIDE EFFECTS

CNS: Fatigue, fever, mood alteration, neuropathy

CV: **Thrombosis/embolism,** *chest pain*

P

GI: Nausea, vomiting, anorexia, diarrhea, ulcerative stomatitis, constipation, dysphagia, dehydration
GU: **Renal failure,** creatinine elevation
HEMA: **Neutropenia, leukopenia, thrombocytopenia, myelosuppression, anemia**
INTEG: Rash, desquamation
RESP: Dyspnea
SYST: **Infection with/without neutropenia, radiation recall reaction**

Contraindications: Pregnancy (D), hypersensitivity, ANC <1500 cells/mm^3, CCr <45 ml/min, thrombocytopenia (<100,000/mm^3), anemia

Precautions: Breastfeeding, children, renal/hepatic disease

PHARMACOKINETICS

Not metabolized; excreted in urine (unchanged 70%-90%); not known if it is excreted in breast milk; half-life 3.5 hr, 81% protein binding

INTERACTIONS

- Do not use with mannitol

Increase: bleeding risk—NSAIDs, anticoagulants

Decrease: pemetrexed's clearance—nephrotoxic products (NSAIDs)

NURSING CONSIDERATIONS

Assess:

⚠ For previous radiation treatments; radiation recall reactions have occurred (erythema, exfoliative dermatitis, pain, burning)

⚠ CBC, differential, platelet count, monitor for nadir and recovery; a new cycle should not begin if ANC <1500 cells/mm^3, platelets are <100,000 cells/mm^3, CCr <45 ml/min

- Renal studies: BUN, serum uric acid, urine CCr, electrolytes before, during therapy
- I&O ratio; report fall in urine output to <30 ml/hr
- Monitor temp q4hr; fever may indicate beginning infection; no rectal temps
- Bleeding time, coagulation time during treatment; bleeding: hematuria, guaiac, bruising or petechiae, mucosa or orifices q8hr
- Buccal cavity q8hr for dryness, sores, ulceration, white patches, oral pain, bleeding, dysphagia

⚠ Symptoms indicating severe allergic reaction: rash, urticaria, itching, flushing

Administer:

- Vit B_{12} and low-dose folic acid as a prophylactic measure to treat related hematologic, GI toxicity; at least 5 daily doses of folic acid must be taken in the 7 days preceding first dose
- Premedicate with a corticosteroid (dexamethasone) given PO bid the day before, day of, and day after administration of pemetrexed

IV route

- Use aseptic technique during reconstitution, dilution
- Reconstitute 500-mg vial/20 ml 0.9% NaCl inj (preservative free) = 25 mg/ml, swirl until dissolved, further dilute with 100 ml 0.9% NaCl inj (preservative free), give as IV inf over 10 mg
- Use only 0.9% NaCl inj (preservative free) for reconstitution, dilution

Perform/provide:

- Strict medical asepsis and protective isolation if WBC levels are low
- Liquid diet: carbonated beverage, Jell-O; dry toast, crackers may be added when patient is not nauseated or vomiting
- Rinsing of mouth tid-qid with water, club soda; brushing of teeth bid-tid with soft brush or cotton-tipped applicators for stomatitis; use unwaxed dental floss
- Storage at 77° F, excursions permitted 59° F-86° F, not light sensitive, discard unused portions

Evaluate:

- Therapeutic response: decreased spread of malignancy

Teach patient/family:

- To report any complaints, side effects to nurse or prescriber: black tarry stools, chills, fever, sore throat, bleeding, bruising, cough, shortness of breath, dark or bloody urine

- To avoid foods with citric acid, hot or rough texture if stomatitis is present
- To report stomatitis: any bleeding, white spots, ulcerations in mouth to prescriber; tell patient to examine mouth daily, report symptoms to nurse, use good oral hygiene
- That contraceptive measures are recommended during therapy and for at least 8 wk after cessation of therapy, to discontinue breastfeeding; toxicity to infant may occur
- To avoid alcohol, salicylates, live vaccines
- To avoid use of razors, commercial mouthwash
- To eat foods high in folic acid and take supplements as prescribed

penciclovir topical

See Appendix B

PENICILLINS

penicillin G benzathine (℞)

(pen-i-sill'in)

Bicillin L-A, Megacillin ✦, Permapen

penicillin G (℞)

Pfizerpen

penicillin G procaine (℞)

Ayercillin ✦, Wycillin

penicillin V (℞)

Apo-Pen-VK ✦, Beepen-VK, Nadopen-V ✦, Novopen-VK ✦, Pen-Vee K ✦, PVF K ✦, Veetids

Func. class.: Broad-spectrum antiinfective

Chem. class.: Natural penicillin

Action: Interferes with cell wall replication of susceptible organisms; lysis is mediated by cell wall autolytic enzymes, results in cell death

Uses: Respiratory infections, scarlet fever, erysipelas, otitis media, pneumonia, skin and soft tissue infections, gonorrhea; effective for gram-positive cocci *(Staphylococcus, Streptococcus pyogenes, S. viridans, S. faecalis, S. bovis, S. pneumoniae)*, gram-negative cocci *(Neisseria gonorrhoeae)*, gram-positive bacilli *(Actinomyces, Bacillus anthracis, Clostridium perfringens, C. tetani, Corynebacterium diphtheriae, Listeria monocytogenes)*, gram-negative bacilli *(Escherichia coli, Proteus mirabilis, Salmonella, Shigella, Enterobacter, Streptobacillus moniliformis)*, spirochetes *(Treponema pallidum)*

DOSAGE AND ROUTES

Penicillin G benzathine

Early syphilis

- *Adult:* **IM** 2.4 million units in single dose

Congenital syphilis

- *Child <2 yr:* **IM** 50,000 units/kg in single dose

Prophylaxis of rheumatic fever, glomerulonephritis

- *Adult and child:* **IM** 1.2 million units in single dose q 3-4 wk or 600,000 units q2wk

Upper respiratory infections (group A streptococcal)

- *Adult:* **IM** 1.2 million units in single dose
- *Child >27 kg:* **IM** 900,000 units in single dose
- *Child <27 kg:* **IM** 300,000-600,000 units in single dose

Available forms: Inj 300,000, 600,000 units/ml

Penicillin G

Pneumococcal/streptococcal infections (serious)

- *Adult:* **IM/IV** 5-24 million units in divided doses q4-6hr
- *Child <12 yr:* **IV** 150,000-300,000 units/kg/day in 4-6 divided doses; max 24 million units/day

Renal dose

- CCr <10 ml/min, give full loading dose, then ½ of loading dose q8-10hr

P

Available forms: Powder for inj 1, 5, 20 million units/vial; inj 1, 2, 3 million units/50 ml

Penicillin G procaine

Moderate to severe pneumococcal infections

- *Adult and child:* **IM** 600,000-1.2 million units in 1 or 2 doses/day for 10 days to 2 wk
- *Newborn:* Avoid use in newborns

Pneumococcal pneumonia

- *Adult and child >12 yr:* **IM** 600,000-1.2 million units/day × 7-10 days

Available forms: Inj 600,000, 1,200,000 units/unit dose

Penicillin V

Pneumococcal/staphylococcal infections

- *Adult:* **PO** 250-500 mg q6hr
- *Child <12 yr:* **PO** 25-50 mg/kg/day in divided doses q6-8hr; max 3 g/day

Streptococcal infections

- *Adult:* **PO** 250 mg q6-8hr × 10 days

Prevention of recurrence of rheumatic fever/chorea

- *Adult:* **PO** 125-250 mg bid continuously

Vincent's gingivitis/pharyngitis

- *Adult:* **PO** 250-500 mg q6-8hr

Renal dose

- Dosage reduction indicated in renal impairment (CCr <50 ml/min) based on clinial response, degree of impairment

Available forms: Tabs 250, 500 mg; powder for oral sol 125, 250 mg/5 ml

SIDE EFFECTS

CNS: Lethargy, hallucinations, anxiety, depression, twitching, **coma, seizures,** hyperreflexia

GI: Nausea, vomiting, diarrhea, increased AST, ALT, abdominal pain, glossitis, colitis, **pseudomembranous colitis**

GU: **Oliguria, proteinuria, hematuria,** *vaginitis, moniliasis,* **glomerulonephritis, renal tubular damage**

HEMA: Anemia, increased bleeding time, **bone marrow depression, granulocytopenia, hemolytic anemia**

META: Hypo/hyperkalemia, alkalosis, hypernatremia

MISC: **Anaphylaxis, serum sickness, Stevens-Johnson syndrome,** *local pain,* tenderness and fever with IM inj

Contraindications: Hypersensitivity to penicillins, corn; neonates

Precautions: Pregnancy (B), breastfeeding, hypersensitivity to cephalosporins/carbapenem/sulfite, severe renal disease, GI disease, asthma

PHARMACOKINETICS

Penicillin G benzathine:

IM: Very slow absorption; time to peak 12-24 hr; duration 21-28 days; excreted in urine, feces, breast milk; crosses placenta

Penicillin G:

IV: Peak immediate

IM: Peak ¼-½ hr

PO: Peak 1 hr, duration 6 hr

Excreted in urine unchanged, excreted in breast milk, crosses placenta, half-life 30-60 min

Penicillin G procaine:

IM: Peak 1-4 hr, duration 15 hr, excreted in urine ***Penicillin V:***

PO: Peak 30-60 min, half-life 30 min, excreted in urine, breast milk

INTERACTIONS

Increase: penicillin concentrations—aspirin, probenecid

Increase: effect of heparin, methotrexate

Decrease: effect of oral contraceptives, typhoid vaccine

Decrease: antimicrobial effect of penicillin—tetracyclines

Drug/Herb

- Do not use acidophilus with antiinfectives; separate by several hours

Decrease: absorption of penicillin—khat

Drug/Lab Test

False positive: urine glucose, urine protein

NURSING CONSIDERATIONS

Assess:

- For infection: temp; characteristics of sputum; wounds; urine; stools before, during, and after treatment
- I&O ratio; report hematuria, oliguria, since penicillin in high doses is nephrotoxic

⚠ Any patient with compromised renal system, since product is excreted slowly in poor renal system function; toxicity may occur rapidly

- Hepatic studies: AST, ALT
- Blood studies: WBC, RBC, Hct, Hgb, bleeding time
- Renal tests: urinalysis, protein, blood
- C&S before therapy; product may be given as soon as culture is taken

⚠ For pseudomembranous colitis: diarrhea, mucus, pus; bowel pattern before and during treatment

- Skin eruptions after administration of penicillin to 1 wk after discontinuing product
- Respiratory status: rate, character, wheezing, tightness in chest

⚠ Allergies before initiation of treatment, reaction of each medication; because of prolonged action, allergic reaction may be prolonged and severe; watch for anaphylaxis: rash, dyspnea, pruritus, laryngeal edema

Administer:

Penicillin G benzathine

- Product after C&S completed
- After shaking well, deep IM inj in large muscle mass; avoid intravascular inj; aspirate; do not give IV

Penicillin G

- Product after C&S

Y-site compatibilities: Acyclovir, amiodarone, cyclophosphamide, diltiazem, enalaprilat, esmolol, fluconazole, foscarnet, heparin, hydromorphone, labetalol, magnesium sulfate, meperidine, morphine, perphenazine, potassium chloride, tacrolimus, theophylline, verapamil, vit B/C

Penicillin G procaine

- Product after C&S
- Deep IM inj; avoid intravascular inj
- Aspirate; do not give IV

Penicillin V

- Orally on empty stomach for best absorption
- Product after C&S

Perform/provide:

- Epinephrine, suction, tracheostomy set, endotracheal intubation equipment
- Adequate fluid intake (2 L) during diarrhea episodes
- Scratch test to assess allergy after securing order from prescriber; usually done when penicillin is only product of choice
- Storage in dry, tight container; oral susp refrigerated 2 wk

Evaluate:

- Therapeutic response: absence of fever, draining wounds
- Allergies before initiation of treatment, reaction of each medication; highlight allergies on chart; hypersensitivity reaction may be delayed

Teach patient/family:

- To report sore throat, fever, fatigue; may indicate superinfection; CNS effects: depression, hallucinations, seizures
- To wear or carry emergency ID if allergic to penicillins
- To report diarrhea, prevent dehydration
- To shake susp well before each dose; store in refrigerator for up to 2 wk
- To use all medication prescribed
- To use additional contraception if using any of these products

Treatment of anaphylaxis: Withdraw product; maintain airway; administer epinephrine, aminophylline, O_2, IV corticosteroids

pentamidine (℞)

(pen-tam'i-deen)

Nebupent, Pentam 300, Pentacarinat ♣, Pneumopent ♣

Func. class.: Antiprotozoal

Chem. class.: Aromatic diamide derivative

Action: Interferes with DNA/RNA synthesis in protozoa

Uses: Treatment/prevention of *Pneumocystis jiroveci* infections

Unlabeled uses: *Leishmania* infections, *Trypanosoma* infections

DOSAGE AND ROUTES

- *Adult and child ≥4 mo:* **IV/IM** 4 mg/kg/day × 2-3 wk; **NEB** 300 mg via specific nebulizer given q4wk for prevention

Available forms: Inj, aerosol 300 mg/vial; sol for aerosol 60 mg/vial ♣

SIDE EFFECTS

CNS: Disorientation, hallucinations, *dizziness,* confusion, drowsiness

CV: Hypotension, ventricular tachycardia, **QT prolongation, dysrhythmias**

GI: Nausea, vomiting, anorexia; increased AST, ALT; **acute pancreatitis,** metallic taste

GU: **Acute renal failure, increased serum creatinine, renal toxicity,** decreased urination

HEMA: Anemia, **leukopenia, thrombocytopenia**

INTEG: Sterile abscess, pain at injection site, pruritus, urticaria, *rash*

META: Hyperkalemia, hypocalcemia, hypoglycemia, hypomagnesemia

MISC: Fatigue, fever, chills, night sweats, **anaphylaxis, Stevens-Johnson syndrome**

RESP: Cough, shortness of breath, **bronchospasm** (with aerosol), sore throat

Contraindications: Hypersensitivity

Precautions: Pregnancy (C), breastfeeding, children, blood dyscrasias, cardiac/renal/hepatic disease, diabetes mellitus, hypocalcemia, hypo/hypertension, anemia

PHARMACOKINETICS

Excreted unchanged in urine (66%)

INTERACTIONS

- Nephrotoxicity: aminoglycosides, amphotericin B, cisplatin, NSAIDs, vancomycin

⚠ Fatal dysrhythmias: erythromycin IV

Increase: QT prolongation—class IA, class III antidysrhythmics; phenothiazines; any agent that increases QT interval

Increase: myelosuppression—antineoplastics, radiation

NURSING CONSIDERATIONS

Assess:

- Blood tests, blood glucose, CBC, platelets, calcium, magnesium
- I&O ratio; report hematuria, oliguria
- ECG for cardiac dysrhythmias
- Patient should be lying down when receiving product; severe hypotension may develop; monitor B/P during administration and until B/P stable

⚠ Any patient with compromised renal system; product is excreted slowly in poor renal system function; toxicity may occur rapidly

- Hepatic studies: AST, ALT
- Renal studies: urinalysis, BUN, creatinine; nephrotoxicity may occur
- Signs of infection, anemia
- Bowel pattern before, during treatment
- Sterile abscess, pain at inj site
- Respiratory status: rate, character, wheezing, dyspnea
- Dizziness, confusion, hallucination
- Allergies before treatment, reaction of each medication; place allergies on chart in bright red letters; notify all people giving products
- Diabetic patients, hypoglycemia may occur, then hyperglycemia with prolonged therapy

Administer:

Inhalation route

- Through nebulizer, using Raspirgard II jet nebulizer; mix contents in 6 ml of sterile H_2O; do not use low pressure (<20 psi); flow rate should be 5-7 L/min

(40-50 psi) air or O_2 source over 30-45 min until chamber is empty

IM route

- 300 mg diluted in 3 ml sterile H_2O; give deep IM by Z-track; painful by this route

IV route

- Reconstitute 300 mg/3-5 ml of sterile water for inj, D_5W, withdraw dose and further dilute in 50-250 ml D_5W, give over 1-2 hr

Y-site compatibilities: Alfentanil, atracurium, atropine, benztropine, buprenorphine, calcium gluconate, carboplatin, caspofungin, chlorpromazine, cimetidine, cisplatin, cyclophosphamide, cycloSPORINE, cytarabine, dactinomycin, diltiazem, gatifloxacin, zidovudine

Perform/provide:

- Storage in refrigerator protected from light

Evaluate:

- Therapeutic response: decreased temp, increased ability to breathe

Teach patient/family:

- To report sore throat, fever, fatigue (may indicate superinfection)
- To maintain adequate fluid intake

⚠ High Alert

pentazocine (℞)

(pen-taz'oh-seen)

Talwin, Talwin NX

Func. class.: Opiate analgesic, antagonist

Chem. class.: Synthetic benzomorphan

Controlled Substance Schedule IV

Action: Inhibits ascending pain pathways in CNS, increases pain threshold, alters pain perception

Uses: Moderate to severe pain

DOSAGE AND ROUTES

- *Adult:* **PO** 50-100 mg q3-4hr prn, max 600 mg/day; **IV/IM/SUBCUT** 30 mg q3-4hr prn, max 360 mg/day

Labor

- *Adult:* **IM** 30-60 mg; **IV** 30 mg q2-3hr when contractions are regular

Renal dose

- CCr 10-50 ml/min reduce dose by 25%; CCr <10 ml/min reduce dose by 50%

Available forms: Inj 30 mg/ml; tabs 50 mg

SIDE EFFECTS

CNS: Drowsiness, dizziness, confusion, headache, sedation, euphoria, hallucinations, dreaming, insomnia, lightheadedness

CV: Palpitations, bradycardia, change in B/P, tachycardia, increased B/P (high doses), hypotension, syncope, flushing

EENT: Tinnitus, blurred vision, miosis, diplopia

GI: Nausea, vomiting, anorexia, constipation, *cramps,* dry mouth

GU: Increased urinary output, dysuria, urinary retention

HEMA: **Eosinophilia, decreased WBC**

INTEG: Rash, urticaria, bruising, flushing, diaphoresis, pruritus, severe irritation at inj sites, **Stevens-Johnson syndrome**

RESP: **Respiratory depression**

Contraindications: Hypersensitivity to this product or sulfites, addiction (opiate)

Precautions: Pregnancy (C), breastfeeding, children <18 yr, addictive personality, increased intracranial pressure, MI (acute), severe heart disease, respiratory depression, renal/hepatic disease, seizure disorder, head trauma, bowel impaction, geriatric patients

PHARMACOKINETICS

Metabolized by liver, excreted by kidneys, crosses placenta, half-life 2-3 hr, extensive first-pass metabolism with less than 20% entering circulation

IM/SUBCUT: Onset 15-30 min, peak 1-2 hr, duration 2-4 hr

IV: Onset 2-3 min, duration 4-6 hr

P

INTERACTIONS

⚠ Unpredictable reactions: MAOIs

Increase: effects—CNS depressants; alcohol, sedative/hypnotics, antipsychotics, skeletal muscle relaxants

Decrease: effects—opiates

Drug/Lab Test

Increase: amylase

NURSING CONSIDERATIONS

Assess:

- For pain: intensity, duration, location prior to and 1 hr after dose
- I&O ratio; check for decreasing output; may indicate urinary retention
- Bowel status: constipation; may need stimulant laxatives/stool softeners
- For withdrawal symptoms in opiate-dependent patients
- Abscesses, ulcerations, WBC
- CNS changes: dizziness, drowsiness, hallucinations, euphoria, LOC, pupil reaction
- Allergic reactions: rash, urticaria
- Respiratory dysfunction: respiratory depression, character, rate, rhythm; notify prescriber if respirations are <10/min
- Need for pain medication, physical dependence

Administer:

- With antiemetic if nausea, vomiting occur
- When pain is beginning to return; determine dosage interval by patient response

IM/SUBCUT route

- Give IM deeply into large muscle mass, rotate sites; SUBCUT may cause necrosis with repeated inj

IV route

- Undiluted or diluted 5 mg/ml of sterile H_2O for inj; give 5 mg or less over 1 min

Syringe compatibilities: Atropine, benzquinamide, butorphanol, chlorproMAZINE, cimetidine, dimenhyDRINATE, diphenhydrAMINE, droperidol, fentanyl, hydromorphone, hydrOXYzine, meperidine, metoclopramide, morphine, perphenazine, prochlorperazine, promazine, promethazine, ranitidine, scopolamine

Y-site compatibilities: Heparin, hydrocortisone, potassium chloride, vit B/C

Perform/provide:

- Storage in light-resistant area at room temperature
- Assistance with ambulation
- Safety measures: night-light, call bell within easy reach

Evaluate:

- Therapeutic response: decrease in pain

Teach patient/family:

- To report any symptoms of CNS changes, allergic reactions
- That physical dependency may result from extended use
- That withdrawal symptoms may occur: nausea, vomiting, cramps, fever, faintness, anorexia
- To avoid CNS depressants, alcohol
- To avoid driving, operating machinery if drowsiness occurs

Treatment of overdose: Naloxone (Narcan) 0.2-0.8 mg IV, O_2, IV fluids, vasopressors

⚠ High Alert

pentobarbital (℞)

(pen-toe-bar′bi-tal)

Nembutal, Novopentobarb ✱, Nova-Rectal ✱, pentobarbital sodium

Func. class.: Sedative/hypnotic barbiturate; anticonvulsant, anesthetic adjunct

Chem. class.: Barbitone, short acting

Controlled Substance Schedule II (USA), Schedule G (CDSA IV) (Canada)

Do not confuse:

pentobarbital/phenobarbital

Action: Depresses activity in brain cells, primarily in reticular activating system in brain stem; selectively depresses neurons in posterior hypothalamus, limbic structures

Uses: Insomnia, sedation, preoperative medication, increased intracranial pressure, dental anesthetic, status epilepticus

DOSAGE AND ROUTES

Insomnia

• *Adult:* **PO** 100-200 mg at bedtime; **IM** 150-200 mg at bedtime; **IV** 100 mg initially, then up to 500 mg; **RECT** 120-200 mg at bedtime

• *Child:* **IM** 2-6 mg/kg, max 100 mg; **PO** 2-6 mg/kg/day in divided doses; **PO** preoperatively 2-6 mg/kg, max 100 mg/dose; **IV** 100 mg (hypnotic/anticonvulsant)

Status epilepticus

• *Adult, child, infant:* **IV** 15-18 mg/kg, then 10 mg/kg, then 5 mg/kg q30-60min after 1st dose

Available forms: Caps 50, 100 mg; elix 20 mg/5 ml; rect supp 30, 60, 120, 200 mg; inj 50 mg/ml

SIDE EFFECTS

CNS: Lethargy, drowsiness, hangover, dizziness, paradoxical stimulation in geriatric patients and children, lightheadedness, dependence, **CNS depression,** mental depression, slurred speech, agitation

CV: Hypotension, bradycardia

GI: Nausea, vomiting, diarrhea, constipation, **hepatic injury**

HEMA: **Agranulocytosis, thrombocytopenia, megaloblastic anemia** (long-term treatment)

INTEG: Rash, urticaria, pain, abscesses at inj site, **angioedema, thrombophlebitis, Stevens-Johnson syndrome**

RESP: **Respiratory depression, apnea, laryngospasm, bronchospasm**

Contraindications: Pregnancy (D), hypersensitivity to barbiturates, respiratory depression, addiction to barbiturates; severe renal/hepatic impairment; porphyria, uncontrolled pain

Precautions: Breastfeeding, geriatric patients, anemia, renal/hepatic disease, hypertension, acute/chronic pain, suicidal ideation, depression, angioedema

PHARMACOKINETICS

Metabolized by liver, excreted by kidneys (metabolites); half-life 15-48 hr

PO: Onset 15-30 min, duration 4-6 hr

RECT: Onset slow, duration 4-6 hr

INTERACTIONS

• Avoid use with voriconazole, cycloSPORINE

Increase: CNS depression—alcohol, MAOIs, sedatives, other CNS depressants, antihistamines, opiates

Increase: half-life of doxycycline

Decrease: effect of oral anticoagulants, corticosteroids, griseofulvin, quinidine

Drug/Herb

Increase: pentobarbital levels—eucalyptus, Jamaican dogwood, kava, lemon balm nettle, pill-bearing spurge, poppy, quinine, senega, valerian

Drug/Lab Test

False increase: sulfobromophthalein

NURSING CONSIDERATIONS

Assess:

• VS q30min after parenteral route for 2 hr

• Blood studies: Hct, Hgb, RBCs, serum folate, vit D (long-term therapy); PT in patients receiving anticoagulants

• Hepatic studies: AST, ALT, bilirubin; if increased, product is usually discontinued

• Mental status: mood, sensorium, affect, memory (long, short)

• Physical dependency: more frequent requests for medication, shakes, anxiety

⚠ Barbiturate toxicity: hypotension; pupillary constriction; cold, clammy skin; cyanosis of lips; insomnia; nausea; vomiting; hallucinations; delirium; weakness; coma; mild symptoms may occur in 8-12 hr without product

• Respiratory changes: respiratory depression, character, rate, rhythm; hold product if respirations are <10/min or if pupils are dilated

• Blood dyscrasias: fever, sore throat, bruising, rash, jaundice, epistaxis

Administer:

• For <14 days, since not effective after that; tolerance develops

• After removal of cigarettes to prevent fires

• After trying conservative measures for insomnia

P

• Avoid use with CNS depressants; serious CNS depression may result

PO route

• Use elixir alone or diluted in fluids
• ½-1 hr before bedtime for sleeplessness
• On empty stomach for best absorption
• Crushed or whole
• Alone; do not mix with other products or inject if there is precipitate

IM route

• Inject deep in large muscle mass to prevent tissue sloughing and abscesses; do not inject more than 5 ml in one site

IV route

• IV undiluted or dilute in sterile H_2O, LR, NaCl, give 50 mg or less/min; titrate to patient response; use only clear sol; avoid extravasation
• IV only with resuscitative equipment available; administer at <100 mg/min (only by qualified personnel)

Additive compatibilities: Amikacin, aminophylline, calcium chloride, cephapirin, chloramphenicol, dimenhyDRINATE, erythromycin lactobionate, lidocaine, thiopental, verapamil

Syringe compatibilities: Aminophylline, ephedrine, hydromorphone, neostigmine, scopolamine, sodium bicarbonate, thiopental

Y-site compatibilities: Acyclovir, insulin (regular), propofol

Perform/provide:

• Assistance with ambulation after receiving dose
• Safety measures: night-light, call bell within easy reach
• Checking to see if PO medication has been swallowed
• Storage of suppositories in refrigerator; do not use aqueous solutions that contain precipitate

Evaluate:

• Therapeutic response: ability to sleep at night, less early morning awakening if taking product for insomnia, or decrease in number, severity of seizures if taking product for seizure disorder

Teach patient/family:

• That hangover is common
• That product is indicated only for short-term treatment of insomnia; probably ineffective after 2 wk
• That physical dependency may result from extended use (45-90 days depending on dose)
• To avoid driving, other activities requiring alertness
• To avoid alcohol ingestion
• Not to discontinue medication quickly after long-term use; product should be tapered over 1-2 wk
• To tell all prescribers that a barbiturate is being taken
• That withdrawal insomnia may occur after short-term use; not to start using product again; insomnia will improve in 1-3 nights
• That effects may take 2 nights for benefits to be noticed
• Alternative measures to improve sleep (reading, exercise several hr before bedtime, warm bath, warm milk, TV, self-hypnosis, deep breathing)

Treatment of overdose: Lavage, activated charcoal, warming blanket, vital signs, hemodialysis, I&O ratio

⚠ High Alert

pentostatin (℞)

(pen-toh-stat′in)

Nipent

Func. class.: Antineoplastic, enzyme inhibitor

Chem. class.: Streptomyces antibioticus derivative

Action: Inhibits the enzyme adenosine deaminase (ADA), which is able to block DNA synthesis and some RNA synthesis

Uses: α-Interferon-refractory hairy cell leukemia

Unlabeled uses: Chronic lymphocytic leukemia, non-Hodgkin's lymphoma, cutaneous T-cell lymphoma, graft-versus-host disease/prophylaxis, mycosis fungoides, stem cell transplant preparation

DOSAGE AND ROUTES

• *Adult:* **IV** 4 mg/m^2 every other wk; may be given **IV BOL,** or diluted in a larger volume and given over 20-30 min

Available forms: Powder for inj 10 mg/vial

SIDE EFFECTS

CNS: Headache, anxiety, confusion, depression, dizziness, insomnia, nervousness, paresthesia

GI: Nausea, vomiting, anorexia, diarrhea, constipation, flatulence, stomatitis, elevated LFTs

GU: **Hematuria,** dysuria, increased BUN/creatinine, **acute renal failure**

HEMA: **Leukopenia, anemia, thrombocytopenia,** *ecchymosis,* **lymphadenopathy,** petechiae

INTEG: Rash, eczema, dry skin, pruritus, sweating, herpes simplex/zoster

RESP: Cough, upper respiratory infection, bronchitis, dyspnea, epistaxis, pneumonia, pharyngitis, rhinitis, sinusitis, **pulmonary edema**

SYST: Fever, infection, fatigue, pain, allergic reaction, chills, **death, sepsis,** chest pain, flulike symptoms

Contraindications: Pregnancy (D), hypersensitivity to this product or mannitol

Precautions: Breastfeeding, children, renal disease, bone marrow depression

Black Box Warning: Hepatic disease, pulmonary edema, renal failure, seizures

PHARMACOKINETICS

IV: Elimination half-life 5.7 hr, low protein binding, 90% excreted in urine unchanged or as metabolites

INTERACTIONS

Black Box Warning: Fatal pulmonary toxicity: fludarabine

Increase: adverse reactions—vidarabine

Increase: bleeding—NSAIDs, anticoagulants

Drug/Lab Test

Increase: uric acid

NURSING CONSIDERATIONS

Assess:

• CBC, differential, platelet count q wk; withhold product if WBC is <2000/mm^3 or platelet count is <75,000/mm^3; notify prescriber

• Renal studies; BUN, serum uric acid, urine CCr, electrolytes before, during therapy

• I&O ratio; report fall in urine output to <30 ml/hr

• Monitor temp q4hr; fever may indicate beginning infection

• Hepatic studies before, during therapy: bilirubin, AST, ALT, alk phos, prn or q mo; check for jaundiced skin and sclera, dark urine, clay-colored stools, itchy skin, abdominal pain, fever, diarrhea

• Bleeding: hematuria, guaiac stools, bruising, petechiae, mucosa or orifices q8hr

• Effects of alopecia on body image; discuss feelings about body changes

• Inflammation of mucosa, breaks in skin

• Buccal cavity q8hr for dryness, sores, ulceration, white patches, oral pain, bleeding, dysphagia

• Local irritation, pain, burning at inj site

• Symptoms of severe allergic reaction: rash, pruritus, urticaria, purpuric skin lesions, itching, flushing

• GI symptoms: frequency of stools, cramping

• Acidosis, signs of dehydration; rapid respiration, poor skin turgor, decreased urine output, dry skin, restlessness, weakness

Administer:

• Antiemetic 30-60 min before giving product to prevent vomiting

• Allopurinol to prevent uric acid increases

• Avoid use of higher doses than recommended, toxicity can occur

IV route

• Hydrate with 500-1000 ml D_5½ NS or equivalent before administration; administer another 500 ml D_5 or equivalent after pentostatin

P

After diluting, use with 5 ml sterile H_2O for injection and mix thoroughly (2 mg/ml); may be given by bolus or diluted in 25-50 ml 5% dextrose, or 0.9% NaCl (0.33 or 0.18 mg/ml)
Solution compatibilities: D_5W, 0.9% NaCl, LR
Y-site compatibilities: Fludarabine, melphalan, ondansetron, paclitaxel, sargramostim
Perform/provide:
• Strict hand-washing technique, gloves, protective covering
• Liquid diet: carbonated beverages; gelatin may be added if patient is not nauseated or vomiting
• Rinsing of mouth tid-qid with water, club soda; brushing of teeth bid-qid with soft brush or cotton-tipped applicators for stomatitis; use unwaxed dental floss
• Storage in refrigerator; reconstituted or diluted sol may be stored at room temperature up to 8 hr
Evaluate:
• Therapeutic response: decrease in tumor size, spread of malignancy
Teach patient/family:
• To report any complaints, side effects to nurse or prescriber
• That hair may be lost during treatment and wig or hairpiece may make patient feel better; tell patient that new hair may be different in color, texture
• To avoid foods with citric acid, hot or rough texture
• To report any bleeding, white spots, ulcerations in mouth to prescriber; tell patient to examine mouth daily
• To avoid crowds and sources of infection when granulocyte count is low

pentoxifylline (℞)
(pen-tox'ih-fill-in)
Pentoxil, Trental
Func. class.: Hemorrheologic agent
Chem. class.: Dimethylxanthine derivative

Action: Decreases blood viscosity, stimulates prostacyclin formation, increases blood flow by increasing flexibility of RBCs; decreases RBC hyperaggregation; reduces platelet aggregation, decreases fibrinogen concentration
Uses: Intermittent claudication related to chronic occlusive vascular disease
Unlabeled uses: Behçet's syndrome, Kawasaki disease to reduce coronary artery lesions, diabetic neuropathies, sickle cell anemia

DOSAGE AND ROUTES

• *Adult:* **PO** 400 mg tid with meals, may decrease to bid if side effects occur; must be taken for ≥8 wk for maximal effect
Behçet's syndrome (unlabeled)
• *Adult:* **PO** 300 mg bid × 2 wk, then 300 mg/day
Acute claudication in sickle cell disease/diabetic neuropathy (unlabeled)
• *Adult:* **PO** 400 mg tid
Kawasaki disease (unlabeled)
• *Child:* **PO** 20 mg/kg/day in 3 divided doses with aspirin and IVIG
Available forms: Cont release tabs 400 mg; ext rel tabs 400 mg

SIDE EFFECTS

CNS: ***Headache,*** anxiety, ***tremors,*** confusion, ***dizziness***
CV: Angina, dysrhythmias, palpitation, hypotension, chest pain, dyspnea, edema
EENT: Blurred vision, earache, increased salivation, sore throat, conjunctivitis
GI: ***Dyspepsia, nausea, vomiting,*** anorexia, bloating, belching, constipation, cholecystitis, dry mouth, thirst, bad taste, flatulence
INTEG: Rash, pruritus, urticaria, brittle fingernails
MISC: Epistaxis, flulike symptoms, laryngitis, nasal congestion, **leukopenia,** malaise, weight changes
Contraindications: Hypersensitivity to this product or xanthines, retinal/cerebral hemorrhage
Precautions: Pregnancy (C), breastfeeding, children, angina pectoris, impaired renal function, recent surgery, pep-

tic ulceration, cardiac disease, bleeding disorders

PHARMACOKINETICS

PO: Peak 2-4 hr, half-life ½-1 hr, degradation in liver, excreted in urine

INTERACTIONS

Increase: bleeding risk—warfarin, salicylates, NSAIDs, thrombolytics, abciximab, eptifibatide, tirofiban, ticlopidine, clopidogrel, heparins, thrombin inhibitor
Increase: theophylline level—theophylline
Increase: hypotension—antihypertensives, nitrates
Increase: pentoxifylline—cimetidine, ciprofloxacin
Drug/Herb
Increase: bleeding potential—anise, arnica, chamomile, clove, dong quai, fenugreek, feverfew, garlic, ginger, ginkgo, ginseng *(Panax)*, licorice

NURSING CONSIDERATIONS

Assess:
- B/P, respirations of patient also taking antihypertensives; intermittent claudication baseline and throughout
- PT, Hgb, Hct in patients at risk for hemorrhage

Administer:
- Do not break, crush, or chew ext rel tabs
- With meals to prevent GI upset

Evaluate:
- Therapeutic response: decreased pain, cramping, increased ambulation

Teach patient/family:
- That therapeutic response may take 2-4 wk, 8-12 wk to reach full benefit
- To observe feet for arterial insufficiency
- To use cotton socks, well-fitted shoes; not to go barefoot
- To watch for bleeding, bruises, petechiae, epistaxis
- To avoid smoking, to prevent blood vessel constriction
- That there are many drug, herb interactions

perindopril (℞)

(per-in'doe-pril)
Aceon
Func. class.: Antihypertensive
Chem. class.: Angiotensin-converting enzyme inhibitor

Action: Selectively suppresses renin-angiotensin-aldosterone system; inhibits ACE; prevents conversion of angiotensin I to angiotensin II, dilation of arterial, venous vessels
Uses: Hypertension, stable artery disease
Unlabeled uses: Heart failure

DOSAGE AND ROUTES

Hypertension
- *Adult:* **PO** 4 mg/day, may increase or decrease to desired response range 4-8 mg/day; may give in 2 divided doses or as a single dose, max 16 mg/day

Patients on diuretics
- Discontinue diuretic 2-3 days prior to perindopril then resume diuretic if needed

Renal dose
- *Adult:* **PO** CCr 16-29 ml/min, 2 mg every other day; CCr 30-59 ml/min, 2 mg/day

Stable CAD
- *Adult:* **PO** 4 mg/day × 2 wk then increase as tolerated to 8 mg/day

Available forms: Tabs scored 2, 4, 8 mg

SIDE EFFECTS

CNS: Insomnia, dizziness, paresthesias, headache, fatigue, anxiety, depression
CV: Hypotension, chest pain, tachycardia, dysrhythmias, syncope
EENT: Tinnitus; visual changes; sore throat; double vision; dry, burning eyes
GI: Nausea, vomiting, colitis, cramps, diarrhea, constipation, flatulence, dry mouth, loss of taste
GU: **Proteinuria, renal failure,** increased frequency of polyuria or oliguria
HEMA: **Agranulocytosis, neutropenia**

P

INTEG: Rash, purpura, alopecia, hyperhidrosis
META: Hyperkalemia
RESP: Dyspnea, *dry cough,* crackles
SYST: **Angioedema**

Contraindications: Hypersensitivity, history of angioedema

Black Box Warning: Pregnancy (D)

Precautions: Breastfeeding, renal disease, hyperkalemia, hepatic failure, dehydration, bilateral renal artery stenosis, cough, angioedema, severe CHF

PHARMACOKINETICS

Bioavailability 75%; peak 1 hr parent product, 3-7 hr prodrug; protein binding 68%; metabolized by liver (active metabolite perindoprilat); half-life 0.8-10 hr; excreted in urine

INTERACTIONS

Increase: effects of neuromuscular blocking agents, antihypertensives, lithium
Increase: antihypertensive effect—diuretics
Increase: hypersensitivity—allopurinol
Increase: severe hypotension—diuretics, other antihypertensives
Increase: hyperkalemia—salt substitutes, potassium-sparing diuretics, potassium supplements
Decrease: effects of NSAIDs
Decrease: antihypertensive effect—NSAIDs, salicylates

Drug/Herb

Increase: toxicity, death—aconite
Increase: antihypertensive effect—barberry, betony, black catechu, black cohosh, bloodroot, broom, burdock, cat's claw, dandelion, goldenseal, hawthorn, Irish moss, Jamaican dogwood, kelp, khella, mistletoe, parsley
Increase or decrease: antihypertensive effect—astragalus, cola tree
Decrease: antihypertensive effect—coltsfoot, guarana, khat, licorice, yohimbe

Drug/Lab Test

Interference: glucose/insulin tolerance tests

NURSING CONSIDERATIONS

Assess:

- B/P, pulse q4hr; note rate, rhythm, quality
- Electrolytes: K, Na, Cl during 1st 2 wk of therapy
- Baselines in renal, hepatic studies before therapy begins and 1 wk into therapy
- Edema in feet, legs daily
- Skin turgor, dryness of mucous membranes for hydration status, dry mouth
- Symptoms of CHF: edema, dyspnea, wet crackles

Administer:

- As a single dose or in 2 divided doses

Evaluate:

- Therapeutic response: decreased B/P

Teach patient/family:

- Not to use OTC (cough, cold, or allergy) products unless directed by prescriber; to avoid salt substitutes
- To avoid sunlight or wear sunscreen for photosensitivity
- To comply with dosage schedule, even if feeling better
- To notify prescriber of mouth sores, sore throat, fever, swelling of hands or feet, irregular heartbeat, chest pains, signs of angioedema
- That excessive perspiration, dehydration, vomiting, diarrhea may lead to fall in B/P; consult prescriber if these occur
- That product may cause dizziness, fainting; light-headedness may occur during 1st few days of therapy
- That product may cause skin rash or impaired perspiration; angioedema may occur and to discontinue if it occurs
- Not to discontinue product abruptly
- To rise slowly to sitting or standing position to minimize orthostatic hypotension

Treatment of overdose: Lavage, IV atropine for bradycardia, IV theophylline for bronchospasm, digoxin, O_2, diuretic for cardiac failure

perphenazine (℞)

(per-fen′a-zeen)

Apo-Perphenazine ♣, perphenazine, PMS Perphenazine ♣

Func. class.: Antipsychotic, neuroleptic

Chem. class.: Phenothiazine piperidine

Action: Depresses cerebral cortex, hypothalamus, limbic system, which control activity, aggression; blocks neurotransmission produced by DOPamine at synapse; exhibits strong α-adrenergic, anticholinergic blocking action; as antiemetic inhibits medullary chemoreceptor trigger zone; receptor affinity DOPamine D_2, histamine H_1, α-adrenergic

Uses: Psychotic disorders, schizophrenia, nausea, vomiting

Unlabeled uses: Agitation, dementia, hiccups

DOSAGE AND ROUTES

Nausea/vomiting

- *Adult and child >12 yr:* **PO** 8-16 mg/day in divided doses, up to 24 mg; **IV** max 5 mg, give diluted or slow IV drip

Psychiatric use in hospitalized patients

- *Adult:* **PO** 4-16 mg bid-qid, gradually increased to desired dose, max 64 mg/day
- *Child >12 yr:* **PO** 6-12 mg in divided doses
- *Geriatric:* **PO** 2-4 mg daily-bid, increase by 2-4 mg/wk to desired dose

Nonhospitalized patients

- *Adult:* **PO** 4-8 mg tid

Available forms: Tabs 2, 4, 8, 16 mg

SIDE EFFECTS

CNS: EPS: pseudoparkinsonism, akathisia, dystonia, tardive dyskinesia, **seizures,** *headache,* **neuroleptic malignant syndrome,** dizziness

CV: Orthostatic hypotension (geriatric patients), **cardiac arrest,** ECG changes, **tachycardia**

EENT: Blurred vision, glaucoma

GI: Dry mouth, nausea, vomiting, anorexia, constipation, diarrhea, jaundice, weight gain

GU: Urinary retention, urinary frequency, enuresis, impotence, amenorrhea, gynecomastia, ejaculatory dysfunction

HEMA: Anemia, **leukopenia, leukocytosis, agranulocytosis**

INTEG: Rash, photosensitivity, dermatitis

RESP: **Laryngospasm,** dyspnea, **respiratory depression**

Contraindications: Children <12 yr, hypersensitivity, blood dyscrasias, coma, brain damage, bone marrow depression, CNS depression

Precautions: Pregnancy (C), breastfeeding, geriatric patients, seizure disorders, hypertension, hepatic/cardiac disease, closed-angle glaucoma, renal failure

Black Box Warning: Dementia

PHARMACOKINETICS

Bioavailability 20%; metabolized by liver (sulfoxidation, hydroxylation, dealkylation; glucuronidation by CYP2D6); excreted in urine, breast milk; crosses placenta, half-life 9-12 hr, 91%-99% protein binding

PO: Onset erratic, peak 4-8 hr

INTERACTIONS

- Oversedation: other CNS depressants, alcohol, anesthetics
- Toxicity: epinephrine

Increase: risk of EPS—lithium

Increase: effects of both products—β-adrenergic blockers, alcohol

Increase: anticholinergic effects—anticholinergics

Increase: perphenazine effect—ritonavir

Increase: hypotension—thiazide diuretics, meperidine

Decrease: absorption—aluminum hydroxide or magnesium hydroxide antacids

Decrease: antiparkinson effect—levodopa
Decrease: oral anticoagulant effect—oral anticoagulants

Drug/Herb

Increase: anticholinergic effect—henbane leaf
Increase: EPS—betel palm, kava
Increase: action—cola tree, hops, nettle, nutmeg

Drug/Lab Test

Increase: LFTs, cardiac enzymes, cholesterol, blood glucose, prolactin, bilirubin, PBI, cholinesterase, ^{131}I
Decrease: hormones (blood, urine)
False positive: pregnancy tests, PKU
False negative: urinary steroids, 17-OHCS

NURSING CONSIDERATIONS

Assess:

- Mental status before initial administration
- Swallowing of PO medication; check for hoarding or giving of medication to other patients
- I&O ratio; palpate bladder if urinary output is low, urinary retention may be the cause
- Bilirubin, CBC, LFTs q mo
- Urinalysis is recommended before and during prolonged therapy
- Affect, orientation, LOC, reflexes, gait, coordination, sleep pattern disturbances
- B/P standing and lying; also include pulse, respirations q4hr during initial treatment; establish baseline before starting treatment; report drops of 30 mm Hg
- Dizziness, faintness, palpitations, tachycardia on rising
- EPS including akathisia (inability to sit still, no pattern to movements), tardive dyskinesia (bizarre movements of jaw, mouth, tongue, extremities), pseudoparkinsonism (rigidity, tremors, pill rolling, shuffling gait)
- Skin turgor daily

⚠ For neuroleptic malignant syndrome: hyperthermia, altered mental status, increased CPK, muscle rigidity

- Constipation, urinary retention daily; increase bulk, water in diet

Administer:

- Antiparkinsonian agent on order from prescriber for EPS
- Avoid use with CNS depressants

Perform/provide:

- Supervised ambulation until stabilized on medication; do not involve in strenuous exercise program because fainting is possible; patient should not stand still for long periods
- Increased fluids, bulk in diet to prevent constipation
- Sips of water, sugarless candy, gum, ice chips for dry mouth
- Storage in tight, light-resistant container

Evaluate:

- Therapeutic response: decrease in emotional excitement, hallucinations, delusions, paranoia, reorganization of patterns of thought, speech

Teach patient/family:

- That orthostatic hypotension occurs frequently and to rise from sitting or lying position gradually; to avoid hazardous activities until stabilized on medication
- To avoid hot tubs, hot showers, tub baths, since hypotension may occur; that in hot weather, heat stroke may occur; take extra precautions to stay cool
- To avoid abrupt withdrawal of this product, or EPS may result; product should be withdrawn slowly
- To avoid OTC preparations (cough, hay fever, cold) unless approved by prescriber, since serious product interactions may occur; avoid use with alcohol; increased drowsiness may occur
- To use a sunscreen to prevent burns
- About compliance with product regimen
- About necessity for meticulous oral hygiene, since oral candidiasis may occur
- To report sore throat, malaise, fever, bleeding, mouth sores; if these occur, CBC should be drawn and product discontinued
- That urine may turn reddish-brown

Treatment of overdose: Lavage if orally ingested; provide an airway; *do not induce vomiting*

phenazopyridine
(℞, OTC)
(fen-az-oh-peer'i-deen)
Azo-100, Azo-Gesic, Azo-Standard, Baridium, Eridium, Geridium, Phenazo ✤, phenazopyridine, Phenazodine, Prodium, Pyridiate, Pyridium, Urinary Analgesic, Urodine, Urogesic, Walgreens Urinary Pain Relief
Func. class.: Urinary analgesic
Chem. class.: Azodye

Action: Exerts analgesic, anesthetic action on the urinary tract mucosa
Uses: Urinary tract irritation, infection used with a urinary antiinfective

DOSAGE AND ROUTES
- *Adult:* **PO** 200 mg tid × 2 days or less when used with antibacterial for UTI
- *Child 6-12 yr:* **PO** 4 mg/kg tid × 2 days

Renal dose
- *Adult:* **PO** CCr 50-80 ml/min, give dose 8-16 hr; do not use in CCr <50 ml/min

Available forms: Tabs 95, 97.2, 100, 200 mg

SIDE EFFECTS
CNS: Headache, **aseptic meningitis**
GI: Nausea, vomiting, diarrhea, heartburn, anorexia, **hepatic toxicity**
GU: **Renal toxicity,** *orange-red urine*
HEMA: **Thrombocytopenia, agranulocytosis, leukopenia, neutropenia, hemolytic anemia, methemoglobinemia**
INTEG: Rash, skin pigmentation, pruritus
SYST: **Anaphylaxis,** body fluid staining
Contraindications: Hypersensitivity, renal insufficiency, hepatic disease, uremia
Precautions: Pregnancy (B), breastfeeding, children <12 yr, geriatric patients, contact lens

PHARMACOKINETICS
Metabolized by liver, excreted by kidneys, crosses placenta, duration 6-8 hr

INTERACTIONS
Drug/Lab Test
Interference: urinalysis

NURSING CONSIDERATIONS
Assess:
- Urinary status: burning, pain, itching, urgency, frequency, hematuria, before/after treatment completed
- Hepatic studies: AST, ALT, bilirubin if patient is on long-term therapy

⚠ Hepatotoxicity: dark urine, clay-colored stools, jaundiced skin and sclera, itching, abdominal pain, fever, diarrhea if patient is on long-term therapy
- Allergic reactions: rash, urticaria; product may have to be discontinued

Administer:
- To patient crushed or whole; chewable tablets may be chewed
- With food or milk to decrease gastric symptoms

Evaluate:
- Therapeutic response: decrease in urinary pain

Teach patient/family:
- Not to exceed recommended dosage and to take with meals
- To discontinue after pain is relieved but continue to take concurrent prescribed antiinfective until finished
- That urine may turn red-orange; may stain clothing or contact lenses

Treatment of overdose: Methylene blue 1-2 mg/kg IV or 100-200 mg vit C PO

⚠ High Alert

phenobarbital (℞)

(fee-noe-bar′bi-tal)
Ancalixir ♣, Luminal,
phenobarbital sodium
Func. class.: Anticonvulsant
Chem. class.: Barbiturate

Controlled Substance Schedule IV

Do not confuse:
phenobarbital/pentobarbital

Action: Decreases impulse transmission; increases seizure threshold at cerebral cortex level

Uses: All forms of epilepsy, status epilepticus, febrile seizures in children, sedation, insomnia

Unlabeled uses: Neonatal hyperbilirubinemia, chronic cholestasis, neonatal abstinence syndrome, febrile seizures in children

DOSAGE AND ROUTES

Seizures

- *Adult:* **PO** 1-3 mg/kg/day in divided doses tid or total dose at bedtime
- *Child 5-12 yr:* **PO** 3-6 mg/kg/day in 1-2 divided doses
- *Child 1-5 yr:* **PO** 6-8 mg/kg/day in 1-2 divided doses
- *Infant:* **PO** 5-6 mg/kg/day in 1-2 divided doses
- *Neonate:* **PO** 3-4 mg/kg/day as a single dose

Status epilepticus

- *Adult:* **IV INF** 10 mg/kg; run no faster than 50 mg/min; may give up to 30 mg/kg
- *Child:* **IV INF** 5-10 mg/kg; may repeat q10-15min up to 20 mg/kg; run no faster than 50 mg/min

Insomnia

- *Adult:* **PO/IM/SUBCUT** 100-200 mg
- *Child (unlabeled):* **PO/IM/SUBCUT** 3-5 mg/kg

Sedation

- *Adult:* **PO/IM** 30-120 mg/day in 2-3 divided doses
- *Child:* **PO** 3-5 mg/kg/day in 3 divided doses

Preoperative sedation

- *Adult:* **IM** 100-200 mg 1-1½ hr before surgery
- *Child:* **PO/IM/IV** 1-3 mg/kg 1-1½ hr before surgery

Available forms: Caps 15 mg; elix 20 mg/5 ml; tabs 15, 30, 32, 60, 65, 100 mg; inj 30, 60, 65, 130 mg/ml

SIDE EFFECTS

CNS: Paradoxic excitement (geriatric patients), drowsiness, lethargy, hangover headache, flushing, hallucinations, **coma**

GI: Nausea, vomiting, diarrhea, constipation

HEMA: **Agranulocytosis, megaloblastic anemia, thrombocytopenia, thrombophlebitis**

INTEG: Rash, urticaria, **Stevens-Johnson syndrome, angioedema,** local pain, swelling, necrosis, scaling eczema

Contraindications: Pregnancy (D), breastfeeding, geriatric patients, hypersensitivity to barbiturates, porphyria, hepatic/respiratory disease, nephritis, hyperthyroidism, diabetes mellitus

Precautions: Anemia, renal disease

PHARMACOKINETICS

Metabolized by liver; crosses placenta; excreted in urine, breast milk; half-life 53-118 hr

PO: Onset 20-60 min, duration 6-10 hr

IM/SUBCUT: Onset 10-30 min, duration 4-6 hr

IV: Onset 5 min, peak 30 min, duration 4-6 hr

INTERACTIONS

Increase: effects—CNS depressants, alcohol, chloramphenicol, valproic acid, disulfiram, nondepolarizing skeletal muscle relaxants, sulfonamides, MAOIs

Increase: orthostatic hypotension—furosemide

Decrease: effects—theophylline, oral anticoagulants, corticosteroids, metronidazole, doxycycline, quinidine, estrogens, hormonal contraceptives

Drug/Herb

Increase: phenobarbital levels—quinine

Increase: CNS depression—chamomile, eucalyptus, hops, Jamaican dogwood, kava, lemon balm, nettle, pill-bearing spurge, poppy, senega, skullcap, valerian

Decrease: barbiturate effect—St. John's wort

NURSING CONSIDERATIONS

Assess:

- Mental status: mood, sensorium, affect, memory (long, short)
- For respiratory depression
- Blood dyscrasias: fever, sore throat, bruising, rash, jaundice
- Convulsion activity: type, duration, precipitating factors
- Blood studies, LFTs during long-term treatment
- Therapeutic blood level periodically: 15-40 mcg/ml
- Respiratory status: rate, rhythm, depth

Administer:

- Avoid use with other CNS depressants

IM route

- IM inj deep in large muscle mass to prevent tissue sloughing; use <5 ml in each site

IV route

- Slow IV after dilution with at least 10 ml sterile H_2O for inj regardless of dose; give 50 mg or less/min; titrate to patient response

Additive compatibilities: Amikacin, aminophylline, calcium chloride, calcium gluconate, cephapirin, colistimethate, dimenhyDRINATE, meropenem, polymyxin B, sodium bicarbonate, thiopental, verapamil

Solution compatibilities: D_5W, $D_{10}W$, 0.45% NaCl, 0.9% NaCl, Ringer's, dextrose/saline combinations, dextrose/Ringer's, dextrose/LR combinations, sodium lactate

Syringe compatibilities: Heparin

Y-site compatibilities: Enalaprilat, meropenem, propofol, sufentanil

Perform/provide:

- Supervision of ambulation for dizziness, drowsiness

Evaluate:

- Therapeutic response: decreased seizures, increased sedation

Teach patient/family:

- To use exactly as ordered
- To avoid alcohol use
- To avoid hazardous activities until stabilized on product; drowsiness may occur
- Never to withdraw product abruptly; withdrawal symptoms may occur
- That therapeutic effects (PO) may not be seen for 2-3 wk

Treatment of overdose: Lavage, activated charcoal, warming blanket, vital signs, hemodialysis, I&O ratio

phentolamine (℞)

(fen-tole'a-meen)

Func. class.: Antihypertensive

Chem. class.: α-Adrenergic blocker

Do not confuse:

phentolamine/phentermine

Action: α-Adrenergic blocker, binds to α-adrenergic receptors, dilating peripheral blood vessels, lowering peripheral resistances, lowering blood pressure

Uses: Hypertension; pheochromocytoma; prevention/treatment of dermal necrosis following extravasation of norepinephrine, DOPamine, epinephrine

Unlabeled uses: Impotence, hypertensive crisis due to MAOIs, sympathomimetic amines, heart failure

DOSAGE AND ROUTES

Treatment of hypertensive episodes in pheochromocytoma

- *Adult:* **IM/IV** 5 mg, repeat if necessary
- *Child:* **IV** 0.05-0.1 mg/kg/dose, repeat if necessary; max 5 mg

Diagnosis of pheochromocytoma

- *Adult:* **IV** 2.5 mg; if negative, repeat with 5 mg IV
- *Child:* **IV** 0.05 mg/kg; if negative, repeat with 0.1 mg/kg IV

P

Treatment of necrosis
• *Adult:* 5-10 mg/10 ml **NS** injected into area of norepinephrine extravasation within 12 hr
• *Child:* 0.1-0.2 mg/kg, max 5 mg
Prevention of necrosis
• *Adult:* 10 mg/L of norepinephrine-containing sol
• *Child:* **IV** 0.1-0.2 mg/kg, max 5 mg
Left ventricular heart failure (unlabeled)
• *Adult:* **IV** 0.17-0.4 mg/min
Erectile dysfunction (unlabeled)
• *Adult:* **PO** 40-80 mg
Hypertensive emergency due to MAOIs, sympathomimetic amines (unlabeled)
• *Adult:* **IV BOL** 5-15 mg
Available forms: Inj 5 mg/ml

SIDE EFFECTS

CNS: Dizziness, flushing, weakness, **cerebrovascular spasm**
CV: Hypotension, tachycardia, angina, dysrhythmias, **MI**
EENT: Nasal congestion
GI: Dry mouth, nausea, vomiting, diarrhea, abdominal pain
Contraindications: Hypersensitivity, MI, coronary insufficiency, angina
Precautions: Pregnancy (C), breastfeeding, dysrhythmia

PHARMACOKINETICS

Metabolized in liver, excreted in urine
IM: Peak 15-20 min, duration 3-4 hr
IV: Peak 2 min, duration 10-15 min

INTERACTIONS

Increase: effects of epinephrine, antihypertensives
Drug/Herb
Increase: toxicity, death—aconite
Increase: antihypertensive effect—barberry, betony, black catechu, black cohosh, bloodroot, broom, burdock, cat's claw, dandelion, goldenseal, hawthorn, Irish moss, Jamaican dogwood, kelp, khella, mistletoe, parsley
Increase or decrease: antihypertensive effect—astragalus, cola tree
Decrease: antihypertensive effect—coltsfoot, guarana, khat, licorice, yohimbe

NURSING CONSIDERATIONS

Assess:
• Weight daily, I&O
• B/P lying, standing before starting treatment, q4hr after
• Nausea, vomiting, diarrhea, edema in feet, legs daily; skin turgor, dryness of mucous membranes for hydration status, postural hypotension, cardiac system: pulse, ECG
Administer:
• Gum, frequent rinsing of mouth, or hard candy for dry mouth
• With vasopressor available
• After discontinuing all medication for 24 hr
• Treatment during required bed rest, 1 hr after
IV route
• After diluting 5 mg/1 ml sterile H_2O for inj; give 5 mg or less/min; patient to remain recumbent during administration
CONT IV INF route
• Dilute 5-10 mg/500 ml D_5W, titrate to patient response
• 10 mg/L may be added to norepinephrine in IV sol for prevention of dermal necrosis
Additive compatibilities: DOBUTamine, verapamil
Syringe compatibilities: Papaverine
Y-site compatibilities: Amiodarone
Evaluate:
• Therapeutic response: decreased B/P
Teach patient/family:
• That bed rest is required during treatment, 1 hr after
Treatment of overdose: Administer norepinephrine; discontinue product

phenylephrine (℞)

(fen-ill-ef′rin)

Neo-Synephrine

Func. class.: Adrenergic, direct-acting

Chem. class.: Substituted phenylethylamine

Action: Powerful and selective (α_1) receptor agonist causing contraction of blood vessels

Uses: Hypotension, paroxysmal supraventricular tachycardia, shock, maintain B/P for spinal anesthesia

DOSAGE AND ROUTES

Hypotension

- *Adult:* **SUBCUT/IM** 2-5 mg; may repeat q10-15min if needed; do not exceed initial dose; **IV** 0.1-0.5 mg; may repeat q10-15min if needed; do not exceed initial dose
- *Child:* **IM/SUBCUT** 0.1 mg/kg/dose q1-2hr prn

Supraventricular tachycardia

- *Adult:* **IV BOL** max 0.5 mg; max single dose 1 mg

Shock

- *Adult:* **IV INF** 10 mg/500 ml D_5W given 100-180 mcg/min (if 20 gtt/ml inf device), then maintenance of 40-60 mcg/min; use inf device
- *Child:* **IV BOL** 5-20 mcg/kg/dose q10-15min; **IV INF** 0.1-0.5 mcg/kg/min

Available forms: Inj 1% (10 mg/ml)

SIDE EFFECTS

CNS: Headache, anxiety, tremor, insomnia, dizziness

CV: Palpitations, tachycardia, hypertension, ectopic beats, angina, reflex bradycardia, **dysrhythmias**

GI: Nausea, vomiting

INTEG: Necrosis, tissue sloughing with extravasation, **gangrene**

SYST: **Anaphylaxis**

Contraindications: Hypersensitivity, ventricular fibrillation, tachydysrhythmias, pheochromocytoma, closed-angle glaucoma, severe hypertension

Precautions: Pregnancy (C), breastfeeding, geriatric patients, arterial embolism, peripheral vascular disease, hyperthyroidism, bradycardia, myocardial disease, severe arteriosclerosis, partial heart block

Black Box Warning: Cardiac disease, extravasation

PHARMACOKINETICS

IM/SUBCUT: Onset 10-15 min, duration 45-60 min

IV: Onset immediate, duration 20-30 min

INTERACTIONS

- Dysrhythmias: general anesthetics, digoxin, bretylium

⚠ Do not use within 2 wk of MAOIs, or hypertensive crisis may result

Increase: in B/P—oxytocics

Increase: pressor effect—tricyclics, β-blockers, H_1 antihistamines

Decrease: phenylephrine action—α-blockers

NURSING CONSIDERATIONS

Assess:

- I&O ratio; notify prescriber if output <30 ml/hr
- ECG during administration continuously; if B/P increases, product is decreased
- B/P and pulse q5min after parenteral route
- CVP or PWP during inf if possible
- For paresthesias and coldness of extremities; peripheral blood flow may decrease

Administer:

IV route

- Plasma expanders for hypovolemia
- IV after diluting 1 mg/9 ml sterile H_2O for inj; give dose over ½-1 min; may be diluted 10 mg/500 ml of D_5W or NS; titrate to response (normal B/P); check for extravasation, check site for infiltration, use inf pump

P

Additive compatibilities: Chloramphenicol, DOBUTamine, lidocaine, potassium chloride, sodium bicarbonate
Y-site compatibilities: Amiodarone, amrinone, cisatracurium, famotidine, haloperidol, remifentanil, zidovudine
Perform/provide:
• Storage of reconstituted sol if refrigerated for no longer than 24 hr
• Discard discolored sol
Evaluate:
• Therapeutic response: increased B/P with stabilization
Teach patient/family:
• The reason for administration
• To report pain at inf site or other adverse reactions immediately
Treatment of overdose: Administer an α-blocker

phenylephrine nasal agent
See Appendix B

phenylephrine ophthalmic
See Appendix B

phenytoin (℞)
(fen'i-toh-in)
Dilantin, Dilantin Infatab, Phenytek
Func. class.: Anticonvulsant; antidysrhythmic (IB)
Chem. class.: Hydantoin

Action: Inhibits spread of seizure activity in motor cortex by altering ion transport; increases AV conduction
Uses: Generalized tonic-clonic seizures; status epilepticus; nonepileptic seizures associated with Reye's syndrome or after head trauma; Bell's palsy, complex partial seizures
Unlabeled uses: Migraines, diabetic neuropathy, neuropathic pain, paroxysmal atrial tachycardia, ventricular tachycardia

DOSAGE AND ROUTES
Seizures
• *Adult:* **PO** 1 g or 20 mg/kg (ext rel) in 3-4 divided doses given q2hr, or 400 mg, then 300 mg q2hr × 2 doses, maintenance 300-400 mg/day, max 600 mg/day; **IV** 15-20 mg/kg, max 25-50 mg/min, then 100 mg q6-8hr
• *Child:* **PO** 5 mg/kg/day in 2-3 divided doses, maintenance 4-8 mg/kg/day in 2-3 divided doses, max 300 mg/day; **IV** 15-20 mg/kg at 1-3 mg/kg/min
Status epilepticus
• *Adult:* **IV** 10-15 mg/kg, max 25-50 mg/min, may give 100 mg q6-8hr thereafter
• *Child:* **IV** 15-20 mg/kg, max in divided doses 1-3 mg/kg/min
Ventricular dysrhythmias
• *Adult:* **PO** Loading dose 1 g divided over 24 hr, then 500 mg/day × 2 days; **IV** 250 mg over 5 min until dysrhythmias subside or until 1 g is given, or 100 mg q15min until dysrhythmias subside or until 1 g is given
• *Child:* **PO** 3-8 mg/kg or 250 mg/m^2/day as single dose or 2 divided doses; **IV** 3-8 mg/kg over several min, or 250 mg/m^2/day as single dose or 2 divided doses
Renal dose
• Do not use loading dose CCr <10 ml/min or hepatic failure
Neuropathic pain/diabetic neuropathy (unlabeled)
• *Adult:* **PO** 300 mg/day in divided doses
Migraine prophylaxis (unlabeled)
• *Adult:* **PO** 200-400 mg/day
Available forms: Susp 25 mg/5 ml; chewable tabs 50 mg; inj 50 mg/ml; ext rel caps 100, 200, 300 mg; prompt rel caps 100 mg

SIDE EFFECTS
CNS: Drowsiness, dizziness, insomnia, paresthesias, depression, **suicidal tendencies,** aggression, headache, confusion, slurred speech, peripheral neuropathy
CV: Hypotension, **ventricular fibrillation**

EENT: Nystagmus, diplopia, blurred vision
ENDO: Diabetes insipidus
GI: Nausea, vomiting, constipation, anorexia, weight loss, **hepatitis,** jaundice, gingival hyperplasia
GU: **Nephritis,** urine discoloration
HEMA: **Agranulocytosis, leukopenia, aplastic anemia, thrombocytopenia, megaloblastic anemia**
INTEG: Rash, **lupus erythematosus, Stevens-Johnson syndrome,** hirsutism, **toxic epidermal necrolysis**
SYST: Hypocalcemia, **purple glove syndrome (IV)**
Contraindications: Pregnancy (D), hypersensitivity, psychiatric condition, bradycardia, SA and AV block, Stokes-Adams syndrome, hepatic failure, acute intermittent porphyria
Precautions: Geriatric patients, allergies, renal/hepatic disease, petit mal seizures, hypotension, myocardial insufficiency, Asian patients positive for HLA-B1502

PHARMACOKINETICS

Metabolized by liver, excreted by kidneys, protein binding 90%-95%, half-life 7-42 hr, dose dependent
PO: Onset 2-24 hr, peak 1½-2½ hr, duration 6-12 hr
PO-ER: Onset 2-24 hr, peak 4-12 hr, duration 12-36 hr
IV: Onset 1-2 hr, duration 12-24 hr

INTERACTIONS

Increase: phenytoin effect—benzodiazepines, cimetidine, tricyclics, salicylates, valproate, cycloSERINE, diazepam, chloramphenicol
Decrease: phenytoin effects—alcohol (chronic use), antacids, barbiturates, carbamazepine, diazoxide, rifampin, folic acid

Drug/Herb
Increase: potassium loss, increase antidysrhythmic action—aloe, buckthorn, cascara sagrada, senna
Increase: action—ginkgo
Decrease: anticonvulsant effect—ginseng, santonica, valerian

Drug/Lab Test
Increase: glucose, alk phos, BSP
Decrease: dexamethasone, metyrapone test serum, PBI, urinary steroids

NURSING CONSIDERATIONS

Assess:

⚠ For phenytoin hypersensitivity syndrome 3-12 wk after start of treatment: rash, temp, lymphadenopathy; may cause hepatotoxicity, renal failure, rhabdomyolysis

⚠ For beginning rash that may lead to Stevens-Johnson syndrome or toxic epidermal necrolysis; phenytoin should not be used again

⚠ For purple glove syndrome with IV use

- Product level: toxic level 30-50 mcg/ml, therapeutic level: 7.5-20 mcg/ml, wait ≥1 wk to draw levels
- For seizures: duration, type, intensity precipitating factors
- Blood studies: CBC, platelets q2wk until stabilized, then q mo × 12, then q3mo; discontinue product if neutrophils <1600/mm^3; renal function: albumin conc

⚠ Mental status: mood, sensorium, affect, memory (long, short), suicidal thoughts/behaviors

- Respiratory depression; rate, depth, character
- Blood dyscrasias: fever, sore throat, bruising, rash, jaundice

Administer:

- Do not interchange chewable product with caps, not equivalent; only ext rel caps are to be used for once-a-day dosing
- Shake susp well before each dose G tube/NG tube; dilute susp prior to administration; flush tube with 20 ml H_2O after dose
- Allow 7-10 days between dosage changes
- Divided PO doses with or after meals to decrease adverse effects
- 2 hr before or after antacid or antidiarrheal use

P

IV route

• After diluting with diluent provided (2.2 ml/100 mg, 5.2 ml/250 mg, 1 ml/50 mg); shake; give through Y-tube or 3-way stopcock; inject slowly <50 mg/min; clear IV tubing first with NS sol; use in-line filter; discard 4 hr after preparation; inject into large veins to prevent purple glove syndrome; if hypotensive/bradycardia episodes develop during inf, slow inf rate

Additive compatibilities: Bleomycin, sodium bicarbonate, verapamil

Y-site compatibilities: Esmolol, famotidine, fluconazole, foscarnet, tacrolimus

Evaluate:

• Therapeutic response; decrease in severity of seizures, ventricular dysrhythmias

Teach patient/family:

• That if diabetic, urine glucose should be monitored

• That urine may turn pink

• Not to discontinue product abruptly; seizures may occur

• Proper brushing of teeth using a soft toothbrush, flossing to prevent gingival hyperplasia; need to see dentist frequently

• To avoid hazardous activities until stabilized on product

• To carry emergency ID stating product use

• That heavy use of alcohol may diminish effect of product; to avoid OTC medications

• Not to change brands or forms once stabilized on therapy; brands may vary

physostigmine ophthalmic

See Appendix B

phytonadione (vit K_1) (℞)

(fye-toe-na-dye′one)

Mephyton

Func. class.: Vit K_1, fat-soluble vitamin

Action: Needed for adequate blood clotting (factors II, VII, IX, X)

Uses: Vit K malabsorption, hypoprothrombinemia, prevention of hypoprothrombinemia caused by oral anticoagulants, prevention of hemorrhagic disease of the newborn

DOSAGE AND ROUTES

Hypoprothrombinemia caused by vit K malabsorption

• *Adult:* **PO/IM** 2.5-25 mg, may repeat or increase to 50 mg

• *Child:* **PO** 2.5-5 mg

• *Infant:* **PO/IM** 2 mg

Prevention of hemorrhagic disease of the newborn

• *Neonate:* **IM** 0.5-1 mg within 1 hr after birth, repeat in 2-3 wk if required

Hypoprothrombinemia caused by oral anticoagulants

• *Adult and child:* **PO/SUBCUT/IM** 1-10 mg, may repeat 12-48 hr after **PO** dose or 6-8 hr after **SUBCUT/IM** dose, based on INR

Available forms: Tabs 5 mg; inj 2 m/10 ml aqueous colloidal; inj aqueous dispersion 10 mg/ml (IM), 1 mg/0.5 ml

SIDE EFFECTS

CNS: Headache, **brain damage** (large doses)

GI: Nausea, decreased LFTs

HEMA: **Hemolytic anemia, hemoglobinuria, hyperbilirubinemia**

INTEG: Rash, urticaria

RESP: **Bronchospasm,** dyspnea, feeling of chest constriction, **respiratory arrest**

Contraindications: Hypersensitivity, severe hepatic disease, last few weeks of pregnancy

Precautions: Pregnancy (C), neonates, hepatic disease

Black Box Warning: IV use

PHARMACOKINETICS

PO/INJ: Metabolized, crosses placenta

INTERACTIONS

Decrease: action of phytonadione—cholestyramine, mineral oil
Decrease: action of oral anticoagulants

Drug/Food

- Olestra, decreased vit K levels

NURSING CONSIDERATIONS

Assess:

- For bleeding: emesis, stools, urine
- PT during treatment (2-sec deviation from control time, bleeding time, and clotting time); monitor for bleeding, pulse, and B/P
- Nutritional status: liver (beef), spinach, tomatoes, coffee, asparagus, broccoli, cabbage, lettuce, greens

Administer:

IV route

- After diluting with D_5NS 10 ml or more; give 1 mg/min or more

⚠ IV only when other routes not possible (deaths have occurred)

Additive compatibilities: Amikacin, calcium gluconate, chloramphenicol, cimetidine, netilmicin, sodium bicarbonate

Syringe compatibilities: Doxapram

Y-site compatibilities: Alfentanil, amikacin, aminophylline, ampicillin, epinephrine, famotidine, heparin, hydrocortisone, potassium chloride, tolazoline, vit B/C

Perform/provide:

- Storage in tight, light-resistant container

Evaluate:

- Therapeutic response: decreased bleeding tendencies, decreased PT, decreased clotting time

Teach patient/family:

- Not to take other supplements unless directed by prescriber
- The necessary foods for diet
- To avoid IM inj, use soft toothbrush, do not floss, use electric razor until coagulation defect corrected
- To report symptoms of bleeding
- Not to use OTC medications unless approved by prescriber
- The importance of frequent lab tests to monitor coagulation factors

pilocarpine ophthalmic

See Appendix B

pimecrolimus topical

See Appendix B

pindolol (℞)

(pin'doe-lole)

Novo-Pindol ♣, Syn-Pindolol ♣, Visken

Func. class.: Antihypertensive

Chem. class.: Nonselective β-blocker

Do not confuse:
pindolol/Parlodel/Plendil

Action: Competitively blocks stimulation of β-adrenergic receptor within vascular smooth muscle; decreases rate of SA node discharge, increases recovery time, slows conduction of AV node, decreases heart rate, which decreases O_2 consumption in myocardium; also decreases renin-aldosterone-angiotensin system, at high doses inhibits β_2 receptors in bronchial system

Uses: Mild to moderate hypertension

Unlabeled uses: Chronic stable angina

DOSAGE AND ROUTES

- *Adult:* **PO** 5 mg bid, usual dose 15 mg/day (5 mg tid), may increase by 10 mg/day q3-4wk to a max of 60 mg/day
- *Geriatric:* **PO** 5 mg/day, increase by 5 mg q3-4wk

Available forms: Tabs 5, 10 mg

SIDE EFFECTS

CNS: Insomnia, dizziness, hallucinations, anxiety, fatigue, headache, depression
CV: Hypotension, bradycardia, **CHF,** edema, chest pain, palpitation, claudication, tachycardia, **AV block, pulmonary edema, bradycardia, dysrhythmias**
EENT: Visual changes, sore throat, *double vision;* dry, burning eyes, nasal stuffiness
GI: Nausea, vomiting, **ischemic colitis,** diarrhea, *abdominal pain,* **mesenteric arterial thrombosis,** flatulence, constipation
GU: Impotence, urinary frequency
HEMA: **Agranulocytosis, thrombocytopenia, purpura**
INTEG: Rash, alopecia, pruritus, fever
MISC: Joint pain, muscle pain
RESP: **Bronchospasm,** *dyspnea,* cough, crackles

Contraindications: Hypersensitivity to β-blockers, cardiogenic shock; 2nd-/3rd-degree heart block; sinus bradycardia; sick sinus syndrome; acute bronchospasm

Precautions: Pregnancy (B), breastfeeding, major surgery, diabetes mellitus, thyroid disease, COPD, well-compensated heart failure, CAD, nonallergic bronchospasm, peripheral vascular disease, renal/hepatic disease

Black Box Warning: Abrupt discontinuation

PHARMACOKINETICS

Peak 1-3 hr; half-life 3-4 hr, excreted 30%-50% unchanged; 60%-65% metabolized by liver; excreted in breast milk; protein binding 40%-60%

INTERACTIONS

- May alter hypoglycemic effect: insulin, oral hypoglycemics

Increase: hypotension, bradycardia—reserpine, hydrALAZINE, methyldopa, prazosin, anticholinergics, β-adrenergic agonists, calcium channel blockers

Increase: effects of β-blockers, calcium channel blockers

Decrease: antihypertensive effects—NSAIDs, salicylates, sympathomimetics, thyroid

Decrease: bronchodilation—theophyllines, β_2-agonists

Drug/Herb

Increase: toxicity, death—aconite

Increase: antihypertensive effect—barberry, betony, black catechu, black cohosh, bloodroot, broom, burdock, cat's claw, dandelion, goldenseal, hawthorn, Irish moss, Jamaican dogwood, kelp, khella, mistletoe, parsley

Increase or decrease: antihypertensive effect—astragalus, cola tree

Decrease: antihypertensive effect—coltsfoot, guarana, khat, licorice, St. John's wort, yohimbe

Drug/Lab Test

Increase: renal, hepatic studies

Interference: glucose, insulin tolerance test

NURSING CONSIDERATIONS

Assess:

- I&O, weight daily
- B/P during initial treatment, periodically thereafter; pulse q4hr, note rate, rhythm, quality; apical, radial pulse before administration; notify prescriber of any significant changes
- Baselines in renal, hepatic studies before therapy begins
- Skin turgor, dryness of mucous membranes for hydration status; edema in feet, legs daily

Administer:

- Before meals, at bedtime; tablet may be crushed or swallowed whole

Perform/provide:

- Storage in dry area at room temperature; do not freeze

Evaluate:

- Therapeutic response: decreased B/P after 1-2 wk

Teach patient/family:

- To take with or immediately after meals if GI symptoms occur

⚠ Not to discontinue product abruptly; taper over 2 wk; may cause precipitate angina

• Not to use OTC products containing α-adrenergic stimulants (nasal decongestants, OTC cold preparations) unless directed by prescriber
• To report bradycardia, dizziness, confusion, depression, fever, sore throat, shortness of breath to prescriber
• To take pulse at home; to notify prescriber if pulse <60 bpm
• To avoid alcohol, smoking, sodium
• To comply with weight control, dietary adjustments, modified exercise program
• To carry emergency ID to identify product, allergies
• To be alert that diabetic symptoms (hypoglycemia, sweating, dizziness) may be masked by product
• To avoid hazardous activities if dizziness is present
• To report symptoms of CHF: difficult breathing, especially on exertion or when lying down, night cough, swelling of extremities
• To take medication at bedtime to prevent orthostatic hypotension
• To wear support hose to minimize effects of orthostatic hypotension

Treatment of overdose: Lavage, IV atropine for bradycardia, IV theophylline for bronchospasm, digoxin, O_2, diuretic for cardiac failure, hemodialysis, hypotension; give vasopressor (norepinephrine)

pioglitazone (℞)

(pie-oh-glye'ta-zone)
Actos
Func. class.: Antidiabetic, oral
Chem. class.: Thiazolidinedione

Action: Specifically targets insulin resistance, an insulin sensitizer; regulates the transcription of a number of insulin responsive genes
Uses: Type 2 diabetes mellitus

DOSAGE AND ROUTES

Monotherapy
• *Adult:* **PO** 15-30 mg/day, may increase to 45 mg/day

Combination therapy
• *Adult:* **PO** 15-30 mg/day with a sulfonylurea, metformin, or insulin; decrease sulfonylurea dose if hypoglycemia occurs; decrease insulin dose by 10%-25% if hypoglycemia occurs or if plasma glucose is <100 mg/dl, max 45 mg/day

Hepatic dose
• Do not use in active hepatic disease or if ALT >2.5 times ULN

Available forms: Tabs 15, 30, 45 mg

SIDE EFFECTS

CNS: Headache
CV: **MI, heart failure, death (geriatric patients)**
ENDO: Hypo/hyperglycemia
MISC: Myalgia, sinusitis, upper respiratory tract infection, pharyngitis, **hepatotoxicity**, edema, weight gain, anemia, macular edema
MS: Fractures (females), myalgia

Contraindications: Breastfeeding, children, hypersensitivity to thiazolidinedione, diabetic ketoacidosis

Black Box Warning: CHF

Precautions: Pregnancy (C), geriatric patients, geriatric patients with CV disease, renal/hepatic/thyroid disease, edema

PHARMACOKINETICS

Maximal reduction in FBS after 12 wk; half-life 3-7 hr, terminal 16-24 hr

INTERACTIONS

• Poor glucose control: gatifloxacin; avoid concurrent use
Decrease: effect of oral contraceptives, use an alternative contraceptive method
Decrease: pioglitazone effect—CYP2C8 inducers (ketoconazole, fluconazole, itraconazole, miconazole, voriconazole)

Drug/Herb
• Poor blood glucose control: glucosamine
Increase: hypoglycemia—chromium, coenzyme Q10, fenugreek
Increase: antidiabetic effect—alfalfa, aloe, basil, bay, bilberry, bitter melon,

P

black catechu, buchu, burdock, coriander, dandelion, eyebright (po), fenugreek, garlic, ginseng, glucomannan, glucosamine, goat's rue, gymnema, horehound, horse chestnut, jambul, myrrh, myrtle
Decrease: antidiabetic effect—bee pollen, blue cohosh, broom, chromium, elecampane, eucalyptus, gotu kola

NURSING CONSIDERATIONS

Assess:

- For hypoglycemic reactions (sweating, weakness, dizziness, anxiety, tremors, hunger), hyperglycemic reactions soon after meals (rare)
- Check LFTs periodically AST, LDH
- FBS, glycosylated Hgb, plasma lipids/lipoproteins, B/P, body weight during treatment

Administer:

- Once a day; give with meals to decrease GI upset
- Tabs crushed and mixed with food or fluids for patients with difficulty swallowing

Perform/provide:

- Conversion from other oral hypoglycemic agents; change may be made with gradual dosage change; monitor serum glucose during conversion
- Storage in tight container in cool environment

Evaluate:

- Therapeutic response: decrease in polyuria, polydipsia, polyphagia; clear sensorium; absence of dizziness; stable gait; blood glucose A1c improvement

Teach patient/family:

- To self-monitor using a blood glucose meter
- The symptoms of hypo/hyperglycemia, what to do about each
- That the product must be continued on daily basis; explain consequence of discontinuing product abruptly
- To avoid OTC medications or herbal preparations unless approved by prescriber
- That diabetes is lifelong illness; that this product is not a cure; only controls symptoms
- To notify prescriber if oral contraceptives are used
- Not to use if breastfeeding
- To report symptoms of hepatic dysfunction (nausea, vomiting, abdominal pain, fatigue, anorexia, dark urine, jaundice)
- To report weight gain, edema

piperacillin (℞)

(pip′er-ah-sill′in)

Func. class.: Broad-spectrum antiinfective
Chem. class.: Extended-spectrum penicillin

Action: Lysis mediated by cell wall autolytic enzymes

Uses: Respiratory, skin, urinary tract, bone infections; gonorrhea; pneumonia; effective for gram-positive cocci *(Staphylococcus aureus, Streptococcus pyogenes, Streptococcus viridans, Streptococcus faecalis, Streptococcus bovis, Streptococcus pneumoniae),* gram-negative cocci *(Neisseria gonorrhoeae, Neisseria meningitidis),* gram-positive bacilli *(Acinetobacter, Clostridium perfringens, Clostridium tetani),* gram-negative bacilli *(Bacteroides, Citrobacter, Enterobacter, Escherichia coli, Eubacterium, Fusobacterium nucleatum, Klebsiella, Morganella morganii, Peptococcus, Peptostreptococcus, Proteus mirabilis, Proteus vulgaris, Providencia rettgeri, Pseudomonas aeruginosa, Serratia)*

DOSAGE AND ROUTES

Urinary tract infections

- *Adult:* **IM/IV** 6-8 g/day (100-125 mg/kg/day) in divided doses q6-12hr, max 24 g/day

Serious systemic infections

- *Adult and child >12 yr:* **IM/IV** 2-4 g q4-6hr (2 g/site **IM**)
- *Child <12 yr:* **IM/IV** 200-300 mg/kg/day in divided doses q4-6hr

Prophylaxis of surgical infections
• *Adult:* **IV** 2 g ½-1 hr before procedure; may be repeated during surgery or after surgery
Renal dose
• *Adult:* **IV** CCr 20-40 ml/min extend dose to q8hr; CCr <20 ml/min extend dose to q12hr
Available forms: Powder for inj 2, 3, 4, 40 g

SIDE EFFECTS

CNS: Lethargy, hallucinations, anxiety, depression, twitching, **coma, seizures**
GI: Nausea, vomiting, diarrhea; increased AST, ALT; abdominal pain; glossitis; **pseudomembranous colitis;** hepatitis
GU: **Oliguria, proteinuria, hematuria,** *vaginitis, moniliasis,* **glomerulonephritis, acute renal failure**
HEMA: Anemia, increased bleeding time, **bone marrow depression,** thrombocytopenia, hemolytic anemia
META: Hypokalemia, hypernatremia
SYST: **Serum sickness, anaphylaxis, Stevens-Johnson syndrome, exfoliative dermatitis, toxic epidermal necrolysis**
Contraindications: Neonates, hypersensitivity to penicillins
Precautions: Pregnancy (B), breastfeeding, children, hypersensitivity to cephalosporins/carbapenems, CHF, GI/renal disease, seizures

PHARMACOKINETICS

Half-life 0.7-1.33 hr; excreted in urine, bile, breast milk; crosses placenta
IM: Peak 30-50 min
IV: Peak 20-30 min

INTERACTIONS

Increase: piperacillin concentrations—aspirin, probenecid
Increase: levels of methotrexate, neuromuscular blockers
Decrease: antimicrobial effect of piperacillin—tetracyclines (with high concentrations of piperacillin), aminoglycosides
Decrease: effect of oral contraceptives
Drug/Herb
• Do not use acidophilus with antiinfectives; separate by several hours
Decrease: absorption—khat
Drug/Lab Test
False positive: urine glucose, urine protein, Coombs' test

NURSING CONSIDERATIONS

Assess:
• For infection: temp, WBC, sputum, stools, urine, wounds
• I&O ratio; report hematuria, oliguria, since penicillin in high doses is nephrotoxic
⚠ Any patient with compromised renal system, since product is excreted slowly in poor renal system function; toxicity may occur rapidly
• Hepatic studies: AST, ALT
• Blood studies: WBC, RBC, Hct, Hgb, bleeding time prior to and periodically during treatment
• Renal studies: urinalysis, protein, blood, BUN, creatinine prior to and periodically during treatment
• C&S before product therapy; product may be taken as soon as culture is taken
• Bowel pattern before and during treatment
• Skin eruptions after administration of penicillin to 1 wk after discontinuing product
• Respiratory status: rate, character, wheezing, tightness in chest
• Allergies before initiation of treatment, reaction of each medication
Administer:
• Product after C&S completed
IM route
• 2 g/4 ml, 3 g/6 ml, 4 g/8 ml of sterile water, 0.9% NaCl max 2 g/site
IV route
• After diluting 1 g or less/5 ml or more sterile H_2O or 0.9% NaCl; shake; give dose over 3-5 min; may further dilute to 50-100 ml with D_5W, 0.9% NS, and give over ½ hr; discontinue primary IV

P

Additive compatibilities: Ciprofloxacin, clindamycin, fluconazole, hydrocortisone, ofloxacin, potassium chloride, verapamil

Syringe compatibilities: Heparin

Y-site compatibilities: Acyclovir, allopurinol, amifostine, aztreonam, ciprofloxacin, cyclophosphamide, diltiazem, DOXOrubicin liposome, enalaprilat, esmolol, famotidine, fludarabine, foscarnet, gallium, granisetron, heparin, hydromorphone, IL-2, labetalol, lorazepam, magnesium sulfate, melphalan, meperidine, midazolam, morphine, perphenazine, propofol, ranitidine, remifentanil, tacrolimus, teniposide, theophylline, thiotepa, verapamil, zidovudine

Perform/provide:

- Epinephrine, suction, tracheostomy set, endotracheal intubation equipment on unit
- Adequate intake of fluids (2 L) during diarrhea episodes
- Scratch test to assess allergy after securing order from prescriber; usually done when penicillin is only product of choice
- Storage of reconstituted sol 24 hr at room temperature or 7 days refrigerated

Evaluate:

- Therapeutic response: absence of fever, purulent drainage, redness, inflammation

Teach patient/family:

- That culture may be taken after completed course of medication
- To report sore throat, fever, fatigue; may indicate superinfection; CNS effects (anxiety, depression, hallucinations, seizures)
- To wear or carry emergency ID if allergic to penicillins
- To notify nurse of diarrhea

Treatment of anaphylaxis: Withdraw product, maintain airway, administer epinephrine, aminophylline, O_2, IV corticosteroids

piperacillin/ tazobactam (℞)

(pip′er-ah-sill′in/ ta-zoe-bak′tam)

Zosyn

Func. class.: Antiinfective, broad-spectrum

Chem. class.: Extended-spectrum penicillin, β-lactamase inhibitor

Action: Interferes with cell wall replication of susceptible organisms; osmotically unstable cell wall swells and bursts from osmotic pressure; tazobactam is a β-lactamase inhibitor, protects piperacillin from enzymatic degradation

Uses: Moderate to severe infections: piperacillin-resistant, β-lactamase–producing strains causing infections in respiratory, skin, urinary tract, bone, gonorrhea, pneumonia; effective for resistant *Staphylococcus aureus,* resistant *Escherichia coli, Bacteroides fragilis, Bacteroides ovatus, Bacteroides thetaiotaomicron, Bacteroides vulgatus, Haemophilus influenzae*

DOSAGE AND ROUTES

Nosocomial pneumonia

- *Adult:* **IV** 4.5 g q6hr or 3.375 g q4hr with an aminoglycoside × 1-2 wk; continue aminoglycoside only if *Pseudomonas aeruginosa* is isolated

Other infections

- *Adult:* **IV INF** 6-12 g/day given 2.25 g q8hr to 3.375 g q6hr over 30 min × 7-10 days

Renal dose

- *Adult:* **IV** CCr 20-40 ml/min give 2.25 g q6hr; CCr <20 ml/min give 2.25 g q8hr

Available forms: Powder for inj 2 g piperacillin/0.25 g tazobactam, 3 g piperacillin/0.375 g tazobactam, 4 g piperacillin/0.5 g tazobactam, 36 g piperacillin/4.5 g tazobactam

SIDE EFFECTS

CNS: Lethargy, hallucinations, anxiety, depression, twitching, insomnia, headache, fever, dizziness, **seizures,** vertigo
CV: **Cardiac toxicity**
GI: *Nausea, vomiting, diarrhea;* increased AST, ALT; abdominal pain, glossitis, **pseudomembranous colitis,** constipation
GU: **Oliguria, proteinuria, hematuria,** *vaginitis, moniliasis,* **glomerulonephritis, renal failure**
HEMA: Anemia, increased bleeding time, **bone marrow depression, agranulocytosis, hemolytic anemia**
INTEG: Rash, pruritus, **exfoliative dermatitis**
META: Hypokalemia, hypernatremia
SYST: **Serum sickness, anaphylaxis, Stevens-Johnson syndrome**
Contraindications: Hypersensitivity to penicillins; neonates; carbapenem allergy
Precautions: Pregnancy (B), breastfeeding, renal insufficiency in children, hypersensitivity to cephalosporins, CHF, seizures, GI disease, electrolyte imbalances

PHARMACOKINETICS

Half-life 0.7-1.2 hr; excreted in urine, bile, breast milk; crosses placenta; 33% bound to plasma proteins
IV: Peak completion of IV

INTERACTIONS

Increase: effect of neuromuscular blockers, oral anticoagulants, methotrexate
Increase: piperacillin concentrations—aspirin, probenecid
Decrease: antimicrobial effect of piperacillin—tetracyclines, aminoglycosides IV
Decrease: effect of oral contraceptives
Drug/Herb
• Do not use acidophilus with antiinfectives; separate by several hours
Decrease: absorption—khat
Drug/Lab Test
Increase: platelet count, eosinophilia, neutropenia, leukopenia, serum creatinine, PTT, AST, ALT, alk phos, bilirubin, BUN, electrolytes
Decrease: Hct, Hgb, electrolytes
False positive: urine glucose, urine protein, Coombs' test

NURSING CONSIDERATIONS

Assess:
• For infection: temp, stools, urine, sputum, wounds
• I&O ratio; report hematuria, oliguria, since penicillin in high doses is nephrotoxic
⚠ Any patient with compromised renal system, since product is excreted slowly in poor renal system function; toxicity may occur rapidly
• Hepatic studies: AST, ALT prior to and periodically thereafter
• Blood studies: WBC, RBC, Hct, Hgb, bleeding time prior to and periodically thereafter
• Renal studies: urinalysis, protein, blood, BUN, creatinine prior to and periodically thereafter
• C&S before product therapy; product may be given as soon as culture is taken
• Bowel pattern before and during treatment
• Skin eruptions after administration of penicillin to 1 wk after discontinuing product
• Respiratory status: rate, character, wheezing, tightness in chest
• Allergies before initiation of treatment, reaction of each medication
Administer:
• Separate aminoglycoside from piperacillin to avoid inactivation
• Product after C&S is complete
IV route
• After diluting 5 ml 0.9% NaCl for inj or sterile H_2O for inj, dextran 6% in NS, dextrose 5%, KCl 40 mEq, bacteriostatic saline/parabens, bacteriostatic saline/benzyl alcohol, bacteriostatic H_2O/benzyl alcohol per 1 g piperacillin; shake well; further dilute in at least 50 ml compatible IV sol and run as int inf over at least 30 min

P

Y-site compatibilities: Aminophylline, aztreonam, bleomycin, bumetanide, buprenorphine, butorphanol, calcium gluconate, carboplatin, carmustine, cefepime, cimetidine, clindamycin, cyclophosphamide, cytarabine, dexamethasone, diphenhydrAMINE, DOPamine, enalaprilat, etoposide, floxuridine, fluconazole, fludarabine, fluorouracil, furosemide, gallium, granisetron, heparin, hydrocortisone, hydromorphone, ifosfamide, leucovorin, lorazepam, magnesium sulfate, mannitol, meperidine, mesna, methotrexate, methylPREDNISolone, metoclopramide, metronidazole, morphine, ondansetron, plicamycin, potassium chloride, ranitidine, remifentanil, sargramostim, sodium bicarbonate, thiotepa, trimethoprim-sulfamethoxazole, vinBLAStine, vinCRIStine, zidovudine

Perform/provide:

- EpINEPHrine, suction, tracheostomy set, endotracheal intubation equipment on unit
- Adequate intake of fluids (2 L) during diarrhea episodes
- Scratch test to assess allergy on order from prescriber; usually when penicillin is only product of choice
- Discard after 24 hr if stored at room temperature or after 48 hr if refrigerated; use single-dose vials immediately after reconstitution; stable in ambulatory IV pump for 12 hr

Evaluate:

- Therapeutic response: absence of fever, purulent drainage, redness, inflammation; culture shows decreased organisms

Teach patient/family:

- That culture may be taken after completed course of medication
- To report sore throat, fever, fatigue (may indicate superinfection); CNS effects (anxiety, depression, hallucinations, seizures)
- To wear or carry emergency ID if allergic to penicillins
- To notify nurse of diarrhea

Treatment of overdose: Withdraw product, maintain airway, administer epinephrine, aminophylline, O_2, IV corticosteroids for anaphylaxis

pirbuterol (℞)

(peer-byoo′ter-ole)

Maxair

Func. class.: Bronchodilator

Chem. class.: β-Adrenergic agonist

Action: Causes bronchodilation with little effect on heart rate by action on β-receptors, causing increased cAMP and relaxation of smooth muscle

Uses: Reversible bronchospasm (prevention, treatment) including asthma; may be given with theophylline or steroids

DOSAGE AND ROUTES

- *Adult and child >12 yr:* **INH** 1-2 puffs (0.4 mg) q4-6hr; max 12 **INH**/day

Available forms: Aerosol delivery 0.2 mg pirbuterol/actuation

SIDE EFFECTS

CNS: Tremors, anxiety, insomnia, headache, dizziness, stimulation, restlessness, hallucinations, drowsiness, irritability

CV: Palpitations, tachycardia, hypertension, angina, hypotension, dysrhythmias

EENT: Dry nose and mouth, irritation of nose, throat

GI: Gastritis, nausea, vomiting, anorexia

MS: Muscle cramps

RESP: **Paradoxical bronchospasm,** dyspnea, coughing

Contraindications: Hypersensitivity to sympathomimetics, tachycardia

Precautions: Pregnancy (C), breastfeeding, cardiac disorders, hyperthyroidism, hypertension, diabetes mellitus, prostatic hypertrophy

PHARMACOKINETICS

INH: Onset 3 min, peak ½-1 hr, duration 5 hr, terminal half-life 2 hr

INTERACTIONS

⚠ Hypertensive crisis: MAOIs

Increase: action of other aerosol bronchodilators

Increase: pirbuterol action—tricyclics, antihistamines, levothyroxine

Decrease: pirbuterol action—β-blockers

Drug/Herb

Increase: action of both—cola nut, guarana, yerba maté

Increase: effect—green tea (large amounts), guarana

NURSING CONSIDERATIONS

Assess:

- Respiratory function: vital capacity, forced expiratory volume, ABGs, B/P, lung sounds, pulse, characteristics of sputum

⚠ Paradoxical bronchospasm, that can occur rapidly, hold product, notify prescriber

Administer:

- After shaking; exhale; place mouthpiece in mouth; inhale slowly; hold breath; remove; exhale slowly
- Gum, sips of water for dry mouth

Perform/provide:

- Storage in light-resistant container; do not expose to temperatures over 86° F (30° C)
- Fluid intake >2 L/day to liquefy thick secretions

Evaluate:

- Therapeutic response: absence of dyspnea, wheezing over 1 hr

Teach patient/family:

- Not to use OTC medications; extra stimulation may occur
- Use of inhaler; review package insert with patient
- To avoid getting aerosol in eyes
- Actuator is for Maxair autoinhaler; do not use with other inhaler canister
- About all aspects of product; avoid smoking, smoke-filled rooms, persons with respiratory infections
- To keep fluid intake >2 L/day to liquefy thick secretions

Treatment of overdose: Administer a β-adrenergic blocker

piroxicam (℞)

(peer-ox′i-kam)

Apo-Piroxicam ✱, Feldene, Gen-Piroxicam ✱, Novopirocam ✱, PMS-Piroxicam ✱

Func. class.: Nonsteroidal antiinflammatory

Chem. class.: Oxicam derivative

Action: Inhibits prostaglandin synthesis by decreasing an enzyme needed for biosynthesis; has analgesic, antiinflammatory, antipyretic properties

Uses: Mild to moderate pain, osteoarthritis, rheumatoid arthritis

DOSAGE AND ROUTES

- *Adult:* **PO** 20 mg/day or 10 mg bid

Available forms: Caps 10, 20 mg

SIDE EFFECTS

CNS: Dizziness, ***drowsiness,*** fatigue, tremors, confusion, insomnia, anxiety, depression, ***headache***

CV: Tachycardia, peripheral edema, palpitations, dysrhythmias, hypertension, **MI, stroke, CHF**

EENT: Tinnitus, hearing loss, blurred vision

GI: ***Nausea, anorexia, vomiting, diarrhea,*** jaundice, **cholestatic hepatitis,** constipation, flatulence, cramps, dry mouth, peptic ulcer, **bleeding, ulceration, perforation,** dyspepsia

GU: **Nephrotoxicity: dysuria, hematuria, oliguria, azotemia**

HEMA: **Blood dyscrasias**

INTEG: Purpura, rash, pruritus, sweating, photosensitivity

MISC: Hyperkalemia, hypoglycemia

SYST: **Anaphylaxis**

P

Contraindications: Pregnancy (D) (3rd trimester), hypersensitivity to this product, NSAIDs, salicylates; asthma

Black Box Warning: Perioperative pain in CABG surgery

Precautions: Pregnancy (C), avoid in late pregnancy, breastfeeding, children, bleeding/GI/cardiac disorders, hypersensitivity to other antiinflammatory agents, CHF

Black Box Warning: GI bleeding, MI, stroke

PHARMACOKINETICS

Peak 3-5 hr; duration 48-72 hr, half-life 50 hr; metabolized in liver; excreted in urine (metabolites), breast milk; 99% protein binding

INTERACTIONS

Increase: hypoglycemia—oral antidiabetics

Increase: toxicity—cycloSPORINE, methotrexate, lithium, alcohol, oral anticoagulants, aspirin, corticosteroids

Increase: bleeding risk—anticoagulants, antiplatelets, thrombin inhibitors, NSAIDs, SSRIs

Decrease: effects of antihypertensives, diuretics

Drug/Herb

Increase: gastric irritation—arginine, gossypol

Increase: NSAIDs effect—bearberry, bilberry

Increase: bleeding risk—bogbean, chondroitin

NURSING CONSIDERATIONS

Assess:

⚠ Cardiac status: CV thrombotic events, MI, stroke; may be fatal

⚠ GI status: ulceration, bleeding, perforation; may be fatal

- For pain: location, duration, type, ROM before and 1-2 hr after administration
- Renal, hepatic, blood studies: BUN, creatinine, AST, ALT, Hgb, before treatment, periodically thereafter
- Audiometric, ophthalmic exam before, during, after treatment
- For eye, ear problems: blurred vision, tinnitus (may indicate toxicity)

⚠ Those with aspirin sensitivity, asthma, nasal polyps may develop allergic reactions

Administer:

- Do not break, crush, or chew caps
- With food to decrease GI symptoms; take on empty stomach to facilitate absorption; take product same time daily

Perform/provide:

- Storage at room temperature in light-resistant container
- At least 6-8 glasses of water/day

Evaluate:

- Therapeutic response: decreased pain, stiffness, swelling in joints; ability to move more easily

Teach patient/family:

- To report blurred vision or ringing, roaring in ears (may indicate toxicity)
- To avoid driving, other hazardous activities if dizzy or drowsy
- That patient should drink at least 6-8 glasses of water/day unless contraindicated
- To report change in urine pattern, weight increase, edema, pain increase in joints, fever, blood in urine (indicates nephrotoxicity)
- That therapeutic effects may take up to 1 mo
- To avoid ASA, other OTC meds, alcohol
- To report if pregnancy is suspected or planned; avoid breastfeeding
- To report bruising; bleeding; black, tarry stools
- To avoid prolonged sun exposure; wear sunscreen, protective clothing
- To inform all health care providers about product use

pitavastatin (℞)
(pit′a-va-stat′-in)
Livalo
Func. class.: Antilipidemic
Chem. class.: HMG-CoA reductase inhibitor

Action: Inhibits HMG-CoA reductase enzyme, which reduces cholesterol synthesis; high doses lead to plaque regression
Uses: As an adjunct in primary hypercholesterolemia (types Ia, Ib), dysbetalipoproteinemia, elevated triglyceride levels, prevention of CV disease by reduction of heart risk in those with mildly elevated cholesterol
Unlabeled Uses: Atherosclerosis

DOSAGE AND ROUTES

• *Adult:* **PO** 2 mg/day, usual range 1-4, max 4 mg/day
Renal dose
• *Adult:* **PO** CCr 30-<60 ml/min, 1 mg daily, max 2 mg daily; CCr <30 ml/min on hemodialysis 1 mg daily, max 2 mg daily; CCr <30 ml/min not recommended
Atherosclerosis (unlabeled)
• *Adult:* **PO** 4 mg/day
Available forms: Tabs 1, 2, 4 mg

SIDE EFFECTS

CNS: Headache
GI: Constipation, diarrhea
INTEG: Rash, pruritus, alopecia
MS: Arthralgia, myalgia, **rhabdomyolysis**
RESP: Pharyngitis
Contraindications: Pregnancy (X), breastfeeding, hypersensitivity, active hepatic disease, cholestasis
Precautions: Past hepatic disease, alcoholism, severe acute infections, trauma, severe metabolic disorders, electrolyte imbalance, seizures, surgery, organ transplant, endocrine disease, females, hypotension, renal disease

PHARMACOKINETICS

Peak 1 hr; metabolized in liver, excreted in urine, feces; half-life 12 hr; protein binding 99%

INTERACTIONS

• Risk for possible rhabdomyolysis: azole antifungals, cycloSPORINE, erythromycin, niacin, gemfibrozil, clofibrate
Increase: levels of pitavastatin—erythromycin, red yeast rice
Increase: effects of warfarin
Drug/Lab Test
Increase: bilirubin, alk phos
Interference: thyroid function tests

NURSING CONSIDERATIONS

Assess:
• Diet, obtain diet history including fat, cholesterol in diet
• Cholesterol triglyceride levels periodically during treatment; check lipid panel 6 wk after changing dose
• Hepatic studies q1-2mo during the first 1½ yr of treatment; AST, ALT, LFTs may be increased
• Renal studies in patients with compromised renal system: BUN, I&O ratio, creatinine
• For muscle pain, tenderness, obtain CPK baseline and if markedly increased, product may need to be discontinued
Administer:
• Total daily dose any time of day without regard to meals
Perform/provide:
• Storage in cool environment in tight container protected from light
Evaluate:
• Therapeutic response: decrease in cholesterol to desired level after 6 wk
Teach patient/family:
• That blood work will be necessary during treatment
• To report blurred vision, severe GI symptoms, headache, muscle pain, weakness

• That previously prescribed regimen will continue: low-cholesterol diet, exercise program, smoking cessation
• Not to take product if pregnant

plasma protein fraction (℞)

Plasmanate

Func. class.: Hematological agent
Chem. class.: Plasma volume expander

Action: Exerts similar oncotic pressure as human plasma, expands blood volume

Uses: Hypovolemic shock, hypoproteinemia, ARDS, preoperative cardiopulmonary bypass, acute hepatic failure, nephrotic syndrome, cardiogenic shock

DOSAGE AND ROUTES

Hypovolemia

• *Adult:* **IV INF** 250-500 ml (12.5-25 g protein), max 10 ml/min
• *Child:* **IV INF** 10-30 ml/kg at max 5-10 ml/min

Hypoproteinemia

• *Adult:* **IV INF** 1000-1500 ml/day, max 8 ml/min

Available forms: Inj 5%

SIDE EFFECTS

CNS: Fever, chills, headache, paresthesias, flushing
CV: **Fluid overload,** hypotension, erratic pulse
GI: Nausea, vomiting, increased salivation
INTEG: Rash, urticaria, cyanosis
RESP: Altered respirations, dyspnea, **PE**

Contraindications: Hypersensitivity to this product or albumin, CHF, severe anemia, renal insufficiency, hyponatremia, cardiopulmonary bypass

Precautions: Pregnancy (C), decreased salt intake, decreased cardiac reserve, lack of albumin deficiency, hepatic disease

PHARMACOKINETICS

Metabolized as a protein/energy source

INTERACTIONS

Drug/Lab Test

False increase: alk phos

NURSING CONSIDERATIONS

Assess:

• Blood studies: Hct, Hgb, electrolytes, serum protein; if serum protein declines, dyspnea, hypoxemia can result
• B/P (decreased), pulse (erratic), respiration during inf
• I&O ratio; urinary output may decrease
• CVP, pulmonary wedge pressure (increases if overload occurs), jugular vein distention
• Allergy: fever, rash, itching, chills, flushing, urticaria, nausea, vomiting, or hypotension requires discontinuation of inf; use new lot if therapy reinstituted, premedicate with diphenhydrAMINE

⚠ Increased CVP reading: distended neck veins indicate circulatory overload; shortness of breath, anxiety, insomnia, expiratory crackles, frothy blood-tinged cough, cyanosis indicate pulmonary overload

Administer:

IV route

• IV access at distant site from infection or trauma; no dilution required; use inf pump, use large-gauge needle ($\geq$20 G); discard unused portion; infuse slowly to prevent hypotension
• Within 4 hr of opening, discard partially used vials
• Do not use sol that has been frozen
• Adjust rate to changes in B/P

Additive compatibilities: Carbohydrate and electrolyte sol, whole blood, packed RBCs, chloramphenicol, tetracycline

Perform/provide:

• Adequate hydration before administration
• Storage—at room temperature, max 86° F

Evaluate:
• Therapeutic response: increased B/P, decreased edema, increased serum albumin

plerixafor
See Appendix A—Selected New Drugs

porfimer (℞)
(pour′fih-mur)
Photofrin
Func. class.: Antineoplastic—miscellaneous
Chem. class.: Photosensitizing agent—hematoporphyrin derivative

Action: Used in photodynamic treatment of tumors (PDT); antitumor and cytotoxic actions are light and O_2 dependent; used with 630-nm laser light
Uses: Esophageal cancer (completely obstructing), endobronchial non–small cell lung cancer, Barrett's esophagus
Unlabeled uses: AIDS-related cutaneous Kaposi's sarcoma; basal cell, squamous cell carcinoma; bladder cancer

DOSAGE AND ROUTES
Refer to Optiguide for complete instructions
• *Adult:* **IV** 2 mg/kg over 3-5 min, then illumination with laser light 40-50 hr after inj; a second laser light application may be given 96-120 hr after inj; may repeat q30days × 3
Endobronchial cancer
• *Adult:* 200 joules/cm of tumor length
Available forms: Cake/powder for inj 75 mg; 15, 75 mg vials

SIDE EFFECTS
CNS: Anxiety, confusion, insomnia
CV: Hypo/hypertension, atrial fibrillation, **cardiac failure,** *tachycardia,* chest pain
GI: Abdominal pain, constipation, diarrhea, dyspepsia, dysphagia, eructation, esophageal edema/bleeding, hematemesis, melena, nausea, vomiting, anorexia
MISC: Dehydration, weight decrease, anemia, photosensitivity reaction, UTI, moniliasis
RESP: **Pleural effusion,** pneumonia, dyspnea, respiratory insufficiency, **tracheoesophageal fistula/stricture/ulceration**
Contraindications: Porphyria, porphyrin allergy (porfimer); tracheoesophageal, bronchoesophageal fistula; major blood vessels with eroding tumors (PDT)
Precautions: Pregnancy (C), breastfeeding, children, geriatric patients

PHARMACOKINETICS
Half-life 250 hr, 90% protein bound, peak 5-10 hr in tissues, cleared through biliary excretion

INTERACTIONS
Increase: photosensitivity—tetracyclines, sulfonamides, phenothiazines, sulfonylureas, thiazides
Decrease: porfimer effect—anticoagulants, NSAIDs, platelet inhibitors, thrombolytics, corticosteroids, calcium channel blockers

P

NURSING CONSIDERATIONS
Assess:
• Ocular sensitivity: sensitivity to sun, bright lights, car headlights, patients should wear dark sunglasses with an average light transmittance of <4%
• Chest pain: may be so severe as to necessitate opiate analgesics
• For extravasation at inj site: take care to protect from light
Administer:
• As a single slow IV inj over 3-5 min at 2 mg/kg; reconstitute each vial with 31.8 ml D_5 or 0.9% NaCl (2.5 mg/ml), shake well; do not mix with other products or sol; protect from light and use immediately

• Laser light is initiated 630-nm wave length laser light, 40-50 hr after inj, 2nd laser if indicated 96-120 hr

Perform/provide:

• Wiping of spills with damp cloth, avoid skin/eye contact, use rubber gloves, eye protection, dispose of material in polyethylene bag according to policy

Teach patient/family:

• To report chest pain, eye sensitivity, bleeding, signs/symptoms of infection, or respiratory distress

• To wear sunglasses; avoid exposure to sunlight or bright light for 30 days, report severe sunburn, blistering

posaconazole (℞)

(poe'sa-kon'a-zole)

Noxafil

Func. class.: Antifungal—systemic

Chem. class.: Triazole derivative

Action: Inhibits a portion of cell wall synthesis; alters cell membranes and inhibits several fungal enzymes

Uses: Prevention of aspergillus, candida infection, oropharyngeal candidiasis in the immunocompromised

DOSAGE AND ROUTES

• *Adult:* **PO** 800 mg/day in 2-4 divided doses

• *Child:* **PO** 100 mg tid

Available forms: Oral susp 200 mg/5 ml

SIDE EFFECTS

CNS: Headache, dizziness, insomnia, fever, rigors, weakness, anxiety

CV: Hypo/hypertension, tachycardia, anemia

GI: Nausea, vomiting, anorexia, diarrhea, cramps, abdominal pain, flatulence, **GI bleeding, hepatotoxicity**

GU: Gynecomastia, impotence, decreased libido

INTEG: Pruritus, fever, *rash,* **toxic epidermal necrolysis**

MISC: Edema, fatigue, malaise, hypokalemia, tinnitus, **rhabdomyolysis**

Contraindications: Hypersensitivity to this product or other systemic antifungal or azoles, fungal meningitis, onchomycosis or dermatomycosis in cardiac dysfunction

Precautions: Pregnancy (C), breastfeeding, children, cardiac/hepatic disease

PHARMACOKINETICS

Well absorbed, enhanced by food, protein binding 98%-99%, peak 4-11 hr, half-life 19-35 hr, metabolized in liver, excreted in feces (77% unchanged)

INTERACTIONS

⚠ Life-threatening reactions: pimozide, quinidine, dofetilide, ergots

Increase: tinnitus, hearing loss—quinidine

Increase: hepatotoxicity—other hepatotoxic products

Increase: edema—calcium channel blockers

Increase: severe hypoglycemia—oral hypoglycemics

Increase: sedation—triazolam, oral midazolam

Increase: levels, toxicity—busPIRone, busulfan, clarithromycin, cycloSPORINE, diazepam, digoxin, felodipine, indinavir, isradipine, niCARdipine, niFEDipine, nimodipine, phenytoin, quinidine, ritonavir, saquinavir, tacrolimus, warfarin

Decrease: effect of oral contraceptives

Decrease: posaconazole action—antacids, H_2-receptor antagonists, rifamycin, didanosine

Drug/Herb

• Nephrotoxicity: gossypol

Drug/Food

• Food increases absorption

NURSING CONSIDERATIONS

Assess:

• For type of infection; may begin treatment prior to obtaining results

• For infection: temp, WBC, sputum, baseline and periodically

• I&O ratio, potassium levels

• Hepatic studies (ALT, AST, bilirubin) if on long-term therapy
• For allergic reaction: rash, photosensitivity, urticaria, dermatitis
⚠ For hepatotoxicity: nausea, vomiting, jaundice, clay-colored stools, fatigue

Administer:
• Shake well; use calibrated measuring device; take only with a full meal or liquid nutritional supplements such as Ensure; rinse measuring device after each use

Perform/provide:
• Storage in a tight container in refrigerator; do not freeze

Evaluate:
• Therapeutic response: decreased fever, malaise, rash, negative C&S for infecting organism

Teach patient/family:
• That long-term therapy may be needed to clear infection (1 wk-6 mo depending on infection)
• To avoid hazardous activities if dizziness occurs
• To take 2 hr before administration of other products that increase gastric pH (antacids, H_2-blockers, omeprazole, sucralfate, anticholinergics); to notify health care provider of all medications taken
• The importance of compliance with product regimen; to use alternative method of contraception
• To notify prescriber of GI symptoms, signs of hepatic dysfunction (fatigue, nausea, anorexia, vomiting, dark urine, pale stools)

potassium acetate
potassium bicarbonate (OTC, ℞)
K+ Care ET, K-Electrolyte, K-Ide, Klor-Con EF, K-Lyte, K-Vescent

potassium bicarbonate and potassium chloride (OTC, ℞)
Klorvess, Klorvess Effervescent Granules, K-Lyte/Cl, Neo-K ✱

potassium bicarbonate and potassium citrate (OTC, ℞)
Effer-K, K-Lyte DS

potassium chloride (OTC, ℞)
Apo-K ✱, Cena-K, Gen-K, K+ Care, K+ 10, Kalium Durules ✱, Kaochlor, Kaochlor S-F, Kaon-Cl, Kay Ciel, KCl, K-Dur, K-Lease, K-Long ✱, K-Lor, Klor-Con, Klorvess, Klotrix, K-Lyte/C1 powder, K-med, K-Norm, K-Sol, K-tab, Micro-K, Micro-LS, Potasalan, Roychlor, Rum-K, Slow-K, Ten-K

potassium chloride/ potassium bicarbonate/ potassium citrate (OTC, ℞)
Kaochlor Eff

potassium gluconate (OTC, ℞)
Kaon, Kaylixir, K-G Elixir, Potassium-Rougier ✱

potassium gluconate/ potassium chloride (OTC, ℞)
Kolyum

potassium gluconate/ potassium citrate (OTC, ℞)
Twin-K

Func. class.: Electrolyte, mineral replacement
Chem. class.: Potassium

Action: Needed for adequate transmission of nerve impulses and cardiac con-

P

traction, renal function, intracellular ion maintenance

Uses: Prevention and treatment of hypokalemia

DOSAGE AND ROUTES

Potassium acetate—hypokalemia

- *Adult and child:* **PO** 40-100 mEq/day in divided doses 2-4 days

Potassium bicarbonate

- *Adult:* **PO** Dissolve 25-50 mEq in water daily-qid

Hypokalemia (prevention)

- *Adult and child:* **PO** 20 mEq/day in 2-4 divided doses

Potassium chloride

- *Adult:* **PO** 40-100 mEq in divided doses tid-qid; **IV** 20 mEq/hr when diluted as 40 mEq/1000 ml, max 150 mEq/day
- *Child:* **PO** 1-2 mEq/kg/day

Potassium gluconate

- *Adult:* **PO** 40-100 mEq in divided doses tid-qid

Potassium phosphate

- *Adult:* **IV** 1 mEq/hr in sol of 60 mEq/L, max 150 mEq/day; **PO** 40-100 mEq/day in divided doses
- *Child:* **IV** Max rate of inf 1 mEq/kg/hr

Available forms: Tabs for sol 6.5, 25 mEq; ext rel caps 8, 10 mEq; powder for sol 3.3, 5, 6.7, 10, 13.3 mEq/5 ml; tabs 2, 4, 5, 13.4 mEq; ext rel tabs 6.7, 8, 10 mEq; elix 6.7 mEq/5 ml; oral sol 2.375 mEq/5 ml; inj for prep of IV 1.5, 2, 2.4, 3, 3.2, 4.4, 4.7 mEq/ml

SIDE EFFECTS

CNS: Confusion

CV: Bradycardia, **cardiac depression, dysrhythmias, arrest, peaking T waves, lowered R and depressed RST, prolonged P-R interval, widened QRS complex**

GI: Nausea, vomiting, cramps, pain, *diarrhea,* ulceration of small bowel

GU: Oliguria

INTEG: Cold extremities, rash

Contraindications: Renal disease (severe), severe hemolytic disease, Addison's disease, hyperkalemia, acute dehydration, extensive tissue breakdown

Precautions: Pregnancy (C), cardiac disease, potassium-sparing diuretic therapy, systemic acidosis

PHARMACOKINETICS

PO: Excreted by kidneys and in feces; onset of action ≈30 min

IV: Immediate onset of action

INTERACTIONS

- Hyperkalemia: potassium phosphate IV and products containing calcium or magnesium; potassium-sparing diuretic, or other potassium products, ACE inhibitors

NURSING CONSIDERATIONS

Assess:

- ECG for peaking T waves, lowered R, depressed RST, prolonged P-R interval, widening QRS complex, hyperkalemia; product should be reduced or discontinued
- Potassium level during treatment (3.5-5 mg/dl is normal level)
- I&O ratio; watch for decreased urinary output; notify prescriber immediately
- Cardiac status: rate, rhythm, CVP, PWP, PAWP, if being monitored directly

Administer:

PO route

- Do not break, crush, or chew ext rel tabs/caps or enteric products
- With or after meals; dissolve effervescent tabs, powder in 8 oz cold water or juice; do not give IM, SUBCUT
- Caps with full glass of liquid

IV route

- Through large-bore needle to decrease vein inflammation; check for extravasation
- In large vein, avoiding scalp vein in child (IV)
- IV after diluting in large volume of IV sol and give as an inf, slowly by IV inf to prevent toxicity; never give IV bolus or IM

Potassium acetate

Additive compatibilities: Metoclopramide

Y-site compatibilities: Ciprofloxacin

Potassium chloride

Additive compatibilities: Aminophylline, amiodarone, atracurium, bretylium, calcium gluconate, cefepime, cephalothin, cephapirin, chloramphenicol, cimetidine, ciprofloxacin, cisatracurium, clindamycin, cloxacillin, corticotropin, cytarabine, dimenhyDRINATE, DOPamine, DOXOrubicin liposome, enalaprilat, erythromycin, floxacillin, fluconazole, fosphenytoin, furosemide, heparin, hydrocortisone, isoproterenol, lidocaine, metaraminol, methicillin, methyldopate, metoclopramide, mitoxantrone, nafcillin, netilmicin, norepinephrine, oxacillin, penicillin G potassium, phenylephrine, piperacillin, ranitidine, sodium bicarbonate, thiopental, vancomycin, verapamil, vit B/C

Y-site compatibilities: Acyclovir, aldesleukin, allopurinol, amifostine, aminophylline, amiodarone, ampicillin, amrinone, atropine, aztreonam, betamethasone, calcium gluconate, cephalothin, cephapirin, chlordiazepoxide, chlorproMAZINE, ciprofloxacin, cladribine, cyanocobalamin, dexamethasone, digoxin, diltiazem, diphenhydrAMINE, DOBUTamine, DOPamine, droperidol, edrophonium, enalaprilat, epinephrine, esmolol, estrogens, ethacrynate, famotidine, fentanyl, filgrastim, fludarabine, fluorouracil, furosemide, gallium, granisetron, heparin, hydrALAZINE, idarubicin, indomethacin, insulin (regular), isoproterenol, kanamycin, labetalol, lidocaine, lorazepam, magnesium sulfate, melphalan, meperidine, methicillin, methoxamine, methylergonovine, midazolam, minocycline, morphine, neostigmine, norepinephrine, ondansetron, oxacillin, oxytocin, paclitaxel, penicillin G potassium, pentazocine, phytonadione, piperacillin/tazobactam, prednisoLONE, procainamide, prochlorperazine, propofol, propranolol, pyridostigmine, remifentanil, sargramostim, scopolamine, sodium bicarbonate, succinylcholine, tacrolimus, teniposide, theophylline, thiotepa, trimethaphan, trimethobenzamide, vinorelbine, warfarin, zidovudine

Perform/provide:
- Storage at room temperature

Evaluate:
- Therapeutic response: absence of fatigue, muscle weakness; decreased thirst and urinary output; cardiac changes

Teach patient/family:
- To add potassium-rich foods to diet: bananas, orange juice, avocados; whole grains, broccoli, carrots, prunes, cocoa after this medication is discontinued
- To avoid OTC products: antacids, salt substitutes, analgesics, vitamin preparations, unless specifically directed by prescriber; avoid licorice in large amounts, may cause hypokalemia, sodium retention
- To report hyperkalemia symptoms (lethargy, confusion, diarrhea, nausea, vomiting, fainting, decreased output) or continued hypokalemia symptoms (fatigue, weakness, polyuria, polydipsia, cardiac changes)
- To dissolve powder or tablet completely in at least 120 ml water or juice
- Importance of regular follow-up visits
- That potassium levels will need to be monitored periodically

P

potassium iodide (℞)

Pima, saturated solution (SSKI), strong iodine solution (Lugol's solution), Thyro-Block

Func. class.: Thyroid hormone antagonist

Chem. class.: Iodine product

Action: Inhibits secretion of thyroid hormone, fosters colloid accumulation in thyroid follicles, decreases vascularity of gland

Uses: Preparation for thyroidectomy, thyrotoxic crisis, neonatal thyrotoxicosis, radiation protectant, thyroid storm

Unlabeled uses: Erythema multiforme, erythema nodosum leprosum (ENL), sporotrichosis, thyroid involution induction

DOSAGE AND ROUTES

Thyrotoxic crisis

• *Adult and child:* **PO** 250 mg tid × 10-14 days pre-op

Preparation for thyroidectomy

• *Adult and child:* **PO** 3-5 gtt strong iodine sol tid, or 1-5 drops SSKI in water tid after meals for 10 days prior to surgery

Available forms: Oral sol (Lugol's solution) iodine 5%/potassium iodide 10%; oral sol (SSKI) 1 g/ml; syr 325 mg/5 ml; tabs 130 mg

SIDE EFFECTS

CNS: Headache, confusion, paresthesias

EENT: Metallic taste, stomatitis, salivation, periorbital edema, sore teeth and gums, cold symptoms

ENDO: Hypothyroidism, hyperthyroid adenoma

GI: Nausea, diarrhea, vomiting, small-bowel lesions, upper gastric pain, metallic taste

INTEG: Rash, urticaria, **angioneurotic edema,** acne, mucosal hemorrhage, fever

MS: Myalgia, arthralgia, weakness

Contraindications: Pregnancy (D), pulmonary edema, pulmonary TB, bronchitis, hypersensitivity to iodine

Precautions: Breastfeeding, children

PHARMACOKINETICS

PO: Onset 24-48 hr, peak 10-15 days after continuous therapy, uptake by thyroid gland or excreted in urine; crosses placenta

INTERACTIONS

• Hypothyroidism: lithium, other antithyroid agents

Increased: hyperkalemia—angiotensin II receptor antagonist, ACE inhibitors, potassium salts, potassium-sparing diuretics

Drug/Lab Test

Interference: urinary 17-OHCS

NURSING CONSIDERATIONS

Assess:

• Pulse, B/P, temp; serum potassium

• I&O ratio; check for edema: puffy hands, feet, periorbit; indicate hypothyroidism

• Weight daily; same clothing, scale, time of day

• T_3, T_4, which is increased; serum TSH, which is decreased; free thyroxine index, which is increased if dosage is too low; discontinue product 3-4 wk before RAIU

⚠ Overdose: peripheral edema, heat intolerance, diaphoresis, palpitations, dysrhythmias, severe tachycardia, fever, delirium, CNS irritability

• Hypersensitivity: rash; enlarged cervical lymph nodes may indicate product should be discontinued

• Hypoprothrombinemia: bleeding, petechiae, ecchymosis

• Clinical response: after 3 wk should include increased weight, pulse; decreased T_4

Administer:

• Strong iodine solution after diluting with water or juice to improve taste

• Through straw to prevent tooth discoloration

• With meals to decrease GI upset

• At same time each day to maintain product level

• Lowest dose that relieves symptoms, discontinue before RAIU

Perform/provide:

• Fluids to 3-4 L/day, unless contraindicated

Evaluate:

• Therapeutic response: weight gain, decreased pulse, T_4, size of thyroid gland

Teach patient/family:

• To abstain from breastfeeding after delivery

• To keep graph of weight, pulse, mood

• To avoid OTC products that contain iodine

• That seafood, other iodine products may be restricted

• Not to discontinue this medication abruptly; thyroid crisis may occur; stress response
• That response may take several mo if thyroid is large
• To discontinue product, notify prescriber of fever, rash, metallic taste, swelling of throat; burning of mouth, throat; sore gums, teeth; severe GI distress, enlargement of thyroid, cold symptoms

⚠ High Alert

pralatrexate

(pra-luh-treks′ate)
Folotyn
Func. class.: Antineoplastic-antimetabolite
Chem. class.: Folate analog

Action: Inhibits an enzyme that reduces folic acid, which is needed for nucleic acid synthesis in all cells; S phase of cell cycle specific; immunosuppressive
Uses: Non-Hodgkin's lymphoma (NHL)

DOSAGE AND ROUTES

• *Adult:* **IV** direct 30 mg/m^2 as a slow push over 3-5 min, via the side port of free-flowing 0.9% NaCL qwk × 6 wk in a 7 wk cycle
Available forms: Inj 20 mg/ml, 40 mg/2 ml

SIDE EFFECTS

CNS: Fatigue, fever, asthenia
CV: Sinus tachycardia
GI: *Nausea, vomiting, anorexia, diarrhea, stomatitis,* constipation, abdominal pain, mucositis
HEMA: **Leukopenia, thrombocytopenia, myelosuppression, anemia, epistaxis, neutropenia**
INTEG: *Rash, pruritus*
META: Hypokalemia
MS: Back pain
RESP: Cough, dyspnea
SYST: **Edema, infection, night sweats**
Contraindications: Pregnancy (D), hypersensitivity, leukopenia (<3500/mm^3), thrombocytopenia (<100,000/mm^3), anemia, bone marrow suppression
Precautions: Breastfeeding, children, renal/hepatic disease

PHARMACOKINETICS

Excreted in urine 34%; crosses placenta, blood-brain barrier; 67% plasma protein bound; terminal half-life 12-18 hr

INTERACTIONS

Increase: toxicity—salicylates, sulfa products, other antineoplastics, radiation, NSAIDs, trimethoprim, SMX-TMP
Decrease: effect of—oral vaccines, toxoids
Decrease: effect of pralatrexate—folic acid supplements

NURSING CONSIDERATIONS

Assess:

⚠ CBC, differential, platelet count weekly; withhold product if WBC is <3500/mm^3 or platelet count is <100,000/mm^3; notify prescriber; WBC, platelet nadirs occur on day 7
• Renal studies: BUN, serum uric acid, urine CCr, electrolytes before, during therapy
• Monitor temp; fever may indicate beginning infection; no rectal temps
• Hepatic studies before and during therapy: bilirubin, alk phos, AST, ALT; liver biopsy should be done before start of therapy (psoriasis patients)
• Buccal cavity for dryness, sores, ulceration, white patches, oral pain, bleeding, dysphagia
⚠ Symptoms indicating severe allergic reaction: rash, urticaria, itching, flushing

Administer:

• Antiemetic 30-60 min before giving product
• Use cytotoxic handling precautions
• Supplement patients with vit B_{12} IM 1 mg q8-10wk, and folic acid PO 1-1.25 mg daily

P

IV route

- Do not dilute
- Inspect for particulate/discoloration, it should be clear yellow
- After withdrawing calculated dose, discard remaining drug

Perform/provide:

- Strict medical asepsis and protective isolation if WBC levels are low
- Liquid diet: carbonated beverage, Jell-O; dry toast, crackers may be added when patient is not nauseated or vomiting
- Rinsing of mouth tid-qid with water, club soda; brushing of teeth bid-tid with soft brush or cotton-tipped applicators for stomatitis; use unwaxed dental floss
- Nutritious diet with iron, vitamin supplements, no folic acid
- Protect from light, refrigerate until use

Evaluate:

- Therapeutic response: decreased tumor size, spread of malignancy

Teach patient/family:

- To report any complaints, side effects to nurse or prescriber: chills, fever, sore throat, bleeding, bruising, cough, dark or bloody urine
- To avoid foods with citric acid, hot or rough texture if stomatitis is present
- To report stomatitis: any bleeding, white spots, ulcerations in mouth to prescriber; tell patient to examine mouth daily, report symptoms to nurse, use good oral hygiene
- That contraceptive measures are recommended during therapy and for at least 8 wk following cessation of therapy, to discontinue breastfeeding; toxicity to infant may occur
- To drink 10-12 glasses of fluid/day
- To avoid alcohol, salicylates, live vaccines
- To avoid use of razors, commercial mouthwash
- To use sunblock to prevent burns

pramipexole (℞)

(pra-mi-pex′ol)

Mirapex, Mirapex ER

Func. class.: Antiparkinson agent

Chem. class.: DOPamine-receptor agonist, non-ergot

Action: Selective agonist for D_2 receptors (presynaptic/postsynaptic sites); binding at D_3 receptor contributes to antiparkinson effects

Uses: Parkinson's disease, restless leg syndrome

DOSAGE AND ROUTES

Initial treatment

- *Adult:* **PO** From a starting dose of 0.375 mg/day given in 3 divided doses; increase gradually by 0.125 mg/dose at 5-7 day intervals until total daily dose of 4.5 mg/day is reached; ER 0.375 mg daily initially, then up to 0.75 mg/day, may increase by 0.75 mg/day q5-7days as needed, max 4.5 mg/day

Maintenance treatment

- *Adult:* **PO** 1.5-4.5 mg/day in 3 divided doses

Restless leg syndrome

- *Adult:* **PO** 0.125 mg 2-3 hr prior to bedtime, increase gradually

Renal dose

- *Adult:* **PO** CCr 35-59 ml/min-0.125 mg bid, may increase q5-7days to 1.5 mg bid if required; CCr 15-34 ml/min 0.125 mg/day, increase q5-7days to 1.5 mg/day

Available forms: Tabs 0.125, 0.25, 0.5, 1, 1.5 mg; ER tab 0.375, 0.75, 1.5, 3.0, 4.5 mg

SIDE EFFECTS

CNS: Agitation, insomnia, psychosis, hallucination, depression, dizziness, headache, confusion, amnesia, dream disorder, asthenia, dyskinesia, hypersomnolence, sudden sleep onset

CV: Orthostatic hypotension, edema, syncope, tachycardia

EENT: Blurred vision

GI: Nausea, anorexia, constipation, dysphagia, dry mouth

GU: Impotence, urinary frequency
HEMA: **Hemolytic anemia, leukopenia, agranulocytosis**
Contraindications: Hypersensitivity
Precautions: Pregnancy (C), cardiac/renal disease, MI with dysrhythmias, affective disorders, psychosis, preexisting dyskinesias, history of falling asleep during daily activities

PHARMACOKINETICS

Minimally metabolized, peak 2 hr, half-life 8 hr, 8.5-12 hr in geriatric

INTERACTIONS

Increase: pramipexole levels—levodopa, cimetidine, ranitidine, diltiazem, triamterene, verapamil, quinidine
Decrease: pramipexole levels—DOPamine antagonists, phenothiazines, metoclopramide, butyrophenones
Drug/Herb
Decrease: effect of pramipexole—chaste tree fruit, kava

NURSING CONSIDERATIONS

Assess:
- Renal studies
- Involuntary movements in parkinsonism: bradykinesia, tremors, staggering gait, muscle rigidity, drooling
- B/P, ECG, respiration during initial treatment; hypo/hypertension should be reported
- Mental status: affect, mood, behavioral changes, depression; complete suicide assessment

⚠ For sleep attacks: may fall asleep during activities without warning; may need to discontinue medication

Administer:
- Adjust dosage to patient response, titrate slowly
- With meals to minimize GI symptoms
- Do not crush, chew, or break ER product

Perform/provide:
- Assistance with ambulation during beginning therapy
- Testing for diabetes mellitus, acromegaly if on long-term therapy

Evaluate:
- Therapeutic response: movement disorder improves

Teach patient/family:
- That therapeutic effects may take several weeks to a few months
- To change positions slowly to prevent orthostatic hypotension
- To use product exactly as prescribed: if product is discontinued abruptly, parkinsonian crisis may occur, avoid alcohol, OTC sleeping products
- To notify prescriber if pregnancy is planned or suspected

pramlintide (℞)

(pram′lin-tide)
Symlin
Func. class.: Antidiabetic
Chem. class.: Synthetic human amylin analog

Action: Modulates and slows stomach emptying, prevents postprandial rise in plasma glucagon, decreases appetite, leads to decreased caloric intake and weight loss
Uses: As an adjunct to insulin therapy with uncontrolled type 1 or type 2 diabetes

DOSAGE AND ROUTES

Type 1 diabetes
- *Adult:* **SUBCUT** Prior to each meal (≥30 g CHO), titrate up from 15 mcg to target dose of 60 mcg/dose, each dose titration should occur after no nausea for 3 days

Type 2 diabetes
- *Adult:* **SUBCUT** 60 mcg prior to each meal (≥30 g CHO), titrate up to 120 mcg **SUBCUT** with each meal after no nausea for 3-7 days

Available forms: Inj 5-ml vials (0.6 mg/ml)

SIDE EFFECTS

CNS: Headache, fatigue, dizziness
GI: Nausea, vomiting, anorexia, abdominal pain
INTEG: Inj site reactions

P

META: Hypoglycemia
MS: Arthralgia
RESP: *Cough,* pharyngitis
SYST: *Systemic allergy*

Contraindications: Hypersensitivity to this product or cresol, gastroparesis

Black Box Warning: Hypoglycemia

Precautions: Pregnancy (C), breastfeeding

PHARMACOKINETICS

Absorption 30%-40%, extensively bound to blood cells or albumin, half-life 48 min, metabolized by kidneys

INTERACTIONS

• Do not use with erythromycin, metoclopramide

Increase: effect of acetaminophen

Increase: pramlintide action—antimuscarinics, α-glucosidase inhibitors, diphenoxylate, loperamide, octreotide, opiate agonist, tricyclics

Increase: hypoglycemia—ACE inhibitors, disopyramide, anabolic steroids, androgens, fibric acid derivatives, alcohol, corticosteroids, insulin

Increase: hyperglycemia—phenothiazines

Decrease: hypoglycemia—niacin, dextrothyroxine, thiazide diuretics, triamterene, estrogens, progestins, oral contraceptives, MAOIs

NURSING CONSIDERATIONS

Assess:

• Fasting blood glucose, 2 hr PP (80-150 mg/dl, normal fasting level; 70-130 mg/dl, normal 2 hr level); A1c may also be drawn to identify treatment effectiveness; also monitor weight, appetite

• For hypoglycemic reaction (sweating; weakness; dizziness; chills; confusion; headache; nausea; rapid, weak pulse; fatigue; tachycardia; memory lapses; slurred speech; staggering gait; anxiety; tremors; hunger)

• For hyperglycemia: acetone breath; polyuria; fatigue; polydipsia; flushed, dry skin; lethargy

Administer:

• Pre-meal insulin should be decreased by 50% when starting and adjusted to therapeutic dose to prevent hypoglycemia

SUBCUT route

• Take immediately before mealtime, or if 30 g of carbohydrates will be consumed

• Do not use if a meal is skipped

• Do not use if discolored; do not give in arm; absorption is variable

Syringe compatibilities: Do not mix with insulin, give separately

Perform/provide:

• Storage at room temperature for up to 30 days, keep away from heat and sunlight; refrigerate all other supply

Evaluate:

• Therapeutic response: decrease in polyuria, polydipsia, polyphagia; clear sensorium; absence of dizziness; stable gait; improving blood glucose, A1c

Teach patient/family:

• That product does not cure diabetes but controls symptoms

• To carry emergency ID as diabetic

• To recognize hypoglycemia reaction: headache, fatigue, weakness

• The dosage, route, mixing instructions, if any diet restrictions, disease process

• To carry a glucose source (candy or lump sugar) to treat hypoglycemia

• The symptoms of ketoacidosis: nausea; thirst; polyuria; dry mouth; decreased B/P; dry, flushed skin; acetone breath; drowsiness; Kussmaul respirations

• That a plan is necessary for diet, exercise; all food on diet should be eaten; exercise routine should not vary

• About blood glucose testing; make sure patient is able to determine glucose level

• To avoid OTC products unless directed by prescriber, alcohol

• Not to operate machinery or drive until effect is known

Treatment of overdose: Glucose 25 g IV, via dextrose 50% sol, 50 ml or glucagon 1 mg SUBCUT

pramoxine topical
See Appendix B

prasugrel (℞)
(pra'soo-grel)
Effient
Func. class.: Platelet aggregation inhibitor
Chem. class.: ADP receptor antagonist

Action: Inhibits ADP-induced platelet aggregation
Uses: Reducing the risk of stroke, MI, vascular death, peripheral arterial disease in high-risk patients

DOSAGE AND ROUTES

- *Adult/geriatric <75 yr and ≥60 kg:* **PO** 60 mg loading dose, then 10 mg daily with aspirin (75-325 mg/day)
- *Adult/geriatric <75 yr and <60 kg:* **PO** 60 mg loading dose then 5 mg daily
- *Geriatric >75 yr:* not recommended

Available forms: Tabs 5, 10 mg

SIDE EFFECTS

CNS: Headache, dizziness
CV: Edema, atrial fibrillation, bradycardia, chest pain, hyper/hypotension
GI: Nausea, vomiting, diarrhea
HEMA: Epistaxis, **leukopenia, thrombocytopenia, neutropenia, anaphylaxis, angioedema, anemia**
INTEG: Rash, hypercholesterolemia
MISC: Fatigue, **intracranial hemorrhage, secondary malignancy**
MS: Back pain
Contraindications: Hypersensitivity, stroke, TIA

Black Box Warning: Active bleeding

Precautions: Pregnancy (B), breastfeeding, children, geriatric patients, hepatic disease, increased bleeding risk, neutropenia, agranulocytosis, renal disease, surgery, trauma, thrombotic thrombocytopenic purpura, Asian patients, weight <60 kg, CABG

Black Box Warning: Abrupt discontinuation

PHARMACOKINETICS

Rapidly absorbed; peak 30 min; metabolized by liver (CYP3A4; CYP2B6); excreted in urine, feces; half-life 7 hr

INTERACTIONS

Increase: bleeding risk—anticoagulants, aspirin, NSAIDs, abciximab, eptifibatide, tirofiban, thrombolytics, ticlopidine, SSRIs, treprostinil, rifampin
Drug/Herb
Increase: prasugrel effect—bogbean, dong quai, feverfew, garlic, ginger, ginkgo biloba, green tea, horse chestnut

NURSING CONSIDERATIONS

Assess:
⚠ Thrombotic/thrombocytic purpura: fever, thrombocytopenia, neurolytic anemia
- For symptoms of stroke, MI during treatment
- Hepatic studies: AST, ALT, bilirubin, creatinine (long-term therapy)
- Blood studies: CBC, differential, Hct, Hgb, PT, cholesterol (long-term therapy)

Administer:
- With food to decrease gastric symptoms
- Do not break tablets
- Do not discontinue therapy abruptly

Evaluate:
- Therapeutic response: absence of stroke, MI

Teach patient/family:
- That blood work will be necessary during treatment
- To report any unusual bruising, bleeding to prescriber, that it may take longer to stop bleeding
- To take with food or just after eating to minimize GI discomfort
- To report diarrhea, skin rashes, subcutaneous bleeding, chills, fever, sore throat

• To tell all health care providers that prasugrel is used; may be held before surgery

pravastatin (℞)

(pra'va-sta-tin)

Pravachol

Func. class.: Antilipidemic

Chem. class.: HMG-CoA reductase enzyme

Do not confuse:
Pravachol/**Prevacid**

Action: Inhibits HMG-CoA reductase enzyme, which reduces cholesterol synthesis

Uses: As an adjunct in primary hypercholesterolemia (types IIa, IIb, III, IV), to reduce the risk of recurrent MI, atherosclerosis, primary/secondary CV events, reduce stroke, TIAs

DOSAGE AND ROUTES

• *Adult:* **PO** 40-80 mg/day at bedtime (range 20-80 mg/day), start at 10 mg/day if also on immunosuppressants
• *Adolescent 14-18 yr:* **PO** 40 mg/day
• *Child 8-13 yr:* **PO** 20 mg/day
• *Geriatric/renal/hepatic disease:* **PO** 10 mg/day initially

Available forms: Tabs 10, 20, 40, 80 mg

SIDE EFFECTS

CNS: Headache, dizziness, fatigue, **ALS (Lou Gehrig's disease)**
CV: Chest pain
EENT: Lens opacities
GI: Nausea, constipation, diarrhea, flatus, abdominal pain, heartburn, **hepatic dysfunction,** pancreatitis, **hepatitis**
INTEG: Rash, pruritus, photosensitivity
MS: Muscle cramps, myalgia, **myositis, rhabdomyolysis**
RESP: Common cold, rhinitis, cough

Contraindications: Pregnancy (X), breastfeeding, hypersensitivity, active hepatic disease

Precautions: Past hepatic disease, alcoholism, severe acute infections, trauma, severe metabolic disorders, electrolyte imbalances

PHARMACOKINETICS

Peak 1-1½ hr; metabolized by the liver, protein binding 80%; excreted in urine 20%, feces 70%, breast milk; crosses placenta

INTERACTIONS

Increase: myopathy risk—erythromycin, niacin, cycloSPORINE, gemfibrozil, clofibrate, clarithromycin, itraconazole, protease inhibitors
Increase: effects of warfarin, digoxin
Decrease: bioavailability of pravastatin —bile acid sequestrants

Drug/Herb
Increase: effect—glucomannan
Decrease: effect—gotu kola, oat bran, St. John's wort

Drug/Lab Test
Increase: CPK, LFTs
Altered: thyroid function tests

NURSING CONSIDERATIONS

Assess:
• Fasting lipid profile: LDL, HDL, triglycerides, cholesterol q8wk, then q3-6mo when stable; obtain diet history
• Hepatic studies: baseline, q6wk during the first 3 mo, q8wk for remainder of yr, then q6mo; AST, ALT, LFTs may increase
• Renal studies in patients with compromised renal system: BUN, I&O ratio, creatinine

⚠ For muscle tenderness, pain, obtain CPK baseline and if these occur; rhabdomyolysis may occur, therapy should be discontinued

Administer:
• Without regard to meals, at bedtime
• Give 1 hr before or 4 hr after bile acid sequestrants

Perform/provide:
• Storage in cool environment in tight container protected from light

Evaluate:
- Therapeutic response: decrease in cholesterol to desired level after 8 wk

Teach patient/family:
- That blood work will be necessary during treatment

⚠ To report blurred vision, severe GI symptoms, dizziness, headache, muscle pain, weakness, fever
- That regimen will continue: low-cholesterol diet, exercise program
- To report suspected, planned pregnancy; not to use during pregnancy; pregnancy category (X)
- To use sunscreen, protective clothing to prevent burns

prazosin (℞)

(pray'zoe-sin)

Minipress, prazosin

Func. class.: Antihypertensive

Chem. class.: α_1-Adrenergic blocker

Action: Blocks α-mediated vasoconstriction of adrenergic receptors, inducing peripheral vasodilation

Uses: Hypertension, refractory CHF, Raynaud's vasospasm

Unlabeled uses: Benign prostatic hypertrophy to decrease urine outflow obstruction, heart failure, hypertensive urgency, Raynaud's phenomenon

DOSAGE AND ROUTES

Hypertension
- *Adult:* **PO** 1 mg bid or tid, increasing to 20 mg/day in divided doses if required; usual range 6-15 mg/day, max 1 mg initially; max 20-40 mg/day
- *Child:* **PO** 5 mcg/kg q6hr; max 400 mcg/kg/day or 15 mg/day

Benign prostatic hyperplasia (unlabeled)
- *Adult:* **PO** 2 mg bid

Raynaud's phenomenon (unlabeled)
- *Adult:* **PO** 0.5-3 mg bid

CHF (unlabeled)
- *Adult:* **PO** 1 mg bid-tid, may gradually increase to max 20 mg/day
- *Child:* **PO** 5 mcg/kg q6hr, may gradually increase to 25 mcg/kg q6hr

Hypertensive urgency (unlabeled)
- *Adult:* **PO** 10-20 mg, may repeat in 30 min

Available forms: Caps 1, 2, 5 mg

SIDE EFFECTS

CNS: Dizziness, headache, drowsiness, anxiety, depression, vertigo, weakness, fatigue

CV: Palpitations, orthostatic hypotension, tachycardia, edema, rebound hypertension

EENT: Blurred vision, epistaxis, tinnitus, dry mouth, red sclera

GI: Nausea, vomiting, diarrhea, constipation, abdominal pain

GU: Urinary frequency, incontinence, impotence, priapism, H_2O, sodium retention

Contraindications: Hypersensitivity

Precautions: Pregnancy (C), breastfeeding, children, geriatric patients, renal/hepatic disease, prostate cancer, ocular surgery, orthostatic hypotension

PHARMACOKINETICS

Onset 2 hr, peak 2-4 hr, duration 6-12 hr; half-life 2 hr, metabolized in liver, excreted via bile, feces (>90%), in urine (<10%), protein binding 97%

INTERACTIONS

Increase: hypotensive effects—β-blockers, nitroglycerin, alcohol, verapamil

Decrease: antihypertensive effect—NSAIDs, clonidine, salicylates

Drug/Herb

Increase: toxicity, death—aconite

Increase: antihypertensive effect—barberry, betony, black catechu, black cohosh, bloodroot, broom, burdock, cat's claw, dandelion, goldenseal, hawthorn, Irish moss, Jamaican dogwood, kelp, khella, mistletoe, parsley

Increase or decrease: antihypertensive effect—astragalus, cola tree

Decrease: antihypertensive effect—coltsfoot, guarana, khat, licorice, yohimbe

Drug/Lab Test

Increase: urinary norepinephrine, VMA

NURSING CONSIDERATIONS

Assess:

- B/P (sitting, standing) during initial treatment, periodically thereafter; pulse, jugular venous distention q4hr
- BUN, uric acid if on long-term therapy
- Weight daily, I&O; edema in feet, legs daily
- Skin turgor, dryness of mucous membranes for hydration status
- Crackles, dyspnea, orthopnea q30min

Administer:

- 1st dose at bedtime to avoid fainting

Perform/provide:

- Storage in tight container in cool environment

Evaluate:

- Therapeutic response: decreased B/P

Teach patient/family:

- That fainting occasionally occurs after 1st dose; take 1st dose at bedtime or do not drive or operate machinery for 4 hr after 1st dose; that full effect may take 4-6 wk
- To change positions slowly, to prevent orthostatic hypotension
- To avoid OTC medications unless approved by prescriber

Treatment of overdose: Administer volume expanders or vasopressors, discontinue product, place in supine position

*prednisoLONE (℞)

(pred-niss′oh-lone)

Articulose-50, Delta-Cortef, Hydeltrasol, Hydeltra-T.B.A., Key-Pred 25, Key-Pred 50, Key-Pred-SP, Orapred, Pediapred, Predaject-50, Predalone 50, Predalone-T.B.A., Predcor-25, Predcor-50, prednisoLONE, PrednisoLONE Acetate, Prednisol TBA, Prelone

Func. class.: Corticosteroid, synthetic

Chem. class.: Glucocorticoid, immediate acting

Do not confuse:

prednisoLONE/**predniSONE**

Action: Decreases inflammation by suppression of migration of polymorphonuclear leukocytes, fibroblasts; reversal to increase capillary permeability and lysosomal stabilization

Uses: Severe inflammation, immunosuppression, neoplasms

DOSAGE AND ROUTES

Rheumatic disorders

- *Adult:* **PO** 5-60 mg/day or in divided doses

Asthma/antiinflammatory

- *Adult:* **PO** 40-80 mg/day in 1-2 divided doses
- *Child:* **PO** 1 mg/kg/day in 2 divided doses

Available forms: Tabs 5 mg; syr 5 mg/5 ml, 15 mg/15 ml; oral liquid 5 mg/ml, tabs 1, 2.5, 5, 10, 20, 50 mg, oral sol 5 mg/ml, 5 mg/5 ml, syr 5 mg/5 ml; oral dissolving tab 10, 15, 30 mg

SIDE EFFECTS

CNS: Depression, flushing, sweating, headache, mood changes

CV: Hypertension, **circulatory collapse, thrombophlebitis, embolism,** tachycardia

EENT: Fungal infections, increased intraocular pressure, blurred vision
GI: Diarrhea, nausea, abdominal distention, **GI hemorrhage,** increased appetite, **pancreatitis**
HEMA: **Thrombocytopenia**
INTEG: Acne, poor wound healing, ecchymosis, petechiae
MS: Fractures, osteoporosis, weakness, arthralgia, myopathy, tendon rupture
Contraindications: Children <2 yr, psychosis, hypersensitivity, idiopathic thrombocytopenia, acute glomerulonephritis, amebiasis, fungal infections, nonasthmatic bronchial disease, measles, varicella, Cushing's syndrome
Precautions: Pregnancy (C), breastfeeding, children, diabetes mellitus, glaucoma, osteoporosis, seizure disorders, ulcerative colitis, CHF, myasthenia gravis

PHARMACOKINETICS

PO: Peak 1-2 hr, duration 2 days

INTERACTIONS

Increase: side effects—alcohol, salicylates, indomethacin, amphotericin B, digitalis, cycloSPORINE, diuretics
Increase: prednisoLONE action—salicylates, estrogens, indomethacin, oral contraceptives, ketoconazole, macrolide antibiotics
Decrease: prednisoLONE action—cholestyramine, colestipol, barbiturates, rifampin, ephedrine, phenytoin, theophylline
Decrease: effects of anticoagulants, anticonvulsants, antidiabetics, ambenonium, neostigmine, isoniazid, toxoids, vaccines, anticholinesterases, salicylates, somatrem

Drug/Herb

- Hypokalemia: aloe, buckthorn, cascara sagrada, Chinese rhubarb, senna

Increase: effect—aloe, licorice, perilla

Drug/Lab Test

Increase: cholesterol, sodium, blood glucose, uric acid, calcium, urine glucose
Decrease: calcium, potassium, T_4, T_3, thyroid ^{131}I uptake test, urine 17-OHCS, 17-KS, PBI
False negative: skin allergy tests

NURSING CONSIDERATIONS

Assess:

- Potassium, blood glucose, urine glucose while on long-term therapy; hypokalemia and hyperglycemia
- Weight daily; notify prescriber if weekly gain >5 lb
- B/P q4hr, pulse; notify prescriber if chest pain occurs
- I&O ratio; be alert for decreasing urinary output, increasing edema
- Plasma cortisol levels (long-term therapy) (normal level: 138-635 nmol/L SI units when drawn at 8 AM)
- Infection: increased temp, WBC, even after withdrawal of medication; product masks infection
- Potassium depletion: paresthesias, fatigue, nausea, vomiting, depression, polyuria, dysrhythmias, weakness
- Edema, hypertension, cardiac symptoms
- Mental status: affect, mood, behavioral changes, aggression

Administer:

- Oral sol: use calibrated measuring device
- Orally disintegrating tabs: place on tongue; allow to dissolve; swallow or swallow whole; do not cut, split

Perform/provide:

- Assistance with ambulation of patient with bone tissue disease to prevent fractures

Evaluate:

- Therapeutic response: ease of respirations, decreased inflammation

Teach patient/family:

- That emergency ID as steroid user should be carried
- To notify prescriber if therapeutic response decreases; dosage adjustment may be needed
- Not to discontinue abruptly; adrenal crisis can result; take exactly as prescribed
- To avoid OTC products: salicylates, cough products with alcohol, cold preparations unless directed by prescriber
- About cushingoid symptoms

P

• The symptoms of adrenal insufficiency: nausea, anorexia, fatigue, dizziness, dyspnea, weakness, joint pain

*prednisoLONE ophthalmic

See Appendix B

*predniSONE (℞)

(pred′ni-sone)

Apo-Prednisone ♣, Deltasone ♣, Liquid Pred, Meticorten, Orasone, Panasol-S, Prednicen-M, PredniSONE, Sterapred, Winpred

Func. class.: Corticosteroid

Chem. class.: Intermediate-acting glucocorticoid

Do not confuse:
predniSONE/methylPREDNISolone/prednisoLONE/Prilosec

Action: Decreases inflammation by suppression of migration of polymorphonuclear leukocytes, fibroblasts, reversal to increase capillary permeability, and lysosomal stabilization, minimal mineralocorticoid activity

Uses: Severe inflammation, immunosuppression, neoplasms, multiple sclerosis, collagen disorders, dermatologic disorders

Unlabeled uses: Adjunct in refractory seizures, infantile spasms

DOSAGE AND ROUTES

• *Adult:* **PO** 5-60 mg/day or divided bid-qid

• *Child:* **PO** 0.05-2 mg/kg/day divided 1-4×/day

Nephrosis

• *Child:* **PO** 2 mg/kg/day in divided doses, max 28 days, then 1-1.5 mg/kg/day every other day × 4 wk

Multiple sclerosis

• *Adult:* **PO** 200 mg/day × 1 wk, then 80 mg every other day × 1 mo

Available forms: Tabs 1, 2.5, 5, 10, 20, 50 mg; oral sol 5 mg/5 ml; syr 5 mg/5 ml

SIDE EFFECTS

CNS: Depression, flushing, sweating, headache, mood changes

CV: Hypertension, **circulatory collapse, thrombophlebitis, embolism,** tachycardia

EENT: Fungal infections, increased intraocular pressure, blurred vision

GI: Diarrhea, nausea, abdominal distention, **GI hemorrhage,** increased appetite, pancreatitis

HEMA: **Thrombocytopenia**

INTEG: Acne, poor wound healing, ecchymosis, petechiae

META: Hyperglycemia

MS: Fractures, osteoporosis, weakness

Contraindications: Children <2 yr, psychosis, hypersensitivity, idiopathic thrombocytopenia, acute glomerulonephritis, amebiasis, fungal infections, nonasthmatic bronchial disease, AIDS, TB, measles

Precautions: Pregnancy (C), diabetes mellitus, glaucoma, osteoporosis, seizure disorders, ulcerative colitis, CHF, myasthenia gravis, renal disease, esophagitis, peptic ulcer, cataracts, coagulopathy

PHARMACOKINETICS

PO: Well absorbed PO, peak 1-2 hr, duration 1-1½ days, half-life 3½-4 hr, biologic terminal half-life 18-36 hr, crosses placenta, enters breast milk, metabolized by liver after conversion, excreted in urine

INTERACTIONS

Increase: side effects—alcohol, salicylates, indomethacin, amphotericin B, digoxin, cycloSPORINE, diuretics

Increase: predniSONE action—salicylates, estrogens, indomethacin, oral contraceptives, ketoconazole, macrolide antiinfectives

Decrease: predniSONE action—cholestyramine, colestipol, barbiturates, rifampin, ephedrine, phenytoin, theophylline

Decrease: effects of anticoagulants, anticonvulsants, antidiabetics, ambenonium, neostigmine, isoniazid, toxoids, vaccines, anticholinesterases, salicylates, somatrem

Drug/Herb

- Hypokalemia: aloe, buckthorn, Chinese rhubarb, senna

Increase: effect—aloe, licorice, perilla

Decrease: prednisone effect—ephedra (ma huang)

Drug/Lab Test

Increase: cholesterol, sodium, blood glucose, uric acid, calcium, urine glucose

Decrease: calcium, potassium, T_4, T_3, thyroid ^{131}I uptake test, urine 17-OHCS, 17-KS, PBI

False negative: skin allergy tests

NURSING CONSIDERATIONS

Assess:

- Adrenal insufficiency: nausea, vomiting, anorexia, confusion, hypotension
- Potassium, blood glucose, urine glucose while on long-term therapy; hypokalemia and hyperglycemia
- Weight daily; notify prescriber of weekly gain >5 lb
- B/P q4hr, pulse; notify prescriber of chest pain; monitor for crackles, dyspnea if edema is present
- I&O ratio; be alert for decreasing urinary output, increasing edema
- Plasma cortisol (long-term therapy) (normal: 138-635 nmol/L SI units drawn at 8 AM)
- Infection: increased temp, WBC, even after withdrawal of medication; product masks infection
- Potassium depletion: paresthesias, fatigue, nausea, vomiting, depression, polyuria, dysrhythmias, weakness
- Edema, hypertension, cardiac symptoms
- Mental status: affect, mood, behavioral changes, aggression

Administer:

- For long-term use, alternate-day therapy is recommended to decrease adverse reactions
- Titrated dose; use lowest effective dose
- With food or milk to decrease GI symptoms

Perform/provide:

- Assistance with ambulation to patient with bone tissue disease to prevent fractures

Evaluate:

- Therapeutic response: ease of respirations, decreased inflammation

Teach patient/family:

- That emergency ID as corticosteroid user should be carried; information on product being taken and condition
- To notify prescriber if therapeutic response decreases; dosage adjustment may be needed
- To avoid vaccinations

⚠ Not to discontinue abruptly, or adrenal crisis can result

- To avoid OTC products: salicylates, cough products with alcohol, cold preparations unless directed by prescriber
- About cushingoid symptoms: moon face, weight gain
- That product causes immunosuppression; to report any symptoms of infection (fever, sore throat, cough)
- The symptoms of adrenal insufficiency: nausea, anorexia, fatigue, dizziness, dyspnea, weakness, joint pain

P

pregabalin (℞)

(pre-gab′a-lin)

Lyrica

Func. class.: Anticonvulsant

Chem. class.: Gamma aminobutyric acid (GABA) analog

Controlled Substance Schedule V

Action: Binds to high-voltage–gated calcium channels in CNS tissues; this may lead to anticonvulsant action, similar to the inhibitory neurotransmitter GABA, anxiolytic, analgesics, and antiepileptic properties

Uses: Neuropathic pain associated with diabetic peripheral neuropathy, partial-onset seizures, postherpetic neuralgia, fibromyalgia

Unlabeled uses: Generalized anxiety disorder (GAD), moderate pain, social anxiety disorder

DOSAGE AND ROUTES

Diabetic peripheral neuropathic pain

• *Adult:* **PO** 50 mg tid, may increase to 300 mg/day (max) within 1 wk, adjust in renal disease

Partial-onset seizures

• *Adult:* **PO** 75 mg bid or 50 mg tid; may increase to 600 mg/day (max)

Postherpetic neuralgia

• *Adult:* **PO** 150 mg/day divided in 2-3 doses, may increase to 300 mg/day in 2-3 divided doses, if higher dose is required in 2-4 wk may increase to 600 mg/day in 2-3 divided doses

Fibromyalgia

• *Adult:* **PO** 75 mg bid, may increase to 150 mg bid within 1 wk, and 225 mg bid after 1 wk

Renal dose

• *Adult:* **PO** CCr 30-60 ml/min 75-300 mg/day in 2-3 divided doses; CCr 15-30 ml/min 25-150 mg/day in 1-2 divided doses; CCr <15 ml/min 25-75 mg/day in a single dose

Generalized anxiety disorder/social phobia (unlabeled)

• *Adult:* **PO** 150-600 mg/day in 3 divided doses

Available forms: Caps 25, 50, 75, 100, 150, 200, 225, 300 mg

SIDE EFFECTS

CNS: Dizziness, fatigue, confusion, euphoria, incoordination, nervousness, neuropathy, tremor, vertigo, somnolence, ataxia, amnesia, abnormal thinking

EENT: Dry mouth, blurred vision, nystagmus, amblyopia, sinusitis

GI: Constipation, flatulence, abdominal pain, weight gain

HEMA: Ecchymosis, **thrombocytopenia**

MS: Back pain, **rhabdomyolysis,** myopathy

OTHER: Pruritus, impotence, peripheral edema, **angioedema, suicidal ideation**

RESP: Dyspnea

Contraindications: Hypersensitivity, abrupt discontinuation

Precautions: Pregnancy (C), breastfeeding, children <12 yr, geriatric patients, renal disease, PR interval prolongation, creatine kinase elevations, CHF (class III, IV), decreased platelets, substance abuse, dependence, glaucoma, myopathy, angioedema history, suicidal behavior

PHARMACOKINETICS

Well absorbed, absorption decreased with food; peak 1.5 hr; 90% recovered in urine unchanged; negligible metabolism; not bound to plasma proteins; half-life 6 hr

INTERACTIONS

Increase: weight gain/fluid retention—thiazolidinedione, avoid use if possible

Increase: CNS depression—anxiolytics, sedatives, hypnotics, barbiturates, general anesthetics, opiate agonists, phenothiazines, sedating H_1 blockers, thiazolidinediones, tricyclics, alcohol

Drug/Herb

Increase: CNS depression—gotu kola, kava, St. John's wort, valerian

Drug/Lab Test

Increase: creatine kinase

Decrease: platelets

NURSING CONSIDERATIONS

Assess:

• Seizures: aura, location, duration, activity at onset

• Pain: location, duration, characteristics if using for diabetic neuropathy

• Renal studies: urinalysis, BUN, urine creatinine q3mo, creatine kinase; if markedly increased, discontinue

• Mental status: mood, sensorium, affect, behavioral changes; if mental status changes, notify prescriber

Administer:

• Do not crush or chew caps; caps may be opened and contents put in applesauce or dissolved in juice

- Give without regard to meals
- Gradually withdraw over 7 days; abrupt withdrawal may precipitate seizures

Perform/provide:

- Storage at room temperature away from heat and light
- Hard candy, frequent rinsing of mouth, gum for dry mouth
- Assistance with ambulation during early part of treatment; dizziness occurs
- Seizure precautions: padded side rails; move objects that may harm patient
- Increased fluids, bulk in diet for constipation

Evaluate:

- Therapeutic response: decreased seizure activity; decrease in neuropathic pain

Teach patient/family:

- To carry emergency ID stating patient's name, products taken, condition, prescriber's name, and phone number
- To avoid driving, other activities that require alertness: dizziness, drowsiness may occur
- Not to discontinue medication quickly after long-term use, taper over ≥1 wk; withdrawal-precipitated seizures may occur, not to double doses if dose is missed, take if 2 hr or more before next dose
- To notify prescriber if pregnancy planned or suspected; avoid breastfeeding
- To report muscle pain, tenderness, weakness, when accompanied by fever, malaise
- To avoid alcohol

Treatment of overdose: Lavage, VS, hemodialysis

primaquine (℞)

(prim'a-kween)

Func. class.: Antimalarial

Chem. class.: Synthetic 8-aminoquinolone

Action: Unknown; thought to destroy exoerythrocytic forms by gametocidal action

Uses: Malaria caused by *Plasmodium vivax,* in combination with clindamycin for *Pneumocystis jiroveci* pneumonia

DOSAGE AND ROUTES

- *Adult:* **PO** 15-30 mg (base)/day × 2 wk or 45 mg (base) daily × 8 wk; 26.3-mg tab is 15-mg base
- *Child:* **PO** 0.5 mg/kg (0.3 mg/base/day) daily × 2 wk

Available forms: Tabs 26.3 mg

SIDE EFFECTS

CNS: Headache, dizziness

CV: Hypertension, dysrhythmias

EENT: Blurred vision, difficulty focusing

GI: Nausea, vomiting, anorexia, cramps

HEMA: **Agranulocytosis, granulocytopenia, leukopenia, hemolytic anemia, leukocytosis,** mild anemia, **methemoglobinemia**

INTEG: Pruritus, skin eruptions, pallor, weakness

Contraindications: Lupus erythematosus, rheumatoid arthritis, hypersensitivity to this product or idoquinol

Precautions: Pregnancy (C), breastfeeding, methemoglobin reductase deficiency

Black Box Warning: Bone marrow suppression, hemolytic anemia, G6PD deficiency

PHARMACOKINETICS

PO: Metabolized by liver (metabolites), half-life 3.7-9.6 hr

INTERACTIONS

- Toxicity: quinacrine

Decrease: effect of carbamazepine, phenobarbital, phenytoins, rifamycins, nafcillin

NURSING CONSIDERATIONS

Assess:

- Ophthalmic test if long-term treatment or product dosage >150 mg/day
- Hepatic studies q wk: AST, ALT, bilirubin, if on long-term therapy

P

• Blood studies: CBC; blood dyscrasias occur
• Allergic reactions: pruritus, rash, urticaria
• Blood dyscrasias: malaise, fever, bruising, bleeding (rare)
• For renal status: dark urine, hematuria, decreased output
⚠ For hemolytic reaction: chills, fever, chest pain, cyanosis; product should be discontinued immediately

Administer:

PO route

• Before or after meals at same time each day to maintain product level; take with food to decrease GI upset

Evaluate:

• Therapeutic response: decreased symptoms of malaria

Teach patient/family:

• To report visual problems, fever, fatigue, dark urine, bruising, bleeding; may indicate blood dyscrasias
• To complete full course of therapy

primidone (℞)

(pri′mi-done)

Apo-Primidone ✱, Mysoline, PMS-Primidone ✱, primidone, Sertan ✱

Func. class.: Anticonvulsant

Chem. class.: Barbiturate derivative

Action: Raises seizure threshold by conversion of product to phenobarbital, decreases neuron firing

Uses: Generalized tonic-clonic (grand mal), complex seizures

Unlabeled uses: Benign familial tremor (essential tremor)

DOSAGE AND ROUTES

• *Adult and child >8 yr:* **PO** 125-250 mg at bedtime, increase by 125-250 mg/day q3-7days, usual dose 750-1500 mg/day in 3-4 divided doses, max 2 g/day in divided doses
• *Child <8 yr:* **PO** 50-125 mg at bedtime, increase by 50-125 mg/day q3-7days, usual dose 10-25 mg/kg/day in 3-4 divided doses
• *Neonate:* **PO** 12-20 mg/kg/day in 2-4 divided doses, start at lower dose and titrate

Benign familial tremor/essential tremor (unlabeled)

• *Adult:* **PO** 50-62.5 mg, increase as tolerated up to 750 mg/day in 3 divided doses

Renal dose

• *Adult:* **PO** CCr 10-50 ml/min increase—interval between doses to 8-12 hr; CCr <10 ml/min increase interval to 12-24 hr

Available forms: Tabs 50, 250 mg; susp 250 mg/5 ml ✱; chew tabs 125 mg ✱

SIDE EFFECTS

CNS: Stimulation, drowsiness, irritability, psychosis, ataxia, vertigo, fatigue, emotional disturbances, mood changes, paranoia, **suicidal ideation**

EENT: Diplopia, nystagmus, edema of eyelids

GI: Nausea, vomiting, anorexia, **hepatitis**

GU: Impotence

HEMA: **Thrombocytopenia, leukopenia, neutropenia, eosinophilia, megaloblastic anemia,** decreased serum folate level, lymphadenopathy

INTEG: Rash, edema, alopecia, lupuslike syndrome

Contraindications: Pregnancy (D), breastfeeding, hypersensitivity, porphyria, hepatic encephalopathy

Precautions: Hyperactive children, COPD, renal/hepatic disease, suicidal ideation/behavior

PHARMACOKINETICS

PO: Peak 4 hr; metabolized in liver; excreted by kidneys, in breast milk; half-life 10-12 hr (primidone)

INTERACTIONS

• Primidone levels are decreased by acetaZOLAMIDE, succinimides

• May decrease effect of oral contraceptives, acebutolol, metoprolol, propranolol, tricyclics, phenothiazines, lamotrigine
Increase: primidone levels—alcohol, heparin, CNS depressants, isoniazid, nicotinamide
Increase: toxicity—CYP3A4 inhibitors (aprepitant, antiretroviral protease inhibitors, delavirdine, fluconazole, imatinib, voriconazole)
Decrease: primidone effect—CYP3A4 inducers (barbiturates, carbamazepine, efavirenz, phenytoins, nevirapine)
Drug/Herb
• Avoid use with kava, St. John's wort, valerian
Increase: effect—ginkgo
Decrease: effect—ginseng, santonica

NURSING CONSIDERATIONS

Assess:
• For seizures: location, duration, type; folic acid deficiency; fatigue, weakness, neuropathy, depression
• Product level: therapeutic level 5-15 mcg/ml; CBC, LFTs should be done q6mo
⚠ Mental status: mood, sensorium, affect, memory (long, short), suicidal thoughts/behaviors
• Respiratory depression, wheezing
• Blood dyscrasias: fever, sore throat, bruising, rash, jaundice
Administer:
PO route
• After shaking liquid susp well
• With food for GI upset
• Tablets crushed and mixed with food or fluid for swallowing difficulties
• Avoid use with CNS depressants
Evaluate:
• Therapeutic response: decreased seizures
Teach patient/family:
• Not to withdraw product quickly; withdrawal symptoms may occur
• To avoid hazardous activities until stabilized on product; drowsiness, dizziness may occur
• To carry emergency ID with condition and medication
• To recognize the signs of blood dyscrasias; when to notify prescriber
• To avoid alcohol

probenecid (℞)
(proe-ben'e-sid)
Benuryl ✤, probenecid
Func. class.: Uricosuric, antigout agent
Chem. class.: Sulfonamide derivative

Action: Inhibits tubular reabsorption of urates, with increased excretion of uric acids
Uses: Hyperuricemia in gout, gouty arthritis, adjunct to cephalosporin, cidofovir, or penicillin treatment

DOSAGE AND ROUTES

Gonorrhea
• *Adult:* **PO** 1 g with 3.5 g ampicillin or 1 g ½ hr before 4.8 million units of aqueous penicillin G procaine injected into 2 sites **IM**
Gout/gouty arthritis
• *Adult:* **PO** 250 mg bid for 1 wk, then 500 mg bid, max 2 g/day; maintenance 500 mg/day × 6 mo
Adjunct in penicillin/cephalosporin treatment
• *Adult and child >50 kg:* **PO** 500 mg qid
• *Child <50 kg:* **PO** 25 mg/kg, then 40 mg/kg in divided doses qid
Minimize nephrotoxicity in cidofovir therapy
• *Adult:* **PO** 2 g 3 hr prior to cidofovir dose, followed by 1 g at 2 and 8 hr after end of cidofovir inf
Renal dose
• Avoid use if CCr <50 ml/min
Available forms: Tabs 0.5 g

SIDE EFFECTS

CNS: Drowsiness, headache
CV: Bradycardia
GI: Gastric irritation, nausea, vomiting, anorexia, **hepatic necrosis**

GU: Glycosuria, thirst, frequency, **nephrotic syndrome**
INTEG: Rash, dermatitis, pruritus, fever
META: *Acidosis, hypokalemia, hyperchloremia,* hyperglycemia
RESP: **Apnea,** irregular respirations
Contraindications: Hypersensitivity, severe renal/hepatic disease, CCr <50 mg/min, history of uric acid calculus
Precautions: Pregnancy (B), children <2 yr, sulfonamide hypersensitivity

PHARMACOKINETICS

Peak 2-4 hr, duration 8 hr, half-life 5-8 hr; metabolized by liver; excreted in urine

INTERACTIONS

Increase: effect of acyclovir, barbiturates, allopurinol, benzodiazepines, dyphylline, zidovudine
Increase: toxicity—sulfa products, dapsone, clofibrate, indomethacin, rifampin, naproxen, methotrexate
Decrease: action of probenecid—salicylates
Drug/Lab Test
Increase: BSP/urinary PSP, theophylline levels
False positive: urine glucose with copper sulfate test (Clinitest)

NURSING CONSIDERATIONS

Assess:
- Uric acid levels (3-7 mg/dl); mobility, joint pain, swelling
- Respiratory rate, rhythm, depth; notify prescriber of abnormalities
- Electrolytes; CO_2 before, during treatment
- Urine pH, output, glucose during beginning treatment

⚠ For CNS symptoms: confusion, twitching, hyperreflexia, stimulation, headache; may indicate overdose

Administer:
- After meals or with milk if GI symptoms occur
- Increase fluid intake to 2-3 L/day to prevent urinary calculi

Evaluate:
- Therapeutic response: absence of pain, stiffness in joints

Teach patient/family:
- To avoid OTC preparations (aspirin) unless directed by prescriber; increase water intake, avoid alcohol, caffeine

procainamide (℞)

(proe-kane-ah'mide)
Func. class.: Antidysrhythmic (Class IA)
Chem. class.: Procaine HCl amide analog

Action: Depresses excitability of cardiac muscle to electrical stimulation and slows conduction in atrium, bundle of His, and ventricle increases refractory period
Uses: Life-threatening ventricular dysrhythmias
Unlabeled uses: Atrial fibrillation, flutter

DOSAGE AND ROUTES

Atrial fibrillation/PAT
- *Adult:* **PO** 1-1.25 g; may give another 750 mg if needed; if no response, 500 mg-1 g q2hr until desired response; maintenance 50 mg/kg in divided doses q6hr

Ventricular tachycardia
- *Adult:* **PO** 1 g; maintenance 50 mg/kg/day given in 3-hr intervals

Other dysrhythmias
- *Adult:* **IV BOL** 100 mg q5min, given 25-50 mg/min, max 500 mg; or 17 mg/kg total then **IV INF** 2-6 mg/min

Renal dose
- *Adult:* **IV** 35-59 ml/min give 70% maintenance dose; CCr 15-34 ml/min give 40%-60% maintenance dose; CCr <15 ml/min individualize dose

Available forms: Caps 250, 375, 500 mg; tabs 250, 500 mg; inj 100, 500 mg/ml

SIDE EFFECTS

CNS: Headache, dizziness, confusion, psychosis, restlessness, irritability, weakness, depression

CV: Hypotension, **heart block, cardiovascular collapse, arrest**
GI: Nausea, vomiting, anorexia, diarrhea, hepatomegaly, pain, bitter taste
HEMA: SLE syndrome, **agranulocytosis, thrombocytopenia, neutropenia, hemolytic anemia**
INTEG: Rash, urticaria, edema, swelling (rare), pruritus, flushing, **angioedema**
SYST: SLE
Contraindications: Hypersensitivity, severe heart block, torsade de pointes

Black Box Warning: Lupus erythematosus

Precautions: Pregnancy (C), breastfeeding, children, renal/hepatic disease, CHF, respiratory depression, cytopenia, dysrhythmia associated with digoxin toxicity, myasthenia gravis, digoxin toxicity

Black Box Warning: Bone marrow failure, cardiac arrhythmias

PHARMACOKINETICS

Metabolized in liver to active metabolites, excreted unchanged by kidneys (60%)
PO: Peak 1-2 hr, duration 3 hr (8 hr extended)
IM: Peak 10-60 min, duration 3 hr; half-life 3 hr

INTERACTIONS

Increase: effects of neuromuscular blockers
Increase: procainamide effects—cimetidine, quinidine, trimethoprim, β-blockers, ranitidine
Increase: toxicity—other antidysrhythmics, thioridazine, quinolones
Drug/Herb
Increase: anticholinergic effect—henbane
Increase: toxicity, death—aconite
Increase: effect—aloe, broom, chronic buckthorn use, cascara sagrada (chronic use), Chinese rhubarb, figwort, fumitory, goldenseal, kudzu, licorice
Increase: serotonin effect—horehound
Decrease: effect—coltsfoot
Drug/Lab Test
Increase: ALT, AST, alk phos, LDH, bilirubin

NURSING CONSIDERATIONS

Assess:
⚠ ECG continuously if using IV to determine increased PR or QRS segments; discontinue immediately; watch for increased ventricular ectopic beats, maximum need to rebolus
- Blood levels, 3-10 mcg/ml or NAPA levels 10-20 mcg/ml

⚠ CBC q2wk × 3 mo; leukocyte, neutrophil, platelet counts may be decreased, treatment may need to be discontinued
- I&O ratio; electrolytes (K, Na, Cl), weigh weekly, report gain >2 lb

⚠ Toxicity: confusion, drowsiness, nausea, vomiting, tachydysrhythmias, oliguria
- ANA titer, during long-term treatment, watch for lupuslike symptoms
- Cardiac rate, rhythm, character, B/P continuously for fluctuations
- Respiratory status: rate, rhythm, character, lung fields; bilateral crackles may occur in CHF patient; watch for respiratory depression

⚠ CNS effects: dizziness, confusion, psychosis, paresthesias, seizures; product should be discontinued

Administer:
IM route
- IM inj in deltoid; aspirate to avoid intravascular administration

IV route
- After diluting 100 mg/ml of D_5W or sterile H_2O for inj; give 20 mg or less/1 min; may dilute 1 g/250-500 ml D_5W, run at 2-6 mg/min
- Check IV site q8hr for infiltration or extravasation

Additive compatibilities: Amiodarone, atracurium, DOBUTamine, flumazenil, lidocaine, netilmicin, verapamil
Solution compatibilities: D_5W, D_5/0.9% NaCl, 0.45% NaCl, 0.9% NaCl, water for inj
Y-site compatibilities: Amiodarone, cisatracurium, famotidine, heparin, hy-

P

drocortisone, potassium chloride, ranitidine, remifentanil, vit B/C

Evaluate:

- Therapeutic response: decreased dysrhythmias

Teach patient/family:

- That wax matrix may appear in stools
- Not to discontinue without health care provider's advice
- ⚠ To notify prescriber immediately if lupuslike symptoms appear (joint pain, butterfly rash, fever, chills, dyspnea)
- ⚠ To notify prescriber of leukopenia (sore mouth, gums, throat) or thrombocytopenia (bleeding, bruising)
- How to take pulse and when to report to prescriber
- To avoid driving, other hazardous activities until effect is known

Treatment of overdose: O_2, artificial ventilation, ECG, administer DOPamine for circulatory depression, diazepam or thiopental for seizures, isoproterenol

procaine (℞)

(proe'kane)

Novocain

Func. class.: Local anesthetic

Chem. class.: Ester

Action: Competes with calcium for sites in nerve membrane that control sodium transport across cell membrane; decreases rise of depolarization phase of action potential

Uses: Spinal anesthesia, epidural, peripheral nerve block, perineum, lower extremities, infiltration, dental anesthesia

DOSAGE AND ROUTES

Spinal anesthesia

- *Adult:* 50-200 mg

Perineum anesthesia

- *Adult:* 50-100 mg (0.5-1 ml of a 10% solution)

Available forms: Inj 1%, 2%, 10%

SIDE EFFECTS

CNS: Anxiety, restlessness, **seizures, loss of consciousness,** drowsiness, disorientation, tremors, shivering

CV: **Myocardial depression, cardiac arrest, dysrhythmias,** bradycardia, hypotension, hypertension, fetal bradycardia

EENT: Blurred vision, tinnitus, pupil constriction

GI: Nausea, vomiting

INTEG: Rash, urticaria, allergic reactions, edema, burning, skin discoloration at inj site, tissue necrosis

RESP: **Status asthmaticus, respiratory arrest, anaphylaxis**

Contraindications: Children <12 yr, hypersensitivity, sulfite allergy, myasthenia gravis, severe hepatic disease

Precautions: Pregnancy (C), geriatric patients, severe product allergies

PHARMACOKINETICS

Onset 2-5 min, duration 1 hr; metabolized by liver, excreted in urine (metabolites)

INTERACTIONS

- Dysrhythmias: epinephrine, halothane, enflurane
- Hypertension: tricyclics, phenothiazines, class IA/III dysrhythmias, other products that prolong QT interval
- Hypotension: MAOIs

Decrease: action of aminosalicylic acid, sulfonamides

Decrease: action of procaine—chloroprocaine

NURSING CONSIDERATIONS

Assess:

- B/P, pulse, respiration during treatment
- Fetal heart tones if product is used during labor
- Allergic reactions: rash, urticaria, itching
- Cardiac status: ECG for dysrhythmias, pulse, B/P during anesthesia

Administer:
- Only products that are not cloudy, do not contain precipitate
- Only with crash cart, resuscitative equipment nearby
- Only products without preservatives for epidural or caudal anesthesia

Additive compatibilities: Ascorbic acid, hydrocortisone, penicillin G, penicillin G sodium, vit B/C

Syringe compatibilities: Ampicillin, cloxacillin, glycopyrrolate, hydroxyzine, gentamicin

Solution compatibilities: D_5, D_{10}, NS, LR, Y_2, 0.45 NaCl

Perform/provide:
- Use of new sol; discard unused portions, protect from light

Evaluate:
- Therapeutic response: anesthesia necessary for procedure

Treatment of overdose: Airway, O_2, vasopressor, IV fluids, anticonvulsants for seizures

procarbazine (℞)

(proe-kar′ba-zeen)

Matulane, Natulan ♣

Func. class.: Antineoplastic, alkylating agent

Chem. class.: Hydrazine derivative

Action: Inhibits DNA, RNA, protein synthesis; has multiple sites of action; a nonvesicant

Uses: Lymphoma, Hodgkin's disease, cancers resistant to other therapy

Unlabeled uses: Brain, lung malignancies, other lymphomas, multiple myeloma, malignant melanoma, polycythemia vera

DOSAGE AND ROUTES

- *Adult:* **PO** 2-4 mg/kg/day for first wk; maintain dosage of 4-6 mg/kg/day until platelets and WBC fall; after recovery, 1-2 mg/kg/day
- *Child:* **PO** 50 mg/m^2/day for 7 days, then 100 mg/m^2 until desired response, leukopenia, or thrombocytopenia occurs; 50 mg/m^2/day is maintenance after bone marrow recovery

Available forms: Caps 50 mg

SIDE EFFECTS

CNS: Headache, dizziness, insomnia, hallucinations, confusion, **coma,** pain, chills, fever, sweating, paresthesias, **seizures,** peripheral neuropathy

EENT: Retinal hemorrhage, nystagmus, photophobia, diplopia, dry eyes

GI: Nausea, vomiting, anorexia, diarrhea, constipation, dry mouth, stomatitis, elevated hepatic enzymes

GU: Azoospermia, cessation of menses

HEMA: **Thrombocytopenia, anemia, leukopenia, myelosuppression, bleeding tendencies,** purpura, petechiae, epistaxis, **hemolysis**

INTEG: Rash, pruritus, dermatitis, alopecia, herpes, hyperpigmentation

MS: Arthralgias, myalgias

RESP: Cough, pneumonitis

SYST: **Secondary malignancy**

Contraindications: Pregnancy (D), breastfeeding, hypersensitivity, thrombocytopenia

Black Box Warning: Bone marrow depression

Precautions: Cardiac/renal/hepatic disease, radiation therapy, seizure disorder, anemia

PHARMACOKINETICS

Half-life 1 hr; concentrates in liver, kidney, skin; metabolized in liver, excreted in urine

INTERACTIONS

- Hypotension: meperidine, do not use together
- Disulfiram-like reaction: alcohol, MAOIs, tricyclics, tyramine foods, sympathomimetic products
- Hypertension: guanethidine, levodopa, methyldopa, reserpine, caffeine

⚠ Life-threatening hypertension: sympathomimetics

P

Increase: bleeding risk—NSAIDs, anticoagulants, platelet inhibitors, thrombolytics
Increase: confusion, seizures, hypertensive SSRIs
Increase: CNS depression—barbiturates, antihistamines, opioids, hypotensive agents, phenothiazines

Drug/Food
- Hypertensive crisis: tyramine foods

NURSING CONSIDERATIONS

Assess:
- CBC, differential, platelet count q wk; withhold product if WBC is <4000/mm^3 or platelet count is <100,000/mm^3; notify prescriber
- Renal studies: BUN; serum uric acid; urine CCr; electrolytes before, during therapy
- I&O ratio, report fall in urine output to <30 ml/hr
- Monitor temp; fever may indicate beginning infection
- Hepatic studies before, during therapy: bilirubin, AST, ALT, alk phos, LDH prn or q mo
- CNS changes: confusion, paresthesias, neuropathies, product should be discontinued

⚠ For tyramine foods in diet, hypertensive crisis can occur

⚠ Toxicity: facial flushing, epistaxis, increased PT, thrombocytopenia; product should be discontinued
- Bleeding: hematuria, guaiac stools, bruising or petechiae, mucosa or orifices q8hr
- Effects of alopecia on body image; discuss feelings about body changes
- Jaundiced skin, sclera; dark urine, clay-colored stools, itchy skin, abdominal pain, fever, diarrhea
- Buccal cavity for dryness, sores or ulceration, white patches, oral pain, bleeding, dysphagia
- Alkalosis if vomiting is severe
- GI symptoms: frequency of stools, cramping
- Acidosis, signs of dehydration: rapid respirations, poor skin turgor, decreased urine output, dry skin, restlessness, weakness

Administer:
- In divided doses and at bedtime to minimize nausea and vomiting
- Nonphenothiazine antiemetic 30-60 min before giving product and 4-10 hr after treatment to prevent vomiting

Perform/provide:
- Storage in tight, light-resistant container in cool environment

Evaluate:
- Therapeutic response: decreasing malignancy

Teach patient/family:
- To report any complaints, side effects to nurse or prescriber, CNS changes, diarrhea; cough, SOB, fever, chills, sore throat, bleeding, bruising, vomiting blood; black, tarry stools
- That hair may be lost during treatment and wig or hairpiece may make patient feel better; tell patient that new hair may be different in color, texture
- To avoid sunlight or UV exposure, wear sunscreen or protective clothing
- To avoid foods with citric acid, hot, or rough texture
- To report any bleeding, white spots, ulcerations in mouth to prescriber; tell patient to examine mouth daily
- To avoid driving, activities requiring alertness; dizziness may occur
- To use effective contraception, avoid breastfeeding; may cause infertility
- To avoid ingestion of alcohol, caffeine, tyramine-containing foods; cold, hay fever, weight-reducing products may cause serious product interactions; avoid smoking
- To avoid crowds, persons with infections if granulocytes are low
- To avoid receiving vaccines

prochlorperazine (℞)

(proe-klor-pair′a-zeen)

Compro

Func. class.: Antiemetic, antipsychotic

Chem. class.: Phenothiazine, piperazine derivative

Do not confuse:
prochlorperazine/**chlorproMAZINE**

Action: Decreases DOPamine neurotransmission by increasing DOPamine turnover through blockade of the D_2 somatodendritic autoreceptor in the mesolimbic system

Uses: Nausea, vomiting, psychotic disorders

Unlabeled uses: Migraine

DOSAGE AND ROUTES

Postoperative nausea/vomiting

- *Adult:* **IM** 5-10 mg 1-2 hr before anesthesia; may repeat in 30 min; **IV** 5-10 mg 15-30 min before anesthesia; **IV INF** 20 mg/L D_5W or **NS** 15-30 min before anesthesia, max 40 mg/day

Severe nausea/vomiting

- *Adult:* **PO** 5-10 mg tid-qid; **SUS REL** 15 mg/day in AM or 10 mg q12hr; **RECT** 25 mg/bid; **IM** 5-10 mg q3-4hr prn, max 40 mg/day
- *Child 18-39 kg:* **PO** 2.5 mg tid or 5 mg bid; **IM** 0.132 mg/kg q3-4hr prn, max 15 mg/day
- *Child 14-17 kg:* **PO/RECT** 2.5 mg bid-tid; **IM** 0.132 mg/kg q3-4hr prn, max 10 mg/day
- *Child 9-13 kg:* **PO/RECT** 2.5 mg/day-bid; **IM** 0.132 mg/kg q3-4hr prn, max 7.5 mg/day

Antipsychotic

- *Adult and child ≥12 yr:* **PO** 5-10 mg tid-qid; may increase q2-3days, max 150 mg/day; **IM** 10-20 mg q2-4hr up to 4 doses, then 10-20 mg q4-6hr, max 200 mg/day; **RECT** 10 mg tid-qid, may increase by 5-10 mg q2-3days as needed
- *Child 2-12 yr:* **PO** 2.5 mg bid-tid; **IM** 0.132 mg/kg

Antianxiety

- *Adult and child ≥12 yr:* **PO** 5 mg tid-qid, max 20 mg/day or >12 wk; **IM** 5-10 mg q3-4hr, max 40 mg/day; **IV** 2.5-10 mg; max 40 mg/day
- *Child 2-12 yr:* **IM** 132 mcg/kg

Available forms: Syr 5 mg/ml; inj 5 mg/ml; tabs 5, 10, 25 mg; sus rel caps 10, 15 mg; supp 2.5, 5, 25 mg

SIDE EFFECTS

CNS: **Neuroleptic malignant syndrome,** *extrapyramidal reactions, tardive dyskinesia, euphoria,* **depression,** *drowsiness,* restlessness, tremor, dizziness, headache

CV: **Circulatory failure, tachycardia,** hypotension, ECG changes

EENT: Blurred vision

GI: Nausea, vomiting, anorexia, dry mouth, diarrhea, constipation, weight loss, metallic taste, cramps

HEMA: **Agranulocytosis**

MISC: Impotence

RESP: **Respiratory depression**

Contraindications: Hypersensitivity to phenothiazines, coma, infants/neonates, children <2 yr, surgery

Precautions: Pregnancy (C), breastfeeding, geriatric patients, seizure, encephalopathy, glaucoma, hepatic disease, Parkinson's disease, BPH

Black Box Warning: Dementia

PHARMACOKINETICS

Metabolized by liver; excreted in urine, breast milk; crosses placenta; 91%-99% protein binding

PO: Onset 30-40 min, duration 3-4 hr

SUS REL: Onset 30-40 min, duration 10-12 hr

RECT: Onset 60 min, duration 3-4 hr

IM: Onset 10-20 min, duration 12 hr

P

INTERACTIONS

Increase: anticholinergic action—anticholinergics, antiparkinson products, antidepressants

Increase: CNS depression—CNS depressants

Decrease: prochlorperazine effect—barbiturates, antacids

Drug/Herb

Increase: CNS depression—chamomile, cola nut, hops, kava, nettle, nutmeg, skullcap, St. John's wort, valerian

Increase: anticholinergic effect—henbane, jimsonweed, scopolia

Increase: EPS—betel palm, kava

- Avoid use with dong quai

Drug/Lab Test

Increase: LFTs, cardiac enzymes, cholesterol, blood glucose, prolactin, bilirubin, PBI, ^{131}I, alk phos, leukocytes, granulocytes, platelets

Decrease: hormones (blood and urine)

False positive: pregnancy tests, urine bilirubin

False negative: urinary steroids, 17-OHCS, pregnancy tests

NURSING CONSIDERATIONS

Assess:

- EPS: abnormal movement, tardive dyskinesia, akathisia
- VS, B/P; check patients with cardiac disease more often

⚠ For neuroleptic malignant syndrome: seizures, hypo/hypertension, fever, tachycardia, dyspnea, fatigue, muscle stiffness, loss of bladder control; notify prescriber immediately

⚠ CBC, LFTs during course of treatment, blood dyscrasias, hepatotoxicity may occur

- Respiratory status before, during, after administration of emetic; check rate, rhythm, character; respiratory depression can occur rapidly with geriatric or debilitated patients

Administer:

- Avoid other CNS depressants

IM route

- IM inj in large muscle mass; aspirate to avoid IV administration
- Keep patient recumbent for ½ hr

IV route

- IV after diluting 5 mg/9 ml of NaCl for inj (0.5 mg/ml); give 5 mg or less/min; may dilute 10-20 mg/L NaCl and give as inf; can cause contact dermatitis

Additive compatibilities: Amikacin, ascorbic acid, dexamethasone, dimenhyDRINATE, erythromycin, ethacrynate, lidocaine, nafcillin, sodium bicarbonate, vit B/C

Syringe compatibilities: Atropine, butorphanol, chlorproMAZINE, cimetidine, diamorphine, diphenhydrAMINE, droperidol, fentanyl, glycopyrrolate, hydrOXYzine, meperidine, metoclopramide, nalbuphine, pentazocine, perphenazine, promazine, promethazine, ranitidine, scopolamine, sufentanil

Y-site compatibilities: Amsacrine, calcium gluconate, cisatracurium, cisplatin, cladribine, cyclophosphamide, cytarabine, DOXOrubicin, DOXOrubicin liposome, fluconazole, granisetron, heparin, hydrocortisone, melphalan, methotrexate, ondansetron, paclitaxel, potassium chloride, propofol, remifentanil, sargramostim, sufentanil, teniposide, thiotepa, vinorelbine, vit B/C

Evaluate:

- Therapeutic response: absence of nausea, vomiting; reduced anxiety, agitation, excitability

Teach patient/family:

- To avoid hazardous activities, activities requiring alertness; dizziness may occur
- To avoid alcohol
- Not to double or skip doses
- That urine may be pink to reddish brown
- Suppositories may contain coconut/palm oil
- To report dark urine, clay-colored stools, bleeding, bruising, rash, blurred vision
- To avoid sun or wear sunscreen, protective clothing

progesterone (℞)

(proe-jess'ter-one)

Crinone, Endometrin, First-Progesterone, progesterone, Prochieve, Prometrium

Func. class.: Progestogen

Chem. class.: Progesterone derivative

Action: Inhibits secretion of pituitary gonadotropins, which prevents follicular maturation, ovulation; stimulates growth of mammary tissue; antineoplastic action against endometrial cancer

Uses: Contraception, amenorrhea, premenstrual syndrome, abnormal uterine bleeding, endometrial hyperplasia prevention, assisted reproductive technology (ART) gel

Unlabeled uses: Corpus luteum insufficiency, early pregnancy failure, PMS, preterm delivery prophylaxis

DOSAGE AND ROUTES

Infertility

• *Adult:* **VAG** 90 mg/day (micronized gel); 100 mg 2-3 times/day starting day after oocyte retrieval and up to 10 wk total (insert)

Amenorrhea/functional uterine bleeding

• *Adult:* **IM** 5-10 mg/day × 6-8 doses

Endometrial hyperplasia prevention

• *Adult:* **PO** 200 mg/day × 12 days

Assisted Reproductive Therapy

• *Adult:* **GEL** 90 mg (8%) vaginally daily, for supplementation; 90 mg (8%) vaginally bid for replacement, if pregnancy occurs continue × 10-12 wk

Corpus luteum insufficiency (unlabeled)

• *Adult:* **VAG INSERT** 100 mg bid-tid starting at oocyte retrieval and continuing up to 10-12 wk gestation

Available forms: Inj 50 mg/ml; vag gel 4%, 8%; caps 100, 200 mg; vag insert 100 mg; vag supp 25, 100, 200, 500 mg; compounding kit 25, 50, 100, 200, 400 mg

SIDE EFFECTS

CNS: Dizziness, headache, migraines, depression, fatigue, mood swings, dementia

CV: Hypotension, **thrombophlebitis,** edema, **thromboembolism, stroke, pulmonary embolism, MI**

EENT: Diplopia, retinal thrombosis

GI: Nausea, vomiting, anorexia, cramps, increased weight, **cholestatic jaundice,** constipation

GU: Amenorrhea, cervical erosion, breakthrough bleeding, dysmenorrhea, vaginal candidiasis, breast changes, *gynecomastia, testicular atrophy, impotence,* endometriosis, **spontaneous abortion,** breast pain, ectopic pregnancy

INTEG: Rash, urticaria, acne, hirsutism, alopecia, oily skin, seborrhea, purpura, melasma

META: Hyperglycemia

SYST: **Angioedema, anaphylaxis**

Contraindications: Pregnancy (D), ectopic pregnancy, hypersensitivity to this product or peanut oil, thromboembolic disorders, reproductive cancer, genital bleeding (abnormal, undiagnosed), cerebral hemorrhage, PID, STDs

Black Box Warning: Breast cancer

Precautions: Breastfeeding, hypertension, asthma, blood dyscrasias, CHF, diabetes mellitus, bone disease, depression, migraine headache, seizure disorders, gallbladder/renal/hepatic disease, family history of breast or reproductive tract cancer

Black Box Warning: Cardiac disease, dementia

PHARMACOKINETICS

Excreted in urine, feces; metabolized in liver

IM/RECT/VAG: Duration 24 hr

INTERACTIONS

Increase: progesterone effect—CYP3A4 inhibitors (ketoconazole, cimetidine, clarithromycin, danazol, diltiazem, erythromycin, fluconazole, itraconazole, troleandomycin, verapamil, voriconazole)

P

Decrease: progesterone effect—barbiturates, phenytoin

Drug/Herb

Increase: hormonal effect—alfalfa

Drug/Lab Test

Increase: alk phos, nitrogen (urine), pregnanediol, amino acids, factors VII, VIII, IX, X

Decrease: GTT, HDL

NURSING CONSIDERATIONS

Assess:

- Cervical cytology
- Weight daily; notify prescriber of weekly weight gain >5 lb
- B/P at beginning of treatment and periodically
- I&O ratio; be alert for decreasing urinary output, increasing edema
- Hepatic studies: ALT, AST, bilirubin periodically during long-term therapy
- Edema, hypertension, cardiac symptoms, jaundice, thromboembolism
- Mental status: affect, mood, behavioral changes, depression
- Hypercalcemia

Administer:

- At least 6 hr after any vaginal treatment before using vaginal gel
- Do not break, crush, or chew caps
- Titrated dose; use lowest effective dose
- After warming to dissolve crystals
- In one dose in AM
- With food or milk to decrease GI symptoms
- Start progesterone 14 days after estrogen dose, if given concomitantly

Perform/provide:

- Storage in dark area

Evaluate:

- Therapeutic response: decreased abnormal uterine bleeding, absence of amenorrhea

Teach patient/family:

⚠ To report breast lumps, vaginal bleeding, edema, jaundice, dark urine, clay-colored stools, dyspnea, headache, blurred vision, abdominal pain, numbness or stiffness in legs, chest pain

- To report suspected pregnancy
- To monitor blood glucose if diabetic

promethazine (℞)

(proe-meth′a-zeen)

Histanil ♣, Phenadoz, Phenergan, promethazine HCl

Func. class.: Antihistamine, H_1-receptor antagonist

Chem. class.: Phenothiazine derivative

Do not confuse:

Phenergan/Theragran

Action: Acts on blood vessels, GI, respiratory system by competing with histamine for H_1-receptor site; decreases allergic response by blocking histamine

Uses: Motion sickness, rhinitis, allergy symptoms, sedation, nausea, preoperative and postoperative sedation

DOSAGE AND ROUTES

Nausea

- *Adult:* **PO/IM/IV/RECT** 12.5-25 mg; q4-6hr prn
- *Child >2 yr:* **PO/IM/IV/RECT** 0.25-0.5 mg/kg q4-6hr prn

Motion sickness

- *Adult:* **PO** 25 mg bid, give ½-1 hr before departure and q8-12hr prn
- *Child ≥2 yr:* **PO/IM/RECT** 12.5-25 mg bid, give ½-1 hr before departure and q8-12hr prn

Allergy/rhinitis (unlabeled)

- *Adult:* **PO** 12.5 mg qid, or 25 mg at bedtime
- *Child ≥2 yr:* **PO** 6.25-12.5 mg tid or 25 mg at bedtime

Sedation

- *Adult:* **PO/IM** 25-50 mg at bedtime
- *Child ≥2 yr:* **PO/IM/RECT** 12.5-25 mg at bedtime

Sedation (preoperative/postoperative)

- *Adult:* **PO/IM/IV** 25-50 mg
- *Child >2 yr:* **PO/IM/IV** 0.5-1.1 mg/kg

Available forms: Tabs 12.5, 25, 50 mg; supp 12.5, 25, 50 mg; inj 25, 50 mg/ml, syr 6.25 mg/5 ml

SIDE EFFECTS

CNS: *Dizziness, drowsiness,* poor coordination, fatigue, anxiety, euphoria, confusion, paresthesia, neuritis, EPS, **neuroleptic malignant syndrome**
CV: Hypo/hypertension, palpitations, tachycardia
EENT: Blurred vision, dilated pupils, tinnitus, nasal stuffiness; dry nose, throat, mouth; photosensitivity
GI: *Constipation,* dry mouth, nausea, vomiting, anorexia, diarrhea
GU: *Urinary retention,* dysuria, frequency
HEMA: **Thrombocytopenia, agranulocytosis, hemolytic anemia**
INTEG: Rash, urticaria, photosensitivity
RESP: Increased thick secretions, wheezing, chest tightness, **apnea in neonates, infants, young children**

Contraindications: Hypersensitivity, breastfeeding, agranulocytosis, bone marrow suppression, coma, jaundice, Reye's syndrome

Black Box Warning: Infants, neonates, children, intraarterial administration, SUBCUT administration

Precautions: Pregnancy (C), cardiac/renal/hepatic disease, asthma, seizure disorder, prostatic hypertrophy, bladder obstruction, glaucoma, COPD, GI obstruction, ileus, CNS depression, diabetes, sleep apnea, urinary retention

Black Box Warning: IV use

PHARMACOKINETICS

Metabolized in liver; excreted by kidneys, GI tract (inactive metabolites)
PO: Onset 20 min, duration 4-12 hr
IV: Onset 3-5 min

INTERACTIONS

Increase: CNS depression—barbiturates, opioids, hypnotics, tricyclics, alcohol
Increase: promethazine effect—MAOIs
Decrease: oral anticoagulants effect—heparin

Drug/Herb
Increase: anticholinergic effect—henbane, jimsonweed, scopolia

Drug/Lab Test
False negative: skin allergy test
False positive: urine pregnancy test
Interference: blood grouping (ABO), GTT

NURSING CONSIDERATIONS

Assess:
- I&O ratio; be alert for urinary retention, frequency, dysuria; product should be discontinued

⚠ CBC during long-term therapy; blood dyscrasias may occur
- Respiratory status: rate, rhythm, increase in bronchial secretions, wheezing, chest tightness
- Cardiac status: palpitations, increased pulse, hypo/hypertension, VS

Administer:
- Avoid use with other CNS depressants

PO route
- With meals for GI symptoms; absorption may slightly decrease
- When used for motion sickness, 30 min–1 hr before travel

IM route
- IM inj deep in large muscle; rotate site

IV route
- Do not use if precipitate is present
- Rapid administration may cause transient decrease in B/P
- After diluting each 25-50 mg/9 ml of NaCl for inj; give 25 mg or less/2 min

Additive compatibilities: Amikacin, ascorbic acid, chloroquine, hydromorphone, netilmicin, vit B/C

Syringe compatibilities: Atropine, butorphanol, chlorproMAZINE, cimetidine, diphenhyDRAMINE, droperidol, fentanyl, glycopyrrolate, hydromorphone, hydrOXYzine, meperidine, metoclopramide, midazolam, pentazocine, perphenazine, prochlorperazine, promazine, ranitidine, scopolamine

Y-site compatibilities: Amifostine, amsacrine, aztreonam, ciprofloxacin, cisatracurium, cisplatin, cladribine, cyclophosphamide, cytarabine, DOXOrubicin, filgrastim, fluconazole, fludarabine, granisetron, melphalan, ondansetron, remifen-

P

tanil, sargramostim, teniposide, thiotepa, vinorelbine

Perform/provide:

- Hard candy, gum, frequent rinsing of mouth for dryness
- Storage in tight, light-resistant container

Evaluate:

- Therapeutic response: absence of running, congested nose; rashes; absence of motion sickness, nausea; sedation

Teach patient/family:

- That product may cause photosensitivity; to avoid prolonged sunlight
- To notify prescriber of confusion, sedation, hypotension, jaundice, fever
- To avoid driving, other hazardous activity if drowsy
- To avoid concurrent use of alcohol
- May reduce sweating, risk of heat stroke

propafenone (℞)

(pro-paff′e-nown)

Rythmol, Rythmol SR

Func. class.: Antidysrhythmic (Class IC)

Action: Slows conduction velocity; reduces membrane responsiveness; inhibits automaticity; increases ratio of effective refractory period to action potential duration; β-blocking activity

Uses: Life-threatening dysrhythmias, sustained ventricular tachycardia, atrial fibrillation (single dose)

DOSAGE AND ROUTES

- *Adult:* **PO** 150 mg q8hr; allow a 3-4 day interval before increasing dose, max 900 mg/day

Atrial fibrillation

- *Adult:* **PO** 450 or 600 mg as a single dose; SR 225 mg q12hr, may increase to 325 q12hr, max 425 mg q12hr

Available forms: Tabs 150, 225, 300 mg; SR cap 225, 325, 425 mg

SIDE EFFECTS

CNS: Headache, dizziness, abnormal dreams, syncope, confusion, **seizures,** insomnia, tremor, anxiety, fatigue

CV: **Supraventricular dysrhythmia, ventricular dysrhythmia, bradycardia,** prodysrhythmia, palpitations, AV block, intraventricular conduction delay, AV dissociation, hypotension, chest pain

EENT: Blurred vision, altered taste, tinnitus

GI: Nausea, vomiting, constipation, dyspepsia, cholestasis, abnormal hepatic studies, dry mouth, diarrhea, anorexia

HEMA: **Leukopenia, agranulocytosis, granulocytopenia, thrombocytopenia,** anemia, bruising

INTEG: Rash

RESP: Dyspnea

Contraindications: 2nd/3rd-degree AV block, right bundle branch block, cardiogenic shock, hypersensitivity, bradycardia, uncontrolled CHF, sick-sinus syndrome, marked hypotension, bronchospastic disorders

Precautions: Pregnancy (C), breastfeeding, children, geriatric patients, CHF, hypo/hyperkalemia, nonallergic bronchospasm, renal/hepatic disease, hematologic disorders

Black Box Warning: Recent MI, cardiac arrhythmias, QT prolongation, torsade de pointes

PHARMACOKINETICS

Peak 3-8 hr, half-life 2-10 hr; metabolized in liver; excreted in urine (metabolite)

INTERACTIONS

Increase: anticoagulation—warfarin

Increase: CNS effects—local anesthetics

Increase: digoxin level—digoxin

Increase: β-blocker effect—propranolol, metoprolol

Increase: cycloSPORINE levels—cycloSPORINE

Decrease: propafenone effect—rifampin, cimetidine, quinidine

Drug/Herb
• Hypokalemia, increased antidysrhythmic action: aloe, buckthorn, cascara sagrada, senna pod/leaf
Increase: toxicity, death—aconite
Increase: effect—aloe, broom, chronic buckthorn use, cascara sagrada (chronic use), Chinese rhubarb, figwort, fumitory, goldenseal, kudzu, licorice
Increase: serotonin effect—horehound
Decrease: effect—coltsfoot
Drug/Lab Test
Increase: CPK

NURSING CONSIDERATIONS

Assess:
• GI status: bowel pattern, number of stools
⚠ Cardiac status: rate, rhythm, quality; ECG or Holter monitor prior to and during therapy; watch for PR, QT prolongation
• CBC, ANA titer, LFTs
• Chest x-ray film, pulmonary function test during treatment
• I&O ratio; check for decreasing output; daily weight
• B/P for fluctuations
• Lung fields; bilateral crackles, dyspnea, peripheral edema, weight gain, jugular venous distention may occur in CHF patient
⚠ Toxicity: fine tremors, dizziness, hypotension, drowsiness, abnormal heart rate
• Cardiac function: respiratory rate, rhythm, character continuously
Administer:
• Do not break, crush, or chew tabs; swallow whole
• To hospitalized patients, since heart monitoring is required
• After hypo/hyperkalemia is corrected
• Dosage adjustment q3-4days
Evaluate:
• Therapeutic response: absence of dysrhythmias
Teach patient/family:
• To avoid hazardous activities until response is known
• To report fever, chills, sore throat, bleeding, SOB, chest pain, palpitations, blurred vision
• Take tab with food
• To carry emergency ID identifying medication and prescriber
• To avoid abrupt discontinuation of product; take as prescribed; do not miss or double doses

Treatment of overdose: O_2, artificial ventilation, defibrillation ECG; administer DOPamine for circulatory depression, diazepam or thiopental for seizures, isoproterenol

propantheline (℞)

(proe-pan'the-leen)
Func. class.: GI anticholinergic, antiulcer agent
Chem. class.: Synthetic quaternary ammonium compound

Action: Inhibits actions of acetylcholine at postganglionic parasympathetic neuroeffector sites
Uses: Treatment of urinary incontinence, peptic ulcer disease, irritable bowel syndrome, duodenography

DOSAGE AND ROUTES

• *Adult:* **PO** 15 mg tid before meals, 30 mg at bedtime
• *Geriatric/small patients:* **PO** 7.5 mg tid before meals
• *Child:* **PO** 1-2 mg/kg/day in 3-4 divided doses
Available forms: Tabs 7.5, 15 mg

SIDE EFFECTS

CNS: Confusion, stimulation in geriatric patients, headache, insomnia, dizziness, drowsiness, anxiety, weakness, hallucinations
CV: Palpitations, tachycardia, orthostatic hypotension (geriatric patients)
EENT: Blurred vision, photophobia, mydriasis, cycloplegia, increased ocular tension
GI: Dry mouth, constipation, **paralytic ileus,** heartburn, nausea, vomiting, dysphagia, absence of taste
GU: Urinary hesitancy, retention, impotence

P

INTEG: Urticaria, rash, pruritus, anhidrosis, fever, allergic reactions

Contraindications: Hypersensitivity to anticholinergics, closed-angle glaucoma, GI obstruction, myasthenia gravis, paralytic ileus, GI atony, toxic megacolon, urinary tract obstruction

Precautions: Pregnancy (C), geriatric patients, hyperthyroidism, CAD, dysrhythmias, CHF, ulcerative colitis, hypertension, hiatal hernia, renal/hepatic disease, urinary retention, prostatic hypertrophy

PHARMACOKINETICS

Onset 30-45 min, duration 6 hr; metabolized by liver, GI system; excreted in urine, bile

INTERACTIONS

Increase: anticholinergic effect—tricyclics, MAOIs, H_1-antihistamines, belladonna alkaloids, opioids, disopyramide, procainamide, quinidine, phenothiazines

Increase: effect—corticosteroids, β-blockers, amoxapine

Drug/Herb

Increase: anticholinergic effect—henbane, jimsonweed, scopolia

NURSING CONSIDERATIONS

Assess:

- VS, cardiac status: checking for dysrhythmias, increased rate, palpitations
- I&O ratio; check for urinary retention or hesitancy
- GI complaints: pain, bleeding (frank or occult), nausea, vomiting, anorexia

Administer:

- ½-1 hr before meals for better absorption; if taking with an antacid, give 1 hr before or after the antacid
- Decreased dose to geriatric patients; metabolism may be slowed
- Gum, hard candy, frequent rinsing for dry mouth
- Avoid use with other CNS depressants

Perform/provide:

- Storage in tight container protected from light
- Increased fluids, bulk, exercise to decrease constipation

Evaluate:

- Therapeutic response: absence of epigastric pain, bleeding, nausea, vomiting

Teach patient/family:

- To avoid driving, other hazardous activities until stabilized on medication; may cause blurred vision; to use caution when standing due to orthostatic hypotension
- To avoid alcohol; will enhance sedating properties of this product
- To drink plenty of fluids
- To report dysphagia

proparacaine ophthalmic

See Appendix B

⚠ High Alert

propofol (℞)

(pro′poh-fole)

Diprivan, Fresenius Propoven

Func. class.: General anesthetic

Action: Produces dose-dependent CNS depression by activation of GABA receptor

Uses: Induction or maintenance of anesthesia as part of balanced anesthetic technique; sedation in mechanically ventilated patients

DOSAGE AND ROUTES

Induction

- *Adult:* **IV** 2-2.5 mg/kg, approximately 40 mg q10sec until induction onset
- *Child 3-16 yr:* **IV** 2.5-3.5 mg/kg over 20-30 sec
- *Geriatric:* **IV** 1-1.5 mg/kg, approximately 20 mg q10sec until induction onset

Maintenance

- *Adult:* **IV** 0.1-0.2 mg/kg/min (6-12 mg/kg/hr)
- *Child ≥3 yr:* **IV** 0.125-0.3 mg/kg/min (7.5-18 mg/kg/hr)
- *Geriatric:* **IV** 0.05-0.1 mg/kg/min (3-6 mg/kg/hr)

ICU sedation

• *Adult:* **IV** 5 mcg/kg/min over 5 min; may increase by 5-10 mcg/kg/min over 5-10 min until desired response

Available forms: Inj 10 mg/ml in 20-ml ampule, 50-ml and 100-ml vials

SIDE EFFECTS

CNS: Involuntary movement, headache, jerking, fever, dizziness, shivering, tremor, confusion, somnolence, paresthesia, agitation, abnormal dreams, euphoria fatigue, **increased intracranial pressure, impaired cerebral flow, seizures**

CV: Bradycardia, hypotension, hypertension, PVC, PAC, tachycardia, abnormal ECG, ST segment depression, **asystole, bradydysrhythmias**

EENT: Blurred vision, tinnitus, eye pain, strange taste, diplopia

GI: Nausea, vomiting, abdominal cramping, dry mouth, swallowing, hypersalivation, **pancreatitis**

GU: Urine retention, green urine, cloudy urine, oliguria

INTEG: Flushing, phlebitis, hives, burning/stinging at inj site, rash, pain of extremities

MS: Myalgia

RESP: **Apnea,** *cough, hiccups,* dyspnea, hypoventilation, sneezing, wheezing, tachypnea, hypoxia, respiratory acidosis

Contraindications: Hypersensitivity to product or soybean oil, egg, benzyl alcohol (some products)

Precautions: Pregnancy (B), breastfeeding, children, geriatric patients, respiratory depression, severe respiratory disorders, cardiac dysrhythmias, labor and delivery, renal disease, hyperlipidemia

PHARMACOKINETICS

Onset 15-30 sec, rapid distribution, half-life 1-8 min, terminal half-life 3-12 hr; 70% excreted in urine; metabolized in liver by conjugation to inactive metabolites, 95%-99% protein binding

INTERACTIONS

• Do not use within 10 days of MAOIs

Increase: CNS depression—alcohol, opioids, sedative/hypnotics, antipsychotics, skeletal muscle relaxants, inhalational anesthetics

Drug/Herb

Increase: propofol effect—St. John's wort

NURSING CONSIDERATIONS

Assess:

• Inj site: phlebitis, burning, stinging

• ECG for changes: PVC, PAC, ST segment changes; monitor VS

• CNS changes: movement, jerking, tremors, dizziness, LOC, pupil reaction

• Allergic reactions: hives

⚠ Respiratory dysfunction: respiratory depression, character, rate, rhythm; notify prescriber if respirations are <10/min

Administer:

IV route

• Shake well before use; if diluted, use only D_5W to not less than 2 mg/ml; give over 3-5 min, titrate to needed level of sedation; use only glass containers when mixing, not stable in plastic; use aseptic technique when transferring from original container

• May be given by cont inf; give by inf pump

• Only with resuscitative equipment available

• Only by qualified persons trained in anesthesia

Y-site compatibilities: Acyclovir, alfentanil, aminophylline, ampicillin, aztreonam, bumetanide, buprenorphine, butorphanol, calcium gluconate, carboplatin, cefazolin, cefoperazone, cefotaxime, cefotetan, cefoxitin, ceftizoxime, ceftriaxone, cefuroxime, chlorproMAZINE, cimetidine, cisplatin, clindamycin, cyclophosphamide, cycloSPORINE, cytarabine, dexamethasone, diphenhydrAMINE, DOBUTamine, DOPamine, doxycycline, droperidol, enalaprilat, ephedrine, epinephrine, esmolol, famoti-

P

dine, fentanyl, fluconazole, fluorouracil, furosemide, ganciclovir, glycopyrrolate, granisetron, haloperidol, heparin, hydrocortisone, hydromorphone, hydrOXYzine, ifosfamide, imipenem/cilastatin, inamrinone, regular insulin, isoproterenol, ketamine, labetalol, levorphanol, lidocaine, lorazepam, magnesium sulfate, mannitol, meperidine, mezlocillin, miconazole, morphine, nafcillin, nalbuphine, naloxone, nitroglycerin, norepinephrine, ofloxacin, paclitaxel, pentobarbital, phenobarbital, piperacillin, potassium chloride, prochlorperazine, propranolol, ranitidine, scopolamine, sodium bicarbonate, sodium nitroprusside, succinylcholine, sufentanil, thiopental ticarcillin, ticarcillin/clavulanate, vecuronium, verapamil

Solution compatibilities: (If given together via Y-site) D_5W, D_5LR, LR, D_5/0.45% NaCl, D_5/0.2% NaCl

Perform/provide:

- Storage in light-resistant area at room temperature, use within 6 hr of opening
- If transferred from original container to another container, complete inf within 12 hr (Dipravan), 6 hr (generic propofol)

Evaluate:

- Therapeutic response: induction of anesthesia

Teach patient/family:

- That this medication will cause dizziness, drowsiness, sedation

Treatment of overdose: Discontinue product; administer vasopressor agents or anticholinergics, artificial ventilation

⚠ High Alert

propoxyphene (℞)

(proe-pox′i-feen)

Darvon, Darvon-N, Dolene, Novopropoxyn 🍁

Func. class.: Opiate analgesic

Chem. class.: Synthetic opiate

Controlled Substance Schedule IV

Action: Depresses pain impulse transmission at the spinal cord level by interacting with opioid receptors

Uses: Mild to moderate pain

DOSAGE AND ROUTES

- *Adult:* **PO** (HCl) 65 mg q4hr prn, max 390 mg/day
- *Adult:* **PO** (napsylate) 100 mg q4hr prn, max 600 mg/day

Available forms: Caps (propoxyphene HCl) 32, 65 mg; tabs (propoxyphene napsylate) 100 mg; oral susp 50 mg/5 ml

SIDE EFFECTS

CNS: Drowsiness, dizziness, confusion, **increased intracranial pressure,** *headache, sedation,* euphoria, **seizures, hyperthermia (geriatric patients)**

CV: Palpitations, bradycardia, change in B/P, **dysrhythmias**

EENT: Tinnitus, blurred vision, miosis, diplopia

GI: Nausea, vomiting, anorexia, constipation, cramps, abdominal pain, jaundice

GU: Urinary retention, dysuria

INTEG: Rash, urticaria, bruising, flushing, diaphoresis, pruritus

RESP: **Respiratory depression, pulmonary edema**

Contraindications: Hypersensitivity to ASA products (some preparations)

Black Box Warning: Alcoholism, substance abuse, suicidal ideation

Precautions: Pregnancy (C), breastfeeding, children <18 yr, geriatric patients, addictive personality, increased intracranial pressure, MI (acute), severe heart disease, respiratory depression, renal/hepatic disease

Black Box Warning: Potential for overdose/poisoning

PHARMACOKINETICS

Metabolized by liver, excreted by kidneys (as metabolites), crosses placenta, excreted in breast milk, half-life 6-12 hr (metabolites)

PO: Onset ½-1 hr, peak 2-3 hr, duration 4-6 hr

INTERACTIONS

⚠ Possible fatal reactions: MAOIs, alcohol

Increase: effects with other CNS depressants—opioids, sedative/hypnotics, antipsychotics, skeletal muscle relaxants

Drug/Herb

Increase: CNS depression—chamomile, hops, Jamaican dogwood, kava, lavender, mistletoe, nettle, pokeweed, poppy, senega, skullcap, valerian

Increase: anticholinergic effect—corkwood

Drug/Lab Test

Increase: amylase

False positive: methadone test

NURSING CONSIDERATIONS

Assess:

- For pain: duration, location, type
- I&O ratio; check for decreasing output; may indicate retention
- Bowel status: constipation; may need stimulant laxative
- CNS changes: dizziness, drowsiness, hallucinations, euphoria, loss of consciousness, pupil reaction
- Allergic reactions: rash, urticaria
- Respiratory dysfunction: respiratory depression, character, rate, rhythm; notify prescriber if respirations are <10/min
- Need for pain medication; physical dependence

Administer:

- May be given with food/milk for GI upset
- With antiemetic for nausea, vomiting
- When pain is beginning to return; determine dosage interval by response

Perform/provide:

- Storage in light-resistant area at room temperature
- Assistance with ambulation, falling precautions

Evaluate:

- Therapeutic response: decrease in pain

Teach patient/family:

- To report any symptoms of CNS changes, allergic reactions
- That physical dependency may result when used for extended periods; not to exceed dose, significant potential for overdose exists
- That withdrawal symptoms may occur: nausea, vomiting, cramps, fever, faintness, anorexia; do not withdraw abruptly
- To avoid CNS depressants, alcohol
- To avoid driving, operating machinery if drowsiness occurs

Treatment of overdose: Naloxone (Narcan) 0.2-0.8 mg IV, O_2, IV fluids, vasopressors

propranolol (℞)

(proe-pran′oh-lole)

Apo-Propranolol ✦, Betaclinron E-R ✦, Detensol ✦, Inderal, Inderal LA, InnoPran XL, NovoPranol ✦, propranolol HCl, PMS-Propranolol ✦

Func. class.: Antihypertensive, antianginal, antidysrhythmic (class II)

Chem. class.: β-Adrenergic blocker

Do not confuse:

propranolol/**Pravachol**

Inderal/**Toradol/Inderide/Adderall/**
Imuran

Action: Nonselective β-blocker with negative inotropic, chronotropic, dromotropic properties

Uses: Chronic stable angina pectoris, hypertension, supraventricular dysrhythmias, migraine prophylaxis, pheochromocytoma, cyanotic spells related to hypertrophic subaortic stenosis

Unlabeled uses: Anxiety, Parkinson's tremor, prevention of variceal bleeding caused by portal hypertension, akathisia induced by antipsychotics, acute MI, portal hypertension, sclerodermal renal crisis, unstable angina, infantile capillary hemangioma

P

DOSAGE AND ROUTES

Dysrhythmias

• *Adult:* **PO** 10-30 mg tid-qid; **IV BOL** 0.5-3 mg give 1 mg/min; may repeat in 2 min, may repeat q4hr thereafter

• *Child:* **PO** 1 mg/kg/day divided in 2 doses; **IV** 0.01-0.1 mg/kg over 5 min

Hypertension

• *Adult:* **PO** 40 mg bid or 80 mg/day (ext rel) initially; usual dose 120-240 mg/day bid-tid or 120-160 mg/day (ext rel)

• *Child:* **PO** 0.5-1 mg/kg/day divided q6-12hr

Angina

• *Adult:* **PO** 80-320 mg in divided doses bid-qid or 80 mg/day (ext rel); usual dose 160 mg/day (ext rel)

MI prophylaxis

• *Adult:* **PO** 180-240 mg/day tid-qid starting 5 days to 2 wk after MI

Pheochromocytoma

• *Adult:* **PO** 60 mg/day × 3 days preoperatively in divided doses or 30 mg/day in divided doses (inoperable tumor)

Migraine

• *Adult:* **PO** 80 mg/day (ext rel) or in divided doses; may increase to 160-240 mg/day in divided doses

• *Child >35 kg (unlabeled):* **PO** 20-40 mg tid

Essential tremor

• *Adult:* **PO** 40 mg bid; usual dose 120 mg/day

Acute MI (unlabeled)

• *Adult:* **PO** 180-320 mg/day in 3-4 divided doses

Anxiety (unlabeled)

• *Adult:* **PO** 10-80 mg given 1 hr prior to anxiety-producing event

Scleroderma renal crisis (unlabeled)

• *Adult:* **PO** 40 mg bid, may increase q3-7days, max 160-480 mg/day

Esophageal varices (portal hypertension) (unlabeled)

• *Adult:* **PO** 40 mg bid, titrate to heart rate reduction of 25%

Infantile capillary hemangioma (unlabeled)

• *Infant:* **PO** 2-3 mg/kg/day

Available forms: Ext rel caps 60, 80, 120, 160 mg; tabs 10, 20, 40, 60, 80, 90 mg; inj 1 mg/ml; oral sol 4 mg/ml, 8 mg/ml; conc oral sol 80 mg/ml

SIDE EFFECTS

CNS: Depression, hallucinations, dizziness, *fatigue,* lethargy, paresthesias, bizarre dreams, disorientation

CV: **Bradycardia,** hypotension, **CHF,** palpitations, AV block, peripheral vascular insufficiency, vasodilation, cold extremities, **pulmonary edema, dysrhythmias**

EENT: Sore throat, **laryngospasm,** blurred vision, dry eyes

GI: Nausea, vomiting, diarrhea, colitis, constipation, cramps, dry mouth, hepatomegaly, gastric pain, acute pancreatitis

GU: Impotence, decreased libido, UTIs

HEMA: **Agranulocytosis, thrombocytopenia**

INTEG: Rash, pruritus, fever

META: Hyperglycemia, hypoglycemia

MISC: Facial swelling, weight change, Raynaud's phenomenon

MS: Joint pain, arthralgia, muscle cramps, pain

RESP: Dyspnea, respiratory dysfunction, *bronchospasm,* cough

Contraindications: Hypersensitivity to this product; cardiogenic shock, AV heart block; bronchospastic disease; sinus bradycardia; bronchospasm; asthma

Precautions: Pregnancy (C), breastfeeding, children, diabetes mellitus, hyperthyroidism, COPD, renal/hepatic disease, myasthenia gravis, peripheral vascular disease, hypotension, cardiac failure, Raynaud's disease, sick sinus syndrome, vasospastic angina, smoking, Wolff-Parkinson-White syndrome

Black Box Warning: Abrupt discontinuation

PHARMACOKINETICS

Metabolized by liver; crosses placenta, blood-brain barrier; excreted in breast milk, protein binding 90%

PO: Onset 30 min, peak 1-1½ hr, duration 12 hr

PO-ER: Peak 6 hr, duration 24 hr, half-life 8-11 hr
IV: Onset 2 min, peak 1 min, duration 5 min

INTERACTIONS

Increase: toxicity—phenothiazines
Increase: propranolol level—propafenone
Increase: effect of calcium channel blockers, neuromuscular blocker
Increase: negative inotropic effects—disopyramide
Increase: β-blocking effect—cimetidine
Increase: hypotension—quinidine, haloperidol, prazosin
Decrease: β-blocking effects—barbiturates
Decrease: propranolol levels—smoking

Drug/Herb

Increase: toxicity, death—aconite
Increase: antihypertensive effect—barberry, betony, black catechu, black cohosh, bloodroot, broom, burdock, cat's claw, dandelion, goldenseal, Irish moss, Jamaican dogwood, kelp, khella, mistletoe, parsley
Increase or decrease: antihypertensive effect—astragalus, cola tree
Decrease: antihypertensive effect—coltsfoot, guarana, khat, licorice, betel palm, ma huang

Drug/Lab Test

Increase: serum potassium, serum uric acid, ALT, AST, alk phos, LDH
Decrease: blood glucose
Interference: glaucoma testing

NURSING CONSIDERATIONS

Assess:

- B/P, pulse, respirations during beginning therapy; notify prescriber if pulse <50 bpm or systolic B/P <90 mm Hg
- Weight daily; report gain of 5 lb
- ⚠ I&O ratio, CCr if kidney damage is diagnosed; watch for fluid overload: fatigue, weight gain, jugular distention, dyspnea, peripheral edema, crackles
- ⚠ ECG continuously if using as antidysrhythmic, IV, PCWP, CVP
- Hepatic enzymes: AST, ALT, bilirubin
- Angina pain: duration, time started, activity being performed, character
- Tolerance (long-term use)
- Headache, light-headedness, decreased B/P; may indicate a need for decreased dosage; may aggrevate symptoms of arterial insufficiency

Administer:

PO route

- Do not break, crush, chew, or open ext rel cap
- Do not use ext rel cap for essential tremor, MI, cardiac dysrhythmias; do not use InnoPran XL in hypertropic subaortic stenosis, migraine, angina pectoris
- Ext rel caps should be taken daily; InnoPran XL should be taken at bedtime
- May mix oral sol with liquid or semisolid food; rinse container to get entire dose
- With 8 oz water with food; food enhances bioavailability
- Do not give with aluminum-containing antacid; may decrease GI absorption

IV route

- IV undiluted or diluted 10 ml D_5W for inj; give 1 mg or less/min; may be diluted in 50 ml NaCl and run 1 mg over 10-15 min

Additive compatibilities: DOBUTamine, verapamil

Solution compatibilities: 0.9% NaCl, 0.45 NaCl, Ringer's, D_5W, D_5/0.9% NaCl, D_5/0.45% NaCl

Syringe compatibilities: Inamrinone, milrinone

Y-site compatibilities: Alteplase, amrinone, heparin, hydrocortisone, meperidine, milrinone, morphine, potassium chloride, propofol, tacrolimus, vit B/C

Perform/provide:

- Protection from light

Evaluate:

- Therapeutic response: decreased B/P, dysrhythmias

Teach patient/family:

- ⚠ Not to discontinue abruptly, may precipitate life-threatening dysrhythmias, exacerbation of angina, MI; to take product at same time each day, either with or without food consistently, to decrease dosage over 2 wk

- To avoid OTC products unless approved by prescriber; avoid alcohol
- To avoid hazardous activities if dizzy
- The importance of compliance with complete medical regimen; monitor blood glucose, may mask symptoms of hypoglycemia
- To make position changes slowly to prevent fainting
- That sensitivity to cold may occur
- How to take pulse, B/P; withhold if <50 bpm or systolic B/P <90 mm Hg

propylhexadrine nasal agent

See Appendix B

propylthiouracil (℞)

(proe-pill-thye-oh-yoor′a-sill)
PIV, propylthiouracil,
Propyl-Thyracil ✱, PTU
Func. class.: Thyroid hormone antagonist (antithyroid)
Chem. class.: Thioamide

Action: Blocks synthesis peripherally of T_3, T_4 (triiodothyronine, thyroxine), inhibits organification of iodine

Uses: Preparation for thyroidectomy, thyrotoxic crisis, hyperthyroidism, thyroid storm

DOSAGE AND ROUTES

Thyrotoxic crisis

- *Adult and child:* **PO** Same as hyperthyroidism with iodine and propranolol

Preparation for thyroidectomy

- *Adult:* **PO** 600-1200 mg/day
- *Child:* **PO** 10 mg/kg/day in divided doses

Hyperthyroidism

- *Adult:* **PO** 100 mg tid increasing to 300 mg q8hr if condition is severe; continue to euthyroid state, then 100 mg daily-tid
- *Child >10 yr:* **PO** 100 mg tid; continue to euthyroid state, then 25 mg tid to 100 mg bid
- *Child 6-10 yr:* **PO** 50-150 mg in divided doses q8hr
- *Neonate (unlabeled):* **PO** 5-10 mg/kg/day in divided doses q8hr

Available forms: Tabs 50 mg

SIDE EFFECTS

CNS: Drowsiness, headache, vertigo, fever, paresthesias, neuritis

GI: Nausea, diarrhea, vomiting, **jaundice, hepatitis,** loss of taste, **liver failure, death**

GU: **Nephritis**

HEMA: **Agranulocytosis, leukopenia, thrombocytopenia, hypothrombinemia, lymphadenopathy,** bleeding, vasculitis, periarteritis

INTEG: Rash, urticaria, pruritus, alopecia, hyperpigmentation, lupuslike syndrome

MS: Myalgia, arthralgia, nocturnal muscle cramps, osteoporosis

Contraindications: Pregnancy (D), breastfeeding, hypersensitivity, agranulocytosis, hepatitis, jaundice

Precautions: Infants, bone marrow depression, hepatic disease, fever

PHARMACOKINETICS

Onset up to 3 wk, peak 6-10 wk, duration 1 wk to 1 mo, half-life 1-2 hr; excreted in urine, bile, breast milk; crosses placenta; concentration in thyroid gland

INTERACTIONS

- Bone marrow depression: radiation, antineoplastics
- Agranulocytosis: phenothiazines

Increase: effects—potassium/sodium iodide, lithium

Decrease: anticoagulant effect—heparin, oral anticoagulants

Drug/Lab Test

Increase: PT, AST, ALT, alk phos

NURSING CONSIDERATIONS

Assess:
- Pulse, B/P, temp
- I&O ratio; check for edema: puffy hands, feet, periorbits; indicates hypothyroidism
- Weight daily; same clothing, scale, time of day
- T_3, T_4, which are increased; serum TSH, which is decreased; free thyroxine index, which is increased if dosage is too low; discontinue product 3-4 wk before RAIU

⚠ Blood studies: CBC for blood dyscrasias: leukopenia, thrombocytopenia, agranulocytosis; LFTs

⚠ Overdose: peripheral edema, heat intolerance, diaphoresis, palpitations, dysrhythmias, severe tachycardia, increased temp, delirium, CNS irritability

⚠ Hypersensitivity: rash, enlarged cervical lymph nodes; product may have to be discontinued

- Hypoprothrombinemia: bleeding, petechiae, ecchymosis
- Clinical response: after 3 wk should include increased weight, pulse; decreased T_4
- Bone marrow depression: sore throat, fever, fatigue

Administer:
- With meals to decrease GI upset
- At same time each day to maintain product level
- Lowest dose that relieves symptoms

Perform/provide:
- Storage in light-resistant container
- Fluids to 3-4 L/day, unless contraindicated

Evaluate:
- Therapeutic response: weight gain, decreased pulse, decreased T_4, decreased B/P

Teach patient/family:
- To abstain from breastfeeding after delivery
- To take pulse daily
- To report redness, swelling, sore throat, mouth lesions, which indicate blood dyscrasias
- To keep graph of weight, pulse, mood
- To avoid OTC products that contain iodine
- That seafood, other iodine products may be restricted
- Not to discontinue this medication abruptly; thyroid crisis may occur; stress response
- That response may take several months if thyroid is large
- The symptoms/signs of overdose: periorbital edema, cold intolerance, mental depression
- The symptoms of inadequate dose: tachycardia, diarrhea, fever, irritability
- To take medication as prescribed; not to skip or double dose; missed doses should be taken when remembered up to 1 hr before next dose
- To carry emergency ID listing condition, medication

protamine (℞)

(proe′ta-meen)

Func. class.: Heparin antagonist

Chem. class.: Low-molecular-weight protein

Action: Binds heparin, making it ineffective

Uses: Heparin overdose, hemorrhage

P

DOSAGE AND ROUTES

- *Adult and child:* **IV** 1 mg of protamine/100 units heparin given or 100 anti-Xa units of LMWH; administer slowly 1-3 min; max 50 mg/10 min

Available forms: Inj 10 mg/ml

SIDE EFFECTS

CNS: Lassitude, flushing

CV: Hypotension, bradycardia, **circulatory collapse,** capillary leak

GI: Nausea, vomiting, anorexia

HEMA: Bleeding

INTEG: *Rash,* dermatitis, urticaria

RESP: Dyspnea, **pulmonary edema, severe respiratory distress,** bronchospasm

SYST: **Anaphylaxis, angioedema**

Contraindications: Hypersensitivity
Precautions: Pregnancy (C), breastfeeding, fish allergy, diabetes, previous exposure to protamine, insulins, heparin rebound or bleeding

PHARMACOKINETICS

IV: Onset 5 min, duration 2 hr

NURSING CONSIDERATIONS

Assess:

⚠ Hypersensitivity: urticaria, cough, wheezing, have emergency equipment nearby

- Blood studies (Hct, platelets, occult blood in stools) q3mo
- Coagulation tests (aPTT, ACT) 15 min after dose, then in several hours
- VS, B/P, pulse after 30 min; plus 3 hr after dose
- Skin rash, urticaria, dermatitis

⚠ Allergy to fish; use with caution; men that have had a vasectomy may be more prone to hypersensitivity

Administer:

IV route

- After diluting 50 mg/5 ml sterile bacteriostatic H_2O for inj; shake, give 20 mg or less over 1-3 min; may further dilute with equal volume of NaCl or D_5W and run over 2-3 hr; titrate to aPTT, ACT; use inf pump
- Too-rapid inf leads to hypotension, anaphylactoid reactions

Additive compatibilities: Cimetidine, ranitidine, verapamil

Perform/provide:

- Storage at 36° F-46° F (2° C-8° C)

Evaluate:

- Therapeutic response: reversal of heparin overdose

Teach patient/family:

- Not to take if allergic to fish

pseudoephedrine

(OTC, ℞)
(soo-doh-eh-fed'rin)
Afrin, Allermed, Cenafed, Children's Congestion Relief, Children's Silfedrine, Congestion Relief, Decofed Syrup, DeFed-60, Dorcol Children's Decongestant, Drixoral Non-Drowsy Formula, Dynafed, Efidac/24, Eltor ♣, Genaphed, Halofed, Mini Thin Pseudo, Pseudo, pseudoephedrine HCl, Pseudogest, Seudotabs, Sinustop Pro, Sudafed, Sudafed 12 Hour, Sudex, Triaminic AM Decongestant Formula
Func. class.: Adrenergic
Chem. class.: Substituted phenylethylamine

Action: Primary activity through α-effects on respiratory mucosal membranes reducing congestion hyperemia, edema; minimal bronchodilation secondary to β-effects
Uses: Nasal decongestant, adjunct in otitis media; with antihistamines

DOSAGE AND ROUTES

- *Adult and child >12 yr:* **PO** 60 mg q6hr; **EXT REL** 120 mg q12hr or 240 mg q24hr
- *Geriatric:* **PO** 30-60 mg q6hr prn
- *Child 6-12 yr:* **PO** 30 mg q6hr, max 120 mg/day
- *Child 2-6 yr:* **PO** 15 mg q6hr, max 60 mg/day

Available forms: Ext rel caps 120, 240 mg; oral sol 15 mg, 30 mg/5 ml; drops 7.5 mg/0.8 ml; tabs 30, 60 mg; caps 60 mg; ext rel tabs 120, 240 mg

SIDE EFFECTS

CNS: Tremors, anxiety, stimulation, insomnia, headache, dizziness, hallucinations, **seizures** (geriatric patients)

CV: Palpitations, tachycardia, hypertension, chest pain, **dysrhythmias, CV collapse**
EENT: Dry nose, irritation of nose and throat
GI: *Anorexia, nausea, vomiting,* dry mouth
GU: Dysuria
Contraindications: Hypersensitivity to sympathomimetics, closed-angle glaucoma
Precautions: Pregnancy (C), breastfeeding, cardiac disorders, hyperthyroidism, diabetes mellitus, prostatic hypertrophy, hypertension

PHARMACOKINETICS

PO: Onset 15-30 min; duration 4-6 hr, 8-12 hr (ext rel); metabolized in liver; excreted in feces and breast milk; terminal half-life 9-16 hr

INTERACTIONS

⚠ Do not use with MAOIs or tricyclics; hypertensive crisis may occur
Increase: effect of this product—urinary alkalizers
Decrease: effect of this product—methyldopa, urinary acidifiers, rauwolfia alkaloids

NURSING CONSIDERATIONS

Assess:
- For nasal congestion; auscultate lung sounds; check for tenacious bronchial secretions
- B/P, pulse throughout treatment
- For CNS side effects in the geriatric patients: excitation, seizures, hallucinations

Administer:
- Near bedtime; stimulation can occur

Perform/provide:
- Storage at room temperature

Evaluate:
- Therapeutic response: decreased nasal congestion

Teach patient/family:
- The reason for product administration
- Not to use continuously, or more than recommended dose; rebound congestion may occur

⚠ To notify prescriber immediately of anxiety; slow, fast heart rate; dyspnea; seizures
- To check with prescriber before using other products, as product interactions may occur
- To avoid taking near bedtime; stimulation can occur
- Not to use if stimulation, restlessness, or tremors occur
- That use in children may cause excessive agitation

pseudoephedrine nasal agent

See Appendix B

psyllium (OTC, ℞)

(sill′ee-um)
Fiberall, Fiberall Natural Flavor and Orange Flavor, Genfiber, Hydrocil Instant, Karacil ✱, Konsyl, Konsyl Orange, Maalox Daily Fiber Therapy, Metamucil, Metamucil Lemon Lime, Metamucil Orange Flavor, Metamucil Sugar Free, Metamucil Sugar Free Orange Flavor, Modane Bulk, Mylanta Natural Fiber Supplement, Natural Fiber Laxative, Natural Fiber Laxative Sugar Free, Natural Vegetable Reguloid, Prodiem Plain ✱, Reguloid Natural, Reguloid Orange, Reguloid Sugar Free Orange, Reguloid Sugar Free Regular, Restore, Restore Sugar Free, Serutan, Syllact
Func. class.: Bulk laxative
Chem. class.: Psyllium colloid

Action: Bulk-forming laxative
Uses: Chronic constipation, ulcerative colitis, irritable bowel syndrome

DOSAGE AND ROUTES

• *Adult:* **PO** 1-2 tsp in 8 oz H_2O bid or tid, then 8 oz H_2O or 1 premeasured packet in 8 oz H_2O bid or tid, then 8 oz H_2O

• *Child >6 yr:* **PO** 1 tsp in 4 oz H_2O at bedtime

Available forms: Chew pieces 1.7, 3.4 g/piece; effervescent powder 3.4, 3.7 g/packet; powder 3.3, 3.4, 3.5, 4.94 g/tsp; wafers 3.4 g/wafer

SIDE EFFECTS

GI: Nausea, vomiting, anorexia, diarrhea, cramps, intestinal esophageal blockage

Contraindications: Hypersensitivity, intestinal obstruction, abdominal pain, nausea/vomiting, fecal impaction

Precautions: Pregnancy (C)

PHARMACOKINETICS

Onset 12-72 hr, excreted in feces, not absorbed in GI tract

INTERACTIONS

Decrease: absorption of cardiac glycosides, oral anticoagulants, salicylates

Drug/Herb

Increase: laxative effect—flax, senna

NURSING CONSIDERATIONS

Assess:

• Blood, urine electrolytes if used often

• I&O ratio to identify fluid loss

• Cause of constipation; fluids, bulk, exercise missing

• Cramping, rectal bleeding, nausea, vomiting; product should be discontinued

Administer:

PO route

• Alone for better absorption, separate from other products by 1-2 hr

• In morning or evening (oral dose)

• Immediately after mixing with H_2O

• With 8 oz H_2O or juice followed by another 8 oz of fluid

Evaluate:

• Therapeutic response: decrease in constipation or decreased diarrhea in colitis

Teach patient/family:

• To maintain adequate fluid consumption

• That normal bowel movements do not always occur daily

• Not to use in presence of abdominal pain, nausea, vomiting

• To notify prescriber if constipation unrelieved or if symptoms of electrolyte imbalance occur: muscle cramps, pain, weakness, dizziness, excessive thirst

pyrantel (OTC)

(pie-ran'tel)

Antiminth, Ascarel, Combantrin ✦, Pin-Rid, Pin-X, Reese's Pinworm

Func. class.: Anthelmintic

Chem. class.: Pyrimidine derivative

Action: Causes paralysis in worm by neuroblockade via stimulation of ganglionic receptors; worms expelled by normal peristalsis

Uses: Pinworms (enterobiasis), roundworms, hairworms, trichinosis

Unlabeled uses: Ascariasis, trichostrongyliasis uncinariasis (hookworm)

DOSAGE AND ROUTES

• *Adult and child ≥2 yr and ≥25 lb:* **PO** 11 mg/kg as single dose (pinworms); × 3 days (hookworms); max 1 g; repeat in 2 wk for pinworms; 10 mg/kg/day × 4 days (trichinosis)

Available forms: Oral susp 50 mg/ml, 144 mg/ml; liquid 50 mg/ml; tabs 180, 250 mg

SIDE EFFECTS

CNS: Dizziness, headache, drowsiness, insomnia, fever, weakness

GI: Nausea, vomiting, anorexia, diarrhea, distention, abdominal cramps

INTEG: Rash

Contraindications: Hypersensitivity

Precautions: Pregnancy (C), children <2 yr, seizure disorders, hepatic disease, dehydration, anemia, malnutrition

PHARMACOKINETICS

PO: Peak 1-3 hr; metabolized in liver; excreted in feces, urine (unchanged/metabolites)

INTERACTIONS

- Antagonizes effect of pyrantel: piperazine

NURSING CONSIDERATIONS

Assess:

- Stools during entire treatment; specimens must be sent to lab while still warm
- For diarrhea during expulsion of worms
- For allergic reaction: rash

Administer:

- Without regard to food
- After shaking suspension

Perform/provide:

- Storage in tight, light-resistant container in cool environment

Evaluate:

- Therapeutic response: expulsion of worms, 3 negative stool cultures after completion of treatment

Teach patient/family:

- Proper hygiene after BM, including hand-washing technique; tell patient not to put fingers in mouth
- That infected person should sleep alone; not to shake bed linen; to change bed linen daily, wash in hot water; that all family members should be treated for pinworms; treat dogs/cats; keep children away from animal's feces
- To clean toilet daily with disinfectant (green soap solution)
- The need for compliance with dosage schedule, duration of treatment
- To drink fruit juice to help expel worms
- To wear shoes, wash all fruits, vegetables well before eating

pyrazinamide (℞)

(peer-a-zin'a-mide)
PMS Pyrazinamide ♣, pyrazinamide, Tebrazid ♣

Func. class.: Antitubercular agent
Chem. class.: Pyrazinoic acid amine, nicoturimide analog

Action: Bactericidal interference with lipid, nucleic acid biosynthesis

Uses: Tuberculosis, as an adjunct when other products are not feasible

DOSAGE AND ROUTES

HIV negative

- *Adult:* **PO** 15-30 mg/kg/day, max 2 g/day
- *Child:* **PO** 7.5-15 mg/kg bid or 15-30 mg/kg/day, max 2 g

HIV positive

- *Adult:* **PO** 15-30 mg/kg/day, max 2 g × 2 mo used with a rifamycin
- *Child:* **PO** 20-40 mg/kg/day, max 2 g/day × 2 mo given with a rifamycin

Renal dose

- *Adult:* **PO** CCr 10-50 ml/min, give dose q48-72hr; CCr <10 ml/min, give dose q72hr

Available forms: Tabs 500 mg

SIDE EFFECTS

CNS: Headache
GI: **Hepatotoxicity,** abnormal hepatic studies, peptic ulcer, nausea, vomiting, anorexia, cramps, diarrhea
GU: Urinary difficulty, increased uric acid
HEMA: **Hemolytic anemia**
INTEG: Photosensitivity, urticaria

Contraindications: Hypersensitivity, severe hepatic damage, acute gout

Precautions: Pregnancy (C), children <13 yr, renal failure, diabetes, porphyria, chronic gout

PHARMACOKINETICS

Peak 2 hr, half-life 9-10 hr; metabolized in liver, excreted in urine (metabolites/unchanged product)

INTERACTIONS

Drug/Lab Test

Increase: PBI

Decrease: 17-KS

NURSING CONSIDERATIONS

Assess:

- Signs of anemia: Hct, Hgb, fatigue
- Temp; if >101° F (38° C), product should be reduced

⚠ Hepatic studies q wk: ALT, AST, bilirubin

- Renal status before, q mo: BUN, creatinine, output, specific gravity, urinalysis, uric acid
- Hepatic status: decreased appetite, jaundice, dark urine, fatigue

Administer:

- With meals for GI symptoms
- After C&S is completed; q mo to detect resistance

Evaluate:

- Therapeutic response: decreased symptoms of TB, culture negative

Teach patient/family:

- That compliance with dosage schedule, length is necessary
- To avoid alcohol
- To report fever, loss of appetite, malaise, nausea, vomiting, darkened urine, pale stools

pyridostigmine (℞)

(peer-id-oh-stig′meen)

Mestinon, Mestinon SR, Mestinon Timespan, Regonol

Func. class.: Cholinergic; anticholinesterase

Chem. class.: Tertiary amine carbamate

Action: Inhibits destruction of acetylcholine, which increases concentration at sites where acetylcholine is released; this facilitates transmission of impulses across myoneural junction

Uses: Nondepolarizing muscle relaxant antagonist, myasthenia gravis

DOSAGE AND ROUTES

Myasthenia gravis

- *Adult:* **PO** 600 mg/day in 5-6 divided doses, max 1.5 g/day; **IM/IV** 2 mg or 1/30 of **PO** dose; **SUS REL** 180-540 mg/day or bid at intervals of at least 6 hr
- *Child:* **PO** 7 mg/kg/day in 5-6 divided doses; **IM/IV** 0.05-0.15 mg/kg/dose

Nondepolarizing neuromuscular blocker antagonist

- *Adult:* 0.6-1.2 mg **IV** atropine, then 0.1-0.25 mg/kg/dose
- *Child:* **IV** 0.1-0.25 mg/kg/dose

Available forms: Tabs 60 mg; ext rel tabs 180 mg; syr 60 mg/5 ml; inj 5 mg/ml

SIDE EFFECTS

CNS: Dizziness, headache, sweating, weakness, **seizures,** incoordination, **paralysis,** drowsiness, LOC

CV: Tachycardia, dysrhythmias, bradycardia, AV block, hypotension, ECG changes, **cardiac arrest,** syncope

EENT: Miosis, blurred vision, lacrimation, visual changes

GI: Nausea, diarrhea, vomiting, cramps, increased salivary and gastric secretions, peristalsis

GU: Urinary frequency, incontinence, urgency

INTEG: Rash, urticaria, flushing

RESP: **Respiratory depression, bronchospasm, constriction, laryngospasm, respiratory arrest**

SYST: **Cholinergic crisis**

Contraindications: Bradycardia; hypotension; obstruction of intestine, renal system; bromide, benzyl alcohol sensitivity; adrenal insufficiency; cholinesterase inhibitor toxicity

Precautions: Pregnancy (C), seizure disorders, bronchial asthma, coronary occlusion, hyperthyroidism, dysrhythmias, peptic ulcer, megacolon, poor GI motility

PHARMACOKINETICS

Metabolized in liver, excreted in urine (unchanged)

PO: Onset 20-30 min, duration 3-6 hr

PO-EXT REL: Onset 30-60 min, duration 6-12 hr
IM/IV/SUBCUT: Onset 2-15 min, duration 2½-4 hr

INTERACTIONS

Increase: action—decamethonium, succinylcholine
Decrease: action—gallamine, metocurine, pancuronium, tubocurarine, atropine
Decrease: pyridostigmine action—aminoglycosides, anesthetics, procainamide, quinidine, mecamylamine, polymyxin, magnesium, corticosteroids, antidysrhythmics, quinolones
Drug/Herb
Increase: effect—jaborandi tree, pill-bearing spurge

NURSING CONSIDERATIONS

Assess:
- VS, respiration q8hr
- I&O ratio; check for urinary retention or incontinence
- Bradycardia, hypotension, bronchospasm, headache, dizziness, seizures, respiratory depression; product should be discontinued if toxicity occurs

Administer:
- Do not break, crush, or chew sus rel tabs
- Only with atropine sulfate available for cholinergic crisis
- Only after all other cholinergics have been discontinued
- Increased doses for tolerance, as ordered
- Larger doses after exercise or fatigue, as ordered
- On empty stomach for better absorption

IV route
- Undiluted, give through Y-tube or 3-way stopcock, give 0.5 mg or less/min

Syringe compatibilities: Glycopyrrolate
Y-site compatibilities: Heparin, hydrocortisone, potassium chloride, vit B/C

Perform/provide:
- Storage at room temperature

Evaluate:
- Therapeutic response: increased muscle strength, hand grasp, improved gait, absence of labored breathing (if severe)

Teach patient/family:
- That product is not a cure, only relieves symptoms
- To wear emergency ID specifying myasthenia gravis, products taken
- To avoid driving, other hazardous activities until effect is known
- To report muscle weakness (cholinergic crisis or underdosage), bradycardia
- Not to drink alcohol
- To take with food to decrease gastric side effects

Treatment of overdose: Discontinue product, atropine 1-4 mg IV

pyridoxine (vit B_6)

(℞, OTC)
(peer-i-dox′een)
Beesix, Doxine, Nestrex, pyridoxine HCl, Pyri, Rodex, Vitabee 6, vitamin B_6
Func. class.: Vit B_6, water soluble

P

Action: Needed for fat, protein, carbohydrate metabolism; enhances glycogen release from liver and muscle tissue; needed as coenzyme for metabolic transformations of a variety of amino acids
Uses: Vit B_6 deficiency of inborn errors of metabolism, seizures, isoniazid therapy, oral contraceptives, alcoholic polyneuritis
Unlabeled uses: Palmar-Plantar erythrodysesthesia syndrome

DOSAGE AND ROUTES

RDA
- *Adult:* **PO** (male) 1.7-2 mg; (female) 1.4-1.6 mg
- *Child 1-3 yr:* **PO** 0.5 mg/day
- *Child 4-8 yr:* **PO** 0.6 mg/day
- *Child 9-13 yr:* **PO** 1 mg/day

• *Infant 7-12 mo:* **PO** 0.3 mg

Vit B_6 deficiency

• *Adult:* **PO/IM/IV** 5-25 mg/day × 3 wk

• *Child:* **PO/IM/IV** 10 mg until desired response

Deficiency caused by isoniazid, cycloSERINE, hydrALAZINE, penicillamine

• *Adult:* **PO** 100-300 mg/day

• *Child:* **PO** 10-50 mg/day

Prevention of deficiency caused by isoniazid, cycloSERINE, hydrALAZINE, penicillamine

• *Adult:* **PO** 25-100 mg/day

• *Child:* **PO** 1-2 mg/kg/day

Palmar-Plantar erythrodysesthesia syndrome (unlabeled)

• *Adult:* **PO** 50-150 mg/day

Available forms: Tabs 10, 25, 50, 100 mg; ext rel tabs 100 mg; inj 100 mg/ml; ext rel caps 150 mg

SIDE EFFECTS

CNS: Paresthesia, flushing, warmth, lethargy (rare with normal renal function)

INTEG: Pain at inj site

Contraindications: Hypersensitivity

Precautions: Pregnancy (A), breastfeeding, children, Parkinson's disease, patients taking levodopa should avoid supplemental vitamins with >5 mg pyridoxine

PHARMACOKINETICS

PO/INJ: Half-life 2-3 wk, metabolized in liver, excreted in urine

INTERACTIONS

Decrease: effects of levodopa

Decrease: effects of pyridoxine—oral contraceptives, isoniazid, cycloSERINE, hydrALAZINE, penicillamine, chloramphenicol, immunosuppressants

NURSING CONSIDERATIONS

Assess:

• Pyridoxine levels throughout treatment

• Nutritional status: yeast, liver, legumes, bananas, green vegetables, whole grains

• Neurologic status: paresthesia, lethargy

• Blood studies: Hct, Hgb

Administer:

PO route

• Do not break, crush, or chew ext rel tabs/caps

IM route

• Rotate sites; burning or stinging at site may occur

• Z-track to minimize pain

IV route

• Undiluted or added to most IV sol; give 50 mg or less/1 min if undiluted

Syringe compatibilities: Doxapram

Perform/provide:

• Storage in tight, light-resistant container

Evaluate:

• Therapeutic response: absence of nausea, vomiting, anorexia, skin lesions, glossitis, stomatitis, edema, seizures, restlessness, paresthesia

Teach patient/family:

• To avoid vitamin supplements unless directed by prescriber

• To keep out of children's reach

• To increase meat, bananas, potatoes, lima beans, whole grain cereals in diet

• To discuss birth control status with prescriber

pyrimethamine (℞)

(peer-i-meth'a-meen)

Daraprim, Fansidar (with sulfadoxine)

Func. class.: Antimalarial, antiprotozoal

Chem. class.: Folic acid antagonist

Action: Inhibits folic acid metabolism in parasite, prevents transmission by stopping growth of fertilized gametes

Uses: Malaria prophylaxis, *Plasmodium vivax, Pneumocystis jiroveci*

Unlabeled uses: Isosporiasis

DOSAGE AND ROUTES

Prophylaxis of malaria

Begin 2 wk before entering endemic area and continue for 6-10 wk after return

- *Adult and child >10 yr:* **PO** 25 mg q wk
- *Child 4-10 yr:* **PO** 12.5 mg q wk
- *Child <4 yr:* **PO** 6.25 mg q wk

Toxoplasmosis
- *Adult:* **PO** 50-75 mg, then reduce by about 50% for 4-5 wk, with 1-4 g sulfadoxine × 1-3 wk, then reduce by 50% for 4-5 wk
- *Child:* **PO** 1 mg/kg/day in 2 divided doses or 2 mg/kg/day × 3 days, then 1 mg/kg/day or divided twice daily × 4 wk, max 25 mg/day

Toxoplasmosis in AIDS patients
- *Adult:* **PO** 100-200 mg/day × 1-2 days, then 50-100 mg/day × 3-6 wk, then 25-50 mg/day for life (given with clindamycin or sulfADIAZINE)

Isosporiasis (unlabeled)
- *Adult:* **PO** 75 mg/day with leucovorin 10 mg/day × 14 days

Available forms: Tabs 25 mg; combo tabs 500 mg sulfadoxine/25 mg pyrimethamine

SIDE EFFECTS

CNS: Stimulation, irritability, **seizures,** tremors, ataxia, fatigue, fever
CV: **Dysrhythmias**
GI: Nausea, vomiting, cramps, anorexia, diarrhea, atrophic glossitis, gastritis
HEMA: **Thrombocytopenia, leukopenia, pancytopenia, megaloblastic anemia,** decreased folic acid, **agranulocytosis**
INTEG: Skin eruptions, photosensitivity, **Stevens-Johnson syndrome**
RESP: **Respiratory failure**

Contraindications: Hypersensitivity, chloroquine-resistant malaria, megaloblastic anemia caused by folate deficiency
Precautions: Pregnancy (C), breastfeeding, geriatric patients, blood dyscrasias, seizure disorder, G6PD disease, renal/hepatic disease

PHARMACOKINETICS

PO: Peak 2 hr, half-life 96 hr, half-life accelerated to 23 hr in AIDS patients, metabolized in liver, highly protein bound, excreted in urine (metabolites)

INTERACTIONS

- Synergistic action: folic acid

Increase: risk of megaloblastic anemia, agranulocytosis, thrombocytopenia—zidovudine
Increase: bone marrow suppression—bone marrow depressants, folate antagonists, radiation therapy

NURSING CONSIDERATIONS

Assess:
- Folic acid level; megaloblastic anemia occurs
- ⚠ Blood studies, CBC, platelets, since blood dyscrasias occur; twice weekly if dosage is increased
- ⚠ For toxicity: vomiting, anorexia, seizure, blood dyscrasia, glossitis; product should be discontinued immediately

Administer:
- Leucovorin IM 3-9 mg/day × 3 days if folic acid deficiency occurs
- Before or after meals at same time each day to maintain product level, to decrease GI symptoms

Perform/provide:
- Storage in tight, light-resistant container

Evaluate:
- Therapeutic response: decreased symptoms of malaria

Teach patient/family:
- To report visual problems, fever, fatigue, bruising, bleeding; may indicate blood dyscrasias
- To report immediately skin rash; stop use

Treatment of overdose: Gastric lavage, short-acting barbiturate, leucovorin, respiratory support if needed

quetiapine (℞)
(kwe-tie′a-peen)
Seroquel, Seroquel XR
Func. class.: Antipsychotic
Chem. class.: Dibenzodiazepine

Action: Functions as an antagonist at multiple neurotransmitter receptors in the brain including $5HT_{1A}$, $5HT_2$, DOPamine

Q

D_1, D_2, H_1, and adrenergic α_1, α_2 receptors

Uses: Bipolar disorder, bipolar I disorder, depression, mania, schizophrenia

Unlabeled uses: Agitation, dementia, OCD

DOSAGE AND ROUTES

Bipolar I disorder

• *Adult:* **PO** (Monotherapy or as adjunct to lithium or divalproex) 50 mg bid on day 1, 100 mg on day 2 in 2 divided doses as tolerated to 400 mg/day on day 4, range 400-800 mg/day

Psychotic disorders

• *Adult:* **PO** 25 mg bid, titrate upward; (XR) 300 mg/day in PM, range 400-800 mg/day

Available forms: Tabs 25, 50, 100, 200, 300, 400 mg; ext rel tab 200, 300, 400 mg

SIDE EFFECTS

CNS: EPS, pseudoparkinsonism, akathisia, dystonia, tardive dyskinesia; *drowsiness,* insomnia, agitation, anxiety, *headache,* **seizures, neuroleptic malignant syndrome,** *dizziness,* dystonia, restless legs

CV: Orthostatic hypotension, **tachycardia, QT prolongation,** CV disease, Parkinson's disease, cardiomyopathy, myocarditis

ENDO: SIADH, hyperglycemia

GI: Nausea, anorexia, constipation, abdominal pain, dry mouth

HEMA: **Leukopenia, agranulocytosis**

INTEG: Rash

META: Hyponatremia

MISC: Asthenia, back pain, fever, ear pain

MS: **Rhabdomyolysis**

RESP: Rhinitis

SYST: **Stevens-Johnson syndrome, anaphylaxis**

Contraindications: Hypersensitivity

Precautions: Pregnancy (C), breastfeeding, geriatric patients, hepatic/cardiac disease, breast cancer, long-term use, seizures, QT prolongation, brain tumor, hematological disease, torsade de pointes, cataracts, dehydration

Black Box Warning: Children (suicide), dementia

PHARMACOKINETICS

Extensively metabolized by liver half-life ≥6 hr, peak 1½ hr, inhibits P450 CYP3A4 enzyme system, 83% protein binding

INTERACTIONS

⚠ ***Increase:*** QT prolongation—class IA/III antidysrhythmics, some phenothiazines, β-agonists, local anesthetics, tricyclics, bepridil, haloperidol, methadone, chloroquine, clarithromycin, droperidol, erythromycin, grepafloxacin, halofantrine, pentamidine, probucol, sparfloxacin

Increase: CNS depression—alcohol, opioid analgesics, sedative/hypnotics, antihistamines

Increase: quetiapine clearance—phenytoin, thioridazine, barbiturates, glucocorticoids, carbamazepine, rifampin

Increase: quetiapine action—fluconazole, itraconazole, ketoconazole (CYP3A4 inhibitors)

Increase: effects of erythromycin

Decrease: quetiapine clearance—cimetidine

Decrease: effects of DOPamine agonists, levodopa, lorazepam

Drug/Herb

Increase: action—cola tree, hops, nettle, nutmeg

Increase: EPS—betel palm, kava

NURSING CONSIDERATIONS

Assess:

⚠ CV status: QT prolongation, tachycardia, orthostatic B/P

• Mental status before initial administration, AIMS assessment

• Swallowing of PO medication: check for hoarding or giving of medication to other patients

• Baseline blood glucose, LFTs, neurostatus, ophthalmologic exam, cholesterol profile, weight

• Affect, orientation, LOC, reflexes, gait, coordination, sleep pattern disturbances
• B/P standing and lying; also pulse, respirations; take these q4hr during initial treatment; establish baseline before starting treatment; report drops of 30 mm Hg; watch for ECG changes
• Dizziness, faintness, palpitations, tachycardia on rising
• EPS, including akathisia (inability to sit still, no pattern to movements), tardive dyskinesia (bizarre movements of the jaw, mouth, tongue, extremities), pseudoparkinsonism (rigidity, tremors, pill rolling, shuffling gait)

⚠ For neuroleptic malignant syndrome: hyperthermia, increased CPK, altered mental status, muscle rigidity, seizures, tachycardia, diaphoresis, hypo/hypertension, fatigue; notify prescriber immediately if symptoms occur
• Skin turgor daily
• Constipation, urinary retention daily; if these occur, increase bulk and water in the diet

Administer:
• Reduced dose in geriatric patients
• Anticholinergic agent on order from prescriber, to be used for EPS
• Avoid use of CNS depressants

Perform/provide:
• Decreased stimulus by dimming lights, avoiding loud noises
• Supervised ambulation until patient is stabilized on medication; do not involve in strenuous exercise program because fainting is possible; patient should not stand still for a long time
• Sips of water, sugarless candy, gum for dry mouth
• Storage in tight, light-resistant container

Evaluate:
• Therapeutic response: decrease in emotional excitement, hallucinations, delusions, paranoia; reorganization of patterns of thought, speech

Teach patient/family:
• To rise slowly, to prevent orthostatic hypotension
• To take medication only as prescribed
• If drowsiness occurs, avoid hazardous activities such as driving
• To avoid use of OTC meds unless directed by prescriber
• To notify prescriber if pregnancy is planned, suspected
• To notify prescriber immediately of fever, difficulty breathing, fatigue

quinapril (℞)

(kwin′a-pril)
Accupril
Func. class.: Antihypertensive
Chem. class.: Angiotensin-converting enzyme (ACE) inhibitor

Action: Selectively suppresses renin-angiotensin-aldosterone system; inhibits ACE, prevents conversion of angiotensin I to angiotensin II; results in dilation of arterial, venous vessels

Uses: Hypertension, alone or in combination with thiazide diuretics; systolic CHF

DOSAGE AND ROUTES

Hypertension (monotherapy)
• *Adult:* **PO** 10-20 mg/day initially, then 20-80 mg/day divided bid or daily
• *Geriatric:* **PO** 10 mg/day, titrate to desired response

Congestive heart failure
• *Adult:* **PO** 5 mg bid, may increase q wk until 20-40 mg/day in 2 divided doses

Renal dose
• *Adult:* **PO** CCr 30-60 ml/min 5 mg/day initially; CCr <30 ml/min 2.5 mg/day initially

Available forms: Tabs 5, 10, 20, 40 mg

SIDE EFFECTS

CNS: Headache, dizziness, fatigue, somnolence, depression, malaise, nervousness, vertigo

CV: Hypotension, postural hypotension, syncope, palpitations, angina pectoris, **MI, tachycardia,** vasodilation, chest pain

GI: Nausea, diarrhea, constipation, *vomiting,* gastritis, **GI hemorrhage,** dry mouth

GU: Increased BUN, creatinine, decreased libido, impotence
HEMA: **Thrombocytopenia, agranulocytosis**
INTEG: **Angioedema,** rash, sweating, photosensitivity, pruritus
META: Hyperkalemia
MISC: Back pain, amblyopia
MS: Myalgia
RESP: *Cough,* pharyngitis, dyspnea

Contraindications: Children, hypersensitivity to ACE inhibitors, angioedema

Black Box Warning: Pregnancy (D)

Precautions: Breastfeeding, geriatric patients, impaired renal/hepatic function, dialysis patients, hypovolemia, blood dyscrasias, COPD, bilateral renal stenosis, asthma, cough

PHARMACOKINETICS

Bioavailability ≥60%, onset <1 hr, peak 1-2 hr, duration 24 hr, serum protein binding 97%, half-life 2 hr, metabolized by liver (active metabolites quinaprilat), metabolites excreted in urine (60%)/feces (37%)

INTERACTIONS

• Use caution with vasodilators, hydrALAZINE, prazosin, potassium-sparing diuretics, sympathomimetics, potassium supplements

Increase: hypotension—diuretics, other antihypertensives, ganglionic blockers, adrenergic blockers, phenothiazines, nitrates, acute alcohol ingestion
Increase: toxicity of lithium, digoxin
Decrease: absorption of tetracycline
Decrease: hypotensive effect of quinapril—indomethacin

Drug/Herb

Increase: toxicity, death—aconite
Increase: antihypertensive effect—barberry, betony, black catechu, black cohosh, bloodroot, broom, burdock, cat's claw, dandelion, goldenseal, hawthorn, Irish moss, Jamaican dogwood, kelp, khella, mistletoe, parsley
Increase or decrease: antihypertensive effect—astragalus, cola tree
Decrease: antihypertensive effect—coltsfoot, guarana, khat, licorice, yohimbe

Drug/Lab Test

False positive: urine acetone, ANA titer

NURSING CONSIDERATIONS

Assess:

⚠ Blood studies: neutrophils, decreased platelets; WBC with differential baseline and periodically q3mo; if neutrophils <1000/mm^3, discontinue treatment (recommended in collagen-vascular disease)
• B/P, orthostatic hypotension, syncope
• Renal studies: protein, BUN, creatinine; watch for increased levels; may indicate nephrotic syndrome
• Baselines in renal, hepatic studies before therapy begins and periodically; increased LFTs; uric acid and glucose may be increased
• Potassium levels; hyperkalemia is rare
• Edema in feet, legs daily, weight daily in CHF
⚠ Allergic reactions: rash, fever, pruritus, urticaria; product should be discontinued if antihistamines fail to help
• Renal symptoms: oliguria, urinary frequency, dysuria

Administer:

• Tabs may be crushed if necessary
• Take 1-2 hr before food or antacids; avoid high-potassium foods

Evaluate:

• Therapeutic response: decrease in B/P

Teach patient/family:

• Not to discontinue product abruptly
• Not to use OTC products (cough, cold, allergy); not to use salt substitutes containing potassium unless directed by prescriber
• To comply with dosage schedule, even if feeling better
• To rise slowly to sitting or standing position to minimize orthostatic hypotension
• To notify prescriber of mouth sores, sore throat, fever, swelling of hands or feet, irregular heartbeat, chest pain, persistent dry cough

- To report excessive perspiration, dehydration, vomiting, diarrhea; may lead to fall in B/P
- That product may cause dizziness, fainting, light-headedness; may occur during first few days of therapy
- That product may cause skin rash or impaired taste perception
- How to take B/P, and normal readings for age-group

Treatment of overdose: 0.9% NaCl IV inf

quinidine (℞)
(kwin'i-deen)

quinidine gluconate (℞)
Quinaglute Dura-Tabs, Quinalan, Quinate ✤

quinidine polygalacturonate (℞)
Cardioquin

quinidine sulfate (℞)
Apo-Quinidine ✤, Cin-Quin, Novoquinidine ✤, Quinidex Extentabs, Quinora

Func. class.: Antidysrhythmic (Class IA)
Chem. class.: Quinine dextroisomer

Action: Prolongs duration of action potential and effective refractory period, thus decreasing myocardial excitability; anticholinergic properties

Uses: PVCs, atrial fibrillation, PAT, ventricular tachycardia, atrial flutter, malaria/IV quinidine gluconate

DOSAGE AND ROUTES

Quinidine gluconate

- *Adult:* **PO** (sus rel) 324-648 mg q8-12hr; **IM** 600 mg, then 400 mg q2hr; **IV** give 16 mg/min

Quinidine sulfate

Atrial fibrillation/flutter

- *Adult:* **PO** 200 mg q2-3hr × 5-8 doses; may increase daily until sinus rhythm is restored; max 4 g/day given only after digitalization; maintenance 200-300 mg tid-qid or **SUS REL** 300-600 mg q8-12hr

Paroxysmal supraventricular tachycardia

- *Adult:* **PO** 400-600 mg q2-3hr, then 200-300 mg q6-8hr or **SUS REL** 300-600 mg q8-12hr

Premature atrial/ventricular contraction

- *Adult:* **PO** 200-300 mg q6-8hr or **SUS REL** 300-600 mg q8-12hr; max 4 g/day
- *Child:* **PO** 30 mg/kg/day or 900 mg/m^2/day in 5 divided doses

Available forms: *Gluconate:* sus rel tabs 324, 330 mg; inj gluconate 80 mg/ml; *sulfate:* tabs 200, 300 mg; sus rel tabs 300 mg; *polygalacturonate:* tabs 275 mg

SIDE EFFECTS

CNS: Headache, dizziness, involuntary movement, confusion, psychosis, restlessness, irritability, syncope, excitement, depression, ataxia

CV: **Hypotension,** *bradycardia,* PVCs, **heart block, CV collapse, arrest,** torsades de pointes, widening QRS complex, **ventricular tachycardia**

EENT: Cinchonism: tinnitus, blurred vision, hearing loss, mydriasis, disturbed color vision

GI: Nausea, vomiting, anorexia, abdominal pain, *diarrhea,* **hepatotoxicity**

HEMA: **Thrombocytopenia,** hemolytic anemia, **agranulocytosis,** hypoprothrombinemia

INTEG: Rash, urticaria, **angioedema,** swelling, photosensitivity, flushing with severe pruritus

RESP: Dyspnea, **respiratory depression**

Contraindications: Hypersensitivity, or idiosyncratic response, digoxin toxicity, blood dyscrasias, myasthenia gravis

Black Box Warning: History of long QT syndrome, product-induced torsades de pointes, severe heart block

Precautions: Pregnancy (C), breastfeeding, children, geriatric patients, potassium imbalance, renal/hepatic disease,

Q

CHF, respiratory depression, bradycardia, hypotension, syncope

Black Box Warning: Cardiac arrhythmias, MI

PHARMACOKINETICS

PO: Peak 0.5-6 hr, duration 6-8 hr, half-life 6-7 hr, metabolized in liver, excreted unchanged (10%-50%) by kidneys, protein bound (80%-90%)

INTERACTIONS

- Additive vagolytic effect: anticholinergic blockers
- Additive cardiac depression: other antidysrhythmics, phenothiazines, reserpine

Increase: effects of neuromuscular blockers, digoxin, warfarin, tricyclics, propranolol

Increase: quinidine effects—cimetidine, sodium bicarbonate, carbonic anhydrase inhibitors, antacids, hydroxide suspensions, amiodarone, verapamil, nifedipine

Decrease: quinidine effects—barbiturates, phenytoin, rifampin, sucralfate, cholinergics

Drug/Herb

- Hypokalemia, increased antidysrhythmic action: aloe, buckthorn, cascara sagrada, senna

Increase: toxicity, death—aconite

Increase: effect—aloe, broom, chronic buckthorn use, cascara sagrada (chronic use), Chinese rhubarb, figwort, fumitory, goldenseal, kudzu, licorice

Increase: serotonin effect—horehound

Decrease: effect—coltsfoot

Drug/Food

- Delayed absorption, decreased metabolism: grapefruit juice

Drug/Lab Test

Increase: CPK

Interference: triamterene therapy interferes with quinidine test levels

NURSING CONSIDERATIONS

Assess:

⚠ ECG continuously to determine increased PR or QRS segments, QT interval; discontinue or reduce dose

- Blood levels (therapeutic level 2-7 mcg/ml), CBC, LFTs
- B/P continuously for fluctuations

⚠ For cinchonism: tinnitus, headache, nausea, dizziness, fever, vertigo, tremor; may lead to hearing loss

- Cardiac status: rate, rhythm, character, continuously
- Respiratory status: rate, rhythm, lung fields for crackles; increased respiration, increased pulse; product should be discontinued
- CNS effects: dizziness, confusion, psychosis, paresthesias, seizures; product should be discontinued

Administer:

- AV node blocker (digoxin) before starting quinidine to avoid increased ventricular rate

PO route

- Do not break, crush, or chew ext rel products
- With a full glass of water, on empty stomach; if GI upset occurs, may take with food
- Sus rel forms not interchangeable

IM route

- IM inj in deltoid; aspirate to avoid intravascular administration

IV route

- After diluting 800 mg/50 ml or more D_5; give 16 mg or less over 1 min as inf; use inf pump

Additive compatibilities: Bretylium, cimetidine, milrinone, ranitidine, verapamil

Y-site compatibilities: Diazepam, milrinone

Evaluate:

- Therapeutic response: decreased dysrhythmias

Teach patient/family:

- That if dizziness, drowsiness occur, avoid driving or hazardous activities
- To use sunglasses; may cause sensitivity to light
- To carry emergency ID stating disease and medication use
- How to take pulse and when to notify prescriber

- To avoid OTC meds unless approved by prescriber
- To report signs of cinchonism
- To avoid using with grapefruit

quinine (℞)

(kwye'nine)

Novoquine ✦, Qualaquin, quinine sulfate

Func. class.: Antimalarial

Chem. class.: Cinchona tree alkaloid

Action: Inhibits parasite replications, transcription of DNA to RNA by forming complexes with DNA of parasite

Uses: *Plasmodium falciparum,* malaria

DOSAGE AND ROUTES

- *Adult:* **PO** 648 mg q8hr × 3 days or 7 days in SE Asia; given with tetracycline 250 mg q5hr × 7 days, or clindamycin 900 mg q8hr × 7 days or doxycycline 100 mg q12hr × 7 days
- *Child:* **PO** 25 mg/kg/day divided q8hr for 3-7 days in conjunction with another agent

Available forms: Tabs 325 mg

SIDE EFFECTS

CNS: Headache, stimulation, fatigue, irritability, **seizures,** bad dreams, dizziness, fever, confusion, anxiety

CV: Angina, dysrhythmias, tachycardia, hypotension, **acute circulatory failure**

EENT: Blurred vision, corneal changes, retinal changes, difficulty focusing, tinnitus, vertigo, deafness, photophobia, diplopia, night blindness

ENDO: Hypoglycemia

GI: Nausea, vomiting, anorexia, diarrhea, epigastric pain

GU: Renal tubular damage, **anuria**

HEMA: **Thrombocytopenia, purpura, hypothrombinemia, hemolysis**

INTEG: Pruritus, pigmentary changes, skin eruptions, lichen planuslike eruptions, flushing, facial edema, sweating

MISC: **Hemolytic uremic syndrome**

RESP: Dyspnea

Contraindications: Hypersensitivity, G6PD deficiency, retinal field changes, myasthenia gravis

Precautions: Pregnancy (C), breastfeeding, blood dyscrasias, severe GI/hepatic disease, neurologic disease, psoriasis, cardiac dysrhythmias, tinnitus, hypoglycemia, nocturnal leg cramps

PHARMACOKINETICS

Peak 1-3 hr, metabolized in liver, excreted in urine, half-life 4-11 hr

INTERACTIONS

Increase: toxicity—$NaHCO_3$, acetaZOLAMIDE

Increase: levels of digoxin, digitoxin, neuromuscular blockers, other anticoagulants

Increase: treatment failure—rifampin

Decrease: absorption—magnesium or aluminum salts (antacids)

Drug/Lab Test

Increase: 17-KS

Interference: 17-OHCS

NURSING CONSIDERATIONS

Assess:

- B/P, pulse, watch for hypotension, tachycardia
- Hepatic studies q wk: ALT, AST, bilirubin
- Blood studies, CBC, since blood dyscrasias occur
- For cinchonism: nausea, blurred vision, tinnitus, headache, difficulty focusing

Administer:

- Take with food to decrease GI upset; if a dose is missed, do not double
- Oral caps are not approved for prevention of malaria, treatment of severe malaria, or treatment/prevention of leg cramps

Perform/provide:

- Storage in tight, light-resistant container

Evaluate:

- Therapeutic response: decreased symptoms of malaria

Teach patient/family:

- Not to breastfeed while taking medication
- To avoid OTC preparations: cold preparations, tonic water

Treatment of overdose: Multiple dosages of activated charcoal

rabeprazole (℞)

(rah-bep'rah-zole)

Aciphex

Func. class.: Antiulcer, proton pump inhibitor

Chem. class.: Benzimidazole

Action: Suppresses gastric secretion by inhibiting hydrogen/potassium ATPase enzyme system in gastric parietal cell; characterized as gastric acid pump inhibitor, since it blocks final step of acid production

Uses: Gastroesophageal reflux disease (GERD), severe erosive esophagitis, poorly responsive systemic GERD, pathologic hypersecretory conditions (Zollinger-Ellison syndrome, systemic mastocytosis, multiple endocrine adenomas); treatment of active duodenal ulcers with or without antiinfectives for *Helicobacter pylori;* daytime, nighttime heartburn

Unlabeled uses: Gastric ulcer, heartburn, *H. pylori* eradication in children

DOSAGE AND ROUTES

Healing of duodenal ulcers

- *Adult:* **PO** 20 mg/day × ≤4 wk to be taken after breakfast

Healing of erosive esophagitis or ulcerative GERD

- *Adult:* **PO** 20 mg/day × 4-8 wk
- *Adolescent:* **PO** 20 mg/day up to 8 wk

Pathologic hypersecretory conditions

- *Adult:* **PO** 60 mg/day; may increase to 120 mg in 2 divided doses

Gastric ulcer (unlabeled)

- *Adult:* **PO** 20 mg/day after AM meal × 3-6 wk

Heartburn (unlabeled)

- *Adult:* **PO** 20 mg/day × up to 14 days

Available forms: Del rel tabs 20 mg

SIDE EFFECTS

CNS: Headache, dizziness, asthenia

CV: Chest pain, angina, tachycardia, bradycardia, palpitations, peripheral edema

EENT: Tinnitus, taste perversion

GI: Diarrhea, abdominal pain, vomiting, nausea, constipation, flatulence, acid regurgitation, abdominal swelling, anorexia, irritable colon, esophageal candidiasis, dry mouth

GU: UTI, urinary frequency, increased creatinine, **proteinuria, hematuria,** testicular pain, glycosuria

HEMA: **Pancytopenia, thrombocytopenia, neutropenia, leukocytosis,** anemia

INTEG: Rash, dry skin, urticaria, pruritus, alopecia

META: Hypoglycemia, increased hepatic enzymes, weight gain

MISC: Back pain, fever, fatigue, malaise

RESP: Upper respiratory tract infections, cough, epistaxis, **pneumonia**

Contraindications: Hypersensitivity

Precautions: Pregnancy (C), breastfeeding, children

PHARMACOKINETICS

Eliminated in urine as metabolites and in feces, terminal half-life 1-2 hr

INTERACTIONS

Increase: bleeding risk—warfarin

Increase: serum levels of rabeprazole—benzodiazepines, phenytoin, clarithromycin

Decrease: levels of rabeprazole—sucralfate, calcium carbonate, vit B_{12}

NURSING CONSIDERATIONS

Assess:

- GI system: bowel sounds q8hr, abdomen for pain, swelling, anorexia
- Hepatic studies: AST, ALT, alk phos during treatment

Administer:

- Do not break, crush, or chew del rel tab
- After breakfast daily with a full glass of water

Evaluate:

- Therapeutic response: absence of epigastric pain, swelling, fullness

Teach patient/family:

- To report severe diarrhea, product may have to be discontinued
- That diabetic patient should know hypoglycemia may occur
- To avoid hazardous activities; dizziness may occur
- To avoid alcohol, salicylates, NSAIDs; may cause GI irritation
- To wear sunscreen, protective clothing to prevent burns
- To use as directed for length of time prescribed

radioactive iodine (sodium iodide) ^{131}I (℞)

Func. class.: Antithyroid
Chem. class.: Radiopharmaceutical

Action: Converted to protein-bound iodine by thyroid gland for use when needed

Uses:
High dose: Thyroid cancer, hyperthyroidism
Low dose: Visualization to determine thyroid cancer, diagnostic aid in thyroid function studies

DOSAGE AND ROUTES

Thyroid cancer

- *Adult:* **PO** 50-150 mCi, may repeat depending on clinical status

Hyperthyroidism

- *Adult:* **PO** 4-10 mCi, depending on serum thyroxine level

Available forms: Caps 1-50, 0.8-100 mCi; oral sol 7.05 mCi/ml, 3.5-150 mCi/vial

SIDE EFFECTS

EENT: Sore throat, cough
ENDO: Hypothyroidism, **hyperthyroid adenoma,** transient thyroiditis, goiter
GI: Nausea, diarrhea, vomiting
HEMA: **Eosinophilia, lymphedema, leukemia, bone marrow depression, leukopenia,** anemia, lymph node swelling
INTEG: Alopecia

Contraindications: Pregnancy (X), breastfeeding, age <30 yr, recent MI, large nodular goiter, vomiting/diarrhea, acute hyperthyroidism, use of thyroid products

PHARMACOKINETICS

PO: Onset 3-6 days; excreted in urine, sweat, feces, breast milk; crosses placenta; excreted in 56 days

INTERACTIONS

- Hypothyroidism: lithium

Decrease: effect of I^{131}—amiodarone
Decrease: uptake if recent intake of stable iodine, thyroid, antithyroid products

NURSING CONSIDERATIONS

Assess:

- Weight daily with same clothing, scale, time of day
- Blood work, including CBC for blood dyscrasias (leukopenia, thrombocytopenia, agranulocytosis)
- Overdose: peripheral edema, heat intolerance, diaphoresis, palpitations, dysrhythmias, severe tachycardia, increased temp, delirium, CNS irritability
- Hypersensitivity: rash, enlarged cervical lymph nodes; product may have to be discontinued
- Hypoprothrombinemia: bleeding, petechiae, ecchymosis
- Clinical response: after 3 wk should include increased weight, pulse; decreased T_4
- Bone marrow depression: sore throat, fever, fatigue

Administer:

- Only after discontinuing all other antithyroid agents × 5-7 days

R

• After NPO overnight, food delays action
• During or within 10 days after menstruation
• Do not take antithyroid agents except propranolol, which decreases hyperthyroid symptoms, until total effect of taking ^{131}I has occurred (about 6 wk)

Perform/provide:

• Limited contact with patient ½ hr/day for each person
• Adequate rest after treatment
• Fluids to 3-4 L/day for 48 hr to remove agent from body

Evaluate:

• Therapeutic response: weight gain, decreased pulse, decreased T_4, B/P

Teach patient/family:

• To empty bladder often during treatment; avoid irradiation of gonads
• To report redness, swelling, sore throat, mouth lesions; indicate blood dyscrasias
• To avoid extended contact with children, spouse for 1 wk
• That bathroom may be used by entire family
• To avoid coughing, expectorating for 24 hr (saliva and vomitus are highly radioactive for 6-8 hr)

raloxifene (℞)

(ral-ox′ih-feen)

Evista

Func. class.: Hormone modifier, selective estrogen receptor modulator (SERM)

Chem. class.: Benzothiophene

Action: Tissue-selective estrogen agonist/antagonist; agonist activity in bone and lipid metabolism; antagonist activity on breast and uterus; reduces resorption of bone and decreases bone turnover

Uses: Prevention, treatment of osteoporosis in postmenopausal women; breast cancer prophylaxis

Unlabeled uses: Uterine leiomyomata in postmenopausal women with osteoporosis or in postmenopausal women who are at high risk for developing the disease

DOSAGE AND ROUTES

• *Adult:* **PO** 60 mg/day, max 60 mg/day

Available forms: Tabs 60 mg

SIDE EFFECTS

CNS: Insomnia, **CVA**

CV: Hot flashes, peripheral edema, **thromboembolism**

EENT: Retinal vein occlusion (rare)

GI: *Nausea,* vomiting, diarrhea, dyspepsia

GU: Vaginitis, leukorrhea, cystitis, *hot flashes,* vaginal bleeding

INTEG: Rash, sweating

META: Weight gain, peripheral edema

MS: Arthralgia, myalgia, *leg cramps,* arthritis

RESP: Sinusitis, pharyngitis, increased cough, pneumonia, laryngitis, bronchitis, **pulmonary embolism,** flulike symptoms

Contraindications: Pregnancy (X), breastfeeding, hypersensitivity

Black Box Warning: Women with active or history of venous thromboembolic events

Precautions: CV/hepatic disease, cervical/uterine cancer, elevated triglycerides, pulmonary embolism

Black Box Warning: Stroke

PHARMACOKINETICS

Elimination half-life 28-32 hr, excreted in feces, excreted in breast milk, highly bound to plasma proteins

INTERACTIONS

• Administer cautiously with other highly protein-bound products

Decrease: action of anticoagulants, thyroid replacement hormones

Decrease: action of raloxifene—ampicillin, cholestyramine

Drug/Food

Decrease: raloxifene—soy

NURSING CONSIDERATIONS

Assess:

- Weight daily, notify prescriber of weekly weight gain >5 lb
- B/P, watch for increase caused by H_2O and sodium retention
- I&O ratio; decreasing urinary output, increasing edema
- Hepatic studies, including AST, ALT, bilirubin, alk phos
- Bone density test baseline and throughout treatment, bone-specific alk phos

Administer:

- Without regard to meals, vit D
- Add calcium supplement if inadequate

Evaluate:

- Therapeutic response: prevention, treatment of osteoporosis

Teach patient/family:

- To weigh weekly, report gain >5 lb
- To discontinue 72 hr before prolonged bedrest; advise to avoid one position for long periods
- To take calcium supplements, vit D if intake is inadequate
- To increase exercise using weights
- To stop smoking and to decrease alcohol consumption
- That this product does not help control hot flashes
- To report fever, acute migraine, insomnia, emotional distress; urinary tract infection, or vaginal burning/itching; swelling, warmth, or pain in calves

raltegravir (℞)

(ral-teg′ra-vir)

Isentress

Func. class.: Antiretroviral

Chem. class.: HIV integrase strand transfer inhibitor (ISTIs)

Action: Inhibits catalytic activity of HIV integrase, which is an HIV encoded enzyme needed for replication

Uses: HIV in combination with other antiretrovirals

DOSAGE AND ROUTES

- *Adult and adolescent ≥16 yr:* **PO** 400 mg bid, max 800 mg/day with or without food

Available forms: Tabs 400 mg

SIDE EFFECTS

CNS: Fatigue, fever, *dizziness, headache,* asthenia, **suicidal ideation**

CV: **MI**

GI: Nausea, vomiting, diarrhea, abdominal pain, asthenia, gastritis, **hepatitis**

GU: **Oliguria, proteinuria, hematuria, glomerulonephritis, acute renal failure, renal tubular necrosis**

HEMA: **Anemia, neutropenia**

INTEG: Rash, urticaria, pruritus, pain or phlebitis at IV site, unusual sweating, alopecia

META: Hyperamylasia, hyperglycemia

MS: Myopathy, **rhabdomyolysis**

Contraindications: Breastfeeding, hypersensitivity

Precautions: Pregnancy (C), children, geriatric patients, hepatic disease, immune reconstitution syndrome, hepatitis, antimicrobial resistance, lactase deficiency

PHARMACOKINETICS

Max absorption 3 hr if taken on an empty stomach; terminal half-life 9 hr; metabolized in the liver, excreted feces 51%, urine 32%

INTERACTIONS

Increase: raltegravir effect—proton pump inhibitors, H_2 blockers

Increase: rhabdomyolysis, myopathy, elevated CPK—fibric acid derivatives, HMG-CoA reductase inhibitors

Decrease: raltegravir levels—rifampin, efavirenz, emtricitabine, tenofovir

NURSING CONSIDERATIONS

Assess:

- Signs of infection, anemia
- Resistance testing prior to therapy and at treatment failure

• Blood studies: CD4, T-cell count, plasma HIV RNA, viral load
• Skin eruptions: rash, urticaria, itching
• Allergies before treatment, reaction of each medication; place allergies on chart in bright red letters

Administer:
• Do not break, crush, or chew tabs
• May give without regard to meals, with 8 oz of water

Perform/provide:
• Storage at room temperature

Evaluate:
• Therapeutic response: improvement in CD4 counts

Teach patient/family:
• To take as prescribed; if dose is missed, take as soon as remembered up to 1 hr before next dose; do not double dose
• That sexual partners need to be told that patient has HIV
• That product does not cure infection, just controls symptoms and does not prevent infecting others
⚠ To report sore throat, fever, fatigue (may indicate superinfection)
• That product must be taken in equal intervals around the clock to maintain blood levels for duration of therapy

ramelteon (℞)

(rah-mel'tee-on)
Rozerem
Func. class.: Sedative/hypnotic, antianxiety
Chem. class.: Melatonin receptor agonist

Action: Binds selectively to melatonin receptors (MT_1, MT_2); thought to be involved in circadian rhythm and the normal sleep/wake cycle

Uses: Insomnia

DOSAGE AND ROUTES

• *Adult:* **PO** 8 mg at bedtime

Hepatic dose
• Do not use in severe hepatic disease; use with caution in mild to moderate hepatic disease

Available forms: Tabs 8 mg

SIDE EFFECTS

CNS: Dizziness, somnolence, fatigue, headache, insomnia, depression, complex sleep-related reactions: sleep driving, sleep eating
GI: Nausea, diarrhea, dysgeusia, vomiting
MISC: Myalgia, arthralgia, decreased blood cortisol, influenza, upper RI
SYST: **Severe allergic reactions, angioedema**

Contraindications: Breastfeeding, children, infants, hypersensitivity, alcohol intoxication, hepatic encephalopathy

Precautions: Pregnancy (C), hepatic disease, alcoholism, COPD, seizure disorder, sleep apnea, suicidal ideation, angioedema, depression, sleep-related behaviors (sleepwalking), schizophrenia, bipolar disorder

PHARMACOKINETICS

Absorbed rapidly; peak 0.75 hr; protein binding 82%; rapid first pass metabolism via liver; 84% excreted in urine, 4% feces; half-life 2-5 hr

INTERACTIONS

• Possible toxicity: antiretroviral protease inhibitors

Increase: ramelteon effect—alcohol; CYP1A2 inhibitors, azole antifungals (ketoconazole, fluconazole), fluvoxamine, anxiolytics, sedatives, hypnotics, barbiturates, ciprofloxacin

Decrease: effect of ramelteon—rifampin

Drug/Herb
• Do not use with melatonin

Increase: CNS depression—catnip, chamomile, clary, cowslip, hops, kava, lavender, mistletoe, nettle, pokeweed, poppy, Queen Anne's lace, senega, skullcap, valerian

Drug/Food
• Prolonged absorption, sleep onset reduced: high-fat/heavy meal

NURSING CONSIDERATIONS

Assess:

- Mental status: mood, sensorium, affect, memory (long, short)
- Type of sleep problem: falling asleep, staying asleep

Administer:

- After removal of cigarettes to prevent fires
- After trying conservative measures for insomnia
- Within 30 min of bedtime for sleeplessness
- On empty stomach for fast onset

Perform/provide:

- Assistance with ambulation after receiving dose
- Safety measure: night-light, call bell within easy reach
- Checking to see if PO medication has been swallowed
- Storage in tight container in cool environment

Evaluate:

- Therapeutic response: ability to sleep at night, decreased amount of early morning awakening

Teach patient/family:

- To avoid driving or other activities requiring alertness until product is stabilized
- To avoid alcohol ingestion or CNS depressants
- Alternative measures to improve sleep: reading, exercise several hr before bedtime, warm bath, warm milk, TV, self-hypnosis, deep breathing
- To take immediately before going to bed
- Not to ingest a high-fat/heavy meal before taking
- To report cessation of menses, galactorrhea (women), decreased libido, infertility; worsening of insomnia, or behavioral changes

ramipril (℞)

(ra-mi′pril)

Altace

Func. class.: Antihypertensive

Chem. class.: Angiotensin-converting enzyme inhibitor (ACE)

Do not confuse:

ramipril/enalapril

Altace/alteplase/Artane

Action: Selectively suppresses renin-angiotensin-aldosterone system; inhibits ACE, prevents conversion of angiotensin I to angiotensin II; results in dilation of arterial, venous vessels

Uses: Hypertension, alone or in combination with thiazide diuretics; CHF (post MI), reduction in risk for MI, stroke, death from CV disorders

Unlabeled uses: Proteinuria due to diabetic nephropathy

DOSAGE AND ROUTES

Hypertension

- *Adult:* **PO** 2.5 mg/day initially, then 2.5-20 mg/day divided bid or daily

CHF post-MI

- *Adult:* **PO** 1.25-2.5 mg bid; may increase to 5 mg bid

Reduction in risk for MI, stroke, death

- *Adult:* **PO** 2.5 mg/day × 7 days, then 5 mg/day × 21 days; then may increase to 10 mg/day

Renal dose

- *Adult:* **PO** CCr <40 ml/min reduce by 50%, titrate upward to max 5 mg/day

Proteinuria due to diabetic nephropathy (unlabeled)

- *Adult:* **PO** 2.5 mg/day

Available forms: Caps 1.25, 2.5, 5, 10 mg

SIDE EFFECTS

CNS: Headache, dizziness, anxiety, insomnia, paresthesia, *fatigue,* depression, malaise, vertigo, **seizures**

R

CV: Hypotension, chest pain, palpitations, angina, syncope, dysrhythmia
EENT: Hearing loss
GI: Nausea, constipation, vomiting, dyspepsia, dysphagia, anorexia, diarrhea, abdominal pain
GU: **Proteinuria,** increased BUN, creatinine, impotence
HEMA: Decreased Hct, Hgb, **eosinophilia, leukopenia**
INTEG: Rash, sweating, photosensitivity, pruritus
META: Hyperkalemia
MISC: **Angioedema**
MS: Arthralgia, arthritis, myalgia
RESP: Cough, dyspnea

Contraindications: Breastfeeding, children, hypersensitivity to ACE inhibitors, history of angioedema

Black Box Warning: Pregnancy (D)

Precautions: Geriatric patients, impaired renal/hepatic function, dialysis patients, hypovolemia, blood dyscrasias, CHF, COPD, asthma, renal artery stenosis, cough

PHARMACOKINETICS

Bioavailability >50%-60%, onset 1-2 hr, peak 3-6 hr, duration 24 hr, protein binding 73%, half-life 1-2 hr, 9-18 hr for active metabolite, metabolized by liver (metabolites excreted in urine, feces)

INTERACTIONS

Increase: hypotension—diuretics, other antihypertensives, ganglionic blockers, adrenergic blockers, nitrates, acute alcohol ingestion
Increase: toxicity—vasodilators, hydrALAZINE, prazosin, potassium-sparing diuretics, sympathomimetics, potassium supplements
Increase: serum levels of digoxin, lithium
Decrease: absorption—antacids
Decrease: antihypertensive effect—indomethacin, NSAIDs, salicylates

Drug/Herb
Increase: toxicity, death—aconite
Increase: antihypertensive effect—barberry, betony, black catechu, black cohosh, bloodroot, broom, burdock, cat's claw, dandelion, goldenseal, hawthorn, Irish moss, Jamaican dogwood, kelp, khella, mistletoe, parsley
Increase or decrease: antihypertensive effect—astragalus, cola tree
Decrease: antihypertensive effect—coltsfoot, guarana, khat, licorice, yohimbe

Drug/Lab Test
False positive: urine acetone, ANA titer

NURSING CONSIDERATIONS

Assess:

⚠ Blood studies: neutrophils, decreased platelets; WBC with differential baseline and periodically q3mo, if neutrophils <1000/mm^3, discontinue treatment (recommended in collagen-vascular disease)
- B/P, orthostatic hypotension, syncope
- Renal studies: protein, BUN, creatinine; increased levels may indicate nephrotic syndrome
- Baselines in renal, hepatic function tests before therapy begins and periodically; increased LFTs; uric acid and glucose may be increased
- Potassium levels, although hyperkalemia rarely occurs
- Dipstick of urine for protein daily in first morning specimen; if protein is increased, a 24-hr urinary protein should be collected
- Edema in feet, legs daily, weight daily in CHF

⚠ Allergic reactions: rash, fever, pruritus, urticaria; product should be discontinued if antihistamines fail to help
- Renal symptoms: polyuria, oliguria, urinary frequency, dysuria

Administer:
- Caps can be opened and added to food

Perform/provide:
- Storage in tight container at 86° F (30° C) or less
- Supine position for severe hypotension

Evaluate:
- Therapeutic response: decrease in B/P

Teach patient/family:

- Not to discontinue product abruptly
- Not to use OTC products (cough, cold, allergy) unless directed by prescriber; not to use salt substitutes containing potassium without consulting prescriber
- To comply with dosage schedule, even if feeling better
- To rise slowly to sitting or standing position to minimize orthostatic hypotension
- To notify prescriber of mouth sores, sore throat, fever, swelling of hands or feet, irregular heartbeat, chest pain
- To report excessive perspiration, dehydration, vomiting, diarrhea; may lead to fall in B/P
- That product may cause dizziness, fainting, light-headedness; may occur during first few days of therapy
- That product may cause skin rash or impaired perspiration
- How to take B/P, and normal readings for age-group

Treatment of overdose: 0.9% NaCl IV infusion, hemodialysis

ranibizumab (℞)

(ran-ih-biz′oo-mab)
Lucentis
Func. class.: Ophthalmic
Chem. class.: Selective vascular endothelial growth factor antagonist

Action: Binds to receptor-binding site of active forms of vascular endothelial growth factor A (VEGF-A) that causes angiogenesis and cell proliferation

Uses: Macular degeneration (neovascular) (wet)

Unlabeled uses: Diabetic macular edema

DOSAGE AND ROUTES

- *Adult:* **INTRAVITREAL** 0.5 mg (0.05 ml) q mo

Diabetic macular edema (unlabeled)

- *Adults:* **INTRAVITREAL** 0.3-0.5 mg q mo × 2-3 inj then bimonthly and/or as needed

Available forms: Sol for inj 0.5 mg/0.05 ml

SIDE EFFECTS

CNS: Dizziness, headache

EENT: Blepharitis, cataract, conjunctival hemorrhage/hyperemia, detachment of the retinal pigment epithelium, dry/irritation/pain in the eye, visual impairment, vitreous floaters, ocular infection

GI: Constipation, nausea

MISC: Hypertension, UTI, **thromboembolism, non-ocular bleeding**

RESP: Bronchitis, cough, sinusitis, URI

Contraindications: Hypersensitivity, ocular infections

Precautions: Pregnancy (C), breastfeeding, children, retinal detachment, increased intraocular pressure

PHARMACOKINETICS

Elimination half-life 9 days

INTERACTIONS

Increase: severe inflammation—verteporfin photodynamic therapy (PDT)

NURSING CONSIDERATIONS

Assess:

- For eye changes: redness; sensitivity to light, vision change; increased intraocular pressure change; report infection to ophthalmologist immediately

Administer:

- By ophthalmologist via intravitreal injection using adequate anesthesia; use 19-gauge filter

Perform/provide:

- Storage in refrigerator; do not freeze
- Protect from light

Evaluate:

- Therapeutic response: prevention of increasing macular degeneration

Teach patient/family:

- That if eye becomes red, sensitive to light, painful, or if there is a change in vision, seek immediate care from ophthalmologist
- Reason for treatment, expected results

ranitidine (℞, OTC)

(ra-nit′i-deen)

Apo-Ranitidine ♣, Equaline, Gen-Ranitidine ♣, Leader Ranitidine, Novo-Ranidine ♣, Nu-Ranit ♣, PMS-Ranitidine ♣, Wal-zan, Zantac, Zantac C ♣, Zantac EFFER-dose, Zantac GELdose

ranitidine bismuth citrate

Tritec

Func. class.: H_2-Histamine receptor antagonist

Do not confuse:
ranitidine/amantadine
Zantac/Xanax/Zofran

Action: Inhibits histamine at H_2-receptor site in parietal cells, which inhibits gastric acid secretion

Uses: Duodenal ulcer, Zollinger-Ellison syndrome, gastric ulcers, hypersecretory conditions, gastroesophageal reflux disease, stress ulcers, erosive esophagitis (maintenance), active duodenal ulcers with *Helicobacter pylori* in combination with clarithromycin, systemic mastocytosis, multiple endocrine adenoma syndrome, heartburn

Unlabeled uses: Prevention of aspiration pneumonitis, stress ulcers (treatment/prophylaxis), upper GI bleeding, angioedema, gastritis, urticaria, NSAID-induced ulcer prophylaxis

DOSAGE AND ROUTES

Ranitidine

Duodenal ulcer

• *Adult:* **PO** 150 mg bid, or 300 mg/day after PM meal or at bedtime; maintenance 150 mg at bedtime

• *Infant and child:* **PO** 2-4 mg/kg bid, max 300 mg/day

Zollinger-Ellison syndrome

• *Adult:* **PO** 150 mg bid, may increase if needed

Gastric ulcer

• *Adult:* **PO** 150 mg bid × 6 wk, then 150 mg at bedtime

• *Infant and child:* **PO** 2-4 mg/kg bid, max 300 mg/day

GERD

• *Adult:* **PO** 150 mg bid

Erosive esophagitis

• *Adult:* **PO** 150 mg qid for up to 12 wk

• *Child ≥1 mo:* **PO** 5-10 mg/kg/day in 2-3 divided doses

Renal dose

• *Adult:* CCr <50 ml/min give 50% of dose or extend dosing interval

NSAID-induced ulcer prophylaxis (unlabeled)

• *Adult:* **PO** 150 mg bid

Stress gastritis prophylaxis (unlabeled)

• *Adult:* **IM/INT IV INF** 50 mg q6-8hr

Severe, acute urticaria/angioedema (unlabeled)

• *Adult:* **INT IV INF** 50 mg with H_1-blocker

Ranitidine bismuth citrate

• *Adult:* **PO** 400 mg bid × 4 wk with clarithromycin 500 mg tid × 1st 2 wk

Available forms: *Ranitidine:* tabs 75, 150, 300 mg; sol for inj 25 mg/ml; effervescent tabs 25 mg; caps 150, 300 mg; syr 15 mg/ml; *ranitidine bismuth citrate:* tabs 400 mg

SIDE EFFECTS

CNS: Headache, sleeplessness, dizziness, confusion, agitation, depression, hallucination (geriatric patients)

CV: Tachycardia, bradycardia, PVCs

EENT: Blurred vision, increased ocular pressure

GI: Constipation, abdominal pain, diarrhea, nausea, vomiting, **hepatotoxicity**

GU: Impotence, gynecomastia, **acute interstitial nephritis (rare)**

INTEG: Urticaria, rash, fever

RESP: **Pneumonia**

SYST: **Anaphylaxis (rare)**

Contraindications: Hypersensitivity

Precautions: Pregnancy (B), breastfeeding, children <12 yr, renal/hepatic disease

PHARMACOKINETICS

PO: Peak 2-3 hr; duration 8-12 hr; metabolized by liver; excreted in urine (30% unchanged, PO), breast milk; half-life 2-3 hr; protein binding 15%

INTERACTIONS

Increase: absorption, toxicity—anticoagulants, sulfonylureas, procainamide
Increase: effects of benzodiazepines, calcium channel blockers
Decrease: absorption of ranitidine—antacids, diazepam, anticholinergics, metoclopramide
Decrease: effects of cephalosporins, iron salts, ketoconazole

Drug/Lab Test
Increase: AST, ALT, alk phos, creatinine, LDH, bilirubin
False positive: urine protein

NURSING CONSIDERATIONS

Assess:

- Gastric pH (>5 should be maintained)
- I&O ratio, BUN, creatinine
- Mental status: confusion, dizziness, depression, anxiety, weakness, tremors, psychosis, diarrhea, abdominal discomfort, jaundice; report immediately
- GI complaints: nausea, vomiting, diarrhea, cramps

Administer:

PO route

- With meals for prolonged effect
- Antacids 1 hr before or 1 hr after ranitidine

IV route

- IV after diluting 50 mg/20 ml 0.9% NaCl, D_5W, $D_{10}W$, LR, $NaCO_3$ 5% and give 50 mg or less/5 min or more; may dilute 50 mg/50-100 ml of 0.9% NaCl, D_5W, $D_{10}W$, LR, $NaCO_3$ 5% and give over 15-20 min

Additive compatibilities: AcetaZOLAMIDE, amikacin, aminophylline, chloramphenicol, chlorothiazide, ciprofloxacin, colistimethate, dexamethasone, digoxin, DOBUTamine, DOPamine, doxycycline, epinephrine, erythromycin, floxacillin, fluconazole/ondansetron, flumazenil, furosemide, gentamicin, heparin, insulin (regular), isoproterenol, lidocaine, lincomycin, meropenem, methylPREDNISolone, moxalactam, penicillin G potassium, penicillin G sodium, polymyxin B, potassium chloride, protamine, quinidine, sodium nitroprusside, ticarcillin, tobramycin, vancomycin

Syringe compatibilities: Atropine, cyclizine, dexamethasone, dimenhyDRINATE, diphenhydrAMINE, DOBUTamine, DOPamine, fentanyl, glycopyrrolate, hydromorphone, isoproterenol, meperidine, metoclopramide, morphine, nalbuphine, oxymorphone, pentazocine, perphenazine, prochlorperazine, promethazine, scopolamine

Y-site compatibilities: Acyclovir, aldesleukin, allopurinol, amifostine, aminophylline, amsacrine, atracurium, aztreonam, bretylium, cefepime, ceftazidime, ciprofloxacin, cisatracurium, cisplatin, cladribine, cyclophosphamide, cytarabine, diltiazem, DOBUTamine, DOPamine, DOXOrubicin, DOXOrubicin liposome, enalaprilat, epinephrine, esmolol, fentanyl, filgrastim, fluconazole, fludarabine, foscarnet, furosemide, gallium, granisetron, heparin, hydromorphone, idarubicin, labetalol, lorazepam, melphalan, meperidine, methotrexate, midazolam, milrinone, morphine, niCARdipine, nitroglycerin, norepinephrine, ondansetron, paclitaxel, pancuronium, piperacillin, piperacillin/tazobactam, procainamide, propofol, remifentanil, sargramostim, tacrolimus, teniposide, theophylline, thiopental, thiotepa, vecuronium, vinorelbine, warfarin, zidovudine

Perform/provide:

- Storage at room temperature

Evaluate:

- Therapeutic response: decreased abdominal pain, heartburn

Teach patient/family:

- That gynecomastia, impotence may occur but are reversible
- To avoid driving, other hazardous activities until stabilized on this medication
- That product must be continued for prescribed time to be effective
- To avoid breastfeeding

• Not to take the maximum OTC daily dose for longer than 2 wk

ranolazine (℞)

(ruh-no'luh-zeen)
Ranexa
Func. class: Antianginal

Action: Antianginal, antiischemic; unknown, may work by inhibiting portal fatty-acid oxidation

Uses: Chronic stable angina pectoris; use in those who have not responded to other treatment options; should be used in combination with other antianginals such as amlodipine, β-blockers, or nitrates

DOSAGE AND ROUTES

• *Adult:* **PO** 500 mg bid and increased to 1000 mg bid based on response; max 1000 mg bid

Available forms: Ext rel tabs 500 mg

SIDE EFFECTS

CNS: Headache, dizziness
CV: Palpitations, **QT prolongation**
GI: Nausea, vomiting, constipation, dry mouth
MISC: Peripheral edema
RESP: Dyspnea

Contraindications: Preexisting QT prolongation, hepatic disease (Child-Pugh class A, B, C), hypersensitivity, hypokalemia, renal failure, torsades de pointes, ventricular dysrhythmia, ventricular tachycardia

Precautions: Pregnancy (C), breastfeeding, children, geriatric patients, hypotension, renal disease

PHARMACOKINETICS

Absorption varied; peak 2-5 hr; half-life 7 hr; metabolized by CYP3A, and lesser by CYP2D6; excreted in urine (75%), feces (25%); protein binding 62%

INTERACTIONS

Increase: ranolazine action—diltiazem, ketoconazole, macrolide antibiotics, dofetilide, paroxetine, protease inhibitors, quinidine, sotalol, thioridazine, verapamil, ziprasidone

Increase: action of digoxin, simvastatin

Increase: ranzolazine action and QT prolongation; do not use concurrently—CYP3A4 inhibitors (ketoconazole, fluconazole, itraconazole, IV miconazole, voriconazole, diltiazem, verapamil)

Increase: QTc interval—macrolides (clarithromycin, erythromycin, troleandomycin)

Increase: ranolazine absorption, toxicity—antiretroviral protease inhibitors

Increase: QT prolongation and torsades de pointes—class IA/III antidysrythmics, arsenic trioxide, chloroquine, droperidol, halofantrine, haloperidol, levomethadyl, methadone, pentamidine, chlorpromazine, mesoridazine, thioridazine, pimozide, probucol

Drug/Food

• Do not use with grapefruit or grapefruit juice

NURSING CONSIDERATIONS

Assess:

• Cardiac status: B/P, pulse, respiration, ECG; watch for prolongation of QT

Administer:

• Do not break, crush, or chew tabs; to take products as prescribed; do not double or skip dose
• Bid, without regard to meals

Evaluate:

• Therapeutic response: decreased anginal pain

Teach patient/family:

• To avoid hazardous activities until stabilized on product, dizziness is no longer a problem
• To avoid OTC drugs, grapefruit juice, products prolonging QTc (quinidine, dofetilide, sotalol, erythromycin, thioridazine, ziprasidone or protease inhibitors, diltiazem, ketoconazole, macrolide antibiotics, verapamil) unless directed by prescriber
• To comply in all areas of medical regimen

• To notify prescriber of palpitations, fainting
• To notify all health care providers of this product use

rasagiline (℞)

(ra-sa'ji-leen)
Azilect
Func. class.: Antiparkinson agent
Chem. class.: MAOI, type B

Action: Inhibits MAOI type B; may increase DOPamine levels
Uses: Idiopathic Parkinson's disease monotherapy or with levodopa

DOSAGE AND ROUTES

Monotherapy
• *Adult:* **PO** 1 mg/day
Adjunctive therapy
• *Adult:* **PO** 0.5 mg/day, may increase 1 mg/day; change of levodopa dose in adjunct therapy; reduce levodopa dose may be needed
Hepatic dose
• *Adult:* **PO** 0.5 mg in mild hepatic disease
Concomitant ciprofloxacin, other CYP1A2 inhibitors
• *Adult:* **PO** 0.5 mg; plasma concentrations of rasagiline may double
Available forms: Tabs 0.5, 1 mg

SIDE EFFECTS

CNS: Drowsiness, hallucinations, depression, headache, malaise, paresthesia, vertigo, syncope
CV: Angina, **hypertensive crisis** (ingestion of tyramine products), orthostatic hypotension
GI: Nausea, diarrhea, dry mouth, dyspepsia
GU: Impotence, decreased libido
MISC: Conjunctivitis, fever, flu syndrome, neck pain, allergic reaction, alopecia
MS: Arthralgia, arthritis, dyskinesia, fall
RESP: Rhinitis
Contraindications: Breastfeeding; hypersensitivity to this product or MAOIs; pheochromocytoma
Precautions: Pregnancy (C), children, psychiatric disorders, moderate/severe hepatic disorders

PHARMACOKINETICS

Onset, peak, duration is unknown; well-absorbed; protein binding >88%-94%; metabolized by CYP1A2 in the liver; excreted by the kidneys

INTERACTIONS

⚠ Do not give with meperidine, other analgesics, serious reaction including coma and death may occur; do not give with sympathomimetics
Increase: levels of rasagiline up to 2-fold—ciprofloxacin, CYP1A2 inhibitors (atazanavir, mexiletine, taurine)
Increase: severe CNS toxicity with antidepressants (tricyclics, SSRIs, SNRIs, mirtazapine, cyclobenzaprine)
⚠ ***Increase:*** hypertensive crisis—MAOIs
Drug/Herb
• Do not give with St. John's wort

NURSING CONSIDERATIONS

Assess:
• For Parkinson's symptoms: tremor, ataxia, muscle weakness and rigidity; baseline and periodically
• Mental status: hallucinations, confusion, notify prescriber
• For hypertensive crisis: severe headache, blurred vision, seizures, chest pain, difficulty thinking, nausea/vomiting, signs of stroke; any unexplained severe headache should be considered to be hypertensive crisis
• For increased dyskinesia and postural hypotension if used in combination with levodopa
• For melanomas frequently, perform periodic skin exams by a dermatologist
• Cardiac status: B/P, ECG; periodically during beginning treatment
Administer:
• With meals to prevent nausea; continuing therapy usually reduces or eliminates nausea
• Reduced dose of carbidopa/levodopa, cautiously

Evaluate:

• Therapeutic response: improved symptoms in those with Parkinson's disease

Teach patient/family:

• To change positions slowly to prevent orthostatic hypotension

• To avoid hazardous activities until stabilized; dizziness can occur

• To rinse mouth frequently, use sugarless gum to alleviate dry mouth

• To take as prescribed, not to miss dose or double doses; take missed dose as soon as remembered, if several hours before next dose

• To prevent hypertensive crisis by avoiding tyramine foods

• To report signs of hypertensive crisis

rasburicase (℞)

(rass-burr′i-case)

Elitek

Func. class.: Enzyme

Chem. class.: Recombinant urate-oxidase enzyme

Action: Catalyzes enzymatic oxidation of uric acid into an inactive and a soluble metabolite (allantoin)

Uses: To reduce uric acid levels in children with leukemia, lymphoma, solid tumor malignancies who are receiving chemotherapy

DOSAGE AND ROUTES

• *Adult/adolescent/infant:* **IV INF** 0.2 mg/kg as a single daily dose given as **IV INF** over ½ hr × 5 days

Available forms: Powder for inj 1.5 mg/vial

SIDE EFFECTS

CNS: Headache, fever

CV: Chest pain, hypotension

GI: Nausea, vomiting, anorexia, diarrhea, abdominal pain, constipation, dyspepsia, mucositis

HEMA: **Neutropenia with fever, hemolysis methemoglobinemia**

INTEG: Rash

MISC: Edema

RESP: **Bronchospasm,** wheezing, dyspnea

SYST: **Anaphylaxis, hemolysis, methemoglobinemia, sepsis**

Contraindications: Hypersensitivity

Black Box Warning: G6PD deficiency, hemolytic reactions, or methemoglobinemia reactions to this product

Precautions: Pregnancy (C), breastfeeding, children <2 yr, anemia

Black Box Warning: Acute bronchospasm, angina, angioedema, atony, African-American and Mediterranean patients, hypotension, urticaria

PHARMACOKINETICS

Elimination half-life 16-21 hr

INTERACTIONS

Increase: toxicity—allopurinol

NURSING CONSIDERATIONS

Assess:

• Blood studies: BUN, serum uric acid, urine creatinine clearance, electrolytes, CBC with differential before and during therapy

• Monitor temp; fever may indicate beginning infection; no rectal temps

• Anaphylaxis, have emergency equipment nearby

• For G6PD deficiency, hemolytic reactions, methemoglobinemia; these patients should not be given this agent

• GI symptoms: frequency of stools, cramping, if severe diarrhea occurs, fluid and electrolytes may need to be given

Administer:

• Reconstitute with diluent provided, add 1 ml of diluent/each vial, swirl, may dilute further prior to administration

• Infuse over 30 min, do not filter, do not give as bolus

• Antiemetic 30-60 min before giving product and prn

Evaluate:

• Therapeutic response: decreased uric acid levels

Teach patient/family:

- Reason for therapy, expected results
- To report trouble breathing, jaundice, chest pain

⚠ High Alert

remifentanil (℞)

(rem-ih-fin'ta-nill)

Ultiva

Func. class.: Opiate agonist analgesic

Chem. class.: μ-Opioid agonist

Controlled Substance Schedule II

Action: Inhibits ascending pain pathways in limbic system, thalamus, midbrain, hypothalamus

Uses: In combination with other products in general anesthesia to provide analgesia

DOSAGE AND ROUTES

- *Adult:* Induction **IV** 0.5-1 mcg/kg/min with a hypnotic or volative agent; maintenance with isoflurane (0.4-1.5 MAC) or propofol (100-200 mcg/kg/min); **CONT INF** 0.25-0.4 mcg/kg/min
- *Child 1-12 yr:* **CONT IV INF** 0.25 mcg/kg/min with isoflurane
- *Full-term neonate and infant up to 2 mo:* **CONT IV INF** 0.4 mcg/kg/min with nitrous oxide

Available forms: Powder for inj lyophilized 1 mg/ml after reconstitution

SIDE EFFECTS

CNS: Drowsiness, *dizziness,* confusion, *headache,* sedation, euphoria, delirium, agitation, anxiety

CV: Palpitations, *bradycardia,* change in B/P, facial flushing, syncope, **asystole**

EENT: Tinnitus, blurred vision, miosis, diplopia

GI: Nausea, vomiting, anorexia, constipation, cramps, dry mouth

GU: Urinary retention, dysuria

INTEG: Rash, urticaria, bruising, flushing, diaphoresis, pruritus

MS: Rigidity

RESP: **Respiratory depression, apnea**

Contraindications: Hypersensitivity

Precautions: Pregnancy (C), breastfeeding, children <12 yr, geriatric patients, increased intracranial pressure, acute MI, severe heart disease, GI/renal/hepatic disease, asthma, respiratory conditions, seizures disorders, bradyarrhythmias

PHARMACOKINETICS

70% protein binding, terminal half-life 3-10 min

INTERACTIONS

- Respiratory depression, hypotension, profound sedation: alcohol, sedatives, hypnotics, or other CNS depressants; antihistamines, phenothiazines

Drug/Herb

Increase: CNS depression—kava

NURSING CONSIDERATIONS

Assess:

- I&O ratio, check for decreasing output; may indicate urinary retention, especially in geriatric patients
- CNS changes; dizziness, drowsiness, hallucinations, euphoria, LOC, pupil reaction
- GI status: nausea, vomiting, anorexia, constipation
- Allergic reactions: rash, urticaria
- Respiratory dysfunction: respiratory depression, character, rate, rhythm; notify prescriber if respirations are <12/min; CV status; bradycardia, syncope
- Use pain scoring to determine pain perception

Administer:

- Add 1 ml diluent per mg remifentanil
- Interruption of infusion results in rapid reversal (no residual opioid effect within 5-10 min)

Y-site compatibilities: Acyclovir, alfentanil, amikacin, aminophylline, ampicillin, ampicillin/sulbactam, aztreonam, bretylium, bumetanide, buprenorphine, butorphanol, calcium gluconate, cefazolin, cefepine, cefotaxime, cefotetan, cefoxitin, ceftazidime, ceftizoxime, ceftriaxone, cefuroxime, cimetidine, ciprofloxacin, cisatracurium, cisplatin, clindamycin, dactinomycin, dexamethasone, digoxin, diltiazem, diphenhydrAMINE, DOBUTamine, docetaxel, DOPamine, doxacurium, doxycycline, droperidol, enalaprilat, epinephrine, esmolol, etoposide, famotidine, fentanyl, fluconazole, furosemide, ganciclovir, gatiflexacin, gemcitabine, gentamicin, granisetron, haloperidol, heparin, hetastarch, hydrocortisone sodium succinate, hydromorphone, hydrOXYzine, imipenem/cilastatin, inamrinone, isoproterenol, ketorolac, levofloxacin, lidocaine, lorazepam, magnesium sulfate, mannitol, meperidine, methylPREDNISolone sodium succinate, metoclopramide, metronidazole, midazolam, minocycline, morphine, nalbuphine, netilmicin, nitroglycerin, norepinephrine, ofloxacin, ondansetron, paclitaxel, palonsetron, phenylephrine, piperacillin, potassium chloride, procainamide, prochlorperazine, promethazine, ranitidine, sulfentanil, sulfamethoxazole, teniposide, theophylline, thiopental, thiotepa, ticarcillin, ticarcillin/clavulanale, tobramycin, trimethoprim, vancomycin, voriconazole, zidovudine

Solution compatibilities: D_5, 0.45% NaCl, LR, D_5 LR, 0.9% NaCl

Perform/provide:

- Storage in light-resistant area at room temperature

Evaluate:

- Therapeutic response: maintenance of anesthesia

Teach patient/family:

- To call for assistance when ambulating or smoking; drowsiness, dizziness may occur
- To make position changes slowly to prevent orthostatic hypotension

repaglinide (℞)

(re-pag′lih′nide)

Gluco Norm ♣, Prandin

Func. class.: Antidiabetic

Chem. class.: Meglitinide

Action: Causes functioning β-cells in pancreas to release insulin, leading to drop in blood glucose levels; closes ATP-dependent potassium channels in the β-cell membrane; this leads to opening of calcium channels; increased calcium influx induces insulin secretion

Uses: Type 2 diabetes mellitus

DOSAGE AND ROUTES

- *Adult:* **PO** 1-2 mg with each meal, max 16 mg/day, adjust at weekly intervals; oral hypoglycemic–naive patients or patients with A1c <8% should start with 0.5 mg with each meal

Renal/hepatic dose

- *Adult:* **PO** CCr 20-39 ml/min 0.5 mg/day; titrate upward cautiously

Available forms: Tabs 0.5, 1, 2 mg

SIDE EFFECTS

CNS: Headache, weakness, paresthesia

ENDO: **Hypoglycemia**

GI: Nausea, vomiting, diarrhea, constipation, dyspepsia

INTEG: Rash, allergic reactions

MISC: Chest pain, UTI, allergy

MS: Back pains, arthralgia

RESP: URI, sinusitis, rhinitis, bronchitis

Contraindications: Hypersensitivity to meglitinides, diabetic ketoacidosis, type 1 diabetes

Precautions: Pregnancy (C), breastfeeding, children, geriatric patients, thyroid/cardiac disease, severe renal/hepatic disease, severe hypoglycemic reactions

PHARMACOKINETICS

Competely absorbed by GI route; onset 30 min; peak 1-1½ hr; duration <4 hr; half-life 1 hr; metabolized in liver;

excreted in urine, feces (metabolites); crosses placenta; 98% plasma protein bound

INTERACTIONS

Increase: in both—levonorgestrel/ethinyl estradiol

Increase: repaglinide metabolism—CYP450 inducers: rifampin, barbiturates, carbamazepine

Increase: repaglinide effect—NSAIDs, salicylates, sulfonamides, chloramphenicol, MAOIs, coumarins, β-blockers, probenecid, gemfibrozil, simvastatin, fenofibrate

Decrease: repaglinide metabolism—CYP450 inhibitors: antifungals (ketoconazole, miconazole), erythromycin, macrolides

Decrease: repaglinide action—calcium channel blockers, corticosteroids, oral contraceptives, thiazide diuretics, thyroid preparations, estrogens, phenothiazines, phenytoin, rifampin, isoniazid, phenobarbital, sympathomimetics

Drug/Herb

Increase: antidiabetic effect—alfalfa, aloe, basil, bay, bilberry, bitter melon, black catechu, buchu, burdock, coriander, dandelion, eyebright (po), fenugreek, garlic, ginseng, glucomannan, glucosamine, goat's rue, gymnema, horehound, horse chestnut, jambul, myrrh, myrtle

Increase or decrease: hypoglycemic effect—chromium, fenugreek, ginseng

Decrease: hypoglycemic effect—broom, buchu, dandelion, juniper

Decrease: glucose tolerance—karela

Decrease: antidiabetic effect—bee pollen, blue cohosh, broom, chromium, elecampane, eucalyptus, gotu kola

Drug/Food

Decrease: repaglinide level, give before meals

NURSING CONSIDERATIONS

Assess:

⚠ Hypo/hyperglycemic reaction that can occur soon after meals: dizziness, weakness, headache, tremor, anxiety, tachycardia, hunger, sweating, abdominal pain

- A1c, fasting, postprandial glucose during treatment

Administer:

- Up to 15 min before meals; 2, 3, or 4×/day preprandially
- Skip dose if meal is skipped; add dose if meal is added

Perform/provide:

- Storage in tight container at room temperature

Evaluate:

- Therapeutic response: decrease in polyuria, polydipsia, polyphagia; clear sensorium; absence of dizziness; stable gait; blood glucose, A1c improvement

Teach family/patient:

- Technique of blood glucose monitoring; use blood glucose meter
- The symptoms of hypo/hyperglycemia; what to do about each
- That product must be continued on daily basis; explain consequences of discontinuing product abruptly
- To avoid OTC medications unless ordered by prescriber
- That diabetes is a lifelong illness; product will not cure disease
- That all food included in diet plan must be eaten to prevent hypoglycemia; to have glucagon emergency kit available; take before meals 2, 3, or 4×/day
- To carry emergency ID

Treatment of overdose: Glucose 25 g IV via dextrose 50% solution, 50 ml or 1 mg glucagon

R

retapamulin topical

See Appendix B

Rh_o(D) immune globulin standard dose IM (℞)

BayRho (HyperRHO SD), Rho Gam Ultra Filtered Plus Solution for Injection

Rh_o(D) immune globulin microdose IM (℞)

MICRhoGAM Ultra Filtered Plus Solution for Injection

Rh_o(D) immune globulin IV (℞)

Rhophylac Pre-Filled Syringes, WinRho SDF

Func. class.: Immune globulins

Action: Suppresses immune response of nonsensitized Rh_o(D or D^u)-negative patients who are exposed to Rh_o(D or D^u)-positive blood

Uses: Prevention of isoimmunization in Rh-negative women given Rh-positive blood after abortions, miscarriages, amniocentesis; chronic idiopathic thrombocytopenia purpura (Rhophylac)

DOSAGE AND ROUTES

To reduce risk of Rh isoimmunization antepartum/suppression of Rh isoimmunization postpartum following delivery of full-term infant

- *Adult and adolescent ≥16 yr:* **IM** (BayRho-D [HyperRHO SD] full dose only) 300 mcg (1500 international units) at 28 wk gestation, repeat within 72 hr of delivery of confirmed Rho(D) positive infant; a dose is not needed after delivery, if delivery is within 3 wk of last dose and no fetal maternal hemorrhage of >15 ml of RBC; **IM** (RhoGam only) 300 mcg (1500 international units) at 26-28 wk gestation, repeat within 72 hr even if status of Rho is unknown or if 72 hr have passed; **IM/IV** (WinRho SDF only) 300 mcg (1500 international units) at 28 wk gestation; if given earlier in pregnancy, give at 12 wk intervals during pregnancy, a 120 mcg (600 international units) dose; IM/IV should be given as soon as possible and preferably within 72 hr of delivery of a confirmed Rho(D) positive infant and even if status is unknown, give up to 28 days after delivery

Known or suspected massive fetomaternal hemorrhage (>15 ml of fetal RBC or >30 ml of fetal whole blood)

- *Adult and adolescent ≥16 yr:* **IM** (BayRho-D [HyperRHO SD] full dose only) 300 mcg (1500 international units) per every 15 ml of fetal blood cells or 30 ml of whole blood, multiple syringes may be injected IM at the same time in different sites, give within 72 hr of exposure, repeat dose within 72 hr of delivery; **IM** (RhoGAM only) 300 mcg (1500 international units) for every 15 ml of fetal blood cells or 30 ml of whole blood, give total dose within 72 hr of exposure; **IM/IV** (WinRho SDF only) if large fetomaternal hemorrhage is suspected, give **IV** 9 mcg (45 international units) or **IM** 12 mcg (60 international units) for every ml of fetal whole blood, give **IV** 600 mcg (3000 international units) q8hr or **IM** 1200 mcg (6000 international units) q12hr until total dose is given, total dose should be given within 72 hr of exposure

Threatened abortion at any stage of pregnancy

- *Adult and adolescent ≥16 yr:* **IM** (BayRho-D [HyperRHO SD] full dose only) 300 mcg (1500 international units) as soon as possible; if given 13-18 wk gestation, give another 300 mcg (1500 international units) at 26-28 wk gestation; repeat dose within 72 hr of delivery; **IM** (RhoGam only) 300 mcg (1500 international units) as soon as possible and within 72 hr of exposure; **IM/IV** (Rhophylac only) 300 mcg (1500 international units) as soon as possible and within 72 hr; **IM/IV** (WinRho SDF only) 300 mcg (1500 international units) as soon as possible and within 72 hr, repeat dose at 12 wk intervals during pregnancy and 120 mcg (600 international units) as soon as possible after delivery and within 72 hr

Following spontaneous abortion, induced termination of pregnancy or ectopic pregnancy that occurs ≤12 wk gestation

• *Adult and adolescent ≥16 yr:* **IM** (BayRho-D Minidose, HYperRHO Minidose, MICRhoGAM only) 50 mcg (250 international units) as soon as possible, give within 3 hr of spontaneous or surgical removal, if possible within 72 hr

Following spontaneous abortion, induced termination or pregnancy, or ruptured tubal pregnancy that occur ≥13 wk

• *Adult and adolescent ≥16 yr:* **IM** (BayRho-D [HyperRHO SD] full dose, RhoGAM only) 300 mcg (1500 international units) as soon as possible and within 72 hr of event

Following spontaneous abortion, induced termination of pregnancy, amniocentesis, chorionic villus sampling, abdominal trauma, ruptured tubal pregnancy, or percutaneous umbilical cord sampling up to 34 wk gestation

• *Adult and adolescent ≥16 yr:* **IM/IV** (WinRho SDF only) 300 mcg (1500 international units) within 72 hr, repeat at 12 wk intervals during pregnancy, give 120 mcg (600 international units) as soon as possible and preferably within 72 hr of delivery

Available forms: BayRho-D solution for injection 300 mcg/ml (HyperRHO SD solution for injection), MICRhoGAM Ultra Filtered Plus Solution for injection 50 mcg/ml; RhoGam Ultra Filtered Plus Solution for injection 50 mcg; Rhophylac Pre-Filled Syringes Solution for injection 300 mcg/2 ml; WinRho SDF Liquid for injection; WinRho powder for injection

SIDE EFFECTS

CNS: Lethargy

INTEG: Irritation at inj site, fever

MS: Myalgia

Contraindications: Previous immunization with this product, Rh_o(O)-positive/D^u-positive patient

Precautions: Pregnancy (C)

INTERACTIONS

Decrease: antibody response—live virus vaccines (measles, mumps, rubella)

NURSING CONSIDERATIONS

Assess:

⚠ Allergies, reactions to immunizations; previous immunization with this product

⚠ For intravascular hemolysis: back pain, chills, hemoglobinuria, renal insufficiency

• Type, crossmatch mother and newborn's cord blood; if mother is Rh_o(D) negative, D^u-negative and newborn Rh_o(D) positive, this medication should be given

Administer:

• BayRho-D is being changed to HyperRHO SD

• BayRho-D (HyperRHO SD), MICRhoGAM, RhoGAM are given by IM only, do not give IV

• WinRhoSDF and Rhophylac can be given IM or IV

• Inspect for particulate matter; do not use if particulate matter is present

• Reconstitute/dilution: no reconstitution or dilution is needed for BayRho-D (HyperRHO SD); Rhophylac, MICRhoGAM, RhoGAM, or the liquid formulation of WinRho SDF

• WinRho SDF powder for IV use: if giving IV, reconstitute 600 international units or 1500 international units immediately before use with 2.5 ml of sterile diluent; reconstitute 5000 international units with 8.5 ml sterile diluent; add diluent to vial slowly down the wall of the vial; gently swirl until powder is dissolved; do not shake

• WinRho SDF powder for IM use: IV giving IM, reconstitute 600 international units or 1500 international units immediately before use with 1.25 ml of sterile diluent; 5000 international units with 8.5 ml of sterile diluent; add diluent to the vial slowly down the wall of the vial; gently swirl until powder is dissolved; do not shake

R

IM route
- Use aseptic technique, observe for 20 min after administration
- Bring Rhophylac to room temperature before using
- Inject into the deltoid muscle of upper arm or anterolateral portion of the upper thigh; do not inject into gluteal muscle
- If dose calculated will need multiple vials or syringes, use different sites at the same time

IV route
- Use aseptic technique
- WinRhoSDF: remove entire contents of vial to obtain calculated dose; if partial vial is required for dosage calculation, withdraw the entire vial contents to ensure correct calculation; infuse correct calculated dose over 3-5 min; do not infuse with other fluids or products
- Rhophylac: bring to room temperature; infuse by slow IV; observe for 20 min

Perform/provide:
- Storage in refrigerator

Evaluate:
- Rh_o(D) sensitivity in transfusion error, prevention of erythroblastosis fetalis for normal vision

Teach patient/family:
- How product works; that product must be given after subsequent deliveries if subsequent babies are Rh positive

riboflavin (vit B_2)
(OTC)
(rye'boh-flay-vin)
Func. class.: Vit B_2, water soluble

Action: Needed for respiratory reactions by catalyzing proteins
Uses: Vit B_2 deficiency or polyneuritis; cheilosis adjunct with thiamine
Unlabeled uses: Migraine prophylaxis

DOSAGE AND ROUTES

Deficiency
- *Adult:* **PO** 5-30 mg/day
- *Child ≥12 yr:* **PO** 3-10 mg/day, then 0.6 mg/1000 calories ingested

RDA
- *Adult:* **PO** (males) 1.3 mg, (females) 1.1 mg

Migraine prophylaxis (unlabeled)
- *Adult:* **PO** 400 mg/day × 3 mo

Available forms: Tabs 5, 10, 25, 50, 100, 250 mg

SIDE EFFECTS

GU: Yellow discoloration of urine
Precautions: Pregnancy (A)

PHARMACOKINETICS

Half-life 65-85 min, 60% protein bound, unused amounts excreted in urine (unchanged)

INTERACTIONS

Increase: riboflavin need—alcohol, probenecid, tricyclics, phenothiazines
Decrease: action of tetracyclines

Drug/Lab Test
- May cause false elevations of urinary catecholamines

NURSING CONSIDERATIONS

Assess:
- Nutritional status: liver, eggs, dairy products, yeast, whole grain, green vegetables

Administer:
- With food for better absorption

Perform/provide:
- Storage in airtight, light-resistant container

Evaluate:
- Therapeutic response: absence of headache, GI problems, cheilosis, skin lesions, depression, burning, itchy eyes, anemia

Teach patient/family:
- That urine may turn bright yellow
- About addition of needed foods that are rich in riboflavin
- To avoid alcohol

rifabutin (℞)
(riff'a-byoo-ten)
Mycobutin
Func. class.: Antimycobacterial agent
Chem. class.: Rifamycin S derivative

Do not confuse:
rifabutin/rifampin
Action: Inhibits DNA-dependent RNA polymerase in susceptible strains of *Escherichia coli* and *Bacillus subtilis;* mechanism of action against *Mycobacterium avium* unknown
Uses: Prevention of *M. avium* complex (MAC) in patients with advanced HIV infection
Unlabeled uses: *Helicobacter pylori* that has not responded to other treatment

DOSAGE AND ROUTES

- *Adult:* **PO** 300 mg/day (may take as 150 mg bid); max 600 mg/day

Renal dose

- *Adult:* **PO** CCr <30 ml/min reduce by 50%

Available forms: Caps 150 mg

SIDE EFFECTS

CNS: Headache, fatigue, anxiety, confusion, insomnia
GI: Nausea, vomiting, anorexia, diarrhea, heartburn, **hepatitis,** discolored saliva
GU: Hematuria, *discolored urine*
HEMA: **Hemolytic anemia, eosinophilia, thrombocytopenia, leukopenia**
INTEG: Rash
MISC: Flulike symptoms, shortness of breath, chest pressure
MS: Asthenia, arthralgia, myalgia
Contraindications: Hypersensitivity, active TB, WBC <1000/mm^3 or platelet count <50,000/mm^3
Precautions: Pregnancy (B), breastfeeding, children, hepatic disease, blood dyscrasias

PHARMACOKINETICS

53% absorbed, peak 2-3 hr, duration >24 hr, half-life 45 hr, metabolized in liver (active/inactive metabolites), excreted in urine primarily as metabolites

INTERACTIONS

Increase: levels of rifabutin: ritonavir
Decrease: action of amprenavir, anticoagulants, β-blockers, barbiturates, busPIRone, clofibrate, corticosteroids, cycloSPORINE, dapsone, delavirdine, digoxin, disopyramide, doxycycline, efavirenz, estrogens, fluconazole, indinavir, ketoconazole, losartan, nelfinavir, nevirapine, opioid analgesic, oral contraceptives, phenytoin, quinidine, saquinavir, sulfonylureas, theophylline, tocainide, tricyclics, verapamil, zidovudine, zolpidem
Drug/Food

- High-fat diet decreases absorption

Drug/Lab Test
Interference: folate level, vit B_{12}, BSP, gallbladder studies

NURSING CONSIDERATIONS

Assess:

- CBC for neutropenia, thrombocytopenia, eosinophilia
- For acute TB: chest x-ray, sputum culture, blood culture, biopsy of lymph nodes, PPD; product should not be given for active TB
- Signs of anemia: Hct, Hgb, fatigue
- Hepatic studies q wk: ALT, AST, bilirubin
- Renal status before, q mo: BUN, creatinine, output, specific gravity, urinalysis
- Hepatic status: decreased appetite, jaundice, dark urine, fatigue

Administer:

- With food if GI upset occurs; better to take on empty stomach 1 hr before or 2 hr after meals; high-fat foods slow absorption; may take in 2 divided doses
- Antiemetic if vomiting occurs
- After C&S is completed; q mo to detect resistance

R

Evaluate:
• Therapeutic response: not used for active TB because of risk of development of resistance to rifampin; culture negative

Teach patient/family:
• That patients using oral contraceptives should consider using nonhormonal methods of birth control, since rifabutin may decrease their efficacy
• That compliance with dosage schedule, duration is necessary
• That scheduled appointments must be kept; relapse may occur
• That urine, feces, saliva, sputum, sweat, tears may be colored red-orange; soft contact lenses may be permanently stained
• To report flulike symptoms: excessive fatigue, anorexia, vomiting, sore throat; unusual bleeding, yellowish discoloration of skin, eyes
• To report myositis: muscle or bone pain

rifampin (℞)
(rif'am-pin)
Rifadin, Rofact ✦
Func. class.: Antitubercular
Chem. class.: Rifamycin B derivative

Do not confuse:
rifampin/rifabutin

Action: Inhibits DNA-dependent polymerase, decreases tubercle bacilli replication

Uses: Pulmonary TB, meningococcal carriers (prevention)

Unlabeled uses: Endocarditis, *Haemophilus influenzae type B prophylaxis,* Hansen's disease, *Mycobacterium avium* complex (MAC), orthopedic device-related infection, pruritus

DOSAGE AND ROUTES

Tuberculosis
• *Adult:* **PO/IV** Max 600 mg/day as single dose 1 hr before meals or 2 hr after meals, or 10 mg/kg/day 2-3×/wk
• *Child >5 yr:* **PO/IV** 10-20 mg/kg/day as single dose 1 hr before meals or 2 hr after meals, max 600 mg/day, with other antituberculars
• *6-mo regimen:* 2 mo treatment of isoniazid, rifampin, pyrazinamide, and possibly streptomycin or ethambutol; then rifampin and isoniazid × 4 mo
• *9-mo regimen:* Rifampin and isoniazid supplemented with pyrazinamide, or streptomycin, or ethambutol

Meningococcal carriers
• *Adult:* **PO/IV** 600 mg bid × 2 days, max 600 mg/dose
• *Child >5 yr:* **PO/IV** 10-20 mg/kg × 2 days, max 600 mg/dose
• *Infant 3 mo-1 yr:* 5 mg/kg **PO** bid for 2 days

Prevention of* H. influenzae *type B infection (unlabeled)
• *Adult:* **PO** 600 mg/day × 4 days
• *Child:* **PO** 20 mg/kg/day × 4 days

MAC (unlabeled)
• *Adult:* **PO/IV** 600 mg/day used with ≥3 other active microbials
• *Child:* **PO/IV** 10-20 mg/kg/day used with ≥3 other active microbials

Endocarditis with prosthetic valves (unlabeled)
• *Adult:* **PO** 300 mg q8hr with gentamicin and vancomycin
• *Child:* **PO** 20 mg/kg/day in 2 divided doses with gentamicin and vancomycin, max 900 mg/day

Available forms: Caps 150, 300 mg; powder for inj 600 mg/vial

SIDE EFFECTS

CNS: Headache, fatigue, anxiety, drowsiness, confusion
EENT: Visual disturbances
GI: Nausea, vomiting, anorexia, diarrhea, **pseudomembranous colitis,** *heartburn,* sore mouth and tongue, **pancreatitis,** increased LFTs
GU: **Hematuria, acute renal failure, hemoglobinuria**
HEMA: **Hemolytic anemia, eosinophilia, thrombocytopenia, leukopenia**
INTEG: Rash, pruritus, urticaria

MISC: Flulike symptoms, menstrual disturbances, edema, SOB
MS: Ataxia, weakness
Contraindications: Hypersensitivity to this product or rifamycins, active *Neisseria meningitidis* infection
Precautions: Pregnancy (C), breastfeeding, children <5 yr, hepatic disease, blood dyscrasias

PHARMACOKINETICS

PO: Peak 1-4 hr, duration >24 hr, half-life 3 hr, metabolized in liver (active/inactive metabolites), excreted in urine as free product (30% crosses placenta) and breast milk

INTERACTIONS

- Lithium toxicity: lithium
- Hepatotoxicity: isoniazid
- Incompatible with sodium lactate

Decrease: action of acetaminophen, alcohol, anticoagulants, antidiabetics, β-blockers, barbiturates, benzodiazepines, chloramphenicol, clofibrate, corticosteroids, cycloSPORINE, dapsone, digoxin, diltiazem, doxycycline, fluoroquinolones, haloperidol, hormones, imidazole antifungals, NIFEdipine, oral contraceptives, phenytoin, protease inhibitors, sulfonamides, theophylline, verapamil, zidovudine

Drug/Lab Test
Interference: folate level, vit B_{12}, gallbladder studies, dexamethasone suppression test
False positive: direct Coombs' test

NURSING CONSIDERATIONS

Assess:
- For infection: sputum culture, lung sounds
- Signs of anemia: Hct, Hgb, fatigue
- Hepatic studies q mo: ALT, AST, bilirubin
- Renal status before, q mo: BUN, creatinine, output, specific gravity, urinalysis
- Hepatic status: decreased appetite, jaundice, dark urine, fatigue

Administer:
- After C&S is completed; q mo to detect resistance
- Do not give IM or SUBCUT

PO route
- On empty stomach, 1 hr before or 2 hr after meals with a full glass of water
- Antiemetic if vomiting occurs

IV route
- After diluting each 600 mg/10 ml of sterile water for inj (60 mg/ml), agitate, withdraw dose and dilute in 100 ml or 500 ml of D_5W or 0.9% NaCl given as an inf over 3 hr, or if diluted in 100 ml, give over ½ hr; do not admix with other sol or medications

Evaluate:
- Therapeutic response: decreased symptoms of TB, culture negative

Teach patient/family:
- That compliance with dosage schedule, duration is necessary
- That scheduled appointments must be kept; relapse may occur
- To avoid alcohol, hepatotoxicity may occur
- That urine, feces, saliva, sputum, sweat, tears may be colored red-orange; soft contact lenses may be permanently stained
- To report flulike symptoms: excessive fatigue, anorexia, vomiting, sore throat; unusual bleeding, yellowish discoloration of skin, eyes
- To use nonhormonal form of birth control

R

rifapentine (℞)
(riff'ah-pen-teen)
Priftin
Func. class.: Antitubercular
Chem. class.: Rifamycin derivative

Action: Inhibits DNA-dependent polymerase, decreases tubercle bacilli replication
Uses: Pulmonary TB, must be used with at least one other antitubercular agent
Unlabeled uses: *Haemophilus influenzae* (β-lactamase negative/positive),

Legionella pneumophila, *Mycobacterium avium,* MAC, *M. bovis, M. fortuitum, M. intracellulare, M. kansasii, M. leprae, M. marinum, Neisseria meningitidis, Staphylococcus aureus* (MSSA)

DOSAGE AND ROUTES

Intensive phase

• *Adult:* **PO** 600 mg (four 150-mg tabs) 2×/wk, with an interval of 72 hr between doses × 2 mo; must be given with at least one other antitubercular agent

Continuation phase

• *Adult:* **PO** 600 mg q wk × 4 mo in combination with isoniazid or other appropriate antitubercular

Available forms: Tabs 150 mg

SIDE EFFECTS

CNS: Headache, fatigue, anxiety, dizziness

EENT: Visual disturbances

GI: Nausea, vomiting, anorexia, diarrhea, bilirubinemia, hepatitis, increased ALT, AST, *heartburn,* **pancreatitis**

GU: **Hematuria,** pyuria, proteinuria, urinary casts, urine discoloration

HEMA: **Thrombocytopenia, leukopenia, neutropenia, lymphopenia,** anemia, **leukocytosis,** purpura, hematoma

INTEG: Rash, pruritus, urticaria, acne

MISC: Edema, aggressive reaction, increased B/P

MS: Gout, arthrosis

Contraindications: Hypersensitivity to rifamycins, porphyria

Precautions: Pregnancy (C), breastfeeding, children <12 yr, geriatric patients, hepatic disease, blood dyscrasias, HIV

PHARMACOKINETICS

Peak 5-6 hr, half-life 13 hr, metabolized in liver (active/inactive metabolites), excreted in urine and feces, excreted in breast milk, protein binding 97%, steady state 10 days, CYP450 3A4, 2C8/9 inducer

INTERACTIONS

• Use with extreme caution with protease inhibitors

Decrease: action of amitriptyline, anticoagulants, antidiabetics, barbiturates, β-blockers, chloramphenicol, clarithromycin, clofibrate, corticosteroids, cycloSPORINE, dapsone, delavirdine, diazepam, digoxin, diltiazem, disopyramide, doxycycline, fentanyl, fluconazole, fluoroquinolones, haloperidol, indinavir, itraconazole, ketoconazole, methadone, mexiletine, nelfinavir, NIFEdipine, nortriptyline, oral contraceptives, phenothiazines, phenytoin, progestins, quinidine, quinine, ritonavir, saquinavir, sildenafil, tacrolimus, theophylline, thyroid preparations, tocainide, verapamil, warfarin, zidovudine

Drug/Food

Increase: absorption with food

Drug/Lab Test

Interference: folate level, vit B_{12}

NURSING CONSIDERATIONS

Assess:

• Baselines in CBC, AST, ALT, bilirubin, platelets

• For infection: sputum culture, lung sounds

• Signs of anemia: Hct, Hgb, fatigue

• Hepatic studies q mo: ALT, AST, bilirubin

• Renal status q mo: BUN, creatinine, output, specific gravity, urinalysis

• Hepatic status: decreased appetite, jaundice, dark urine, fatigue

Administer:

• May give with food for GI upset

• Antiemetic if vomiting occurs

• After C&S is completed; q mo to detect resistance

Evaluate:

• Therapeutic response: decreased symptoms of TB, culture negative

Teach patient/family:

• That compliance with dosage schedule, duration is necessary

• That scheduled appointments must be kept; relapse may occur

• That urine, feces, saliva, sputum, sweat, tears may be colored red-orange; soft contact lenses, dentures may be permanently stained
• To use alternative method of contraception, oral contraceptive action may be decreased
• To report flulike symptoms: excessive fatigue, anorexia, vomiting, sore throat; unusual bleeding, yellowish discoloration of skin, eyes

rifaximin (℞)

(rif-ax′i-min)
Xifaxan
Func. class.: Antiinfective—miscellaneous
Chem. class.: Analog of rifampin

Action: Binds to bacterial DNA–dependent RNA polymerase, thereby inhibiting bacterial RNA synthesis
Uses: Traveler's diarrhea in those ≥12 yr, caused by *E. coli*
Unlabeled uses: Crohn's disease, diverticulitis, hepatic encephalopathy

DOSAGE AND ROUTES

• *Adult and child ≥12 yr:* **PO** 200 mg tid × 3 days without regard to meals
Crohn's disease (unlabeled)
• *Adult:* **PO** 200 mg tid × 16 wk
Diverticulitis (unlabeled)
• *Adult:* **PO** 400 mg bid with mesalamine 800 mg tid × 7 days, then 7 days/mo
Hepatic encephalopathy (unlabeled)
• *Adult:* **PO** 400 mg q8hr × 5-21 days
Available forms: Tabs 200 mg

SIDE EFFECTS

CNS: Abnormal dreams, dizziness, insomnia
GI: Abdominal pain, constipation, defecation urgency, flatulence, nausea, rectal tenesmus, vomiting
MISC: Headache, pyrexia, motion sickness, tinnitus, rash, photosensitivity, **exfoliative dermatitis**

Contraindications: Hypersensitivity, diarrhea with fever, blood in stool
Precautions: Pregnancy (C), breastfeeding, children

PHARMACOKINETICS

Half-life 6 hr, induces P4503A4 (CYP3A4), excreted in feces

INTERACTIONS

Drug/Herb
• Do not use acidophilus with antiinfectives; separate by several hours

NURSING CONSIDERATIONS

Assess:
• For GI symptoms: amount, character of diarrhea, abdominal pain, nausea, vomiting
⚠ For overgrowth of infection and pseudomembranous colitis
Administer:
• Without regard to food
Evaluate:
• Therapeutic response: absence of infection
Teach patient/family:
• To discontinue rifaximin and notify prescriber if diarrhea persists for more than 24-48 hr, if diarrhea worsens, or if blood is in stools and fever is present
• That headache, rash, insomnia, abnormal dreams, tinnitus may occur

R

rilonacept (℞)

(ril-on′a-sept)
Arcalyst
Func. class.: Biologic response modifier
Chem. class.: Interleukin-1 inhibitor

Action: Inhibits interleukin-1 by binding IL-1 and preventing its interaction with receptors, thus reducing inflammation
Uses: Cryopyrin-associated periodic syndromes (CAPS) including familial cold autoinflammatory syndrome (FCAS) and

Muckle-Wells syndrome (MWS) in adults and children ≥12 yr

DOSAGE AND ROUTES

- *Adult:* **SUBCUT** 320 mg given as two 2-ml inj of 160 mg on the same day at two different sites, continue q wk with 160 mg as a single 2 ml inj starting on day 8, max 320 mg q wk
- *Child 12-17 yr:* **SUBCUT** 4.4 mg/kg (max 320 mg) given as 1 or 2 inj with no more volume than 2 ml, then 2.2 mg/kg (max 160 mg) once/wk starting on day 8

Available forms: Inj, lyophilized powder, vial 220 mg

SIDE EFFECTS

EENT: Sinusitis

GI: Nausea, vomiting, abdominal pain, stomach discomfort

HEMA: **Neutropenia, bleeding**

INTEG: Inj site reactions, rash, pruritus, ecchymosis

META: Hypercholesterolemia, hypertriglyceridemia

RESP: Upper respiratory infection, cough

SYST: **Malignancies,** meningitis

Contraindications: Hypersensitivity, IM/IV administration

Precautions: Pregnancy (C), breastfeeding, children <12 yr, geriatric patients, hepatic/renal disease, HIV/AIDS, asthma, bone-marrow suppression, diabetes mellitus, hamster protein hypersensitivity, hepatitis, hypercholesterolemia, hypertriglyceridemia, immunosuppression, infection, TB, live vaccines

PHARMACOKINETICS

Steady state 8 days

INTERACTIONS

- Avoid concurrent use with anakinra, adalimumab, tumor necrosis factor modifiers
- Do not use with vaccines, toxoids
- Change in effect: warfarin

Increase: infections—immunosuppressives

NURSING CONSIDERATIONS

Assess:

- Serum cholesterol/serum triglycerides baseline and periodically during treatment
- For symptoms of CAPS: fever, chills, rash, fatigue, joint pain, eye redness

Administer:

- As SUBCUT injection only
- Reconstitute each vial with 2.3 ml of supplied sterile water for inj (80 mg/ml); shake for 1 min and let stand for 1 min; do not use if particulate is present or if color is anything other than clear to pale yellow; use a new syringe/needle to withdraw needed amount; discard unused amount
- Maximum single inj is 2 ml (160 mg); if giving 4 ml (320 mg), give in two divided inj
- Rotate inj sites; do not use areas that are hard, bruised, red, or tender

Perform/provide:

- Storage of reconstituted solution for up to 3 hr at room temperature

Evaluation:

- Therapeutic response: absence of joint pain, fever, chills, fatigue, rash, eye redness

Teach patient/family:

- Reason for use and expected result

riluzole (℞)

(rill'you-zole)

Rilutek

Func. class.: ALS agent

Chem. class.: Benzathiazole

Action: May act by modulating the release of glutamate and inactivating voltage-dependent sodium channels

Uses: Amyotropic lateral sclerosis (ALS)

DOSAGE AND ROUTES

- *Adult:* **PO** 50 mg q12hr, take 1 hr before or 2 hr after meals

Available forms: Tabs 50 mg

SIDE EFFECTS

CNS: Hypertonia, depression, dizziness, insomnia, somnolence, vertigo, paresthesia
CV: Hypertension, tachycardia, phlebitis, palpitation, postural hypertension
GI: Nausea, vomiting, dyspepsia, anorexia, diarrhea, flatulence, stomatitis, dry mouth, increased LFTs, jaundice, abdominal pain
GU: UTI, dysuria
HEMA: **Neutropenia**
INTEG: Pruritus, eczema, alopecia, **exfoliative dermatitis**
MS: Arthralgia
RESP: Decreased lung function, rhinitis, increased cough, pneumonia
Contraindications: Hypersensitivity
Precautions: Pregnancy (C), breastfeeding, children, geriatric patients, neutropenia, renal/hepatic disease, cigarette smoking, febrile illness, pneumonia

PHARMACOKINETICS

Well absorbed, extensively metabolized by the liver, excretion in urine/feces

INTERACTIONS

Increase: elimination of riluzole—cigarette smoking, rifampin, omeprazole, charcoal-broiled food
Increase: hepatic injury—allopurinol, methyldopa, sulfasalazine, leflunomide, methotrexate, tacrine
Increase: LFTs—barbiturates, carbamazepine
Decrease: elimination of riluzole—caffeine, theophylline, amitriptyline, quinolones
Drug/Food
Decrease: absorption—high fat meal

NURSING CONSIDERATIONS

Assess:
- For clinical improvement in neurologic function
- Hepatic studies: AST, ALT, bilirubin, GGT, baseline and q mo × 3 mo, then q3mo; monitor LFTs
- For neutropenia <500/mm

Administer:
- 1 hr before or 2 hr after meals; a high-fat meal decreases absorption

Evaluate:
- Therapeutic response: improvement in neurologic status

Teach patient/family:
- To report febrile illness, signs of infection, cardiac/respiratory changes, which may indicate neutropenia
- The reason for product and expected results

rimantadine (℞)

(ri-man'tah-deen)
Flumadine
Func. class.: Synthetic antiviral
Chem. class.: Tricyclic amine

Do not confuse:
rimantadine/amantadine/ranitidine
Action: Prevents uncoating of nucleic acid in viral cell, preventing penetration of virus to host; causes release of DOPamine from neurons
Uses: Prophylaxis or treatment of influenza type A

DOSAGE AND ROUTES

Influenza type A
Prophylaxis
- *Adult and child >10 yr:* **PO** 100 mg bid
- *Child 1-10 yr:* **PO** 5 mg/kg/day, max 150 mg

Treatment
- *Adult:* **PO** 100 mg bid; start treatment at onset of symptoms, continue for at least 1 wk
- *Child ≥10 yr (unlabeled):* **PO** 200 mg/day either as a single dose or in 2 divided doses
- *Child 1-9 yr (unlabeled):* **PO** 6.6 mg/kg/day in 2 divided doses, max 150 mg/day in 2 divided doses
- *Geriatric:* **PO** 100 mg/day

Renal/hepatic dose
- *Adult:* **PO** ≤10 ml/min 100 mg daily

Available forms: Tabs 100 mg; syr 50 mg/5 ml

R

SIDE EFFECTS

CNS: ***Headache, dizziness,*** fatigue, depression, hallucinations, tremors, **seizures,** insomnia, poor concentration, asthenia, gait abnormalities, *anxiety,* confusion
CV: Pallor, palpitations, edema
EENT: Tinnitus, taste abnormality, eye pain
GI: ***Nausea, vomiting,*** constipation, ***dry mouth, anorexia, abdominal pain,*** diarrhea, dyspepsia
INTEG: Rash

Contraindications: Hypersensitivity to products of adamantine class (this product, amantadine)

Precautions: Pregnancy (C), breastfeeding, children <1 yr, seizure disorders, renal/hepatic disease

PHARMACOKINETICS

PO: Peak 6 hr, elimination half-life 13-65 hr, plasma protein binding (40%)

INTERACTIONS

Increase: rimantadine concentration—cimetidine

Decrease: peak concentration of rimantadine—acetaminophen, aspirin; intranasal influenza vaccine (separate by at least 48 hr)

NURSING CONSIDERATIONS

Assess:

• Assess for seizures; if seizures occur, product should be discontinued
• Bowel pattern before, during treatment
• CNS effect in geriatric patients or patients with severe renal, hepatic disease
• Skin eruptions, photosensitivity after administration of product
• Respiratory status: rate, character, wheezing, tightness in chest
• Allergies before initiation of treatment, reaction of each medication; list allergies on chart in bright red letters
• Signs of infection

Administer:

• Within 48 hr of exposure to influenza; continue for 10 days after contact
• At least 4 hr before bedtime to prevent insomnia
• After meals for better absorption, to decrease GI symptoms
• In divided doses to prevent CNS disturbances: headache, dizziness, fatigue, drowsiness

Perform/provide:

• Storage in tight, dry container

Evaluate:

• Therapeutic response: absence of fever, malaise, cough, dyspnea in infection

Teach patient/family:

• About aspects of product therapy: need to report dyspnea, dizziness, poor concentration, behavioral changes
• To avoid hazardous activities if dizziness occurs

rimexolone ophthalmic

See Appendix B

risedronate (℞)

(rih-sed′roh-nate)
Actonel
Func. class.: Bone resorption inhibitor
Chem. class.: Bisphosphonate

Action: Inhibits bone resorption, absorbs calcium phosphate crystal in bone and may directly block dissolution of hydroxyapatite crystals of bone

Uses: Paget's disease; prevention, treatment of osteoporosis in postmenopausal women; glucocorticoid-induced osteoporosis; osteoporosis in men

Unlabeled uses: Osteolytic metastases

DOSAGE AND ROUTES

Paget's disease

• *Adult:* **PO** 30 mg/day × 2 mo; patients with Paget's disease should receive calcium and vit D if dietary intake is lacking; if relapse occurs, retreatment is advised

Treatment/prevention of postmenopausal osteoporosis
• *Adult:* **PO** 5 mg/day or 35 mg q wk or 75 mg/day × 2 consecutive days 2× monthly or 150 mg q mo
Glucocorticoid osteoporosis
• *Adult:* **PO** 5 mg/day
Osteoporosis in men
• *Adult:* **PO** 35 mg q wk
Osteolytic metastases (unlabeled)
• *Adult:* **PO** 30 mg/day × 6 mo
Renal dose
• *Adult:* **PO** CCr <30 ml/min, avoid use
Available forms: Tabs 5, 30, 35, 75, 150 mg

SIDE EFFECTS

CNS: Dizziness, headache, depression
CV: *Chest pain,* hypertension, **atrial fibrillation**
GI: *Abdominal pain, diarrhea, nausea,* constipation, esophagitis
MISC: Rash, UTI, pharyngitis, hypocalcemia, hypophosphatemia, increase PTH
MS: Osteonecrosis of the jaw, severe muscle/joint/bone pain
SYST: Angioedema
Contraindications: Hypersensitivity to bisphosphonates, inability to stand or sit upright for ≥30 min
Precautions: Pregnancy (C), breastfeeding, children, renal disease, active upper GI disorders, dental disease

PHARMACOKINETICS

Rapidly cleared from circulation, taken up mainly by bones (50%), eliminated primarily through kidneys, absorption decreased by food, terminal half-life 220 hr

INTERACTIONS

Increase: GI irritation—NSAIDs, salicylates
Decrease: absorption of risedronate—aluminum, calcium, iron, magnesium salts, antacids
Drug/Food
Decrease: bioavailability—take ½ hr before food or drinks other than water
Drug/Lab Test
Interference: bone-imaging agents

NURSING CONSIDERATIONS

Assess:
• Symptoms of Paget's disease: headache, bone pain, increased head circumference
• Phosphate, alk phos, calcium; creatinine, BUN (renal disease)
• For hypocalcemia: paresthesia, twitching, laryngospasm, Chvostek's, Trousseau's signs
⚠ For serious skin reactions: angioedema
• For dental health; cover with antiinfectives prior to dental extraction
⚠ For atrial fibrillation
Administer:
• For 2 months to be effective in Paget's disease
• With a full glass of water, patient should be in upright position for ½ hr
• Supplemental calcium and vit D in Paget's disease if instructed by prescriber
• Give daily ≥30 min before meals
• For osteoporosis: bone density test before and after treatment
Perform/provide:
• Storage in cool environment, out of direct sunlight
Evaluate:
• Therapeutic response: increased bone mass, absence of fractures
Teach patient/family:
• To sit upright for ½ hr after dose to prevent irritation
• To comply with diet
• To notify prescriber if pregnancy is suspected or if breastfeeding
• Maintain good oral hygiene

R

risperidone (℞)

(ris-pehr′ih-dohn)

Risperdal, Risperdal Consta, Risperdal M-TAB

Func. class.: Antipsychotic

Chem. class.: Benzisoxazole derivative

Do not confuse:
Risperdal/reserpine

Action: Unknown; may be mediated through both DOPamine type 2 (D_2) and serotonin type 2 (5-HT_2) antagonism

Uses: Irritability associated with autism, bipolar disorder, mania, schizophrenia

Unlabeled uses: Acute psychosis, agitation, ADHD, dementia, psychotic depression, Tourette's syndrome

DOSAGE AND ROUTES

- *Adult:* **PO** 1 mg bid, with incremental increases of 1 mg bid on days 2 and 3 to a dose of 3 mg bid by day 3; then do not increase dose for at least 1 wk; **IM** 25 mg q2wk, may increase to max 50 mg q2wk
- *Geriatric:* **PO** 0.5 mg daily-bid, increase by 1 mg q wk

Hepatic/renal dose

- *Adult:* **PO** 0.5 mg bid, increase by 0.5 mg bid, increase to 1.5 mg bid

Available forms: Tabs 0.25, 0.5, 1, 2, 3, 4 mg; oral sol 1 mg/ml; orally disintegrating tabs 0.5, 1, 2, 3, 4 mg; long-acting inj kit (Risperidal Consta) 12.5, 25, 37.5, 50 mg; oral sol 1 mg/ml (30 ml)

SIDE EFFECTS

CNS: EPS, pseudoparkinsonism, akathisia, dystonia, tardive dyskinesia; drowsiness, insomnia, agitation, anxiety, headache, **seizures, neuroleptic malignant syndrome,** dizziness

CV: Orthostatic hypotension, **tachycardia; heart failure, sudden death (geriatric patients)**

EENT: Blurred vision

GI: Nausea, vomiting, *anorexia, constipation,* jaundice, weight gain

GU: Hyperprolactinemia, gynecomastia

MISC: **Renal artery occlusion;** weight gain, hyperprolactinemia (child)

RESP: Rhinitis; sinusitis, upper respiratory infection, cough

Contraindications: Hypersensitivity

Precautions: Pregnancy (C), children, geriatric patients, cardiac/renal/hepatic disease, breast cancer, Parkinson's disease, CNS depression, brain tumor, dehydration, diabetes, hematologic disease, seizure disorders, breastfeeding

Black Box Warning: Dementia with Lewy bodies

PHARMACOKINETICS

PO: Extensively metabolized by liver to a major active metabolite, plasma protein binding 90%, peak 1-2 hr, excreted 90% urine, terminal half-life 3-24 hr

INTERACTIONS

⚠ Possible death in dementia-related psychosis: furosemide

Increase: sedation—other CNS depressants, alcohol

Increase: EPS—CYP2D6 inhibitors (SSRIs)

Increase: EPS—other antipsychotics

Increase: risperidone excretion—carbamazepine

⚠ ***Increase:*** QT prolongation—class IA/III antidysrhythmics, some phenothiazines, β-agonists, local anesthetics, tricyclics, bepridil, haloperidol, methadone, chloroquine, clarithromycin, droperidol, erythromycin, grepafloxacin, halofantrine, pentamidine, probucol, sparfloxacin

Decrease: risperidone action—CYP2D6 inducers (carbamazepine, barbiturates, phenytoins, rifampin)

Decrease: levodopa effect—levodopa

Drug/Herb

Increase: CNS depression—kava

Increase: action—cola tree, hops, nettle, nutmeg

Increase: EPS—betel palm, kava

Drug/Lab Test

Increase: prolactin levels

NURSING CONSIDERATIONS

Assess:

- Mental status before initial administration
- Swallowing of PO medication; check for hoarding or giving of medication to other patients
- I&O ratio; palpate bladder if urinary output is low
- Bilirubin, CBC, hepatic studies q mo
- Urinalysis before, during prolonged therapy
- Affect, orientation, LOC, reflexes, gait, coordination, sleep pattern disturbances
- B/P standing and lying; also pulse, respirations; take these q4hr during initial treatment; establish baseline before starting treatment; report drops of 30 mm Hg; watch for ECG changes; QT prolongation may occur
- Dizziness, faintness, palpitations, tachycardia on rising
- EPS, including akathisia, tardive dyskinesia (bizarre movements of the jaw, mouth, tongue, extremities), pseudoparkinsonism (rigidity, tremors, pill rolling, shuffling gait)

⚠ For serious reactions in the geriatric patient: fatal pneumonia, heart failure, sudden death

⚠ For neuroleptic malignant syndrome: hyperthermia, increased CPK, altered mental status, muscle rigidity

- Skin turgor daily
- Constipation, urinary retention daily; if these occur, increase bulk and water in diet
- Weight gain, hyperglycemia, metabolic changes in diabetes

Administer:

- Reduced dose in geriatric patients
- Anticholinergic agent on order from prescriber, to be used for EPS
- Avoid use with CNS depressants
- Oral disintegrating tab: do not open blister pack until ready to use; tear 1 of the 4 units apart at perforation; bend corner where indicated; peel back foil; do not push tab through foil; remove from pack and place on tongue; tab disintegrates in seconds and can be swallowed with or without liquids

IM route

- Only use diluent and needle provided; do not substitute
- Do not give IV
- Inject deeply in gluteal or deltoid area of arm
- When switching from oral to inj, give oral dose with first inj and continue for 3 wk, then discontinue

Perform/provide:

- Decreased stimulus by dimming lights, avoiding loud noises
- Supervised ambulation until patient is stabilized on medication; do not involve in strenuous exercise program because fainting is possible; patient should not stand still for a long time
- Increased fluids to prevent constipation
- Sips of water, candy, gum for dry mouth
- Storage in tight, light-resistant container (PO); unopened vials in refrigerator, protect from light; do not freeze

Evaluate:

- Therapeutic response: decrease in emotional excitement, hallucinations, delusions, paranoia; reorganization of patterns of thought, speech

Teach patient/family:

- That orthostatic hypotension may occur and to rise from sitting or lying position gradually
- To avoid hot tubs, hot showers, tub baths; hypotension may occur
- To avoid abrupt withdrawal of this product; EPS may result; product should be withdrawn slowly
- To avoid OTC preparations (cough, hay fever, cold) unless approved by prescriber; serious product interactions may occur; avoid use of alcohol; increased drowsiness may occur
- To avoid hazardous activities if drowsy or dizzy
- Compliance with product regimen
- To report impaired vision, tremors, muscle twitching

R

• That heat stroke may occur in hot weather; take extra precautions to stay cool
• To use contraception, inform prescriber if pregnancy is planned or suspected
Treatment of overdose: Lavage if orally ingested; provide airway; *do not induce vomiting*

ritodrine (℞)
(rih'toh-dreen)
ritodrine, Yutopar
Func. class.: Tocolytic, uterine relaxant
Chem. class.: β_2-Adrenergic agonist

Action: Reduces frequency, intensity of uterine contractions by stimulation of the β_2-receptors in uterine smooth muscle
Uses: Management of preterm labor

DOSAGE AND ROUTES
• *Adult:* **IV INF** 150 mg/500 ml (0.3 mg/ml) given 0.1 mg/min, increase gradually by 0.05 mg/min q10min until desired response, max 0.35 mg/min
Available forms: Inj 10 mg/ml, 15 mg/ml

SIDE EFFECTS
CNS: Headache, restlessness, anxiety, nervousness, sweating, chills, drowsiness, tremor
CV: Altered maternal, fetal heart rate, B/P, dysrhythmias, palpitations, chest pain, maternal pulmonary edema
GI: Nausea, vomiting, anorexia, malaise, bloating, constipation, diarrhea
META: Hyperglycemia, hypokalemia
MISC: Erythema, rash, dyspnea, hyperventilation, glycosuria, **lactic acidosis**
Contraindications: Hypersensitivity, eclampsia, hypertension, dysrhythmias, thyrotoxicosis, before 20th wk of pregnancy, antepartum hemorrhage, intrauterine fetal death, maternal cardiac disease, pulmonary hypertension, uncontrolled diabetes, pheochromocytoma, bronchial asthma
Precautions: Pregnancy (B), migraine, sulfite sensitivity, pregnancy-induced hypertension, diabetes

PHARMACOKINETICS
IV: Immediate, distribution half-life 6 min, 2nd phase 1½-2½ hr, elimination phase >10 hr, metabolized in liver, 90% excreted in urine, crosses placenta

INTERACTIONS
Increase: pulmonary edema—corticosteroids
Increase: systemic hypertension—atropine
Increase: CV effects of ritodrine—magnesium sulfate, diazoxide, meperidine, potent general anesthetics
Increase: effects of sympathomimetic amines
Decrease: action of ritodrine—β-blockers
Drug/Lab Test
Increase: blood glucose, free fatty acids, insulin, GTT
Decrease: potassium

NURSING CONSIDERATIONS
Assess:
• Maternal, fetal heart tones during inf; maternal ECG to determine CV disease
• Intensity, length of uterine contractions
• Fluid intake to prevent fluid overload; discontinue if this occurs
• Blood glucose in diabetics
Administer:
• Only clear sol
• After dilution: 150 mg/500 ml D_5W or NS, give at 0.3 mg/ml
• Using inf pump; product should be continued for 12 hr after contractions stop
• Considered incompatible with any product in sol or syringe
• In bed during inf
Perform/provide:
• Positioning of patient in left lateral recumbent position to decrease hypotension, increase renal blood flow

Evaluate:
- Therapeutic response: decreased intensity, length of contraction, absence of preterm labor, decreased B/P

ritonavir (℞)
(ri-toe'na-veer)
Norvir
Func. class.: Antiretroviral
Chem. class.: Protease inhibitor

Do not confuse:
ritonavir/Retrovir

Action: Inhibits human immunodeficiency virus (HIV-1) protease and prevents maturation of the infectious virus

Uses: HIV-1 in combination with other antiretrovirals

DOSAGE AND ROUTES
- *Adult and adolescent >16 yr:* **PO** 600 mg bid; if nausea occurs begin dose at ½ and gradually increase
- *Adolescent ≤16 yr and child, infant:* **PO** 400 mg/m^2 bid up to 1200 mg/day, may start lower and escalate

Available forms: Caps 100 mg; oral sol 80 mg/ml

SIDE EFFECTS
CNS: Paresthesia, headache, **seizures,** fever, dizziness, insomnia, asthenia, **intracranial bleeding**
CV: **QT, PR interval prolongation**
GI: Diarrhea, buccal mucosa ulceration, *abdominal pain, nausea, taste perversion,* dry mouth, *vomiting, anorexia*
INTEG: Rash
MISC: Asthenia, **angioedema, anaphylaxis, Stevens-Johnson syndrome,** increase lipids, lipodystrophy
MS: Pain

Contraindications: Hypersensitivity

Black Box Warning: Coadministration with other drugs

Precautions: Pregnancy (B), breastfeeding, hepatic disease, pancreatitis, diabetes, hemophilia, AV block, hypercholesterolemia, immune reconstitution syndrome, neonates, cardiomyopathy

PHARMACOKINETICS
Well absorbed, 98% protein binding, hepatic metabolism, peak 2-4 hr, terminal half-life 3-5 hr

INTERACTIONS
⚠ Toxicity: amiodarone, astemizole, azole antifungals, benzodiazepines, bepridil, buPROPion, cisapride, clozapine, desipramine, dihydroergotamine, encainide, ergotamine, flecainide, HMG-CoA reductase inhibitors, interleukins, meperidine, midazolam, pimozide, piroxicam, propafenone, propoxyphene, quinidine, ranolazine, saquinavir, terfenadine, triazolam, zolpidem

Increase: ritonavir levels—fluconazole

Increase: level of both products—clarithromycin, ddI

Increase: levels of—bosentan

Decrease: ritonavir levels—rifamycins, nevirapine, barbiturates, phenytoin

Decrease: levels of anticoagulants, atovaquone, divalproex, ethinyl estradiol, lamotrigine, phenytoin, sulfamethoxazole, theophylline, voriconazole, zidovudine

Drug/Herb

Decrease: ritonavir levels—St. John's wort; avoid concurrent use
- Avoid use with red yeast rice

Drug/Lab Test

Increase: AST, ALT, CPK, cholesterol, GGT, triglycerides, uric acid

Decrease: Hct, Hgb, RBC, neutrophils, WBC

R

NURSING CONSIDERATIONS
Assess:
⚠ For QT, PR prolongation, ECG
- Signs of infection, anemia
- Hepatic studies: ALT, AST
- Viral load and CD4 baseline and throughout therapy; blood glucose, plasma HIV RNA, serum cholesterol/lipid profile
- Resistance testing prior to starting therapy and after treatment failure
- C&S before product therapy; product may be taken as soon as culture is taken; repeat C&S after treatment; determine the

presence of other sexually transmitted diseases

• Bowel pattern before, during treatment; if severe abdominal pain with bleeding occurs, discontinue product; monitor hydration

• Skin eruptions; rash

• Allergies before treatment, reaction to each medication

Administer:

• Shake oral solution well

• Store caps in refrigerator

• That product must be taken in equal intervals around the clock to maintain blood levels for duration of therapy

• To take with food; mix liquid formulation with chocolate milk or liquid nutritional supplement

Evaluate:

• Therapeutic response: improvement in HIV symptoms; improving viral load, CD4+ T cells

Teach patient/family:

• To take as prescribed; if dose is missed, take as soon as remembered up to 1 hr before next dose; do not double dose

• That product is not a cure for HIV; opportunistic infections may continue to be acquired

• That redistribution of body fat or accumulation of body fat may occur

• That others may continue to contract HIV from the patient

• Not to use St. John's wort; that it decreases this product's effect

rituximab (℞)

(rih-tuks'ih-mab)

Rituxan

Func. class.: Antineoplastic—miscellaneous; DMARDs

Chem. class.: Murine/human monoclonal antibody

Action: Directed against the CD20 antigen that is found on malignant B lymphocytes; CD20 regulates a portion of cell-cycle initiation/differentiation

Uses: Non-Hodgkin's lymphoma (CD20 positive, B-cell), bulky disease (tumors >10 cm), rheumatoid arthritis

Unlabeled uses: Acquired blood factor deficiency, acute lymphocytic leukemia (ALL), Burkitt's lymphoma, chronic lymphocytic leukemia (CLL), hemolytic anemia, human herpesvirus 8, mantle cell lymphoma (MCL), multicentric Castleman's disease, peripheral blood stem cell (PBSC) mobilization, refractory pemphigus vulgaris, relapsing–remitting MS, ITP with dexamethasone

DOSAGE AND ROUTES

Non-Hodgkin's lymphoma (NHL), chronic lymphocytic leukemia (CLL)

• *Adult:* **IV INF** 375 mg/m^2 q wk × 4 doses; give at 50 mg/hr for 1st inf; if hypersensitivity does not occur, increase rate by 50 mg/hr q½hr, max 400 mg/hr; slow/interrupt inf if hypersensitivity occurs; other inf can be given at 100 mg/hr and increased by 100 mg/hr, max 400 mg/hr

Rheumatoid arthritis; relapsing–remitting MS (unlabeled)

• *Adult:* **IV** 1000 mg on days 1, 15

Available forms: Inj 10 mg/ml

SIDE EFFECTS

CNS: **Life-threatening brain infection**

CV: **Cardiac dysrhythmias, heart failure, hypertension, MI, supraventricular tachycardia,** angina

GI: *Nausea, vomiting, anorexia,* **GI obstruction/perforation**

GU: **Renal failure**

HEMA: **Leukopenia, neutropenia, thrombocytopenia,** anemia

INTEG: *Irritation at site, rash,* **fatal mucocutaneous infections (rare)**

MISC: *Fever,* chills, asthenia, *headache,* **angioedema,** hypotension, myalgia, **bronchospasm, ARDs**

SYST: **Toxic epidermal necrolysis, tumor lysis syndrome, Stevens-Johnson syndrome, exfoliative dermatitis**

Contraindications: Hypersensitivity, murine proteins

Precautions: Pregnancy (C), breastfeeding, children, geriatric patients, pulmonary/cardiac/renal conditions

Black Box Warning: Exfoliative dermatitis, infusion-related reactions, progressive multifocal leukoencephalopathy

PHARMACOKINETICS

Half-life 31-152 hr

INTERACTIONS

Increase: bleeding—anticoagulants
- Avoid with vaccines, toxoids

NURSING CONSIDERATIONS

Assess:

⚠ For signs of fatal inf reaction: hypoxia, pulmonary infiltrates, ARDS, MI, ventricular fibrillation, cardiogenic shock; most fatal inf reactions occur with first inf; potentially fatal

⚠ For signs of severe mucocutaneous reactions: Stevens-Johnson syndrome, lichenoid dermatitis, toxic epidermal lysis; occur 1-13 wk after product is given

⚠ Tumor lysis syndrome: acute renal failure requiring hemodialysis, hyperkalemia, hypocalcemia, hyperuricemia, hyperphosphatemia

- CBC, differential, platelet count weekly; withhold product if WBC is <3500/mm^3, or platelet count <100,000/mm^3; notify prescriber of these results; product should be discontinued
- ECG, serum creatinine/BUN, electrolytes, uric acid
- GI symptoms: frequency of stools
- Signs of dehydration: rapid respirations, poor skin turgor, decreased urine output, dry skin, restlessness, weakness

Administer:

Intermittent IV INF route
- Hold antihypertensives 12 hr prior to administration
- After diluting to a final conc. of 1-4 mg/ml; use 0.9% NaCl, D_5W, gently invert bag to mix; do not mix with other products

Perform/provide:
- Increase fluid intake to 2-3 L/day for dehydration unless contraindicated
- Nutritious diet with iron, vitamin supplement, low fiber, few dairy products
- Storage of vials at 36° F-40° F, protect vials from direct sunlight, inf sol is stable at 36° F-46° F × 24 hr and room temperature for another 12 hr

Evaluate:
- Therapeutic response: prevention of increasing cancer progression

Teach patient/family:
- Avoid with vaccines, toxoids
- Use contraception during and up to 12 mo after therapy
- To report adverse reactions
- To avoid OTC products
- To avoid crowds, those with known infections
- To maintain fluid intake

rivastigmine (℞)

(riv-as-tig′mine)

Exelon, Exelon Patch

Func. class.: Anti-Alzheimer agent

Chem. class.: Cholinesterase inhibitor

Action: Potent, selective inhibitor of brain acetylcholinesterase (AChE) and butyrylcholinesterase (BChE)

Uses: Mild to moderate Alzheimer's dementia, dementia associated with Parkinson's disease

Unlabeled use: Vascular dementia, dementia with Lewy bodies, Pick's disease

DOSAGE AND ROUTES

- *Adult:* **PO** 1.5 mg bid with food; after 4 wk or more, may increase to 3 mg bid after 4 wk or more; may increase to 4.5 mg bid and thereafter 6 mg bid, max 12 mg/day; **TRANSDERMAL** apply 4.6 mg/24 hr/day, after 4 wk or more may increase to 9.5 mg/24 hr/day

Available forms: Caps 1.5, 3, 4.5, 6 mg; solution 2 mg/ml; transdermal patch 4.6, 9.5 mg/24 hr

R

SIDE EFFECTS

CNS: Tremors, confusion, insomnia, psychosis, hallucination, depression, dizziness, headache, anxiety, somnolence, fatigue, syncope, EPS, exacerbation of Parkinson's disease

GI: Nausea, vomiting, anorexia, abdominal distress, flatulence, diarrhea, constipation, dyspepsia

MISC: Urinary tract infection, asthenia, increased sweating, hypertension, flulike symptoms, weight change

Contraindications: Hypersensitivity to this product, other carbamates; GI bleeding; jaundice

Precautions: Pregnancy (B), breastfeeding, children, respiratory/cardiac/renal/hepatic disease, seizure disorder, peptic ulcer, urinary obstruction, asthma, increased intracranial pressure, surgery

PHARMACOKINETICS

Rapidly and completely absorbed, metabolized to decarbamylated metabolite, half-life is 1.5 hr, excreted via kidneys (metabolites), clearance is lowered in the geriatric patient, hepatic disease, and increased in nicotine use; 40% protein binding

INTERACTIONS

Increase: synergistic effect—cholinergic agonists, other cholinesterase inhibitors

Increase: metabolism—nicotine

Increase: GI effects—NSAIDs

Decrease: rivastigmine effect—anticholinergics, sedating H_1 blockers, tricyclics, phenothiazines

NURSING CONSIDERATIONS

Assess:

- Hepatic studies: AST, ALT, alk phos, LDH, bilirubin, CBC
- For severe GI effects: nausea, vomiting, anorexia, weight loss, diarrhea
- B/P, heart rate, respiration during initial treatment; hypo/hypertension should be reported
- Mental status: affect, mood, behavioral changes, depression, insomnia; complete suicide assessment

Administer:

- With meals; take with morning and evening meal even though absorption may be decreased
- Discontinue treatment for several doses and restart at same or next lower dosage level, if adverse reactions cause intolerance
- If treatment is interrupted for longer than several days, treatment should be initiated with lowest daily dose and titrated as indicated above

Transdermal route

- To hairless, clean, dry skin not in an area that clothing will rub; rotate sites daily; remove liner; apply firmly; may be used during bathing, swimming; avoid saunas

Perform/provide:

- Assistance with ambulation during beginning therapy; dizziness may occur

Evaluate:

- Therapeutic response: improved mood/confusion

Teach patient/family:

- The procedure for giving oral solution; use instruction sheet provided
- To notify prescriber of severe GI effects
- That product may cause dizziness, anorexia, weight loss

rizatriptan (℞)

(rye-zah-trip'tan)

Maxalt, Maxalt-MLT

Func. class.: Migraine agent

Chem. class.: 5-HT_{1D} receptor agonist, abortive agent-triptan

Action: Binds selectively to the vascular 5-$HT_{1B/1D}$ receptor subtype, exerts antimigraine effect; causes vasoconstriction in cranial arteries

Uses: Acute treatment of migraine

DOSAGE AND ROUTES

- *Adult:* **PO** 5-10 mg single dose, redosing separate by 2 hr or more, max 30 mg/24 hr; use 5 mg in patient on propranolol, max 15 mg/24 hr

Available forms: Tabs (Maxalt) 5, 10 mg; orally disintegrating tabs (Maxalt-MLT) 5, 10 mg

SIDE EFFECTS

CNS: Dizziness, drowsiness, headache, fatigue, warm/cold sensations, flushing

CV: **MI, ventricular fibrillation, ventricular tachycardia, coronary artery vasospasm**

ENDO: Hot flashes, mild increase in growth hormone

GI: Nausea, dry mouth, diarrhea, abdominal pain

RESP: Chest tightness, pressure, dyspnea

Contraindications: Angina pectoris, history of MI, documented silent ischemia, Prinzmetal's angina, ischemic heart disease, concurrent ergotamine-containing preparations, uncontrolled hypertension, hypersensitivity, basilar or hemiplegic migraine

Precautions: Pregnancy (C), breastfeeding, children, geriatric patients, postmenopausal women, men >40 yr, risk factors for CAD, hypercholesterolemia, obesity, diabetes, impaired renal/hepatic function

PHARMACOKINETICS

Onset of pain relief 10 min-2 hr; peak 1-1½ hr; duration 14-16 hr; 14% plasma protein binding; metabolized in the liver (metabolite); excreted in urine (82%), feces (12%); half-life 2-3 hr

INTERACTIONS

• Weakness, hyperreflexia, incoordination: SSRIs

Increase: levels of sibutramine

Increase: rizatriptan action—cimetidine, oral contraceptives, MAOIs, nonselective MAOI (type A and B), isocarboxazide, pargyline, phenelzine, propranolol, tranylcypromine

Increase: vasospastic effects—ergot, ergot derivatives, other 5-HT receptor agonists

Drug/Herb

• Serotonin syndrome: SAM-e, St. John's wort

Increase: effect—butterbur, feverfew

NURSING CONSIDERATIONS

Assess:

• For migraine symptoms: visual disturbances, aura

• For stress level, activity, recreation, coping mechanisms

• Neurologic status: LOC, blurring vision, nausea, vomiting, tingling in extremities preceding headache

• Ingestion of tyramine foods (pickled products, beer, wine, aged cheese), food additives, preservatives, colorings, artificial sweeteners, chocolate, caffeine, which may precipitate these types of headaches

• Renal status: urine output

Administer:

• Oral disintegrating tab: do not open blister until use; peel blister open with dry hands; place tab on tongue, where it will dissolve, and swallow with saliva (contains phenylalanine)

Perform/provide:

• Quiet, calm environment with decreased stimulation for noise, bright light, excessive talking

Evaluate:

• Therapeutic response: decrease in frequency, severity of headache

Teach patient/family:

• Use of orally disintegrating tab: instruct patient not to open blister until use, to peel blister open with dry hands, to place tab on tongue, where it will dissolve, and to swallow with saliva (contains phenylalanine)

• To report any side effects to prescriber

• To use alternative contraception while taking product if oral contraceptives are being used

• That product does not prevent or reduce number of migraines, main action is abortive

R

⚠ High Alert

rocuronium (℞)
(ro-kyur-oh′nium)
Zemuron
Func. class.: Neuromuscular blocker (nondepolarizing)
Chem. class.: Biquaternary ammonium ester

Action: Inhibits transmission of nerve impulses by binding with cholinergic receptor sites, antagonizing action of acetylcholine

Uses: Facilitation of endotracheal intubation, skeletal muscle relaxation during mechanical ventilation, surgery, or general anesthesia

DOSAGE AND ROUTES

• *Adult (intubation):* **IV** 0.6 mg/kg, max blockade within 4 min; median relaxation time 31 min; 0.45 mg/kg provides about 22 min relaxation
• *Child 1-12 yr:* **IV** 0.6 mg/kg; onset 1 min; median relaxation time 27 min
• *Child 3 mo-1 yr:* **IV** 0.6 mg/kg; onset 1 min; median relaxation time 41 min

Rapid-sequence intubation
• *Adult/geriatric:* **IV** 0.6-1.2 mg/kg

Available forms: Inj 10 mg/ml

SIDE EFFECTS

CV: Bradycardia, tachycardia, change in B/P, edema
GI: Nausea, vomiting
INTEG: Rash, flushing, pruritus, urticaria
MS: Myopathy
RESP: **Prolonged apnea, bronchospasm, cyanosis, respiratory depression,** dyspnea, **pulmonary vascular resistance**
SYST: Tolerance

Contraindications: Hypersensitivity

Precautions: Pregnancy (C), breastfeeding, children, geriatric patients, electrolyte imbalances, dehydration, respiratory/neuromuscular/cardiac/renal/hepatic disease

PHARMACOKINETICS

Terminal half-life 60-70 min, duration ½ hr, metabolized in liver

INTERACTIONS

• Theophylline increases risk of dysrhythmias

Increase: neuromuscular blockade caused by amphotericin B, verapamil, aminoglycosides, clindamycin, enflurane, isoflurane, lincomycin, lithium, opiates, local anesthetics, polymyxin, antiinfectives, quinidine, thiazides

NURSING CONSIDERATIONS

Assess:
• For electrolyte imbalances (K, Mg), before product is used; electrolyte imbalances may lead to increased action of this product
• VS (B/P, pulse, respirations, airway) until fully recovered; rate, depth, pattern of respirations, strength of hand grip; patient should be intubated before use
• Recovery: decreased paralysis of face, diaphragm, leg, arm, rest of body; residual weakness and respiratory problems may occur during recovery
• Allergic reactions: rash, fever, respiratory distress, pruritus; product should be discontinued

Administer:
• Using peripheral nerve stimulator by anesthesiologist to determine neuromuscular blockade; deep tendon reflexes should be monitored during extended use
• Undiluted direct IV over 2 min (only by qualified person, usually anesthesiologist); do not administer IM
• Maintenance q20-45min after 1st dose; titrate to response

Perform/provide:
• Storage in light-resistant area, refrigerate; stable for 30 days at room temperature
• Reassurance if communication is difficult during recovery from neuromuscular blockade

Evaluate:

- Therapeutic response: paralysis of jaw, eyelid, head, neck, rest of body as evaluated by peripheral nerve stimulator

Teach patient/family:

- About all procedures or treatments; patient will remain conscious if anesthesia is not given also

Treatment of overdose: Edrophonium or neostigmine, atropine, monitor VS; may require mechanical ventilation

romiplostim (℞)

(roe-mi-ploe'stim)

Nplate

Func. class.: Thrombopoietin receptor agonist

Action: A thrombopoietin-like fusion protein produced by DNA recombinant technology

Uses: Chronic idiopathic thrombocytopenic purpura in patients who have had an insufficient response to corticosteroids, immunoglobulins, or splenectomy

DOSAGE AND ROUTES

- *Adult:* **SUBCUT** 1 mcg/kg q wk, increase q wk by 1 mcg/kg until platelets ≥50,000/mm^3, max 10 mcg/kg/wk

Available forms: Inj vials 250, 500 mcg

SIDE EFFECTS

CNS: ***Dizziness, insomnia, headache,*** fatigue

GI: Abdominal pain, dyspepsia, diarrhea

HEMA: **Thromboembolism, thrombosis,** bleeding, myelofibrosis

MS: Myalgia

SYST: **Secondary malignancy,** antibody formation

Contraindications: Hypersensitivity to this product or mannitol

Precautions: Pregnancy (C), breastfeeding, children, malignancies, bleeding, bone marrow suppression

PHARMACOKINETICS

Peak 7-50 hr, half-life 1-34 days

INTERACTIONS

- Possible bleeding risk: anticoagulants, NSAIDs, platelet inhibitors, thrombolytics, salicylates

NURSING CONSIDERATIONS

Assess:

- Blood studies: CBC during treatment weekly and for 2 wk after discontinuing

Administer:

- Romiplastin is only available through Nplate NEXUS Program; call 1-877-675-2831 to enroll

SUBCUT route

- Use 0.01 ml graduations syringe
- Discard any unused portion in vial; do not pool unused portions from vials
- Dilute 250 mcg/0.72 preservative-free sterile water for inj; 500 mcg/1.2 preservative-free sterile water for inj; final concentration 500 mcg/ml
- Gently swirl until dissolved; do not shake
- Do not use if discolored or if particulate matter is present
- Inject into outer aspect of upper arm or abdomen except for 2 inches around navel or front aspect of middle thigh; do not use areas that are bruised, scratched, or scarred
- Rotate inj sites

Perform/provide:

- Storage of vials refrigerated, do not freeze; protect from light; diluted sol is stable refrigerated or at room temperature for 24 hr

Evaluate:

- Therapeutic response: increase in platelet counts, absence of bleeding

Teach patient/family:

- To report bleeding
- The reason for product and expected results
- To report a missed dose to prescriber due to increased risk of bleeding

R

ropinirole (℞)

(roh-pin'ih-role)

Requip, Requip XL

Func. class.: Antiparkinson agent

Chem. class.: DOPamine-receptor agonist, nonergot

Action: Selective agonist for D_2 receptors (presynaptic/postsynaptic sites); binding at D_3 receptor contributes to antiparkinson effects

Uses: Parkinson's disease, restless leg syndrome (RLS)

DOSAGE AND ROUTES

• *Adult:* **PO** 0.25 mg tid, titrate weekly to a max of 24 mg/day; (XL) 2 mg/day × 1-2 wk, may increase by 2 mg/day q wk

Restless leg syndrome

• *Adult:* **PO** 0.25 mg 1-3 hr before bedtime; may increase until symptoms resolve

Available forms: Tabs 0.25, 0.5, 1, 2, 3, 4, 5 mg; ext rel tab 2, 4, 8, 12 mg

SIDE EFFECTS

CNS: Agitation, insomnia, psychosis, hallucination, dystonia, depression, dizziness, somnolence, **sleep attacks**

CV: Orthostatic hypotension, tachycardia, hypo/hypertension, syncope, palpitations

EENT: Blurred vision

GI: Nausea, vomiting, anorexia, dry mouth, constipation, dyspepsia, flatulence

GU: Impotence, urinary frequency

HEMA: **Hemolytic anemia, leukopenia, agranulocytosis**

INTEG: Rash, sweating

RESP: Pharyngitis, rhinitis, sinusitis, bronchitis, dyspnea

Contraindications: Hypersensitivity

Precautions: Pregnancy (C), dysrhythmias, affective disorder, psychosis, cardiac/renal/hepatic disease

PHARMACOKINETICS

Peak 1-2 hr, half-life 6 hr, extensively metabolized by the liver by P450 CYP1A2 enzyme system, protein binding 40%

INTERACTIONS

Increase: ropinirole effect—cimetidine, ciprofloxacin, diltiazem, enoxacin, erythromycin, fluvoxamine, mexiletine, norfloxacin, tacrine, digoxin, theophylline, L-dopa

Decrease: ropinirole effects—butyrophenones, metoclopramide, phenothiazines, thioxanthenes

Drug/Herb

Decrease: ropinirole action—chaste tree fruit, kava

NURSING CONSIDERATIONS

Assess:

• Involuntary movements in parkinsonism: akinesia, tremors, staggering gait, muscle rigidity, drooling

• B/P, respiration during initial treatment; hypo/hypertension should be reported

⚠ For sleep attacks, drowsiness, falling asleep without warning even during hazardous activities

• Mental status: affect, mood, behavioral changes, depression; complete suicide assessment

Administer:

• Product until NPO before surgery

• Adjust dosage to patient response

• With meals to reduce nausea

Perform/provide:

• Testing for diabetes mellitus, acromegaly if on long-term therapy

Evaluate:

• Therapeutic response: improvement in movement disorder

Teach patient/family:

• That therapeutic effects may take several weeks to a few months

• To change positions slowly to prevent orthostatic hypotension

• To use product exactly as prescribed; if product is discontinued abruptly, parkinsonian crisis may occur

ropivacaine (℞)
(roe-pi'va-kane)
Naropin
Func. class.: Local anesthetic
Chem. class.: Amide

Action: Competes with calcium for sites in nerve membrane that control sodium transport across cell membrane; decreases rise of depolarization phase of action potential

Uses: Peripheral nerve block, caudal anesthesia, central neural block, vaginal, epidural, spinal block

DOSAGE AND ROUTES

Lumbar epidural block for cesarean section
- *Adult:* 20-30 ml of 0.5% sol
- *Adult:* 15-20 ml of 0.75% sol

Thoracic epidural
- *Adult:* 5-15 ml of 0.5% to 0.75% sol

Major nerve block
- *Adult:* 35-50 ml of 0.5% sol
- *Adult:* 10-40 ml of 0.75% sol

Labor pain (epidural)
- *Adult:* 10-20 ml 0.2% sol then 6-14 ml/1 hr

Postop (lumbar or thoracic epidural)
- *Adult:* 6-14 ml/hr of 0.2% sol

Infiltration/minor nerve block
- *Adult:* 1-100 ml of 0.2% sol
- *Adult:* 1-40 ml of 0.5% sol

Available forms: Inj 2, 5, 7.5 mg/ml

SIDE EFFECTS

CNS: Anxiety, restlessness, **seizures, loss of consciousness,** drowsiness, disorientation, tremors, shivering, *paresthesia*

CV: **Myocardial depression, cardiac arrest, dysrhythmias,** bradycardia, *hypo*/hypertension, ***fetal bradycardia***

EENT: Blurred vision, tinnitus, pupil constriction

ENDO: Hypokelamia

GI: Nausea, vomiting

GU: Urinary retention

INTEG: Rash, urticaria, allergic reactions, edema, burning, skin discoloration at inj site, tissue necrosis

RESP: **Status asthmaticus, respiratory arrest, anaphylaxis**

Contraindications: Children <12 yr, geriatric patients, hypersensitivity to amide local anesthetics, severe hepatic disease, severe hypotension, complete heart block

Precautions: Pregnancy (B), severe product allergies, hyperthyroidism, neurologic/CV/hepatic disease

PHARMACOKINETICS

Onset varies with inj site, duration varies with inj site, metabolized by liver, excreted in urine (metabolites)

INTERACTIONS

- Dysrhythmias: epinephrine, halothane, enflurane
- Hypertension: MAOIs, tricyclics, phenothiazines

Increase: effect—amiodarone, cimetidine, ciprofloxacin, fluvoxamine, azole antifungals, theophylline, imipramine

Decrease: action of ropivacaine—chloroprocaine

NURSING CONSIDERATIONS

Assess:
- B/P, pulse, respiration during treatment
- Fetal heart tones during labor
- Allergic reactions: rash, urticaria, itching
- Cardiac status: ECG for dysrhythmias, pulse, B/P during anesthesia

Administer:
- Only with crash cart, resuscitative equipment nearby
- Only products without preservatives for epidural or caudal anesthesia

Perform/provide:
- Use of new sol; discard unused portions

Evaluate:
- Therapeutic response: anesthesia necessary for procedure

R

Treatment of overdose: Airway, O_2, vasopressor, IV fluids, anticonvulsants for seizures

rosiglitazone (℞)

(ros-ih-glit′ah-zone)
Avandia
Func. class.: Antidiabetic, oral
Chem. class.: Thiazolidinedione

Action: Improves insulin resistance by hepatic glucose metabolism, insulin receptor kinase activity, insulin receptor phosphorylation

Uses: Type 2 diabetes mellitus, alone or in combination with sulfonylureas, metformin, or insulin

Unlabeled uses: Increased ovulation frequency in those with polycystic ovary syndrome; reduced in-stent restenosis in those with diabetes

DOSAGE AND ROUTES

• *Adult:* **PO** 4 mg/day or in 2 divided doses, may increase to 8 mg/day or in 2 divided doses after 12 wk; may be added to metformin, sulfonylurea at the adult dose

• *Adults with CHF class I/II:* **PO** 2 mg daily, may increase slowly

Available forms: Tabs 2, 4, 8 mg

SIDE EFFECTS

CNS: Fatigue, ***headache***

CV: **MI, CHF, death (geriatric patients)**

ENDO: Hypo/hyperglycemia

GI: Weight gain, **hepatotoxicity**

MISC: Accidental injury, URI, sinusitis, anemia, back pain, diarrhea, edema, bone fractures (female)

SYST: **Anaphylaxis, Stevens-Johnson syndrome**

Contraindications: Breastfeeding, children, hypersensitivity to thiazolidinediones, diabetic ketoacidosis, jaundice, CAD, T1 DM

Precautions: Pregnancy (C), geriatric patients, thyroid disease, renal/hepatic disease, heart failure

Black Box Warning: MI

PHARMACOKINETICS

Maximal reductions in FBS after 6-12 wk; protein binding 99.8%; excreted in urine, feces; elimination half-life 3-4 hr; may be excreted in breast milk

INTERACTIONS

• Avoid concurrent use with insulin, nitrates

• May increase or decrease level: CYP2C5 inducer/inhibitors

Drug/Herb

• Hypoglycemia: chromium, coenzyme Q10, fenugreek

• Poor glucose control: glucosamine

Increase: antidiabetic effect—alfalfa, aloe, basil, bay, bilberry, bitter melon, black catechu, buchu, burdock, coriander, dandelion, eyebright (po), fenugreek, garlic, ginseng, glucomannan, glucosamine, goat's rue, gymnema, horehound, horse chestnut, jambul, myrrh, myrtle

Decrease: antidiabetic effect—bee pollen, blue cohosh, broom, chromium, elecampane, eucalyptus, gotu kola

NURSING CONSIDERATIONS

Assess:

⚠ For CV status, those with CV disease should be monitored carefully

• For hypoglycemic reactions (sweating, weakness, dizziness, anxiety, tremors, hunger), hyperglycemic reactions soon after meals

⚠ Systemic reactions: anaphylaxis, Stevens-Johnson syndrome

• Check LFTs periodically AST, ALT (if ALT >2.5 × ULN, do not use)

• Fasting blood sugar, A1c, plasma lipids/lipoproteins, B/P, body weight during treatment

Administer:

• Once or in 2 divided doses

• Tabs crushed and mixed with food or

fluids for patients with difficulty swallowing

Perform/provide:

- Conversion from other oral hypoglycemic agents if needed; change may be made without gradual dosage change; monitor blood glucose during conversion
- Storage in tight container in cool environment

Evaluate:

- Therapeutic response: decrease in polyuria, polydipsia, polyphagia; clear sensorium; absence of dizziness; stable gait; blood glucose, A1c improvement

Teach patient/family:

- To monitor blood glucose; that periodic LFTs mandatory; report edema, weight gain
- The symptoms of hypo/hyperglycemia, what to do about each
- That the product must be continued on daily basis: explain consequences of discontinuing product abruptly
- To avoid OTC medications, herbal preparations, nitrates, or insulin unless approved by prescriber
- That diabetes is lifelong illness; that this product is not a cure; only controls symptoms
- That all food included in diet plan must be eaten to prevent hypoglycemia
- To carry emergency ID and glucagon emergency kit for emergencies
- To report symptoms of hepatic dysfunction (nausea, vomiting, abdominal pain, fatigue, anorexia, dark urine, jaundice)
- That 2 wk is needed to see a reduction in blood glucose and 2-3 mo to see full effect
- To notify prescriber if oral contraceptives are used
- Not to use if breastfeeding, may be secreted in breast milk
- That a medication guide should be dispensed with each prescription/refill

rosuvastatin (℞)

(roe-soo'va-sta-tin)

Crestor

Func. class.: Antilipemic

Chem. class.: HMG-CoA reductase inhibitor

Action: Inhibits HMG-CoA reductase enzyme, which reduces cholesterol synthesis

Uses: As an adjunct in primary hypercholesterolemia (types IIa, IIb) and mixed dyslipidemia elevated serum triglycerides, homozygous familial hypercholesterolemia (FH), slowing of atherosclerosis

Unlabeled uses: MI, stroke prophylaxis (normal LDL)

DOSAGE AND ROUTES

Patient should first be placed on a cholesterol-lowering diet

Hypercholesterolemia

- *Adult:* **PO** 5-40 mg/day; initial dose 10 mg/day, reanalyze lipid levels at 2-4 wk and adjust dosage accordingly

Homozygous FH

- *Adult:* **PO** 20 mg/day, max 40 mg

Dose in patients taking cycloSPORINE

- *Adult:* **PO** 5 mg/day

Dose when taken with gemfibrozil

- *Adult:* **PO** Max 10 mg/day

Asian patients/predisposition for myopathy

- *Adult:* **PO** 5 mg/day

Atherosclerosis slowing

- *Adult:* **PO** 10 mg/day (for those not taking cycloSPORINE or gemfibrozil)

MI/stroke prophylaxis (unlabeled)

- *Adult:* **PO** 20 mg daily

Renal dose

- *Adult:* **PO** CCr <30 ml/min 5 mg/day; max 10 mg/day

Available forms: Tabs 5, 10, 20, 40 mg

SIDE EFFECTS

CNS: *Headache, dizziness,* insomnia, paresthesia, **ALS (Lou Gehrig's disease)**

R

GI: Nausea, constipation, abdominal pain, flatus, diarrhea, dyspepsia, heartburn, **kidney failure, liver dysfunction,** vomiting

HEMA: **Thrombocytopenia, hemolytic anemia, leukopenia**

INTEG: Rash, pruritus, photosensitivity

MS: Asthenia, muscle cramps, arthritis, arthralgia, myalgia, **myositis, rhabdomyolysis,** leg, shoulder or localized pain

RESP: Rhinitus, sinusitis, *pharyngitis,* bronchitis, increased cough

Contraindications: Pregnancy (X), breastfeeding, hypersensitivity, active hepatic disease

Precautions: Children, geriatric patients, past hepatic disease, alcoholism, severe acute infections, trauma, hypotension, uncontrolled seizure disorders, severe metabolic disorders, electrolyte imbalances, severe renal impairment, hypothyroidism

PHARMACOKINETICS

Peak 3-5 hr, minimal live metabolism (about 10%), 88% protein bound, excreted primarily in feces (90%), crosses placenta, half-life 19 hr, not dialyzable

INTERACTIONS

Increase: effects of rosuvastatin—bile acid sequestrants

Increase: myalgia, myositis—cycloSPORINE, gemfibrozil, niacin, clofibrate, azole antifungals

Increase: bleeding—warfarin

Drug/Herb

Decrease: rosuvastatin effect—St. John's wort

Drug/Food

- Possible toxicity: grapefruit juice

Drug/Lab Test

Increase: CPK, LFTs

NURSING CONSIDERATIONS

Assess:

- Diet, obtain diet history including fat, cholesterol in diet
- Fasting cholesterol, LDL, HDL, triglycerides periodically during treatment
- LFTs q1-2mo during the first 1½ yr of treatment; AST, ALT, LFTs may increase
- Renal function in patients with compromised renal system: BUN, creatinine, I&O ratio

⚠ For muscle pain, tenderness, obtain CPK; if these occur, product may need to be discontinued

Administer:

- May be taken at any time of day, with or without food

Perform/provide:

- Storage in cool environment in airtight, light-resistant container

Evaluate:

- Therapeutic response: cholesterol at desired level after 8 wk

Teach patient/family:

- To report suspected pregnancy, to use contraception while taking this product; pregnancy category (X)
- That blood work and ophthalmic exam will be necessary during treatment
- To report blurred vision, severe GI symptoms, dizziness, headache, muscle pain, weakness
- To use sunscreen or stay out of the sun to prevent photosensitivity
- That previously prescribed regimen will continue: low-cholesterol diet, exercise program, smoking cessation

rufinamide (℞)

(roo-fin′a-mide)

Banzel

Func. class.: Anticonvulsant

Chem. class.: Triazole derivative

Action: May act through action at sodium channels; exact action is unknown

Uses: Lennox-Gastaut syndrome

Unlabeled uses: Partial seizures

DOSAGE AND ROUTES

- *Adult:* **PO** 400-800 mg/day divided bid, increase by 400-800 mg/day q2days to 3200 mg/day

• *Child ≥4 yr:* **PO** 10 mg/kg/day divided equally bid; increase by 10 mg/kg/day every other day to 45 mg/kg/day or 3200 mg/day, whichever is less

Available forms: Tabs 200, 400 mg

SIDE EFFECTS

CNS: Dizziness, ataxia, drowsiness, fever, seizures, tremor, fatigue, headache, gait disturbance

EENT: Diplopia, blurred vision, nystagmus

GI: Nausea, hepatitis, vomiting

HEMA: **Anemia, leukopenia, neutropenia, thrombocytopenia,** lymphadenopathy

INTEG: Rash, urticaria

MISC: Edema, hematuria, influenzae, nephrolithiasis

Contraindications: Hypersensitivity

Precautions: Pregnancy (C), breastfeeding, children <16 yr, geriatric patients, renal/hepatic disease, depression, dialysis, hazardous activities, suicidal ideation

PHARMACOKINETICS

Peak 4-6 hr, half-life 6-10 hr, metabolized by liver, excreted by kidneys

INTERACTIONS

Increase: rufinamide effect—valproate

Decrease: effect of hormonal contraceptives

Decrease: effect of rufinamide—carbamazepine, phenytoin, primidone, phenobarbital

Drug/Lab Test

Increase: LFTs

NURSING CONSIDERATIONS

Assess:

• For seizures: duration, type, intensity precipitating factors

⚠ Mental status: mood, sensorium, affect, memory (long, short), increased suicidal thoughts/actions

Evaluate:

• Therapeutic response: decrease in severity of seizures

Teach patient/family:

• Not to discontinue product abruptly; seizures may occur

• To avoid hazardous activities until stabilized on product

• To carry emergency ID stating product use

• To notify prescriber if pregnancy is planned or suspected

• To use alternative form of contraception; hormonal contraceptives may be decreased

• To take adequate fluids

salicylic acid topical

See Appendix B

salmeterol (℞)

(sal-met′er-ole)

Serevent, Serevent Diskus

Func. class.: β_2-Adrenergic agonist, bronchodilator

Action: Causes bronchodilation by action on β_2 (pulmonary) receptors by increasing levels of cAMP, which relaxes smooth muscle with very little effect on heart rate, maintains improvement in FEV from 3 to 12 hr; prevents nocturnal asthma symptoms

Uses: Prevention of exercise-induced asthma, bronchospasm, COPD

DOSAGE AND ROUTES

• *Adult:* **INH** 50 mcg (one inhalation as dry powder); exercise-induced bronchospasm 50 mcg (2 inh) ½-1 hr prior to exercise

• *Child 4-12 yr:* **INH** 50 mcg as dry powder bid; exercise-induced bronchospasm 50 mcg as dry powder ½-1 hr prior to exercise

Available forms: Inhalation powder 50 mcg/blister

SIDE EFFECTS

CNS: Tremors, anxiety, insomnia, headache, dizziness, stimulation, restlessness, hallucinations, flushing, irritability

CV: Palpitations, tachycardia, hypo/hypertension, angina, dysrhythmias
EENT: Dry nose, irritation of nose and throat
GI: Heartburn, nausea, vomiting, abdominal pain
MS: Muscle cramps
RESP: **Bronchospasm**

Contraindications: Hypersensitivity to sympathomimetics, tachydysrhythmias, severe cardiac disease

Precautions: Pregnancy (C), breastfeeding, cardiac disorders, hyperthyroidism, diabetes mellitus, hypertension, prostatic hypertrophy, closed-angle glaucoma, seizures, acute asthma, as a substitute to corticosteroids

Black Box Warning: Respiratory insufficiency

PHARMACOKINETICS

INH: Onset 30-50 min; peak 4 hr; duration 12 hr; metabolized in liver; excreted in urine, breast milk; crosses placenta; blood-brain barrier; protein binding 94%-98%; terminal half-life 3-5 hr

INTERACTIONS

Increase: action of aerosol bronchodilators
Increase: action of salmeterol—tricyclics, MAOIs
Decrease: salmeterol action—other β-blockers

Drug/Herb
Increase: stimulation—betel palm, butterbur, coffee, cola nut, figwort, fumitory, guarana, hawthorn, lily of the valley, motherwort, plantain, tea (black/green), yerba maté

NURSING CONSIDERATIONS

Assess:
- Respiratory function: vital capacity, forced expiratory volume, ABGs, lung sounds, heart rate and rhythm

Administer:
- Gum, sips of water for dry mouth

Perform/provide:
- Storage in foil pouch; do not expose to temperatures over 86° F (30° C); discard 6 wk after removal from foil pouch

Evaluate:
- Therapeutic response: absence of dyspnea, wheezing

Teach patient/family:
- Not to use OTC medications; extra stimulation may occur
- Review package insert with patient
- To avoid getting powder in eyes
- To avoid smoking, smoke-filled rooms, persons with respiratory infections
- Not for treatment of acute exacerbation

Treatment of overdose: β_2-Adrenergic blocker

salsalate (℞)

(sal'sah-late)
Amigesic, Anaflex, Disalcid, Marthritic, Mono-Gesic, Salflex, salsalate, Salgesic, Salsitab
Func. class.: Nonopioid analgesic, nonsteroidal antiinflammatory
Chem. class.: Salicylate

Action: Blocks formation of peripheral prostaglandins, which cause pain and inflammation; antipyretic action results from inhibition of hypothalamic heat-regulating center; does not inhibit platelet aggregation

Uses: Mild to moderate pain or fever, including arthritis (osteoarthritis, rheumatoid arthritis)

DOSAGE AND ROUTES

- *Adult:* **PO** 3 g/day in divided doses

Available forms: Caps 500 mg; tabs 500, 750 mg

SIDE EFFECTS

CNS: Stimulation, drowsiness, dizziness, confusion, **seizures,** headache, flushing, hallucinations, **coma**
CV: Rapid pulse, **pulmonary edema**
EENT: Tinnitus, hearing loss

ENDO: Hypoglycemia, hyponatremia, hypokalemia, alteration in acid-base balance
GI: Nausea, vomiting, GI bleeding, diarrhea, heartburn, anorexia, **hepatotoxicity**
HEMA: **Thrombocytopenia, agranulocytosis, leukopenia, neutropenia, hemolytic anemia,** increased PT
INTEG: Rash, urticaria, bruising
RESP: Wheezing, hyperpnea
Contraindications: Children <3 yr, hypersensitivity to salicylates, NSAIDs, GI bleeding, bleeding disorders, vit K deficiency
Precautions: Pregnancy (C) 1st trimester, breastfeeding, geriatric patients, anemia, renal/hepatic disease, Hodgkin's disease

PHARMACOKINETICS

Full benefit 3-4 days, metabolized by liver, excreted by kidneys, half-life 1 hr, highly protein bound, crosses blood-brain barrier and placenta slowly

INTERACTIONS

- Toxic effects: PABA

Increase: blood loss—alcohol, heparin, NSAIDs, warfarin
Increase: effects of anticoagulants, insulin, methotrexate, probenecid, penicillins, phenytoin, NSAIDs, thrombolytics, platelet inhibitors
Decrease: effects of spironolactone, sulfinpyrazone, sulfonamides, loop diuretics
Decrease: effects of salsalate—antacids, steroids, urinary alkalizers
Decrease: blood glucose levels—salicylates

Drug/Herb
Decrease: levels of feverfew

Drug/Food
- Foods that cause acidic urine, may increase salsalate levels

Drug/Lab Test
Increase: coagulation studies, hepatic studies, serum uric acid, amylase, CO_2, urinary protein
Decrease: serum potassium, cholesterol, blood glucose
Interference: urine catecholamines, pH, pregnancy test

NURSING CONSIDERATIONS

Assess:
- Pain: frequency, intensity, characteristics; relief of pain after medication

⚠ For asthma, aspirin hypersensitivity, nasal polyps; may develop hypersensitivity to this product
- Hepatic studies: AST, ALT, bilirubin (long-term therapy)
- Renal studies: BUN, urine creatinine (long-term therapy)
- Blood studies: CBC, Hct, Hgb, PT, stool guaiac, serum salicylate (long-term therapy)
- I&O ratio; decreasing output may indicate renal failure (long-term therapy)
- Hepatotoxicity: dark urine, clay-colored stools; jaundiced skin, sclera; itching, abdominal pain, fever, diarrhea (long-term therapy)
- Allergic reactions: rash, urticaria; product may have to be discontinued
- Ototoxicity: tinnitus, ringing, roaring in ears; audiometric testing is needed before, after long-term therapy
- Visual changes
- Edema in feet, ankles, legs
- Product history; many interactions

Administer:
- With food or milk to decrease gastric symptoms

Evaluate:
- Therapeutic response: decreased pain, fever

Teach patient/family:
- To report any symptoms of hepatotoxicity, renal toxicity, visual changes, ototoxicity, allergic reactions (long-term therapy)
- Not to exceed recommended dosage; acute poisoning may result
- To read label on other OTC products; many contain aspirin and should avoid
- That therapeutic response takes 2 wk (arthritis)

• To avoid alcohol ingestion; GI bleeding may occur
• To watch for signs of bleeding: dark stools

Treatment of overdose: Lavage, activated charcoal, monitor electrolytes, VS

saquinavir (℞)

(sa-quen'ah-veer)
Invirase
Func. class.: Antiretroviral
Chem. class.: Protease inhibitor

Action: Inhibits human immunodeficiency virus (HIV-1) protease, which prevents maturation of the infectious virus

Uses: HIV-1 in combination with other antiretrovirals

DOSAGE AND ROUTES

• *Adult:* **PO** 1000 mg bid with 100 mg ritonavir

Available forms: Caps 200, 500 mg

SIDE EFFECTS

CNS: Paresthesia, headache, **seizures**
GI: Diarrhea, buccal mucosa ulceration, *abdominal pain, nausea,* vomiting
INTEG: Rash
MISC.: Asthenia, hyperglycemia, **Stevens-Johnson syndrome**
MS: Pain

Contraindications: Hypersensitivity

Precautions: Pregnancy (B), breastfeeding, children, hepatic disease, diabetes, pancreatitis, immune reconstitution syndrome, hemophilia, hyperlipidemia

PHARMACOKINETICS

Absorption increased with food, protein binding 98%, extensive first-pass hepatic metabolism, terminal half-life 12 hr

INTERACTIONS

• Avoid use with HMG-CoA reductase inhibitors

Increase: toxicity—ergots, midazolam, triazolam, dapsone, quinidine, calcium channel blockers, clindamycin

⚠ ***Increase:*** vasoconstriction—ergots, do not use concurrently

⚠ ***Increase:*** CNS depression—midazolam, triazolam, do not use concurrently

Increase: saquinavir levels—ketoconazole, indinavir, delaviridine, nelfinavir, ritonavir, clarithromycin

Decrease: saquinavir levels—rifamycins, carbamazepine, phenobarbital, phenytoin, nevirapine, dexamethasone

Drug/Herb

• St. John's wort, garlic may decrease saquinavir levels; avoid concurrent use

Drug/Food

Increase: bioavailability after high-fat meal; grapefruit juice increases levels

Drug/Lab Test

• Interference: CPK, glucose

NURSING CONSIDERATIONS

Assess:

• Signs of infection, anemia
• Blood glucose, viral load, CD4+ T cell count, plasma HIV RNA, serum cholesterol/lipid profile
• Resistance testing at start of therapy and at treatment failure
• Hepatic studies: ALT, AST
• C&S before product therapy; product may be taken as soon as culture is taken; repeat C&S after treatment; determine the presence of other sexually transmitted diseases
• Bowel pattern before, during treatment; if severe abdominal pain with bleeding occurs, product should be discontinued; monitor hydration
• Skin eruptions, rash, urticaria, itching
• Allergies before treatment, reaction of each medication

Administer:

• Within 2 hr of meal

Teach patient/family:

• To take as prescribed within 2 hr of a full meal; if dose is missed, take as soon as remembered up to 1 hr before next dose; do not double dose

• That product must be taken in equal intervals around the clock to maintain blood levels for duration of therapy; product is not a cure
• To take precautions to prevent transmission
• There are significant product interactions

sargramostim (℞)

(sar-gram'oh-stim)
Leukine, rhu GM-CSF
Func. class.: Biologic modifier
Chem. class.: Granulocyte macrophage colony-stimulating factor (GM-CSF)

Do not confuse:
Leukine/leucovorin/Leukeran

Action: Stimulates proliferation and differentiation of hematopoietic progenitor cells (granulocytes, macrophages)

Uses: Acceleration of myeloid recovery in patients with non-Hodgkin's lymphoma, acute lymphoblastic leukemia, acute myelogenous leukemia, autologous bone marrow transplantation in Hodgkin's disease; bone marrow transplantation failure or engraftment delay, mobilization and transplant of peripheral blood progenitor cells (PBPCs)

Unlabeled uses: Aplastic anemia, Crohn's disease, HIV, ganciclovir- or zidovudine-induced neutropenia, malignant melanoma

DOSAGE AND ROUTES

Myeloid reconstitution after autologous bone marrow transplantation
• *Adult:* **IV** 250 mcg/m²/day × 3 wk; give over 2 hr, begin 2-4 hr after bone marrow inf, not less than 24 hr after last dose of antineoplastics and 12 hr after last dose of radiotherapy, bone marrow transplantation failure, or engraftment delay

Acceleration of myeloid recovery
• *Adult:* **IV** 250 mcg/m²/day × 14 days; give over 2 hr; may repeat in 7 days, may repeat 500 mcg/m²/day × 14 days after another 7 days if no improvement

Mobilization of PBPCs
• *Adult:* **IV/SUBCUT** 250 mcg/m²/day during collection of PBPCs

After PBPC transplantation
• *Adult:* **IV/SUBCUT** 250 mcg/m²/day until ANC >1500 cells/mm³ × 3 days

Aplastic anemia (unlabeled)
• *Adult:* **SUBCUT** 250-500 mcg/day or 5 mcg/kg/day × 14-90 days, used with erythropoietin or immunosuppressive therapy

Malignant melanoma (unlabeled)
• *Adult:* **SUBCUT** 125 mcg/m²/day × 14 days, alternate with 14 days off

HIV (unlabeled)
• *Adult:* **SUBCUT** 250 mcg/day 3×/wk for up to 20 mo

Available forms: Powder for inj lyophilized 250 mcg

SIDE EFFECTS

CNS: Fever, malaise, CNS disorder, weakness, chills, dizziness, syncope, headache
CV: **Transient supraventricular tachycardia,** peripheral edema, **pericardial effusion,** hypotension, tachycardia
GI: Nausea, vomiting, diarrhea, anorexia, **GI hemorrhage,** stomatitis, **liver damage,** hyperbilirubinemia
GU: Urinary tract disorder, abnormal kidney function
HEMA: **Blood dyscrasias, hemorrhage**
INTEG: Alopecia, rash, peripheral edema
MS: Bone pain, myalgia
RESP: Dyspnea

Contraindications: Neonates, hypersensitivity to GM-CSF, benzyl alcohol, yeast products; excessive leukemic myeloid blast in bone marrow, peripheral blood

Precautions: Pregnancy (C), breastfeeding, children; lung/cardiac/renal/hepatic disease; pleural, pericardial effusions, peripheral edema, leukocytosis, mannitol hypersensitivity, hepatic/renal disease

PHARMACOKINETICS

Half-life elimination: IV 60 min, SUBCUT 2-3 hr; detected within 5 min after administration, peak 2 hr

S

INTERACTIONS

• Do not use this product concomitantly with antineoplastics

Increase: myeloproliferation—lithium, corticosteroids

NURSING CONSIDERATIONS

Assess:

⚠ Blood studies: CBC, differential count before treatment and twice weekly; leukocytosis may occur (WBC >50,000 cells/mm^3, ANC >20,000 cells/mm^3), platelets; if ANC >20,000/mm^3 or 10,000/mm^3 after nadir has occurred, or platelets >500,000/mm^3 reduce dose by ½ or discontinue; if blast cells occur, discontinue

• Renal, hepatic studies before treatment: BUN, creatinine, urinalysis; AST, ALT, alk phos; twice weekly monitoring is needed in renal, hepatic disease

• For hypersensitivity, rashes, local inj site reactions; usually transient

• Body weight, hydration status; increased fluid retention in cardiac disease; pulmonary function

• For myalgia, arthralgia in legs, feet, use analgesics

Administer:

SUBCUT route

• Use reconstituted sol

IV route

• After reconstituting with 1 ml sterile water for inj without preservative; do not reenter vial; discard unused portion; direct reconstitution sol at side of vial; rotate contents; do not shake

• Dilute in 0.9% NaCl inj to prepare IV inf; if final concentration is <10 mcg/ml, add human albumin to make a final concentration of 0.1% to NaCl before adding sargramostim to prevent adsorption; for a final concentration of 0.1% albumin, add 1 mg human albumin/1 ml 0.9% NaCl inj run over 2 hr (bone marrow transplant or failure of graft); over 4 hr (chemotherapy for AML); over 24 hr as cont inf (PBPCs); give within 6 hr after reconstitution

Y-site compatibilities: Amikacin, aminophylline, aztreonam, bleomycin, butorphanol, calcium gluconate, carboplatin, carmustine, cefazolin, cefepime, cefotaxime, cefotetan, ceftizoxime, ceftriaxone, cefuroxime, cimetidine, cisplatin, clindamycin, cyclophosphamide, cycloSPORINE, cytarabine, dacarbazine, dactinomycin, dexamethasone, diphenhydrAMINE, DOPamine, DOXOrubicin, doxycycline, droperidol, etoposide, famotidine, fentanyl, floxuridine, fluconazole, fluorouracil, furosemide, gentamicin, granisetron, heparin, idarubicin, ifosfamide, immune globulin, magnesium sulfate, mannitol, mechlorethamine, meperidine, mesna, methotrexate, metoclopramide, metronidazole, minocycline, mitoxantrone, netilmicin, pentostatin, piperacillin/tazobactam, potassium chloride, prochlorperazine, promethazine, ranitidine, teniposide, ticarcillin, ticarcillin/clavulanate, trimethoprim-sulfamethoxazole, vinBLAStine, vinCRIStine, zidovudine

Perform/provide:

• Storage in refrigerator; do not freeze

Evaluate:

• Therapeutic response: WBC and differential recovery

saxagliptin (℞)

(sax-a-glip'tin)

Onglyza

Func. class.: Antidiabetic, oral

Chem. class.: Dipeptidyl-peptidase-4 inhibitor (DPP-4 inhibitor)

Action: Slows the inactivation of incretin hormones; improves glucose homeostasis, improves glucose-dependent insulin synthesis, lowers glucagon secretions, and slows gastric emptying time

Uses: In adults, type 2 diabetes mellitus as monotherapy or in combination with other antidiabetic agents

DOSAGE AND ROUTES

• *Adult:* **PO** 2.5-5 mg; may use with other antidiabetic agents other than insulin

Renal Dose

- *Adult:* **PO** CCr ≤50 ml/min 2.5 mg daily

Available forms: Tabs 2.5, 5 mg

SIDE EFFECTS

CNS: Headache

ENDO: Hypoglycemia

GI: Nausea, vomiting, abdominal pain

INTEG: Urticaria, **angioedema**

MISC: Lymphopenia, peripheral edema

Contraindications: Hypersensitivity, diabetic ketoacidosis (DKA), type 1 diabetes

Precautions: Pregnancy (B), geriatric patients, GI obstruction, surgery, thyroid/renal/hepatic disease, trauma

PHARMACOKINETICS

Rapidly absorbed, excreted by the kidneys (unchanged 24%), terminal half-life 2.5 hr, 3.1 hr metabolite, peak 2 hr

INTERACTIONS

Increase: sitagliptan level—cimetidine, disopyramide

Increase: levels of digoxin

Increase: hypoglycemia—androgens, insulins, β-blockers, cimetidine, corticosteroids, salicylates, MAOIs, fibric acid derivatives, fluoxetine

Decrease: antidiabetic effect—thiazide diuretics, ACE inhibitors, protease inhibitors, sympathomimetics, aripiprazole, clozapine, olanzapine, quetiapine, risperidone, ziprasidone, phenytoin, fosphenytoin, phenothiazines, estrogens, progestins, oral contraceptives

Drug/Herb

Increase: hyperglycemia—glucosamine

Increase: hypoglycemia—chromium, coenzyme Q-10, fenugreek

Increase: antidiabetic effect—alfalfa, aloe, basil, bay, bilberry, bitter melon, black catechu, buchu, burdock, coriander, dandelion, eyebright (po), fenugreek, garlic, ginseng, glucomannan, glucosamine, goat's rue, gymnema, horehound, horse chestnut, jambul, myrrh, myrtle

Decrease: antidiabetic effect—bee pollen, blue cohosh, broom, chromium, elecampane, eucalyptus, gotu kola

NURSING CONSIDERATIONS

Assess:

- For hypoglycemic reactions (sweating, weakness, dizziness, anxiety, tremors, hunger), hyperglycemic reactions soon after meals
- CBC (baseline, q3mo) during treatment; check LFTs periodically, AST, LDH, renal studies: BUN, creatinine during treatment; A1c
- Monitor blood glucose as needed

Administer:

- May be taken with or without food

Perform/provide:

- Conversion from other antidiabetic agents; change may be made with gradual dosage change
- Storage in tight container at room temperature

Evaluate:

- Therapeutic response: decrease in polyuria, polydipsia, polyphagia; clear sensorium; absence of dizziness; stable gait, blood glucose at normal level

Teach patient/family:

- To use regular self-monitoring of blood glucose using blood glucose meter
- The symptoms of hypo/hyperglycemia; what to do about each
- That product must be continued on daily basis; explain consequence of discontinuing product abruptly
- To avoid OTC medications, alcohol, digoxin, exenatide, insulins, nateglinide, repaglinide and other products that lower blood glucose, unless approved by prescriber
- That diabetes is a lifelong illness; that this product is not a cure, only controls symptoms
- That all food included in diet plan must be eaten to prevent hypo/hyperglycemia
- To carry emergency ID

S

scopolamine (℞)

(skoe-pol'a-meen)

Maldemar, Scopace, Scopolamine Hydrobromide Injection

Func. class.: Cholinergic blocker

Chem. class.: Belladonna alkaloid

Action: Inhibits acetylcholine at receptor sites in autonomic nervous system, which controls secretions, free acids in stomach; blocks central muscarinic receptors, which decreases involuntary movements

Uses: Preoperatively to produce amnesia, sedation and to decrease secretions; motion sickness, parkinsonian symptoms

DOSAGE AND ROUTES

Parkinsonian symptoms

- *Adult:* **PO** 0.4-0.8 mg q8hr

Preoperatively

- *Adult:* **IM/IV/SUBCUT** 0.32-0.65 mg

Nausea and vomiting

- *Adult:* **SUBCUT** 0.6-1 mg
- *Child:* **SUBCUT** 0.006 mg/kg; max 0.3 mg/dose

Available forms: Inj 0.3, 0.4, 0.86, 1 mg/ml

SIDE EFFECTS

CNS: Confusion, anxiety, restlessness, irritability, delusions, hallucinations, headache, sedation, depression, incoherence, dizziness, excitement, delirium, flushing, weakness, fatigue, loss of memory

CV: Palpitations, tachycardia, postural hypotension, paradoxic bradycardia

EENT: Blurred vision, photophobia, dilated pupils, difficulty swallowing, mydriasis, cycloplegia

GI: Dryness of mouth, constipation, nausea, vomiting, abdominal distress, **paralytic ileus**

GU: Urinary hesitancy, retention

INTEG: Urticaria, dry skin

MISC: Suppression of breastfeeding, nasal congestion, decreased sweating

Contraindications: Hypersensitivity, closed-angle glaucoma, myasthenia gravis, GI/GU obstruction, hypersensitivity to belladonna, barbiturates

Precautions: Pregnancy (C), breastfeeding, children, geriatric patients, prostatic hypertrophy, CHF, hypertension, dysrhythmia, gastric ulcer, renal/hepatic disease, hiatal hernia, GERD, ulcerative colitis, hyperthyroidism

PHARMACOKINETICS

Excreted in urine, bile, feces (unchanged)

SUBCUT/IM: Peak 30-60 min, duration 7 hr

IV: Peak 10-15 min, duration 2 hr

INTERACTIONS

Increase: anticholinergic effect—alcohol, opioids, antihistamines, phenothiazines, tricyclics

Drug/Herb

Increase: anticholinergic effects—henbane, jimsonweed, scopolia

NURSING CONSIDERATIONS

Assess:

- VS periodically
- I&O ratio; retention commonly causes decreased urinary output
- Parkinsonism, EPS: shuffling gait, muscle rigidity, involuntary movements if using for Parkinson symptoms
- Urinary hesitancy, retention; palpate bladder if retention occurs
- Constipation; increase fluids, bulk, exercise if this occurs
- For tolerance over long-term therapy; dose may have to be increased or changed
- Mental status: affect, mood, CNS depression, worsening of mental symptoms during early therapy if using for Parkinson symptoms

Administer:

- Parenteral dose with patient recumbent to prevent postural hypotension
- Parenteral dose slowly; keep in bed for at least 1 hr after dose

• With or after meals for GI upset; may give with fluids other than H_2O
• At bedtime to avoid daytime drowsiness in patient with parkinsonism
• With analgesic to avoid behavioral changes when given as a preop

IV route
• Give over 2-3 min, 30-60 min prior to anesthesia

Additive compatibilities: Floxacillin, furosemide, meperidine, succinylcholine

Syringe compatibilities: Atropine, benzquinamide, butorphanol, chlorproMAZINE, cimetidine, diamorphine, dimenhyDRINATE, diphenhydrAMINE, droperidol, fentanyl, glycopyrrolate, hydromorphone, hydrOXYzine, meperidine, metoclopramide, midazolam, morphine, nalbuphine, pentazocine, pentobarbital, perphenazine, prochlorperazine, promazine, promethazine, ranitidine, sufentanil, thiopental

Y-site compatibilities: Heparin, hydrocortisone, potassium chloride, propofol, sufentanil, vit B/C

Perform/provide:
• Storage at room temperature in light-resistant container
• Hard candy, frequent drinks, sugarless gum to relieve dry mouth

Evaluate:
• Therapeutic response: decreased secretions

Teach patient/family:
• Not to discontinue this product abruptly; to taper off over 1 wk
• To avoid driving, other hazardous activities; drowsiness may occur
• To avoid OTC medication: cough, cold preparations with alcohol, antihistamines unless directed by prescriber

scopolamine ophthalmic

See Appendix B

scopolamine (transdermal) (℞)

(skoe-pol'-a-meen)
Transderm-Scop, Transderm-V
Func. class.: Antiemetic, anticholinergic
Chem. class.: Belladonna alkaloid

Action: Competitive antagonism of acetylcholine at receptor site in eye, smooth muscle, cardiac muscle, glandular cells; inhibition of vestibular input to the CNS, resulting in inhibition of vomiting reflex

Uses: Prevention of motion sickness

Unlabeled uses: Drooling

DOSAGE AND ROUTES

• *Adult:* **PATCH** 1 placed behind ear 4-5 hr before travel, reapply q3days, alternate ears
• Not recommended for children

Drooling (unlabeled)
• *Adult:* **TRANSDERMAL** 1.5 mg patch q3days

Available forms: Patch, 1, 1.5 mg delivered in 72 hr

SIDE EFFECTS

CNS: Dizziness, drowsiness, confusion, disorientation, memory disturbances, hallucinations

EENT: Blurred vision, altered depth perception, *dilated pupils,* photophobia, *dry mouth;* dry, itchy, red eyes; acute closed-angle glaucoma

GU: Difficult urination

INTEG: Rash, erythema

Contraindications: Hypersensitivity, glaucoma

Precautions: Pregnancy (C), children, geriatric patients; pyloric, urinary, bladder neck, intestinal obstruction; renal/hepatic disease

PHARMACOKINETICS

Patch: Onset 4-5 hr, duration 72 hr

S

INTERACTIONS

Increase: anticholinergic effects—antihistamines, antidepressants

NURSING CONSIDERATIONS

Administer:

• With clean, dry hands; wash, dry hands before and after applying to surface behind ear, press patch firmly

Teach patient/family:

• To avoid hazardous activities, activities requiring alertness; dizziness may occur
• To change patch q72hr
• To apply at least 4 hr before traveling
• If blurred vision, severe dizziness, drowsiness occurs, to discontinue use, use another type of antiemetic or rotate the patch to other ear
• To read label of all OTC medications; if any scopolamine is found in product, avoid use
• To keep out of children's reach

selegiline (℞)
(se-le′ji-leen)
Carbex, Eldepryl, Emsam, Novo-Selegiline ✦, Zelapar
Func. class.: Antiparkinson agent
Chem. class.: MAOI, type B

Do not confuse:
Eldepryl/enalapril

Action: Increased dopaminergic activity by inhibition of MAO type B activity; not fully understood

Uses: Adjunct management of Parkinson's disease in patients being treated with levodopa/carbidopa who had poor response to therapy

Unlabeled uses: Alzheimer's disease, depression

DOSAGE AND ROUTES

• *Adult:* **PO** 10 mg/day given with levodopa/carbidopa in divided doses 5 mg at breakfast and lunch; after 2-3 days begin to reduce dose of levodopa/carbidopa 10%-30%; **ORAL DISINTEGRATING** 1.25 mg (1 tab) × 6 wk or more initially, then 2.5 mg (2 tabs) dissolved on tongue daily before breakfast; max 2.5 mg/day; **TRANSDERMAL** 6 mg/24 hr initially, increase by 3 mg/24 hr at ≥2 wk, up to 12 mg/24 hr if needed

Alzheimer's disease (unlabeled)

• *Adult:* **PO** 5 mg bid AM, PM

Available forms: Tabs 5 mg; caps 5 mg; oral disintegrating tabs 1.25 mg; transdermal 6 mg/24 hr (20 mg/20 cm^2), 9 mg/24 hr (30 mg/30 cm^2), 12 mg/24 hr (40 mg/40 cm^2)

SIDE EFFECTS

CNS: Increased tremors, chorea, restlessness, blepharospasm, increased bradykinesia, grimacing, tardive dyskinesia, dystonic symptoms, involuntary movements, increased apraxia, hallucinations, *dizziness,* mood changes, nightmares, delusions, lethargy, apathy, overstimulation, sleep disturbances, headache, migraine, numbness, muscle cramps, confusion, anxiety, tiredness, vertigo, personality change, back/leg pain, **suicide in child/adolescent, suicidal ideations in adults**

CV: Orthostatic hypotension, hypo/hypertension, dysrhythmia, palpitations, angina pectoris, **tachycardia,** edema, **sinus bradycardia,** syncope, **hypertensive crisis (children)**

EENT: Diplopia, dry mouth, blurred vision, tinnitus

GI: Nausea, vomiting, constipation, weight loss, anorexia, diarrhea, heartburn, rectal bleeding, poor appetite, dysphagia, xerostomia

GU: Slow urination, nocturia, prostatic hypertrophy, urinary hesitation, retention, frequency, sexual dysfunction

INTEG: Increased sweating, alopecia, hematoma, rash, photosensitivity, facial hair

RESP: Asthma, SOB

Contraindications: Children/adolescents (suicide/hypertensive crisis), hypersensitivity, breastfeeding

Precautions: Pregnancy (C)

PHARMACOKINETICS

Absorption (tab) 40-90 min, (oral disintegrating tab) 10-15 min; peak ½-2 hr; rapidly metabolized (active metabolites: *N*-desmethyldeprenyl, amphetamine, methamphetamine); metabolites excreted in urine; half-life 10 hr; protein binding up to 85%

INTERACTIONS

⚠ Fatal interaction: opioids (especially meperidine); do not administer together

⚠ Serotonin syndrome (confusion, seizures, fever, hypertension, agitation); death—fluoxetine, paroxetine, sertraline, fluvoxamine (discontinue 5 wk prior to selegiline); do not use together

⚠ Fatal interaction: do not use with tricyclics

Increase: side effects of levodopa/carbidopa

Increase: unusual behavior, psychosis—dextromethorphan

Increase: hypotension—antihypertensives

Drug/Herb

Decrease: selegiline action—chaste tree fruit, kava

Drug/Lab Test

Decrease: VMA

False positive: urine ketones, urine glucose

False negative: urine glucose (glucose oxidase)

False increase: uric acid, urine protein

NURSING CONSIDERATIONS

Assess:

- Decreased parkinsonian symptoms: rigidity, unsteady gait, weakness, tremors
- Cardiac status: tachycardia/bradycardia; B/P, respiration throughout treatment
- Mental status: affect, mood behavioral changes, depression; perform suicide assessment on all patients, suicide ideation may occur

⚠ For opioids; if patient has received, do not administer selegiline, fatal reactions have occurred

Administer:

PO route

⚠ Do not use in children due to risk for hypertensive crisis

- Product until NPO before surgery
- Adjust dosage to response
- With meals; limit protein taken with product
- Dosing bid in AM and afternoon; avoid PM or bedtime dosing
- At doses <10 mg/day, because of risks associated with nonselective inhibition of MAO
- Oral disintegrating tab: peel back foil; remove tab, do not push through foil; place tab on tongue; allow to dissolve, swallow with saliva

Transdermal route

- Apply to dry, intact skin on upper torso, upper thigh, or outer surface of upper arm q12hr

Perform/provide:

- Assistance with ambulation during beginning therapy

Evaluate:

- Therapeutic response: decrease in akathisia, improved mood

Teach patient/family:

- To change positions slowly to prevent orthostatic hypotension
- To report side effects: twitching, eye spasms; indicate overdose
- To use product exactly as prescribed; if discontinued abruptly, parkinsonian crisis may occur
- To avoid foods high in tyramine: cheese, pickled products, wine, beer, large amounts of caffeine
- Not to exceed recommended dose of 10 mg (PO); might precipitate hypertensive crisis; report severe headache, other unusual symptoms

Treatment of overdose: IV fluids for hypertension, IV dilute pressure agent for B/P titration

selenium topical

See Appendix B

S

senna, sennosides

(OTC)
(sen′na)
Black Draught, Dr. Caldwell Dosalax, Ex-Lax Gentle, Fletcher's Castoria, Gentlax, Senexon, Senna-Gen, Senokot, Senokotxtra, Senolax
Func. class.: Laxative-stimulant
Chem. class.: Anthraquinone

Action: Stimulates peristalsis by action on Auerbach's plexus; softens feces by increasing water, electrolytes in large intestine

Uses: Acute constipation, bowel preparation for surgery or examination, prevention of constipation in those taking opiates long term

DOSAGE AND ROUTES

- *Adult:* **PO** (Senokot) 1-8 tabs/day or ½ to 4 tsp of granules (1 tsp-4 ml) added to water or juice; **RECT SUPP** 1-2 at bedtime; **SYR** 1-4 tsp at bedtime, 7.5-15 ml (Black Draught) ¾ oz dissolved in 2.5 oz liquid given between 2-4 PM the day before procedure (X-Prep)
- *Child >27 kg:* **PO** ½ adult dose; do not use Black Draught for children
- *Child 1 mo-1 yr:* **SYR** (Senokot) 1.25-2.5 ml at bedtime

Available forms: Tabs 6, 8.6, 15, 25 mg; granules 15, 20 mg/5 ml; syr 8.8 mg/5 ml; liquid 33.3 mg/ml

SIDE EFFECTS

GI: Nausea, vomiting, anorexia, cramps, diarrhea, flatulence
GU: Pink, red or brown, black urine
META: Hypocalcemia, enteropathy, alkalosis, hypokalemia, **tetany**

Contraindications: Breastfeeding, hypersensitivity, GI bleeding, obstruction, CHF, abdominal pain, nausea/vomiting, appendicitis, acute surgical abdomen

Precautions: Pregnancy (C)

PHARMACOKINETICS

PO: Onset 6-24 hr, metabolized by liver, excreted in feces

INTERACTIONS

- Do not use with disulfiram (Antabuse)

Drug/Herb

Increase: laxative effect—flax, senna

NURSING CONSIDERATIONS

Assess:

- Stool: color, consistency, amount
- Blood, urine electrolytes if product is used often
- I&O ratio to identify fluid loss
- Cause of constipation; fluids, bulk, exercise missing, constipating products
- Cramping, rectal bleeding, nausea, vomiting; product should be discontinued

Administer:

- In morning or evening (oral dose) with full glass of water
- Dissolve granules in water or juice before administration
- On empty stomach for more rapid results
- Shake oral sol before giving

Evaluate:

- Therapeutic response: decrease in constipation

Teach patient/family:

- That urine, feces may turn yellow-brown to red
- Not to use laxatives for long-term therapy; bowel tone will be lost
- That normal bowel movements do not always occur daily
- Not to use in presence of abdominal pain, nausea, vomiting
- To notify prescriber if constipation unrelieved or of symptoms of electrolyte imbalance: muscle cramps, pain, weakness, dizziness, excessive thirst

sertraline (℞)
(ser′tra-leen)
Zoloft
Func. class.: Antidepressant
Chem. class.: SSRI

Do not confuse:
Zoloft/Zocor

Action: Inhibits serotonin reuptake in CNS; increases action of serotonin; does not affect DOPamine, norepinephrine

Uses: Major depressive disorder, obsessive-compulsive disorder (OCD), posttraumatic stress disorder (PTSD), panic disorder, social anxiety disorder, premenstrual dysphoric disorder (PMDD)

Unlabeled uses: Premature ejaculation, pruritus in cholestatic liver disease, hot flashes

DOSAGE AND ROUTES

- *Adult/adolescent:* **PO** 25-50 mg/day; may increase to max of 200 mg/day; do not change dose at intervals of <1 wk; administer daily in AM or PM
- *Geriatric:* **PO** 25 mg/day, increase by 25 mg q3days to desired dose
- *Child 6-12 yr:* **PO** 25 mg/day, max 200 mg/day

Premenstrual disorders

- *Adult:* **PO** 50-150 mg nightly

Premature ejaculation (unlabeled)

- *Adult:* **PO** 50 mg/day

Pruritus (unlabeled)

- *Adult:* **PO** 50-100 mg/day

Hot flashes (unlabeled)

- *Adult:* **PO** 50 mg/day × 4 wk

Available forms: Tabs 25, 50, 100 mg; oral conc 20 mg/ml

SIDE EFFECTS

CNS: Insomnia, agitation, somnolence, dizziness, headache, tremor, fatigue, paresthesia, twitching, confusion, ataxia, gait abnormality (geriatric patients), **seizures, neuroleptic malignant syndrome–like reaction**

CV: Palpitations, chest pain

EENT: Vision abnormalities, yawning

ENDO: SIADH (geriatric patients)

GI: Diarrhea, nausea, constipation, anorexia, dry mouth, dyspepsia, *vomiting, flatulence*

GU: Male sexual dysfunction, micturition disorder

INTEG: Increased sweating, rash, hot flashes

MISC: Hyponatremia

Contraindications: Hypersensitivity to this product or SSRIs

Precautions: Pregnancy (C), breastfeeding, geriatric patients, renal/hepatic disease, epilepsy, recent MI, latex sensitivity (dropper of oral conc)

Black Box Warning: Children, suicidal ideation

PHARMACOKINETICS

PO: Peak 4.5-8.4 hr; steady state 1 wk; plasma protein binding 99%; elimination half-life 26 hr; extensively metabolized; metabolite excreted in urine, bile

INTERACTIONS

- Altered lithium levels: lithium
- Sertraline is contraindicated with pimozide
- Disulfiram reaction: disulfiram and oral conc due to alcohol content

⚠ Fatal reactions: MAOIs

Increase: sertraline levels—cimetidine, warfarin, other highly protein-bound products

Increase: effects of antidepressants (tricyclics), diazepam, TOLBUTamide, warfarin, benzodiazepines, sumatriptan

Drug/Herb

- Hypertensive crisis: ephedra

Increase: of SSRI, serotonin syndrome—St. John's wort, SAM-e; do not use together

Increase: anticholinergic effect—corkwood, jimsonweed

Increase: CNS effect—hops, lavender

Drug/Lab Test

Increase: AST, ALT

S

NURSING CONSIDERATIONS

Assess:

- Mental status: mood, sensorium, affect, suicidal tendencies, increase in psychiatric symptoms, depression, panic
- B/P (lying/standing), pulse q4hr; if systolic B/P drops 20 mm Hg, hold product, notify prescriber; VS q4hr in patients with CV disease
- Weight q wk; appetite may decrease with product
- Urinary retention, constipation, especially in geriatric patients
- Alcohol consumption; hold dose until morning

Administer:

- Increased fluids, bulk in diet for constipation, urinary retention
- With food, milk for GI symptoms
- Crushed if patient is unable to swallow medication whole
- Sugarless gum, hard candy, frequent sips of water for dry mouth
- Oral conc: dilute prior to use with 4 oz (½ cup) of water, orange juice, ginger ale or lemon/lime soda; do not mix with other liquids
- Avoid use with other CNS depressants

Perform/provide:

- Storage at room temperature; do not freeze
- Assistance with ambulation during therapy, since drowsiness, dizziness occur
- Safety measures, including raised side rails, primarily for geriatric patients
- Checking to see that PO medication is swallowed

Evaluate:

- Therapeutic response: significant improvement in depression, OCD

Teach patient/family:

- That therapeutic effect may take 1 wk or longer
- To use caution in driving, other activities requiring alertness; drowsiness, dizziness, blurred vision may occur
- Not to discontinue medication quickly after long-term use; may cause nausea, headache, malaise
- To avoid alcohol
- To notify prescriber if pregnant or plan to become pregnant or breastfeed
- That suicidal thoughts/behavior may occur in children/adolescents

sildenafil (℞)

(sil-den′a-fill)

Revatio, Viagra

Func. class.: Erectile agent, antihypertensive, peripheral vasodilator

Chem. class.: Selective inhibitor of cGMP-PDE5

Action: Enhances the effect of nitric oxide (NO) by inhibiting phosphodiesterase type 5 (PDE5), which is necessary for degrading cGMP in the corpus cavernosum

Uses: Treatment of erectile dysfunction, improvement in exercise ability, pulmonary hypertension

Unlabeled uses: Sexual dysfunction (women); lower urinary tract symptoms and erectile dysfunction (with alfuzosin); pediatrics with primary/secondary pulmonary hypertension, altitude sickness, Raynaud's disease

DOSAGE AND ROUTES

Erectile dysfunction (Viagra only)

- *Adult:* **PO** 50 mg 1 hr before sexual activity, may be taken ½-4 hr before sexual activity; may be increased to 100 mg or decreased to 25 mg; max once/day

Renal/hepatic dose

- *Adult:* **PO** (Child Pugh A, B) 25 mg, take 1 hr before sexual activity; max 1×/day; CCr <30 ml/min 25 mg starting dose

Pulmonary hypertension (Revatio only)

- *Infant/child/adolescent (unlabeled):* **PO** 0.25-0.5 mg/kg/dose tid qid
- *Adult:* **PO** 20 mg tid; take 4-6 hr apart

Pulmonary hypertension induced by altitude sickness (unlabeled)

- *Adult:* **PO** 40 mg 6-8 hr after arriving at 14,272 ft, then 40 mg tid × 6 days

Anorgasmy in antidepressant therapy/sexual dysfunction in women (unlabeled)

• *Adult:* **PO** 50 mg 60-90 min prior to sexual activity

Available forms: Tabs 20, 25, 50, 100 mg

SIDE EFFECTS

CNS: Headache, flushing, dizziness, transient global amnesia

CV: **MI, sudden death, CV collapse**

MISC.: Dyspepsia, nasal congestion, UTI, abnormal vision, diarrhea, rash, **non-arteritic ischemic optic neuropathy,** hearing loss, priapism

Contraindication: Hypersensitivity to this product or nitrates

Precautions: Pregnancy (B), anatomical penile deformities, sickle cell anemia, leukemia, multiple myeloma, retinitis pigmentosa, bleeding disorders, active peptic ulceration, CV/renal/hepatic disease, multiproduct antihypertensive regimens

PHARMACOKINETICS

Rapidly absorbed; bioavailability 40%; metabolized by P45 CYP3A4, 2C9 in the liver (active metabolites); terminal half-life 4 hr; peak ½-1½ hr; reduced absorption with high-fat meal; excreted feces, urine

INTERACTIONS

⚠ Do not use with nitrates; fatal fall in B/P

Increase: sildenafil levels—cimetidine, erythromycin, ketoconazole, itraconazole, antiretroviral protease inhibitors

Decrease: sildenafil levels—rifampin, barbiturates, antacids, bosentan

Decrease: B/P—α-blockers, alcohol, amlodipine, angiotensin II receptor blockers

NURSING CONSIDERATIONS

Assess:

⚠ For any severe loss of vision while taking this or any similar products; these products should not be used

⚠ Use of organic nitrates that should not be used with this product

• Cardiac status in pulmonary hypertension: B/P, pulse

Administer:

• Approximately 1 hr before sexual activity; do not use more than once a day

Evaluate:

• Therapeutic response: decreasing pulmonary hypertension; ability to perform sexually (male)

Teach patient/family:

• That product does not protect against sexually transmitted diseases, including HIV

• That product absorption is reduced with a high-fat meal

• That product should not be used with nitrates in any form

• That tabs may be split

• To notify prescriber immediately and stop taking product if vision loss occurs, or erection >4 hr

silodosin (℞)

(si-lo′do-seen)

Rapaflo

Func. class.: Selective α_1 adrenergic blocker

Chem. class.: Sulfamoylphenethylamine derivative

Action: Binds preferentially to α_{1A}-adrenoceptor subtype located mainly in the prostate

Uses: Symptoms of benign prostatic hyperplasia (BPH)

DOSAGE AND ROUTES

• *Adult:* **PO** 8 mg/day with a meal; max 8 mg/day

Available forms: Tabs 8 mg

SIDE EFFECTS

CNS: Dizziness, headache, asthenia, insomnia, syncope

CV: Orthostatic hypotension

EENT: Nasal congestion, rhinorrhea, sinusitis

GI: Diarrhea, abdominal pain, jaundice

S

GU: Abnormal ejaculation, priapism, urinary incontinence
HEMA: Purpura
Contraindications: Hypersensitivity, renal failure
Precautions: Pregnancy (B), breastfeeding, children, females, geriatric patients, renal/hepatic disease, hypotension, ocular surgery, orthostatic hypotension, prostate cancer, syncope

PHARMACOKINETICS

Decreased absorption with high-fat/high-calorie meal, half-life of metabolite is 24 hr, metabolized in liver, excreted via urine, extensively protein bound (97%)

INTERACTIONS

Increase: silodosin effect—CYP3A4 inhibitors (clarithromycin, itraconazole, ritonavir, antiretroviral protease inhibitors, aprepitant, chloramphenicol, conivaptan, dalfopristin, danazol, delavirdine, efavirenz, fosaprepitant, fluconazole, fluvoxamine, imatinib, isoniazid, mifepristone, nefazodone, tamoxifen, telithromycin, troleandomycin, voriconazole, zileuton, zafirlukast

Drug/Food

Increase: silodosin effect—grapefruit juice

Drug Lab/Test

Increase: LFTs

NURSING CONSIDERATIONS

Assess:

- Prostatic hyperplasia: change in urinary patterns, baseline and throughout treatment
- CBC with differential and LFTs; B/P and heart rate
- BUN, uric acid, urodynamic studies (urinary flow rates, residual volume)
- I&O ratios, weight daily, edema, report weight gain or edema

Administer:

- Give with meal at same time of day

Perform/provide:

- Storage at room temperature; protect from light and moisture

Evaluate:

- Therapeutic response: decreased symptoms of BPH

Teach patient/family

- Not to drive or operate machinery until effect is known
- Not to use with grapefruit juice

silver nitrate 1% ophthalmic

See Appendix B

silver nitrate sulfacetamide sodium ophthalmic

See Appendix B

*silver sulfADIAZINE topical

See Appendix B

simethicone (OTC, ℞)

(si-meth′i-kone)
Extra Strength Gas-X, Extra Strength Maalox Anti-Gas, Extra Stength Maalox GRF Gas Relief Formula ❖, Flatulex, Gas-Relief, Gas-X, Genasyme, Maalox Anti-Gas, Maalox GRF Gas Relief Formula ❖, Maximum Strength Gas Relief, Maximum Strength Mylanta Gas Relief, Maximum Strength Phazyme, Mylanta Gas, Mylicon, Ovol ❖, Phazyme, Phazyme 95, Phazyme 125

Func. class.: Antiflatulent

Do not confuse:
Mylicon/Mylanta Gas

Action: Disperses, prevents mucus gas

pockets in GI system, lowers surface tension of gas bubbles
Uses: Flatulence
Unlabeled uses: Dyspepsia

DOSAGE AND ROUTES

- *Adult and child >12 yr:* **PO** 40-125 mg after meals and at bedtime prn, max 500 mg/day
- *Child 2-12 yr:* **PO** 40-50 mg after meals and at bedtime prn, max 240 mg/day
- *Child <2 yr:* **PO** 20 mg qid prn

Available forms: Chew tabs 40, 150, 166 mg; tabs 60, 80, 95, 125 mg; drops 20 mg/0.3 ml, 95 mg/1.425 ml; caps 95, 180 mg; soft gel caps 125, 180 mg; oral dissolving film 62.5 mg

SIDE EFFECTS

GI: Belching, rectal flatus, diarrhea
Contraindications: Hypersensitivity, GI obstruction/perforation
Precautions: Pregnancy (C), abdominal pain, fistula, hiatal hernia

NURSING CONSIDERATIONS

Assess:
- Reason for excess gas production, decreased bowel sounds, recent surgery, other GI conditions

Administer:
- After meals, at bedtime; shake susp well before giving; chew tabs should be chewed

Evaluate:
- Therapeutic response: reduction of abdominal gas, discomfort

Teach patient/family:
- That tablets must be chewed
- To shake suspension well before pouring

simvastatin (℞)

(sim-va-sta'tin)
Zocor
Func. class.: Antilipidemic
Chem. class.: HMG-CoA reductase inhibitor

Do not confuse:
Zocor/Cozaar/Zoloft

Action: Inhibits HMG-CoA reductase enzyme, which reduces cholesterol synthesis
Uses: As an adjunct in primary hypercholesterolemia (types IIa, IIb), isolated hypertriglyceridemia (Frederickson type IV) and type III hyperlipoproteinemia, CAD

DOSAGE AND ROUTES

- *Adult:* **PO** 20 mg/day in PM initially; usual range 5-40 mg/day in PM, not to exceed 80 mg/day; dosage adjustments may be made in 4-wk intervals or more; those taking verapamil and amiodarone max 20 mg/day

Renal disease/those taking cycloSPORINE, gemfibrozil, danazol
- *Adult:* **PO** 5 mg/day, initially; CCr <20 ml/min 5 mg daily in the evening

Cardiac/renal transplantation
- *Adult:* **PO** 5 mg/day; max 10 mg/day

With amiodarone or verapamil
- *Adult:* **PO** max 20 mg/day

With fibrates or niacin
- *Adult:* **PO** max 10 mg/day

Available forms: Tabs 5, 10, 20, 40, 80 mg

SIDE EFFECTS

CNS: Headache, **ALS (Lou Gehrig's disease)**
EENT: Lens opacities
GI: Nausea, constipation, diarrhea, dyspepsia, flatus, abdominal pain, **liver dysfunction,** pancreatitis
INTEG: Rash, pruritus, photosensitivity
MS: Muscle cramps, myalgia, **myositis, rhabdomyolysis**
RESP: Upper respiratory tract infection
Contraindications: Pregnancy (X), breastfeeding, hypersensitivity, active hepatic disease
Precautions: Past hepatic disease, alcoholism, severe acute infections, trauma, severe metabolic disorders, electrolyte imbalances

S

PHARMACOKINETICS

Metabolized in liver (active metabolites); highly protein bound; excreted primarily in bile, feces (60%), kidneys (15%)

INTERACTIONS

Increase: effects of warfarin
Increase: myalgia, myositis—cycloSPORINE, gemfibrozil, niacin, erythromycin, clofibrate, clarithromycin, ketoconazole, itraconazole, protease inhibitors
Increase: serum level of digoxin

Drug/Herb

Increase: effect—glucomannan
Decrease: effect—gotu kola, St. John's wort

Drug/Lab Test

Increase: CPK, LFTs

NURSING CONSIDERATIONS

Assess:

- 12-hr fasting lipid profile: LDL, HDL, TG, cholesterol at 6-8 wk, and q6mo
- Hepatic studies q1-2mo during the first 1½ yr of treatment; AST, ALT, LFTs may increase
- ⚠ For rhabdomyolysis: muscle tenderness, increased CPK levels; therapy should be discontinued
- Renal studies in patients with compromised renal system: BUN, I&O ratio, creatinine

Administer:

- Total daily dose in evening

Perform/provide:

- Storage in cool environment in tight container protected from light

Evaluate:

- Therapeutic response: decrease in cholesterol to desired level after 8 wk

Teach patient/family:

- That blood work and eye exam will be necessary during treatment
- To report blurred vision, severe GI symptoms, dizziness, headache
- That previously prescribed regimen will continue: low-cholesterol diet, exercise program

sirolimus (℞)

(seer-oh-lie'mus)
Rapamune
Func. class.: Immunosuppressant
Chem. class.: Macrolide

Action: Produces immunosuppression by inhibiting T-lymphocyte activation and proliferation

Uses: Organ transplants to prevent rejection, recommended use is with cycloSPORINE and corticosteroids

DOSAGE AND ROUTES

- *Adult:* **PO** 2 mg/day with a 6 mg loading dose
- *Child >13 yr weighing <40 kg (88 lb):* to 1 mg/m^2/day, 3 mg/m^2 loading dose

Hepatic dose

- *Adult and child ≥13 yr/<40 kg:* **PO** Reduce by 33% in maintenance dose (mild-moderate hepatic impairment); reduce by 50% in maintenance dose (severe hepatic impairment)

Available forms: Oral sol 1 mg/ml; tabs 1 mg, 2 mg

SIDE EFFECTS

CNS: Tremors, headache, insomnia, paresthesia, chills, fever

CV: Hypertension, *atrial fibrillation, CHF, hypotension, palpitation, tachycardia,* peripheral edema

EENT: Blurred vision, photophobia

GI: Nausea, vomiting, diarrhea, constipation, **hepatotoxicity**

GU: UTIs, **albuminuria, hematuria, proteinuria, renal failure, nephrotic syndrome,** increased creatinine

HEMA: **Anemia, leukopenia, thrombocytopenia, purpura**

INTEG: Rash, acne, photosensitivity

META: Hyperglycemia, increased creatinine, edema, hypercholesterolemia, *hyperlipemia,* hypophosphatemia, weight gain, hypo/hyperkalemia, hyperuricemia, hypomagnesemia

MS: Arthralgia

RESP: **Pleural effusion, atelectasis,** *dyspnea*
SYST: **Lymphoma, exfoliative dermatitis**

Contraindications: Breastfeeding, hypersensitivity to this product or to components of the product

Precautions: Pregnancy (C), children <13 yr, severe cardiac/renal/hepatic disease; diabetes mellitus, hyperkalemia, hyperuricemia, hypertension, interstitial lung disease, hyperlipidemia

Black Box Warning: Lymphomas, infection, other malignancies

PHARMACOKINETICS

Rapidly absorbed; peak 1 hr single dose, 2 hr multiple dosing; protein binding 92%; extensively metabolized by CYP3A4 enzyme system

INTERACTIONS

⚠ ***Increase:*** angioedema—ACE inhibitors, angiotensin II–receptor antagonists, cephalosporins, iodine-containing radiopaque contrast media, neuromuscular blockers, NSAIDs, penicillins, salicylates, thrombolytics

Increase: blood levels—antifungals, calcium channel blockers, cimetidine, danazol, erythromycin, cycloSPORINE, metoclopramide, bromocriptine, HIV-protease inhibitors

Decrease: blood levels—carbamazepine, phenobarbital, phenytoin, rifamycin, rifapentine

Decrease: effect of vaccines

Drug/Herb

- St. John's wort: may decrease the effect of sirolimus

Increase: effect—ginseng, maitake, mistletoe

Decrease: immunosuppression—astragalus, echinacea, melatonin

Drug/Food

- Alters bioavailability; use consistently with or without food; do not use with grapefruit juice

NURSING CONSIDERATIONS

Assess:

- Blood levels in those that may have altered metabolism, trough level ≥15 ng/ml are associated with increased adverse reactions; monitor trough concentrations in all patients
- Lipid profile: cholesterol, triglycerides, a lipid-lowering agent may be needed

⚠ For infection and development of lymphoma

⚠ Blood studies: Hgb, WBC, platelets during treatment q mo; if leukocytes <3000/mm^3 or platelets <100,000/mm^3, product should be discontinued or reduced; decreased hemoglobulin level may indicate bone marrow suppression

- Hepatic studies: alk phos, AST, ALT, amylase, bilirubin, and for hepatotoxicity: dark urine, jaundice, itching, light-colored stools; product should be discontinued

Administer:

- Prophylaxis for *Pneumocystis jiroveci* pneumonia for 1 yr after transplantation; prophylaxis for CMV is recommended for 90 days after transplantation in those at increased risk for CMV
- All medications PO if possible, avoiding IM inj; bleeding may occur
- For 3 days before transplant surgery; patients should be placed in protective isolation
- Use amber oral dose syringe and withdraw amount oral sol needed from the bottle, empty correct dose into plastic/glass container holding 60 ml of water/orange juice, stir vigorously and have patient drink at once, refill container with additional 120 ml water/orange juice, stir vigorously and drink at once, if using a pouch squeeze entire contents into container and follow above directions
- Store protected from light, refrigerate, stable for 24 mo

Evaluate:

- Therapeutic response: absence of graft rejection; immunosuppression in autoimmune disorders

Teach patient/family:

- To report fever, rash, severe diarrhea, chills, sore throat, fatigue; serious infections may occur; clay-colored stools, cramping (hepatotoxicity)
- To avoid crowds, persons with known infections to reduce risk of infection
- To use contraception before, during, and 12 wk after product has been discontinued, avoid breastfeeding
- Use sunscreen, protective clothing to prevent burns
- Not to use with grapefruit juice
- To avoid vaccines

sitagliptin (℞)

(sit-a-glip′tin)

Januvia

Func. class.: Antidiabetic, oral

Chem. class.: Dipeptidyl-peptidase-4 inhibitor (DPP-4 inhibitor)

Action: Slows the inactivation of incretin hormones; improves glucose homeostasis, improves glucose-dependent insulin secretion, lowers glucagon secretions, and slows gastric emptying time

Uses: Type 2 diabetes mellitus as monotherapy or in combination with other antidiabetic agents

DOSAGE AND ROUTES

- *Adult:* **PO** 100 mg/day; may use with other antidiabetic agents other than insulin

Renal dose

- *Adult:* **PO** CCr 30-50 ml/min 50 mg daily; CCr <30 ml/min 25 mg daily

Available forms: Tabs 25, 50, 100 mg

SIDE EFFECTS

CNS: Headache

ENDO: Hypoglycemia

GI: Nausea, vomiting, abdominal pain, diarrhea

SYST: **Anaphylaxis, Stevens-Johnson syndrome, angioedema**

Contraindications: Hypersensitivity, diabetic ketoacidosis (DKA)

Precautions: Pregnancy (C), geriatric patients, hypersensitivity, GI obstruction, surgery, thyroid/renal/hepatic disease, trauma

PHARMACOKINETICS

Rapidly absorbed, excreted by the kidneys (unchanged 79%), terminal half-life 12.4 hr, peak 1-4 hr

INTERACTIONS

Increase: sitagliptan level—cimetidine, disopyramide

Increase: levels of digoxin

Increase: hypoglycemia—androgens, insulins, β-blockers, cimetidine, corticosteroids, salicylates, MAOIs, fibric acid derivatives, fluoxetine

Decrease: antidiabetic effect—thiazide diuretics, ACE inhibitors, protease inhibitors, sympathomimetics, aripiprazole, clozapine, olanzapine, quetiapine, risperidone, ziprasidone, phenytoin, fosphenytoin, phenothiazines, estrogens, progestins, oral contraceptives

Drug/Herb

Increase: hyperglycemia—glucosamine

Increase: hypoglycemia—chromium, coenzyme Q-10, fenugreek

Increase: antidiabetic effect—alfalfa, aloe, basil, bay, bilberry, bitter melon, black catechu, buchu, burdock, coriander, dandelion, eyebright (po), fenugreek, garlic, ginseng, glucomannan, glucosamine, goat's rue, gymnema, horehound, horse chestnut, jambul, myrrh, myrtle

Decrease: antidiabetic effect—bee pollen, blue cohosh, broom, chromium, elecampane, eucalyptus, gotu kola

NURSING CONSIDERATIONS

Assess:

- For hypoglycemic reactions (sweating, weakness, dizziness, anxiety, tremors, hunger), hyperglycemic reactions soon after meals
- CBC (baseline, q3mo) during treatment; check LFTs periodically, AST, LDH,

renal studies: BUN, creatinine during treatment; glycosylated hemoglobin A1c
• Monitor blood glucose (BG) as needed

Administer:
• May be taken with or without food

Perform/provide:
• Conversion from other antidiabetic agents; change may be made with gradual dosage change
• Storage in tight container at room temperature

Evaluate:
• Therapeutic response: decrease in polyuria, polydipsia, polyphagia; clear sensorium; absence of dizziness; stable gait, blood glucose, A1c improvement

Teach patient/family:
• To use regular self-monitoring of blood glucose using blood glucose meter
• The symptoms of hypo/hyperglycemia; what to do about each
• That product must be continued on daily basis; explain consequence of discontinuing product abruptly
• To avoid OTC medications, alcohol, digoxin, exenatide, insulins, nateglinide, repaglinide and other products that lower blood glucose, unless approved by prescriber
• That diabetes is a lifelong illness; that this product is not a cure, only controls symptoms
• That all food included in diet plan must be eaten to prevent hypo/hyperglycemia
• To carry emergency ID

sodium bicarbonate (℞, OTC)

Baking Soda, Brioschi-Neut, Citrocarbonate, Neut, Sellymin ✦

Func. class.: Alkalinizer
Chem. class.: $NaHCO_3$

Action: Orally neutralizes gastric acid, which forms water, NaCl, CO_2; increases plasma bicarbonate, which buffers H^+-ion concentration; reverses acidosis IV

Uses: Acidosis (metabolic), cardiac arrest, alkalinization (systemic/urinary) antacid, salicylate poisoning

Unlabeled uses: Contrast media nephrotoxicity prevention

DOSAGE AND ROUTES

Acidosis, metabolic
• *Adult and child:* **IV INF** 2-5 mEq/kg over 4-8 hr depending on CO_2, pH

Cardiac arrest
• *Adult and child:* **IV BOL** 1 mEq/kg of 7.5% or 8.4% sol, then 0.5 mEq/kg q10min, then doses based on ABGs
• *Infant:* **IV INF** Max 8 mEq/kg/day based on ABGs (4.2% sol)

Alkalinization of urine
• *Adult:* **PO** 325 mg-2 g qid or 48 mEq (4 g), then 12-24 mEq q4hr
• *Child:* **PO** 84-840 mg/kg/day (1-10 mEq/kg) in divided doses q4-6hr

Antacid
• *Adult:* **PO** 300 mg-2 g chewed, taken with H_2O daily-qid

Available forms: Tabs 300, 325, 600, 650 mg; inj 4.2%, 5%, 7.5%, 8.4%

SIDE EFFECTS

CNS: Irritability, headache, confusion, stimulation, tremors, *twitching, hyperreflexia,* **tetany,** weakness, **seizures** of alkalosis
CV: Irregular pulse, **cardiac arrest,** water retention, edema, weight gain
GI: Flatulence, *belching, distention,* **paralytic ileus,** acid rebound, nausea
GU: Calculi
META: Alkalosis
MS: Muscular twitching, tetany, irritability
RESP: Shallow, slow respirations; cyanosis, **apnea**

Contraindications: Metabolic/respiratory alkalosis, hypochloremia, hypocalcemia

Precautions: Pregnancy (C), CHF, cirrhosis, toxemia, renal disease, hypertension, hypokalemia, breastfeeding, hypernatremia

S

PHARMACOKINETICS

PO: Onset rapid, duration 10 min
IV: Onset 15 min, duration 1-2 hr, excreted in urine

INTERACTIONS

Increase: effects—amphetamines, mecamylamine, quinine, quinidine, pseudoephedrine, flecainide, anorexiants, sympathomimetics
Increase: sodium and decrease potassium—corticosteroids
Decrease: effects—lithium, chlorpropamide, barbiturates, salicylates, benzodiazepines, ketoconazoles, corticosteroids

Drug/Herb

Decrease: action of sodium bicarbonate—oak bark

Drug/Lab Test

Increase: urinary urobilinogen, sodium, lactate
Decrease: potassium
False positive: urinary protein, blood lactate

NURSING CONSIDERATIONS

Assess:

- Respiratory and pulse rate, rhythm, depth, lung sounds; notify prescriber of abnormalities
- Fluid balance (I&O, weight daily, edema); notify prescriber of fluid overload
- Electrolytes, blood pH, PO_2, HCO_3^-, during treatment; ABGs frequently during emergencies
- Urine pH, urinary output, during beginning treatment
- Extravasation with IV administration (tissue sloughing, ulceration, and necrosis)
- Weight daily with initial therapy
- Alkalosis: irritability, confusion, twitching, hyperreflexia stimulation, slow respirations, cyanosis, irregular pulse
- Milk-alkali syndrome: confusion, headache, nausea, vomiting, anorexia, urinary stones, hypercalcemia
- For GI perforation secondary to CO_2 in GI tract; may lead to perforation if ulcer is severe enough

Administer:

- Chew antacid tablets and drink 8 oz water
- Do not take antacid with milk or milk-alkali syndrome may result

IV route

- In prepared sol or diluted in an equal amount of compatible sol given 2-5 mEq/kg over 4-8 hr, not to exceed 50 mEq/hr; slower rate in children

Additive compatibilities: Amikacin, aminophylline, amobarbital, amphotericin B, atropine, bretylium, calcium gluceptate, cefoxitin, ceftazidime, cephalothin, cephapirin, chloramphenicol, chlorothiazide, cimetidine, clindamycin, cytarabine, droperidol/fentanyl, ergonovine, erythromycin, esmolol, floxacillin, furosemide, heparin, hyaluronidase, hydrocortisone, kanamycin, lidocaine, mannitol, metaraminol, methotrexate, methyldopate, multivitamins, nafcillin, nalmefene, netilmicin, nizatidine, ofloxacin, oxacillin, oxytocin, phenobarbital, phenylephrine, phenytoin, phytonadione, potassium chloride, prochlorperazine, thiopental, verapamil

Syringe compatibilities: Milrinone, pentobarbital

Y-site compatibilities: Acyclovir, amifostine, asparaginase, aztreonam, cefepime, cefmetazole, ceftriaxone, cladribine, cyclophosphamide, cytarabine, DAUNOrubicin, dexamethasone, dexchlorpheniramine, DOXOrubicin, etoposide, famotidine, filgrastim, fludarabine, gallium, granisetron, heparin, ifosfamide, indomethacin sodium trihydrate, insulin, melphalan, mesna, methylPREDNISolone, morphine, paclitaxel, piperacillin/tazobactam, potassium chloride, propofol, remifentanil, tacrolimus, teniposide, thiotepa, tolazoline, vancomycin, vit B/C

Evaluate:

- Therapeutic response: ABGs, electrolytes, blood pH, HCO_3^- WNL

Teach patient/family:
- Not to take antacid with milk, or milk-alkali syndrome may result
- Not to use antacid for more than 2 wk
- To notify prescriber if indigestion is accompanied by chest pain; trouble breathing; diarrhea; dark, tarry stools; coffee-grounds-looking vomit; swelling of feet/ankles
- About sodium-restricted diet; to avoid use of baking soda for indigestion

sodium biphosphate/ sodium phosphate

(OTC)

Fleet Enema, Phospho-Soda

Func. class.: Laxative, saline

Action: Increases water absorption in the small intestine by osmotic action, laxative effect occurs by increased peristalsis and water retention

Uses: Constipation, bowel or rectal preparation for surgery, exam

DOSAGE AND ROUTES

- *Adult:* **PO** 20-30 ml (Phospho-Soda)
- *Child:* **PO** 5-15 ml (Phospho-Soda)
- *Adult and child >12 yr:* **RECT** 1 enema (118 ml)
- *Child 2-12 yr:* **RECT** ½ enema (59 ml)

Available forms: Enema 7 g phosphate/19 g biphosphate/118 ml; oral sol 18 g phosphate/48 g biphosphate/100 ml

SIDE EFFECTS

CV: **Dysrhythmias, cardiac arrest,** hypotension, widening QRS complex

GI: Nausea, cramps, diarrhea

META: Electrolyte, fluid imbalances

Contraindications: Hypersensitivity, rectal fissures, abdominal pain, nausea/vomiting, appendicitis, acute surgical abdomen, ulcerated hemorrhoids, sodium-restricted diets, renal failure, hyperphosphatemia, hypocalcemia, hypokalemia, hypernatremia, Addison's disease, CHF, ascites, bowel perforation, megacolon, imperforate anus

Black Box Warning: GI obstruction, renal failure

Precautions: Pregnancy (C)

Black Box Warning: Colitis, geriatric hypovolemia, renal disease

PHARMACOKINETICS

Onset 30 min-3 hr, excreted in feces

NURSING CONSIDERATIONS

Assess:
- Stools: color, amount, consistency
- Bowel pattern, bowel sounds, flatulence, distention, fever, dietary patterns, exercise
- Blood, urine electrolytes if product is used often by patient
- Cramping, rectal bleeding, nausea, vomiting; if these symptoms occur, product should be discontinued

Administer:
- Alone for better absorption; do not take within 1-2 hr of other products

Evaluate:
- Therapeutic response: decrease in constipation

Teach patient/family:
- Not to use laxatives for long-term therapy; bowel tone will be lost
- That normal bowel movements do not always occur daily
- Not to use in presence of abdominal pain, nausea, vomiting
- To notify prescriber if constipation unrelieved or if symptoms of electrolyte imbalance occur: muscle cramps, pain, weakness, dizziness, excessive thirst
- To maintain fluid consumption

S

sodium polystyrene sulfonate (℞)

(po-lee-stye′reen)

Kayexalate, K-Exit ✤, Kionex, PMS Sodium Polystyrene Sulfonate ✤, SPS

Func. class.: Potassium-removing resin

Chem. class.: Cation exchange resin

Action: Removes potassium by exchanging sodium for potassium in body primarily in large intestine

Uses: Hyperkalemia in conjunction with other measures

DOSAGE AND ROUTES

• *Adult:* **PO** 15 g daily-qid; **RECT** enema 30-50 g q1-2hr initially prn, then q6hr prn

• *Child (unlabeled):* **PO** 1 g/kg q6hr prn; **RECT** 1 g/kg q2-6hr prn

Available forms: Powder for susp 453.6 g, 454 g; oral susp 15 g/60 ml; rectal enema susp 15 g/60 ml

SIDE EFFECTS

GI: Constipation, anorexia, nausea, vomiting, diarrhea (sorbitol), fecal impaction, gastric irritation

META: Hypocalcemia, hypokalemia, hypomagnesemia, sodium retention

Contraindications: Hypersensitivity to saccharin or parabens that may be in some products, ileus

Precautions: Pregnancy (C), geriatric patients, renal failure, CHF, severe edema, severe hypertension, sodium restriction, constipation

INTERACTIONS

Increase: hypokalemia—loop diuretics

Decrease: effect of sodium polystyrene—antacids, laxatives

NURSING CONSIDERATIONS

Assess:

• Hyperkalemia: confusion, dyspnea, weakness, dysrhythmias

• ECG for spiked T waves, depressed ST segments, prolonged QT and widening QRS complex

• Bowel function daily, note consistency of stools, times/day

• Hypotension: confusion, irritability, muscular pain, weakness

• Serum K, Ca, Mg, Na, acid-base balance

• I&O ratio, weight daily

• For digoxin; toxicity in those receiving digoxin

Administer:

• Oral dose as susp mixed with H_2O or syr (20-100 ml)

• Mild laxative as ordered to prevent constipation, fecal impaction

• Sorbitol as ordered to prevent constipation

• Retention enema after mixing with warm water; introduce by gravity, continue stirring, flush with 100 ml of fluid, clamp, and leave in place

Perform/provide:

• Retention of enema for at least ½-1 hr

• Irrigation of colon after enema with 1-2 qt nonsodium sol, drain

• Storage of freshly prepared sol 24 hr at room temperature

Evaluate:

• Therapeutic response: potassium level 3.5-5 mg/dl

Teach patient/family:

• Reason for medication and expected results

solifenacin (℞)

(sol-i-fen′a-sin)

VESIcare

Func. class.: Overactive bladder product, anticholinergic

Chem. class.: Muscarinic receptor antagonist

Action: Relaxes smooth muscles in urinary tract by inhibiting acetylcholine at postganglionic sites

Uses: Overactive bladder (urinary frequency, urgency, incontinence)

DOSAGE AND ROUTES

• *Adult:* **PO** 5 mg/day, max 10 mg/day

Renal/hepatic dose

• *Adult:* **PO** (Child-Pugh B) max 5 mg/day

• *Adult:* **PO** CCr <30 ml/min 5 mg/day

Available forms: Tabs 5, 10 mg

SIDE EFFECTS

CNS: Anxiety, paresthesia, fatigue, *dizziness,* headache

CV: Chest pain, hypertension, **QTc prolongation,** peripheral edema

EENT: Vision abnormalities, xerophthalmia, nasal dryness

GI: Nausea, vomiting, anorexia, abdominal pain, *constipation, dry mouth,* dyspepsia

GU: Dysuria, urinary retention, frequency, UTI

INTEG: Rash, pruritus

RESP: Bronchitis, cough, pharyngitis, upper respiratory tract infection

Contraindications: Hypersensitivity, uncontrolled closed-angle glaucoma, urinary retention, gastric retention

Precautions: Pregnancy (C), breastfeeding, children, geriatric patients, renal/hepatic disease, controlled closed-angle glaucoma, bladder outflow obstruction, GI obstruction, decreased GI motility, history of QT prolongation

PHARMACOKINETICS

Rapidly absorbed, 98% highly protein bound, extensively metabolized by CYP3A4, excreted in urine/feces, terminal half-life 45-68 hr

INTERACTIONS

Increase: CNS depression—sedatives, hypnotics, benzodiazepines, opioids

Increase: effects—CYP3A4 inhibitors (ketoconazole, clarithromycin, diclofenac, doxycycline, erythromycin, isoniazid, nefazodone, propofol, protease inhibitors, verapamil), with max dose 5 mg

Decrease: effects—CYP3A4 inducers (carbamazepine, nevirapine, phenobarbital, phenytoin)

Drug/Herb

Increase: effects—henbane, jimsonweed, scopolia

Decrease: effects—St. John's wort

Drug/Food

Increase: effect—grapefruit juice

NURSING CONSIDERATIONS

Assess:

• Urinary patterns: distention, nocturia, frequency, urgency, incontinence

• Allergic reactions: rash; if this occurs, product should be discontinued

Evaluate:

• Urinary status: dysuria, frequency, nocturia, incontinence

Teach patient/family:

• To avoid hazardous activities; dizziness may occur

• Constipation, blurred vision may occur

• Call prescriber if severe abdominal pain or constipation lasts for 3 or more days

• Heat prostration may occur if used in a hot environment

somatropin (℞)

(soe-ma-troe'pin)

Accretropin, Genotropin, Genotropin-MiniQuick, Humatrope, Norditropin, Nutropin, Nutropin AQ, Nutropin Depot, Omnitrope, Saizen, Serostim, Tev-Tropin, Zorbtive

Func. class.: Pituitary hormone

Chem. class.: Growth hormone

Do not confuse:

somatropin/sumatriptan

Action: Stimulates growth; somatropin similar to natural growth hormone; both preparations developed by recombinant DNA

Uses: Pituitary growth hormone deficiency (hypopituitary dwarfism), children with human growth hormone deficiency/growth failure, AIDS wasting syndrome, cachexia, adults with somatropin deficiency syndrome (SDS), short stature in

S

Noonan syndrome, SHOX deficiency, Turner's syndrome, Prader-Willi syndrome

DOSAGE AND ROUTES

Genotropin

• *Child:* **SUBCUT** 0.16-0.24 mg/kg/wk divided into 6 or 7 daily inj, give in abdomen, thigh, buttocks

• *Adult:* **SUBCUT** 0.4-0.8 mg/kg/wk divided in 6-7 daily doses

Humatrope

• *Adult:* **IM** 0.018 units/kg/day, max 0.0125 units/kg/day

• *Child:* **SUBCUT/IM** 0.18 mg/kg divided into equal doses either on 3 alternate days or 6×/wk, max wk dose is 0.3 mg/kg

Nutropin/Nutropin AQ (growth hormone deficiency)

• *Child:* **SUBCUT** 0.3 mg/kg/wk

Serostim

• *Adult:* **SUBCUT** at bedtime >55 kg, 6 mg; 45-55 kg, 5 mg; 35-45 kg, 4 mg

Norditropin

• *Child:* **SUBCUT** 0.024-0.034 mg/kg 6-7×/wk

Accretropin

• *Child:* **SUBCUT** 0.18-0.3 mg/kg/wk divided into 6 or 7 equal daily inj

Replacement of GH in GH deficiency

• *Adult:* **SUBCUT** (Saizen) 0.005 mg/kg/day; may increase after 4 wk to max 0.01 mg/kg/day

Available forms: Powder for inj (lyophilized) 1.5 mg (4 international units/ml), 4 mg (12 international units/vial), 5 mg (13 international units/vial), 5 mg (15 international units/vial) rDNA origin, 5.8 mg (15 international units/ml), 6 mg (18 international units/ml), 8 mg (24 international units/vial), 10 mg (26 international units/vial); inj 10 mg (30 international units/vial), 5 mg/1.5 ml, 10 mg/1.5 ml, 15 mg/1.5 ml

SIDE EFFECTS

CNS: Headache, growth of intracranial tumor, fever, aggressive behavior

ENDO: **Hyperglycemia, ketosis, hypothyroidism**

GI: Nausea, vomiting

GU: Hypercalciuria

INTEG: Rash, urticaria, pain; inflammation at inj site, hematoma

MS: Tissue swelling, joint and muscle pain

SYST: **Antibodies to growth hormone**

Contraindications: Hypersensitivity to benzyl alcohol, closed epiphyses, intracranial lesions, acute respiratory failure, Prader-Willi syndrome with obesity, trauma

Precautions: Pregnancy (C), breastfeeding, newborn, geriatric patients, diabetes mellitus, hypothyroidism, intracranial lesions, prolonged treatment in adults, scoliosis, sleep apnea, chemotherapy, diabetes, respiratory disease

PHARMACOKINETICS

Half-life 15-60 min, duration 7 days, metabolized in liver

INTERACTIONS

• Epiphyseal closure: androgens, thyroid hormones

Decrease: growth—glucocorticosteroids

NURSING CONSIDERATIONS

Assess:

• For signs/symptoms of diabetes

• Growth hormone antibodies if patient fails to respond to therapy

• Thyroid function tests: T_3, T_4, T_7, TSH to identify hypothyroidism

• Allergic reaction: rash, itching, fever, nausea, wheezing

• Hypercalciuria: urinary stones; groin, flank pain; nausea, vomiting, urinary frequency, hematuria, chills

• Growth rate, bone age of child at intervals during treatment

Administer:

IM route

• Rotate inj site

• Accretropin: does not require reconstitution

• Norditropin: after reconstituting 4 or 8 mg/2 ml diluent

• Humatrope: 5 mg/1.5-5 ml diluent, do not shake

• Nutropin/Nutropin AQ: reconstitute 5 mg/1-5 ml or 10 mg/1-10 ml bacteriostatic water for inj (benzyl alcohol preserved)
• Zorbtive: reconstitute 4, 5, 6 mg with 0.5-1 ml of sterile water for inj; reconstitute each 8.8 mg with 1-2 ml bacteriostatic water for inj

Perform/provide:
• Storage in refrigerator for <1 mo, if reconstituted <1 wk; do not use discolored or cloudy sol

Evaluate:
• Therapeutic response: growth in children

Teach patient/family:
• That treatment may continue for years; regular assessments are required
• Maintain a growth record; report knee, hip pain, or limping
• That treatment is very expensive

sorafenib (℞)
(sore-ah-fen′ib)
Nexavar
Func. class.: Antineoplastic—miscellaneous
Chem. class.: Multikinase inhibitor, signal transduction inhibitor

Action: Multikinase inhibitor that decreases tumor cell proliferation
Uses: Advanced/metastatic murine renal cell carcinoma, unresectable hepatocellular cancer
Unlabeled uses: Metastatic, malignant melanoma

DOSAGE AND ROUTES

• *Adult:* **PO** 400 mg bid without food, continue until no longer benefiting or until unacceptable toxicity occurs
Available forms: Tabs 200 mg

SIDE EFFECTS

CNS: Fatigue, weight loss, headache
CV: **Hypertension, cardiac ischemia, infarction, hypertensive crisis, cardiotoxicity, MI**
GI: Nausea, diarrhea, vomiting, anorexia, **pancreatitis,** mouth ulceration, *abdominal pain,* constipation, **GI perforation**
HEMA: **Hemorrhage, leukopenia, lymphopenia, anemia, neutropenia, thrombocytopenia, pancytopenia**
INTEG: Rash, pruritus, *dry skin,* erythema, *hand-foot syndrome,* **exfoliative dermatitis**, acne, flushing, *alopecia*
META: Hypophosphatemia
MS: Arthralgia, myalgia
RESP: Hoarseness
Contraindications: Pregnancy (D), hypersensitivity
Precautions: Breastfeeding, children, geriatric patients, cardiac/renal/hepatic disease, GI bleeding infection, surgery, dental disease/work

PHARMACOKINETICS

Bioavailability 38%-49%, elimination half-life 1-2 days, peak 3 hr, high-fat meal decreases bioavailability, plasma protein binding 99.5%, metabolized in the liver, oxidative metabolism by CYP3A4, glucuronidation by UGT1A9, 77% excreted in feces

INTERACTIONS

• May decrease sorafenib effect: CYP3A4 inducers (barbiturates, bosentan, carbamazepine, efavirenz, phenytoins, nevirapine, rifabutin, rifampin); use cautiously
Increase: bleeding risk—NSAIDs, anticoagulants, platelet inhibitors, thrombolytics
Increase: effect of UGT1A1 substrates (irinotecan, DOXOrubicin, morphine, naltrexone, estradiol, buprenorphine)
Decrease: sorafenib levels—phenytoin, rifampin, cimetidine, ranitidine, sodium bicarbonate, carbamazepine, dexamethasone, phenobarbital

Drug/Herb
• Avoid use with St. John's wort

Drug/Lab Test
Increase: lipase, amylase, TSH, bilirubin transaminase
Decrease: RBC, WBC, platelets

S

NURSING CONSIDERATIONS

Assess:

- CBC with differential, LFTs
- For skin toxicities: grade 1, continue therapy, topical treatment for relief; grade 2 (1st episode), continue therapy, if no improvement after 7 days, delay treatment until resolved to grade ≤1, resume dose by one dose level; grade 2 (2nd or 3rd episode), delay treatment until resolved to grade ≤1, resume dose by one dose level; grade 2 (4th episode), discontinue therapy; grade 3 (1st or 2nd episode), delay treatment until resolved to grade ≤1, resume dose by one dose level; grade 3 (3rd episode), discontinue therapy
- B/P weekly × 6 wk (hypertension); cardiac ischemia; bleeding, bruising
- Hand-foot reactions during first 6 wk of therapy
- PT, INR (bleeding)

Administer:

- Swallow tab whole; do not break, crush, or chew
- On empty stomach 1 hr before or 2 hr after meal

Perform/provide:

- Storage in room temperature, in dry place

Evaluate:

- Therapeutic response: stabilization in renal cell carcinoma progression

Teach patient/family:

⚠ To report adverse reactions immediately

- Reason for treatment, expected results
- Use contraception during treatment, birth defects may occur, avoid breastfeeding
- To not double dose if missed
- To avoid OTC products without approval of prescriber

sotalol (℞)

(sot'ah-lahl)

Betapace, Betapace AF, Sorine Sotalol AF, Sotocar ✤

Func. class.: Antidysrhythmic group III

Chem. class.: Nonselective β-blocker

Action: Blockade of β_1- and β_2-receptors leads to antidysrhythmic effect, prolongs action potential in myocardial fibers without affecting conduction, prolongs QT interval, no effect on QRS duration

Uses: Life-threatening ventricular dysrhythmias; Betapace AF: to maintain sinus rhythm in symptomatic atrial fibrillation/flutter

Unlabeled uses: Atrial fibrillation prophylaxis, cardiac surgery, PSVT, Wolff-Parkinson-White (WPW) syndrome

DOSAGE AND ROUTES

- *Adult:* **PO** Initial 80 mg bid, may increase to 240-320 mg/day

Renal dose

- *Adult:* **PO** CCr 30-60 ml/min, give q24hr; CCr 10-29 ml/min, give q36-48hr; CCr <10 ml/min, individualize dose

Betapace AF

- *Adult:* **PO** Initial 80 mg bid, titrate upward to 120 mg bid during initial hospitalization

Renal dose (Betapace AF)

- *Adult:* **PO** CCr >60 ml/min, give q12hr; CCr 40-60 ml/min, give q24hr; CCr <40 ml/min, do not use

Available forms: Tabs 80, 120, 160, 240 mg; (Betapace AF) 80, 120, 160 mg; inj 150 mg/10 ml (15 mg/ml)

SIDE EFFECTS

CNS: Dizziness, mental changes, drowsiness, fatigue, headache, catatonia, depression, anxiety, nightmares, paresthesia, lethargy, insomnia, decreased concentration

CV: **Prodysrhythmia, prolonged QT,** orthostatic hypotension, bradycardia,

CHF, chest pain, ventricular dysrhythmias, AV block, peripheral vascular insufficiency, palpitations, torsades de pointes; **life-threatening ventricular dysrhythmias (Betapace AF)**

EENT: Tinnitus, visual changes, sore throat, double vision; dry, burning eyes

GI: Nausea, vomiting, diarrhea, dry mouth, flatulence, constipation, anorexia, indigestion

GU: Impotence, dysuria, ejaculatory failure, urinary retention

HEMA: **Agranulocytosis, thrombocytopenic purpura** (rare), **thrombocytopenia, leukopenia**

INTEG: Rash, alopecia, urticaria, pruritus, fever, diaphoresis

MISC: Facial swelling, decreased exercise tolerance, weight change, Raynaud's disease

MS: Joint pain, arthralgia, muscle cramps, pain

RESP: **Bronchospasm,** dyspnea, wheezing, nasal stuffiness, pharyngitis

Contraindications: Hypersensitivity to β-blockers, cardiogenic shock, heart block (2nd/3rd degree), sinus bradycardia, CHF, bronchial asthma, CCr <40 ml/min

Black Box Warning: Congenital or acquired long QT syndrome, hypokalemia

Precautions: Pregnancy (B), breastfeeding, major surgery, diabetes mellitus, renal/thyroid disease, COPD, well-compensated heart failure, CAD, nonallergic bronchospasm, electrolyte disturbances, bradycardia, peripheral vascular disease

Black Box Warning: Cardiac dysrhythmias, torsade de pointes, ventricular dysrhythmias, ventricular fibrillation

PHARMACOKINETICS

PO: Onset 1-2 hr, peak 2-4 hr, duration 8-12 hr, half-life 12 hr, excreted unchanged in urine, crosses placenta, excreted in breast milk, protein binding 0%

INTERACTIONS

Increase: hypoglycemia effect—insulin

Increase: effects of lidocaine

Increase: hypotension—diuretics, other antihypertensives, nitroglycerin

Decrease: β-blocker effects—sympathomimetics

Decrease: bronchodilating effects of theophylline, β_2-agonists

Decrease: hypoglycemic effects of sulfonylureas

Drug/Herb

- Hypokalemia, increased antidysrhythmic effect: aloe, buckthorn, cascara sagrada, senna

Increase: toxicity, death—aconite

Increase: effect—aloe, broom, chronic buckthorn use, cascara sagrada (chronic use), Chinese rhubarb, figwort, fumitory, goldenseal, kudzu, licorice

Increase: serotonin effect—horehound

Decrease: effect—coltsfoot

Drug/Lab Test

False increase: urinary catecholamines

Interference: glucose, insulin tolerance tests

NURSING CONSIDERATIONS

Assess:

- I&O, weight daily; edema in feet, legs daily
- B/P, pulse q4hr; note rate, rhythm, quality
- Potassium, magnesium levels

⚠ Apical/radial pulse before administration: notify prescriber of any significant changes; monitor ECG continuously (Betapace AF); use QT interval to determine patient eligibility; baseline QT must be ≤450 msec

- Baselines in renal studies before therapy begins
- Skin turgor, dryness of mucous membranes for hydration status

Administer:

PO route

- Before, at bedtime; tablet may be crushed or swallowed whole, give 1 hr before or 2 hr after meals
- Reduced dosage in renal dysfunction

S

• Betapace and Betapace AF are not interchangeable
• Do not give within 2 hr of antacids

IV route
• Dilute to a volume of either 120 ml or 300 ml with D_5W, LR
• 75 mg dose: withdraw 6 ml sotalol inj (90 mg) add 114 ml dilute to make 120 ml (0.75 mg/ml) or withdraw 6 ml sotalol inj (90 mg) add 294 ml, dilute to make 300 ml (0.3 mg/ml)
• 112.5 mg dose: withdraw 9 ml sotalol inj (135 ml) add 111 ml, dilute to 120 ml (1.125 mg/ml; or withdraw 9 ml sotalol (135 mg) and add 291 ml dilute to 300 ml (0.45 mg/ml)
• 150 mg dose: withdraw 12 ml of sotalol (180 mg) add 108 ml to 120 ml (1.5 mg/ml) or withdraw 12 ml sotalol (180 mg) add 288 ml to 300 ml (0.6 mg/ml)
• Use inf pump

Perform/provide:
• Storage in dry area at room temperature; do not freeze

Evaluate:
• Therapeutic response: absence of life-threatening dysrhythmias

Teach patient/family:
• Not to discontinue product abruptly; taper over 2 wk or may precipitate angina, take exactly as prescribed
• Not to use antacids or OTC products containing α-adrenergic stimulants (nasal decongestants, OTC cold preparations) unless directed by prescriber
• To report bradycardia, dizziness, confusion, depression, fever
• To take pulse at home; advise when to notify prescriber
• To avoid alcohol, smoking, sodium intake
• To carry emergency ID to identify product being taken, allergies
• To avoid hazardous activities if dizziness is present
• To report symptoms of CHF including: difficulty in breathing, especially on exertion or when lying down; night cough, swelling of extremities
• To wear support hose to minimize effects of orthostatic hypotension
• To monitor blood glucose if diabetic

Treatment of overdose: Lavage, IV atropine for bradycardia, IV theophylline for bronchospasm, digoxin, O_2, diuretic for cardiac failure; hemodialysis is useful for removal; administer vasopressor (norepinephrine) for hypotension, isoproterenol for heart block

spironolactone (℞)

(speer′on-oh-lak′tone)
Aldactone, Novo-Spiroton ♣
Func. class.: Potassium-sparing diuretic
Chem. class.: Aldosterone antagonist

Action: Competes with aldosterone at receptor sites in distal tubule, resulting in excretion of sodium chloride, water, retention of potassium, phosphate

Uses: Edema of CHF, hypertension, diuretic-induced hypokalemia, primary-hyperaldosteronism (diagnosis, short-term treatment, long-term treatment), edema of nephrotic syndrome, cirrhosis of the liver with ascites

Unlabeled uses: CHF, hirsutism in women, bronchopulmonary dysplasia (BPD), PMS, polycystic ovary syndrome, acne vulgaris, premenstrual syndrome

DOSAGE AND ROUTES

Edema/hypertension
• *Adult:* **PO** 25-200 mg/day in 1-2 divided doses

CHF
• *Adult:* **PO** 12.5-25 mg/day; max 50 mg/day

Edema
• *Child:* **PO** 1.5-3.3 mg/kg/day in single or divided doses

Hypertension
• *Child (unlabeled):* **PO** 1.5-2 mg/kg/day in divided doses

Hypokalemia
• *Adult:* **PO** 25-100 mg/day; if **PO**, potassium supplements must not be used

Primary hyperaldosteronism diagnosis

• *Adult:* **PO** 400 mg/day × 4 days or 4 wk depending on test, then 100-400 mg/day maintenance

Edema (nephrotic syndrome, CHF, hepatic disease)

• *Adult:* **PO** 100 mg/day given as a single dose or in divided doses, titrate to response

• *Child:* **PO** 1.5-3.3 mg/kg/day or 60 mg/m^2/day given daily or in 2-4 divided doses

Renal dose

• *Adult:* **PO** CCr 10-50 ml/min; give dose q12-24hr; CCr <10 ml/min, avoid use

Polycystic ovary syndrome/ hirsutism in women (unlabeled)

• *Adult:* **PO** 50-200 mg in 1-2 divided doses

Acne vulgaris (unlabeled)

• *Adult:* **PO** 50-200 mg/day

Available forms: Tabs 25, 50, 100 mg

SIDE EFFECTS

CNS: *Headache,* confusion, drowsiness, lethargy, ataxia

ELECT: Hyperchloremic metabolic acidosis, **hyperkalemia,** hyponatremia

ENDO: Impotence, gynecomastia, irregular menses, amenorrhea, postmenopausal bleeding, hirsutism, deepening voice, breast pain

GI: *Diarrhea,* cramps, **bleeding,** gastritis, *vomiting,* anorexia, nausea, **hepatocellular toxicity**

HEMA: **Agranulocytosis**

INTEG: *Rash, pruritus,* urticaria

Contraindications: Pregnancy (D), hypersensitivity, anuria, severe renal disease, hyperkalemia

Precautions: Breastfeeding, dehydration, hepatic disease, renal impairment, electrolyte imbalances, metabolic acidosis, gynecomastia

Black Box Warning: Secondary malignancy

PHARMACOKINETICS

Onset 24-48 hr, peak 48-72 hr, metabolized in liver, excreted in urine, crosses placenta

INTERACTIONS

Increase: action of antihypertensives, digoxin, lithium

Increase: hyperchloremic acidosis in cirrhosis—cholestyramine

Increase: hyperkalemia—potassium-sparing diuretics, potassium products, ACE inhibitors, salt substitutes

Decrease: effect of anticoagulants

Decrease: effect of spironolactone—ASA, NSAIDs

Drug/Herb

⚠ Fatal hypokalemia: arginine

Increase: hypokalemia—bearberry, gossypol

Increase: severe photosensitivity—St. John's wort

Increase: effect—cucumber, dandelion, horsetail, licorice, nettle, pumpkin, Queen Anne's lace

Increase: hypotension—khella

Drug/Lab Test

Interference: 17-OHCS, 17-KS, radioimmunoassay, digoxin assay

NURSING CONSIDERATIONS

Assess:

• Electrolytes: Na, Cl, K, BUN, serum creatinine, ABGs, CBC, signs of hyperkalemia

• Weight, I&O daily to determine fluid loss; effect of product may be decreased if used daily; ECG periodically (long-term therapy)

• Signs of metabolic acidosis: drowsiness, restlessness

• Rashes, temp daily

• Confusion, especially in geriatric patients; take safety precautions if needed

• Hydration: skin turgor, thirst, dry mucous membranes

Administer:

• In AM to avoid interference with sleep

• With food; if nausea occurs, absorption may be decreased slightly

S

Evaluate:
• Therapeutic response: improvement in edema of feet, legs, sacral area daily if medication is being used in CHF

Teach patient/family:
• To avoid foods with high potassium content: oranges, bananas, salt substitutes, dried apricots, dates; avoid potassium salt substitutes
• That drowsiness, ataxia, mental confusion may occur; observe caution in driving
• To notify prescriber of cramps, diarrhea, lethargy, thirst, headache, skin rash, menstrual abnormalities, deepening voice, breast enlargement

Treatment of overdose: Lavage if taken orally; monitor electrolytes, administer IV fluids, monitor hydration, renal, CV status

stavudine (℞)

(sta'vyoo-deen)
d4t, Zerit
Func. class.: Antiretroviral
Chem. class.: Nucleoside reverse transcriptase inihibitor

Action: Prevents replication of HIV by the inhibition of the enzyme reverse transcriptase, causes DNA chain termination
Uses: Treatment of HIV-1 in combination with other antiretrovirals

DOSAGE AND ROUTES

• *Adult >60 kg:* **PO** 40 mg q12hr
• *Adult <60 kg:* **PO** 30 mg q12hr
• *Child <30 kg:* **PO** 1 mg/kg q12hr
• *Child ≥30 kg ≤60 kg:* **PO** 30 mg q12hr
• *Child >60 kg:* **PO** 40 mg q12hr

Renal dose
• *Adult: >60 kg:* **PO** CCr 26-50 ml/min 20 mg q12hr; CCr 10-25 ml/min 20 mg q24hr
• *Adult: <60 kg:* **PO** CCr 26-50 ml/min 15 mg q12hr; CCr 10-25 ml/min 15 mg q24hr

Available forms: Caps 15, 20, 30, 40 mg; powder for oral sol 1 mg/ml

SIDE EFFECTS

CNS: Peripheral neuropathy, insomnia, anxiety, depression, dizziness, confusion, *headache,* chills/fever, malaise, neuropathy
CV: Chest pain, vasodilation, hypertension
EENT: Conjunctivitis, abnormal vision
GI: **Hepatotoxicity,** *diarrhea, nausea, vomiting,* anorexia, dyspepsia, constipation, stomatitis, **pancreatitis**
HEMA: **Bone marrow suppression**
INTEG: Rash, sweating, pruritus, benign neoplasms
MISC: **Lactic acidosis,** asthenia, lipodystrophy
MS: Myalgia, arthralgia
RESP: Dyspnea, pneumonia, asthma

Contraindications: Hypersensitivity to this product or zidovudine, didanosine, zalcitabine; severe peripheral neuropathy

Black Box Warning: Lactic acidosis

Precautions: Breastfeeding, advanced HIV infection, bone marrow suppression, renal disease, peripheral neuropathy, osteoporosis, obesity

Black Box Warning: Pregnancy (C), hepatic disease, pancreatitis

PHARMACOKINETICS

Excreted in urine, breast milk; peak 1 hr; half-life: elimination 1-1.6 hr, intracellular 3-3.5 hr

INTERACTIONS

Increase: myelosuppression—other myelosuppressants
Increase: peripheral neuropathy—lithium, dapsone, chloramphenicol didanosine, ethambutol, hydrALAZINE, phenytoin, vinCRIStine, zalcitabine
Increase: stavudine levels—probenecid
Decrease: stavudine effect—methadone

NURSING CONSIDERATIONS

Assess:
⚠ For lactic acidosis and severe hepatomegaly with steatosis, death may result

• Blood studies: WBC, differential, RBC, Hct, Hgb, platelets, serum amylase, lipase
• Renal tests: urinalysis, protein, blood, serum creatinine
• C&S before product therapy; product may be given as soon as culture is taken
• Bowel pattern before, during treatment
• Weakness, tremors, confusion, dizziness; product may have to be decreased or discontinued
• Viral load and CD4 counts, plasma HIV RNA, baseline and throughout treatment
• For peripheral neuropathy: tingling, pain in extremities; discontinue product
⚠ For pancreatitis: severe upper abdominal pain, nausea, vomiting throughout treatment, discontinue product

Administer:

• With or without meals; absorption does not appear to be lowered when taken with food
• Every 12 hr around the clock
• Shake suspension well before using

Evaluate:

• Therapeutic response: decreased symptoms of HIV

Teach patient/family:

• The signs of peripheral neuropathy: burning, weakness, pain, prickling feeling in the extremities
• That product should not be given with antineoplastics
• That product is not a cure for AIDS, but will control symptoms
• To call prescriber if sore throat, swollen lymph nodes, malaise, fever occur; other products may be needed to prevent other infections
• That even with this product, patient may pass AIDS virus to others
• That follow-up visits are necessary; serious toxicity may occur; blood counts must be done q2wk
• That serious product interactions may occur if other medications are ingested; see prescriber before taking chloramphenicol, dapsone, cisplatin, didanosine, ethambutol, lithium, antifungals, antineoplastics
• That product may cause fainting or dizziness

⚠ High Alert

streptokinase (℞)

(strep-toe-kye′nase)
Streptase
Func. class.: Thrombolytic enzyme
Chem. class.: β-Hemolytic streptococcus filtrate (purified)

Action: Activates conversion of plasminogen to plasmin (fibrinolysin): plasmin breaks down clots (fibrin), fibrinogen, factors V, VII; occlusion of venous access lines

Uses: Deep vein thrombosis, PE, arterial thrombosis, arterial embolism, lysis of coronary artery thrombi after acute MI, acute evolving transmural MI

Unlabeled uses: Arteriovenous cannula occlusion

DOSAGE AND ROUTES

Lysis of coronary artery thrombi

• *Adult:* **IC** 20,000 international units, then 2000 international units/min over 1 hr as **IV INF**

Thrombosis/embolism/deep vein thrombosis/pulmonary embolism

• *Adult:* **IV INF** 250,000 international units over ½ hr, then 100,000 international units/hr for 72 hr for deep vein thrombosis; 100,000 international units/hr over 24-72 hr for PE; 100,000 international units/hr × 24-72 hr for arterial thrombosis or embolism

Acute evolving transmural MI

• *Adult:* **IV INF** 1,500,000 international units diluted to a volume of 45 ml; give within 1 hr via inf pump; intracoronary **INF** 20,000 international units by **BOL,** then 2000 international units/min × 1 hr, total dose 140,000 international units

Arteriovenous cannula occlusion (unlabeled)

• *Adult:* **IV INF** 10,000 international units/3 ml sol into occluded limb of cannula; clamp for 1 hr distally; aspirate con-

S

tents; flush with NaCl sol and reconnect (serious reactions have been reported)
Available forms: Powder for inj, lyophilized, 250,000, 750,000, 1,500,000 international units/vial

SIDE EFFECTS

CNS: Headache, fever, **Guillain-Barré syndrome**
CV: Dysrhythmias, hypotension, noncardiogenic pulmonary edema, **PE**
EENT: Periorbital edema
GI: Nausea
HEMA: Decreased Hct, **bleeding,** anemia
INTEG: Rash, urticaria, phlebitis at IV inf site, itching, flushing
MS: Low back pain, arthralgia, myalgia
RESP: Altered respirations, SOB, **bronchospasm,** pulmonary bleeding
SYST: **GI, GU, intracranial, retroperitoneal bleeding, surface bleeding, anaphylaxis**
Contraindications: Breastfeeding, children, hypersensitivity, active internal bleeding, recent CVA, intracranial or intrapleural surgery, intraspinal surgery, CNS neoplasms, uncontrolled severe hypertension
Precautions: Pregnancy (C), arterial emboli from left side of heart, ulcerative colitis, enteritis, severe renal disease, hepatic disease, hypocoagulation, COPD, subacute bacterial endocarditis, rheumatic valvular disease, cerebral embolism/thrombosis/hemorrhage, recent intraarterial diagnostic procedure or surgery (10 days), recent major surgery

PHARMACOKINETICS

IV: Onset immediate; duration <12 hr; half-life 20-80 min; excreted in bile, urine; fibrolytic effect <12 hr, anticoagulant effect 12-24 hr

INTERACTIONS

• Bleeding potential: aspirin, indomethacin, phenylbutazone, anticoagulants, other NSAIDs, abciximab, eptifibatide, tirofiban, clopidogrel, ticlopidine, some cephalosporins, plicamycin, valproic acid, dipyridamole, GP IIb, IIIa inhibitors

Drug/Lab Test
Increase: PT, aPTT, TT
Decrease: plasminogen, fibrinogen

NURSING CONSIDERATIONS

Assess:

• Allergy: fever, rash, itching, chills; mild reaction may be treated with antihistamines

⚠ For bleeding during 1st hr of treatment; hematuria, hematemesis, bleeding from mucous membranes, epistaxis, ecchymosis; may require tranfusion (rare), continue to assess for bleeding for 24 hr

• Blood studies (Hct, platelets, PTT, PT, TT, aPTT) before starting therapy; PT or aPTT must be less than 2× control before starting therapy; PTT or PT q3-4hr during treatment

⚠ For hypersensitive reactions: fever, rash, dyspnea, facial swelling; product should be discontinued; for streptokinase reactions previously; notify prescriber immediately, stop product, keep resuscitative equipment nearby

• VS, B/P, pulse, respirations, neurologic signs, temp at least q4hr; temp >104° F (40° C) indicates internal bleeding; systolic pressure increase >25 mm Hg should be reported to prescriber; assess neurologic status, neurologic change may indicate intracranial bleeding

⚠ For neurologic changes that may indicate intracranial bleeding

⚠ Retroperitoneal bleeding: back pain, leg weakness, diminished pulses

• For Guillain-Barré syndrome that may occur after treatment with this product

• ECG continuously, cardiac enzymes, radionuclide myocardial scanning/coronary angiography

• For respiratory depression

Administer:

IV route

• As soon as thrombi identified; not useful for thrombi over 1 wk old

• Cryoprecipitate or fresh frozen plasma if bleeding occurs

• Loading dose at beginning of therapy; may require increased loading doses
• Heparin after fibrinogen level >100 mg/dl; heparin inf to increase PTT to 1.5-2 × baseline for 3-7 days; IV heparin with loading dose is recommended after discontinuing streptokinase to prevent redevelopment of thrombi
• After reconstituting with 5 ml NS or D_5W; do not shake; further dilute to total volume of 45 ml; may be diluted to 500 ml in 45 ml increments; may dilute vial in 15 ml NS, further dilute 750,000 international units/50 ml NS or D_5W; further dilute 1,500,000 international units dose/100 ml or more
• About 10% patients have high streptococcal antibody titers requiring increased loading doses
• IV therapy using 0.8-µm filter

Y-site compatibilities: DOBUTamine, DOPamine, heparin, lidocaine, nitroglycerin, morphine

Perform/provide:
• Storage of reconstituted sol in refrigerator; discard after 24 hr
• Bed rest during entire course of treatment
• Avoid venous or arterial puncture, inj, rectal temp; any invasive treatment
• Treatment of fever with acetaminophen or aspirin
• Pressure for 30 sec to minor bleeding sites; inform prescriber if this does not attain hemostasis; apply pressure dressing

Evaluate:
• Therapeutic response: resolution of thrombosis, embolism

Teach patient/family:
• Reason for medication and expected results

streptomycin (℞)

(strep-toe-mye′sin)
Func. class.: Antiinfective/antitubercular
Chem. class.: Aminoglycoside

Action: Interferes with protein synthesis in bacterial cell by binding to ribosomal 30 S, causing inaccurate peptide sequence to form in protein chain, causing bacterial death

Uses: Sensitive strains of *Mycobacterium tuberculosis,* nontuberculous infections caused by sensitive strains of *Yersinia pestis, Brucella, Haemophilus influenzae, Klebsiella pneumoniae, Escherichia coli, Enterobacter aerogenes, Streptococcus viridans, Francisella tularensis, Proteus*

DOSAGE AND ROUTES

Tuberculosis (HIV negative)
• *Adult:* **IM** 15 mg/kg/day (1 g) × 2-3 mo, then 1 g 2-3×/week with other antitubercular products
• *Child:* **IM** 20-40 mg/kg/day max 1 g/day

Streptococcal endocarditis
• *Adult:* **IM** 15 mg/kg/day divided q12hr

Enterococcal endocarditis
• *Adult:* **IM** 1 g q12hr × 2 wk, then 500 mg q12hr × 4 wk with penicillin

Available forms: Inj 500 mg ✤, 1 g/ml

S

SIDE EFFECTS

CNS: Confusion, depression, numbness, tremors, **seizures,** muscle twitching, **neurotoxicity,** dizziness, headache
CV: Hypotension, myocarditis, palpitations
EENT: **Ototoxicity,** deafness, visual disturbances, tinnitus
GI: Nausea, vomiting, anorexia, increased ALT, AST, bilirubin; hepatomegaly, **hepatic necrosis,** splenomegaly
GU: **Oliguria, hematuria, renal damage, azotemia, renal failure, nephrotoxicity**

HEMA: **Agranulocytosis, thrombocytopenia, leukopenia, eosinophilia, anemia**

INTEG: *Rash,* burning, urticaria, dermatitis, alopecia

MS: Arthralgia, weakness

Contraindications: Hypersensitivity

Black Box Warning: Pregnancy (D), severe renal disease

Precautions: Breastfeeding, neonates, geriatric patients, mild renal disease, myasthenia gravis, Parkinson's disease, hepatic disease

Black Box Warning: Hearing deficit, neuromuscular disease

PHARMACOKINETICS

IM: Onset rapid, peak 1-2 hr, plasma half-life 2-2½ hr, not metabolized, excreted unchanged in urine, crosses placental barrier, poor penetration into CSF, small amounts enter breast milk

INTERACTIONS

Increase: ototoxicity, neurotoxicity, nephrotoxicity—other aminoglycosides, amphotericin B, polymyxin, vancomycin, ethacrynic acid, furosemide, mannitol, methoxyflurane, cisplatin, cephalosporins, cidofovir

Increase: streptomycin effects—nondepolarizing muscle relaxants, succinylcholine, warfarin, NSAIDs

Drug/Herb

• Do not use acidophilus with antiinfectives; separate by several hours

Increase: toxicity—lysine (large amounts)

NURSING CONSIDERATIONS

Assess:

• Weight before treatment; calculation of dosage is usually based on ideal body weight, but may be calculated on actual body weight

• I&O ratio, urinalysis daily for proteinuria, cells, casts; report sudden change in urine output

• Serum peak 20-30 min after IM inj, trough level drawn 8 hr; acceptable levels—peak 5-25 mcg/ml, trough should not be >5 mcg/ml

• Renal impairment by collecting urine for CCr testing, BUN, serum creatinine; lower dosage should be given in renal impairment (CCr <80 ml/min), monitor electrolytes: K, Na, Cl, Mg

• Deafness by audiometric testing, ringing, roaring in ears, vertigo; assess hearing before, during, after treatment

• Dehydration: high specific gravity, decrease in skin turgor, dry mucous membranes, dark urine

• Overgrowth of infection: fever, malaise, redness, pain, swelling, perineal itching, diarrhea, stomatitis, change in cough, sputum

• C&S before starting treatment to identify infecting organism; use only for susceptible bacteria to prevent development of drug-resistant bacteria

• Vestibular dysfunction: nausea, vomiting, dizziness, headache; product should be discontinued if severe

• Inj sites for redness, swelling, abscesses; use warm compresses at site

Administer:

• IM inj in large muscle mass; rotate inj sites

• Product in evenly spaced doses to maintain blood level

Additive compatibilities: Bleomycin

Syringe compatibilities: Penicillin G sodium

Y-site compatibilities: Esmolol

Perform/provide:

• Adequate fluids of 2-3 L/day unless contraindicated to prevent irritation of tubules

• Supervised ambulation, other safety measures with vestibular dysfunction

Evaluate:

• Therapeutic effect: absence of fever, draining wounds, negative C&S after treatment

Teach patient/family:

- To report headache, dizziness, symptoms of overgrowth of infection, renal impairment
- To report loss of hearing, ringing, roaring in ears, fullness in head

Treatment of overdose: Hemodialysis; monitor serum levels of product

succimer (℞)

(sux'i-mer)

Chemet

Func. class.: Heavy metal chelator antagonist

Chem. class.: Chelating agent

Action: Binds with ions of lead to form a water-soluble complex excreted by kidneys

Uses: Lead poisoning in children with lead levels above 45 mcg/dl; may be beneficial in mercury, arsenic poisoning

Unlabeled uses: Adults with lead levels >45 mcg/dl

DOSAGE AND ROUTES

- *Adult:* **PO** 10-30 mg/kg/day × 5 days
- *Child with lead level >45 mcg/dl:* **PO** 10 mg/kg or 350 mg/m^2 q8hr × 5 days, then 10 mg/kg or 350 mg/m^2 q12hr × 2 wk; another course may be required depending on lead levels; allow 2 wk between courses

Available forms: Caps 100 mg

SIDE EFFECTS

CNS: Drowsiness, dizziness, paresthesia, sensorimotor neuropathy

EENT: Otitis media, watery eyes, film in eyes, plugged ears

GI: Nausea, vomiting, diarrhea, metallic taste, anorexia

GU: **Proteinuria,** decreased urination, voiding difficulties

HEMA: **Increased platelets, intermittent eosinophilia**

INTEG: Rash, urticaria, pruritus

META: Increased AST, ALT, alk phos, cholesterol

RESP: Sore throat, rhinorrhea, nasal congestion, cough

SYST: Back, stomach, head, rib, flank pain; abdominal cramps, chills, fever, flulike symptoms, head cold, headache

Contraindications: Hypersensitivity

Precautions: Pregnancy (C), breastfeeding, children <1 yr, renal/hepatic disease

PHARMACOKINETICS

Peak 1-2 hr, 49% excreted (39% in feces, 25% urine, 1% as CO_2 from lungs), terminal half-life 48 hr

INTERACTIONS

- Not recommended concurrently with other chelating agents

NURSING CONSIDERATIONS

Assess:

- Renal, hepatic studies: ALT, AST, alk phos, BUN, creatinine, serum lead level
- I&O
- For lead sources in home, school
- Allergic reactions: rash, pruritus, urticaria; product should be discontinued if antihistamines fail to help

Administer:

- To children who cannot swallow capsule by separating the capsule and sprinkling content on food or in a spoon followed by a drink; administer immediately after preparation

Perform/provide:

- Adequate fluids; check hydration status daily

Evaluate:

- Therapeutic response: decrease in serum lead level

Teach patient/family:

- That therapeutic effect may take 1-3 mo
- To report urticaria, rash
- To increase fluid intake

S

⚠ High Alert

succinylcholine (℞)
(suk-sin-ill-koe'leen)
Anectine, Anectine Flo-Pack, Quelicin, succinylcholine chloride, Sucostrin, Suxamethonium

Func. class.: Neuromuscular blocker (depolarizing–ultra short)

Action: Inhibits transmission of nerve impulses by binding with cholinergic receptor sites, antagonizing action of acetylcholine; causes release of histamine

Uses: Facilitation of endotracheal intubation, skeletal muscle relaxation during orthopedic manipulations

DOSAGE AND ROUTES

• *Adult:* **IV** 0.3-1.1 mg/kg, max 150 mg, maintenance 0.04-0.07 mg/kg q5-10min as needed; **CONT IV INF** dilute to concentration of 1-2 mg/ml in D_5W or NS 10-100 mcg/kg/min

• *Child:* **IV** Initially 1-2 mg/kg; **CONT IV INF** not recommended

Available forms: Inj 20, 50, 100 mg/ml; powder for inj 100, 500 mg/vial, 1 g/vial

SIDE EFFECTS

CV: Bradycardia, tachycardia; increased, decreased B/P; **sinus arrest, dysrhythmias,** edema

EENT: Increased secretions, increased intraocular pressure

HEMA: **Myoglobulinemia**

INTEG: Rash, flushing, pruritus, urticaria

MS: Weakness, muscle pain, fasciculations, prolonged relaxation, myalgia, **rhabdomyolysis**

RESP: **Prolonged apnea, bronchospasm, cyanosis, respiratory depression,** wheezing, dyspnea

SYST: **Anaphylaxis, angioedema**

Contraindications: Hypersensitivity, malignant hyperthermia, trauma

Precautions: Pregnancy (C), breastfeeding, geriatric or debilitated patients, cardiac disease, severe burns, fractures—fasciculations may increase damage—electrolyte imbalances, dehydration, neuromuscular/respiratory/cardiac/renal/hepatic disease, collagen diseases, glaucoma, eye surgery

Black Box Warning: Children <2 yr, hyperkalemia, myopathy, rhabdomyolysis

PHARMACOKINETICS

Hydrolyzed in blood, excreted in urine (active/inactive metabolites)

IM: Onset 2-3 min, duration 10-30 min

IV: Onset 1 min, peak 2-3 min, duration 6-10 min

INTERACTIONS

• Dysrhythmias: theophylline

Increase: neuromuscular blockade—aminoglycosides, β-blockers, cardiac glycosides, clindamycin, lincomycin, procainamide, quinidine, local anesthetics, polymyxin antibiotics, lithium, opioids, thiazides, enflurane, isoflurane, magnesium salts, oxytocin

Drug/Herb

• Blocks succinylcholine: melatonin

NURSING CONSIDERATIONS

Assess:

• For electrolyte imbalances (K, Mg); may lead to increased action of this product

• VS (B/P, pulse, respirations, airway) until fully recovered; rate, depth, pattern of respirations, strength of hand grip

• I&O ratio; check for urinary retention, frequency, hesitancy

• Recovery: decreased paralysis of face, diaphragm, leg, arm, rest of body

• Allergic reactions: rash, fever, respiratory distress, pruritus; product should be discontinued

Administer:

• Deep IM inj, preferably high in deltoid muscle

IV route

• Using nerve stimulator by anesthesiologist to determine neuromuscular blockade

• Anticholinesterase to reverse neuromuscular blockade
• IV inf: dilute 1-2 mg/ml in D_5, isotonic saline sol; give 0.5-10 mg/min; titrate to response; may be given directly over 1 min

Additive compatibilities: Amikacin, cephapirin, isoproterenol, meperidine, methyldopate, morphine, norepinephrine, scopolamine

Syringe compatibilities: Heparin

Y-site compatibilities: Etomidate, heparin, potassium chloride, propofol, vit B/C

Perform/provide:
• Storage in refrigerator, powder at room temperature; close tightly
• Reassurance if communication is difficult during recovery from neuromuscular blockade; postoperative stiffness is normal, soon subsides

Evaluate:
• Therapeutic response: paralysis of jaw, eyelid, head, neck, rest of body

Treatment of overdose: Edrophonium or neostigmine, atropine, monitor VS; may require mechanical ventilation

sucralfate (℞)
(soo-kral′fate)
Carafate, Sulcrate ♣
Func. class.: Protectant, antiulcer
Chem. class.: Aluminum hydroxide, sulfated sucrose

Do not confuse:
Carafate/Cafergot

Action: Forms a complex that adheres to ulcer site, adsorbs pepsin

Uses: Duodenal ulcer, oral mucositis, stomatitis after radiation of head and neck

Unlabeled uses: Gastric/aphthous ulcers, gastroesophageal reflux, NSAID-induced ulcer prophylaxis, proctitis, stomatitis, stress gastritis prophylaxis, *C. difficle*

DOSAGE AND ROUTES

Duodenal ulcers
• *Adult:* **PO** 1 g qid 1 hr before meals, at bedtime
• *Child:* **PO** 40-80 mg/kg/day divided

Aphthous ulcer/stomatitis (unlabeled)
• *Adult:* **PO** 5-10 ml (500 mg-1 g) swished in mouth for several min; spit or swallow qid

Gastric ulcer/NSAID-induced ulcer prophylaxis/esophagitis/GERD (unlabeled)
• *Adult:* **PO** 1 g qid, 1 hr before meals and at bedtime

Available forms: Tabs 1 g; oral susp 1 g/10 ml

SIDE EFFECTS

CNS: Drowsiness, dizziness
GI: *Dry mouth, constipation,* nausea, gastric pain, vomiting
INTEG: Urticaria, rash, pruritus

Contraindications: Hypersensitivity

Precautions: Pregnancy (B), breastfeeding, children, renal failure

PHARMACOKINETICS

PO: Duration up to 6 hr

INTERACTIONS

Decrease: action of tetracyclines, phenytoin, fat-soluble vitamins, cimetidine, digoxin, ketoconazole, ranitidine, theophylline

Decrease: absorption of fluoroquinolones

Decrease: absorption of sucralfate—antacids

NURSING CONSIDERATIONS

Assess:
• Gastric pH (>5 should be maintained); blood in stools

Administer:

PO route
• Do not crush or chew tabs; tabs may be broken or dissolved in water
• Do not take antacids 30 min before or after sucralfate
• On an empty stomach, 1 hr before meals or other medications and at bedtime

Perform/provide:
• Storage at room temperature

S

Evaluate:
• Therapeutic response: absence of pain, GI complaints

Teach patient/family:
• To take on empty stomach
• To take full course of therapy, not to use over 8 wk, to avoid smoking
• To avoid antacids within ½ hr of product

*sulfADIAZINE (℞)

(sul-fa-dye′a-zeen)
sulfADIAZINE
Func. class.: Antiinfective
Chem. class.: Sulfonamide, intermediate acting

Do not confuse:
sulfADIAZINE/sulfiSOXAZOLE
Action: Inhibits folic acid synthesis
Uses: UTIs, rheumatic fever prophylaxis, with pyrimethamine for *Toxoplasma gondii* encephalitis, chancroid, inclusion conjunctivitis, malaria, meningitis, *Haemophilus influenzae,* meningococeal meningitis, nocardiosis, acute otitis media, trachoma, chloroquine-resistant malaria

DOSAGE AND ROUTES

Meningococcal carriers (asymptomatic)
• *Adult:* **PO** 1 g q12hr × 2 days
• *Child 1-12 yr:* **PO** 500 mg q12hr × 2 days
• *Child 2-12 mo:* **PO** 500 mg/day × 2 days

Rheumatic fever prophylaxis
• *Adult and child >30 kg:* **PO** 1 g/day
• *Child <30 kg:* **PO** 500 mg/day

Available forms: Tabs 500 mg, 7.7 g

SIDE EFFECTS

CNS: Headache, insomnia, hallucinations, depression, vertigo, fatigue, anxiety, **seizures,** product fever, chills, drowsiness
CV: **Allergic myocarditis**
GI: Nausea, vomiting, abdominal pain, stomatitis, **hepatitis,** glossitis, pancreatitis, diarrhea, **enterocolitis,** anorexia
GU: **Renal failure, toxic nephrosis,** increased BUN, creatinine, crystalluria, hematuria, proteinuria
HEMA: **Leukopenia, thrombocytopenia, agranulocytosis, hemolytic anemia, aplastic anemia**
INTEG: Rash, dermatitis, urticaria, **Stevens-Johnson syndrome,** erythema, *photosensitivity,* alopecia
SYST: **Anaphylaxis, serum sickness-like symptoms**

Contraindications: Breastfeeding, infants <2 mo (except congenital toxoplasmosis), hypersensitivity to sulfonamides, sulfonylureas, thiazide and loop diuretics, salicylates, sunscreens with PABA, pregnancy at term, porphyria
Precautions: Pregnancy (C), impaired hepatic function, severe allergy, bronchial asthma, renal dysfunction, G6PD deficiency, UV exposure

PHARMACOKINETICS

Rapidly absorbed; onset ½ hr; peak 3-6 hr; 30%-50% bound to plasma proteins; half-life 8-10 hr; excreted in urine, breast milk; crosses placenta; metabolized in liver

INTERACTIONS

Increase: effects of vorconizole, phenytoin
Increase: hypoglycemic response—sulfonylurea agents
Increase: anticoagulant effects—warfarin
Increase: effects of barbiturates, antidiabetics, uricosurics
Increase: free-product concentrations—indomethacin, probenecid, salicylates
Increase: thrombocytopenia—thiazide diuretics
Increase: nephrotoxicity—cycloSPORINE
Decrease: renal excretion of methotrexate, risk of bone marrow suppression
Decrease: hepatic clearance of phenytoin

Drug/Herb
• Do not use acidophilus with antiinfectives; separate by several hours

Drug/Lab Test

False positive: urinary glucose test (Benedict's method, Chemstrip uG)

NURSING CONSIDERATIONS

Assess:

- I&O ratio; note color, character, pH of urine if product administered for UTIs; output should be 800 ml less than intake; if urine is highly acidic, alkalization may be needed
- Renal studies: BUN, creatinine, urinalysis (long-term therapy)
- Blood dyscrasias: skin rash, fever, sore throat, bruising, bleeding, fatigue, joint pain, monitor CBC before and periodically
- Allergic reaction: rash, dermatitis, urticaria, pruritus, dyspnea, bronchospasm

Administer:

- On an empty stomach
- With full glass of H_2O to maintain adequate hydration; increase fluids to 2 L/day to decrease crystallization in kidneys
- Medication after C&S; repeat C&S after full course of medication

Perform/provide:

- Storage in tight, light-resistant container at room temperature

Evaluate:

- Therapeutic response: absence of pain, fever, C&S negative

Teach patient/family:

- To take each oral dose with full glass of water to prevent crystalluria
- To complete full course of treatment to prevent superinfection
- To avoid sunlight or use sunscreen to prevent burns
- To avoid OTC medication (aspirin, vit C) unless directed by prescriber
- To notify prescriber of skin rash, sore throat, fever, mouth sores, unusual bruising, bleeding; CNS effects: anxiety, depression, seizures

sulfamethoxazole (℞)

(sul-fa-meth-ox'a-zole)

Apo-Sulfamethoxazole ✱, Gantanol, Urobak

Func. class.: Antiinfective

Chem. class.: Sulfonamide, intermediate acting

Action: Inhibits folic acid synthesis

Uses: UTIs, chancroid, inclusion conjunctivitis, malaria, meningococcal meningitis, nocardiosis, acute otitis media, toxoplasmosis, trachoma

DOSAGE AND ROUTES

- *Adult:* **PO** 2 g, then 1 g bid or tid for 7-10 days
- *Child >2 mo:* **PO** 50-60 mg/kg × 1 dose then 25-30 mg/kg bid; max 2 g/day

Renal dose

- *Adult:* **PO** CCr <10-30 ml/min give 50% of dose; CCr <10 ml/min give 25% of dose or extend interval

Available forms: Tabs 500 mg; oral susp 500 mg/5 ml

SIDE EFFECTS

CNS: Headache, insomnia, hallucinations, depression, vertigo, fatigue, anxiety, **seizures, product fever,** chills, drowsiness

CV: **Allergic myocarditis**

EENT: Tinnitus

GI: Nausea, vomiting, abdominal pain, stomatitis, **hepatitis,** glossitis, pancreatitis, diarrhea, **enterocolitis,** anorexia

GU: **Renal failure, toxic nephrosis,** increased BUN, creatinine, crystalluria, hematuria, proteinuria

HEMA: **Leukopenia, thrombocytopenia, agranulocytosis, hemolytic anemia, aplastic anemia**

INTEG: Rash, dermatitis, urticaria, **Stevens-Johnson syndrome,** erythema, photosensitivity, alopecia

SYST: **Anaphylaxis**

Contraindications: Pregnancy at term, breastfeeding, infants <2 mo (except congenital toxoplasmosis), hypersensitivity to

S

sulfonamides, sulfonylureas, thiazide and loop diuretics, salicylates, sunscreens with PABA, porphyria, G6PD deficiency
Precautions: Pregnancy (C), geriatric patients, impaired renal/hepatic function, severe allergy, bronchial asthma, UV exposure

PHARMACOKINETICS

PO: Poorly absorbed; peak 3-4 hr; 50%-70% bound to plasma proteins; half-life 7-12 hr; excreted in urine (unchanged 90%), breast milk; crosses placenta

INTERACTIONS

Increase: effects of barbiturates, uricosurics
Increase: product-free concentrations—indomethacin, probenecid, salicylates
Increase: thrombocytopenia—thiazide diuretics
Increase: nephrotoxicity—cycloSPORINE
Increase: hypoglycemic response—sulfonylurea agents
Increase: anticoagulant effects—warfarin
Increase: crystalluria—methenamine
Increase: effects of voriconazole, bosentan, ramelteon
Decrease: renal excretion of methotrexate
Decrease: hepatic clearance of phenytoin
Drug/Herb
• Do not use acidophilus with antiinfectives; separate by several hours
Drug/Lab Test
False positive: urinary glucose test (Benedict's method)

NURSING CONSIDERATIONS

Assess:
• I&O ratio; note color, character, pH of urine if product administered for UTIs; output should be 800 ml less than intake; if urine is highly acidic, alkalization may be needed
• Renal studies: BUN, creatinine, urinalysis (long-term therapy)
• Blood dyscrasias: skin rash, fever, sore throat, bruising, bleeding, fatigue, joint pain, monitor CBC before and periodically
⚠ Allergic reaction: rash, dermatitis, urticaria, pruritus, dyspnea, bronchospasm
Administer:
PO route
• On empty stomach
• With full glass of H_2O to maintain adequate hydration; increase fluids to 2 L/day to decrease crystallization in kidneys
• Medication after C&S; repeat C&S after full course of medication
Perform/provide:
• Storage in tight, light-resistant container at room temperature
Evaluate:
• Therapeutic response: absence of pain, fever, C&S negative
Teach patient/family:
• To take each oral dose with full glass of H_2O to prevent crystalluria
• To complete full course of treatment to prevent superinfection
• To avoid sunlight or use sunscreen to prevent burns
• To avoid OTC medication (aspirin, vit C) unless directed by prescriber
⚠ To notify prescriber of skin rash, sore throat, fever, mouth sores, unusual bruising, bleeding, crystals in urine

sulfasalazine (℞)

(sul-fa-sal′a-zeen)
Azulfidine, Azulfidine EN-tabs, PMS-Sulfasalazine ✱, S.A.S. ✱, Salazopyrin ✱, sulfasalazine
Func. class.: GI antiinflammatory, antirheumatic (DMARD)
Chem. class.: Sulfonamide

Do not confuse:
sulfasalazine/sulfiSOXAZOLE
Action: Prodrug to deliver sulfapyridine and 5-aminosalicylic acid to colon; antiinflammatory in connective tissue also
Uses: Ulcerative colitis; RA; juvenile RA (Azulfidine EN-tabs)
Unlabeled uses: Crohn's disease

DOSAGE AND ROUTES

Bowel disease

- *Adult:* **PO** 3-4 g/day in divided doses; maintenance 2 g/day in divided doses q6hr
- *Child ≥6 yr:* **PO** 40-60 mg/kg/day in 4-6 divided doses, then 30 mg/kg/day in 4 doses, max 2 g/day

Rheumatoid arthritis

- *Adult:* **PO** 0.5-1 g/day, then increase daily dose by 500 mg q wk to 2 g/day in 2-3 divided doses use

Juvenile rheumatoid arthritis

- *Child ≥6 yr:* **PO** 30-50 mg/kg/24 hr, divided into 2 doses

Renal dose

- *Adult:* **PO** CCr 10-30 ml/min give bid; CCr <10 ml/min give daily

Crohn's disease (unlabeled)

- *Adult:* **PO** 1 g/15 kg, max 5 g/day

Available forms: Tabs 500 mg; oral susp 250 mg/5 ml; del rel tabs 500 mg

SIDE EFFECTS

CNS: Headache, confusion, insomnia, hallucinations, depression, vertigo, fatigue, anxiety, **seizures,** product fever, chills

CV: **Allergic myocarditis**

GI: Nausea, vomiting, abdominal pain, stomatitis, **hepatitis,** glossitis, pancreatitis, diarrhea

GU: **Renal failure, toxic nephrosis,** increased BUN, creatinine, crystalluria

HEMA: **Leukopenia, neutropenia, thrombocytopenia, agranulocytosis, hemolytic anemia**

INTEG: Rash, dermatitis, urticaria, **Stevens-Johnson syndrome,** erythema, photosensitivity

SYST: **Anaphylaxis**

Contraindications: Pregnancy at term, children <2 yr, hypersensitivity to sulfonamides or salicylates, intestinal, urinary obstruction, porphyria

Precautions: Pregnancy (B), breastfeeding, impaired renal/hepatic function, severe allergy, bronchial asthma, megaloblastic anemia

PHARMACOKINETICS

PO: Partially absorbed; peak 1½-6 hr; duration 6-12 hr; half-life 6 hr; excreted in urine as sulfasalazine (15%), sulfapyridine (60%), 5-aminosalicylic acid and metabolites (20%-33%), in breast milk; crosses placenta

INTERACTIONS

Increase: leukopenia risk—thiopurines (azathioprine, mercaptopurine)

Increase: hypoglycemic response—oral hypoglycemics

Increase: anticoagulant effects—oral anticoagulants

Decrease: effect of cycloSPORINE, digoxin, folic acid

Decrease: renal excretion of methotrexate

Drug/Food

Decrease: iron/folic acid absorption

Drug/Lab Test

False positive: urinary glucose test

NURSING CONSIDERATIONS

Assess:

- Renal studies: BUN, creatinine, urinalysis (long-term therapy)
- ⚠ Blood dyscrasias: skin rash, fever, sore throat, bruising, bleeding, fatigue, joint pain; monitor CBC before and q3mo
- ⚠ Allergic reaction: rash, dermatitis, urticaria, pruritus, dyspnea, bronchospasm

Administer:

- Do not break, crush, or chew delayed rel tabs
- With full glass of H_2O to maintain adequate hydration; increase fluids to 2 L/day to decrease crystallization in kidneys
- Total daily dose in evenly spaced doses and after meals to help minimize GI intolerance

Perform/provide:

- Storage in tight, light-resistant container at room temperature

Evaluate:

- Therapeutic response: absence of fever, mucus in stools, pain in joints

S

Teach patient/family:
• To take each oral dose with full glass of H_2O to prevent crystalluria
• That contact lens, urine/skin may be yellow-orange
• To avoid sunlight or use sunscreen to prevent burns
• To notify prescriber of skin rash, sore throat, fever, mouth sores, unusual bruising, bleeding

sulfinpyrazone (℞)

(sul-fin-peer′a-zone)
Anturan 🍁, Anturane, sulfinpyrazone
Func. class.: Uricosuric
Chem. class.: Pyrazolone

Action: Inhibits tubular reabsorption of urates, with increased excretion of uric acid; inhibits prostaglandin synthesis, which decreases platelet aggregation
Uses: Gout, gouty arthritis

DOSAGE AND ROUTES

Gout/gouty arthritis
• *Adult:* **PO** 100-200 mg bid × 1 wk, then 200-400 mg bid, max 800 mg/day
• *Child:* **PO** 10 mg/kg/day in 3-4 divided doses

Renal dose
• CCr <50 ml/min; avoid use

Available forms: Tabs 100 mg; caps 200 mg

SIDE EFFECTS

CNS: Dizziness, **seizures, coma**
EENT: Tinnitus
GI: Gastric irritation, nausea, vomiting, anorexia, **hepatic necrosis, GI bleeding**
GU: Renal calculi, hypoglycemia
HEMA: **Agranulocytosis** (rare)
INTEG: Rash, dermatitis, pruritus, fever, photosensitivity
RESP: **Apnea,** irregular respirations

Contraindications: Hypersensitivity to pyrazolone derivatives, salicylates, blood dyscrasias, CCr <50 ml/min, active peptic ulcer, GI inflammation, nephrolithiasis
Precautions: Pregnancy (C), renal disease, NSAIDs hypersensitivity

PHARMACOKINETICS

Peak 1-2 hr, duration 4-6 hr, half-life 4 hr, metabolized by liver, excreted in urine

INTERACTIONS

Increase: toxicity—acetaminophen
Increase: effects of warfarin, TOLBUTamide
Increase: bleeding risk—NSAIDs
Decrease: effects of verapamil, theophylline
Decrease: effects of sulfinpyrazone—salicylates, niacin

Drug/Lab Test
Increase: PSP, aminohippuric acid
False positive: Clinitest

NURSING CONSIDERATIONS

Assess:
• Uric acid levels (3-7 mg/dl); joint mobility, pain, swelling
• Respiratory rate, rhythm, depth; notify prescriber of abnormalities
• Renal function
• Bleeding tendencies, RBC, Hct
• I&O
• Electrolytes, CO_2 before, during treatment
• Urine pH, output, glucose during beginning treatment

Administer:
• With glass of milk
• With food for GI symptoms
• Increased fluids to prevent calculi; alkalinization of urine may be required

Evaluate:
• Therapeutic response: absence of pain, stiffness in joints

Teach patient/family:
• To avoid aspirin, NSAIDs, alcohol, high-purine diet

*sulfiSOXAZOLE (℞)

(sul-fi-sox'a-zole)
Gantrisin, Novo-Soxazole ♣, sulfiSOXAZOLE, Gantrisin Pediatric
Func. class.: Antiinfective
Chem. class.: Sulfonamide, short acting

Do not confuse:
sulfiSOXAZOLE/sulfasalazine/sulfADIAZINE

Action: Inhibits folic acid synthesis

Uses: Urinary tract, systemic infections; chancroid; trachoma; toxoplasmosis; acute otitis media, malaria, *Haemophilus influenzae* meningitis, meningococcal meningitis, nocardiosis, eye infections

DOSAGE AND ROUTES

UTIs, other systemic infections

- *Adult:* **PO** 2-4 g loading dose, then 1-2 g qid × 7-10 days; max 12 g/day
- *Child >2 mo:* **PO** 75 mg/kg or 2 g/m^2 loading dose, then 120-150 mg/kg/day or 4 g/m^2/day in divided doses q6hr, max 6 g/day

Chlamydia trachomatis

- *Adult:* **PO** 500 mg-1 g qid × 3 wk

Renal dose

- *Adult:* **PO** CCr 10-50 ml/min give q8-12hr; CCr <10 ml/min give q12-24hr

Available forms: Tabs 500 mg; *sulfiSOXAZOLE acetyl*: liquid 500 mg/5 ml

SIDE EFFECTS

CNS: Headache, insomnia, hallucinations, depression, vertigo, fatigue, anxiety, **seizures,** product fever, chills, drowsiness

CV: **Allergic myocarditis, tachycardia,** vasculitis

GI: Nausea, vomiting, abdominal pain, stomatitis, **hepatitis,** glossitis, pancreatitis, diarrhea, **enterocolitis,** anorexia, **pseudomembranous colitis**

GU: **Renal failure, toxic nephrosis,** increased BUN, creatinine, crystalluria, hematuria, proteinuria, urinary retention

HEMA: **Leukopenia, thrombocytopenia, agranulocytosis, hemolytic anemia, aplastic anemia**

INTEG: Rash, dermatitis, urticaria, **Stevens-Johnson syndrome,** erythema, photosensitivity, alopecia

SYST: **Anaphylaxis, serum sickness-like symptoms, thyroid dysfunction**

Contraindications: Pregnancy at term, breastfeeding, infants <2 mo (except congenital toxoplasmosis), hypersensitivity to sulfonamides and sulfonylureas, thiazide and loop diuretics, salicylates; sunscreen with PABA, porphyria, G6PD deficiency

Precautions: Pregnancy (C), breastfeeding, geriatric patients, impaired renal/hepatic function, severe allergy, bronchial asthma, UV exposure

PHARMACOKINETICS

PO: Rapidly absorbed, peak 2-4 hr, 85% protein bound, half-life 4-7 hr, excreted in urine, crosses placenta

INTERACTIONS

- Avoid use with PABA

Increase: effects of barbiturates, antidiabetics, uricosurics

Increase: crystalluria risk—methenamine

Increase: free-drug concentrations—indomethacin, probenecid, salicylates

Increase: thrombocytopenia—thiazides

Increase: nephrotoxicity—cycloSPORINE

Increase: hypoglycemic response—sulfonylurea agents

Increase: anticoagulant effect—warfarin

Decrease: renal excretion of methotrexate

Decrease: hepatic clearance of phenytoin

Drug/Herb

- Do not use acidophilus with antiinfectives; separate by several hours

Drug/Lab Test

False positive: urinary glucose test

S

NURSING CONSIDERATIONS

Assess:

- I&O ratio; note color, character, pH of urine if product administered for UTIs; output should be 800 ml less than intake; if urine is highly acidic, alkalization may be needed
- Renal studies: BUN, creatinine, urinalysis (long-term therapy); monitor for crystalluria

⚠ Blood dyscrasias: skin rash, fever, sore throat, bruising, bleeding, fatigue, joint pain, monitor CBC before and periodically

⚠ Allergic reaction: rash, dermatitis, urticaria, pruritus, dyspnea, bronchospasm

Administer:

- On an empty stomach
- With full glass of H_2O to maintain adequate hydration; increase fluids to 2 L/day to decrease crystallization in kidneys
- Medication after C&S; repeat C&S after full course of medication

Perform/provide:

- Storage in tight, light-resistant container at room temperature

Evaluate:

- Therapeutic response: absence of pain, fever, C&S negative

Teach patient/family:

- To take each oral dose with full glass of H_2O to prevent crystalluria
- To complete full course of treatment to prevent superinfection
- To avoid sunlight or use sunscreen to prevent burns; avoid hazardous activities if dizziness occurs
- To avoid OTC medication (aspirin, vit C) unless directed by prescriber
- To notify prescriber of skin rash, sore throat, fever, mouth sores, unusual bruising, bleeding; CNS effects (anxiety, depression, hallucinations, seizures)

sulindac (℞)

(sul-in′dak)

Apo-Sulin ✦, Clinoril, NovoSundac ✦, sulindac

Func. class.: Nonsteroidal antiinflammatory, antirheumatic

Chem. class.: Indene acetic acid derivative

Do not confuse:

Clinoril/Clozaril/Oruvail

Action: Metabolite inhibits COX-1, COX-2 by blocking arachidonate; analgesic, antiinflammatory, antipyretic

Uses: Osteoarthritis; RA, gouty arthritis; ankylosing spondylitis; bursitis, tendinitis

Unlabeled uses: Arthralgia, bone pain, desmoid tumor, headache, juvenile RA

DOSAGE AND ROUTES

Arthritis

- *Adult:* **PO** 150 mg bid, may increase to 200 mg bid, max 400 mg/day
- *Child (unlabeled):* **PO** 2-4 mg/kg/day in divided doses, max 6 mg/kg/day or 200 mg bid whichever is less (safe and effective dose not established)

Bursitis/acute arthritis

- *Adult:* **PO** 200 mg bid × 1-2 wk, then reduce dose

Available forms: Tabs 150, 200 mg

SIDE EFFECTS

CNS: Dizziness, drowsiness, fatigue, tremors, confusion, insomnia, anxiety, depression, headache

CV: Tachycardia, peripheral edema, palpitations, dysrhythmias, **MI, stroke, CHF**

EENT: Tinnitus, hearing loss, blurred vision

GI: Nausea, anorexia, vomiting, diarrhea, jaundice, **cholestatic hepatitis,** constipation, flatulence, cramps, dry mouth, peptic ulcer, **bleeding, ulceration, perforation,** dyspepsia

GU: **Nephrotoxicity: dysuria, hematuria, oliguria, azotemia**

HEMA: **Blood dyscrasias** with prolonged use

INTEG: Purpura, *rash, pruritus,* sweating, photosensitivity
SYST: **Anaphylaxis, Stevens-Johnson syndrome, toxic epidermal necrolysis**

Contraindications: Hypersensitivity, asthma, severe renal/hepatic disease, active ulcers, pregnancy (D) 3rd trimester

Black Box Warning: Perioperative pain in CABG

Precautions: Pregnancy (C) 1st trimester, breastfeeding, children, cardiac disorders, hypersensitivity to other antiinflammatory agents, renal disease

Black Box Warning: GI bleeding, MI, stroke

PHARMACOKINETICS

Peak 2-4 hr; half-life 7.8 hr; metabolized in liver; excreted in urine (metabolites), breast milk; 93% protein binding

INTERACTIONS

- GI side effects: aspirin, corticosteroids, other NSAIDs

Increase: CNS stimulation, seizures—quinolones (norfloxacin, ofloxacin, levofloxacin)
Increase: bleeding risk—anticoagulants, thrombolytics, plicamycin, tirofiban, eptifibatide, clopidogrel, ticlopidine, SSRIs, SNRIs, valproic acid, some cephalosporins
Increase: nephrotoxicity—cycloSPORINE
Increase: toxicity—methotrexate, sulfonamides, sulfonylureas, probenecid, aminoglycosides
Decrease: sulindac effect—diflunisal, antacids
Decrease: effect—antihypertensives

Drug/Herb

Increase: gastric irritation—arginine, gossypol
Increase: NSAIDs effect—bearberry, bilberry
Increase: bleeding risk—bogbean, chondroitin, garlic, ginger, horse chestnut, red clover

NURSING CONSIDERATIONS

Assess:

- ⚠ Cardiac status: CV thrombotic events, MI, stroke; may be fatal
- ⚠ GI status: ulceration, bleeding, perforation; may be fatal
- Pain: frequency, intensity, characteristics, relief after med
- ⚠ Asthma, aspirin hypersensitivity, nasal polyps; increased hypersensitivity; monitor for rash
- Renal, hepatic studies: BUN, creatinine, AST, ALT, Hgb, before treatment, periodically thereafter
- Have B/P checked q mo; product causes sodium retention
- Audiometric, ophthalmic exam before, during, after treatment
- For eye, ear problems: blurred vision, tinnitus may indicate toxicity

Administer:

- With food to decrease GI symptoms; take on empty stomach to facilitate absorption; tablet may be crushed
- With a full glass of water

Perform/provide:

- Storage at room temperature

Evaluate:

- Therapeutic response: decreased pain, stiffness, swelling in joints, ability to move more easily

Teach patient/family:

- To report blurred vision or ringing, roaring in ears (may indicate toxicity)
- To avoid driving, other hazardous activities if dizzy or drowsy
- To report change in urine pattern, weight increase, edema, pain increase in joints, fever, blood in urine (indicates nephrotoxicity)
- That therapeutic effects may take up to 1 mo
- To avoid alcohol and aspirin, NSAIDs
- To take with full glass of water
- To use sunscreen
- To report bruising; black, tarry stools
- To inform all health care providers that this product is used

sumatriptan (℞)

(soo-ma-trip'tan)

Imitrex, Sumavel DosePro

Func. class.: Antimigraine agent

Chem. class.: 5-HT_{1P} receptor agonist, abortive agent, triptan

Do not confuse:

sumatriptan/somatropin

Action: Binds selectively to the vascular 5-HT_{1D} receptor subtype, exerts antimigraine effect; causes vasoconstriction in cranial arteries

Uses: Acute treatment of migraine with or without aura and cluster headache

DOSAGE AND ROUTES

• *Adult:* **SUBCUT** 6 mg or less; may repeat in 1 hr; max 12 mg/24 hr; **PO** 25 mg with fluids, if no relief in 2 hr, give another dose, max 200 mg/day; **NASAL** one dose of 5, 10, or 20 mg in one nostril, may repeat in 2 hr, max 40 mg/24 hr; 1 puff each nostril q2hr

Hepatic dose

• *Adult:* **PO** 25 mg, if no response after 2 hr, give up to 50 mg

Available forms: Inj 12 mg/ml; tabs 25, 50, 100 mg; nasal spray 5 mg/100 mcl-U; dose spray device 20 mg/100 mcl-U

SIDE EFFECTS

CNS: Tingling, hot sensation, burning, feeling of pressure, tightness, numbness, dizziness, sedation, headache, anxiety, fatigue, cold sensation

CV: Flushing, **MI**

EENT: Throat, mouth, nasal discomfort; vision changes

GI: Abdominal discomfort

INTEG: Inj site reaction, sweating

MS: Weakness, neck stiffness, myalgia

RESP: Chest tightness, pressure

Contraindications: Angina pectoris, history of MI, documented silent ischemia, Prinzmetal's angina, ischemic heart disease, IV use, concurrent ergotamine-containing preparations, uncontrolled hypertension, hypersensitivity, basilar or hemiplegic migraine

Precautions: Pregnancy (C), breastfeeding, children <18 yr, geriatric patients, postmenopausal women, men >40 yr, risk factors for CAD, hypercholesterolemia, obesity, diabetes, impaired renal/hepatic function

PHARMACOKINETICS

Onset of pain relief 10 min-2 hr, peak 10-20 min, 10%-20% plasma protein binding, metabolized in the liver (metabolite), excreted in urine/feces, nasal spray half-life 2 hr

INTERACTIONS

• Extended vasospastic effects: ergot, ergot derivatives

Increase: sumatriptan effect—MAOIs, SSRIs

Drug/Herb

• Serotonin syndrome: SAM-e, St. John's wort

Increase: effect—butterbur, feverfew

NURSING CONSIDERATIONS

Assess:

• For migraine: type of pain, aura, alleviating, aggravating factors, sensitivity to light, noise

• B/P; signs/symptoms of coronary vasospasms

• Tingling, hot sensation, burning, feeling of pressure, numbness, flushing, inj site reaction

• For stress level, activity, recreation, coping mechanisms

• Neurologic status: LOC, blurring vision, nausea, vomiting, tingling in extremities preceding headache

• Ingestion of tyramine foods (pickled products, beer, wine, aged cheese), food additives, preservatives, colorings, artificial sweeteners, chocolate, caffeine, which may precipitate these types of headaches

• Renal function, urinary output

Administer:

• Swallow tabs whole; do not break, crush, or chew

• SUBCUT only just below the skin; avoid IM or IV administration; use only for actual migraine attack
• Take tabs with fluids as soon as symptoms appear; may take a second dose >4 hr; max 200 mg/24 hr

Perform/provide:
• Quiet, calm environment with decreased stimulation for noise, bright light, excessive talking

Evaluate:
• Therapeutic response: decrease in frequency, severity of migraine

Teach patient/family:
• To report chest pain, tightness; sudden, severe abdominal pain to prescriber immediately
• To use contraception while taking product
• To use nasal spray: one spray in one nostril, may repeat if headache returns, do not repeat if pain continues after 1st dose
• To have dark, quiet environment
• That product does not reduce number of migraines

sunitinib (℞)

(soo-nit′-in-ib)
Sutent
Func. class.: Antineoplastic—miscellaneous
Chem. class.: Protein-tyrosine kinase inhibitor

Action: Inhibits multiple receptor tyrosine kinases (RTKs), some are responsible for tumor growth

Uses: Gastrointesitnal stromal tumors (GIST) after disease progression or intolerance to imatinib; advanced renal carcinoma

DOSAGE AND ROUTES

• *Adult:* **PO** 50 mg/day × 4 wk, then 2 wk off; may increase or decrease dose by 12.5 mg; if administered with CYP3A4 inducers, give 87.5 mg/day; if given with CYP3A4 inhibitors give 37.5 mg/day

Available forms: Caps 12.5, 25, 50 mg

SIDE EFFECTS

CNS: **CNS hemorrhage**, headache, dizziness, insomnia, **seizures**, fatigue
CV: Hypertension, **left ventricular dysfunction, QT prolongation, cardiotoxicity, torsade de pointes, thrombotic microangiopathy**
ENDO: Hypo/hyperthyroidism
GI: Nausea, **hepatotoxicity, vomiting, dyspepsia,** *anorexia, abdominal pain,* altered taste, *constipation,* stomatitis, mucositis, **pancreatitis**, diarrhea, **GI bleeding/perforation**
GU: **Nephrotic syndrome**
HEMA: **Neutropenia, thrombocytopenia, hemolytic anemia, leukopenia**
INTEG: Rash, skin discoloration, depigmentation of hair or skin, alopecia
MS: Pain, arthralgia, myalgia, **myopathy, rhabdomyolysis**
RESP: Cough, dyspnea, **pulmonary embolism**
SYST: **Bleeding,** electrolyte abnormalities, hand-foot syndrome, **serious infection**

Contraindications: Pregnancy (D), breastfeeding, hypersensitivity

Precautions: Children, geriatric patients, active infections, QT prolongation, torsade de pointes, stroke, heart failure

PHARMACOKINETICS

Protein binding 95%; metabolized by CYP3A4; excreted in feces, small amount in urine; peak plasma levels 6-12 hr; terminal half-life 40-60 hr (sunitnib); active metabolite 80-110 hr

INTERACTIONS

Increase: microangiopathic hemolytic anemia—bevacizumab; avoid concurrent use
Increase: hepatotoxicity—acetaminophen
Increase: sunitinib concentrations—ketoconazole, itraconazole, erythromycin, clarithromycin
Increase: plasma concentrations of simvastatin, calcium channel blockers

Increase: plasma concentration of warfarin; avoid use with warfarin, use low-molecular-weight anticoagulants instead
Decrease: sunitinib concentrations—dexamethasone, phenytoin, carbamazepine, rifampin, phenobarbital
Drug/Herb
Decrease: sunitinib concentration—St. John's wort
Drug/Food
Increase: plasma concentrations—grapefruit juice

NURSING CONSIDERATIONS

Assess:

- ANC and platelets; if ANC $<1 \times 10^9/L$ and/or platelets $<50 \times 10^9/L$, stop until ANC $>1.5 \times 10^9/L$ and platelets $>75 \times 10^9/L$; if ANC $<0.5 \times 10^9/L$ and/or platelets $<10 \times 10^9/L$, reduce dose by 200 mg, if cytopenia continues, reduce dose by another 100 mg; if cytopenia continues for 4 wk, stop product until ANC $\geq 1 \times 10^9/L$
- CV status: hypertension, QT prolongation can occur; monitor left ventricular ejection fraction (LVEF) (MUGA) baseline periodically
- For renal toxicity: if bilirubin $>3 \times$ IULN, withhold sunitinib until bilirubin levels return to $<1.5 \times$ IULN; electrolytes
- For hepatotoxicity: monitor LFTs, before treatment and q mo; if liver transaminases $>5 \times$ IULN, withhold sunitinib until transaminase levels return to $<2.5 \times$ IULN
- For CHF: adrenal insufficiency in those experiencing trauma
- For bleeding: epistaxis rectal, gingival, upper GI, genital and wound bleeding; tumor-related hemorrhage may occur rapidly

Administer:

- With meal and large glass of water to decrease GI symptoms

Perform/provide:

- Nutritious diet with iron, vitamin supplement, low fiber, few dairy products
- Storage at 25° C (77° F)

Evaluate:

- Therapeutic response: decrease in size of tumor

Teach patient/family:

- To report adverse reactions immediately: shortness of breath, bleeding
- Reason for treatment, expected result
- That many adverse reactions may occur: high B/P, bleeding, mouth swelling, taste change, skin discoloration, depigmentation of hair/skin
- Avoid persons with known upper respiratory infections; immunosuppression is common
- Avoid grapefruit juice

suprofen ophthalmic

See Appendix B

tacrolimus (℞)

(tak-roe-li'mus)
Prograf

tacrolimus topical (℞)

Protopic
Func. class.: Immunosuppressant
Chem. class.: Macrolide

Action: Produces immunosuppression by inhibiting T-lymphocytes
Uses: Organ transplants to prevent rejection; topical: atopic dermatitis
Unlabeled uses: Severe recalcitrant psoriasis, contact dermatitis, GVHD prophylaxis/disease, pancreas/heart/kidney/liver/lung/small bowel transplant rejection, uveitis, ulcerative colitis, nephrotic syndrome, lichen sclerosus

DOSAGE AND ROUTES

Kidney transplant rejection prophylaxis

- *Adult:* **IV** 0.03-0.05 mg/kg/day as a **CONT INF**, give no sooner than 6 hr after transplantation

Liver transplant rejection prophylaxis

- *Adult:* **PO** 0.10-0.15 mg/kg/day in 2 divided doses q12hr, give no sooner than 6 hr after transplantation; **IV** 0.03-0.05 mg/kg/day as a **CONT INF**, give no sooner than 6 hr after transplantation

Heart transplant rejection prophylaxis

• *Adult:* **PO** 0.075 mg/kg/day in 2 divided doses q12hr, give no sooner than 6 hr after transplantation; **IV** 0.01 mg/kg/day as a **CONT INF**, give no sooner than 6 hr after transplantation

Atopic dermatitis

• *Adult:* **TOP** use 0.03% or 0.1% ointment, apply bid × 7 days

• *Child ≥ 2-15 yr:* **TOP** 0.03% ointment, apply bid × 7 days

Graft-versus-host disease (unlabeled)

• *Adult and adolescent:* **IV** 0.1 mg/kg/day in 2 divided doses given with other immunosuppressants or **PO** 0.3 mg/kg/day

• *Child:* **CONT IV INF** 0.1 mg/kg/day

Graft-versus-host prophylaxis (unlabeled)

• *Adult:* **CONT IV INF** 0.03 mg/kg/day starting 1-2 days prior to bone marrow transplant; **PO** 0.12 mg/kg/day in 2 divided doses

• *Adolescent and child:* **PO** 0.12 mg/kg/day in 2 divided doses

Heart transplant rejection (unlabeled)

• *Adult:* **IV** 0.05 mg/kg/day or **PO** 0.2-0.3 mg/kg/day in 2 divided doses

Lung transplant rejection (unlabeled)

• *Adult:* **PO** 0.15 mg/kg/day, maintain 12 hr trough whole blood conc 1-1.5 ng/ml

Small bowel transplant rejection (unlabeled)

• *Adult:* **IV** 0.1-0.15 mg/kg/day, then **PO** 0.3 mg/kg/day in divided doses

Contact dermatitis (unlabeled)

• *Adult:* **TOP** 0.1% ointment, apply bid × 8 wk

Available forms: Inj 5 mg/ml; caps 0.5, 1, 5 mg; ointment 0.03%, 0.1%

SIDE EFFECTS

CNS: Tremors, headache, insomnia, paresthesia, chills, fever, **seizures,** posterior reversible encephalopathy syndrome, BK-virus–associated nephropathy

CV: Hypertension, myocardial hypertrophy, **prolonged QT**

EENT: Blurred vision, photophobia

GI: Nausea, vomiting, diarrhea, constipation, **GI bleeding**

GU: UTIs, **albuminuria, hematuria, proteinuria, renal failure**

HEMA: **Anemia, leukocytosis, thrombocytopenia, purpura**

INTEG: Rash, flushing, itching, alopecia

META: Hirsutism, hyperglycemia, hyperuricemia, hypo/hyperkalemia, hypomagnesemia

MS: Back pain, muscle spasms

RESP: **Pleural effusion, atelectasis,** dyspnea, **interstitial lung disease**

SYST: **Anaphylaxis**

Contraindications: Children <2 yr (topical); hypersensitivity to this product or to some kinds of castor oil; long-term use (topical)

Precautions: Pregnancy (C), breastfeeding, severe renal/hepatic disease; diabetes mellitus, hyperkalemia, hyperuricemia, hypertension

Black Box Warning: Children <12, lymphomas, infection, neoplastic disease

PHARMACOKINETICS

PO: Extensively metabolized, half-life 10 hr, 75% protein binding

INTERACTIONS

Increase: toxicity—aminoglycosides, cisplatin, cycloSPORINE

Increase: blood levels—antifungals, calcium channel blockers, cimetidine, danazol, erythromycin, mycophenolate, mofetil

Decrease: blood levels—carbamazepine, phenobarbital, phenytoin, rifamycin

Decrease: effect of vaccines

Drug/Herb

Decrease: immunosuppression—astragalus, echinacea, melatonin

Decrease: effect—ginseng, maitake, mistletoe

T

NURSING CONSIDERATIONS

Assess:

• Blood studies: Hgb, WBC, platelets during treatment q mo; if leukocytes <3000/mm^3 or platelets <100,000/mm^3, product should be discontinued or reduced; decreased hemoglobulin level may indicate bone marrow suppression

• Hepatic studies: alk phos, AST, ALT, amylase, bilirubin, and for hepatotoxicity: dark urine, jaundice, itching, light-colored stools; product should be discontinued

Administer:

⚠ Anaphylaxis: rash, pruritus, wheezing, laryngeal edema; stop infusion, initiate emergency procedures

PO route

• All medications PO if possible, avoiding IM inj; bleeding may occur

• With meals to reduce GI upset; nausea is common

• For several days before transplant surgery, patients should be placed in protective isolation

Topical route

• Do not use occlusive dressings

IV route

• After diluting in 0.9% NaCl or D_5W to 0.004 to 0.02 mg/ml as a continuous inf

Additive compatibilities: Cimetidine

Y-site compatibilities: Acyclovir, aminophylline, amphotericin B, ampicillin, ampicillin/sulbactam, benztropine, calcium gluconate, cefazolin, cefotetan, ceftazidime, ceftriaxone, cefuroxime, chloramphenicol, cimetidine, ciprofloxacin, clindamycin, dexamethasone, digoxin, diphenhydrAMINE, DOBUTamine, DOPamine, doxycycline, erythromycin, esmolol, fluconazole, furosemide, ganciclovir, gentamicin, haloperidol, heparin, hydrocortisone, imipenem/cilastatin, insulin (regular), isoproterenol, leucovorin, lorazepam, methylPREDNISolone, metoclopramide, metronidazole, mezlocillin, multivitamins, nitroglycerin, oxacillin, penicillin G potassium, perphenazine, phenytoin, piperacillin, potassium chloride, propranolol, ranitidine, sodium bicarbonate, sodium nitroprusside, trimethoprim-sulfamethoxazole, vancomycin

Evaluate:

• Therapeutic response: absence of graft rejection; immunosuppression in autoimmune disorders

Teach patient/family:

PO route

• To report fever, rash, severe diarrhea, chills, sore throat, fatigue; serious infections may occur; clay-colored stools, cramping (hepatotoxicity), nephrotoxicity

• To avoid crowds, persons with known infections to reduce risk of infection

• To avoid exposure to natural or artificial sunlight

• Not to breastfeed while taking this medication

• That repeated lab tests will be needed during treatment

• To avoid vaccines

• To not use with alcohol, grapefruit

tadalafil (℞)

(tah-dal'a-fil)

Adcirca, Cialis

Func. class.: Impotence agent

Chem. class.: Phosphodiesterase type 5 inhibitor

Action: Inhibits phosphodiesterase type 5 (PDE5); enhances erectile function by increasing the amount of cGMP, which causes smooth muscle relaxation and increased blood flow into the corpus cavernosum; improves erectile function for up to 36 hr

Uses: Treatment of erectile dysfunction; pulmonary arterial hypertension (PAH) (Adcirca only)

Unlabeled uses: Sexual dysfunction in males receiving antidepressants

DOSAGE AND ROUTES

• *Adult:* **PO** 10 mg taken prior to sexual activity, dose may be reduced to 5 mg or increased to a max of 20 mg; usual max dosing frequency is once per day; once daily dosing 2.5 mg/day at same time each day

Renal dose

• *Adult:* **PO** CCr 31-50 ml/min 5 mg/day, max 10 mg q48hr; CCr <30 ml/min max 5 mg q72hr

Hepatic dose

• *Adult:* **PO** (Child-Pugh A, B) max 10 mg/day; (Child-Pugh C) not recommended

Concomitant medications

• Ketoconazole, itraconazole, ritonavir, max 10 mg q72hr

Pulmonary hypertension

• *Adult:* **PO** (Adcirca only) 40 mg daily

• *Adult taking ritonavir:* **PO** 20 mg daily initially, then increase to 40 mg daily as tolerated

Male sexual dysfunction (from antidepressants) (unlabeled)

• *Adult:* **PO** 10-20 mg prior to sexual activity

Available forms: Tabs 2.5, 5, 10, 20 mg; PO tab (Adcirca) 20 mg

SIDE EFFECTS

CNS: Headache, flushing, dizziness, **seizures,** transient global amnesia

CV: **MI, sudden death, CV collapse,** hypo/hypertension, tachycardia

MISC: Back pain/myalgia, *dyspepsia, nasal congestion, UTI,* blurred vision, changes in color vision, *diarrhea,* pruritus, priapism, **nonarteritic ischemic optic neuropathy (NAION),** hearing loss

Contraindications: Newborns, children, women, hypersensitivity, patients taking organic nitrates either regularly and/or intermittently, patients taking any α-adrenergic antagonist other than 0.4 mg once daily tamsulosin

Precautions: Pregnancy (B) although not indicated for females, anatomical penile deformities, sickle cell anemia, leukemia, multiple myeloma, CV/renal/hepatic disease, bleeding disorders, active peptic ulcer, prolonged erection

PHARMACOKINETICS

Rapidly absorbed; metabolized by liver; terminal half-life 17.5 hr; peak ½-6 hr; excreted primarily as metabolites in feces, urine; plasma concentration 61% in feces, 36% in urine; 94% protein bound; rate and extent of absorption of tadalafil are not influenced by food

INTERACTIONS

⚠ Do not use with nitrates because of unsafe drop in B/P, which could result in MI or stroke

Increase: tadalafil levels—itraconazole, ketoconazole, ritonavir (although not studied, may also include other HIV protease inhibitors)

Decrease: B/P—alcohol, α-blockers, amlodipine, angiotensin II receptor blockers, enalapril

Decrease: effects of tadalafil—bosentan, antacids

NURSING CONSIDERATIONS

Assess:

• Use of organic nitrates that should not be used with this product

• For any severe loss of vision, while taking this or any similar products

Administer:

• That product should not be used with nitrates in any form

• Sexual dysfunction: give prior to sexual activity; do not use more than once a day

• Pulmonary hypertension: give Adcirca with or without meals

Evaluate:

• Therapeutic response: ability to engage in sexual intercourse, improvement in exercise ability in pulmonary hypertension

Teach patient/family:

• That product does not protect against sexually transmitted diseases, including HIV

• To tell physician if patient has a bleeding problem

• That product has no effect in the absence of sexual stimulation

T

• To seek medical help if an erection lasts more than 4 hours
• To tell physician of all medicines, vitamins, and herbs patient is taking, especially ritonavir, indinavir, ketoconozole, itraconazole, erythromycin, nitrates, α-blockers
• That tadalafil is contraindicated for use with α-blockers except 0.4 mg/day tamsulosin
• To notify prescriber immediately, and stop taking product if vision loss occurs, erection >4 hr

tamoxifen (℞)

(ta-mox'i-fen)
Alpha-Tamoxifen ♣, Med Tamoxifen ♣, Nolvadex, Nolvadex-D ♣, Novo-Tamoxifen ♣, Soltamox, Tamofen ♣, Tamone ♣, Tamoplex ♣
Func. class.: Antineoplastic
Chem. class.: Antiestrogen hormone

Action: Inhibits cell division by binding to cytoplasmic estrogen receptors; resembles normal cell complex but inhibits DNA synthesis and estrogen response of target tissue
Uses: Advanced breast carcinoma not responsive to other therapy in estrogen-receptor-positive patients (usually postmenopausal), prevention of breast cancer, following breast surgery/radiation in ductal carcinoma in situ
Unlabeled uses: Mastalgia, to reduce pain/size of gynecomastia, ovulation stimulation, malignant carcinoid tumor, carcinoid syndrome, metastatic melanoma, desmoid tumors, McCune-Albright syndrome (female pediatric patients), osteoporosis, bipolar I disorder, infertility, precocious puberty, gynecomastia, mastalgia

DOSAGE AND ROUTES

Breast cancer
• *Adult:* **PO** 20-40 mg/day for 5 yr; doses >20 mg/day, divide AM/PM
High risk for breast cancer
• *Adult:* **PO** 20 mg/day × 5 yr
DCIS
• *Adult:* **PO** 20 mg/day × 5 yr
McCune-Albright syndrome/ precocious puberty (unlabeled)
• *Child 2-10 yr (girls):* **PO** 20 mg/day for up to 1 yr
Bipolar I disorder (unlabeled)
• *Adult:* **PO** 40 mg bid
Stimulation of ovulation in infertility (unlabeled)
• *Adult:* **PO** 20-80 mg/day × 5 days
Mastalgia (unlabeled)
• *Adult (female):* **PO** 10-20 mg/day × 3-6 mo
Mastalgia/gynecomastia in men with prostate cancer (unlabeled)
• *Adult (male):* **PO** 20 mg/day for up to 1 yr
Available forms: Tabs 10, 20 mg

SIDE EFFECTS

CNS: *Hot flashes, headache, lightheadedness,* depression, mood changes
CV: Chest pain, **stroke,** fluid retention, flushing
EENT: Ocular lesions, retinopathy, cataracts, corneal opacity, blurred vision (high doses)
GI: *Nausea, vomiting,* altered taste (anorexia)
GU: Vaginal bleeding, pruritus vulvae, **uterine malignancies,** *altered menses, amenorrhea*
HEMA: **Thrombocytopenia, leukopenia,** DVT
INTEG: *Rash,* alopecia
META: Hypercalcemia
RESP: **Pulmonary embolism**
Contraindications: Pregnancy (D), breastfeeding, hypersensitivity
Black Box Warning: Thromboembolic disease
Precautions: Women of childbearing age, leukopenia, thrombocytopenia, cataracts
Black Box Warning: Endometrial cancer, stroke

PHARMACOKINETICS

PO: Peak 4-7 hr, half-life 7 days (1 wk terminal), metabolized in liver, excreted primarily in feces

INTERACTIONS

Increase: bleeding—anticoagulants
Increase: tamoxifen levels—bromocriptine
Increase: thromboembolic events—cytotoxics
Increase: toxicity—CYP3A4 inhibitors (aprepitant, antiretroviral protease inhibitors, clarithromycin, danazol, delavirdine, diltiazem, erythromycin, fluconazole, fluoxetine, fluvoxamine, imatinib, ketoconazole, mibefradil, nefazodone, telithromycin, voriconazole)
Decrease: tamoxifen levels—aminoglutethimide, rifamycin
Decrease: letrozole levels—letrozole
Decrease: tamoxifen effect—CYP3A4 inducers (barbiturates, bosentan, carbamazepine, efavirenz, phenytoins, nevirapine, rifabutin, rifampin)
Decrease: tamoxifen effects—CYP2D6 inhibitors (antidepressants)

Drug/Herb
- Avoid use with St. John's wort, dong qui, black cohosh

Drug/Lab Test
Increase: serum calcium, T_4, AST, ALT, cholesterol, triglycerides

NURSING CONSIDERATIONS

Assess:
- CBC, differential, platelet count q wk; withhold product if WBC is <3500 or platelet count is <100,000; notify prescriber; breast exam, mammogram, pregnancy test, bone mineral density, LFTs, serum calcium, serum lipid profile
- Bleeding q8hr: hematuria, guaiac, bruising, petechiae, mucosa, or orifices
- Effects of alopecia on body image; discuss feelings about body changes

⚠ For uterine malignancies, symptoms of stroke, pulmonary embolism that may occur in women with ductal carcinoma in situ (DCIS) and women at high risk for breast cancer

⚠ Symptoms indicating severe allergic reactions: rash, pruritus, urticaria, purpuric skin lesions, itching, flushing
- For bone pain; may give analgesics; pain is usually transient

Administer:
- Do not break, crush, or chew tabs
- Antacid before oral agent; give product after evening meal, before bedtime; give with food or fluids for GI symptoms
- Antiemetic 30-60 min before giving product to prevent vomiting

Perform/provide:
- Nutritious diet with iron, vitamin supplements as ordered
- Storage in light-resistant container at room temperature

Evaluate:
- Therapeutic response: decreased tumor size, spread of malignancy

Teach patient/family:
- To report any complaints, side effects to prescriber, that use may be 5 yr
- To increase fluids to 2 L/day unless contraindicated
- To wear sunscreen, protective clothing, sunglasses
- That vaginal bleeding, pruritus, hot flashes are reversible after discontinuing treatment
- To report immediately decreased visual acuity, which may be irreversible; stress need for routine eye exams; care providers should be told about tamoxifen therapy
- To report vaginal bleeding immediately
- That tumor flare—increase in size of tumor, increased bone pain—may occur and will subside rapidly; may take analgesics for pain
- That premenopausal women must use mechanical birth control because ovulation may be induced
- That hair may be lost during treatment; a wig or hairpiece may make patient feel better; new hair may be different in color, texture

tamsulosin (℞)

(tam-sue-lo′sen)
Flomax
Func. class.: Selective α_1-peripheral adrenergic blocker
Chem. class.: Sulfamoylphenethylamine derivative

Do not confuse:
Flomax/Fosamax/Volmax

Action: Binds preferentially to α_{1A}-adrenoceptor subtype located mainly in the prostate

Uses: Symptoms of benign prostatic hyperplasia (BPH)

DOSAGE AND ROUTES

- *Adult:* **PO** 0.4 mg/day, increasing up to 0.8 mg/day if required

Available forms: Caps 0.4 mg

SIDE EFFECTS

CNS: ***Dizziness, headache,*** asthenia, insomnia
CV: Chest pain
EENT: Amblyopia, floppy iris syndrome
GI: Nausea, diarrhea, dysgeusia
GU: Decreased libido, abnormal ejaculation, **priapism**
INTEG: Rash, pruritus, urticaria
MS: Back pain
RESP: Rhinitis, pharyngitis, cough
SYST: **Angioedema**

Contraindications: Hypersensitivity

Precautions: Pregnancy (B), breastfeeding, children, hepatic disease, CAD, severe renal disease

PHARMACOKINETICS

Peak 4-5 hr, duration 9-15 hr, half-life 14 hr, metabolized in liver, excreted via urine, extensively protein bound (98%)

INTERACTIONS

- Not to be taken with: prazosin, terazosin, doxazosin, β-blockers, vardenafil

Increase: toxicity—cimetidine

Drug/Food

Decrease: absorption with food

NURSING CONSIDERATIONS

Assess:

- Prostatic hyperplasia: change in urinary patterns, baseline and throughout treatment
- CBC with diff and LFTs; B/P and heart rate
- BUN, uric acid, urodynamic studies (urinary flow rates, residual volume)
- I&O ratios, weight daily, edema, report weight gain or edema

Administer:

- Swallow caps whole; do not break, crush, or chew
- Give ½ hr after same meal each day

Perform/provide:

- Storage in tight container in cool environment

Evaluate:

- Therapeutic response: decreased symptoms of benign prostatic hyperplasia

Teach patient/family:

- Not to drive or operate machinery for 4 hr after first dose or after dosage increase
- To continue to take even if feeling better

tapentadol (℞)

(ta-pen′ta-dol)
Nucynta
Func. class.: Analgesic, misc.
Chem. class.: Mu-opiod receptor agonist

Controlled Substance Schedule II

Action: Centrally acting synthetic analgesic, mu-opioid agonist activity is thought to result in analgesia, inhibits norepinephrine uptake

Uses: Moderate to severe pain

DOSAGE AND ROUTES

- *Adult:* **PO** 50-100 mg q4-6hr, may give second dose 1 hr or more after 1st dose, max 700 mg on day 1, 600 mg/day thereafter

Available forms: Tabs 50, 75, 100 mg

SIDE EFFECTS

CNS: ***Drowsiness, dizziness, confusion, headache, euphoria,*** hallucinations, restlessness, syncope, anxiety, flushing, psychological dependence, insomnia, lethargy, tremor, **seizures**
CV: Palpitations, bradycardia, hypo/hypertension, orthostatic hypotension, sinus tachycardia
GI: *Nausea, vomiting, anorexia, constipation, cramps,* gastritis, dyspepsia, biliary spasms
GU: Urinary retention/frequency
INTEG: *Rash,* urticaria, diaphoresis, pruritus
RESP: **Respiratory depression,** cough
SYST: **Anaphylaxis,** infection, serotonin syndrome

Contraindications: Hypersensitivity, asthma, ileus, respiratory depression

Precautions: Pregnancy (C), breastfeeding, children <18 yr, increased intracranial pressure, MI (acute), severe heart disease, respiratory depression, renal/hepatic disease, GI obstruction, ulcerative colitis, sleep apnea, seizure disorder

PHARMACOKINETICS

Bioavailability 32%, extensively metabolized by liver, excreted in urine 99%, terminal half-life 4 hr, protein binding 20%

INTERACTIONS

Increase: effects with other CNS depressants—alcohol, opioids, sedative/hypnotics, antipsychotics, skeletal muscle relaxants

Increase: toxicity—MAOIs

Increase: serotonin syndrome—SSRIs, SNRIs, serotonin-receptor agonists, tricyclics

Drug/Herb

Increase: sedative effect—gotu kola, Jamaican dogwood, kava, lavender, mistletoe, nettle, pokeweed, poppy, senega, St. John's wort, valerian

NURSING CONSIDERATIONS

Assess:

- I&O ratio; check for decreasing output; may indicate urinary retention
- CNS changes: dizziness, drowsiness, hallucinations, euphoria, LOC, pupil reaction
- Allergic reactions: rash, urticaria, anaphylaxis
- Respiratory dysfunction: respiratory depression, character, rate, rhythm; notify prescriber if respirations are <10/min; also B/P, pulse
- For pain: intensity, location, type, characteristics; need for pain medication by pain/sedation scoring; physical dependence

Administer:

- With antiemetic if nausea, vomiting occur
- When pain is beginning to return; determine dosage interval by response

Perform/provide:

- Storage in light-resistant area at room temperature
- Assistance with ambulation
- Safety measures: night-light, call bell within easy reach

Evaluate:

- Therapeutic response: decrease in pain

Teach patient/family:

- To report any symptoms of CNS changes, allergic reactions
- That physical dependency may result from extended use
- That withdrawal symptoms may occur: nausea, vomiting, cramps, fever, faintness, anorexia
- Avoid CNS depressants, alcohol
- Avoid driving, operating machinery if drowsiness occurs

tegaserod (℞)

(teg-as′er-odd)

Zelnorm

Func. class.: 5-HT_4 receptor partial agonist, misc. GI agent, prokinetic

Action: A 5-HT_4 receptor partial agonist that binds 5-HT_4 receptors, stimulating peristalsis and intestinal secretion

Uses: Irritable bowel syndrome (IBS) where primary bowel symptom is constipation, chronic constipation not associated with IBS

DOSAGE AND ROUTES

This product is only available to women ≤55 yr old who meet specific guidelines; it is off the market for the general public

• *Adult (females ≤55 yr):* **PO** 6 mg bid before meals × 4-6 wk

Available forms: Tabs 2, 6 mg

SIDE EFFECTS

CNS: Headache, dizziness, depression, vertigo, fatigue, suicide attempt, poor concentration

CV: Hypotension, angina, ***dysrhythmias, bundle branch block, supraventricular tachycardia***

GI: Nausea, abdominal pain, increased appetite, eructation, increased AST, increased ALT, diarrhea, irritable colon, tenesmus, flatulence

GU: Polyuria, renal pain, ovarian cyst, miscarriage, albuminuria

MISC: Pain, facial edema, increased CPK, asthma, breast carcinoma

MS: Back pain, arthralgia

SYST: ***Anaphylaxis***

Contraindications: Hypersensitivity, severe renal disease, moderate to severe hepatic disease, history of bowel obstruction, gallbladder disease, abdominal adhesions, sphincter of Oddi dysfunction, hypotension

Precautions: Pregnancy (B), breastfeeding, children, diarrhea

PHARMACOKINETICS

Peak 1 hr, 98% protein binding, terminal half-life 11 hr, ⅔ excreted unchanged in feces, remainder in urine as metabolite

INTERACTIONS

Decrease: effect of digoxin

Decrease: tegaserod effect—antimuscarinics

Drug/Food

• Food decreases absorption, but is minimized when taken ½ hr before meal

NURSING CONSIDERATIONS

Assess:

• GI symptoms: nausea, abdominal pain

• CV status: B/P, pulse, chest pain

Administer:

• Before meals, bid

Perform/provide:

• Store at room temperature

Evaluate:

• Therapeutic response: Decreased constipation in IBS

Teach patient/family:

• To notify prescriber of GI symptoms, hypersensitivity reactions

telavancin (℞)

(tel-a-van′sin)

Vibativ

Func. class.: Antiinfective—miscellaneous

Chem. class.: Lipoglycopeptide, a semi-synthetic derivative of vacomycin

Action: Inhibits bacterial cell wall synthesis, blocks glycopeptides

Uses: Skin/skin structure infections caused by *Enterococcus faecalis, E. faecium, Staphylococcus aureus* (MSRA), *S. aureus* (MSSA), *S. epidermidis, S. haemolyticus, Streptococcus agalactiae* (group B), *S. dysgalactiae, S. pyogenes* (group A beta tremolytic), *S. anginosus, S. intermedius, S. constellates*

Unlabeled uses: Nosocomial pneumonia caused by susceptible gram-positive bacteria

DOSAGE AND ROUTES

- *Adult:* **IV INF** 10 mg/kg over 60 min q24hr × 7-14 days

Nosocomial pneumonia (unlabeled)

- *Adult:* **IV INF** 10 mg/kg q24hr × 7-21 days

Available forms: Powder for inj 250, 750 mg

SIDE EFFECTS

CNS: Anxiety, chills, flushing, headache, insomnia

CV: **QT prolongation,** irregular heartbeat

EENT: Hearing loss

GI: **Nausea,** vomiting, **pseudomembranous colitis,** abdominal pain, constipation, diarrhea, metallic taste

GU: **Nephrotoxicity,** *increased BUN, creatinine,* **renal failure,** foamy urine

HEMA: **Leukopenia, eosinophilia, anemia, thrombocytopenia**

INTEG: Chills, fever, rash, thrombophlebitis at inj site, urticaria, pruritus, necrosis (red man syndrome)

SYST: **Anaphylaxis, superinfection**

Contraindications: Hypersensitivity

Precautions: Breastfeeding, children, geriatric patients, renal disease, antimicrobial resistance, diabetes mellitus, diarrhea, GI disease, heart failure, hypertension, pseudomembranous colitis, QT prolongation, vancomycin hypersensitivity

Black Box Warning: Pregnancy (C), females

PHARMACOKINETICS

Onset rapid, half-life 8-9 hr, excreted in urine (76%)

INTERACTIONS

Increase: otoxicity or nephrotoxicity—aminoglycosides, cephalosporins, colistin, polymyxin, bacitracin, cisplatin, amphotericin B, nondepolarizing muscle relaxants, cidofovir

Increase: QT prolongation—Class IA, III antidysrhythmics, some phenothiazines, bepridil, chloroquine, clarithromycin, droperidol, dronedarone, erythromycin, grepafloxacin, halofantrine, haloperidol, levomethadye, methadone, pimozide, probucol, sparfloxacin, ziprasidone

Drug/Herb

- Do not use acidophilus with antiinfectives; separate by several hours

NURSING CONSIDERATIONS

Assess:

- Infection: WBC, urine, stools, sputum, characteristics of wound, throughout treatment
- I&O ratio; report hematuria, oliguria; nephrotoxicity may occur

⚠ Any patient with compromised renal system; product is excreted slowly in poor renal system function; toxicity may occur rapidly; BUN, creatinine

- C&S
- Auditory function during, after treatment, hearing loss, ringing, roaring in ears; product should be discontinued
- B/P during administration; sudden drop may indicate red man syndrome
- Skin eruptions
- Respiratory status: rate, character, wheezing, tightness in chest
- Allergies before treatment, reaction of each medication

Administer:

- Use only for susceptible organisms to prevent drug-resistant bacteria
- Antihistamine if red man syndrome occurs: decreased B/P, flushing of neck, face

Intermittent IV route

- After reconstitution with 15 ml D_5W sterile water for inj; 0.9% NaCl (15 mg/ml) 250 mg vial; add 45 ml to 750 mg vial (15 mg/ml) for dose of 150-800 mg; further dilute with 100-250 ml of compatible solution; for dose <150 mg or >800 mg, further dilute to a conc of 0.6-8 mg/ml with compatible solution; give over 60 min

Solution compatibilities: D_5W, LR, NS

T

Perform/provide:
- Storage in refrigerator
- Epinephrine, suction, tracheostomy set, endotracheal intubation equipment on unit; anaphylaxis may occur
- Adequate intake of fluids (2 L/day) to prevent nephrotoxicity

Evaluate:
- Therapeutic response: negative culture

Teach patient/family:
- All aspects of product therapy; culture may be taken after completed course of medication
- To report sore throat, fever, fatigue; could indicate superinfection

telbivudine (℞)

(tel-bi'vyoo-deen)

Tyzeka

Func. class.: Antiretroviral

Chem. class.: Nucleoside reverse transcriptase inhibitor (NRTI)

Action: Inhibits replication of HBV DNA polymerase, which inhibits HBV replication

Uses: Hepatitis B

DOSAGE AND ROUTES

- *Adult and adolescent >16 yr:* **PO** 600 mg/day; max 600 mg/day

Available forms: Tabs 600 mg

SIDE EFFECTS

CNS: ***Fever, headache, malaise,*** weakness, ***dizziness, insomnia***

EENT: Taste change, hearing loss, photophobia

GI: ***Nausea, vomiting, diarrhea, anorexia,*** abdominal pain, hepatomegaly

INTEG: ***Rash***

MISC: Lactic acidosis

MS: Myalgia, arthralgia, muscle cramps

RESP: Cough

Contraindications: Hypersensitivity, breastfeeding

Precautions: Pregnancy (B), children, severe renal disease, anemia, organ transplant, dialysis, HIV, obesity, alcoholism

Black Box Warning: Impaired hepatic function, lactic acidosis

PHARMACOKINETICS

Excreted by kidneys (unchanged), steady state 5-7 days, protein binding 3.3%, terminal half-life 40-49 hr

INTERACTIONS

- Altered telbivudine levels: any agent altering renal function

Increase: myopathy risk—HMG-CoA reductase inhibitors, fibric acid derivatives, penicillamine, zidovudine, ZDV, cycloSPORINE, erythromycin, niacin, azole antifungals, corticosteroids, hydrochloroquine

NURSING CONSIDERATIONS

Assess:
- LFTs, hepatitis B serology, creatine kinase, periodically

Administer:
- With or without food with a full glass of water

Perform/provide:
- Storage at room temperature

Evaluate:
- Therapeutic response: decreasing hepatitis B serology

Teach patient/family:
- That GI complaints and insomnia may resolve after 3-4 wk of treatment
- That product does not cure hepatitis B and does not stop the spread to others
- That follow-up visits must be continued
- That serious product interactions may occur if OTC products are ingested; check with prescriber before taking
- That product may cause dizziness; avoid hazardous activities until response is known
- To report symptoms of cough, difficulty sleeping, or excessive headache

telithromycin (℞)

(teh-lih-throw-my′sin)

Ketek

Func. class.: Antiinfective

Chem. class.: Ketolides

Action: Binds to 50S ribosomal subunits of susceptible bacteria and suppresses protein synthesis

Uses: Acute bacterial exacerbation of bronchitis, acute bacterial sinusitis, community-acquired pneumonia (mild to moderate)

Unlabeled uses: Acute tonsillitis/pharyngitis

DOSAGE AND ROUTES

Acute bacterial exacerbation of bronchitis

- *Adult:* **PO** 800 mg/day × 5 days

Acute bacterial sinusitis

- *Adult:* **PO** 800 mg/day × 5 days

Community-acquired pneumonia

- *Adult:* **PO** 800 mg/day × 7-10 days

Available forms: Tabs 300, 400 mg

SIDE EFFECTS

CNS: Dizziness, headache, insomnia, increased sweating

CV: **Atrial dysrhythmias, QT prolongation, torsade de pointes**

EENT: Blurred vision, diplopia, difficulty focusing

GI: Nausea, vomiting, diarrhea, hepatitis, abdominal pain/distention, stomatitis, anorexia, **pseudomembranous colitis, pancreatitis**

GU: Vaginitis, moniliasis

INTEG: Rash, urticaria

MS: Muscle cramps

SYST: **Anaphylaxis, superinfection**

Contraindications: Hypersensitivity to this product or macrolide antibiotics, history of hepatitis

Black Box Warning: Myasthenia gravis

Precautions: Pregnancy (C), breastfeeding, children, geriatric patients, ongoing prodysrhythmias, GI/hepatic disease, QT prolongation

PHARMACOKINETICS

Peak 1 hr; metabolized in liver (CYP450 enzyme system); excreted in bile, feces; protein binding 60%-70%; possible P-glycoprotein inhibition; terminal half-life 10 hr

INTERACTIONS

⚠ ***Increase:*** serious dysrhythmias—pimozide, antidysrhythmics (amiodarone, bretylium, disopyramide, dofetilide, procainamide, quinidine, sotalol); do not use together

Increase: action of atorvastatin, digoxin, ergots, lovastatin, metoprolol, midazolam, simvastatin, theophylline, carbamazepine, cycloSPORINE, tacrolimus, sirolimus, phenobarbital, phenytoin

Increase: telithromycin—itraconazole, ketoconazole

⚠ ***Increase:*** QT prolongation—class IA/III antidysrhythmics, some phenothiazines, β-agonists, local anesthetics, tricyclics, bepridil, haloperidol, methadone, chloroquine, clarithromycin, droperidol, erythromycin, grepafloxacin, halofantrine, pentamidine, probucol, sparfloxacin

Increase: cardiotoxicity—verapamil

Decrease: action of telithromycin—rifampin, phenytoin, carbamazepine, phenobarbital

Decrease: action of sotalol

Drug/Herb

- Do not use acidophilus with antiinfectives; separate by several hours

Drug/Lab Test

Increase: AST/ALT

NURSING CONSIDERATIONS

Assess:

- For infection: temp, sputum, WBCs, baseline and periodically

⚠ Cardiac status: ECG for QT prolongation

⚠ GI status: increasing diarrhea, pseudomembranous colitis may occur

⚠ Anaphylaxis: itching, skin rash, inabil-

T

ity to breathe; have emergency equipment available
• Oliguria in renal disease
• Hepatic studies: AST, ALT, if patient is on long-term therapy
• C&S before product therapy; product may be given as soon as culture is taken; C&S may be repeated after treatment

Administer:
• May take without regard to food
• Do not use this product if using class IA or III antidysrhythmics

Perform/provide:
• Storage at room temperature
• Adequate intake of fluids (2 L) during diarrhea episodes

Evaluate:
• Therapeutic response: decreased symptoms of infection

Teach patient/family:
• To report sore throat, fever, fatigue (could indicate superinfection)
• To notify nurse of diarrhea stools, dark urine, pale stools, jaundice of eyes or skin, and severe abdominal pain
• To report blurred vision, if interfering with daily activities
• To inform prescriber of all medications, herbs taking
• To avoid driving, hazardous activities if blurred vision occurs
• To take as prescribed, do not double or skip doses
• To report fainting; not to take if using class IA, III antidysrhythmics, simvastatin, lovastatin, or atorvastatin
• May take without regard to meals

Treatment of hypersensitivity:
• Withdraw product; maintain airway; administer epinephrine, aminophylline, O_2, IV corticosteroids

telmisartan (℞)

(tel-mih-sar′tan)
Micardis
Func. class.: Antihypertensive
Chem. class.: Angiotensin II receptor (Type AT_1) antagonist

Action: Blocks the vasoconstrictor and aldosterone-secreting effects of angiotensin II; selectively blocks the binding of angiotensin II to the AT_1 receptor found in tissues

Uses: Hypertension, alone or in combination

Unlabeled uses: Heart failure

DOSAGE AND ROUTES

• *Adult:* **PO** 40 mg/day; range 20-80 mg/day

Available forms: Tabs 20, 40, 80 mg

SIDE EFFECTS

CNS: Dizziness, insomnia, *anxiety,* headache, fatigue
GI: Diarrhea, dyspepsia, *anorexia, vomiting*
MS: Myalgia, pain
RESP: Cough, *upper respiratory infection,* sinusitis, pharyngitis

Contraindications: Hypersensitivity

Black Box Warning: Pregnancy (D) 2nd/3rd trimesters

Precautions: Pregnancy (C) 1st trimester, breastfeeding, children, geriatric patients; hypersensitivity to ACE inhibitors; renal/hepatic disease, renal artery stenosis, dialysis, CHF

PHARMACOKINETICS

Onset 3 hr, peak 0.5-1 hr, extensively metabolized, terminal half-life 24 hr, protein binding 99.5%, excreted in feces >97%, B/P response is less in African-American patients

INTERACTIONS

Increase: digoxin peak/trough concentrations—digoxin

Increase: antihypertensive action—diuretics, other antihypertensives
Increase: hyperkalemia—potassium-sparing diuretics, potassium salt substitutes
Decrease: antihypertensive effect—NSAIDs, salicylates
Drug/Herb
Increase: toxicity, death—aconite
Increase: antihypertensive effect—barberry, betony, black catechu, black cohosh, bloodroot, broom, burdock, cat's claw, dandelion, goldenseal, hawthorn, Irish moss, Jamaican dogwood, kelp, khella, mistletoe, parsley
Increase or decrease: antihypertensive effect—astragalus, cola tree
Decrease: antihypertensive effect—coltsfoot, guarana, khat, licorice, yohimbe

NURSING CONSIDERATIONS

Assess:
• B/P, pulse q4hr; note rate, rhythm, quality
• Electrolytes: K, Na, Cl
• Baselines in renal, hepatic studies before therapy begins
• Edema in feet, legs daily
• Skin turgor, dryness of mucous membranes for hydration status
Administer:
• Without regard to meals
• Increased dose to African-American patients; B/P response may be reduced
Evaluate:
• Therapeutic response: decreased B/P
Teach patient/family:
• To comply with dosage schedule, even if feeling better; take at same time of day; therapeutic effect may take 2-4 wk
• To notify prescriber of mouth sores, fever, swelling of hands or feet, irregular heartbeat, chest pain, decreased urine output
• That excessive perspiration, dehydration, vomiting, diarrhea may lead to fall in blood pressure; consult prescriber if these occur
• That product may cause dizziness, fainting; light-headedness may occur
• To use contraception while taking this product
• To notify prescriber of all prescriptions, OTC, and supplements taken

temazepam (℞)
(te-maz′e-pam)
Restoril, temazepam
Func. class.: Sedative-hypnotic
Chem. class.: Benzodiazepine, short-intermediate acting

Controlled Substance Schedule IV (USA), Schedule F (Canada)
Action: Produces CNS depression at limbic, thalamic, hypothalamic levels of the CNS; may be mediated by neurotransmitter γ-aminobutyric acid (GABA); results are sedation, hypnosis, skeletal muscle relaxation, anticonvulsant activity, anxiolytic action
Uses: Insomnia

DOSAGE AND ROUTES

• *Adult:* **PO** 7.5-30 mg at bedtime
• *Geriatric:* **PO** 7.5 mg at bedtime
Available forms: Caps 7.5, 15, 22.5, 30 mg

SIDE EFFECTS

CNS: Lethargy, drowsiness, daytime sedation, dizziness, confusion, light-headedness, headache, anxiety, irritability, complex sleep related reactions (sleep driving, sleep eating), fatigue
CV: Chest pain, pulse changes, hypotension
EENT: Blurred vision
GI: Nausea, vomiting, diarrhea, heartburn, abdominal pain, constipation, anorexia
HEMA: **Leukopenia, granulocytopenia (rare)**
SYST: **Severe allergic reactions**
Contraindications: Pregnancy (X), breastfeeding, hypersensitivity to benzodiazepines, intermittent porphyria
Precautions: Children <15 yr, geriatric patients, anemia, renal/hepatic disease, suicidal individuals, drug abuse, psychosis, acute closed-angle glaucoma, seizure disorders, angioedema, sleep-related be-

haviors (sleepwalking), pulmonary disease

PHARMACOKINETICS

Onset 30-60 min, duration 6-8 hr, half-life 10-20 hr, metabolized by liver, excreted by kidneys, crosses placenta, excreted in breast milk, 98% protein binding

INTERACTIONS

Increase: effects of cimetidine, disulfiram, oral contraceptives
Increase: action of both products—alcohol, CNS depressants
Decrease: effect of antacids, theophylline, rifampin

Drug/Herb

Increase: CNS depression—catnip, chamomile, clary, cowslip, hops, kava, lavender, mistletoe, nettle, pokeweed, poppy, Queen Anne's lace, senega, skullcap, valerian
Increase: hypotension—black cohosh

Drug/Lab Test

Increase: ALT, AST, serum bilirubin
Decrease: RAI uptake
False increase: urinary 17-OHCS

NURSING CONSIDERATIONS

Assess:

- Blood studies: Hct, Hgb, RBCs (long-term therapy)
- Hepatic studies: AST, ALT, bilirubin (long-term therapy)
- Mental status: mood, sensorium, affect, memory (long, short)

⚠ Blood dyscrasias: fever, sore throat, bruising, rash, jaundice, epistaxis (rare)

- Type of sleep problem: falling asleep, staying asleep

Administer:

- After removal of cigarettes to prevent fires
- After trying conservative measures for insomnia
- ½-1 hr before bedtime for sleeplessness
- On empty stomach for fast onset, but may be taken with food if GI symptoms occur
- Avoid use with CNS depressants; serious CNS depression may result

Perform/provide:

- Assistance with ambulation after receiving dose
- Safety measures: night-light, call bell within easy reach
- Checking to see if PO medication has been swallowed
- Storage in tight container in cool environment

Evaluate:

- Therapeutic response: ability to sleep at night, decreased early morning awakening if taking product for insomnia

Teach patient/family:

- To avoid driving, other activities requiring alertness until stabilized
- To avoid alcohol ingestion
- That effects may take 2 nights for benefits to be noticed
- Limit to 7-10 days of continuous use
- Alternative measures to improve sleep: reading, exercise several hours before bedtime, warm bath, warm milk, TV, self-hypnosis, deep breathing
- Not to discontinue abruptly, withdraw gradually
- That complex sleep-related behaviors may occur: sleep driving/eating
- That hangover, memory impairment are common in geriatric patients but less common than with barbiturates
- To use contraception while taking this product

Treatment of overdose: Lavage, activated charcoal; monitor electrolytes, VS

temozolomide (℞)

(tem-oh-zole′oh-mide)
Temodar
Func. class.: Antineoplastic-alkylating agent
Chem. class.: Imidazotetrazine derivative

Action: A prodrug that undergoes conversion to MTIC; MTIC action prevents DNA transcription

Uses: Anaplastic astrocytoma with relapse, glioblastoma multiforme, malignant glioma

Unlabeled uses: Metastatic melanoma

DOSAGE AND ROUTES

Anaplastic astrocytoma

• *Adult:* **PO** Adjust dose based on nadir neutrophil and platelet counts 150 mg/m^2/day × 5 days during a 28-day cycle

Glioblastoma multiforme

• *Adult:* **PO/IV** 75 mg/m^2/day × 42 days with focal radiotherapy; then maintenance of 6 cycles

Malignant glioma

• *Adult:* **IV** 150 mg/m^2/day over 90 min, day 1-5, q28days, may increase to 200 mg/m^2/day on days 1-5, q28days if hematologic parameters permit

Available forms: Caps 5, 20, 100, 140, 180, 250 mg; powder for inj 100 mg

SIDE EFFECTS

CNS: **Seizures,** *hemiparesis, dizziness, poor coordination, amnesia, insomnia, paresthesia, somnolence, paresis, ataxia, anxiety, dysphagia, depression, confusion*

GI: Nausea, anorexia, vomiting, abdominal pain, constipation

GU: Urinary incontinence, UTI, frequency

HEMA: **Thrombocytopenia, leukopenia,** anemia, **myelosuppression, neutropenia**

INTEG: Rash, pruritus

MISC: Headache, fatigue, asthenia, fever, edema, back pain, weight increase, diplopia

RESP: URI, pharyngitis, sinusitis, coughing

SYST: **Anaphylaxis, secondary malignancy**

Contraindications: Pregnancy (D), breastfeeding, hypersensitivity to this product, carbazine, or gelatin

Precautions: Geriatric patients, radiation therapy, renal/hepatic disease, bone marrow suppression, infection, myelosuppression

PHARMACOKINETICS

Absorption complete, rapid; crosses blood-brain barrier; excreted in urine/feces; half-life 1.8 hr; peak 1 hr

INTERACTIONS

• Do not use within 24 hr of sargramostim, filgrastim, G-CSF

Increase: myelosuppression—radiation, other antineoplastics

Increase: bleeding risk—NSAIDs, anticoagulants, platelet inhibitors, thrombolytics

Decrease: antibody reaction—live virus vaccines, toxoids

Decrease: action of digoxin

NURSING CONSIDERATIONS

Assess:

• Tumor response during treatment

• CBC on day 22 (21 days after 1st dose), CBC weekly until recovery if ANC is <1.5 × 10^9/L and platelets <100 × 10^9/L, do not administer to patients that do not tolerate 100 mg/m^2, myelosuppression usually occurs late in the treatment cycle

• For seizures throughout treatment; mental status

• Monitor temp (may indicate beginning infection)

• Hepatic studies before, during therapy (bilirubin, AST, ALT, LDH), as needed or monthly

• Bleeding: hematuria, guaiac, bruising or petechiae, mucosa or orifices

Administer:

PO route

• Do not break, crush, chew, or open caps

• Antiemetic 30-60 min before giving product to prevent vomiting

• Caps one at a time with 8 oz of water at same time of day

• Fluids IV or PO before chemotherapy to hydrate patient

• If caps accidentally damaged, do not allow contact with skin, or inhale

• Use proper procedures for handling/disposing of chemotherapy products

• Give on empty stomach at bedtime to prevent nausea/vomiting

IV route

• Bring vial to room temperature

• Inject 41 ml sterile water for inj into vial (2.5 mg/ml)

• Gently swirl, do not shake

Intermittent IV Inf

• Withdraw up to 40 ml from each vial to make total dose and transfer to empty 250 ml PVC inf bag, flush before and after inf

• Run over 90 min

• Use reconstituted sol within 14 hr, including inf time

Perform/provide:

• Storage in light-resistant container, dry area

Evaluate:

• Therapeutic response: decreased tumor size, spread of malignancy

Teach patient/family:

• To report signs of infection: fever, sore throat, flulike symptoms

• To report signs of anemia: fatigue, headache, faintness, SOB, irritability

• To report bleeding; avoid use of razors, commercial mouthwash

temsirolimus (℞)

(tem-sir-oh′li-mus)

Torisel

Func. class.: Biologic response modifier

Chem. class.: Kinase inhibitor, mTOR antagonist

Action: Inhibits mammalian target of rapamycin (mTOR), a protein kinase

Uses: Renal cell carcinoma

Unlabeled uses: Astrocytoma, mantle cell lymphoma

DOSAGE AND ROUTES

• *Adult:* **IV** 25 mg over 30-60 min q wk; treat until disease progression or severe toxicity occurs

Available forms: 25 mg/ml solution for inj kit

SIDE EFFECTS

CNS: Headache, **seizures**

CV: Hypertension, **thrombophlebitis**

ENDO: Hypertriglyceridemia, hyperlipidemia, hyperglycemia

GI: Nausea, vomiting, diarrhea, constipation, **bowel perforation**

GU: UTIs, **albuminuria, hematuria, proteinuria, renal failure,** mucositis

HEMA: **Anemia, leukopenia, thrombocytopenia**

INTEG: Rash, pruritus

META: Metabolic acidosis, hyperglycemia, hyperlipidemia

RESP: **Interstitial lung disease**

SYST: **Lymphoma**

Contraindications: Pregnancy (D), breastfeeding, hypersensitivity to this product or to sirolimus, polysorbate 80

Precautions: Children <13 yr, females, severe pulmonary/renal/hepatic disease, diabetes mellitus, hyperkalemia, hyperuricemia, hypertension, bone marrow suppression, hypertriglyceridemia/hyperlipidemia, surgery, brain tumors

PHARMACOKINETICS

Rapidly absorbed, peak 0.5-2 hr, extensively metabolized via liver by P450 3A4, eliminated via feces

INTERACTIONS

Increase: blood levels—CYP3A4 inhibitors, antifungals, calcium channel blockers, cimetidine, clarithromycin, danazol, erythromycin, cycloSPORINE, metoclopramide, bromocriptine, HIV-protease inhibitors, benzodiazepines, HMG-CoA reductase inhibitors

Increase: toxicity—sunitinib

Decrease: blood levels—CYP3A4 inducers, carbamazepine, dexamethasone, phenobarbital, phenytoin, rifamycin, rifapentine

Decrease: effect of vaccines

• Avoid with vaccines

Drug/Herb

• St. John's wort: may decrease the effect of sirolimus

Increase: effect—ginseng, maitake, mistletoe
Decrease: immunosuppression—astragalus, echinacea, melatonin
Drug/Food
• Alters bioavailability; use consistently with or without food; do not use with grapefruit juice

NURSING CONSIDERATIONS

Assess:
• Cardiac status: B/P, heart rate
• For interstitial lung disease
• Hypersensitive reactions: anaphylaxis
• Lipid profile: cholesterol, triglycerides, a lipid-lowering agent may be needed; blood glucose
⚠ For infection and development of lymphoma
⚠ Blood studies: Hgb, WBC, platelets during treatment q mo
• Renal studies: BUN, creatinine, phosphate potassium; proteinuria, hematuria, albuminemia may indicate renal failure
Administer:
• Using in-line filter ≤5 microns and inf pump
• Premedicate with 25-50 mg diphenhydrAMINE IV 30 min before dose, if reaction occurs, stop for ½-1 hr, may resume at slower rate
• Over 30-60 min, complete inf within 6 hr
• Dilute product with 1.8 ml of provided diluent, the result is 3 ml (10 mg/ml); invert to mix well; withdraw the required amount and inject rapidly into 250 ml of NS; do not use PVC inf bags/sets
• Protect from light during preparation, use only glass
Evaluate:
• Therapeutic response: decreased time of progression of renal cell carcinoma
Teach patient/family:
• To report fever, rash, severe diarrhea, chills, sore throat, fatigue; serious infections may occur; clay-colored stools, cramping (hepatotoxicity); excessive thirst, urinary frequency, new or worsening breathing problems, blood in stool, abdominal pain
• To avoid crowds, persons with known infections to reduce risk of infection
• To use contraception before, during, and 12 wk after product has been discontinued; avoid breastfeeding; men should also use reliable contraception during and 12 wk after cessation of product

⚠ High Alert

tenecteplase (℞)

(ten-ek'ta-place)
TNKase
Func. class.: Thrombolytic enzyme
Chem. class.: Tissue plasminogen activator

Action: Activates conversion of plasminogen to plasmin (fibrinolysin): plasmin breaks down clots (fibrin), fibrinogen, factors V, VII; occlusion of venous access lines
Uses: Acute myocardial infarction

DOSAGE AND ROUTES

• *Adult <60 kg:* **IV BOL** 30 mg, give over 5 sec
• *Adult ≥60-<70 kg:* **IV BOL** 35 mg, give over 5 sec
• *Adult ≥70-<80 kg:* **IV BOL** 40 mg, give over 5 sec
• *Adult ≥80-<90 kg:* **IV BOL** 45 mg, give over 5 sec
• *Adult ≥90 kg:* **IV BOL** 50 mg, give over 5 sec
Available forms: Powder for inj, lyophilized 50 mg

T

SIDE EFFECTS

CV: Dysrhythmias, hypotension, pulmonary edema, **PE, cardiogenic shock, cardiac arrest, heart failure, myocardial reinfarction, myocardial rupture, tamponade, pericarditis, pericardial effusion, thrombosis, CVA**
HEMA: Decreased Hct, **bleeding**
INTEG: Rash, urticaria, phlebitis at IV inf site, itching, flushing

SYST: **GI, GU, intracranial, retroperitoneal bleeding, surface bleeding, anaphylaxis**

Contraindications: Hypersensitivity, arteriovenous malformation, aneurysm, active bleeding, intracranial/intraspinal surgery or trauma within 2 mo, CNS neoplasms, severe hypertension, severe renal/hepatic disease, history of CVA, increased ICP/stroke

Precautions: Pregnancy (C), breastfeeding, children, geriatric patients, arterial emboli from left side of heart, hypocoagulation, subacute bacterial endocarditis, rheumatic valvular disease, cerebral embolism/thrombosis/hemorrhage, intraarterial diagnostic procedure or surgery (10 days), recent major surgery, dysrhythmias, hypertension

PHARMACOKINETICS

IV: Onset immediate, half-life 20-24 min, metabolized by the liver

INTERACTIONS

• Bleeding potential: aspirin, indomethacin, phenylbutazone, anticoagulants, antithrombolytics, glycoprotein IIb/IIIa inhibitors, dipyridamole, clopidogrel, ticlopidine, NSAIDs, cefamandole, cefoperazone, cefotetan

Drug/Herb

Increase: risk of bleeding—agrimony, alfalfa, angelica, anise, basil, bay, bilberry, black haw, bogbean, bromelain, buchu, chondroitin, cinchona bark, dong quai, fenugreek, feverfew, garlic, ginger, ginkgo, ginseng, green tea, horse chestnut, Irish moss, kelp, kelpware, khella, lovage, lungwort, meadowsweet, motherwort, mugwort, nettle, papaya, parsley (large amts), pau d'arco, pineapple, poplar, prickly ash, safflower, saw palmetto, tonka bean, turmeric, wintergreen, yarrow

Decrease: anticoagulant effect—chamomile, coenzyme Q10, flax, glucomannan, goldenseal, guar gum

Drug/Lab Test

Increase: PT, aPTT, TT

Decrease: plasminogen, fibrinogen

NURSING CONSIDERATIONS

Assess:

• Allergy: fever, rash, itching, chills; mild reaction may be treated with antihistamines

⚠ For bleeding during 1st hr of treatment; hematuria, hematemesis, bleeding-from mucous membranes, epistaxis, ecchymosis; may require tranfusion (rare), continue to assess for bleeding for 24 hr

• Blood studies (Hct, platelets, PTT, PT, TT, aPTT) before starting therapy; PT or aPTT must be less than 2× control before starting therapy; PTT or PT q3-4hr during treatment

• For hypersensitive reactions: fever, rash, dyspnea; product should be discontinued

• VS, B/P, pulse, respirations, neurologic signs, temp at least q4hr; temp >104° F (40° C) indicates internal bleeding; systolic pressure increase >25 mm Hg should be reported to prescriber

⚠ For neurologic changes that may indicate intracranial bleeding

⚠ Retroperitoneal bleeding: back pain, leg weakness, diminished pulses

Administer:

IV route

• As soon as thrombi identified; not useful for thrombi over 1 wk old

• Cryoprecipitate or fresh frozen plasma if bleeding occurs

• Heparin after fibrinogen level >100 mg/dl; heparin infusion to increase PTT to 1.5-2 × baseline for 3-7 days; IV heparin with loading dose is recommended

• Aseptically withdraw 10 ml of sterile H_2O for inj from diluent vial, use red cannula syringe-filling device, inject all contents of syringe into product vial, direct into powder, swirl, withdraw correct dose, discard any unused solution; stand the shield with dose vertically on flat surface and passively recap the red cannula, remove entire shield assembly by twisting counter-clockwise, give by IV BOL

• IV therapy: use upper extremity vessel that is accessible to manual compression

If not used immediately refrigerate and use within 8 hr; not compatible with dextrose; flush dextrose containing lines with saline before and after administration

Perform/provide:

- Bed rest during entire course of treatment
- Avoidance of venous or arterial puncture, inj, rectal temp; any invasive treatment
- Treatment of fever with acetaminophen or aspirin
- Pressure for 30 sec to minor bleeding sites; inform prescriber if this does not attain hemostasis; apply pressure dressing

Evaluate:

- Therapeutic response: resolution of myocardial infarction

Teach patient/family:

- Proper tooth brushing to avoid bleeding
- Notify prescriber immediately of sudden severe headache
- Notify prescriber of bleeding, hypersensitivity

tenofovir (℞)

(ten-oh-foh'veer)

Viread

Func. class.: Antiretroviral

Chem. class.: Nucleoside analog reverse transcriptase inhibitor

Action: Inhibits replication of HIV virus by competing with the natural substrate and then incorporating into cellular DNA by viral reverse transcriptase, thereby terminating cellular DNA chain

Uses: HIV-1 infection with other antiretrovirals, hepatitis B

DOSAGE AND ROUTES

- *Adult:* **PO** 300 mg/day with meal; if used with didanosine, give tenofovir 2 hr before or 1 hr after didanosine

Renal dose

- CCr 30-49 ml/min 300 mg q48hr; CCr 10-29 ml/min 300 mg 2×/wk; CCr <10 ml/min not recommended

Available forms: Tabs 300 mg (300 mg of fumarate salt equivalent to 245 mg tenofovir disoproxil)

SIDE EFFECTS

CNS: Headache, asthenia

GI: Nausea, vomiting, diarrhea, anorexia, *flatulence, abdominal pain,* **pancreatitis**

GU: **Renal failure, renal tubular acidosis/necrosis, Fanconi syndrome**

HEMA: Neutropenia, osteopenia

INTEG: Rash, **angioedema**

META: **Lactic acidosis,** hypokalemia, hypophosphatemia

MS: Myopathy, **rhabdomyolysis**

SYST: Lipodystrophy

Contraindications: Hypersensitivity

Black Box Warning: Lactic acidosis

Precautions: Pregnancy (B), breastfeeding, children, geriatric patients, renal disease, CCr <60 ml/min, osteoporosis, immune reconstitution syndrome

Black Box Warning: Hepatic disease, hepatitis

PHARMACOKINETICS

Rapidly absorbed, distributed to extravascular space, excreted unchanged in urine 70%-80%, terminal half-life 17 hr

INTERACTIONS

Increase: tenofovir level—cidofovir, acyclovir, valacyclovir, ganciclovir, valganciclovir

Increase: level of didanosine when given with tenofovir

Increase: tenofovir level—any product that decreases renal function

NURSING CONSIDERATIONS

Assess:

- Viral load, CD4+ T cell count, plasma HIV RNA, serum creatinine/BUN/phosphate
- Resistance testing at start of therapy and at treatment failure

T

• Hepatic studies: AST, ALT, bilirubin; amylase, lipase, triglycerides periodically during treatment
• For bone, renal toxicity: if bone abnormalities are suspected, obtain tests; serum phosphorus, creatinine
⚠ For lactic acidosis, severe hepatomegaly with steatosis

Administer:
• PO daily with meal
• This product 2 hr before or 1 hr after taking didanosine (if used)

Perform/provide:
• Storage at 25° C (77° F)

Evaluate:
• Therapeutic response: decrease in signs/symptoms of HIV

Teach patient/family:
• To take with meal
• That GI complaints resolve after 3-4 wk of treatment
• Not to breastfeed while taking this product
• That product must be taken daily even if patient feels better
• That follow-up visits must be continued because serious toxicity may occur; blood counts must be done q2wk
• That product will control symptoms but is not a cure for HIV; patient is still infectious, may pass HIV virus on to others
• That other products may be necessary to prevent other infections
• That changes in body fat distribution may occur

terazosin (℞)
(ter-ay′zoe-sin)
Hytrin
Func. class.: Antihypertensive
Chem. class.: α-Adrenergic blocker

Action: Decreases total vascular resistance, which is responsible for a decrease in B/P; this occurs by blockade of α_1-adrenoreceptors

Uses: Hypertension, as a single agent or in combination with diuretics or β-blockers, BPH

DOSAGE AND ROUTES

Hypertension
• *Adult:* **PO** 1 mg at bedtime, may increase dose slowly to desired response; max 20 mg/day

Benign prostatic hyperplasia
• *Adult:* **PO** 1 mg at bedtime, gradually increase up to 5-10 mg; max 20 mg

Available forms: Caps 1, 2, 5, 10 mg

SIDE EFFECTS

CNS: Dizziness, headache, drowsiness, anxiety, depression, vertigo, weakness, fatigue
CV: Palpitations, orthostatic hypotension, tachycardia, edema, rebound hypertension
EENT: Blurred vision, epistaxis, tinnitus, dry mouth, red sclera, nasal congestion, sinusitis
GI: Nausea, vomiting, diarrhea, constipation, abdominal pain
GU: Urinary frequency, incontinence, impotence, priapism
RESP: Dyspnea, cough, pharyngitis

Contraindications: Hypersensitivity

Precautions: Pregnancy (C), breastfeeding, children, prostate cancer

PHARMACOKINETICS

Peak 1 hr; half-life 9-12 hr; protein binding 90%-94%; metabolized in liver; excreted in urine, feces

INTERACTIONS

Increase: hypotensive effects—β-blockers, nitroglycerin, verapamil, other antihypertensives, alcohol
Decrease: hypotensive effects—estrogens, NSAIDs, sympathomimetics, salicylates

Drug/Herb
Increase: toxicity, death—aconite
Increase: antihypertensive effect—barberry, betony, black catechu, black cohosh, bloodroot, broom, burdock, cat's claw, dandelion, goldenseal, hawthorn, Irish moss, Jamaican dogwood, kelp, khella, mistletoe, parsley

Increase or decrease: antihypertensive effect—astragalus, cola tree
Decrease: antihypertensive effect—coltsfoot, guarana, khat, licorice, yohimbe

NURSING CONSIDERATIONS

Assess:

- Urinary symptoms associated with BPH
- Orthostatic B/P, pulse, jugular venous distention q4hr
- BUN, uric acid if on long-term therapy
- Weight daily, I&O
- Skin turgor, dryness of mucous membranes for hydration status
- Crackles, dyspnea, orthopnea q30min

Administer

- Dose at bedtime or do not operate machinery; fainting may occur

Perform/provide:

- Cool storage in tight container

Evaluate:

- Therapeutic response: decreased B/P, edema in feet, legs, decreased symptoms of BPH

Teach patient/family:

- That fainting occasionally occurs after first dose; not to drive or operate machinery for 4 hr after first dose or after an increase in dose; or take first dose at bedtime
- To rise slowly from sitting/lying position
- To not discontinue abruptly

terbinafine (℞)

(ter-bin′a-feen)
Lamisil
Func. class.: Antifungal
Chem. class.: Synthetic allylamine derivative

Action: Interferes with cell membrane permeability in fungi such as *Trichophyton rubrum, Trichophyton mentagrophytes, Trichophyton tonsurans, Epidermophyton floccosum, Microsporum canis, Microsporum audouinii, Microsporum gypseum, Candida,* broad-spectrum antifungal

Uses: (Topical) Tinea cruris, tinea corporis, tinea pedis; (oral) onychomycosis of the toenail or fingernail due to dermatophytes
Unlabeled uses: Cutaneous candidiasis, tinea versicolor

DOSAGE AND ROUTES

- *Fingernail:* **PO** 250 mg/day × 6 wk
- *Toenail:* **PO** 250 mg/day × 12 wk

Available forms: Tabs 250 mg

SIDE EFFECTS

GI: Diarrhea, dyspepsia, abdominal pain, nausea, hepatitis
HEMA: **Neutropenia**
INTEG: Rash, pruritus, urticaria, **Stevens-Johnson syndrome**
MISC: Headache, hepatic enzyme changes, taste, visual disturbance
Contraindications: Hypersensitivity, chronic/active hepatic disease, renal disease GFR ≤50 ml/min
Precautions: Pregnancy (B), breastfeeding, children, renal disease

PHARMACOKINETICS

Peak 1-2 hr, >99% protein binding, half-life 36 hr

INTERACTIONS

Increase: levels of dextromethorphan
Increase: terbinafine clearance—rifampin
Increase: clearance of cycloSPORINE
Decrease: terbinafine clearance—cimetidine

Drug/Herb

- Side effects: cola nut, guarana, yerba maté, tea (black, green), coffee

NURSING CONSIDERATIONS

Assess:

- Hepatic studies (ALT, AST) prior to beginning treatment; do not use in presence of hepatic disease
- CBC in treatment >6 wk
- For continuing infection: increased size, number of lesions

Perform/provide:

- Storage below 25° C (77° F)

Evaluate:

- Therapeutic response: decrease in size, number of lesions

Teach patient/family:

- To notify prescriber of nausea, vomiting, fatigue, jaundice, dark urine, clay-colored stool, RUQ pain, that may indicate hepatic dysfunction

terbinafine topical

See Appendix B

terbutaline (℞)

(ter-byoo′te-leen)

Brethine, Bricanye ✦

Func. class.: Selective β_2-agonist; bronchodilator

Chem. class.: Catecholamine

Action: Relaxes bronchial smooth muscle by direct action on β_2-adrenergic receptors through accumulation of cAMP at β-adrenergic receptor sites; bronchodilation, diuresis, CNS, cardiac stimulation occur; relaxes uterine smooth muscle

Uses: Bronchospasm, hyperkalemia

Unlabeled uses: Premature labor, nonresponsive status asthmaticus in children (IV)

DOSAGE AND ROUTES

Bronchodilation

- *Adult and child >15 yr:* **PO** 2.5-5 mg q6hr during the day, max 15 mg/24 hr
- *Child 12-15 yr:* **PO** 2.5 mg tid q6hr

Bronchospasm

- *Adult and child >12 yr:* **PO** 2.5-5 mg q8hr; **SUBCUT** 0.25 mg q15-30min, max 0.5 mg in 4 hr

Renal dose

- *Adult:* **PO** CCr 10-50 ml/min 50% of dose; CCr <10 ml/min avoid use

Severe renal failure

- *Adult:* Avoid GFR if <10 ml/min

Tocolytic (preterm labor) (unlabeled)

- *Adult:* **PO** 2.5 mg q4-6hr until delivery

Available forms: Tabs 2.5, 5 mg; inj 1 mg/ml

SIDE EFFECTS

CNS: Tremors, anxiety, insomnia, headache, dizziness, stimulation

CV: Palpitations, tachycardia, hypertension, dysrhythmias, **cardiac arrest**

GI: Nausea, vomiting

Contraindications: Hypersensitivity to sympathomimetics, closed-angle glaucoma, tachydysrhythmias

Precautions: Pregnancy (B), breastfeeding, geriatric patients, cardiac disorders, hyperthyroidism, diabetes mellitus, prostatic hypertension, hypertension, seizure disorder

PHARMACOKINETICS

PO: Onset ½ hr, peak 1-2 hr, duration 4-8 hr

SUBCUT: Onset 6-15 min, peak ½-1 hr, duration 1½-4 hr

INTERACTIONS

- Incompatible with bleomycin
- Hypertensive crisis: MAOIs

Increase: effects of both products—other sympathomimetics

Decrease: action—β-blockers

Drug/Herb

Increase: effect—green tea (large amounts), guarana

NURSING CONSIDERATIONS

Assess:

- Respiratory function: vital capacity, forced expiratory volume, ABGs, B/P, pulse, respiratory pattern, lung sounds, sputum before and after treatment
- Tolerance over long-term therapy; dose may have to be changed; monitor for rebound bronchospasm

⚠ Paradoxical bronchospasm: dyspnea, wheezing, keep emergency equipment nearby

• Labor: maternal heart rate, B/P, contraction, fetal heart rate

Administer:

• With food; may be crushed

• 2 hr before bedtime to avoid sleeplessness

IV route

• IV after diluting each 5 mg/1 L D_5W for inf

• IV, run 5 mcg/min; may increase 5 mcg q10min, titrate to response; after ½-1 hr taper dose by 5 mcg; switch to PO as soon as possible

Additive compatibilities: Aminophylline

Syringe compatibilities: Doxapram

Y-site compatibilities: Insulin (regular)

Perform/provide:

• Storage at room temperature; do not use discolored sol

• An increase in fluids of >2 L/day

Evaluate:

• Therapeutic response: absence of dyspnea, wheezing

Teach patient/family:

• Not to use OTC medications; extra stimulation may occur

• All aspects of product; avoid smoking, smoke-filled rooms, persons with respiratory infections

• To increase fluids >2 L/day; allow 15 min between inhalation of this product and inhaler containing steroid

• To take on time; if missed, do not make up after 1 hr; wait until next dose

Treatment of overdose: Administer an α-blocker, then norepinephrine for severe hypotension

terconazole vaginal antifungal

See Appendix B

teriparatide (℞)

(tah-ree-par′ah-tide)

Forteo

Func. class.: Parathyroid hormone (rDNA)

Action: Contains human recombinant parathyroid hormone, to stimulate new bone growth

Uses: Postmenopausal women with osteoporosis, men with primary or hypogonadal osteoporosis who are at high risk for fracture, glucocorticoid-induced osteoporosis

Unlabeled uses: Hypoparathyroidism

DOSAGE AND ROUTES

• *Adult:* **SUBCUT** 20 mcg/day up to 2 yr

Available forms: Prefilled pen delivery device (delivers 20 mcg/day)

SIDE EFFECTS

CNS: Dizziness, headache, insomnia, depression, vertigo

CV: Hypertension, angina, syncope

GI: Nausea, diarrhea, dyspepsia, vomiting, constipation

INTEG: Rash, sweating

MISC: Pain, asthenia, hyperuricemia

MS: Arthralgia, leg cramps, back/leg pain, weakness, **osteosarcoma (rare)**

RESP: Rhinitis, cough, pharyngitis, pneumonia, dyspnea

Contraindications: Hypersensitivity, increased baseline risk of osteosarcoma (Paget's disease, open epiphyses; previous bone radiation), bone metastases, history of skeletal malignancies, other metabolic bone diseases, preexisting hypercalcemia

Precautions: Pregnancy (C), breastfeeding, children, urolithiasis, hypotension, use >2 yr, cardiac disease

Black Box Warning: Secondary malignancy

T

PHARMACOKINETICS

SUBCUT: Extensively and rapidly absorbed, metabolized by liver, excreted by kidneys, terminal half-life 1 hr

INTERACTIONS

Increase: digoxin toxicity: digoxin

Drug/Lab Test

Increase: calcium

NURSING CONSIDERATIONS

Assess:

- Uric acid, magnesium, creatinine, BUN, urine pH, vit D, phosphate for normal serum levels; serum calcium may be transiently increased after dosing (max at 4-6 hr post-dose)
- For bone pain, headache, fatigue, changes in LOC, leg cramps
- For signs of persistent hypercalcemia: nausea, vomiting, constipation, lethargy, muscle weakness
- Nutritional status: diet for sources of vit D (milk, some seafood); calcium (dairy products, dark green vegetables), phosphates (dairy products)

Administer:

SUBCUT route

- Give by SUBCUT using disposable pen only; inject in thigh or abdomen; lightly pinch a fold of skin; insert needle; release skin; inject at 90-degree angle over 5 sec; rotate inj sites
- Have patient sit or lie down; orthostatic hypotension may occur

Perform/provide:

- Store refrigerated, do not freeze; may be used for 28 days after first inj

Evaluate:

- Therapeutic response: increased bone mineral density

Teach patient/family:

- The symptoms of hypercalcemia
- About foods rich in calcium, vit D
- How to use delivery device, dispose of needles, not to share pen with others
- To sit or lie down if dizziness or fast heartbeat occurs after the first few doses
- To rotate administration sites
- To store pen in refrigerator

testosterone cypionate (℞)

Andro-Cyp, Andronate, depAndro, Depotest, Depo-Testosterone, Dura-test, T-Cypionate, Testa-C, Testred, Testoject-LA, Virilon IM

testosterone enanthate (℞)

Andro LA, Andropository, Andryl, Delatest, Delatestryl, Everone, Malog-x ♣, Testone LA, Testrin-PA

testosterone gel (℞)

AndroGel 1%, Testim

testosterone, long-acting (℞)

testosterone pellets (℞)

Testopel

testosterone transdermal (℞)

Androderm, Androplex ♣, Testoderm, Testoderm TTS, Testoderm with Adhesive

testosterone buccal (℞)

Striant

Func. class.: Androgenic anabolic steroid

Chem. class.: Halogenated testosterone derivative

Controlled Substance Schedule III

Action: Increases weight by building body tissue, increases potassium, phosphorus, chloride, nitrogen levels, bone development

Uses: Female breast cancer, hypogonadism, eunuchoidism, male climacteric, oligospermia, impotence, osteoporosis, weight loss in AIDS patients, vulvar dystrophies, low testosterone levels, delayed male puberty (inj)

DOSAGE AND ROUTES

Replacement

• *Adult:* **IM** (base or propionate) 25-50 mg 2-3×/wk or (enanthate or cypionate) 50-400 mg q2-4wk

• *Adult (male) and child:* **SUBCUT** (pellets) 150-450 mg (2-6 pellets) inserted q3-6mo

• *Adult:* **TRANSDERMAL** (Testoderm) 4-6 mg applied q24hr; (Androderm) 5 mg applied q24hr; **GEL** (AndroGel) 5 mg applied q24hr, once daily; **BUCCAL** 1 buccal system (30 mg) to the gum region q12hr before meals/PM

Breast cancer

• *Adult:* **IM** 50-100 mg 3×/wk (propionate) or 200-400 mg q2-4wk (cypionate or enanthate)

Delayed male puberty

• *Child >12 yr:* **IM** Up to 100 mg/mo for up to 6 mo

Available forms: *Enanthate:* inj 200 mg/ml; *cypionate:* inj 100, 200 mg/ml; pellets 75 mg; transdermal 2.5, 4, 5, 6 mg/24 hr; gel 1%; buccal system 30 mg

SIDE EFFECTS

CNS: Dizziness, headache, fatigue, tremors, paresthesias, flushing, sweating, anxiety, lability, insomnia, carpal tunnel syndrome

CV: Increased B/P

EENT: Conjunctival edema, nasal congestion

ENDO: Abnormal glucose tolerance test

GI: Nausea, vomiting, constipation, weight gain, **cholestatic jaundice**

GU: Hematuria, amenorrhea, vaginitis, decreased libido, decreased breast size, clitoral hypertrophy, testicular atrophy, gynecomastia

HEMA: Polycythemia

INTEG: Rash, acneiform lesions, oily hair and skin, flushing, sweating, acne vulgaris, alopecia, hirsutism

MS: Cramps, spasms

Contraindications: Pregnancy (X), breastfeeding, severe cardiac/renal/hepatic disease, hypersensitivity, genital bleeding (rare), male breast/prostate cancer

Precautions: Diabetes mellitus, CV disease, MI, urinary tract disorders, prostate cancer

Black Box Warning: Children, accidental exposure

PHARMACOKINETICS

PO: Metabolized in liver; excreted in urine, breast milk; crosses placenta

INTERACTIONS

• Edema: ACTH, adrenal steroids, buPROPion

Increase: effects of oxyphenbutazone

Increase: PT—anticoagulants

Decrease: glucose levels may alter need for oral antidiabetics, insulin

Drug/Lab Test

Increase: serum cholesterol, blood glucose, urine glucose

Decrease: serum calcium, serum potassium, T_4, T_3, thyroid ^{131}I uptake test, urine 17-OHCS, 17-KS, PBI

NURSING CONSIDERATIONS

Assess:

• Weight daily; notify prescriber if weekly weight gain is >5 lb

• B/P q4hr, Hgb/HCT

• I&O ratio; be alert for decreasing urinary output, increasing edema

• Growth rate, bone age in children; growth rate may be uneven (linear/bone growth) with extended use

• Electrolytes: K, Na, Cl, Ca; cholesterol

• Hepatic studies: ALT, AST, bilirubin

• Edema, hypertension, cardiac symptoms, jaundice

• Mental status: affect, mood, behavioral changes, aggression

• Signs of masculinization in female: increased libido, deepening of voice, decreased breast tissue, enlarged clitoris, menstrual irregularities; male: gynecomastia, impotence, testicular atrophy

• Hypercalcemia: lethargy, polyuria, polydipsia, nausea, vomiting, constipation; product may have to be decreased

• Hypoglycemia in diabetics; oral antidiabetic action is increased

Administer:

• Titrated dose; use lowest effective dose

• IM inj deep into upper outer quadrant of gluteal muscle

• Transdermal patches: Testoderm to skin of scrotum; Androderm to skin of back, upper arms, thighs, abdomen; area must be dry-shaved; may be reapplied after bathing, swimming

• Gel: apply daily to clean, dry area on shoulders, upper arms, or abdomen; women, children should not touch skin treated

Buccal system route

• Do not chew or swallow buccal system

• Rotate sites; place above incisor tooth on either side of mouth

• Open packet; place rounded side of surface against the gum and hold firmly in place with finger over lip for 30 sec; if it falls off, replace with new system; discard in trash can away from children or pets

Perform/provide:

• Diet with increased calories, protein; decrease sodium if edema occurs

Evaluate:

• Therapeutic response: 4-6 wk in osteoporosis

Teach patient/family:

• That product must be combined with complete health plan: diet, rest, exercise

• To notify prescriber if therapeutic response decreases; if edema occurs

• About changes in sex characteristics: priapism, gynecomastia, increased libido

• That women should report menstrual irregularities, voice changes, acne, facial hair growth, if pregnancy is planned or suspected

• That 1-3-mo course is necessary for response in breast cancer

• The proper application of patches

tetracaine (℞)

(tet′ra-kane)

Pontocaine

Func. class.: Local anesthetic

Chem. class.: Ester

Action: Competes with calcium for binding sites in nerve membrane that control sodium transport across cell membrane; decreases rise of depolarization phase of action potential

Uses: Spinal anesthesia, epidural and peripheral nerve block, perineum, lower extremities

DOSAGE AND ROUTES

Varies with route of anesthesia

Available forms: Inj 0.2%, 0.3%, 1%; powder

SIDE EFFECTS

CNS: Anxiety, restlessness, **seizures, loss of consciousness,** drowsiness, disorientation, tremors, shivering

CV: **Myocardial depression, cardiac arrest, dysrhythmias,** bradycardia, hypo/hypertension, fetal bradycardia

EENT: Blurred vision, tinnitus, pupil constriction

GI: Nausea, vomiting

INTEG: Rash, urticaria, allergic reactions, edema, burning, skin discoloration at inj site, tissue necrosis

RESP: **Status asthmaticus, respiratory arrest, anaphylaxis**

Contraindications: Hypersensitivity, sulfite allergy, severe hepatic disease, heart block, thrombocytopenia

Precautions: Pregnancy (C), breastfeeding, children ≤12 yr, geriatric patients, severe product allergies, cardiac disease

PHARMACOKINETICS

Onset MS 3 min, spinal 3-8 min; duration 1.5-3 hr; metabolized by liver; excreted in urine (metabolites)

INTERACTIONS

- Dysrhythmias: epinephrine, halothane, enflurane
- Hypertension: tricyclics, phenothiazines
- Hypotension: MAOIs

Decrease: action of tetracaine—chloroprocaine

Decrease: action of sulfonamides

NURSING CONSIDERATIONS

Assess:

- B/P, pulse, respiration during treatment
- Fetal heart tones during labor
- Allergic reactions: rash, urticaria, itching
- Cardiac status: ECG for dysrhythmias, pulse, B/P, during anesthesia

Administer:

- Only if not cloudy, does not contain precipitate
- Only with crash cart, resuscitative equipment nearby
- Only without preservatives for epidural or caudal anesthesia

Perform/provide:

- Use of new sol, discard unused portions, store in refrigerator, avoid freezing

Evaluate:

- Therapeutic response: anesthesia necessary for procedure

Treatment of overdose: Maintain adequate airway, O_2, vasopressor, IV fluids, anticonvulsants for seizures

tetracaine ophthalmic

See Appendix B

tetracaine topical

See Appendix B

tetracycline (℞)

(tet-ra-sye′kleen)

Apo-Tetra ✱, Emtet, Nu-Tetra ✱, tetracycline HCl

Func. class.: Broad-spectrum antiinfective

Chem. class.: Tetracycline

Action: Inhibits protein synthesis and phosphorylation in microorganisms; bacteriostatic

Uses: Syphilis, *Chlamydia trachomatis,* gonorrhea, lymphogranuloma venereum; uncommon gram-positive, gram-negative organisms; rickettsial infections

DOSAGE AND ROUTES

Susceptible gram-positive/gram-negative infections

- *Adult:* **PO** 250-500 mg q6hr
- *Child >8 yr:* **PO** 25-50 mg/kg/day in divided doses q6hr

Chlamydia trachomatis

- *Adult:* **PO** 500 mg qid × 7 days

Syphilis

- *Adult and adolescent:* **PO** 500 mg qid × 2 wk; if syphilis duration >1 yr, must treat 30 days

Brucellosis

- *Adult:* **PO** 500 mg q6hr × 3 wk with **IM** 1 g streptomycin bid × 1st wk, then daily × 2nd wk

***Urethral, endocervical, rectal infections* (C. trachomatis)**

- *Adult:* **PO** 500 mg qid × 7 days

Acne

- *Adult and adolescent:* **PO** 250 mg q6hr, then 125-500 mg/day or every other day

Renal dose

- *Adult:* **PO** CCr 51-90 ml/min give dose q8-12hr; CCr 10-50 ml/min give dose q12-24hr; CCr <10 ml/min give dose q24hr

Available forms: Oral susp 125 mg/5 ml; caps 250, 500 mg

SIDE EFFECTS

CNS: Fever, headache, paresthesia

CV: Pericarditis

EENT: Dysphagia, glossitis, decreased calcification, discoloration of deciduous teeth, oral candidiasis, oral ulcers

GI: *Nausea,* abdominal pain, *vomiting, diarrhea,* anorexia, enterocolitis, **hepatotoxicity,** flatulence, abdominal cramps, epigastric burning, stomatitis, **hepatitis, pseudomembranous colitis**

GU: *Increased BUN,* **azotemia, acute renal failure**

HEMA: **Eosinophilia, neutropenia, thrombocytopenia, leukocytosis, hemolytic anemia**

INTEG: *Rash, urticaria, photosensitivity, increased pigmentation,* **exfoliative dermatitis,** pruritus, **angioedema, Stevens-Johnson syndrome**

MISC: Increased ICP, candidiasis

Contraindications: Pregnancy (D), breastfeeding, children <8 yr, hypersensitivity to tetracyclines

Precautions: Renal/hepatic disease, UV exposure

PHARMACOKINETICS

PO: Peak 2-3 hr; duration 6 hr; half-life 6-12 hr; excreted in urine, breast milk; crosses placenta; 65% protein bound

INTERACTIONS

- Nephrotoxicity: methoxyflurane

Increase: effect of warfarin, digoxin

Decrease: effect of tetracycline—antacids, $NaHCO_3$, dairy products, alkali products, iron, cimetidine

Decrease: effect of penicillins, oral contraceptives

Drug/Herb

- Do not use acidophilus with antiinfectives; separate by several hours
- Photosensitivity: dong quai

Drug/Lab Test

False increase: urinary catecholamines

NURSING CONSIDERATIONS

Assess:

- Signs of anemia: Hct, Hgb, fatigue
- I&O ratio
- Blood studies: PT, CBC, AST, ALT, BUN, creatinine
- Allergic reactions: rash, itching, pruritus, angioedema
- Nausea, vomiting, diarrhea; administer antiemetic, antacids as ordered
- Overgrowth of infection: fever, malaise, redness, pain, swelling, drainage, perineal itching, diarrhea, changes in cough or sputum

Administer:

- After C&S obtained
- 2 hr before or after iron products; hr after antacid products
- Should be given on an empty stomach

Perform/provide:

- Storage in tight, light-resistant container at room temperature

Evaluate:

- Therapeutic response: decreased temp, absence of lesions, negative C&S

Teach patient/family:

- To avoid sun exposure; sunscreen does not seem to decrease photosensitivity
- That all prescribed medication must be taken to prevent superinfection
- To avoid milk products, antacids, or separate by 2 hr; take with a full glass of water
- That tooth discoloration may occur

tetrahydrozoline nasal agent

See Appendix B

tetrahydrozoline ophthalmic

See Appendix B

theophylline (℞)

(thee-off'i-lin)

Accurbron, Aquaphyllin, Asmalix, Bronkodyl, Elixomin, Elixophyllin, Lanophyllin, Quibron-T Dividose, Quibron-T/SR Dividose, Respbid, Slo-bid Gyrocaps, Slo-Phyllin, Sustaire, Theo-24, Theobid Duracaps, Theochron, Theoclear-80, Theoclear L.A., Theo-Dur, Theolair-SR, Theo-Sav, Theospan-SR, Theostat 80, Theovent, Theo-X, T-Phyl, Uni-Dur, Uniphyl

Func. class.: Bronchodilator

Chem. class.: Methylxanthine

Action: Relaxes smooth muscle of respiratory system by blocking phosphodiesterase, which increases cAMP, exact action unknown

Uses: Bronchial asthma, bronchospasm of COPD, chronic bronchitis, emphysema

DOSAGE AND ROUTES

Acute exacerbations of reversible airway obstruction

• *Adult:* **PO** 5 mg/kg loading dose over 20-30 min

COPD, chronic bronchitis

• *Adult:* **IV** 0.4 mg/kg/hr in nonsmokers or 0.7 mg/kg/hr in smokers

• *Adult/child >45 kg maintenance:* **PO** 10 mg/kg/day in divided doses q1-8hr, max 300 mg/day

Apnea of prematurity

• *Neonate:* **IV** 4 mg/kg over 20-30 min, then maintenance

• *Neonate ≥24 days:* **IV/PO** 1.5 mg/kg q12hr

Available forms: Caps 50, 100, 200, 250 mg; tabs 100, 125, 200, 225, 250, 300 mg; time rel tabs 100, 200, 250, 300, 400, 500 mg; time rel caps 50, 65, 100, 125, 130, 200, 250, 260, 300, 400, 500 mg; elix 80, 11.25 mg/15 ml; sol 80 mg/15 ml; liquid 80, 150, 160 mg/15 ml; susp 300 mg/15 ml

SIDE EFFECTS

*CNS: **Anxiety, restlessness, insomnia, dizziness,*** **seizures,** headache, lightheadedness, muscle twitching, tremors

*CV: **Palpitations, sinus tachycardia,*** hypotension, **dysrhythmias,** fluid retention with tachycardia

ENDO: Hyperglycemia

*GI: **Nausea, vomiting, anorexia,*** diarrhea, bitter taste, dyspepsia, gastric distress

INTEG: Flushing, urticaria

MISC: SIADH, urinary frequency

RESP: Increased rate, tachypnea

Contraindications: Hypersensitivity to xanthines, tachydysrhythmias

Precautions: Pregnancy (C), children, geriatric patients, CHF, cor pulmonale, hepatic disease, active peptic ulcer disease, diabetes mellitus, hyperthyroidism, hypertension, seizure disorder

PHARMACOKINETICS

Metabolized in liver, excreted in urine and breast milk, crosses placenta, protein binding 40%, terminal half-life 6.5-10.5 hr

PO: Peak 1-2 hr

SOL: Peak 1 hr

INTERACTIONS

• Cardiotoxicity: β-blockers

Increase: theophylline action—cimetidine, propranolol, erythromycin, oral contraceptives, influenza vaccine, fluoroquinlones, mexiletine, corticosteroids, disulfiram, fluvoxamine, interferons

Increase: effects of anticoagulants

Decrease: theophylline level—phenytoin, phenobarbital, carbamazepine, rifampin, smoking

Decrease: effect of lithium

T

Drug/Herb
• Toxicity: ephedra (ma huang), cola nut, guarana, yerba maté, tea (black, green), coffee
Decrease: theophylline levels—St. John's wort

NURSING CONSIDERATIONS

Assess:
⚠ Theophylline blood levels (therapeutic level is 5-15 mcg/ml); toxicity may occur with small increase above 20 mcg/ml
• Monitor I&O; diuresis occurs; geriatric patients or children may be dehydrated
• Signs of toxicity: irritability, insomnia, restlessness, tremors, nausea, vomiting
• Respiratory rate, rhythm, depth; auscultate lung fields bilaterally; notify prescriber of abnormalities
• Allergic reactions: rash, urticaria; product should be discontinued

Administer:
• Do not break, crush, chew, or dissolve time-release products
• PO with 8 oz of water for GI symptoms; avoid food; absorption may be affected; take dose consistently; do not take Theo-24 with meals
• Contents of bead-filled capsule sprinkled over food for children's use
• Check OTC medications, current prescriptions for ephedrine, which will increase stimulation

IV route
• Loading dose over 20-30 min, max 20-25 mg/min; do not give by rapid IV, use only cont inf

Additive compatibilities: Cefepime, chlorproMAZINE, fluconazole, furosemide, hydrocortisone, lidocaine, methylprednisolone, verapamil

Y-site compatibilities: Acyclovir, ampicillin, ampicillin/sulbactam, aztreonam, cefazolin, cefotetan, ceftazidime, ceftriaxone, cimetidine, cisatracurium, clindamycin, dexamethasone, diltiazem, DOBUTamine, DOPamine, doxycycline, erythromycin, famotidine, fluconazole, gentamicin, haloperidol, heparin, hydrocortisone, lidocaine, methyldopate, methylPREDNISolone, metronidazole, midazolam, nafcillin, nitroglycerin, penicillin G potassium, piperacillin, potassium chloride, ranitidine, remifentanil, sodium nitroprusside, ticarcillin, ticarcillin/clavulanate, tobramycin, vancomycin

Evaluate:
• Therapeutic response: ability to breathe more easily

Teach patient/family:
• To check OTC medications, current prescription medications for ephedrine, which will increase stimulation; to avoid alcohol, caffeine
• To avoid hazardous activities; dizziness may occur
• That if GI upset occurs, to take product with 8 oz H_2O; avoid food; take at same time of day; absorption may be decreased
• To notify prescriber of toxicity: nausea, vomiting, anxiety, insomnia, seizures
• To notify prescriber of change in smoking habit; dosage may have to be changed

thiamine (vit B_1)

(PO-OTC; IV, IM-℞)
Betalin S, Betaxin 🍁, Biamine, Revitonus, Thiamilate, thiamine HCl
Func. class.: Vit B_1
Chem. class.: Water soluble

Do not confuse:
thiamine/Tenormin

Action: Needed for pyruvate metabolism, carbohydrate metabolism

Uses: Vit B_1 deficiency or polyneuritis, cheilosis adjunct with thiamine beriberi, Wernicke-Korsakoff syndrome, pellagra, metabolic disorders, alcoholism

DOSAGE AND ROUTES

RDA
• *Adult:* **PO** (Males) 1.2-1.5 mg; (females) 1.1 mg; (pregnancy) 1.4 mg; (breastfeeding) 1.4 mg
• *Child 9-13 yr:* **PO** 0.9 mg
• *Child 4-8 yr:* **PO** 0.6 mg

- *Child 1-3 yr:* **PO** 0.5 mg
- *Infant 7 mo-1 yr:* **PO** 0.3 mg
- *Neonate and infant to 6 mo:* **PO** 0.2 mg

Beriberi

- *Adult:* **PO** 5-30 mg daily or given in 3 divided doses × 1 mo; **IM/IV** 5-30 mg daily or divided in 3 doses, then convert to **PO**
- *Infant/child:* **PO** 10-50 mg daily × 2 wk, then 5-10 mg daily × 1 mo; **IV/IM** 10-25 mg/day × 2 wk, then 5-10 mg daily × 1 mo

Available forms: Tabs 50, 100, 250, 500 mg; inj 100 mg/ml; enteric coated tabs 20 mg

SIDE EFFECTS

CNS: Weakness, restlessness
CV: **Collapse, pulmonary edema,** hypotension
EENT: Tightness of throat
GI: Hemorrhage, *nausea, diarrhea*
INTEG: **Angioneurotic edema,** cyanosis, sweating, warmth
SYST: **Anaphylaxis**
Contraindications: Hypersensitivity
Precautions: Pregnancy (A)

PHARMACOKINETICS

PO/INJ: Unused amounts excreted in urine (unchanged)

NURSING CONSIDERATIONS

Assess:

- Nutritional status: yeast, beef, liver, whole or enriched grains, legumes

Administer:

IM route

- By IM inj; rotate sites if pain and inflammation occur; do not mix with alkaline sols; Z-track to minimize pain

IV route

- Undiluted over 5 min or diluted with IV sol and given as an inf at 100 mg or less/5 min or more

Syringe compatibilities: Doxapram
Y-site compatibilities: Famotidine

Perform/provide:

- Storage in tight, light-resistant container
- Application of cold to help decrease pain

Evaluate:

- Therapeutic response: absence of nausea, vomiting, anorexia, insomnia, tachycardia, paresthesias, depression, muscle weakness

Teach patient/family:

- The necessary foods to be included in diet: yeast, beef, liver, legumes, whole grain

thiethylperazine (℞)

(thye-eth-il-per′a-zeen)
Norzine, Torecan
Func. class.: Antiemetic
Chem. class.: Phenothiazine, piperazine derivative

Do not confuse:
Torecan/Toradol

Action: Acts centrally by blocking chemoreceptor trigger zone, which in turn acts on vomiting center; DOPamine blocker

Uses: Nausea, vomiting

DOSAGE AND ROUTES

- *Adult:* **PO/IM** 10 mg daily-tid

Available forms: Tabs 10 mg; inj 5 mg/ml

SIDE EFFECTS

CNS: Euphoria, depression, restlessness, tremor, EPS, **seizures,** drowsiness, confusion, **neuroleptic malignant syndrome**
CV: **Circulatory failure, tachycardia,** postural hypotension, ECG changes
GI: Nausea, vomiting, anorexia, dry mouth, diarrhea, constipation, weight loss, metallic taste, cramps
GU: Urinary retention, dark urine
HEMA: **Agranulocytosis, leukopenia**
RESP: **Respiratory depression**
Contraindications: Pregnancy (X); coma; seizure; encephalopathy; bone marrow depression; hypersensitivity to phe-

T

nothiazines, sulfites (inj), tartrazine (tabs)

Precautions: Breastfeeding, children <2 yr, geriatric patients, Parkinson's disease

PHARMACOKINETICS

PO: Onset 45-60 min

RECT: Onset 45-60 min; metabolized by liver; crosses placenta; excreted in urine, breast milk

INTERACTIONS

• Avoid use with phenothiazines; seizures may occur

Increase: anticholinergic action—anticholinergics, antiparkinson products, tricyclics

Increase: sedation—barbiturates, general anesthetics, ethanol, anxiolytics, sedatives, hypnotics, benzodiazepines, opiate agonists

Decrease: effect of thiethylperazine—barbiturates, antacids

NURSING CONSIDERATIONS

Assess:

• VS, B/P; check patients with cardiac disease more often

⚠ For neuroleptic malignant syndrome: dyspnea, fever, seizures, diaphoresis, fatigue, loss of urinary control, tachycardia; have emergency equipment nearby

• Respiratory status before, during, after administration of emetic; check rate, rhythm, character; respiratory depression can occur rapidly with geriatric or debilitated patients

Administer:

• IM inj in large muscle mass; aspirate to avoid IV administration; patient should remain recumbent 1 hr after inj

Syringe compatibilities: Butorphanol, hydromorphone, midazolam, ranitidine

Y-site compatibilities: Aldesleukin

Evaluate:

• Therapeutic response: absence of nausea, vomiting

Teach patient/family:

• To avoid hazardous activities, activities requiring alertness; dizziness may occur

⚠ High Alert

thiopental (℞)

(thye-oh-pen′tal)

Pentothal, thiopental sodium

Func. class.: General anesthetic

Chem. class.: Barbiturate

Controlled Substance Schedule III

Action: Increases membrane ion conduction to chloride, decreases depolarization due to glutamate and increases in GABA

Uses: Short, general anesthesia; narcoanalysis, induction anesthesia before other anesthetics, status epilepticus, increased intracranial pressure

Unlabeled uses: Reduction of intracranial pressure in head trauma

DOSAGE AND ROUTES

Induction and anesthesia

• *Adult:* **IV** 25-75 mg test dose, observe for 60 min; initial dose 50-100 mg given at 20-40 sec interval; additional 25-50 mg as needed

• *Child 1-12 yr:* **IV** 5-6 mg/kg over 10-60 min, maintenance 1 mg/kg as needed

• *Infant:* **IV** 5-8 mg/kg over 10-60 min

• *Neonate:* **IV** 3-4 mg over 10-60 min

Rapid induction

• *Adult:* **IV** 210-280 mg or 3-5 mg/kg in 2-4 divided doses

• *Child:* **IV** 3-5 mg/kg over 20-30 sec, then 1 mg/kg as needed

Narcoanalysis

• *Adult:* **IV** 100 mg/min, max 50 ml/min

Sedation or narcosis

• *Adult:* **RECT** 30 mg/kg

Reduction of intracranial pressure in neurosurgery

• *Adult:* **IV BOL** 1.5-3.5 mg/kg

Reduction of intracranial pressure in head trauma, mechanically ventilated patients only (unlableled)

• *Adult and child:* **IV BOL** Loading dose 10-20 mg/kg, then **CONT IV INF** 3-5 mg/kg/hr

Available forms: Powder for inj 2%, 2.5% (20 mg/ml, 25 mg/ml)

SIDE EFFECTS

CNS: Retrograde amnesia, prolonged somnolence
CV: Tachycardia, hypotension, **myocardial depression, dysrhythmias**
EENT: Sneezing, coughing
INTEG: Chills, *shivering,* necrosis, *pain at inj site*
MISC: **Hemolytic anemia (rare)**
MS: Muscle irritability
RESP: **Respiratory depression, bronchospasm**

Contraindications: Hypersensitivity, status asthmaticus, porphyrias

Precautions: Pregnancy (C), severe CV disease, renal/hepatic disease, hypotension, myxedema, myasthenia gravis, asthma, increased intracranial pressure

PHARMACOKINETICS

IV: Onset 30-60 sec, duration 4-15 min, terminal half-life 3-8 hr, crosses placenta

INTERACTIONS

- Do not use with voriconazole

Increase: hypotension—MAOIs
Increase: action—CNS depressants, probenecid

Drug/Herb

Increase: CNS depression—kava, St. John's wort

NURSING CONSIDERATIONS

Assess:

- VS q3-5min during IV administration, after dose, q4hr postoperatively
- Extravasation; if it occurs, apply moist heat and 1% procaine to affected area
- Dysrhythmias or myocardial depression

Administer:

- Only with crash cart, resuscitative equipment nearby

Intermittent IV INF route

- Dilute to 20-50 mg/ml; give by slow injection over 20-30 sec; max 25 mg/min

CONT IV INF route

- Dilute to 2-4 mg/ml

Additive compatibilities: Chloramphenicol, hydrocortisone sodium succinate, oxytocin, pentobarbital, phenobarbital, potassium chloride, sodium bicarbonate

Solution compatibilities: D_5/0.45% NaCl, D_5W, multiple electrolyte sol, 0.45% NaCl, 0.9% NaCl, 1/6 M sodium lactate

Syringe compatibilities: Aminophylline, hyaluronidase, hydrocortisone sodium succinate, neostigmine, pentobarbital, propofol, scopolamine, tubocurarine

Y-site compatibilities: Doxacurium, fentanyl, heparin, milrinone, mivacurium, nitroglycerin, ranitidine, remifentanil

Evaluate:

- Therapeutic response: maintenance of anesthesia

thioridazine (℞)

(thye-or-rid'a-zeen)
Apo-Thioridazine ♣,
Novo-Ridazine ♣,
PMS-Thioridazine ♣,
thioridazine HCl
Func. class.: Antipsychotic, neuroleptic
Chem. class.: Phenothiazine piperidine

Do not confuse:
thioridazine/thiothixene

Action: Depresses cerebral cortex, hypothalamus, limbic system, which control activity, aggression; blocks neurotransmission produced by DOPamine at synapse; exhibits strong α-adrenergic and anticholinergic blocking action; mechanism for antipsychotic effects is unclear

Uses: Psychotic disorders, schizophrenia, behavioral problems in children, anxiety, major depressive disorders, organic brain syndrome

Unlabeled uses: Behavioral symptoms associated with dementia in geriatric patients

T

DOSAGE AND ROUTES

Psychosis

• *Adult:* **PO** 25-100 mg tid, max 800 mg/day; dose is gradually increased to desired response, then reduced to minimum maintenance

Depression/behavioral problems/organic brain syndrome

• *Adult:* **PO** 25 mg tid, range from 10 mg bid-qid to 50 mg tid-qid, max 800 mg/day for short period

• *Geriatric:* **PO** 10-25 mg daily-bid, increase 4-7 days by 10-25 mg to desired dose, max 300 mg/day for short period

• *Child 2-12 yr:* **PO** 0.5-3 mg/kg/day in divided doses, max 3 mg/kg/day

Available forms: Tabs 10, 15, 25, 50, 100, 150, 200 mg

SIDE EFFECTS

CNS: EPS: pseudoparkinsonism, akathisia, dystonia, tardive dyskinesia, **seizures,** *headache,* confusion, **neuroleptic malignant syndrome,** dizziness, drowsiness

CV: Orthostatic hypotension, **cardiac arrest,** ECG changes, **tachycardia, QT prolongation, torsade de pointes**

EENT: Blurred vision, glaucoma, dry eyes

GI: Dry mouth, nausea, vomiting, anorexia, constipation, diarrhea, jaundice, weight gain

GU: Urinary retention, urinary frequency, enuresis, impotence, amenorrhea, gynecomastia, ejaculation dysfunction, priapism

HEMA: Anemia, **leukopenia, leukocytosis, agranulocytosis**

INTEG: Rash, photosensitivity, dermatitis

RESP: **Laryngospasm,** dyspnea, **respiratory depression**

Contraindications: Children <2 yr, hypersensitivity, coma, CNS depression

Black Box Warning: QT prolongation, cardiac dysrhythmias

Precautions: Pregnancy (C), breastfeeding, seizure disorders, hypertension, hepatic/pulmonary disease, renal failure, BPH, glaucoma, phenothiazine hypersensitivity, suicidal ideation, smoking, Reye's syndrome, Parkinson's disease

Black Box Warning: Cardiac disease, dementia, AV block, bundle-branch block, torsade de pointes

PHARMACOKINETICS

PO: Onset erratic; peak 2-4 hr; metabolized by liver; excreted in urine, breast milk; crosses placenta; half-life 26-36 hr; 91%-99% protein binding

INTERACTIONS

• Oversedation: other CNS depressants, alcohol, barbiturate anesthetics

Increase: anticholinergic effects—anticholinergics

Increase: levels of this product—CYP2D6 inhibitors

Decrease: levels of this product—CYP2D6 inducers

Decrease: antiparkinson's agent effects

Decrease: thioridazine effect—lithium, barbiturates

Decrease: antihypertensive effect—centrally acting antihypertensives

Decrease: absorption—aluminum hydroxide, magnesium hydroxide antacids

Drug/Herb

Increase: CNS depression—kava, St. John's wort, valerian

Increase: EPS—betel palm, kava

Increase: effect—cola tree, hops, nettle, nutmeg

Drug/Lab Test

Increase: LFTs, cardiac enzymes, cholesterol, blood glucose, prolactin, bilirubin, PBI, cholinesterase, ^{131}I

Decrease: hormones (blood, urine)

False positive: pregnancy test, PKU

False negative: urinary steroid, pregnancy test

NURSING CONSIDERATIONS

Assess:

• Mental status before first dose

• Swallowing of PO medication; check for hoarding or giving of medication to other patients

- I&O ratio; palpate bladder if low urinary output occurs, urinary retention may be the cause
- Bilirubin, CBC, LFTs q mo
- Urinalysis is recommended before and during prolonged therapy
- Affect, orientation, LOC, reflexes, gait, coordination, sleep pattern disturbances
- B/P standing and lying; also include pulse and respirations q4hr during initial treatment; establish baseline before starting treatment; report drops of 30 mm Hg
- Dizziness, faintness, palpitations, tachycardia on rising
- EPS including akathisia (inability to sit still, no pattern to movements), tardive dyskinesia (bizarre movements of jaw, mouth, tongue, extremities), pseudoparkinsonism (rigidity, tremors, pill rolling, shuffling gait)

⚠ For neuroleptic malignant syndrome: altered mental status, muscle rigidity, increased CPK, hyperthermia, dyspnea, fatigue

- Skin turgor daily
- Constipation, urinary retention daily; increase bulk, water in diet

Administer:

- Antiparkinsonian agent on order from prescriber for EPS
- Avoid use with CNS depressants
- Antacids separated by 2 hr or more

Perform/provide:

- Decreased sensory input by dimming lights, avoiding loud noises
- Supervised ambulation until stabilized on medication if needed; do not involve in strenuous exercise program because fainting is possible; patient should not stand still for long periods
- Increased fluids to prevent constipation
- Sips of water, candy, gum for dry mouth
- Storage in tight, light-resistant container; avoid contact with skin

Evaluate:

- Therapeutic response: decrease in emotional excitement, hallucinations, delusions, paranoia, reorganization of patterns of thought, speech

Teach patient/family:

- That orthostatic hypotension occurs frequently, to rise from sitting or lying position gradually; to avoid hazardous activities until stabilized on medication
- To avoid hot tubs, hot showers, tub baths; hypotension may occur
- To avoid abrupt withdrawal of thioridazine, or EPS may result; product should be withdrawn slowly
- To avoid OTC preparations (cough, hay fever, cold) unless approved by prescriber; serious product interactions may occur; avoid use with alcohol; increased drowsiness may occur
- To use sunscreen to prevent burns
- About compliance with product regimen
- About the necessity for meticulous oral hygiene, since oral candidiasis may occur
- To report sore throat, malaise, fever, bleeding, mouth sores; if these occur, CBC should be drawn and product discontinued; may cause vision impairment, report to prescriber
- That in hot weather, heat stroke may occur; take extra precautions to stay cool
- May cause discoloration of urine

Treatment of overdose: Lavage if orally ingested, provide an airway; do not induce vomiting, CV monitoring, continuous ECG

thyroid USP (desiccated) (℞)

(thye′roid)

Armour Thyroid, Bio-Throid, Nature Thyroid, Thyroid Strong, Westhroid

Func. class.: Thyroid hormone

Chem. class.: Active thyroid hormone in natural state and ratio

Action: Increases metabolic rates, increases cardiac output, O_2 consumption, body temp, blood volume, growth, development at cellular level

T

Uses: Hypothyroidism, cretinism (juvenile hypothyroidism), myxedema

DOSAGE AND ROUTES

Hypothyroidism

- *Adult:* **PO** 60-65 mg/day, increased by 30 mg q mo until desired response; maintenance dose 60-120 mg/day
- *Geriatric:* **PO** 7.5-15 mg/day, increase dose q6-8wk until desired response

Cretinism/juvenile hypothyroidism

- *Child:* **PO** 15 mg/day, then 30 mg/day after 2 wk, then 60 mg/day after another 2 wk; maintenance dose 60-180 mg/day

Myxedema

- *Adult:* **PO** 15 mg/day, double dose q2wk, maintenance 60-180 mg/day

Available forms: Tabs 16, 32, 60, 65, 98, 130, 195, 260, 325 mg; enteric coated tabs 32, 65, 130 mg; sugarcoated tabs 32, 65, 130, 195 mg; caps 65, 130, 195, 325 mg

SIDE EFFECTS

CNS: Insomnia, tremors, headache, **thyroid storm**

CV: Tachycardia, palpitations, angina, dysrhythmias, hypertension, **cardiac arrest**

GI: Nausea, diarrhea, increased or decreased appetite, cramps

MISC: Menstrual irregularities, weight loss, sweating, heat intolerance, fever

Contraindications: Adrenal insufficiency, MI, thyrotoxicosis, porcine protein hypersensitivity

Black Box Warning: Obesity treatment

Precautions: Pregnancy (A), breastfeeding, geriatric patients, angina pectoris, hypertension, ischemia, cardiac disease

PHARMACOKINETICS

PO: Peak 12-48 hr, half-life 6-7 days

INTERACTIONS

Increase: effects of anticoagulants, sympathomimetics, tricyclics, catecholamines

Decrease: thyroid absorption—bile acid sequestrants, aluminum, magnesium, calcium

Decrease: effects of digoxin, insulin, hypoglycemics

Decrease: thyroid effects—estrogens

Drug/Herb

Decrease: thyroid effect—agar, bugleweed, carnitine, kelpware, soy, spirulina

Drug/Lab Test

Increase: CPK, LDH, AST, PBI, blood glucose

Decrease: thyroid function tests

NURSING CONSIDERATIONS

Assess:

- B/P, pulse before each dose
- I&O ratio
- Weight daily in same clothing, using same scale, at same time of day
- Height, growth rate of child
- T_3, T_4, which are decreased; radioimmunoassay of TSH, which is increased; radio uptake, which is decreased if dosage is too low
- PT may require decreased anticoagulant; check for bleeding, bruising
- Increased nervousness, excitability, irritability; may indicate too high dose of medication, usually after 1-3 wk of treatment
- Cardiac status: angina, palpitation, chest pain, change in VS

Administer:

- In AM if possible as a single dose to decrease sleeplessness; separate iron, calcium products by 4 hr
- At same time each day to maintain product level
- Only for hormone imbalances; not to be used for obesity, male infertility, menstrual disorders, lethargy
- Lowest dose that relieves symptoms

Perform/provide:

- Removal of medication 4 wk before RAIU test

Evaluate:

- Therapeutic response: absence of depression; increased weight loss, diuresis, pulse, appetite; absence of constipation, peripheral edema, cold intolerance; pale, cool, dry skin; brittle nails, alopecia, coarse hair, menorrhagia, night blindness, paresthesias, syncope, stupor, coma, rosy cheeks

Teach patient/family:

- That hair loss will occur in child, is temporary
- To report excitability, irritability, anxiety; indicates overdose
- Not to switch brands unless directed by prescriber
- That strong odor is normal
- That hypothyroid child will show almost immediate behavior/personality change
- That treatment drug is not to be taken to reduce weight
- To avoid OTC preparations with iodine; read labels
- To separate iron, calcium products by 4 hr
- To avoid iodine food, iodized salt, soybeans, tofu, turnips, some seafood, some bread

tiagabine (℞)

(tie-ah-ga'been)

Gabitril

Func. class.: Anticonvulsant

Action: Inhibits reuptake and metabolism of GABA, may increase seizure threshold; structurally similar to GABA; tiagabine binding sites in neocortex, hippocampus

Uses: Adjunct treatment of partial seizures in adults and children ≥12 yr

DOSAGE AND ROUTES

When not given with a CYP3A4 enzyme, effect of tiagabine is doubled; lower doses are indicated

- *Adult:* **PO** 4 mg/day in divided doses, may increase by 4-8 mg q wk until desired response, max 56 mg/day
- *Child 12-18 yr:* **PO** 4 mg/day, may increase by 4 mg at beginning of wk 2; may increase by 4-8 mg q wk until desired response; max 32 mg/day

Available forms: Tabs 2, 4, 12, 16 mg

SIDE EFFECTS

CNS: Dizziness, anxiety, somnolence, ataxia, confusion, *asthenia,* unsteady gait, depression, **suicidal ideation**

CV: Vasodilation

GI: Nausea, vomiting, diarrhea, increased appetite

INTEG: Pruritus, rash, **Stevens-Johnson syndrome**

RESP: Pharyngitis, coughing

Contraindications: Hypersensitivity

Precautions: Pregnancy (C), breastfeeding, children <12 yr, geriatric patients, renal/hepatic disease, suicidal ideation/behavior, status epilepticus, mania, bipolar disorder, abrupt discontinuation, depression

PHARMACOKINETICS

Absorption >95%, peak 45 min, protein binding 96%, metabolized in the liver via CYP3A4; half-life 7-9 hr without enzyme inducers, 2-5 hr with enzyme inducers

INTERACTIONS

- Lower doses may be needed when used with valproate

Increase: CNS depression—CNS depressants

Decrease: tiagabine effect—sevelamer

Decrease: effect—carbamazepine, phenobarbital, phenytoin, primidone

Drug/Food

Decrease: rate of absorption—high-fat meal

NURSING CONSIDERATIONS

Assess:

- Renal studies: urinalysis, BUN, urine creatinine q3mo
- Hepatic studies: ALT, AST, bilirubin
- Description of seizures: location, duration, presence of aura

⚠ Mental status: mood, sensorium, affect, behavioral changes, suicidal thoughts/behaviors; if mental status changes, notify prescriber

Administer:

- With food

Perform/provide:

- Storage at room temperature away from heat and light
- Assistance with ambulation during early part of treatment; dizziness occurs
- Seizure precautions: padded side rails; move objects that may harm patient

Evaluate:

- Therapeutic response: decreased seizure activity; document on patient's chart

Teach patient/family:

- To carry emergency ID stating patient's name, products taken, condition, prescriber's name and phone number
- To avoid driving, other activities that require alertness
- Not to discontinue medication quickly after long-term use
- To take with food

Treatment of overdose: Lavage, VS

ticarcillin (℞)

(tye-kar-sill′in)

Ticar

Func. class.: Broad-spectrum antiinfective

Chem. class.: Extended-spectrum penicillin

Action: Cell wall lysis mediated by cell wall autolytic enzymes

Uses: Respiratory, soft tissue, urinary tract infections, bacterial septicemia; effective for gram-positive cocci *(Staphylococcus aureus, Streptococcus faecalis, Streptococcus pneumoniae)*, gram-negative cocci *(Neisseria gonorrhoeae)*, gram-positive bacilli *(Clostridium perfringens, Clostridium tetani)*, gram-negative bacilli *(Bacteroides, Fusobacterium nucleatum, Escherichia coli, Proteus mirabilis, Salmonella, Morganella morganii, Proteus rettgeri, Enterobacter, Pseudomonas aeruginosa, Serratia)*; and *Peptococcus, Peptostreptococcus, Eubacterium*

DOSAGE AND ROUTES

Bacterial septicemia, respiratory, skin, soft tissue, intraabdominal, reproductive infections

- *Adult:* **IV INF** 200-300 mg/kg/day in divided doses q4-6hr
- *Child <40 kg:* **IV INF** 33.3-50 mg/kg q4hr or 50-75 mg/kg q6hr

Urinary tract complicated infections

- *Adult and child:* **IV INF** 150-200 mg/kg/day in divided doses q4-6hr

Uncomplicated urinary infections

- *Adult:* **IV Direct/IM** 1 g q6hr
- *Child <40 kg:* **IV Direct/IM** 50-100 mg/kg/day q6-8hr

Severe infections

(Pseudomonas, Proteus, E. coli)

- *Neonate <2 kg:* **IM/IV** 75 mg/kg q8-12hr
- *Neonate >2 kg:* **IM/IV** 75-100 mg/kg q8hr

Renal/hepatic dose

- CCr >60 ml/min 3 g q4hr; CCr 30-60 ml/min 2 g q4hr; CCr 10-30 ml/min 2 g q8hr; CCr <10 ml/min 2 g q12hr or 1 g q6hr; CCr <10 ml/min and hepatic dysfunction 2 g q24hr or 1 g q12hr

Available forms: Inj 1, 3, 6, 20, 30 g

SIDE EFFECTS

CNS: Lethargy, hallucinations, anxiety, depression, twitching, **coma, seizures,** confusion

GI: Nausea, vomiting, diarrhea, increased AST/ALT, abdominal pain, glossitis, colitis, **pseudomembranous colitis, hepatotoxicity**

GU: Oliguria, proteinuria, hematuria, *vaginitis, moniliasis,* **glomerulonephritis**

HEMA: Anemia, increased bleeding time, **bone marrow depression, granulocytopenia**

INTEG: Rash, **Stevens-Johnson syndrome**

META: Hypokalemia

SYST: **Anaphylaxis**

Contraindications: Hypersensitivity to penicillins

Precautions: Pregnancy (B), breastfeeding, hypersensitivity to cephalosporins, renal/GI disease, diabetes, electrolyte imbalances

PHARMACOKINETICS

Small amount metabolized in liver; excreted in urine, breast milk

IM: Peak 1 hr, duration 4-6 hr

IV: Peak 30-45 min; duration 4 hr; half-life 70 min

INTERACTIONS

Increase: effect of neuromuscular blockers, anticoagulants, methotrexate

Increase: ticarcillin concentrations—aspirin, probenecid

Decrease: effect—oral contraceptives, erythromycins

Decrease: antimicrobial effect of ticarcillin—tetracyclines, aminoglycosides IV

Drug/Herb

- Do not use acidophilus with antiinfectives; separate by several hours

Drug/Lab Test

False positive: urine glucose, urine protein

NURSING CONSIDERATIONS

Assess:

- I&O ratio; report hematuria, oliguria, since penicillin in high doses is nephrotoxic

⚠ Any patient with compromised renal system, since product is excreted slowly in poor renal system function; toxicity may occur rapidly

⚠ For anaphylaxis: wheezing, rash, pruritus, laryngeal edema, keep emergency equipment nearby

- Hepatic studies: AST, ALT
- Blood studies: WBC, RBC, Hct, Hgb, bleeding time
- Renal tests: urinalysis, protein, blood, BUN, creatinine
- C&S before product therapy; product may be given as soon as culture is taken
- Bowel pattern before, during treatment
- Skin eruptions after administration of penicillin to 1 wk after discontinuing product
- Allergies before initiation of treatment, reaction of each medication

Administer:

- Product after C&S has been completed

IM route

- Inject into well-developed muscle
- Reconstitute ticarcillin 1 g/2 ml sterile water for inj, NaCl inj, 1% lidocaine HCl without epinephrine (385 mg/ml)

IV route

- After diluting 1 g or less/4 ml sterile H_2O for inj; dilute further with 10-20 ml or more D_5W, NS, or sterile H_2O for inj sol; give 1 g or less/5 min or more or by intermittent inf over ½-2 hr or by continuous inf at prescribed rate

Y-site compatibilities: Acyclovir, allopurinol, amifostine, aztreonam, cisatracurium, cyclophosphamide, diltiazem, DOXOrubicin, famotidine, filgrastim, fludarabine, granisetron, heparin, hydromorphone, IL-2, insulin (regular), magnesium sulfate, melphalan, meperidine, morphine, ondansetron, perphenazine, propofol, remifentanil, sargramostim, teniposide, theophylline, thiotepa, verapamil, vinorelbine

Perform/provide:

- Epinephrine, suction, tracheostomy set, endotracheal intubation equipment
- Adequate fluid intake (2 L) during diarrhea episodes
- Scratch test to assess allergy on order from prescriber; done when penicillin is only product of choice
- Storage at room temperature, reconstituted sol 72 hr at room temperature

Evaluate:

- Therapeutic response: absence of fever, purulent drainage, redness, inflammation

Teach patient/family:

- That culture may be taken after completed course of medication
- To report sore throat, fever, fatigue (may indicate superinfection); CNS effects (anxiety, depression, hallucinations, seizures)

T

• To wear or carry emergency ID if allergic to penicillins
• To notify nurse of diarrhea

Treatment of overdose: Withdraw product, maintain airway, administer epinephrine, aminophylline, O_2, IV corticosteroids for anaphylaxis

ticarcillin/clavulanate (℞)

Timentin

Func. class.: Broad-spectrum antiinfective

Chem. class.: Extended-spectrum penicillin

Action: Interferes with cell wall replication of susceptible organisms; osmotically unstable cell wall swells, bursts from osmotic pressure; clavulanate inhibits β-lactamase and protects against enzymatic degradation of ticarcillin

Uses: Respiratory, soft tissue, and urinary tract infections, bacterial septicemia; effective for gram-positive cocci *(Staphylococcus aureus, Streptococcus faecalis, Streptococcus pneumoniae)*, gram-negative cocci *(Neisseria gonorrhoeae)*, gram-positive bacilli *(Clostridium perfringens, Clostridium tetani)*, gram-negative bacilli *(Bacteroides, Fusobacterium nucleatum, Escherichia coli, Proteus mirabilis, Salmonella, Morganella morganii, Proteus rettgeri, Enterobacter, Pseudomonas aeruginosa, Serratia)*; and *Peptococcus, Peptostreptococcus, Eubacterium*

DOSAGE AND ROUTES

Systemic/urinary tract infections, moderate/severe infections

• *Adult ≥60 kg:* **IV INF** 3.1 g q4-6hr
• *Adult <60 kg:* **IV INF** 200-300 mg/kg/day q4-6hr
• *Child >60 kg:* **IV INF** 3.1 g q4hr
• *Child <60 kg:* **IV INF** 300 mg/kg/day q4hr

Mild/moderate infections

• *Child ≥60 kg:* **IV INF** 3.1 g q6hr
• *Child <60 kg:* **IV INF** 200 mg/kg/day q6hr

Renal dose

• *Adult:* **IV INF** Loading dose 3.1 g; CCr 60 ml/min 3.1 g q4hr; CCr 30-60 ml/min 2 g q4hr; CCr 10-30 ml/min 2 g q8hr; CCr <10 ml/min 2 g q12hr; CCr <10 ml/min with hepatic dysfunction 2 g q24hr

Available forms: Inj 3 g ticarcillin, 0.1 g clavulanate; IV inf 3 g ticarcillin, 0.1 g clavulanate; powder for inj 3 g ticarcillin, 0.1 g clavulanate

SIDE EFFECTS

CNS: Lethargy, hallucinations, anxiety, depression, twitching, **coma, seizures,** confusion, drowsiness

GI: *Nausea, vomiting, diarrhea;* increased AST, ALT; abdominal pain, glossitis, colitis, **pseudomembranous colitis, hepatotoxicity**

GU: Oliguria, proteinuria, hematuria, *vaginitis, moniliasis,* **glomerulonephritis**

HEMA: Anemia, increased bleeding time, **bone marrow depression, granulocytopenia**

INTEG: Rash, urticaria, **toxic epidermal necrolysis**

META: Hyperkalemia, hypokalemia, alkalosis, hypernatremia

SYST: **Anaphylaxis, Stevens-Johnson syndrome**

Contraindications: Neonates, hypersensitivity to penicillins

Precautions: Pregnancy (B), hypersensitivity to cephalosporins, renal disease

PHARMACOKINETICS

IV: Peak 30-45 min, duration 4 hr, half-life 64-68 min, excreted in urine

INTERACTIONS

⚠ ***Increase:*** bleeding—anticoagulants

Increase: methotrexate level—methotrexate

Increase: ticarcillin concentrations—probenecid, sulfipyrazone

Decrease: antimicrobial effect of ticarcillin—tetracyclines, aminoglycosides IV, chloramphenicol, macrolides, sulfonamides
Decrease: effect—oral contraceptives, erythromycin
Drug/Herb
• Do not use acidophilus with antiinfectives; separate by several hours
Drug/Lab Test
False positive: urine glucose, urine protein, Coombs' test

NURSING CONSIDERATIONS

Assess:
• I&O ratio; report hematuria, oliguria, since penicillin in high doses is nephrotoxic
⚠ For pseudomembranous colitis; Stevens-Johnson syndrome
⚠ Any patient with compromised renal system, since product is excreted slowly in poor renal system function; toxicity may occur rapidly
⚠ For anaphylaxis: wheezing, rash, laryngeal edema; have emergency equipment nearby
• Hepatic studies: AST, ALT
• Blood studies: WBC, RBC, Hct, Hgb, bleeding time
• Renal studies: urinalysis, protein, blood, BUN, creatinine
• C&S before product therapy; product may be given as soon as culture is taken
• Bowel pattern before, during treatment
• Skin eruptions after administration of penicillin to 1 wk after discontinuing product
• Allergies before initiation of treatment, reaction of each medication
Administer:
• Product after C&S
IV route
• After diluting 3.1 g or less/13 ml of sterile H_2O or NaCl (200 mg/ml), shake; may further dilute in 50-100 ml or more NS, D_5W, or LR sol and run over ½ hr
Y-site compatibilities: Allopurinol, amifostine, aztreonam, cefepime, cyclophosphamide, diltiazem, DOXOrubicin liposome, famotidine, filgrastim, fluconazole, fludarabine, foscarnet, gallium, granisetron, heparin, insulin (regular), melphalan, meperidine, morphine, ondansetron, perphenazine, propofol, remifentanil, sargramostim, teniposide, theophylline, thiotepa, vinorelbine
Perform/provide:
• Epinephrine, suction, tracheostomy set, endotracheal intubation equipment
• Adequate fluid intake (2 L) during diarrhea episodes
• Scratch test to assess allergy on order from prescriber; usually done when penicillin is only product of choice
• Storage of reconstituted sol 12-24 hr at room temperature, or 3-7 days refrigerated
Evaluate:
• Therapeutic response: absence of fever, purulent drainage, redness, inflammation
Teach patient/family:
• To report persistent diarrhea
• That culture may be taken after completed course of medication
• To report sore throat, fever, fatigue (may indicate superinfection); CNS effects (anxiety, depression, hallucinations, seizures)
• To wear or carry emergency ID if allergic to penicillins
• To use alternate birth control method
Treatment of overdose: Withdraw product, maintain airway, administer epinephrine, O_2, IV corticosteroids for anaphylaxis

ticlopidine (℞)

(tye-cloe′pi-deen)
Func. class.: Platelet aggregation inhibitor
Chem. class.: Thienopyridine compound

Action: Irreversible inhibition of platelet aggregation through antagonism of ADP
Uses: Reducing the risk of stroke in high-risk patients

Unlabeled uses: Intermittent claudication, chronic arterial occlusion, subarachnoid hemorrhage, uremic patients with AV shunts/fistulas, open heart surgery, coronary artery bypass grafts, primary glomerulonephritis, sickle cell disease, diabetic retinopathy

DOSAGE AND ROUTES

• *Adult:* **PO** 250 mg bid with food

Available forms: Tabs 250 mg

SIDE EFFECTS

CNS: Dizziness

GI: Nausea, vomiting, *diarrhea,* GI discomfort, **cholestatic jaundice, hepatitis,** increased cholesterol, LDL, VLDL, triglycerides

HEMA: **Bleeding (epistaxis, hematuria, conjunctival hemorrhage, GI bleeding), agranulocytosis, neutropenia, thrombocytopenia, thrombotic thombocytopenic purpura**

INTEG: *Rash,* pruritus

Contraindications: Hypersensitivity, severe hepatic disease, active bleeding, coagulopathy

Black Box Warning: Agranulocytosis, neutropenia, thrombocytopenia, thrombotic thrombocytopenic purpura (TTP)

Precautions: Pregnancy (B), breastfeeding, children, geriatric patients, past hepatic disease, renal disease, increased bleeding risk, peptic ulcer disease, surgery

Black Box Warning: Anemia, hematological disease

PHARMACOKINETICS

Peak 1-3 hr; metabolized by liver; excreted in urine, feces; half-life increases with repeated dosing, initially 12-36 hr; antiplatelet effect 2-5 days; 98% protein binding

INTERACTIONS

Increase: levels of CYP2C19, CYP2DC substrates, phenytoin, fosphenytoin, ambrisentan, theophylline

Increase: bleeding tendencies—anticoagulants, salicylates, thrombolytics, NSAIDs, abciximab, eptifibatide, tirofiban, thrombin inhibitors, SSRIs, aspirin

Increase: effects of ticlopidine—cimetidine

Decrease: plasma levels of ticlopidine—antacids

Decrease: plasma levels of digoxin, cycloSPORINE

Drug/Herb

Increase: bleeding risk—ginger, gingko, garlic, feverfew, horse chestnut, green tea

NURSING CONSIDERATIONS

Assess:

• Hepatic studies: AST, ALT, bilirubin, creatinine (long-term therapy)

▲ Blood studies: CBC; CBC q2wk × 3 mo, Hct, Hgb, PT (long-term therapy)

▲ Bleed time baseline and throughout, levels may be 2-5× normal limit

Administer:

• With food to decrease gastric symptoms

• Discontinue when absolute neutrophil count falls during treatment to <1200/mm^3 or platelets <80,000/mm^3

Evaluate:

• Therapeutic response: absence of stroke

Teach patient/family:

• That blood work will be necessary during treatment

• To report any unusual bleeding to prescriber

• To report side effects such as diarrhea, skin rashes, subcutaneous bleeding, signs of cholestasis (jaundiced skin and sclera, dark urine, light-colored stools)

• That product should be discontinued 10-14 days before surgery; not to double a missed dose

• That there are many product and herb interactions

tigecycline (℞)

(tye-ge-sye'kleen)

Tygacil

Func. class.: Broad-spectrum antiinfective

Chem. class.: Glycylcyclines

Action: Inhibits protein synthesis and phosphorylation in microorganisms; bacteriostatic structurally similar to the tetracyclines

Uses: Complicated skin/skin structure infections *(Escherichia coli, Enterococcus faecalis* [vancomycin-susceptible only] *Staphylococcus aureus, Streptococcus agalactiae, S. anginosus* group, *S. pyogenes, Bacteroides fragilis;* complicated intraabdominal infections *[Citrobacter freundii] Enterobacter cloacae, E. coli, Klebsiella oxytoca, K. pneumoniae, E. faecalis* [vancomycin-susceptible only], *S. aureus* [methicillin-susceptible only], *S. anginosus* group, *B. fragilis, Bacteroides thetaiotaomicron, B. uniformis, B. vulgatus, Clostridium perfringens, Peptostreptococcus micros),* community-acquired pneumonia

DOSAGE AND ROUTES

• *Adult:* **IV** 100 mg, then 50 mg q12hr, **IV INF** is given over 30-60 min q12hr; given for 5-14 days depending on infection

Hepatic dose

• *Adult:* **IV** (Child-Pugh C) 100 mg, then 25 mg q12hr

Available forms: Powder for inj, lyophilized 50 mg

SIDE EFFECTS

CNS: Headache, dizziness, insomnia

CV: Hypo/hypertension, phlebitis

EENT: Tooth discoloration

GI: Nausea, vomiting, diarrhea, anorexia, constipation, dyspepsia, abdominal pain, **hepatotoxicity, hepatic failure**

HEMA: **Anemia, leukocytosis, thrombocytopenia**

INTEG: Rash, pruritus, sweating, photosensitivity

META: Increased ALT, AST, BUN, lactic acid, alk phos, amylase, hyperglycemia, hypokalemia, hypoproteinemia, bilirubinemia

MISC: Back pain, fever, abnormal healing, abdominal pain, abscess, asthenia, infection, pain, peripheral edema, local reactions

RESP: Cough, dyspnea

SYST: **Anaphylaxis**

Contraindications: Pregnancy (D), breastfeeding, children <18 yr, hypersensitivity to tigecycline

Precautions: Renal/hepatic disease, hypersensitivity to tetracyclines, ventilator-associated/hospital-acquired pneumonias

PHARMACOKINETICS

Not extensively metabolized, 22% of unchanged product is excreted in urine, terminal half-life 42 hr, primarily biliary excreted, protein binding 71%-89%

INTERACTIONS

Increase: effect of warfarin

Decrease: effect of oral contraceptives

NURSING CONSIDERATIONS

Assess:

⚠ For pseudomembranous colitis

• Signs of anemia: Hct, Hgb, fatigue

• Blood studies: PT, CBC, AST, ALT, BUN creatinine

• Allergic reactions: rash, itching, pruritus, angioedema

• Nausea, vomiting, diarrhea; administer antiemetic, antacids as ordered

• Overgrowth of infection: fever, malaise, redness, pain, swelling, drainage, perineal itching, diarrhea, changes in cough or sputum

Administer:

• After C&S obtained

IV route

• Reconstitute each vial with 5.3 ml of 0.9% NaCl, or D_5 (10 mg/ml); swirl to dissolve; immediately withdraw 5 ml of

T

the reconstituted sol and add to a 100-ml IV bag for inf (1 mg/ml); may be yellow or orange, if not, sol should be discarded; do not give if particulate matter is present

Perform/provide:

- Storage in tight, light-resistant container at room temperature

Evaluate:

- Therapeutic response: decreased temp, absence of lesions, negative C&S

Teach patient/family:

- To avoid sun exposure; sunscreen does not seem to decrease photosensitivity
- To avoid pregnancy while taking this product; fetal harm may occur
- To report infection, increase in temperature

tiludronate (℞)

(till-oo'droe-nate)

Skelid

Func. class.: Bone resorption inhibitor

Chem. class.: Bisphosphonate

Action: Decreases bone resorption by inhibiting resorption of mineralized bone matrix, inhibits osteoclasts

Uses: Paget's disease in those with alk phos at 2× upper limit, patients at risk for future complications of Paget's disease and those who are symptomatic

DOSAGE AND ROUTES

- *Adult:* **PO** 400 mg/day, with 8 oz water × 3 mo

Renal dose

- *Adult:* **PO** CCr <30 ml/min, do not use

Available forms: Tabs 240 mg (equivalent to 200 mg tiludronic acid)

SIDE EFFECTS

CNS: Headache, dizziness, paresthesia

CV: Chest pain, edema, peripheral edema, **atrial fibrillation**

EENT: Cataracts, ocular hypertension, pain/inflammation, conjunctivitis, visual impairment, sinusitis

ENDO: Hyperparathyroidism

GI: Nausea, diarrhea, dry mouth, vomiting, flatulence, gastric ulcers, gastritis, dyspepsia

GU: **Nephrotoxicity**

INTEG: Rash, epidermal necrosis, pruritus, sweating

MS: Bone pain, osteonecrosis of the jaw

RESP: Rhinitis, sinusitis, upper respiratory tract infection

SYST: **Stevens-Johnson syndrome**

Contraindications: Breastfeeding, hypersensitivity to bisphosphonates, severe renal disease with creatinine <30 ml/min

Precautions: Pregnancy (C), GI/renal disease, restricted vit D/calcium, asthma, anemia coagulopathy, dental disease, GERD, hiatal hernia, hypocalcemia, infection

PHARMACOKINETICS

Bioavailability 6%

Onset up to several wk, protein binding 90%, excreted by kidneys, half-life 150 hr

INTERACTIONS

Increase: tiludronate effect—indomethacin

Decrease: tiludronate absorption—antacids, mineral supplements with magnesium, calcium, iron, aluminum, aspirin, salicylates

NURSING CONSIDERATIONS

Assess:

- GI symptoms, polyuria, flushing, head swelling, tingling, headache—may indicate hypercalcemia; nervousness, irritability, twitching, seizures, spasm, paresthesia indicates hypocalcemia
- Nutritional status; evaluate diet for sources of vit D (milk, some seafood), calcium (dairy products, dark green vegetables), phosphates; dental status
- BUN, creatinine, electrolytes, urinary calcium, magnesium, phosphate, urinalysis (calcium should be kept at 9-10 mg/dl), albumin, alk phos baseline and q3-6mo

• For increased product level—toxic reactions occur rapidly; have calcium chloride or gluconate on hand if calcium level drops too low; check for tetany

Administer:

• On empty stomach to improve absorption (2 hr before meals), with 6-8 oz water; do not use with mineral water, juice, coffee

• Take calcium or mineral supplements 2 hr before or 2 hr after tiludronate

• Take aluminum or magnesium antacids ≥2 hr after tiludronate

• Do not take NSAIDs within 2 hr

• Tabs from foil strip immediately before use

Evaluate:

• Therapeutic response: calcium levels 9-10 mg/dl; decreasing symptoms of Paget's disease

Teach patient/family:

• To notify prescriber of hypercalcemic relapse: renal calculi, nausea, vomiting, thirst, lethargy, deep bone or flank pain

• To follow a low-calcium diet as prescribed (Paget's disease, hypercalcemia)

• To notify prescriber of diarrhea, nausea; dose may be divided to lessen these symptoms

• Maintain good oral hygiene

timolol (℞)

(tye′moe-lole)

Apo-Timol ✦, Novo-Timol ✦, timolol maleate

Func. class.: Antihypertensive

Chem. class.: Nonselective β-blocker

Action: Competitively blocks stimulation of β-adrenergic receptor within vascular smooth muscle (decreases rate of SA node discharge, increases recovery time), slows conduction of AV node, decreases heart rate, which decreases O_2 consumption in myocardium; also decreases renin-aldosterone-angiotensin system, at high doses inhibits β_2-receptors in bronchial system

Uses: Mild to moderate hypertension, migraine prophylaxis

Unlabeled uses: Tremors, angina pectoris

DOSAGE AND ROUTES

Hypertension

• *Adult:* **PO** 10 mg bid, or 20 mg/day, may increase by 10 mg q7days, max 60 mg/day

Myocardial infarction

• *Adult:* **PO** 10 mg bid beginning 1-4 wk after MI

Migraine headache prevention

• *Adult:* **PO** 10 mg bid or 20 mg/day; may increase to 30 mg/day, 20 mg in AM, 10 mg in PM; discontinue if not effective after 8 wk

Available forms: Tabs 5, 10, 20 mg

SIDE EFFECTS

CNS: Insomnia, dizziness, hallucinations, anxiety, fatigue, depression, headache

CV: Hypotension, bradycardia, **CHF,** edema, chest pain, claudication, angina, AV block, ventricular dysrhythmias

EENT: Visual changes; sore throat; *double vision;* dry, burning eyes

GI: Nausea, vomiting, **ischemic colitis,** diarrhea, *abdominal pain,* **mesenteric arterial thrombosis,** flatulence, constipation

GU: Impotence, urinary frequency

HEMA: **Agranulocytosis, thrombocytopenia, purpura**

INTEG: Rash, alopecia, pruritus, fever

META: Hypoglycemia

MUSC: Joint pain, muscle pain

RESP: **Bronchospasm,** *dyspnea,* cough, crackles, nasal stuffiness

Contraindications: Hypersensitivity to β-blockers, cardiogenic shock, heart block (2nd/3rd degree), sinus bradycardia, CHF, cardiac failure, severe COPD, asthma

Precautions: Pregnancy (C), breastfeeding, major surgery, diabetes mellitus, COPD, well-compensated heart failure, CAD, nonallergic bronchospasm, periph-

T

eral vascular disease, thyroid/renal/hepatic disease

Black Box Warning: Abrupt discontinuation

PHARMACOKINETICS

Peak 1-2 hr; half-life 4 hr; metabolized by liver; excreted in urine, breast milk; protein binding <10%

INTERACTIONS

Increase: hypotension, bradycardia—hydrALAZINE, methyldopa, prazosin, anticholinergics, alcohol, reserpine, nitrates
Increase: effects of β-blockers, calcium channel blockers
Decrease: antihypertensive effects—NSAIDs, sympathomimetics, thyroid, salicylates
Decrease: hypoglycemic effects—insulin, sulfonylureas
Decrease: bronchodilation—theophyllines

Drug/Herb

Increase: toxicity, death—aconite
Increase: antihypertensive effect—barberry, betony, black catechu, black cohosh, bloodroot, broom, burdock, cat's claw, dandelion, goldenseal, hawthorn, Irish moss, Jamaican dogwood, kelp, khella, mistletoe, parsley
Increase or decrease: antihypertensive effect—astragalus, cola tree
Decrease: antihypertensive effect—coltsfoot, guarana, khat, licorice, yohimbe

Drug/Lab Test

Increase: renal, hepatic studies, potassium, uric acid
Decrease: Hct, Hgb, HDL
Interference: glucose, insulin tolerance test

NURSING CONSIDERATIONS

Assess:

- Headaches: location, severity, duration, frequency baseline and throughout treatment
- I&O, weight daily
- B/P during initial treatment, periodically thereafter, pulse q4hr; note rate, rhythm, quality
- Apical/radial pulse before administration; notify prescriber of any significant changes
- Baselines in renal, hepatic studies before therapy begins
- Edema in feet, legs daily
- Skin turgor, dryness of mucous membranes for hydration status

Administer:

- PO before or immediately after meals, at bedtime; tab may be crushed or swallowed whole
- Reduced dosage in renal dysfunction

Perform/provide:

- Dry storage at room temperature; do not freeze

Evaluate:

- Therapeutic response: decreased B/P after 1-2 wk

Teach patient/family:

- To take before or immediately after meals
- Not to discontinue product abruptly; taper over 2 wk; may cause precipitate angina
- Not to use OTC products containing α-adrenergic stimulants (nasal decongestants, cold preparations) unless directed by prescriber
- To report bradycardia, dizziness, confusion, depression, fever, sore throat, SOB to prescriber
- To take pulse at home; advise when to notify prescriber
- To avoid alcohol, smoking, sodium intake
- To comply with weight control, dietary adjustments, modified exercise program
- To carry emergency ID to identify product, allergies
- To avoid hazardous activities if dizziness is present
- To report symptoms of CHF: difficulty breathing, especially on exertion or when lying down; night cough; swelling of extremities

• To take medication at bedtime and wear support hose to minimize effect of orthostatic hypotension

Treatment of overdose: Lavage, IV atropine for bradycardia, IV theophylline for bronchospasm, digoxin, O_2, diuretic for cardiac failure, hemodialysis; administer vasopressor (norepinephrine)

timolol ophthalmic

See Appendix B

tinidazole (℞)

(tye-ni′da-zole)

Tindamax

Func. class.: Antiprotozoal

Chem. class.: Nitroimidazole derivative

Action: Interferes with DNA/RNA synthesis in protozoa

Uses: Amebiasis, giardiasis, trichomoniasis

Unlabeled uses: *Bacteroides* sp., *Clostridium* sp., *Eubacterium* sp., *Fusobacterium* sp., *Peptococcus* sp., *Peptostreptococcus* sp., gingivitis, urethritis, *Veillonella* sp.

DOSAGE AND ROUTES

Amebic involvement of the liver

• *Adult:* **PO** 2 g/day × 3-5 days

• *Child ≥3 yr:* **PO** 50 mg/kg/day × 3-5 days, max 2 g

Giardiasis

• *Adult:* **PO** 2 g as a single dose

• *Child ≥3 yr:* **PO** 50 mg/kg as a single dose, max 2 g

Trichomoniasis

• *Adult:* **PO** 2 g as a single dose

Bacterial vaginosis

• *Adult (nonpregnant woman):* **PO** 2 g/day × 2 days with food or 1 g/day × 5 days with food

Prevention of postoperative infections (unlabeled)

• *Adult:* **PO** 2 g (single dose) 12 hr prior to surgery

Anaerobic infections (unlabeled)

• *Adult:* **PO** 2 g on day 1, then 1 g daily or 500 mg bid for 5-6 days

Available forms: Tabs 250, 500 mg

SIDE EFFECTS

CNS: Dizziness, headache, **seizures,** *peripheral neuropathy,* malaise, fatigue

GI: Nausea, vomiting, anorexia, increased AST and ALT, constipation, abdominal pain, indigestion, altered taste

HEMA: **Leukopenia,** neutropenia

INTEG: Pruritus, urticaria, *rash*, oral candidiasis

SYST: **Angioedema,** cramping

Contraindications: Pregnancy, breastfeeding, hypersensitivity to this product or nitroimidazole derivative

Precautions: Children, geriatric patients, hepatic disease, CNS depression, blood dyscrasias, candidiasis, seizures, viral infection, alcoholism

Black Box Warning: Secondary malignancy

PHARMACOKINETICS

Metabolized extensively in the liver; excreted unchanged (20%-25%) in urine, (12%) feces; half-life 12-14 hr; crosses blood-brain barrier

INTERACTIONS

• Do not use within 2 wk of taking disulfiram

• CYP3A4 inducers (phenobarbital, rifampin, phenytoin); cholestyramine, oxytetracycline: decrease action of tinidazole

• CYP3A4 inhibitors (cimetidine, ketoconazole): increase action of tinidazole

Increase: action of anticoagulants, cycloSPORINE, tacrolimus, fluorouracil, hydantoins, lithium

NURSING CONSIDERATIONS

Assess:

• Amebic liver abscess: CBC, ESR, amebic gel diffusion test, ultrasound; also total and differential leukocyte count

• Signs of infection, anemia

• Bowel pattern before, during treatment

T

Administer:

- Tabs can be crushed and mixed with artificial cherry syrup
- To those over 3 yr old
- With food to increase plasma concentrations, minimize epigastric distress and other GI effects

Evaluate:

- Therapeutic response: decreased in infection as evidenced by negative culture

Teach patient/family:

- To take with food to increase plasma concentrations, minimize epigastric distress and other GI effects; not to use alcoholic beverages during or for 3 days afterward
- Trichomoniasis: both partners should be treated at the same time

⚠ High Alert

tinzaparin (℞)

(tin-zay-par′in)

Innohep

Func. class.: Anticoagulant

Chem. class.: Unfractionated porcine heparin

Action: Increases the inhibitory effect of antithrombin factor Xa, thrombin

Uses: Treatment of DVT, PE after abdominal, knee, hip surgery or knee, hip replacement

Unlabeled uses: Antiphospholipid antibody syndrome, arterial thromboembolism prophylaxis, cerebral thromboembolism, DVT prophylaxis, PE prophylaxis, thrombosis prophylaxis

DOSAGE AND ROUTES

Treatment of DVT

- *Adult:* **SUBCUT** 175 anti-Xa international units/kg/day ≥6 days and until adequate anticoagulation with warfarin (therapeutic INR ≥2 for 2 consecutive days)

Prophylaxis of DVT in orthopedic procedures (unlabeled)

- *Adult:* 75 anti-Xa units/kg/day started 12-24 hr after surgery

Prophylaxis of DVT/thromboembolism/PE (unlabeled)

- *Adult:* 3500 anti-Xa units (50 anti-Xa units/kg) daily beginning 1-2 hr prior to surgery and continued for 5-10 days

Available forms: Inj 20,000 international units/1 ml

SIDE EFFECTS

CNS: Fever, confusion, dizziness, insomnia

CV: Angina, dysrhythmias, peripheral edema, tachycardia, hypo/hypertension

GI: Nausea, constipation, flatulence, dyspepsia, **hepatitis**

GU: UTI, hematuria, urinary retention, dysuria

HEMA: Hemorrhage, **anemia, thrombocytopenia,** bleeding

INTEG: Ecchymosis, inj site reaction

MISC: Headache, chest/back pain, hypersensitivity

SYST: **Stevens-Johnson syndrome**

Contraindications: Hypersensitivity to this product, heparin, pork or benzyl alcohol, sulfites; hemophilia, leukemia with bleeding, peptic ulcer disease, thrombocytopenic purpura, heparin-induced thrombocytopenia

Precautions: Pregnancy (B), breastfeeding, children, geriatric patients, alcoholism, severe renal/hepatic disease, blood dyscrasias, severe, uncontrolled hypertension, subacute bacterial endocarditis, acute nephritis; geriatric >70 yr (renal disease with DVT/PE)

Black Box Warning: Spinal/epidural anesthesia, lumbar puncture

PHARMACOKINETICS

Onset 2-3 hr, maximum antithrombin activity (3-5 hr), elimination half-life 4.5 hr

INTERACTIONS

Increase: action of tinzaparin—oral anticoagulants, salicylates, thrombolytics, NSAIDs, platelet inhibitors, ticlopidine

Drug/Herb

Increase: bleeding risk—agrimony, alfalfa, angelica, anise, basil, bay, bilberry, black haw, bogbean, bromelain, buchu, chondroitin, cinchona bark, dong quai, fenugreek, feverfew, garlic, ginger, ginkgo, ginseng, horse chestnut, Irish moss, kelp, kelpware, khella, lovage, lungwort, meadowsweet, motherwort, mugwort, nettle, papaya, parsley (large amts), pau d'arco, pineapple, poplar, prickly ash, safflower, saw palmetto, tonka bean, turmeric, wintergreen, yarrow

Decrease: anticoagulant effect—chamomile, coenzyme Q10, flax, glucomannan, goldenseal, guar gum

NURSING CONSIDERATIONS

Assess:

- Blood studies (Hct, platelets, occult blood in stools), anti-Xa; thrombocytopenia may occur
- Bleeding gums, petechiae, ecchymosis, black tarry stools, hematuria, decreased Hct, Hgb
- For hypersensitivity (fever, urticaria, chills) report to prescriber
- For inj site reactions and neurologic changes in epidural catheters

Administer:

- Only after screening patient for bleeding disorders
- SUBCUT only; do not give IM
- To recumbent patient; give SUBCUT; rotate inj sites (left/right anterolateral, left-right posterolateral abdominal wall)
- Insert whole length of needle into skin fold held with thumb and forefinger

⚠ Only this product when ordered; not interchangeable with heparin or LMWHs

- At same time each day to maintain steady blood levels
- Do not massage area or aspirate when giving SUBCUT inj
- Do not mix with other products or infusion fluids
- Avoiding all IM inj that may cause bleeding

Perform/provide:

- Storage at 77° F (25° C); do not freeze

Evaluate:

- Therapeutic response: resolution of DVT

Teach patient/family:

- To use soft-bristle toothbrush to avoid bleeding gums, to use electric razor
- To report any signs of bleeding: gums, under skin, urine, stools

Treatment of overdose: Protamine 1 mg/100 anti-Xa international units of tinzaparin

tioconazole vaginal antifungal

See Appendix B

tiotropium (℞)

(ty-oh'tro-pee-um)

HandiHaler, Spiriva

Func. class.: Anticholinergic, bronchodilator

Chem. class.: Synthetic quaternary ammonium compound

Action: Inhibits interaction of acetylcholine at receptor sites on the bronchial smooth muscle, resulting in decreased cGMP and bronchodilation

Uses: COPD, for long-term treatment, once-daily maintenance of bronchospasm, associated with COPD, including chronic bronchitis and emphysema

DOSAGE AND ROUTES

- *Adult:* **INH** Content of 1 cap/day using HandiHaler inhalation device

Available forms: Powder for INH 18 mcg in blister packs containing 6 caps with inhaler; 30 caps with inhaler

SIDE EFFECTS

CNS: Depression, paresthesia

CV: Chest pain, increased heart rate

EENT: Dry mouth, blurred vision, glaucoma

GI: Vomiting, abdominal pain, constipation, dyspepsia

INTEG: Rash, **angioedema**

MISC: Urinary difficulty, urinary retention
RESP: *Cough, worsening of symptoms, sinusitis, upper respiratory tract infection,* epistaxis, pharyngitis

Contraindications: Hypersensitivity to this product, atropine or its derivatives

Precautions: Pregnancy (C), breastfeeding, children, geriatric patients, closed-angle glaucoma, prostatic hypertrophy, bladder neck obstruction, renal disease

PHARMACOKINETICS

Half-life 5-6 days in animals, does not cross blood-brain barrier, very little metabolized in the liver, excreted in urine

INTERACTIONS

• Anticholinergics: avoid use with other anticholinergics

Drug/Herb

Increase: constipation—black catechu

Increase: anticholinergic effect—butterbur, jimsonweed

Increase: bronchodilator effect—green tea (large amounts), guarana

Decrease: anticholinergic effect—jaborandi tree, pill-bearing spurge

NURSING CONSIDERATIONS

Assess:

• For tolerance over long-term therapy; dose may have to be increased or changed
• For patient's ability to use HandiHaler

Administer:

• Caps are for INH only; do not swallow
• Immediately before administration, peel back foil until cap is visible and until "stop" line; remove cap from blister cavity; open dust cap of HandiHaler by pulling upward, then open mouthpiece; place cap in center chamber; firmly close mouthpiece until it clicks, leaving dust cap open
• When finished taking dose, remove used capsule and dispose; close the mouthpiece and dust cap; store
• Rinse mouth after use

Evaluate:

• Therapeutic response: ability to breathe easier

Teach patient/family:

• Signs of closed-angle glaucoma
• That product is used for long-term maintenance, not for immediate relief of breathing problems; effect takes 20 min, lasts 24 hr
• To avoid getting the powder in the eyes; may cause blurred vision and pupil dilation
• Hold HandiHaler with mouthpiece upward; press button in once, completely, and release; this allows for medication to be released
• Breathe out completely; do not breathe into mouthpiece at any time
• Raise device to mouth and close lips tightly around mouthpiece
• With head upright, breathe in slowly/deeply, but allow the cap to vibrate; breathe until lungs fill; hold breath and remove mouthpiece; resume normal breathing
• Rinse mouth after use; use hard candy or regular oral hygiene to reduce dry mouth

tipranavir (℞)

(ti-pran′a-veer)
Aptivus
Func. class.: Antiretroviral
Chem. class.: Protease inhibitor

Action: Inhibits human immunodeficiency virus (HIV) protease; this prevents the maturation of virus

Uses: HIV in combination with other antiretrovirals

DOSAGE AND ROUTES

Reduce dose in mild/moderate hepatic impairment and ketoconazole coadministration

• *Adult:* **PO** 500 mg coadministered with ritonavir 200 mg bid with food
• *Adolescent and child* ≥ 2 *yr:* **PO** 14 mg/kg given with ritonavir 6 mg/kg bid or 375 mg/m^2 given with ritonavir 150

mg/m^2 bid, max 500 mg with ritonavir 200 mg bid

Available forms: Caps 250 mg; oral sol 100 mg/ml

SIDE EFFECTS

CNS: *Headache, insomnia,* dizziness, somnolence, fatigue, *fever,* **intracranial bleeding**

GI: *Diarrhea, abdominal pain, nausea, vomiting,* anorexia, dry mouth, **hepatitis B or C, fatalities when given with ritonavir, pancreatitis**

GU: Nephrolithiasis

INTEG: *Rash,* urticaria, lipodystrophy

MS: Pain

OTHER: Asthenia, **insulin-resistant hyperglycemia,** *hyperlipidemia,* **ketoacidosis**

Contraindications: Hypersensitivity

Black Box Warning: Hepatic disease (Child-Pugh B to C)

Precautions: Pregnancy (C), breastfeeding, children, renal disease, history of renal stones, sulfa allergy, hemophilia, diabetes mellitus, pancreatitis, alcoholism, immune reconstitution syndrome, surgery, trauma, infection

Black Box Warning: Intracranial bleeding, hepatitis

PHARMACOKINETICS

Terminal half-life 6 hr, plasma protein binding 99.9%, steady state 7-10 days, metabolism CYP3A4, 80% fecal excretion

INTERACTIONS

⚠ Life-threatening dysrhythmias: amiodarone, astemizole, cisapride, ergots, flecainide, midazolam, pimozide, propafenone, quinidine, rifabutin, rifampin, terfenadine, triazolam

Increase: myopathy, rhabdomyolysis—HMG-CoA reductase inhibitors (lovastatin, simvastatin)

Increase: tipranavir levels—ketoconazole, delavirdine, itraconazole

Increase: levels of both products—clarithromycin, zidovudine

Increase: levels of tipranavir—oral contraception

Decrease: tipranavir levels—rifamycins, fluconazole, nevirapine, efavirenz

Drug/Herb

Decrease: tipranavir levels—St. John's wort; avoid concurrent use

Drug/Food

Decrease: tipranavir absorption—grapefruit juice, high-fat, high-protein foods

Drug/Lab Test

Increase: AST/ALT

NURSING CONSIDERATIONS

Assess:

- For complaints of lower back, flank pain, indicates kidney stones
- Signs of infection, anemia, the presence of other sexually transmitted diseases
- Hepatic studies: ALT, AST; total bilirubin, amylase, all may be elevated
- Viral load, CD4, plasma HIV RNA, serum cholesterol profile, serum triglycerides during treatment
- Bowel pattern before, during treatment; if severe abdominal pain with bleeding occurs, product should be discontinued; monitor hydration
- Skin eruptions; rash, urticaria, itching
- Allergies before treatment, reaction of each medication; place allergies on chart

Administer:

- Swallow cap whole; do not break, crush, or chew
- After meals
- In equal intervals around the clock to maintain blood levels
- Give oral solution using calibrated dosing syringe or the 5 ml oral syringe provided

Perform/provide:

- Storage for caps in refrigerator prior to use; after opening, store at room temperature; use within 60 days
- Storage for oral sol at room temperature; use within 60 days after opening bottle

Evaluate:

- Therapeutic response: improving CD4 counts and viral load

Teach patient/family:
- To take as prescribed; if dose is missed, take as soon as remembered up to 1 hr before next dose; do not double dose
- That product must be taken in equal intervals around the clock to maintain blood levels for duration of therapy
- ⚠ That hyperglycemia may occur; watch for increased thirst, weight loss, hunger, dry, itchy skin; notify prescriber
- To increase fluids to prevent kidney stones, if stone formation occurs, treatment may need to be interrupted
- That product does not cure AIDS, only controls symptoms; not to donate blood

⚠ High Alert

tirofiban (℞)

(tie-roh-fee′ban)

Aggrastat

Func. class.: Antiplatelet

Chem. class.: Glycoprotein IIb/IIIa inhibitor

Action: Antagonist of platelet glycoprotein (GP) IIb/IIIa receptor that prevents binding of fibrinogen and von Willebrand's factor, which inhibits platelet aggregation

Uses: Acute coronary syndrome in combination with heparin

DOSAGE AND ROUTES

- *Adult:* **IV** 0.4 mcg/kg/min × 30 min, then 0.1 mcg/kg/min for 12-24 hr after angioplasty or atherectomy

Renal dose
- *Adult:* **IV** CCr <30 ml/min 0.2 mcg/kg/min × 30 min, then 0.05 mcg/kg/min, during angiography and for up to 24 hr after angioplasty

Available forms: Inj for sol 250 mcg/ml, inj 50 mcg/ml

SIDE EFFECTS

CNS: Dizziness, headache
CV: Bradycardia, hypotension
GI: Nausea, vomiting
HEMA: **Bleeding, thrombocytopenia**
INTEG: *Rash*
MISC: Dissection, edema, pain in legs/pelvis, sweating
SYST: **Anaphylaxis**

Contraindications: Hypersensitivity, active internal bleeding, stroke, major surgery, severe trauma within 30 days, intracranial neoplasm, aneurysm, hemorrhage, acute pericarditis, platelets <100,000/mm^3, history of thrombocytopenia, coagulopathy, systolic B/P >180 mm Hg or diastolic B/P >110 mm Hg

Precautions: Pregnancy (B), breastfeeding, children, geriatric patients, renal disease, bleeding tendencies, hypertension, platelets <150,000/mm^3

PHARMOCOKINETICS

Half-life 2 hr, excretion via urine/feces; plasma clearance 20%-25% lower in geriatric patients with CAD; renal insufficiency decreases plasma clearance

INTERACTIONS

Increase: bleeding—aspirin, heparin, NSAIDs, abciximab, eptifibatide, clopidogrel, ticlopidine, dipyridamole, cefamandole, cefotetan, cefoperazone, valproic acid, heparins, thrombin inhibitors, SSRIs, SNRIs

Drug/Herb

Increase: risk of bleeding—agrimony, alfalfa, angelica, anise, basil, bay, bilberry, black haw, bogbean, bromelain, buchu, chondroitin, cinchona bark, dong quai, fenugreek, feverfew, garlic, ginger, ginkgo, ginseng, green tea, horse chestnut, Irish moss, kelp, kelpware, khella, lovage, lungwort, meadowsweet, motherwort, mugwort, nettle, papaya, parsley (large amts), pau d'arco, pineapple, poplar, prickly ash, safflower, saw palmetto, tonka bean, turmeric, wintergreen, yarrow

Decrease: anticoagulant effect—chamomile, coenzyme Q10, flax, glucomannan, goldenseal, guar gum

NURSING CONSIDERATIONS

Assess:
- ⚠ Platelet counts, Hct, Hgb, prior to treatment, within 6 hr of loading dose and

at least daily thereafter; watch for bleeding from puncture sites, catheters or in stools, urine

• Discontinue if platelets <100,000/mm^3

Administer:

IV route

• Dilute inj: withdraw and discard 100 ml from a 500-ml bag of sterile 0.9% NaCl or D_5W and replace this vol with 100 ml of tirofiban inj from two vials

• Tirofiban inj for sol is premixed in containers of 500-ml 0.9% NaCl (50 mg/ml), infuse over 30 min

• Minimize other arterial/venous punctures; IM inj, catheter use, intubation, to reduce bleeding risk

Y-site compatibility: Heparin, DOBUTamine, DOPamine, morphine, potassium chloride, propranolol

Evaluate:

• Therapeutic response: treatment of acute coronary syndrome

Teach patient/family:

• That it is necessary to quit smoking to prevent excessive vasoconstriction

• Signs/symptoms of bleeding and low platelets

• That there are many product and herb interactions

tizanidine (℞)

(ti-za'nih-deen)

Zanaflex

Func. class.: Skeletal muscle relaxant, α_2-adrenergic agonist

Chem. class.: Imidazoline

Do not confuse:

tizanidine/tiagabine

Action: Increases presynaptic inhibition of motor neurons and reduces spasticity by α_2-adrenergic agonism

Uses: Acute/intermittent management of increased muscle tone associated with spasticity, symptoms of MS

Unlabeled uses: Tension headache, low back pain, trigeminal neuralgia

DOSAGE AND ROUTES

• *Adult:* **PO** 8 mg q6-8hr, max 36 mg/24 hr

Renal dose

• *Adult:* **PO** CCr <25 ml/min start with lower dose

Available forms: Tabs 2, 4 mg; caps 2, 4, 6 mg

SIDE EFFECTS

CNS: Somnolence, dizziness, speech disorder, dyskinesia, nervousness, hallucination, psychosis

CV: Hypotension, bradycardia

GI: Dry mouth, vomiting, increased ALT, abnormal LFTs, constipation

OTHER: Blurred vision, urinary frequency, pharyngitis, rhinitis, tremor, rash, muscle weakness

Contraindications: Hypersensitivity

Precautions: Pregnancy (C), breastfeeding, children, geriatric patients, hypotension, renal/hepatic disease

PHARMACOKINETICS

Completely absorbed, widely distributed, peak 1-2 hr, duration 3-6 hr, half-life 2.5 hr, protein binding 30%, metabolized by liver, excreted in urine/feces

INTERACTIONS

Increase: CNS depression—alcohol, other CNS depressants

Increase: tizanidine levels—amiodarone, famotidine, ciprofloxacin, fluvoxamine; do not use concurrently

Decrease: clearance of tizanidine—oral contraceptives

Drug/Herb

Increase: CNS depression—gotu kola, kava, St. John's wort

Increase: hypotension—black cohosh, California poppy, goldenseal, hawthorn

Drug/Lab Test

Increase: alk phos, AST, ALT, serum glucose

T

NURSING CONSIDERATIONS

Assess:

- For muscle spasticity baseline and throughout treatment
- For hypotension, gradual dosage increase should lessen hypotensive effects; have patient rise slowly from supine to upright; watch those patients receiving antihypertensives for increased effects
- For increased sedation, dizziness, hallucinations, psychosis; product may need to be discontinued
- Vision by ophthalmic exam, corneal opacities may occur
- Hepatic studies: 1, 3, 6 mo during treatment and periodically thereafter

Administer

- Consistently either with or without food; food may affect absorption
- Titrate doses carefully
- Avoid use with other CNS depressants

Evaluate:

- Therapeutic response: decreased muscle spasticity

Teach patient/family:

- To rise slowly from lying or sitting to upright position
- To ask for assistance if dizziness, sedation occur; to avoid drinking alcohol, to avoid operating machinery or driving until effects are known
- To avoid use of alcohol
- Discontinue gradually

tobramycin (℞)

(toe-bra-mye′sin)

TOBI, tobramycin sulfate

Func. class.: Antiinfective

Chem. class.: Aminoglycoside

Action: Interferes with protein synthesis in bacterial cell by binding to ribosomal subunits, causing inaccurate peptide sequence to form in protein chain, causing bacterial death

Uses: Severe systemic infections of CNS, respiratory, GI, urinary tract, bone, skin, soft tissues caused by *Pseudomonas aeruginosa, Escherichia coli, Enterobacter, Providencia, Citrobacter, Staphylococcus, Proteus, Klebsiella, Serratia;* cystic fibrosis (nebulizer) for *Pseudomonas aeruginosa*

DOSAGE AND ROUTES

- *Adult:* **IM/IV** 3 mg/kg/day in divided doses q8hr; may give up to 6 mg/kg/day in divided doses q8-12hr; once daily dosing (pulse dosing) (unlabeled) **IV** 5-7 mg/kg, dosing intervals are determined using a nomogram and are based on random levels drawn 8-12 hr after first dose
- *Child:* **IM/IV** 6-7.5 mg/kg/day in 3-4 equal divided doses
- *Child ≥6 yr:* **NEB** 300 mg bid in repeating cycles of 28 days on/28 days off of product; give **INH** over 10-15 min using a handheld PARI LC PLUS reusable nebulizer with a DeVilbiss Pulmo-Aid compressor
- *Neonate <1 wk:* **IM** Up to 4 mg/kg/day in divided doses q12hr; **IV** up to 4 mg/kg/day in divided doses q12hr diluted in 50-100 mg NS or D_5W; give over 30-60 min

Renal dose

- *Adult:* **IM/IV** 1 mg/kg, then dose determined by blood levels

Available forms: Inj 10, 40 mg/ml; powder for inj 1.2 g; neb sol 300 mg/5 ml

SIDE EFFECTS

CNS: Confusion, depression, numbness, tremors, **seizures,** muscle twitching, **neurotoxicity,** dizziness, vertigo

CV: Hypo/hypertension, palpitation

EENT: **Ototoxicity,** deafness, visual disturbances, tinnitus

GI: Nausea, vomiting, anorexia; increased ALT, AST, bilirubin, hepatomegaly, **hepatic necrosis,** splenomegaly

GU: **Oliguria, hematuria, renal damage, azotemia, renal failure, nephrotoxicity**

HEMA: **Agranulocytosis, thrombocytopenia, leukopenia, eosinophilia,** anemia

INTEG: Rash, burning, urticaria, dermatitis, alopecia

Contraindications: Hypersensitivity to aminoglycosides

Black Box Warning: Pregnancy (D), severe renal disease

Precautions: Breastfeeding, geriatric patients, neonates, mild renal disease, myasthenia gravis, Parkinson's disease

Black Box Warning: Hearing deficits, neuromuscular disease

PHARMACOKINETICS

Plasma half-life 2-3 hr, prolonged in neonates; not metabolized; excreted unchanged in urine; crosses placental barrier; poor penetration into CSF
IM: Onset rapid, peak 1 hr
IV: Onset immediate, peak 1 hr

INTERACTIONS

Increase: ototoxicity, neurotoxicity, nephrotoxicity—other aminoglycosides, amphotericin B, polymyxin, vancomycin, ethacrynic acid, furosemide, mannitol, methoxyflurane, cisplatin, cephalosporins, bacitracin, acyclovir, penicillins, cidofovir

Drug/Herb

- Do not use acidophilus with antiinfectives; separate by several hours
- Toxicity: lysine (large amounts)

NURSING CONSIDERATIONS

Assess:

- Weight before treatment; dosage is usually based on ideal body weight, but may be calculated on actual body weight
- I&O ratio, urinalysis daily for proteinuria, cells, casts; report sudden change in urine output
- VS during inf; watch for hypotension, change in pulse
- IV site for thrombophlebitis, including pain, redness, swelling q30min; change site if needed; apply warm compresses to discontinued site
- Serum aminoglycoside conc; serum peak, drawn at 30-60 min after IV inf or 60 min after IM inj, trough drawn just before next dose, peak 4-10 mcg/ml, trough 0.5-2 mcg/ml
- Renal impairment by securing urine for CCr testing, BUN, serum creatinine; lower dosage should be given in renal impairment (CCr <80 ml/min); monitor electrolytes: potassium, sodium, chloride, magnesium monthly, if patient is on long-term therapy
- Deafness by audiometric testing; ringing, roaring in ears; vertigo; assess hearing before, during, after treatment
- Dehydration: high specific gravity, decrease in skin turgor, dry mucous membranes, dark urine
- Overgrowth of infection: fever, malaise, redness, pain, swelling, perineal itching, diarrhea, stomatitis, change in cough, sputum
- C&S before starting treatment to identify infecting organism
- Vestibular dysfunction: nausea, vomiting, dizziness, headache; product should be discontinued if severe
- Inj sites for redness, swelling, abscesses; use warm compresses at site

Administer:

- Product in evenly spaced doses to maintain blood level; separate aminoglycosides and penicillins by ≥1 hr
- Use only on susceptible organisms to prevent the development of product-resistant bacteria

IM route

- IM inj in large muscle mass; rotate inj sites

Nebulizer route

- Give as close to q12hr apart as possible; do not use <6 hr apart
- Do not mix with dornase alfa in the nebulizer
- Have patient inhale sitting or standing, breathe normally through mouthpiece; may use noseclips

IV route

- Diluted in 50-100 ml 0.9% NaCl or D_5W (adult), infuse over 20-60 min
- Do not admix

Syringe compatibilities: Doxapram

Y-site compatibilities: Acyclovir, amifostine, amiodarone, amsacrine, aztreonam, ciprofloxacin, cisatracurium, cyclophosphamide, diltiazem, doxorubicin

T

liposome, enalaprilat, esmolol, filgrastim, fluconazole, fludarabine, foscarnet, furosemide, granisetron, hydromorphone, IL-2, insulin (regular), labetalol, magnesium sulfate, melphalan, meperidine, midazolam, morphine, perphenazine, remifentanil, tacrolimus, teniposide, theophylline, thiotepa, tolazoline, vinorelbine, zidovudine

Perform/provide:

- Adequate fluids of 2-3 L/day unless contraindicated to prevent irritation of tubules
- Flush of IV line with NS or D_5W after infusion
- Supervised ambulation, other safety measures with vestibular dysfunction

Evaluate:

- Therapeutic response: absence of fever, draining wounds, negative C&S after treatment

Teach patient/family:

- To report headache, dizziness, symptoms of overgrowth of infection, renal impairment
- To report loss of hearing; ringing, roaring in ears; feeling of fullness in head

Nebulizer

- To use multiple therapies first, then tobramycin

Treatment of overdose: Hemodialysis; monitor serum levels of product

tobramycin ophthalmic

See Appendix B

tocainide (℞)

(toe-kay′nide)

Func. class.: Antidysrhythmic (Class Ib)

Chem. class.: Lidocaine analog

Action: Produces dose-dependent decreases in sodium and potassium conduction, thereby decreasing the excitability of myocardial cells; does not affect heart rate or B/P

Uses: Life-threatening ventricular dysrhythmias (multifocal/unifocal PVCs), ventricular tachycardia

Unlabeled uses: Neuropathic pain syndromes

DOSAGE AND ROUTES

- *Adult:* **PO** 400 mg q8hr, may increase to 1.2-1.8 g/day in divided doses q8-12hr

Neuropathic pain (unlabeled)

- *Adult:* **PO** 20 mg/kg/day

Available forms: Tabs 400, 600 mg

SIDE EFFECTS

CNS: Headache, dizziness, involuntary movement, confusion, psychosis, restlessness, irritability, paresthesias, tremors, **seizures**

CV: Hypotension, bradycardia, angina, PVCs, **heart block, CV collapse, sinus arrest, CHF,** chest pain, tachycardia, prodysrhythmia

EENT: Tinnitus, blurred vision, hearing loss

GI: Nausea, vomiting, anorexia, diarrhea, hepatitis, loss of taste

HEMA: **Blood dyscrasias: leukopenia, agranulocytosis, hypoplastic anemia, thrombocytopenia, bone marrow depression**

INTEG: Rash, urticaria, lupus, alopecia, sweating, **Stevens-Johnson syndrome**

RESP: Dyspnea, **respiratory depression, pulmonary fibrosis,** pulmonary edema, interstitial pneumonitis pneumonia

Contraindications: Hypersensitivity to amides, severe heart block

Precautions: Pregnancy (C), breastfeeding, children, geriatric patients, renal/hepatic disease, CHF, myasthenia gravis, hypokalemia, atrial flutter/fibrillation

Black Box Warning: Bone marrow suppression, cardiac arrhythmias, pulmonary fibrosis

PHARMACOKINETICS

Peak 0.5-3 hr; half-life 10-17 hr; metabolized by liver; excreted in urine, 40% unchanged

INTERACTIONS

Increase: tocainide effects—metoprolol
Decrease: tocainide effects—cimetidine, rifampin

Drug/Herb

Increase: toxicity, death—aconite
Increase: effect—aloe, broom, chronic buckthorn use, cascara sagrada (chronic use), Chinese rhubarb, figwort, fumitory, goldenseal, kudzu, licorice
Increase: serotonin effect—horehound
Decrease: effect—coltsfoot

Drug/Lab Test

Increase: CPK
False positive: ANA titer

NURSING CONSIDERATIONS

Assess:

⚠ Chest x-ray film, pulmonary function tests, hepatic enzymes during treatment, monitor for lung sounds, sputum, SOB after 3-18 wk

- CBC, with differential and platelet count during beginning treatment and q3mo
- Renal status: I&O ratio, check for decreasing output
- Blood levels (therapeutic level 4-10 mcg/ml)
- B/P continuously for fluctuations
- Lung fields; bilateral crackles may occur in CHF patient
- Increased respiration, increased pulse; product should be discontinued
- Toxicity: fine tremors, dizziness
- Blood dyscrasias: fatigue, sore throat, fever, bruising
- Cardiac status, respiration: rate, rhythm, character; ECG

Administer:

- With meals to decrease GI symptoms

Evaluate:

- Therapeutic response: decreased dysrhythmia

Teach patient/family:

- Of reason for medication and expected results
- Method for taking pulse at home and what to report to prescriber
- To avoid hazardous activities until product response is known; dizziness, confusion, sedation may occur
- To use a bracelet or other emergency ID indicating medications taken, condition, and prescriber's name and phone number
- To report bleeding, bruising, respiratory symptoms, chills, fever, sore throat to prescriber

Treatment of overdose: O_2, artificial ventilation, ECG; administer DOPamine for circulatory depression, diazepam or thiopental for seizures

tolcapone (℞)

(toll'cah'pone)
Tasmar
Func. class.: Antiparkinson agent
Chem. class.: COMT inhibitor

Action: Inhibits COMT; used as adjunct to levodopa/carbidopa therapy
Uses: Parkinson's disease

DOSAGE AND ROUTES

- *Adult:* **PO** 100-200 mg tid, with levodopa/carbidopa therapy; max 600 mg/day, discontinue if no benefit in 3 wk

Renal dose

- *Adult:* **PO** Use 100 mg tid or less

Available forms: Tabs 100, 200 mg

SIDE EFFECTS

CNS: Dystonia, dyskinesia, dreaming, *fatigue, headache, confusion,* psychosis, hallucination, dizziness, sleep disorders
CV: Orthostatic hypotension, chest pain, hypotension
EENT: Cataract, eye inflammation
GI: Nausea, vomiting, anorexia, abdominal distress, diarrhea, constipation, **fatal hepatic failure,** increased LFTs
GU: UTI, urine discoloration, uterine tumor, micturition disorder, hematuria
HEMA: **Hemolytic anemia, leukopenia, agranulocytosis**
INTEG: Sweating, alopecia
MS: **Rhabdomyolysis**

T

Contraindications: Hypersensitivity
Precautions: Pregnancy (C), breastfeeding, cardiac/renal disease, hypertension, asthma, history of rhabdomyolysis
Black Box Warning: Hepatic disease

PHARMACOKINETICS

Rapidly absorbed, peak 2 hr, protein binding 99%, extensively metabolized, half-life 2-3 hr, excreted in urine (60%)/feces (40%)

INTERACTIONS

• May influence pharmacokinetics of α-methyldopa, DOBUTamine, apomorphine, isoproterenol
• Inhibition of normal catecholamine metabolism: MAOIs, MAO-B inhibitor may be used

Drug/Herb

Decrease: effect—kava

NURSING CONSIDERATIONS

Assess:

⚠ Hepatic studies: AST, ALT, alk phos, LDH, bilirubin, CBC, monitor ALT, AST q2wk × 1 yr, then q4wk × 6 mo, and q8wk thereafter; if LFTs are elevated, this product should not be used
• Involuntary movements in parkinsonism: akinesia, tremors, staggering gait, muscle rigidity, drooling
• B/P, respiration during initial treatment; hypo/hypertension should be reported
• Mental status: affect, mood, behavioral changes

Administer:

• Only to be used if levodopa/carbidopa does not provide satisfactory result

Evaluate:

• Therapeutic response: decrease in akathisia, increased mood

Teach patient/family:

• To change positions slowly to prevent orthostatic hypotension
• That urine, sweat may change color
• That food taken within 1 hr before meals or 2 hr after meals decreases action of product by 20%
⚠ To report signs of hepatic injury: clay-colored stools, jaundice, fatigue, appetite loss, lethargy
• To report nausea, vomiting, anorexia; nausea may occur in the beginning of treatment

tolnaftate topical

See Appendix B

tolterodine (℞)

(toll-tehr′oh-deen)
Detrol, Detrol LA
Func. class.: Overactive bladder product
Chem. class.: Muscarinic receptor antagonist

Action: Relaxes smooth muscles in urinary tract by inhibiting acetylcholine at postganglionic sites
Uses: Overactive bladder (urinary frequency, urgency), urinary incontinence

DOSAGE AND ROUTES

• *Adult and geriatric:* **PO** 2 mg bid; **EXT REL** 4 mg/day, may decrease to 2 mg if needed, max 4 mg/day

Hepatic disease

• *Adult:* **PO** 1 mg bid (50% dose) or **EXT REL** 2 mg/day

Renal dose

• *Adult:* **PO** CCr ≤30 ml/min reduce by 50%

Available forms: Tabs 1, 2 mg; ext rel caps 2, 4 mg

SIDE EFFECTS

CNS: Anxiety, paresthesia, fatigue, *dizziness, headache,* increasing dementia, memory impairment
CV: Chest pain, hypertension, **QT prolongation**
EENT: Vision abnormalities, xerophthalmia
GI: Nausea, vomiting, anorexia, abdominal pain, constipation, dry mouth, dyspepsia

GU: Dysuria, urinary retention, frequency, UTI
INTEG: Rash, pruritus
RESP: Bronchitis, cough, pharyngitis, upper respiratory tract infection
SYST: **Angioedema, Stevens-Johnson syndrome**
Contraindications: Hypersensitivity, uncontrolled closed-angle glaucoma, urinary retention, gastric retention
Precautions: Pregnancy (C), breastfeeding, children, renal/hepatic disease, controlled closed-angle glaucoma, bladder obstruction, QT prolongation, decreased GI motility

PHARMACOKINETICS

Rapidly absorbed, highly protein bound, extensively metabolized, excreted in urine/feces

INTERACTIONS

⚠ ***Increase:*** QT prolongation—class IA/III antidysrhythmics, some phenothiazines, β-agonists, local anesthetics, tricyclics, bepridil, haloperidol, methadone, chloroquine, clarithromycin, droperidol, erythromycin, grepafloxacin, halofantrine, pentamidine, probucol, sparfloxacin
Increase: action of tolterodine—antiretroviral protease inhibitors, macrolide antiinfectives, azole antifungals
Increase: anticholinergic effect—antimuscarinics
Increase: urinary frequency—diuretics
Drug/Food
- Food increases the bioavailability of tolterodine

NURSING CONSIDERATIONS

Assess:
- Urinary patterns: distention, nocturia, frequency, urgency, incontinence
- Allergic reactions: rash; if this occurs, product should be discontinued

Administer:
- Whole; take with liquids

Evaluate:
- Urinary status: dysuria, frequency, nocturia, incontinence

Teach patient/family:
- To avoid hazardous activities; dizziness may occur
- Not to drink liquids before bedtime
- The importance of bladder maintenance

tolvaptan (℞)
(tole-vap'tan)
Samsca
Func. class.: Vasopressin receptor antagonist, V2

Action: Arginine vasopressin (AVP) antagonist with affinity for V2 receptors; level of circulating AVP in circulating blood is critical for regulation of water and electrolyte balance and is usually elevated in euvolemic/hypervolemic hyponatremia
Uses: Hypervolemic/euvolemic hyponatremia in heart failure, cirrhosis, SIADH

DOSAGE AND ROUTES

- *Adult:* **PO** 15 mg daily, after 24 hr, may increase to 30 mg daily, max 60 mg/day

Available forms: Tab 15, 30 mg

SIDE EFFECTS

CNS: Fever
CV: **Ventricular fibrillation, DIC, stroke, thrombosis**
GI: Nausea, vomiting, constipation, colitis
GU: Polyuria
HEMA: **Bleeding**
META: Dehydration, hyperglycemia, hyperkalemia, hypernatremia
MS: **Rhabdomyolysis**
RESP: **Respiratory depression, pulmonary embolism**
Contraindications: Hypersensitivity, hypovolemia, anuria
Precautions: Pregnancy (C), breastfeeding, children, dehydration, geriatric, hepatic disease, hyperkalemia
Black Box Warning: Alcoholism, malnutrition

T

PHARMACOKINETICS

Peak 2-4 hr, protein binding 99%, metabolized by CYP3A4, terminal half-life 12 hr

INTERACTIONS

Increase: plasma concentrations of tolvaptan—CYP3A4 inhibitors (efavirenz, fosamprenavir, quinine); P-gp inhibitors (cycloSPORINE, azithromycin, bepridil, mefloquine, palperidone, propafenone, quinidine, testosterone)

Decrease: plasma concentration of tolvaptan—CYP3A4 inducers (carbamazepine, dexamethasone, etravirine, flutamide, griseofulvin, metyrapsone, modafinil, nafacillin, nevirapine, oxcarbazepine, phenytoin, rifampin, rifabutin, rifapendine, topiramate)

Drug/Herb

Decreased: tolvaptan effect: CYP3A4 inducer (St. John's wort)

NURSING CONSIDERATIONS

Assess:

- Renal, hepatic function
- Frequent sodium volume status; overly rapid correction of sodium concentration (12 mEq/L per 24 hr) may result in osmotic demyelination syndrome
- CV status: ventricular fibrillation, hypertension, monitor B/P, pulse
- Monitor electrolytes (sodium, potassium)

Administer:

- PO with or without food
- Avoid fluid restriction the first 24 hr
- Initiate in hospital setting

Evaluate:

- Therapeutic response: correction of serum sodium levels

Teach patient/family:

- To avoid pregnancy, breastfeeding while taking this product
- Administrations procedure and expected result

topiramate (℞)

(toh-pire'ah-mate)

Topamax, Topamax Sprinkle, Topiragen

Func. class.: Anticonvulsant—miscellaneous

Chem. class.: Monosaccharide derivative

Action: May prevent seizure spread as opposed to an elevation of seizure threshold, increases GABA activity

Uses: Partial seizures in adults and children 2-16 yr old; tonic-clonic seizures; seizures in Lennox-Gastaut syndrome, migraine prophylaxis

Unlabeled uses: Infantile spasms, bipolar disorder, alcohol dependence, absence seizures, neuropathic pain, cluster headache

DOSAGE AND ROUTES

Adjunctive therapy in seizures

- *Adult/adolescent/child ≥10 yr:* **PO** 25-50 mg/day initially, titrate by 25-50 mg/wk, up to 200-400 mg/day in 2 divided doses

Renal dose

- *Adult:* **PO** CCr <70 ml/min give ½ dose

Migraine prophylaxis

- *Adult:* **PO** 25 mg/day initially, increase by 25 mg/day q wk up to 100 mg/day in 2 divided doses

Atonic/atypical absence/myoclonic seizures (unlabeled)

- *Adult and adolescent >16 yr:* **PO** 50 mg/day, titrate slowly by 50 mg/wk to 100-300 mg tid
- *Child 2-16 yr:* **PO** 0.5-1 mg/kg, max 25 mg, initially daily × 7 days, then increase by 0.5-1 mg/kg/day weekly up to 3-6 mg/kg/day in divided doses

Refractory infantile spasms (unlabeled)

- *Child:* **PO** 25 mg/day may increase by 25 mg q2-3days until spasms are controlled, max 24 mg/kg/day

Available forms: Tabs 25, 50, 100, 200 mg; sprinkle caps 15, 25 mg

SIDE EFFECTS

CNS: *Dizziness, fatigue*, cognitive disorder, insomnia, *anxiety*, depression, paresthesia, *memory loss, tremor,* motor retardation, **suicidal ideation**
EENT: Diplopia, *vision abnormality*
GI: Diarrhea, *anorexia, nausea, dyspepsia*, abdominal pain, constipation, dry mouth, **pancreatitis**
GU: Breast pain, dysmenorrhea, menstrual disorder
INTEG: Rash
MISC: Weight loss, leukopenia, metabolic acidosis, increased body temperature
RESP: Upper respiratory tract infection, pharyngitis, sinusitis

Contraindications: Hypersensitivity, metabolic acidosis

Precautions: Pregnancy (C), breastfeeding, children, renal/hepatic disease, acute myopia, secondary closed-angle glaucoma, behavioral disorders

PHARMACOKINETICS

Well absorbed, peak 2 hr, terminal half-life 19-25 hr, excreted in urine (55%-97% unchanged), crosses placenta, excreted in breast milk, protein binding (9%-17%), steady state 4 days

INTERACTIONS

Increase: renal stones—carbonic anhydrase inhibitors
Increase: effect of amitriptyline
Increase: CNS depression—alcohol, CNS depressants
Increase: topiramate levels—metformin, hydrochlorothiazide, lamotrigine
Decrease: levels of oral contraceptives, estrogen, digoxin, valproic acid, lithium, risperidone
Decrease: topiramate levels—phenytoin, carbamazepine, valproic acid, probenecid

Drug/Herb
Increase: effect—ginkgo
Decrease: effect—ginseng, santonica

NURSING CONSIDERATIONS

Assess:

- Renal studies: urinalysis, BUN, urine creatinine q3mo; symptoms of renal colic
- Hepatic studies: ALT, AST, bilirubin if on long-term treatment
- CBC during long-term therapy; serum bicarbonate
- Description of seizures: location, type, duration, aura

⚠ Mental status: mood, sensorium, affect, behavioral changes, suicidal thoughts/behaviors; if mental status changes, notify prescriber

- Body weight, evidence of cognitive disorder

Administer:

- Swallow tabs whole; do not break, crush, or chew tabs; very bitter
- May take without regard to meals
- Sprinkle cap can be given whole or opened and sprinkled on soft food; do not chew

Perform/provide:

- Storage at room temperature away from heat and light
- Assistance with ambulation during early part of treatment; dizziness occurs
- Seizure precautions: padded side rails, move objects that may harm patient

Evaluate:

- Therapeutic response: decreased seizure activity

Teach patient/family:

- To carry emergency ID stating patient's name, products taken, condition, prescriber's name, phone number
- To avoid driving, other activities that require alertness
- Not to discontinue medication quickly after long-term use
- To notify prescriber immediately of blurred vision, periorbital pain
- To maintain adequate fluid intake
- To use nonhormonal contraceptive; effect of oral contraceptives is decreased

⚠ High Alert

topotecan (℞)
(toh-poh-tee'kan)
Hycamtin
Func. class.: Antineoplastic, natural; topoisomerase inhibitor
Chem. class.: Camptothecin analog

Action: Antitumor product with topoisomerase I–inhibitory activity topoisomerase I relieves torsional strain in DNA by causing single-strand breaks; causes double-strand DNA damage

Uses: Metastatic ovarian cancer after failure of traditional chemotherapy, relapsed small cell lung cancer, cervical cancer

Unlabeled uses: Non–small cell lung cancer (NSCLC), rhabdomyosarcoma

DOSAGE AND ROUTES

• *Adult:* **IV INF** 1.5 mg/m^2 over 30 min daily × 5 days starting on day 1 of a 21-day course × 4 courses; may be reduced to 0.25 mg/m^2 for subsequent courses if severe neutropenia occurs; **PO** 2.3 mg/m^2/day on days 1-5 of a 21-day course (relapsed small cell lung cancer in those with prior response)

Renal dose

• *Adult:* **IV** CCr 20-39 ml/min 0.75 mg/m^2/day × 5 days starting on day 1 of a 21-day course

Available forms: Lyophilized powder for inj 4 mg; caps 0.25, 1 mg

SIDE EFFECTS

CNS: Arthralgia, *asthenia, headache,* myalgia, *pain,* weakness

GI: Abdominal pain, constipation, diarrhea, obstruction, *nausea,* stomatitis, *vomiting;* increased ALT, AST; anorexia

HEMA: **Neutropenia, leukopenia, thrombocytopenia, anemia, sepsis**

INTEG: Total alopecia

RESP: Dyspnea, cough, **interstitial lung disease**

Contraindications: Pregnancy (D), breastfeeding, hypersensitivity, severe bone marrow depression

Black Box Warning: Neutropenia

Precautions: Children, renal disease

PHARMACOKINETICS

Rapidly and completely absorbed, excreted in urine and feces as metabolites, half-life 2.8 hr, 7%-35% bound to plasma proteins

INTERACTIONS

• Avoid use with P-glycoprotein, breast cancer resistance protein inhibitors (amiodarone, clarithromycin, diltiazem, erythromycin, indinavir), quinidine, testosterone, verapamil, tamoxifen, itraconazole, mefloquine, RU-486, niCARdipine, vaccines, toxoids

Increase: myelosuppression when used with cisplatin

Increase: bleeding risk—NSAIDs, anticoagulants, thrombolytics, platelet inhibitors

Drug/Food

• Avoid use with grapefruit juice

NURSING CONSIDERATIONS

Assess:

• Hepatic studies: AST, ALT, alk phos, which may be elevated; creatinine, BUN

• CBC, differential, platelet count weekly; withhold product if WBC is $<3500/mm^3$ or platelet count is $<100,000/mm^3$; notify prescriber of these results; product should be discontinued

• Buccal cavity for dryness, sores or ulceration, white patches, oral pain, bleeding, dysphagia

• GI symptoms: frequency of stools, cramping

• Signs of dehydration: rapid respiration, poor skin turgor, decreased urine output, dry skin, restlessness, weakness

Administer:

PO route

• Do not break, crush, chew, or open caps

• Take without regard to food

IV route
- Give as IV INF

Perform/provide:
- Storage of caps in refrigerator; IV INF unopened at room temperature; protect both from light
- Increased fluid intake to 2-3 L/day to prevent dehydration, unless contraindicated
- Rinsing of mouth tid-qid with water, club soda; brushing of teeth bid-tid with soft brush or cotton-tipped applicator for stomatitis; use unwaxed dental floss
- Nutritious diet with iron, vit K supplements, low fiber, few dairy products

Evaluate:
- Therapeutic response: decreased tumor size, spread of malignancy

Teach patient/family:
- That total alopecia may occur; hair grows back, but is different in color and texture
- To avoid foods with citric acid or hot or rough texture if stomatitis is present; to drink adequate fluids
- To report stomatitis; any bleeding, white spots, ulcerations in mouth; tell patient to examine mouth daily; report symptoms
- To report signs of anemia: fatigue, headache, faintness, SOB, irritability
- To use effective contraception during treatment and up to 6 mo after, avoid breastfeeding
- To avoid OTC products without approval of prescriber
- To avoid driving or other activities requiring alertness
- Avoid vaccines, toxoids

toremifene (℞)

(tor-em′ih-feen)
Fareston
Func. class.: Antineoplastic
Chem. class.: Antiestrogen hormone

Action: Inhibits cell division by binding to cytoplasmic estrogen receptors; resembles normal cell complex but inhibits DNA synthesis and estrogen response of target tissue

Uses: Advanced breast carcinoma not responsive to other therapy in estrogen-receptor-positive patients (usually postmenopausal)

Unlabeled uses: Prostate cancer prophylaxis

DOSAGE AND ROUTES

- *Adult:* **PO** 60 mg/day

Available forms: Tabs 60 mg

SIDE EFFECTS

CNS: *Hot flashes, headache, lightheadedness,* depression
CV: **CHF, MI, PE,** chest pain, angina
EENT: Ocular lesions, retinopathy, corneal opacity, blurred vision (high doses)
GI: *Nausea, vomiting,* altered taste (anorexia)
GU: Vaginal bleeding, pruritus vulvae
HEMA: **Thrombocytopenia, leukopenia, thrombosis**
INTEG: Rash, alopecia, *sweating*
META: Hypercalcemia
RESP: **Pulmonary embolism**

Contraindications: Pregnancy (D), hypersensitivity, history of thromboembolism

Precautions: Breastfeeding, children, leukopenia, thrombocytopenia, cataracts, hypercalcemia, hepatic disease, endometrial hyperplasia

PHARMACOKINETICS

Peak 3 hr, excreted primarily in feces, 99.5% protein binding, terminal half-life 5-6 days, metabolized by the liver

INTERACTIONS

- May increase the effect of warfarin

Increase: toxicity—CYP3A4 inhibitors (aprepitant, antiretroviral protease inhibitors, clarithromycin, danazol, delavirdine, diltiazem, erythromycin, fluconazole, fluoxetine, fluvoxamine, imatinib, ketoconazole, mibefradil, nefazodone, telithromycin, voriconazole)

Decrease: toremifene effect—CYP3A4 inducers (barbiturates, bosentan, carba-

T

mazepine, efavirenz, phenytoins, nevirapine, rifabutin, rifampin)

Drug/Herb

• Avoid use with St. John's wort

Drug/Lab Test

Increase: serum calcium

NURSING CONSIDERATIONS

Assess:

• CBC, differential, platelet count q wk; withhold product if WBC is <3500/mm^3 or platelet count is <100,000/mm^3; notify prescriber; LFTs, serum calcium

• Bleeding: hematuria, guaiac, bruising, petechiae, mucosa, or orifices q8hr

• Effects of alopecia on body image; discuss feelings about body changes

⚠ Symptoms indicating severe allergic reactions: rash, pruritus, urticaria, purpuric skin lesions, itching, flushing

Administer:

• Antacid before oral agent; give product after evening meal, before bedtime

• Antiemetic 30-60 min before giving product to prevent vomiting

Perform/provide:

• Increase fluid intake to 2-3 L/day to prevent dehydration

• Nutritious diet with iron, vitamin supplements as ordered; avoid use of herbals

• Storage in light-resistant container at room temperature

Evaluate:

• Therapeutic response: decreased tumor size, spread of malignancy

Teach patient/family:

• To report any complaints, side effects to prescriber

• That vaginal bleeding, pruritus, hot flashes are reversible after discontinuing treatment

• To report immediately decreased visual acuity, which may be irreversible; stress need for routine eye exams; care providers should be told about tamoxifen therapy

• To report vaginal bleeding immediately

• That tumor flare—increase in size of tumor, increased bone pain—may occur and will subside rapidly; may take analgesics for pain

• That premenopausal women must use mechanical birth control because ovulation may be induced

• That hair may be lost during treatment; a wig or hairpiece may make patient feel better; new hair may be different in color, texture

torsemide (℞)

(tor′suh-mide)

Demadex

Func. class.: Loop diuretic

Chem. class.: Sulfonamide derivative

Action: Acts on loop of Henle, proximal, distal tubule by inhibiting absorption of chloride, sodium, water

Uses: Treatment of hypertension and edema in CHF, renal/hepatic disease

DOSAGE AND ROUTES

CHF

• *Adult:* **PO/IV** 10-20 mg/day, may increase as needed, max 200 mg/day

Chronic renal failure

• *Adult:* **PO/IV** 20 mg/day, may increase up to 200 mg/day

Hepatic cirrhosis in combination with aldosterone antagonist/ potassium-sparing diuretic

• *Adult:* **PO/IV** 5-10 mg/day may increase as needed, max 40 mg/day

Hypertension

• *Adult:* **PO** 5 mg/day may increase to 10 mg/day

Available forms: Tabs 5, 10, 20, 100 mg; inj 10 mg/ml

SIDE EFFECTS

CNS: Headache, dizziness, asthenia, insomnia, nervousness

CV: Orthostatic hypotension, chest pain, ECG changes, **circulatory collapse,** ventricular tachycardia, edema

EENT: Loss of hearing, ear pain, tinnitus, blurred vision

ELECT: Hypokalemia, hypochloremic alkalosis, hyponatremia, metabolic alkalosis
ENDO: Hyperglycemia, hyperuricemia
GI: Nausea, diarrhea, dyspepsia, cramps, constipation
GU: Polyuria, **renal failure,** glycosuria
INTEG: Rash, photosensitivity, pruritus
MS: Cramps, stiffness
RESP: Rhinitis, cough increase
Contraindications: Infants, hypersensitivity to sulfonamides, anuria, hypovolemia
Precautions: Pregnancy (B), breastfeeding, diabetes mellitus, dehydration, severe renal disease, electrolyte depletion

PHARMACOKINETICS

PO: Rapidly absorbed; duration 6 hr; excreted in urine, feces, breast milk; crosses placenta; half-life 2-4 hr; plasma protein binding 97%-99%

INTERACTIONS

- Incompatible with any product in syringe

Increase: toxicity—lithium, nondepolarizing skeletal muscle relaxants, digoxin
Increase: action of antihypertensives, oral anticoagulants, nitrates
Increase: ototoxicity—aminoglycosides, cisplatin, vancomycin
Decrease: antihypertensive effect of torsemide—indomethacin, carbamazepine, phenobarbital, phenytoin, rifampin, NSAIDs

Drug/Herb

- Severe photosensitivity: St. John's wort

Increase: effect—aloe, cucumber, dandelion, horsetail, pumpkin, Queen Anne's lace
Increase: hypotension khella

Drug/Lab Test

Interference: GTT

NURSING CONSIDERATIONS

Assess:

- Hearing when giving high doses
- Weight, I&O daily to determine fluid loss; effect of product may be decreased if used daily
- Rate, depth, rhythm of respiration, effect of exertion
- B/P lying, standing; postural hypotension may occur
- Electrolytes: K, Na, Cl; include BUN, blood glucose, CBC, serum creatinine, blood pH, ABGs, uric acid, Ca, Mg
- Glucose in urine of diabetic
- Signs and symptoms of metabolic alkalosis: drowsiness, restlessness
- Signs and symptoms of hypokalemia: postural hypotension, malaise, fatigue, tachycardia, leg cramps, weakness
- Rashes, temp elevation daily
- Confusion, especially in geriatric patients; take safety precautions if needed

Administer:

- In AM to avoid interference with sleep if using product as a diuretic
- Potassium replacement if potassium <3 mg/dl
- With food or milk if nausea occurs; absorption may be decreased slightly

Evaluate:

- Therapeutic response: improvement in edema of feet, legs, sacral area daily if medication is being used in CHF

Teach patient/family:

- To rise slowly from lying, sitting position
- To recognize adverse reactions: muscle cramps, weakness, nausea, dizziness, tinnitus
- To take with food or milk for GI symptoms; to limit alcohol use
- To take early in day to prevent nocturia

Treatment of overdose: Lavage if taken orally; monitor electrolytes, administer dextrose in saline; monitor hydration, CV, renal status

T

trace elements (℞)

Concentrated Multiple Trace Elements, ConTE-PAK-4, M.T.E.-4, M.T.E.-4 Concentrated, M.T.E.-5, M.T.E.-5 Concentrated, M.T.E.-6, M.T.E.-6 Concentrated, M.T.E.-7, MulTE-PAK-4, MulTE-PAK-5, Multiple Trace Element, Multiple Trace Element Neonatal, Multiple Trace Element Pediatric, Neotrace 4, PedTE-PAK-4, Pedtrace-4, P.T.E.-4, P.T.E.-5

Func. class.: Mineral supplements

Action: Needed for adequate absorption and synthesis of amino acids

Uses: Prevention of trace element deficiency

DOSAGE AND ROUTES

Usual dosage may be given in TPN sol

Chromium

- *Adult:* **IV** 10-15 mcg/day
- *Child:* **IV** 0.14-0.20 mcg/kg/day

Copper

- *Adult:* **IV** 0.5-1.5 mg/day
- *Child:* **IV** 0.05-0.2 mg/kg/day

Iodine

- *Adult:* **IV** 1 mcg/kg/day

Manganese

- *Adult:* **IV** 0.15-0.8 mg/day

Selenium

- *Adult:* **IV** 20-40 mcg/day
- *Child:* **IV** 3 mcg/kg/day

Zinc

- *Adult:* **IV** 2-4 mg/day
- *Child:* **IV** 0.05 mg/kg/day

Available forms: Many forms available—see particular elements

SIDE EFFECTS

CHROMIUM: **Seizures, coma,** nausea, vomiting, ulcers, renal/hepatic toxicity

COPPER: Personality changes, diarrhea, weakness, photophobia, muscle weakness

IODINE: Headache, edema of eyelids, acne, metallic taste, sore mouth, runny nose

MANGANESE: Incoordination, headache, irritability, lability, slurred speech, impotence

SELENIUM: Alopecia, depression, vomiting, GI cramping, nervousness, garlic smell

ZINC: Vomiting, oliguria, hypothermia, vision changes, tachycardia, jaundice, **coma**

Precautions: Pregnancy (C), breastfeeding, biliary/hepatic disease, vomiting, diarrhea

NURSING CONSIDERATIONS

Assess:

- Trace element levels; notify prescriber if low; copper 0.07-0.15 mg/ml, zinc 0.05-0.15 mg/100 ml, manganese 4-20 mcg/100 ml, selenium 0.1-0.19 mcg/ml
- Trace element deficiency of patient receiving TPN for extended period

Administer:

- By IV inf, often mixed with TPN solution

Evaluate:

- Therapeutic response: absence of element deficiency

tramadol (℞)

(tram′a-dole)

Ryzolt, Ultram, Ultram ER

Func. class.: Analgesic—miscellaneous

Do not confuse:

tramadol/Toradol

Action: Not completely understood, binds to opioid receptors, inhibits reuptake of norepinephrine, serotonin; does not cause histamine release or affect heart rate

Uses: Management of moderate to severe pain, chronic pain

Unlabeled uses: Restless leg syndrome (RLS), postoperative shivering

DOSAGE AND ROUTES

Mild to moderate pain

• *Adult:* **PO** 50-100 mg prn q4-6hr; max 400 mg/day

• *Geriatric >75 years:* **PO** <300 mg/day in divided doses

Moderate to severe chronic pain

• *Adult:* **PO-ER** (Ultram ER) 100 mg, titrate upward q5days in 100 mg increments, max 300 mg/day; (Ryzolt) 100 mg, titrate upward q2-3days in 100 mg increments, max 300 mg/day; products are not interchangeable

Renal dose

• *Adult:* **PO** CCr <30 ml/min give q12hr, max 200 mg/day, do use ER tab

Hepatic impairment

• *Adult (Child-Pugh C):* **PO** 50 mg q12hr

Restless leg syndrome (RLS) (unlabeled)

• *Adult:* **PO** 50-150 mg/day × 15-24 mo

Available forms: Tabs 50 mg; ext rel tab 100, 200, 300 mg

SIDE EFFECTS

CNS: Dizziness, CNS stimulation, somnolence, headache, anxiety, confusion, euphoria, **seizures,** hallucinations, sedation, **neuroleptic malignant syndrome–like reactions**

CV: Vasodilation, orthostatic hypotension, tachycardia, hypertension, abnormal ECG

EENT: Visual disturbances

GI: Nausea, constipation, vomiting, dry mouth, diarrhea, abdominal pain, anorexia, flatulence, *GI bleeding*

GU: Urinary retention/frequency, menopausal symptoms, dysuria, menstrual disorder

INTEG: Pruritus, rash, urticaria, vesicles, flushing

SYST: **Anaphylaxis, Stevens-Johnson syndrome, toxic epidermal necrolysis,** serotonin syndrome

Contraindications: Hypersensitivity, acute intoxication with any CNS depressant

Precautions: Pregnancy (C), breastfeeding, children, geriatric patients, seizure disorder, renal/hepatic disease, respiratory depression, head trauma, increased intracranial pressure, acute abdominal condition, drug abuse

PHARMACOKINETICS

Rapidly and almost completely absorbed, steady state 2 days, peak 1.5 hr, duration 6 hr, terminal half-life 7.9-8.8 hr, may cross blood-brain barrier, extensively metabolized, 30% excreted in the urine as unchanged product

INTERACTIONS

• Inhibition of norepinephrine and serotonin reuptake: MAOIs, use together with caution

Increase: CNS depression—alcohol, sedatives, hypnotics, opiates

Increase: serotonin syndrome—SSRIs

Increase: tramadol levels—CYP3A4 inhibitors (aprepitant, antiretroviral protease inhibitors, clarithromycin, danazol, delavirdine, diltiazem, erythromycin, fluconazole, fluoxetine, fluvoxamine, imatinib, ketoconazole, mibefradil, nefazodone, telithromycin, voriconazole)

Decrease: tramadol effects—CYP3A4 inducers (barbiturates, bosentan, carbamazepine, efavirenz, phenytoins, nevirapine, rifabutin, rifampin)

Decrease: levels of tramadol—carbamazepine

Drug/Herb

• Avoid use with St. John's wort

Increase: CNS depression—chamomile, hops, kava, skullcap, valerian

Drug/Lab Test

Increase: creatinine, hepatic enzymes

Decrease: Hgb

NURSING CONSIDERATIONS

Assess:

• Pain: location, type, character, give before pain becomes extreme

• I&O ratio: check for decreasing output; may indicate urinary retention

• Need for product; dependency

• Bowel pattern; for constipation increase fluids, bulk in diet

T

- CNS changes: dizziness, drowsiness, hallucinations, euphoria, LOC, pupil reaction
- Allergic reactions: rash, urticaria
- For increased side effects in renal/hepatic disease

Administer:

- Ext rel products (Ryzolt/Utram ER) are not interchangeable
- Do not break, crush, or chew ER product
- With antiemetic for nausea, vomiting
- When pain is beginning to return; determine dosage interval by patient response

Perform/provide:

- Storage in cool environment, protected from sunlight
- Assistance with ambulation
- Safety measures: side rails, night-light, call bell within easy reach

Evaluate:

- Therapeutic response: decrease in pain

Teach patient/family:

- To report any symptoms of CNS changes, allergic reactions
- That drowsiness, dizziness, and confusion may occur, to call for assistance
- To make position changes slowly, orthostatic hypotension may occur
- To avoid OTC medications and alcohol unless approved by prescriber

trandolapril (℞)

(tran-doe′la-prill)

Mavik

Func. class.: Antihypertensive

Chem. class.: Angiotension-converting enzyme inhibitor

Action: Selectively suppresses renin-angiotensin-aldosterone system; inhibits ACE; prevents conversion of angiotensin I to angiotensin II, dilates arterial and venous vessels, lowers B/P

Uses: Hypertension, heart failure, post-MI/left ventricular dysfunction post MI

DOSAGE AND ROUTES

Hypertension

- *Adult:* **PO** 1 mg/day; 2 mg/day in African-Americans; make dosage adjustment ≥ wk; max 8 mg/day

Heart failure post-MI/left ventricular dysfunction post MI

- *Adult:* **PO** 1 mg/day, titrate upward to 4 mg/day if tolerated

Renal/hepatic dose

- *Adult:* **PO** CCr <30 ml/min or hepatic disease give 0.5 mg/day, may increase gradually up to 4 mg/day

Available forms: Tabs 1, 2, 4 mg

SIDE EFFECTS

CNS: *Dizziness, syncope,* paresthesias, headache, fatigue, drowsiness, depression, sleep disturbances, anxiety

CV: *Hypotension,* **MI,** palpitations, angina, TIAs, **stroke,** *bradycardia,* dysrhythmias

GI: Nausea, vomiting, cramps, diarrhea, constipation, **pancreatitis,** *dyspepsia*

GU: **Proteinuria, renal failure**

HEMA: **Agranulocytosis, neutropenia, leukopenia, anemia**

INTEG: Rash, purpura, pruritus

MISC: Hyperkalemia, hyponatremia, impotence, *myalgia,* **angioedema,** muscle cramps, *asthenia,* hypocalcemia, gout

RESP: Dyspnea, *cough*

Contraindications: Breastfeeding, hypersensitivity, history of angioedema

Black Box Warning: Pregnancy (D)

Precautions: Geriatric patients, hyperkalemia, hepatic disease, bilateral renal stenosis, post–kidney transplant, aorta/mitral valve stenosis, cirrhosis, severe renal disease, untreated CHF, autoimmune disease, cough

PHARMACOKINETICS

Peak 4-10 hr, duration 24 hr, half-life 6-10 hr, metabolized by liver (active metabolite trandolaprilat), excreted in urine, protein binding 65%-94%

INTERACTIONS

Increase: effects—phenothiazines, diuretics
Increase: severe hypotension—diuretics, other antihypertensives
Increase: potassium levels—salt substitutes, potassium-sparing diuretics, potassium supplements
Increase: effects of ergots, neuromuscular blocking agents, antihypertensives, hypoglycemics, barbiturates, reserpine, levodopa, lithium
Decrease: effects of trandolapril—antacids, NSAIDs, salicylates

Drug/Herb

Increase: toxicity, death—aconite
Increase: antihypertensive effect—barberry, betony, black catechu, black cohosh, bloodroot, broom, burdock, cat's claw, dandelion, goldenseal, hawthorn, Irish moss, Jamaican dogwood, kelp, khella, mistletoe, parsley
Increase or decrease: antihypertensive effect—astragalus, cola tree
Decrease: antihypertensive effect—coltsfoot, guarana, khat, licorice, yohimbe

NURSING CONSIDERATIONS

Assess:

- B/P, pulse q4hr; note rate, rhythm, quality
- Electrolytes: K, Na, Cl
- Baselines in renal, hepatic studies before therapy begins
- Edema in feet, legs daily
- Skin turgor, dryness of mucous membranes for hydration status
- Symptoms of CHF: edema, dyspnea, wet crackles

Administer:

- Discontinue diuretic 2-3 days before starting this product; if not possible, decrease initial dose to 0.5 ml
- Make dosage changes ≥1 wk

Evaluate:

- Therapeutic response: decreased B/P

Teach patient/family:

- Not to use OTC (cough, cold, or allergy) products unless directed by prescriber
- To avoid sunlight or wear sunscreen for photosensitivity
- To comply with dosage schedule, even if feeling better
- To notify prescriber of mouth sores, sore throat, fever, swelling of hands or feet, irregular heartbeat, chest pain, signs of angioedema
- That excessive perspiration, dehydration, vomiting, diarrhea may lead to fall in blood pressure; consult prescriber if these occur
- That product may cause dizziness, fainting; light-headedness may occur during 1st few days of therapy
- That product may cause skin rash or impaired perspiration
- Not to discontinue product abruptly
- To rise slowly to sitting or standing position to minimize orthostatic hypotension

⚠ High Alert

trastuzumab (℞)

(tras-tuz'uh-mab)
Herceptin
Func. class.: Antineoplastic—miscellaneous
Chem. class.: Humanized monoclonal antibody

Action: DNA-derived monoclonal antibody selectively binds to extracellular portion of human epidermal growth factor receptor 2; it inhibits proliferation of cancer cells

Uses: Breast cancer; metastatic with overexpression of HER2, early breast cancer (adjuvant, neoadjuvant)

Unlabeled uses: Gastric cancer

DOSAGE AND ROUTES

- Several regimens may be used
- *Adult:* **IV** 4 mg/kg given over 90 min, then maintenance 2 mg/kg given over 30 min; do not give as IV push or bol; may be given in combination with other antineoplastics

T

Gastric cancer (unlabeled)

• *Adult:* **IV** 8 mg/kg over 90 min on day 1, then 6 mg/kg over 30-60 min q21days from day 22, give with cisplatin 80 mg/m^2 on day 1 plus 5-fluorouracil 800 mg/m^2 **CONT INF** on days 1-5 or capecitabine 1000 mg/m^2 bid on days 1-14, repeat cycle q3wk

Available forms: Lyophilized powder 440 mg

SIDE EFFECTS

CNS: Dizziness, numbness, paresthesias, depression, *insomnia,* neuropathy, peripheral neuritis

CV: **Tachycardia, CHF**

GI: Nausea, vomiting, *anorexia, diarrhea,* abdominal pain, **hepatotoxicity**

HEMA: Anemia, **leukopenia**

INTEG: Rash, acne, herpes simplex

META: Edema, peripheral edema

MISC: Flulike symptoms; fever, headache, chills

MS: Arthralgia, *bone pain*

RESP: Cough, dyspnea, pharyngitis, rhinitis, sinusitis, **pneumonia**

SYST: **Anaphylaxis, angioedema**

Contraindications: Pregnancy (D), hypersensitivity to this product, Chinese hamster ovary cell protein

Precautions: Breastfeeding, children, geriatric patients, pulmonary disease, anemia, leukopenia

Black Box Warning: Cardiac disease, respiratory distress syndrome, inf-related reactions

PHARMACOKINETICS

Half-life 1-32 days

INTERACTIONS

Increase: bleeding risk—warfarin

Increase: cardiomyopathy—anthracyclines, cyclophosphamide, avoid use

Decrease: immune response—vaccines/toxoids

NURSING CONSIDERATIONS

Assess:

• CBC, HER 2 overexpression

⚠ CHF and other cardiac symptoms: dyspnea, coughing; gallop; obtain a full cardiac workup including ECG, echo, MUGA

• For symptoms of infection; may be masked by product

• CNS reaction: LOC, mental status, dizziness, confusion

⚠ For hypersensitive reactions, anaphylaxis

⚠ For infusion reactions that may be fatal: fever, chills, nausea, vomiting, pain, headache, dizziness, hypotension, discontinue product

Administer:

• Acetaminophen as ordered to alleviate fever and headache

IV route

• After reconstituting vial with 20 ml bacteriostatic water for inj, 1.1% benzyl alcohol preserved (supplied) to yield 21 mg/ml, mark date on vial 28 days from reconstitution date, if patient is allergic to benzyl alcohol, reconstitute with sterile water for inj—use immediately, infuse over 90 min, q3wk give 8 mg/kg loading dose over 90 min, subsequent 6 mg/kg dose may be given over 30-60 min

• Do not mix or dilute with other products or dextrose sol

Perform/provide:

• Increased fluid intake to 2-3 L/day

Evaluate:

• Therapeutic response: decrease in size of tumors

Teach patient/family:

• To take acetaminophen for fever

• To avoid hazardous tasks, since confusion, dizziness may occur

• To report signs of infection: sore throat, fever, diarrhea, vomiting

• Emotional lability is common; notify prescriber if severe or incapacitating

• To use contraception while taking this product; pregnancy category (D); avoid breastfeeding

travoprost ophthalmic
See Appendix B

trazodone (℞)
(tray′zoe-done)
trazodone HCl
Func. class.: Antidepressant—miscellaneous
Chem. class.: Triazolopyridine

Action: Selectively inhibits serotonin, norepinephrine uptake by brain, potentiates behavorial changes
Uses: Depression
Unlabeled uses: Alcoholism, anxiety, panic disorder, insomnia

DOSAGE AND ROUTES
- *Adult:* **PO** 150 mg/day in divided doses, may increase by 50 mg/day q3-4days, max 400 mg/day (outpatient), 600 mg/day (inpatients)
- *Child 6-18 yr:* **PO** 1.5-2 mg/kg/day in divided dose, may increase q3-4days, up to 6 mg/kg/day or 400 mg/day, whichever is less
- *Geriatric:* **PO** 25-50 mg at bedtime, increase by 25-50 mg q3-7days to desired dose, usual 75-150 mg/day

Alcoholism (unlabeled)
- *Adult:* **PO** 50-100 mg/day

Panic disorder (unlabeled)
- *Adult:* **PO** 150 mg in divided doses, may increase by 50 mg/day q3-4days

Insomnia (unlabeled)
- *Adult:* **PO** 50 mg at bedtime

Available forms: Tabs 50, 100, 150, 300 mg

SIDE EFFECTS
CNS: Dizziness, drowsiness, confusion, headache, anxiety, tremors, stimulation, weakness, insomnia, nightmares, EPS (geriatric patients), increase in psychiatric symptoms, **suicide in children/adolescents**
CV: Orthostatic hypotension, ECG changes, tachycardia, **hypertension,** palpitations
EENT: Blurred vision, tinnitus, mydriasis
GI: Diarrhea, dry mouth, nausea, vomiting, **paralytic ileus,** increased appetite, cramps, epigastric distress, jaundice, **hepatitis,** stomatitis, constipation
GU: Urinary retention, **acute renal failure,** priapism
HEMA: **Agranulocytosis, thrombocytopenia, eosinophilia, leukopenia**
INTEG: Rash, urticaria, sweating, pruritus, photosensitivity

Contraindications: Hypersensitivity to tricyclics, recovery phase of MI, seizure disorders, prostatic hypertrophy
Precautions: Pregnancy (C), suicidal patients, severe depression, increased intraocular pressure, closed-angle glaucoma, urinary retention, cardiac/hepatic disease, hyperthyroidism, electroshock therapy, elective surgery

Black Box Warning: Suicidal ideation in children/adolescents

PHARMACOKINETICS
Peak 1 hr without food, 2 hr with food; metabolized by liver (CYP3A4); excreted by kidneys, feces; half-life 4.4-7.5 hr

INTERACTIONS
⚠ Hyperpyretic crisis, seizures, hypertensive episode: MAOIs, do not use within 14 days of trazadone
Increase: toxicity, serotonin syndrome—fluoxetine, nefazodone, other SSRIs
Increase: effects of direct-acting sympathomimetics (epinephrine), alcohol, barbiturates, benzodiazepines, CNS depressants, digoxin, phenytoin, carbamazepine
Increase: effects of trazadone—CYP3A4, 2D6 inhibitors (phenothiazines, protease inhibitors, azole antifungals)
Increase or decrease: effects of warfarin
Decrease: effects of guanethidine, clonidine, indirect-acting sympathomimetics (ephedrine)

T

Drug/Herb

Increase: serotonin syndrome—SAM-e, St. John's wort

Increase: CNS depression—chamomile, hops, kava, lavender, skullcap, valerian

Increase: anticholinergic effect—corkwood, jimsonweed

Drug/Lab Test

Increase: serum bilirubin, blood glucose, alk phos

Decrease: VMA, 5-HIAA

False increase: urinary catecholamines

NURSING CONSIDERATIONS

Assess:

- Pain: location, duration, intensity before and 1-2 hr after medication
- B/P (lying, standing), pulse q4hr; if systolic B/P drops 20 mm Hg, hold product, notify prescriber; take vital signs q4hr in patients with CV disease
- Blood studies: CBC, leukocytes, differential, cardiac enzymes if patient is receiving long-term therapy
- Hepatic studies: AST, ALT, bilirubin
- Weight q wk; appetite may increase with product
- ECG for flattening of T wave, bundle branch block, AV block, dysrhythmias in cardiac patients
- EPS, primarily in geriatric patients: rigidity, dystonia, akathisia

⚠ Mental status changes: mood, sensorium, affect, suicidal tendencies, increase in psychiatric symptoms, depression, panic; observe for suicidal behaviors in children/adolescents

- Urinary retention, constipation; constipation most likely in children
- Withdrawal symptoms: headache, nausea, vomiting, muscle pain, weakness; not usual unless product discontinued abruptly
- Alcohol consumption; hold dose until morning

Administer:

- Increased fluids, bulk in diet if constipation occurs, especially in geriatric patients
- With food, milk for GI symptoms
- Dosage at bedtime for oversedation during day; may take entire dose at bedtime; geriatric patients may not tolerate daily dosing
- Gum, hard candy, frequent sips of water for dry mouth
- Avoid use of CNS depressants

Perform/provide:

- Storage in tight, light-resistant container at room temperature
- Assistance with ambulation during beginning therapy for drowsiness/dizziness
- Safety measures, including side rails, primarily for geriatric patients
- Checking to see if PO medication swallowed

Evaluate:

- Therapeutic response: decreased depression

Teach patient/family:

- That therapeutic effects may take 2-3 wk; to take before bedtime
- To use caution in driving, other activities requiring alertness because of drowsiness, dizziness, blurred vision
- To avoid alcohol ingestion
- Not to discontinue medication quickly after long-term use; may cause nausea, headache, malaise
- To report urinary retention, priapism >4 hr immediately
- To wear sunscreen or large hat, since photosensitivity occurs
- That suicidal thoughts/behavior may occur (adolescents/children)

Treatment of overdose: ECG monitoring; lavage, activated charcoal; administer anticonvulsant

treprostinil (℞)

(treh-prah'stin-ill)

Remodulin, Tyvaso

Func. class.: Antiplatelet agent

Chem. class.: Tricyclic benzidine prostacyclin analog

Action: Direct vasodilation of pulmonary, systemic arterial vascular beds, inhibition of platelet aggregation

Uses: Pulmonary arterial hypertension (PAH) NYHA class II through IV

Unlabeled uses: Pulmonary arterial hypertension in children/adolescents, pediatric patients transitioning from epoprostenol to treprostinil, claudication

DOSAGE AND ROUTES

• *Adult:* **SUBCUT INF** 1.25 ng/kg/min by **CONT INF**, may reduce to 0.625 ng if not tolerated; may increase by 1.25 ng/kg/min q wk for first 4 wk, then 2.5 ng/kg/min/wk for remainder of inf; oral inh 3 breaths via Tyvaso inh system qid

Hepatic dose

• *Adult:* **SUBCUT INF** 0.625 ng/kg ideal body weight/min and increase cautiously

Available forms: Inj 1, 2.5, 5, 10 mg/ml; neb sol 1.74 mg/2.9 ml

SIDE EFFECTS

CNS: Dizziness, headache

CV: Vasodilation, hypotension, edema

GI: Nausea, *diarrhea*

INTEG: *Rash,* pruritus

OTHER: Jaw pain

SYST: Inf site reactions, inf site pain, increased risk of infection

Contraindications: Hypersensitivity to this product or other prostacyclin analogs

Precautions: Pregnancy (B), breastfeeding, children, geriatric patients, past renal/hepatic disease, thromboembolic disease, abrupt discontinuation, IV administration

PHARMACOKINETICS

Metabolized by liver, excreted in urine/feces, terminal half-life 2-4 hr, 90% protein binding

INTERACTIONS

• Excessive hypotension: diuretics, antihypertensives, vasodilators, MAOIs, β-blockers, calcium channel blockers

Increase: bleeding tendencies—anticoagulants, aspirin, NSAIDs, thrombin inhibitors, SSRIs

NURSING CONSIDERATIONS

Assess:

• Hepatic studies: AST, ALT, bilirubin, creatinine (long-term therapy)

⚠ Blood studies: CBC; CBC q2wk × 3 mo, Hct, Hgb, PT (long-term therapy)

⚠ Bleed time baseline and throughout; levels may be 2-5 × normal limit

Administer:

• Sudden decreased doses or abrupt withdrawal may worsen pulmonary arterial hypertension symptoms

SUBCUT INF route

• By continuous inf

• No dilution required

CONT IV INF route

• By surgically placed CV catheter using an ambulatory inf pump

• The IV pump, product, and patient education can be obtained from Priority Healthcare in the United States

• Must be diluted with sterile water for inj or 0.9% NaCl

• The concentration should be calculated using this formula: diluted conc = [dose (ng/kg/min) × weight (kg) × 0.00006] / inf rate (ml/hr)]

Evaluate:

• Therapeutic response: decreased pulmonary arterial hypertension (PAH)

Teach patient/family:

• That blood work will be necessary during treatment

• To report side effects such as diarrhea, skin rashes

• That therapy will be needed for prolonged periods of time, sometimes years

• To prevent infection, aseptic technique must be used in preparing and administration of treprostinil

• There are many product and herb interactions

• Signs/symptoms of bleeding; blood in urine, stools

tretinoin (vit A acid, retinoic acid) (℞)

(tret′i-noyn)

Avita, Renova, Retin-A, Retin-A Micro, Stieva-A ♣

Func. class.: Vit A acid, acne product; antineoplastic (miscellaneous)

Chem. class.: Tretinoin derivative

Action: (Topical) Decreases cohesiveness of follicular epithelium, decreases microcomedone formation; (PO) induces maturation of acute promyelocytic leukemia, exact action is unknown

Uses: (Topical) Acne vulgaris (grades 1-3); (PO) acute promyelocytic leukemia, facial wrinkles, photoaging

Unlabeled uses: Acne rosacea, actinic keratosis, ichthyosis, Kaposi's sarcoma, keloids, keratosis follicularis, melasma

DOSAGE AND ROUTES

• *Adult and child:* **TOP** Cleanse area, apply 0.025%-0.1% cream or 0.05% liquid gel at bedtime, cover lightly

Promyelocytic leukemia

• *Adult:* **PO** 45 mg/m^2/day given as 2 evenly divided doses until remission, discontinue treatment 30 days after remission or 90 days of treatment, whichever is first

Available forms: Cream 0.01%, 0.02%, 0.025%, 0.05%, 0.1%; gel 0.01%, 0.025%, 0.04%, 0.05%, 0.1%; liquid 0.05%; caps 10 mg

SIDE EFFECTS

Oral

CNS: Headache, fever, sweating, fatigue

CV: Cardiac dysrhythmias, pericardial effusion

GI: Nausea, vomiting, **hemorrhage,** *abdominal pain, diarrhea, constipation, dyspepsia, distention, hepatitis*

Topical

INTEG: Rash, stinging, warmth, redness, erythema, blistering, crusting, peeling, contact dermatitis, hypo/hyperpigmentation, dry skin, pruritus, scaly skin

META: Hypercholesterolemia, hypertriglyceridemia

RESP: Pneumonia, upper respiratory tract disease

Contraindications: Hypersensitivity to retinoids or sensitivity to parabens

Black Box Warning: Pregnancy (D) (PO)

Precautions: Pregnancy (C) (topical), breastfeeding, eczema, sunburn, sun exposure

Black Box Warning: Rapid-evolving leukocytosis, respiratory compromise, acute promyelocytic leukemia differentiation syndrome

PHARMACOKINETICS

PO: Terminal half-life 0.5-2 hr

TOPICAL: Poor systemic absorption

INTERACTIONS

• Use with caution: medicated, abrasive soaps, cleansers that have drying effect, products with high concentrations of alcohol astringents (topical)

Increase: peeling—medication containing agents such as sulfur, benzoyl peroxide, resorcinol, salicylic acid (topical)

Increase: plasma concentrations of tretinoin—ketoconazole (PO)

Increase: ICP, risk of pseudotumor cerebri—tetracyclines, do not use together

Increase: photosensitivity—retinoids, quinolones, phenothiazines, sulfonamides, sulfonylureas, thiazide diuretics

Increase: thrombotic complications—aninocaproic acid, aprotinin, tranexamic acid

Drug/Lab Test

Increase: AST, ALT

NURSING CONSIDERATIONS

Assess:

Topical route

• Area of body involved, what helps or aggravates condition; cysts, dryness, itching; lesions may worsen at beginning of treatment

PO route

• Hepatic function, coagulation, hematologic parameters, also cholesterol, triglyceride

Administer:

Topical route

• Once daily before bedtime; cover area lightly using gauze; use gloves to apply

Perform/provide:

Topical route

• Storage at room temperature

• Hand washing after application

Evaluate:

• Therapeutic response: decrease in size and number of lesions

Teach patient/family:

Topical route

• To avoid application on normal skin, getting cream in eyes, nose, other mucous membranes; do not use product on areas with cuts, scrapes

• To use cream/gel by applying a thin layer to affected skin; rub gently; to use liquid, apply with fingertip or cotton swab

• To avoid sunlight, sunlamps, or use protective clothing, sunscreen

• That treatment may cause warmth, stinging, dryness, peeling will occur

• That cosmetics may be used over product; not to use shaving lotions

• That rash may occur during first 1-3 wk of therapy

• That product does not cure condition; only relieves symptoms

• That therapeutic results may be seen in 2-3 wk but may not be optimal until after 6 wk

tretinoin topical

See Appendix B

triamcinolone (℞)

(trye-am-sin'oh-lone)

Amcort, Aristocort, Aristocort Forte, Aristocort Intralesional, Aristospan Intra-Articular, Aristospan Intralesional, Articulose L.A., Atolone, Azmacort, Cenocort A-40, Cenocort Forte, Kenacort, Kenaject-40, Kenalog, Kenalog-10, Kenalog-40, Tac-3, Tac-40, Triam-A, Triam Forte, Triamolone 40, Triamonide 40, Tri-Kort, Trilog, Trilone, Trisoject, Trivaris

Func. class.: Corticosteroid, synthetic

Chem. class.: Glucocorticoid, intermediate-acting

See ophthalmic in Appendix B

Action: Decreases inflammation by suppression of migration of polymorphonuclear leukocytes, fibroblasts, reversal of increased capillary permeability and lysosomal stabilization

Uses: Severe inflammation, immunosuppression, neoplasms, asthma (steroid dependent), collagen, respiratory, dermatologic/rheumatic disorders

DOSAGE AND ROUTES

• *Adult:* **PO** 4-12 mg/day in divided doses daily-qid; **IM** (acetonide, diacetate) 40 mg q wk; (diacetate, acetonide) 5-48 mg into neoplasms; (diacetate, acetonide) 2-40 mg into joint or soft tissue; (hexacetonide) 0.5 mg/in^2 of affected intralesional skin; (hexacetonide) 2-20 mg into joint or soft tissue

• *Child:* **PO** 117 mcg/kg/day in divided doses

Asthma

• *Adult:* **INH** 2 tid-qid, max 16 inh/day

• *Child 6-12 yr:* **INH** 1-2 tid-qid, max 12 inh/day

T

Severe/incapacitating allergic conditions such as asthma

• *Adult:* **IM** (Trivaris) 60 mg, titrate, usual range 40-80 mg

• *Child:* **IM** (Trivaris) 0.11-1.6 mg/kg/day (3.2-48 mg/m^2/day) given in 3-4 divided doses

Available forms: Tabs 1, 2, 4, 8 mg; syr 2 mg/5 ml, 4.85 mg/5 ml; inj 25, 40 mg/ml diacetate; inj 3, 10, 40 mg/ml acetonide; inj 20, 5 mg/ml hexacetonide; aerosol actuation/100 mcg (acetonide)

SIDE EFFECTS

CNS: Depression, flushing, sweating, headache, mood changes

CV: Hypertension, **circulatory collapse, thrombophlebitis, embolism,** tachycardia, edema

EENT: Fungal infections, increased intraocular pressure, blurred vision

GI: Diarrhea, nausea, abdominal distention, **GI hemorrhage,** *increased appetite,* **pancreatitis**

HEMA: **Thrombocytopenia**

INTEG: Acne, poor wound healing, ecchymosis, petechiae

MS: Fractures, osteoporosis, weakness

Contraindications: Children <2 yr, psychosis, hypersensitivity, idiopathic thrombocytopenia, acute glomerulonephritis, amebiasis, fungal infections, nonasthmatic bronchial disease, AIDS, TB, adrenal insufficiency, acute bronchospasm, neonatal prematurity

Precautions: Pregnancy (C), breastfeeding, diabetes mellitus, glaucoma, osteoporosis, seizure disorders, ulcerative colitis, CHF, myasthenia gravis, renal disease, esophagitis, peptic ulcer, acne, cataracts, coagulopathy, head trauma

PHARMACOKINETICS

PO/IM: Peak 1-2 hr, half-life 2-5 hr

INTERACTIONS

Increase: side effects—alcohol, salicylates, indomethacin, amphotericin B, digoxin, cycloSPORINE, diuretics

Increase: action of triamcinolone—salicylates, estrogens, indomethacin, oral contraceptives, ketoconazole, macrolide antiinfectives

Decrease: action of triamcinolone—cholestyramine, colestipol, barbiturates, rifampin, ephedrine, phenytoin, theophylline

Decrease: effects of anticoagulants, anticonvulsants, antidiabetics, ambenonium, neostigmine, isoniazid, toxoids, vaccines, anticholinesterases, salicylates, somatrem

Drug/Herb

• Hypokalemia: aloe, buckthorn, cascara, Chinese rhubarb, senna

Drug/Lab Test

Increase: cholesterol, sodium, blood glucose, uric acid, calcium, urine glucose

Decrease: Ca, K, T_4, T_3, thyroid ^{131}I uptake test, urine 17-OHCS, 17-KS, PBI

False negative: skin allergy tests

NURSING CONSIDERATIONS

Assess:

• Potassium, blood glucose, urine glucose while on long-term therapy; hypokalemia and hyperglycemia

• Weight daily; notify prescriber if weekly gain >5 lb

• B/P q4hr, pulse; notify prescriber if chest pain occurs

• I&O ratio; be alert for decreasing urinary output, increasing edema

• Plasma cortisol levels during long-term therapy (normal level: 138-635 nmol/L SI units when drawn at 8 AM)

• Infection: increased temp, WBC, even after withdrawal of medication; product masks infection

• Potassium depletion: paresthesias, fatigue, nausea, vomiting, depression, polyuria, dysrhythmias, weakness

• Edema, hypertension, cardiac symptoms

• Mental status: affect, mood, behavioral changes, aggression

Administer:

• After shaking susp (parenteral)

• Titrated dose; use lowest effective dose

• IM inj deep in large muscle mass; rotate sites; avoid deltoid; use 21G needle

- In one dose in AM to prevent adrenal suppression; avoid SUBCUT administration; may damage tissue
- With food or milk to decrease GI symptoms, tablet may be crushed
- Mouth should be rinsed after inhalations

Perform/provide:

- Assistance with ambulation for patient with bone tissue disease to prevent fractures
- Use of spacer device for geriatric patients with inhaler

Evaluate:

- Therapeutic response: ease of respirations, decreased inflammation

Teach patient/family:

- That emergency ID as corticosteroid user should be carried
- To notify prescriber if therapeutic response decreases; dosage adjustment may be needed
- Not to discontinue abruptly; adrenal crisis can result
- To avoid OTC products: salicylates, alcohol in cough products, cold preparations unless directed by prescriber
- About cushingoid symptoms
- The symptoms of adrenal insufficiency: nausea, anorexia, fatigue, dizziness, dyspnea, weakness, joint pain

triamcinolone nasal agent

See Appendix B

triamcinolone ophthalmic

See Appendix B

triamcinolone topical

See Appendix B

triamcinolone (topical-oral) (OTC)

(trye-am-sin′oh-lone)

Kenalog in Orabase, Oralone Dental

Func. class.: Topical anesthetic

Chem. class.: Synthetic fluorinated adrenal corticosteroid

Action: Binds with steroid receptors, decreases inflammation

Uses: Oral pain

DOSAGE AND ROUTES

- *Adult and child:* **TOP** Press ¼ inch into affected area until film appears, repeat bid-tid

Available forms: Paste 0.1%

SIDE EFFECTS

INTEG: Rash, irritation, sensitization

Contraindications: Infants <1 yr, hypersensitivity, application to large areas, presence of fungal, viral, or bacterial infections of mouth or throat

Precautions: Pregnancy (C), children <6 yr, sepsis, denuded skin

NURSING CONSIDERATIONS

Assess:

- Allergy: rash, irritation, reddening, swelling
- Infection: if affected area is infected, do not apply

Administer:

- After cleansing oral cavity after meals

Evaluate:

- Therapeutic response: absence of pain in affected area

Teach patient/family:

- To report rash, irritation, redness, swelling
- How to apply paste

T

triamterene (℞)

(trye-am'ter-een)

Dyrenium

Func. class.: Potassium-sparing diuretic

Chem. class.: Pteridine derivative

Action: Acts on distal tubule to inhibit reabsorption of sodium, chloride; increase potassium retention

Uses: Edema, may be used with other diuretics; hypertension

DOSAGE AND ROUTES

- *Adult:* **PO** 50-100 mg bid after meals, max 300 mg/day
- *Geriatric:* **PO** 50 mg/day, max 100 mg/day

Renal dose

- Do not use in CCr <10 ml/min

Available forms: Caps 50, 100 mg

SIDE EFFECTS

CNS: Weakness, ***headache,*** dizziness, fatigue

CV: Hypotension, edema, CHF, bradycardia

ELECT: Hypo/hyperkalemia, hyponatremia, hypochloremia

GI: Nausea, diarrhea, vomiting, dry mouth, jaundice, constipation

GU: **Azotemia, interstitial nephritis,** increased BUN, creatinine, renal stones, bluish discoloration of urine, **nephrotoxicity**

HEMA: **Thrombocytopenia, megaloblastic anemia, agranulocytosis**

INTEG: Photosensitivity, rash

RESP: Dyspnea

Contraindications: Breastfeeding, hypersensitivity, anuria, severe renal/hepatic disease

Black Box Warning: Hyperkalemia

Precautions: Pregnancy (B), dehydration, renal/hepatic disease, cirrhosis, renal stenosis, hyperuricemia, electrolyte abnormalities

PHARMACOKINETICS

Onset 2 hr, duration 7-9 hr, half-life 3 hr, metabolized in liver, excreted in bile and urine

INTERACTIONS

Increase: effects of antihypertensives

Increase: hyperkalemia—other potassium-sparing diuretics, potassium products, ACE inhibitors, salt substitutes

Drug/Herb

Increase: fatal hypokalemia—arginine

Increase: hypokalemia—bearberry, gossypol

Increase: severe photosensitivity—St. John's wort

Increase: diuretic—cucumber, dandelion, horsetail, licorice, nettle, pumpkin, Queen Anne's lace

Drug/Lab Test

Interference: LDH

NURSING CONSIDERATIONS

Assess:

- Weight, I&O daily to determine fluid loss; effect of product may be decreased if used daily
- Electrolytes: K, Na, Cl; include BUN, blood glucose, CBC, serum creatinine, blood pH, ABGs, LFTs
- Improvement in CVP q8hr
- Signs of metabolic acidosis: drowsiness, restlessness
- Rashes, temp daily
- Confusion, especially in geriatric patients; take safety precautions if needed
- Hydration: skin turgor, thirst, dry mucous membranes

Administer:

- In AM to avoid interference with sleep
- After meals if nausea occurs; absorption may be decreased slightly

Evaluate:

- Therapeutic response: improvement in edema of feet, legs, sacral area daily if medication is being used in CHF

Teach patient/family:

- To take medication after meals for GI upset

• To avoid prolonged exposure to sunlight; photosensitivity may occur; may turn urine blue
• To avoid foods high in potassium: oranges, bananas, salt substitutes, dried apricots, dates
• To notify prescriber of weakness, headache, nausea, vomiting, dry mouth, fever, sore throat, mouth sores, unusual bleeding or bruising

Treatment of overdose: Lavage if taken orally; monitor electrolytes; administer IV fluids, dialysis; monitor hydration, CV, renal status

triazolam (℞)

(trye-ay′zoe-lam)
Apo-Triazo ♣, Gen-Triazolam ♣, Halcion, Novo-Triolam ♣, Nu-Triazol ♣
Func. class.: Sedative-hypnotic, antianxiety
Chem. class.: Benzodiazepine, short

Controlled Substance Schedule IV (USA), Targeted (CDSA IV) (Canada)

Action: Produces CNS depression at limbic, thalamic, hypothalamic levels of CNS; may be mediated by neurotransmitter γ-aminobutyric acid (GABA); results are sedation, hypnosis, skeletal muscle relaxation, anticonvulsant activity, anxiolytic action

Uses: Insomnia, sedative, hypnotic

DOSAGE AND ROUTES

• *Adult:* **PO** 0.125-0.5 mg at bedtime, max 0.5 mg
• *Geriatric:* **PO** 0.0625-0.125 mg at bedtime

Available forms: Tabs 0.125, 0.25 mg

SIDE EFFECTS

CNS: Headache, lethargy, drowsiness, daytime sedation, dizziness, confusion, light-headedness, anxiety, irritability, amnesia, poor coordination, complex sleep related reactions: sleep driving, sleep eating

CV: Chest pain, pulse changes

GI: Nausea, vomiting, diarrhea, heartburn, abdominal pain, constipation, **hepatic injury**

HEMA: **Leukopenia, granulocytopenia (rare)**

SYST: **Severe allergic reactions**

Contraindications: Pregnancy (X), breastfeeding, hypersensitivity to benzodiazepines, intermittent porphyria

Precautions: Children <15 yr, geriatric patients, anemia, renal/hepatic disease, suicidal individuals, drug abuse, psychosis, acute closed-angle glaucoma, seizure disorders, angioedema, respiratory disease, depression, sleep-related behaviors (sleep walking)

PHARMACOKINETICS

Onset 30-45 min, duration 6-8 hr, metabolized by liver, excreted by kidneys (inactive metabolites), crosses placenta, excreted in breast milk, half-life 2-3 hr

INTERACTIONS

• Smoking may decrease hypnotic effect

Increase: triazolam levels—CYP3A4 inhibitors, protease inhibitors

⚠ ***Increase:*** effects of cimetidine, disulfiram, erythromycin, clarithromycin, probenecid, isoniazid, oral contraceptives; do not use concurrently

Increase: action of both products—alcohol, CNS depressants

Decrease: effect of antacids, theophylline, rifampin, smoking

Drug/Herb

Increase: CNS depression—catnip, chamomile, clary, cowslip, hops, kava, lavender, mistletoe, nettle, pokeweed, poppy, Queen Anne's lace, senega, skullcap, valerian

Increase: hypotension—black cohosh

Drug/Lab Test

Increase: ALT, AST, serum bilirubin

Decrease: RAI uptake

False increase: urinary 17-OHCS

T

NURSING CONSIDERATIONS

Assess:

- Blood studies: Hct, Hgb, RBC if blood dyscrasias suspected (rare)
- Hepatic studies: AST, ALT, bilirubin if hepatic damage has occurred
- Mental status: mood, sensorium, affect, memory (long, short), insomnia, withdrawal symptoms, excessive sedation, impaired coordination
- Blood dyscrasias: fever, sore throat, bruising, rash, jaundice, epistaxis (rare)
- Type of sleep problem: falling asleep, staying asleep

Administer:

- After removal of cigarettes to prevent fires
- After trying conservative measures for insomnia
- ½ hr before bedtime for sleeplessness
- On empty stomach for fast onset, but may be taken with food if GI symptoms occur
- Avoid use with CNS depressants; serious CNS depression may result

Perform/provide:

- Assistance with ambulation after receiving dose
- Safety measures: side rails, night-light, call bell within easy reach
- Checking to see if PO medication has been swallowed
- Cool storage in tight container

Evaluate:

- Therapeutic response: ability to sleep at night, decreased amount of early morning awakening if taking product for insomnia

Teach patient/family:

- Use reliable contraception, pregnancy category (X)
- That dependence is possible after long-term use
- To avoid driving, other activities requiring alertness until product is stabilized
- To avoid alcohol ingestion
- That effects may take 2 nights for benefits to be noticed; for short-term use only; use for 7-10 continuous nights
- Alternative measures to improve sleep: reading, exercise several hours before bedtime, warm bath, warm milk, TV, self-hypnosis, deep breathing
- That complex sleep related behaviors (sleep eating/driving) may occur
- That hangover is common in geriatric patients but less common than with barbiturates; rebound insomnia may occur for 1-2 nights after discontinuing product; to discontinue, decrease dose by 50% q2 nights until 0.125 mg for 2 nights, then stop

Treatment of overdose: Lavage, activated charcoal; monitor electrolytes, VS

trifluoperazine (℞)

(trye-floo-oh-per′a-zeen)

Apo-Trifluoperazine ♣, Novoflurazine ♣, Solazine ♣, Terfluzine, trifluoperazine HCl

Func. class.: Antipsychotic, neuroleptic

Chem. class.: Phenothiazine, piperazine

Do not confuse:

trifluoperazine/trihexyphenidyl

Action: Depresses cerebral cortex, hypothalamus, limbic system, which control activity, aggression; blocks neurotransmission produced by DOPamine at synapse; exhibits strong α-adrenergic, anticholinergic blocking action; mechanism for antipsychotic effects is unclear

Uses: Psychotic disorders, nonpsychotic anxiety, schizophrenia

DOSAGE AND ROUTES

Psychotic disorders

- *Adult:* **PO** 1-5 mg bid, usual range 15-20 mg/day, may require 40 mg/day or more
- *Geriatric:* **PO** 0.5-1 mg daily-bid, increase q4-7days by 0.5-1 mg/day to desired dose, max 40 mg/day
- *Child >6 yr:* **PO** 1 mg/day or bid

Nonpsychotic anxiety

• *Adult:* **PO** 1-2 mg bid, max 6 mg/day; do not give longer than 12 wk

Available forms: Tabs 1, 2, 5, 10 mg

SIDE EFFECTS

CNS: EPS: pseudoparkinsonism, akathisia, dystonia, tardive dyskinesia, **seizures,** *headache,* **neuroleptic malignant syndrome,** dizziness

CV: Orthostatic hypotension, hypertension, **cardiac arrest,** ECG changes, **tachycardia**

EENT: Blurred vision, glaucoma, dry eyes, pigmentary retinopathy, cornea/lens change

GI: Dry mouth, nausea, vomiting, anorexia, constipation, diarrhea, jaundice, weight gain

GU: Urinary retention, urinary frequency, enuresis, impotence, amenorrhea, gynecomastia, ejaculatory dysfunction, priapism

HEMA: Anemia, **leukopenia, leukocytosis, agranulocytosis**

INTEG: Rash, photosensitivity, dermatitis

RESP: **Laryngospasm,** dyspnea, **respiratory depression**

Contraindications: Children <6 yr, hypersensitivity, CV disease, coma, blood dyscrasias

Precautions: Pregnancy (C), breastfeeding, geriatric patients, breast cancer, seizure disorders, diabetes mellitus, respiratory conditions, prostatic hypertrophy, Parkinson's disease, renal failure, severe hepatic disease, closed-angle glaucoma, severe CNS depression

Black Box Warning: Dementia

PHARMACOKINETICS

Metabolized by liver; excreted in urine, breast milk; crosses placenta; 91%-99% protein binding

PO: Onset rapid, peak 2-3 hr, duration 12 hr

INTERACTIONS

• Oversedation: other CNS depressants, alcohol, anesthetics, sedative-hypnotics, opiate agonists

Increase: effects of both products—β-adrenergic blockers, alcohol

Increase: anticholinergic effects—anticholinergics

Increase: levels of this product—CYP2D6 inhibitors

Decrease: levels of this product—CYP2D6 inducers

Decrease: absorption—aluminum hydroxide, magnesium hydroxide antacids

Decrease: effects of lithium, levodopa, anticonvulsants

Drug/Herb

Increase: EPS—betel palm, kava

Increase: action—cola tree, hops, nettle, nutmeg

Increase: CNS depression—chamomile, hops, kava, skullcap, valerian

Drug/Lab Test

Increase: LFTs, cardiac enzymes, cholesterol, blood glucose, prolactin, bilirubin, PBI, cholinesterase, ^{131}I

Decrease: hormones (blood, urine)

False positive: pregnancy tests, PKU

False negative: urinary steroids, 17-OHCS, pregnancy tests

NURSING CONSIDERATIONS

Assess:

⚠ For neuroleptic malignant syndrome: seizures, hypo/hypertension, dyspnea, diaphoresis, fatigue, muscle stiffness; notify prescriber immediately

• Mental status before initial administration

• Swallowing of PO medication; check for hoarding or giving of medication to other patients

• I&O ratio; palpate bladder if low urinary output occurs, urinary retention may be the cause

• Bilirubin, CBC, LFTs q mo

• Urinalysis is recommended before and during prolonged therapy

• Affect, orientation, LOC, reflexes, gait, coordination, sleep pattern disturbances

- For hypo/hyperglycemia; appetite patterns
- B/P standing and lying; also include pulse, respirations q4hr during initial treatment; establish baseline before starting treatment; report drops of 30 mm Hg
- Dizziness, faintness, palpitations, tachycardia on rising
- EPS including akathisia (inability to sit still, no pattern to movements), tardive dyskinesia (bizarre movements of jaw, mouth, tongue, extremities), pseudoparkinsonism (rigidity, tremors, pill rolling, shuffling gait)
- Skin turgor daily
- Constipation, urinary retention daily; if these occur increase bulk, water in diet

Administer:

- Reduced dose in geriatric patients
- Antiparkinsonian agent on order from prescriber for EPS
- Avoid use with CNS depressants

Perform/provide:

- Decreased stimulus by dimming lights, avoiding loud noises
- Supervised ambulation until stabilized on medication if needed; do not involve in strenuous exercise program because fainting is possible; patient should not stand still for long periods
- Increased fluids and bulk in diet to prevent constipation
- Sips of water, candy, gum for dry mouth
- Storage in tight, light-resistant container

Evaluate:

- Therapeutic response: decrease in emotional excitement, hallucinations, delusions, paranoia, reorganization of patterns of thought, speech

Teach patient/family:

- That orthostatic hypotension occurs frequently, and to rise from sitting or lying position gradually; avoid hazardous activities until stabilized on medication
- To avoid hot tubs, hot showers, tub baths; hypotension may occur
- To avoid abrupt withdrawal of this product or EPS may result; product should be withdrawn slowly
- To avoid OTC preparations (cough, hay fever, cold) unless approved by prescriber, since serious product interactions may occur; avoid use with alcohol; increased drowsiness may occur
- To use sunscreen
- About compliance with product regimen
- About the necessity for meticulous oral hygiene; oral candidiasis may occur
- To report sore throat, malaise, fever, bleeding, mouth sores; CBC should be drawn and product discontinued

⚠ That in hot weather, heat stroke may occur; take extra precautions to stay cool

Treatment of overdose: Lavage if orally ingested; provide an airway; do not induce vomiting

trifluridine ophthalmic

See Appendix B

trihexyphenidyl (℞)

(trye-hex-ee-fen′i-dill)

Apo-Trihex ♣, Novohexidyl ♣, PMS-Trihexyphenidyl ♣, Trihexane, Trihexy-2, Trihexy-5, trihexyphenidyl HCl

Func. class.: Cholinergic blocker

Chem. class.: Synthetic tertiary amine

Do not confuse:

trihexyphenidyl/trifluoperazine

Action: Directly inhibits the parasympathetic nervous system; result is relaxation of smooth muscle by direct action on the muscle itself and indirectly via the parasympathetic nervous system

Uses: Parkinson's symptoms, product-induced EPS

Unlabeled uses: Hypersalivation

DOSAGE AND ROUTES

Parkinson symptoms

- *Adult:* **PO** 1 mg, increase by 2 mg q3-5 days to a total of 5-15 mg/day, given in 3-4 divided doses

Product-induced EPS

• *Adult:* **PO** 1 mg/day; usual dose 5-15 mg/day in 3-4 divided doses

Available forms: Tabs 2, 5 mg; elix 2 mg/5 ml

SIDE EFFECTS

CNS: Confusion, anxiety, restlessness, irritability, delusions, hallucinations, headache, sedation, depression, incoherence, *dizziness,* flushing, weakness

CV: Palpitations, tachycardia, postural hypotension

EENT: Blurred vision, photophobia, dilated pupils, difficulty swallowing, dry eyes, increased intraocular tension, closed-angle glaucoma

GI: Dryness of mouth, constipation, nausea, vomiting, abdominal distress, **paralytic ileus**

GU: Urinary hesitancy, retention, dysuria

INTEG: Urticaria, rash, dry skin, photosensitivity

MISC: Suppression of lactation, nasal congestion, decreased sweating, hyperthermia, heat stroke, numbness of fingers

MS: Weakness, cramping

Contraindications: Hypersensitivity, tardive dyskinesia, closed-angle glaucoma, myasthenia gravis, GI/GU obstruction

Precautions: Pregnancy (C), breastfeeding, children, geriatric patients, tachycardia, abdominal obstruction, infection, gastric ulcer, myocardial ischemia, unstable CV disease, prostatic hypertrophy

PHARMACOKINETICS

PO: Onset 1 hr, peak 2-3 hr, duration 6-12 hr, excreted in urine, half-life 3-4 hr

INTERACTIONS

Increase: anticholinergic effects—antihistamines, phenothiazines, amantadine, tricyclics

Increase: CNS depression—analgesics, alcohol, sedatives/hypnotics, antihistamines, opioids

Increase: levels of digoxin

Decrease: action of haloperidol, levodopa

Decrease: anticholinergic effect—donepezil, rivastigmine, galantamine

Drug/Herb

Increase: this product—henbane, jimsonweed, scopolia

NURSING CONSIDERATIONS

Assess:

• For Parkinson's and EPS baseline and throughout treatment

• I&O ratio; retention commonly causes decreased urinary output

• B/P, pulse frequently while dose is being determined

• Constipation; increase fluids, bulk, exercise

• For tolerance over long-term therapy; dosage may have to be increased or medication changed

• Mental status: affect, mood, CNS depression, worsening of mental symptoms during early therapy

Administer:

• With or after meals for GI upset; may give with fluids other than water

• At bedtime to avoid daytime drowsiness in patient with parkinsonism

Perform/provide:

• Storage at room temperature in light-resistant container

• Hard candy, frequent drinks, sugarless gum to relieve dry mouth

Evaluate:

• Therapeutic response: parkinsonism: shuffling gait, muscle rigidity, involuntary movements

Teach patient/family:

• Not to discontinue this product abruptly; to taper off over 1 wk

• To avoid driving, other hazardous activities; drowsiness may occur

• To avoid OTC medications: cough, cold preparations with alcohol, antihistamines unless directed by prescriber

• To avoid sudden position changes

• To avoid hot climates; overheating may occur

T

trimethobenzamide (℞)

(trye-meth-oh-ben′za-mide)
Tigan, trimethobenzamide
Func. class.: Antiemetic, anticholinergic
Chem. class.: Ethanolamine derivative

Action: Acts centrally by blocking chemoreceptor trigger zone, which in turn acts on vomiting center
Uses: Nausea, vomiting

DOSAGE AND ROUTES

Nausea/vomiting
- *Adult:* **IM** 200 mg 3-4×/day; **PO** 300 mg 3-4×/day

Postoperative
- *Adult:* **IM** 200 mg followed by a second dose 1 hr later

Renal dose
- *Adult:* **IM** CCr 15-30 ml/min, give 50% of dose

Available forms: Caps 300 mg; inj 100 mg/ml

SIDE EFFECTS

CNS: ***Drowsiness,*** headache, dizziness, confusion, disorientation, **coma, seizures,** depression, *vertigo,* EPS
CV: Hypo/hypertension, palpitation, **cardiac dysrhythmias**
EENT: Dry mouth, blurred vision, photosensitivity
GI: Nausea, diarrhea, vomiting, difficulty swallowing
INTEG: Rash, urticaria, fever, chills, flushing, hyperpyrexia
Contraindications: Children (parenterally), hypersensitivity to opioids, shock
Precautions: Pregnancy (C), children, geriatric patients, cardiac dysrhythmias, acute febrile illness, encephalitis, gastroenteritis, dehydration, electrolyte imbalances, Reye's syndrome

PHARMACOKINETICS

Metabolized by liver, excreted by kidneys
PO: Onset 20-40 min, duration 3-4 hr
IM: Onset 15-35 min, duration 2-3 hr

INTERACTIONS

Increase: effect—CNS depressants, alcohol

NURSING CONSIDERATIONS

Assess:
- For nausea, vomiting before, after treatment
- VS, B/P; check patients with cardiac disease more often
- Signs of toxicity of other products or masking of symptoms of disease: brain tumor, intestinal obstruction
- Observe for drowsiness, dizziness

Administer:

PO route
- Capsules may be swallowed whole, chewed, allowed to dissolve

IM route
- Inj in large muscle mass; aspirate to avoid IV administration; inj is not to be used in children or infants

Syringe compatibilities: Butorphanol, glycopyrrolate, hydromorphone, midazolam, nalbuphine
Y-site compatibilities: Heparin, hydrocortisone, potassium chloride, vit B/C

Evaluate:
- Therapeutic response: decreased nausea, vomiting

Teach patient/family:
- To avoid hazardous activities, activities requiring alertness; dizziness may occur; to request assistance with ambulation
- To avoid alcohol, other depressants
- To keep out of children's reach

trimethoprim (℞)

(trye-meth'oh-prim)

Primsol, Proloprim, trimethoprim, Trimpex

Func. class.: Urinary antiinfective

Chem. class.: Folate antagonist

Action: Prevents bacterial synthesis by blocking enzyme reduction of dihydrofolic acid

Uses: *Escherichia coli, Proteus mirabilis, Klebsiella, Enterobacter* UTIs, *Haemophilus influenzae*

DOSAGE AND ROUTES

Urinary tract infection

• *Adult:* **PO** 100 mg q12hr × 10 days

Otitis media

• *Child >6 mo:* **PO** 5 mg/kg q12hr × 10 days

Pneumocystis jiroveci *pneumonia*

• *Adult:* **PO** 20 mg/kg/day in 4 divided doses with 100 mg dapsone × 21 days

Renal dose

• *Adult:* **PO** CCr 15-30 ml/min 50 mg q12hr; CCr <15 ml/min avoid use

Available forms: Tabs 100 mg

SIDE EFFECTS

CNS: Fever

GI: Nausea, vomiting, abdominal pain, abnormal taste, increased AST, ALT, bilirubin, creatinine

HEMA: **Thrombocytopenia, leukopenia, neutropenia, megaloblastic anemia** (rare)

INTEG: **Exfoliative dermatitis, Stevens-Johnson syndrome,** pruritus, rash, candidiasis

Contraindications: Hypersensitivity, CCr <15 ml/min, megaloblastic anemia, hyperkalemia

Precautions: Pregnancy (C), breastfeeding, children <12 yr old, geriatric patients, folate deficiency, fragile X chromosome, renal/hepatic disease

PHARMACOKINETICS

Peak 1-4 hr; half-life 8-11 hr; metabolized in liver; excreted in urine (unchanged 60%), breast milk; crosses placenta

INTERACTIONS

Increase: action of phenytoin, warfarin, dofetilide, procainamide, antidiabetics, CYP2C8 substrates (repaglinide)

Increase: potassium levels—potassium-sparing diuretics; potassium salts, supplements

Drug/Herb

• Do not use acidophilus with antiinfectives; separate by several hours

NURSING CONSIDERATIONS

Assess:

• For symptoms of UTI: fever, frequency, burning or pain when urinating; baseline and throughout

• Nocturia; may indicate product resistance

• Signs of infection, anemia

• AST, ALT, BUN, bilirubin, creatinine, urine cultures

• C&S; product may be given as soon as culture is obtained

• Skin eruptions

Administer:

• With full glass of water

• Product in equal intervals around clock to maintain blood levels

Perform/provide:

• Storage in tight, light-resistant container

• Adequate intake of fluids (2 L) to decrease bacteria in bladder

Evaluate:

• Therapeutic response: absence of pain in bladder area, negative C&S

Teach patient/family:

• All aspects of product therapy: need to complete entire course of medication to ensure organism death (10-14 days); culture may be taken after completed course of medication

• That product must be taken in equal intervals around clock to maintain blood levels

• To notify nurse of nausea, vomiting, rash, severe fatigue, sore throat

trimethoprim-sulfamethoxazole (℞)

(trye-meth′oh-prim–sul-fa-meth-ox′a-zole)

Apo-Sulfatrim ✦, Apo-Sulfatrim DS ✦, Bactrim, Bactrim IV, Bethaprim, Cotrim, Novo-Trimel ✦, Novo-Trimel DS ✦, Nu-Cotrimox ✦, Nu-Cotrimox DS ✦, Roubac ✦, Septra, Septra DS, SMZ/TMP, Sulfatrim

Func. class.: Antiinfective

Chem. class.: Sulfonamide—miscellaneous

Action: Sulfamethoxazole (SMZ) interferes with bacterial biosynthesis of proteins by competitive antagonism of PABA when adequate levels are maintained; trimethoprim (TMP) blocks synthesis of tetrahydrofolic acid; combination blocks 2 consecutive steps in bacterial synthesis of essential nucleic acids, protein

Uses: UTI, otitis media, acute and chronic prostatitis, shigellosis, *Pneumocystis jiroveci* pneumonitis, chronic bronchitis, chancroid, traveler's diarrhea

DOSAGE AND ROUTES

Based on TMP content

UTI

• *Adult:* **PO** 160 mg TMP q12hr × 10-14 days

• *Child:* **PO** 8 mg/kg TMP/day in 2 divided doses q12hr

Otitis media

• *Child:* **PO** 8 mg/kg TMP/day in 2 divided doses q12hr × 10 days

Chronic bronchitis

• *Adult:* **PO** 160 mg TMP q12hr × 10-14 days

Pneumocystis jiroveci *pneumonitis*

• *Adult and child:* **PO** 15-20 mg/kg TMP daily in 4 divided doses q6hr × 14 days; **IV** 15-20 mg/kg/day (based on TMP) in 3-4 divided doses for up to 14 days

• Dosage reduction necessary in moderate to severe renal impairment (CCr <30 ml/min)

Available forms: Tabs 80 mg trimethoprim/400 mg sulfamethoxazole, 160 mg trimethoprim/800 mg sulfamethoxazole; susp 40 mg/200 mg/5 ml; IV 16 mg/80 mg/ml

SIDE EFFECTS

CNS: Headache, insomnia, hallucinations, depression, vertigo, fatigue, anxiety, **seizures, product fever,** chills, **aseptic meningitis**

CV: **Allergic myocarditis**

EENT: Tinnitus

GI: Nausea, vomiting, abdominal pain, stomatitis, **hepatitis**, glossitis, pancreatitis, diarrhea, **enterocolitis,** anorexia, **pseudomembranous colitis**

GU: **Renal failure, toxic nephrosis;** increased BUN, creatinine; crystalluria

HEMA: **Leukopenia, neutropenia, thrombocytopenia, agranulocytosis, hemolytic anemia, hypoprothrombinemia, Henoch-Schönlein purpura, methemoglobinemia, eosinophilia I**

INTEG: Rash, dermatitis, urticaria, **Stevens-Johnson syndrome,** erythema, photosensitivity, pain, inflammation at inj site, **toxic epidermal necrolysis, erythema multiforme**

RESP: Cough, SOB

SYST: **Anaphylaxis, SLE**

Contraindications: Breastfeeding, infants <2 mo, hypersensitivity to trimethoprim or sulfonamides, pregnancy at term, megaloblastic anemia, CCr <15 ml/min, porphyria, hyperkalemia

Precautions: Pregnancy (C), geriatric patients, infants, renal disease, G6PD deficiency, impaired hepatic/renal function, possible folate deficiency, severe allergy, bronchial asthma, UV exposure

PHARMACOKINETICS

PO: Rapidly absorbed; peak 1-4 hr; half-life 8-13 hr; excreted in urine (metabolites and unchanged), breast milk; crosses placenta; 68% bound to plasma proteins; TMP achieves high levels in prostatic tissue and fluid

INTERACTIONS

Increase: thrombocytopenia—thiazide diuretics
Increase: potassium levels—potassium-sparing diuretics, potassium supplements
Increase: hypoglycemic response—sulfonylurea agents
Increase: anticoagulant effects—oral anticoagulants
Increase: levels of dofetilide
Increase: crystalluria—methenamine
Increase: bone marrow depressant effects—methotrexate
Decrease: hepatic clearance of phenytoin, CYP2C9, CYP3A4 inducers
Decrease: response—cycloSPORINE

Drug/Herb

- Do not use acidophilus with antiinfectives; separate by several hours

Drug/Lab Test

Increase: alk phos, creatinine, bilirubin, AST, ALT

NURSING CONSIDERATIONS

Assess:

- Allergic reactions: rash, fever (AIDS patients more susceptible)
- I&O ratio; note color, character, pH of urine if product administered for UTI; output should be 800 ml less than intake; if urine is highly acidic, alkalization may be needed
- Renal studies: BUN, creatinine, urinalysis (long-term therapy)
- Type of infection; obtain C&S before starting therapy
- Blood dyscrasias, skin rash, fever, sore throat, bruising, bleeding, fatigue, joint pain
- Allergic reaction: rash, dermatitis, urticaria, pruritus, dyspnea, bronchospasm

Administer:

PO route

- Medication after C&S; repeat C&S after full course of medication
- With resuscitative equipment, epinephrine available; severe allergic reactions may occur
- On an empty stomach 1 hr before or 2 hr after meals
- With full glass of water to maintain adequate hydration; increase fluids to 2 L/day to decrease crystallization in kidneys

IV route

- After diluting 5 ml of product/125 ml D_5W, run over 1-1½ hr

Syringe compatibilities: Heparin

Y-site compatibilities: Acyclovir, aldesleukin, allopurinol, amifostine, amphotericin B cholesteryl, atracurium, aztreonam, cefepime, cyclophosphamide, diltiazem, DOXOrubicin liposome, enalaprilat, esmolol, filgrastim, fludarabine, gallium, granisetron, hydromorphone, labetalol, lorazepam, magnesium sulfate, melphalan, meperidine, morphine, pancuronium, perphenazine, piperacillin/tazobactam, remifentanil, sargramostim, tacrolimus, teniposide, thiotepa, vecuronium, zidovudine

Perform/provide:

- Storage in tight, light-resistant container at room temperature

Evaluate:

- Therapeutic response: absence of pain, fever, C&S negative

Teach patient/family:

- To take each oral dose with full glass of water to prevent crystalluria; drink 8-10 glasses of water/day; to take on an empty stomach 1 hr before meals, 2 hr after meals
- To complete full course of treatment to prevent superinfection
- To avoid sunlight or use sunscreen to prevent burns
- To avoid OTC medications (aspirin, vit C) unless directed by prescriber
- To use alternative contraceptive measures; decreased effectiveness of oral contraceptives may result

T

• To notify prescriber if skin rash, sore throat, fever, mouth sores, unusual bruising, bleeding occur; CNS effects (anxiety, depression, hallucinations, seizures)

triptorelin (℞)

(trip-toe'rel-in)

Trelstar Depot, Trelstar LA

Func. class.: Gonadotropin-releasing hormone

Chem. class.: Synthetic decapeptide analog of LHRH

Action: Inhibitor of pituitary gonadotropin secretion; initially increases LH and FSH, with increases in testosterone, reduction in sex steroid levels

Uses: Advanced prostate cancer

DOSAGE AND ROUTES

• *Adult:* **IM** 3.75 mg q mo; 11.25 mg q84days

Available forms: Microgranules, depot inj 3.75 mg, 11.25 mg

SIDE EFFECTS

CNS: Headache, insomnia, dizziness, lability, fatigue

CV: *Hypertension,* peripheral edema

ENDO: Gynecomastia, breast tenderness, hot flashes

GI: Nausea, vomiting, diarrhea

GU: Impotence, urinary retention, UTI

INTEG: Rash, pain on inj, pruritus, hypersensitivity

MISC: **Anaphylaxis, angioedema**

MS: Osteoneuralgia

Contraindications: Pregnancy (X), breastfeeding, hypersensitivity to this product or other LHRH agonists or LHRH

Precautions: Metastatic vertebral lesions, urinary tract obstruction, spinal cord compression, renal disease

PHARMACOKINETICS

Metabolism may be by CYP450; eliminated by liver, kidneys; terminal half-life is 3 hr in healthy males

INTERACTIONS

Drug/Lab Test

Increase: alk phos, estradiol, FSH, LH, testosterone levels

Decrease: testosterone levels, progesterone

NURSING CONSIDERATIONS

Assess:

• Severe hypersensitivity: discontinue product and give antihistamines, have emergency equipment nearby

• I&O ratios; palpate bladder for distention in urinary obstruction

• For relief of bone pain (back pain)

• Assess levels of testosterone and PSA

Administer:

• IM using implant, inserted by qualified person

• Using syringe with 20G needle, withdraw 2 ml sterile water for inj, inject into vial, shake well, withdraw vial contents, inject immediately

Evaluate:

• Therapeutic response: more normal levels of prostate-specific antigen, acid phosphatase, alk phos; testosterone level of <25 ng/dl, tumor response

Teach patient/family:

• That postmenopausal symptoms may occur but will decrease after treatment is discontinued

• That disease flare may occur at beginning of therapy

• To report allergic reaction immediately

Rarely Used

tromethamine (℞)

(troe-meth'a-meen)

Tham

Func. class.: Alkalinizer

Uses: Acidosis (metabolic) associated with cardiac disease, COPD, cardiac bypass surgery, neonatal respiratory distress syndrome (RDS)

DOSAGE AND ROUTES

Cardiopulmonary bypass—metabolic acidosis

• *Adult and child:* **IV** 9 ml/kg (324 mg/kg), max 500 mg/kg over <1 hr

Cardiac arrest—metabolic acidosis

• *Adult:* **IV INF** 3.5-6 ml/kg, max 500 mg/kg/dose

Contraindications: Hypersensitivity, anuria, uremia, neonates (chronic respiratory acidosis, salicylate intoxication)

tropicamide ophthalmic

See Appendix B

trospium (℞)

(trose′pee-um)

Sanctura, Sanctura XR

Func. class.: Anticholinergic

Chem. class.: Muscarinic receptor antagonist

Action: Relaxes smooth muscles in bladder by inhibiting acetylcholine effect on muscarinic receptors

Uses: Overactive bladder (urinary frequency, urgency)

DOSAGE AND ROUTES

• *Adult:* **PO** 20 mg bid 1 hr before meals or on empty stomach; ER 60 mg q AM

Renal dose

• *Adult:* **PO** CCr <30 ml/min 20 mg/day at bedtime

• *Geriatric ≥75 yr:* **PO** Titrate down to 20 mg/day based on response and tolerance

Available forms: Tabs 20 mg; caps ER 60 mg

SIDE EFFECTS

CNS: Fatigue, dizziness, headache

CV: Tachycardia

EENT: Dry eyes, vision abnormalities

GI: Flatulence, abdominal pain, *constipation, dry mouth,* dyspepsia

GU: Urinary retention

INTEG: Dry skin

Contraindications: Hypersensitivity, uncontrolled closed-angle glaucoma, urinary retention, gastric retention, myasthenia gravis

Precautions: Pregnancy (C), breastfeeding, children, geriatric patients, renal/hepatic disease, controlled closed-angle glaucoma, ulcerative colitis, intestinal atony, bladder outflow obstruction

PHARMACOKINETICS

Rapidly absorbed (10%), peak 5-6 hr, protein bound (50%-85%), metabolism in humans not fully understood, extensively metabolized, excreted in urine (6%)/feces (85%), excreted in urine by active tubular secretion

INTERACTIONS

Increase: drowsiness—CNS depressants, alcohol

Increase or decrease: products excreted by active renal secretion (amiloride, digoxin, morphine), metformin, quinidine, procainamide, ranitidine, tenofovir, triamterene, vancomycin

Drug/Herb

Increase: effect—henbane, jimsonweed, scopolia

Drug/Food

Decrease: absorption—high-fat meal

NURSING CONSIDERATIONS

Assess:

• Urinary patterns: distention, nocturia, frequency, urgency, incontinence

Administer:

• 1 hr before meals or on empty stomach (reg rel); q AM (ER)

Evaluate:

• Therapeutic response: correction of urinary status: absence of dysuria, frequency, nocturia, incontinence

Teach patient/family:

• To avoid hazardous activities; dizziness may occur

• Alcohol may increase drowsiness

• Define anticholinergic effects that may occur

undecylenic acid topical

See Appendix B

unoprostone ophthalmic

See Appendix B

⚠ High Alert

urokinase (℞)

(yoor-oh-kin′ase)

Kinlytic

Func. class.: Thrombolytic enzyme

Chem. class.: β-Hemolytic streptococcus filtrate (purified)

Action: Promotes thrombolysis by directly converting plasminogen to plasmin

Uses: Pulmonary embolism

Unlabeled uses: Acute MI, arterial thromboembolism, coronary artery thrombosis, DVT, occluded IV catheter, percutaneous coronary intervention, venous thrombosis, arterial embolism

DOSAGE AND ROUTES

Lysis of pulmonary emboli

• *Adult:* **IV** 4400 international units/kg, over 10 min (90 ml/hr), then **CONT IV INF** 4400 international units/kg/hr × 12 hr (15 ml/hr); flush line at end of INF

Coronary artery thrombosis (MI)

• *Adult:* **INSTILL** 6000 international units/min into occluded artery for 1-2 hr after giving **IV BOL** of heparin 2500-10,000 units

• May also give as **IV INF** 2 million-3 million units over 45-90 min

Venous catheter occlusion (unlabeled)

• *Adult and child:* **INSTILL** 5000 international units into line, wait 5 min, then aspirate, repeat aspiration attempts q5min × ½ hr; if occlusion has not been removed, cap line and wait ½-1 hr, then aspirate; may need 2nd dose if still occluded

Available forms: Powder for inj, lyophilized 250,000 international units/vial; powder for catheter clearance

SIDE EFFECTS

CNS: Headache, fever

CV: Hypotension, dysrhythmias

GI: Nausea, vomiting

HEMA: Decreased Hct, **bleeding**

INTEG: Rash, urticaria, phlebitis at IV inf site, itching, flushing

MS: Low back pain

RESP: Altered respirations, SOB, **bronchospasm,** cyanosis

SYST: **GI, GU, intracranial, retroperitoneal bleeding,** surface bleeding, **anaphylaxis** (rare)

Contraindications: Hypersensitivity to this product or other thrombolytic enzymes, internal active bleeding, intraspinal surgery, neoplasms of CNS, ulcerative colitis/enteritis, severe uncontrolled hypertension, renal/hepatic disease, hypocoagulation, COPD, subacute bacterial endocarditis, rheumatic valvular disease, cerebral embolism/thrombosis/hemorrhage, intraarterial diagnostic procedure or surgery (10 days), recent major surgery/trauma, aneurysm AV malformation

Precautions: Pregnancy (B), arterial emboli from left side of heart, hepatic disease

PHARMACOKINETICS

IV: Half-life 10-20 min, small amounts excreted in urine

INTERACTIONS

• Bleeding potential: aspirin, indomethacin, phenylbutazone, anticoagulants, other NSAIDs, abciximab, eptifibatide, tirofiban, clopidogrel, ticlopidine, some cephalosporins, plicamycin, valproic acid, dipyridamole, glycoprotein IIb, IIIa inhibitors

Drug/Lab Test

Increase: PT, APTT, TT

NURSING CONSIDERATIONS

Assess:

- VS, B/P, pulse, resp, neurologic signs, temp at least q4hr; temp >104° F (40° C) is an indicator of internal bleeding; cardiac rhythm following intracoronary administration
- For neurologic changes that may indicate intracranial bleeding
- Retroperitoneal bleeding: back pain, leg weakness, diminished pulses
- Peripheral pulses, lung sounds, respiratory function
- Hypersensitivity: fever, rash, itching, chills, facial swelling, dyspnea; mild reaction may be treated with antihistamines; notify prescriber of severe reactions, stop product, keep resuscitative equipment nearby
- Bleeding during 1st hr of treatment (hematuria, hematemesis, bleeding from mucous membranes, epistaxis, ecchymosis)
- Blood studies (Hct, platelets, PTT, PT, TT, APTT) before starting therapy; PT or APTT must be less than 2× control before starting therapy TT; or PT q3-4hr during treatment
- ECG continuously, cardiac enzymes, radionuclide myocardial scanning/coronary angiography

Administer:

IV route

- Using inf pump, terminal filter (0.45 μm or smaller)
- Reconstituting only with 5 ml sterile water for inj (not bacteriostatic water)/ 250,000 international units urokinase (Kinlytic), and roll (not shake) to enhance reconstitution; further dilute with 190 ml; give as intermittent inf or give to clear cannula by using 1 ml of diluted product; inject into cannula slowly, clamp 5 min, aspirate clot; avoid excessive pressure when urokinase is injected into catheter; force could rupture catheter or expel clot into circulation
- As soon as thrombi identified; not useful for thrombi over 1 wk old

Cryoprecipitate or fresh frozen plasma if bleeding occurs

Loading dose at beginning of therapy; may require increased loading doses

Heparin therapy after thrombolytic therapy is discontinued, TT or APTT less than 2× control (about 3-4 hr)

Y-site compatibilities: TPN 55, 56

Perform/provide:

- Storage in refrigerator; use immediately after reconstitution
- Bed rest during entire course of treatment; use caution in handling patients
- Avoidance of venous, arterial puncture procedures, inj, rectal temp
- Treatment of fever with acetaminophen or aspirin
- Placement of sign above patient's bed stating urokinase therapy
- Pressure for 30 sec to minor bleeding sites; 30 min to sites of arterial puncture followed by pressure dressing; inform prescriber if hemostasis not attained, apply pressure dressing

Evaluate:

- Therapeutic response: decreased clotting, thrombosis, embolism

Teach patient/family:

- To report immediately any sign of bleeding
- That bed rest is needed during treatment
- Reasons for treatment and expected results

ursodiol (℞)

(ur-soh-die′-ohl)

Actigall, Urso

Func. class.: Gallstone solubilizing agent

Chem. class.: Ursodeoxycholic acid

Action: Suppresses hepatic synthesis, secretion of cholesterol; inhibits intestinal absorption of cholesterol

Uses: Dissolution of radiolucent, noncalcified gallbladder stones (<20 mm in diameter) in which surgery is not indicated, biliary cirrhosis, gallstone prophylaxis

Unlabeled uses: Severe pruritus, cholestasis secondary to cystic fibrosis, intrahepatic cholestasis of pregnancy (ICP), nonalcoholic steatosis-hepatitis (NASH)

DOSAGE AND ROUTES

• *Adult:* **PO** 8-10 mg/kg/day in 2-3 divided doses using gallbladder ultrasound q6mo; determine if stones have dissolved; if so, continue therapy, repeat ultrasound within 1-3 mo

Primary biliary cirrhosis

• *Adult:* **PO** (Urso tabs) 13-15 mg/kg/day given in divided doses 2-4×/day

Gallstone prophylaxis in rapid weight loss

• *Adult:* **PO** 300 mg bid morning and bedtime with food

Available forms: Caps 300 mg; tabs 250, 500 mg

SIDE EFFECTS

CNS: Headache, anxiety, depression, insomnia, fatigue

GI: Diarrhea, nausea, vomiting, abdominal pain, constipation, stomatitis, flatulence, dyspepsia, biliary pain

INTEG: Pruritus, rash, urticaria, dry skin, sweating, alopecia

MS: Arthralgia, myalgia, back pain

OTHER: Cough, rhinitis

Contraindications: Calcified cholesterol stones, radiopaque stones, radiolucent bile pigment stones, chronic hepatic disease, hypersensitivity, biliary obstruction, pancreatitis, compelling for cholecystectomy

Precautions: Pregnancy (B), breastfeeding, children

PHARMACOKINETICS

80% excreted in feces, 20% metabolized, excreted into bile, lost in feces

INTERACTIONS

Increase: risk of stone formation—clofibrate, gemfibrozil, estrogens, oral contraceptives

Decrease: action of ursodiol—cholestyramine, colestipol, aluminum-based antacids

NURSING CONSIDERATIONS

Assess:

• GI status: diarrhea, abdominal pain, nausea, vomiting; product may have to be discontinued if side effects are severe

• Skin for pruritus, rash, urticaria, dry skin; provide soothing lotion to lesions

• Musculoskeletal status: aches or stiffness in joints

Administer:

• For up to 6-24 mo; if no improvement is seen, discontinue product; dosing depends on size and composition of stones

Evaluate:

• Therapeutic response: decreasing size of stones on ultrasound

Teach patient/family:

• That anxiety, depression, insomnia are side effects and are reversible after discontinuing product

ustekinumab (℞)

(us'te-kin'ue-mab)

Stelara

Func. class.: Antipsoriatic agent

Action: Interleukin (IL)-12, IL-23 Antagonist

Uses: Plaque psoriasis

DOSAGE AND ROUTES

• *Adult ≥100 kg:* **SUBCUT** 90 mg, repeat in 4 wk, then 90 mg q12wk starting wk 16

• *Adult ≤100 kg:* **SUBCUT** 45 mg, repeat in 4 wk, then 45 mg q12wk starting wk 16

Available forms: Solutions for inj 45 mg/0.5 mc

SIDE EFFECTS

CNS: Headache, leukoencephalopathy

HEMA: Bleeding

INTEG: ***Inj site reaction,*** pruritus, skin irritation, erythema

SYST: **Serious infections, malignancies**

Contraindications: Hypersensitivity, sepsis, active infections

Precautions: Pregnancy (B), breastfeeding, children ≤18 yr, geriatric patients, surgery, TB, diabetes mellitus, immunosuppression

PHARMACOKINETICS

Maximum serum concentration: 13.5 days after a single 45 mg subcut dose, 7 days after a single 90 mg subcut dose; half-life 14.9-45.6 days

INTERACTIONS

- Do not give concurrently with vaccines; immunizations should be brought up to date before treatment
- Avoid use with immunosuppressives

NURSING CONSIDERATIONS

Assess:

- For inj site pain, swelling

Administer:

- Visually inspect for particulate matter or discoloration; solution should be slightly yellow and may contain a few small translucent or white particles; do not use if discolored, cloudy or if foreign particulate matter is present; do not shake
- Use at 27 G, 0.5 inch needle
- May be administered subcut into upper arm, abdomen, or thigh; rotate inj sites

Evaluate:

- Therapeutic response: decreased plaque psoriasis

Teach patient/family:

- That product must be continued for prescribed time to be effective
- Not to receive live vaccinations during treatment
- To notify prescriber of possible infection (upper respiratory or other)

valacyclovir (℞)

(val-a-sye'kloh-vir)

Valtrex

Func. class.: Antiviral

Chem. class.: Acyclic purine nucleoside analog

Do not confuse:

valacyclovir/valganciclovir

Valtrex/Valcyte

Action: Interferes with DNA synthesis by conversion to acyclovir, causing decreased viral replication, time of lesional healing

Uses: Treatment or suppression of herpes zoster (shingles), genital herpes, herpes labialis (cold sores), varicella, varicella-zoster

Unlabeled uses: CMV in advanced HIV, posttransplant patients, Bell's palsy, herpes simplex virus prophylaxis, acute retinal necrosis (ARN), encephalitis

DOSAGE AND ROUTES

Herpes zoster

- *Adult:* **PO** 1 g tid × 1 wk

Genital herpes (suppressive, initial)

- *Adult:* **PO** 1 g bid × 10 days initially

Genital herpes (recurrent episodes)

- *Adult:* **PO** 500 mg bid × 3 days

Genital herpes (suppressive therapy)

- *Adult:* **PO** 1 g/day with normal immune function; 500 mg/day for those with ≤9 recurrences/yr; 500 mg bid in HIV-infected patients with CD4 ≥100

Reduction of transmission

- *Adult:* **PO** 500 mg/day for source partner

Herpes labialis

- *Adult:* **PO** 2 g bid × 1 day

Varicella (chickenpox) in immunocompetent patients

- *Adolescent and child ≥2 yr:* **PO** 20 mg/kg/dose tid × 5 days, max 3 g/day; start at first sign, preferably within 24 hr of rash

Renal dose

- *Adult:* **PO** CCr 30-49 ml/min 1 g q12hr (herpes zoster); 1 g q12hr × 1 day

V

(herpes labialis); CCr 10-29 ml/min 1 g q24hr (genital herpes/herpes zoster); 500 mg q24hr (recurrent genital herpes); CCr <10 ml/min 500 mg q24hr (genital herpes/herpes zoster), 500 mg q24hr (recurrent genital herpes)

Available forms: Tabs 500 mg, 1 g

SIDE EFFECTS

CNS: Tremors, lethargy, *dizziness, headache,* weakness, depression

ENDO: Dysmenorrhea

GI: Nausea, vomiting, diarrhea, abdominal pain, constipation, *increased AST*

HEMA: **Thrombocytopenic purpura, hemolytic uremic syndrome**

INTEG: Rash

Contraindications: Hypersensitivity to this product or acyclovir, valganciclovir

Precautions: Pregnancy (B), breastfeeding, geriatric patients, hepatic/renal disease, electrolyte imbalance, dehydration, penciclovir, famciclovir, ganciclovir, hypersensitivity, varicella

PHARMACOKINETICS

Onset unknown, terminal half-life 2½-3½ hr, converted to acyclovir that crosses placenta and enters breast milk, excreted in urine primarily as acyclovir, protein binding 13.5%-17.9%

INTERACTIONS

Increase: blood levels of valacyclovir—cimetidine, probenecid, only in renal disease is significant

NURSING CONSIDERATIONS

Assess:

- Signs of infection; characteristics of lesions; therapy should be started at first sign or symptom of herpes and is most effective within 72 hr of outbreak

⚠ For thrombocytopenic purpura, hemolytic uremic syndrome; may be fatal

- C&S before product therapy; product may be taken as soon as culture is taken; repeat C&S after treatment; determine the presence of other sexually transmitted diseases
- Bowel pattern before, during treatment
- Skin eruptions: rash
- Allergies before treatment, reaction of each medication

Administer:

- As soon as possible (herpes labialis, genital herpes); within 24 hr of rash (varicella)
- Within 72 hr of outbreak (herpes zoster)
- Without regard to food
- Caps may be made into susp by pharmacy

Perform/provide:

- Storage at room temperature; protect from light, moisture

Evaluate:

- Therapeutic response: absence of itching, painful lesions; crusting and healed lesions

Teach patient/family:

- To take as prescribed; if dose is missed, take as soon as remembered up to 2 hr before next dose; do not double dose
- That product may be taken orally before infection occurs; product should be taken when itching or pain occurs, usually before eruptions
- That partners need to be told that patient has herpes; they can become infected; condoms must be worn to prevent reinfections
- That product does not cure infection, just controls symptoms and does not prevent infection of others

valganciclovir (℞)

(val-gan-sy'kloh-veer)

Valcyte

Func. class.: Antiviral

Chem. class.: Synthetic nucleoside analog

Do not confuse:

valganciclovir/valacyclovir

Valcyte/Valtrex

Action: Valganciclovir is metabolized to ganciclovir; inhibits replication of human cytomegalovirus in vivo and in vitro by selective inhibition of viral DNA synthesis

Uses: Cytomegalovirus (CMV) retinitis in immunocompromised persons, including those with AIDS, after indirect ophthalmoscopy confirms diagnosis; prevention of CMV in transplantation; prevention of CMV in patient at risk going through transplant (kidney, heart, pancreas)

Unlabeled uses: Colitis, Epstein-Barr virus, esophagitis, herpes simplex type 1, 2; human herpesvirus 6, 8; multicentric Castleman's disease, varicella-zoster virus

DOSAGE AND ROUTES

Treatment of CMV

• *Adult and adolescent (unlabeled):* **PO** Induction 900 mg bid × 21 days with food; maintenance 900 mg/day with food

Transplant (CMV prophylaxis)

• *Adult/adolescent >16 yr:* **PO** 900 mg/day with food starting 10 days prior to transplantation until day 100 of posttransplantation

• *Infant ≥4 mg/child/adolescent ≤16 yr:* **PO** give within 10 days of heart/kidney transplant, only calculate dose as 7× BSA × CCr and give as single daily dose

Renal dose

• *Adult:* **PO** CCr ≥60 ml/min same as above; CCr 40-59 ml/min 450 mg bid for 21 days, then 450 mg/day; CCr 25-39 ml/min 450 mg/day, then 450 mg q2days; CCr 10-24 ml/min 450 mg q2days, then 450 mg 2×/week

Available form: Tabs 450 mg, powder for oral sol 50 mg/ml

SIDE EFFECTS

CNS: *Fever,* chills, **coma,** *confusion,* abnormal thoughts, dizziness, bizarre dreams, *headache, insomnia,* psychosis, tremors, somnolence, *paresthesia, weakness,* **seizures**

EENT: Retinal detachment in CMV retinitis

GI: Abnormal LFTs, *nausea, vomiting, anorexia, diarrhea, abdominal pain,* **hemorrhage**

GU: **Hematuria,** increased creatinine, BUN

HEMA: **Granulocytopenia, thrombocytopenia, irreversible neutropenia, anemia, eosinophilia**

INTEG: *Rash,* alopecia, *pruritus,* urticaria, pain at site, phlebitis, **Stevens-Johnson syndrome**

MISC: Local and systemic infections and **sepsis**

Contraindications: Breastfeeding, hypersensitivity to ganciclovir, valacyclovir; absolute neutrophil count <500/mm^3; platelet count <25,000/mm^3; hemodialysis; liver transplantation

Precautions: Pregnancy (C), children, geriatric patients, renal function impairment, hypersensitivity to acyclovir, penciclovir, famciclovir

Black Box Warning: Preexisting cytopenias, secondary malignancy, infertility, anemia

PHARMACOKINETICS

Metabolized to ganciclovir, which has a half-life of 3-4½ hr; excreted by kidneys (unchanged); crosses blood-brain barrier, CSF

INTERACTIONS

• Severe granulocytopenia: zidovudine, antineoplastics, radiation; do not use together

Increase: toxicity—dapsone, pentamidine, flucytosine, vinCRIStine, vinBLAStine, adriamycin, DOXOrubicin, amphotericin B, trimethoprim-sulfamethoxazole combinations or other nucleoside analogs, cycloSPORINE

Increase: seizures—imipenem/cilastatin

Increase: effect of didanosine

Decrease: renal clearance of valganciclovir—probenecid

Drug/Food

Increase: absorption, high-fat meal

NURSING CONSIDERATIONS

Assess:

• For CMV retinitis by ophthalmoscopy before beginning treatment and q2wk

• Culture for CMV retinitis

V

• For infection: sore throat, cough, fever, chills, back pain; notify prescriber
• For leukopenia/neutropenia/thrombocytopenia: WBCs, platelets q2days during 2 ×/day dosing and then q1wk
• For leukopenia with daily WBC count in patients with prior leukopenia with other nucleoside analogs or for whom leukopenia counts are <1000 cells/mm^3 at start of treatment
• Serum creatinine or CCr ≥q2wk

Administer:

PO tab

• With food for better absorption

Oral sol

• Measure 9 ml of purified water in graduated cylinder, shake bottle to loosen powder, add ½ liquid, shake well, add remaining water, shake; remove child-resistant cap and push bottle adapter into neck of bottle, close with cap, give using the dispenser provided

Evaluate:

• Therapeutic response: decreased symptoms of CMV

Teach patient/family:

• That product does not cure condition; regular ophthalmologic and blood tests are necessary
• That major toxicities may necessitate discontinuing product
• To use contraception during treatment and that infertility may occur; men should use barrier contraception for 90 days after treatment
• To take with food
⚠ To report infection: fever, chills, sore throat; blood dyscrasias: bruising, bleeding, petechiae
• To avoid crowds, persons with respiratory infections
• To use sunscreen to prevent burns

valproate (℞)
(val′proh-ate)
Depacon

valproic acid (℞)
(val′proh-ik)
Depakene, Stavzor

divalproex sodium (℞)
(dye-val′proh-ex)
Depakote, Depakote ER, Epival ✤

Func. class.: Anticonvulsant, vascular headache suppressant
Chem. class.: Carboxylic acid derivative

Action: Increases levels of γ-aminobutyric acid (GABA) in brain, which decreases seizure activity

Uses: Simple (petit mal), complex (petit mal) absence, mixed, manic episodes associated with bipolar disorder, prophylaxis of migraine, adjunct in schizophrenia, tardive dyskinesia, aggression in children with ADHD, organic brain syndrome mania, migraines, tonic-clonic (grand mal), myoclonic seizures

Unlabeled uses: Rectal for seizures (valproic acid)

DOSAGE AND ROUTES

Epilepsy

• *Adult and child:* **PO** 10-15 mg/kg/day divided in 2-3 doses, may increase by 5-10 mg/kg/day q wk, max 60 mg/kg/day in 2-3 divided doses; **IV** ≤20 mg/min over 1 hr

Status epilepticus refractory to diazepam IV (unlabeled)

• *Adult:* **RECT** 400-600 mg PR as an enema or wax-based suppository (not commercially available)
• *Child:* **RECT** 20 mg/kg/dose

Mania (divalproex sodium)

• *Adult:* **PO** 750 mg/day in divided doses, max 60 mg/kg/day or 3000 mg/day

Mania (valproic acid-Stavzor)

• *Adult:* **DEL REL CAP** 750 mg/day in divided doses

Migraine (divalproex sodium)
• *Adult:* **PO** 250 mg bid, may increase to 1000 mg/day if needed or 500 mg (Depakote ER) daily × 7 days, then 1000 mg/day

Available forms: *Valproate:* inj 100 mg/ml; *valproic acid:* caps 250 mg; syr 250 mg/5 ml; del rel cap (Stavzor) 125 mg; *divalproex:* del rel tabs 125, 250, 500 mg; ext rel tabs 250, 500 mg; sprinkle cap 125 mg

SIDE EFFECTS

CNS: Sedation, drowsiness, dizziness, headache, incoordination, depression, hallucinations, behavioral changes, tremors, aggression, weakness, **coma, suicidal ideation**

EENT: Visual disturbances, taste perversion

GI: Nausea, vomiting, constipation, diarrhea, dyspepsia, anorexia, cramps, **hepatic failure, pancreatitis, toxic hepatitis,** stomatitis, weight gain

GU: Enuresis, irregular menses

HEMA: **Thrombocytopenia, leukopenia, lymphocytosis,** increased PT, bruising, epistaxis

INTEG: Rash, alopecia, photosensitivity, dry skin

Contraindications: Hypersensitivity, urea cycle disorders

Black Box Warning: Pregnancy (D), hepatic disease, pancreatitis

Precautions: Breastfeeding, geriatric patients

Black Box Warning: Children <2 yr

PHARMACOKINETICS

Metabolized by liver; excreted by kidneys, breast milk; crosses placenta; half-life 6-16 hr; 90% protein binding

PO: Peak 4 hr (regular rel); 4-17 hr (ext rel)

INTERACTIONS

Increase: valproic acid level—erythromycin, felbamate

Increase: CNS depression—alcohol, opioids, barbiturates, antihistamines, MAOIs, sedative/hypnotics

Increase: toxicity of valproic acid—salicylates

Increase: action of phenytoin, tricyclics, carbamazepine, ethosuximide, barbiturates, zidovudine, lorazepam, rufinamide

Increase: bleeding—antiplatelets, NSAIDs, tirofiban, eptifibatide, abciximab, cefoperazone, cefotetan, heparin, thrombolytics

Increase: toxicity of carbamazepine ethosuximide, lamotrigine, zidovudine

Decrease: metabolism of valproic acid—cimetidine

Decrease: valproic acid level—rifampin carbamazepine, lamotrigine

Drug/Lab Test

False positive: ketones, urine

Interference: thyroid function tests

NURSING CONSIDERATIONS

Assess:

• Seizure disorder: location, aura, activity, duration; seizure precautions should be in place

⚠ Mental status: bipolar disorder: mood, activity, sleeping/eating, behavior; suicidal thoughts/behaviors

• Migraines: frequency, intensity, alleviating factor

• Blood studies: Hct, Hgb, RBC, serum folate, PT/PTT, serum ammonia, platelets, vit D if on long-term therapy

⚠ Hepatic studies: AST, ALT, bilirubin; hepatic failure has occurred

• Blood levels: therapeutic level 50-100 mcg/ml, in seizures

• Respiratory dysfunction: respiratory depression, character, rate, rhythm; hold product if respirations are <12/min or if pupils are dilated

⚠ For pancreatitis; may be fatal

Administer:

PO route

• Swallow tabs or caps whole; do not break, crush, or chew ER tabs

• Use sprinkle cap contents on food

V

• Elixir alone; do not dilute with carbonated beverage; do not give syrup to patients on sodium restriction
• Give with food or milk to decrease GI symptoms

Evaluate:
• Therapeutic response: decreased seizures

Teach patient/family:
• That physical dependency may result from extended use
• To avoid driving, other activities that require alertness
• Not to discontinue medication quickly after long-term use; seizures may result
• To report visual disturbances, rash, diarrhea, abdominal pain, light-colored stools, jaundice, protracted vomiting to prescriber
• To use contraception while taking this product; pregnancy category (D)

valsartan (℞)

(val'sahr-tan)
Diovan
Func. class.: Antihypertensive
Chem. class.: Angiotensin II receptor antagonist (Type AT_1)

Action: Blocks the vasoconstrictor and aldosterone-secreting effects of angiotensin II; selectively blocks the binding of angiotensin II to the AT_1 receptor found in tissues

Uses: Hypertension, alone or in combination in patients >6 yr, CHF

DOSAGE AND ROUTES

Hypertension
• *Adult:* **PO** 80-160 mg/day alone or in combination with other antihypertensives, may increase to 320 mg
• *Child and adolescent 6-16 yr:* **PO** 1.3 mg/kg/day, max 40 mg/day

CHF
• *Adult:* **PO** 40 mg bid, up to 160 mg bid

Available forms: Tabs 80, 160, 320 mg

SIDE EFFECTS

CNS: Dizziness, insomnia, drowsiness, vertigo, headache, fatigue
CV: Angina pectoris, 2nd-degree AV block, **cerebrovascular accident,** hypotension, **myocardial infarction,** *dysrhythmias*
EENT: Conjunctivitis
GI: Diarrhea, abdominal pain, nausea, **hepatotoxicity**
GU: Impotence, **nephrotoxicity**
HEMA: Anemia, neutropenia
META: Hyperkalemia
MISC: Vasculitis
MS: Cramps, myalgia, pain, stiffness
RESP: Cough

Contraindications: Hypersensitivity, severe hepatic disease, bilateral renal artery stenosis

Black Box Warning: Pregnancy (D) 2nd/3rd trimester

Precautions: Breastfeeding, children, geriatric patients, hypersensitivity to ACE inhibitors; CHF, hypertrophic cardiomyopathy aortic/mitral valve stenosis, CAD, angioedema, renal/hepatic disease

PHARMACOKINETICS

Onset up to 2 hr; peak 4-6 hr; duration 24 hr; extensively metabolized; protein binding 95%; half-life 6 hr; excreted in feces, urine, breast milk

INTERACTIONS

Increase: effects of lithium
Increase: hyperkalemia—potassium-sparing diuretics, potassium supplements, ACE inhibitors
Decrease: antihypertensive effects—NSAIDs, salicylates

Drug/Herb
Increase: toxicity, death—aconite
Increase: antihypertensive effect—barberry, betony, black catechu, black cohosh, bloodroot, broom, burdock, cat's claw, dandelion, goldenseal, hawthorn, Irish moss, Jamaican dogwood, kelp, khella, mistletoe, parsley
Increase or decrease: antihypertensive effect—astragalus, cola tree

Decrease: antihypertensive effect—coltsfoot, guarana, khat, licorice, yohimbe

NURSING CONSIDERATIONS

Assess:

- B/P, pulse q4hr (lying, sitting, standing); note rate, rhythm, quality, periodically
- Blood studies; BUN, creatinine, LFTs before treatment
- Electrolytes: K, Na, Cl, total CO_2
- Baselines in renal, hepatic studies before therapy begins
- Angioedema: facial swelling; SOB; edema in feet, legs daily
- Skin turgor, dryness of mucous membranes for hydration status; correct volume depletion before initiating therapy

Administer:

- Without regard to meals

Evaluate:

- Therapeutic response: decreased B/P

Teach patient/family:

- To comply with dosage schedule, even if feeling better
- To notify prescriber of fever, swelling of hands or feet, irregular heartbeat, chest pain, dizziness
- That excessive perspiration, dehydration, diarrhea may lead to fall in blood pressure; consult prescriber if these occur
- That product may cause dizziness, fainting; light-headedness may occur
- To rise slowly to sitting or standing position to minimize orthostatic hypotension; to take B/P
- Not to take this medication if pregnant or breastfeeding, or have had an allergic reaction to this product
- That if a dose is missed, to take it as soon as possible, unless it is within an hour before next dose

vancomycin (℞)

(van-koe-mye'sin)
Vancocin, vancomycin HCl
Func. class.: Antiinfective—miscellaneous
Chem. class.: Tricyclic glycopeptide

Action: Inhibits bacterial cell wall synthesis, blocks glycopeptides

Uses: Resistant staphylococcal infections, pseudomembranous colitis, staphylococcal enterocolitis, endocarditis prophylaxis for dental procedures, diphtheroid endocarditis

DOSAGE AND ROUTES

Serious staphylococcal infections

- *Adult:* **IV** 500 mg q6-8hr or 1 g q12hr
- *Child:* **IV** 40-60 mg/kg/day divided q6-8hr
- *Neonate:* **IV** 15 mg/kg initially followed by 10 mg/kg q8-24hr

Pseudomembranous/staphylococcal enterocolitis

- *Adult:* **PO** 125-500 mg/day in divided doses for 7-10 days
- *Child:* **PO** 40 mg/kg/day divided q6hr, max 2 g/day

Endocarditis prophylaxis

- *Adult:* **IV** 1 g over 1 hr, 1 hr before procedure
- *Child:* **IV** 20 mg/kg over 1 hr, 1 hr prior to procedure

Renal dose

- *Adult:* **IV** CCr >70 ml/min no dosage adjustment; CCr 50-70 ml/min loading dose of 15 mg/kg, reduce dose to 750 mg-1 g q18-24 hr; CCr <49 ml/min initial loading dose of 15 mg/kg, with subsequent dosing based on concentration, may be q24-72hr or longer

Available forms: Pulvules 125, 250 mg; powder for oral sol 250 mg/5 ml, 500 mg/6 ml; powder for inj 500 mg, 1, 5, 10 g

SIDE EFFECTS

CV: **Cardiac arrest, vascular collapse (rare)**, hypotension
EENT: *Ototoxicity, permanent deafness,* tinnitus, nystagmus
GI: **Nausea, pseudomembranous colitis**
GU: **Nephrotoxicity,** *increased BUN, creatinine, albumin,* **fatal uremia**
HEMA: **Leukopenia, eosinophilia, neutropenia**
INTEG: Chills, fever, rash, thrombophlebitis at inj site, urticaria, pruritus, necrosis (red man syndrome), skin/subcutaneous tissue disorders
RESP: Wheezing, dyspnea
SYST: **Anaphylaxis, superinfection**

Contraindications: Hypersensitivity, previous hearing loss

Precautions: Pregnancy (B), breastfeeding, neonates, geriatric patients, renal disease

PHARMACOKINETICS

PO: Absorption poor
IV: Onset rapid, peak 1 hr, half-life 4-8 hr, excreted in urine (active form)

INTERACTIONS

Increase: ototoxicity or nephrotoxicity—aminoglycosides, cephalosporins, colistin, polymyxin, bacitracin, cisplatin, amphotericin B, nondepolarizing muscle relaxants, cidofovir

Drug/Herb

- Do not use acidophilus with antiinfectives; separate by several hours

NURSING CONSIDERATIONS

Assess:

- Infection: WBC, urine, stools, sputum, characteristics of wound, throughout treatment
- I&O ratio; report hematuria, oliguria; nephrotoxicity may occur
- ⚠ Any patient with compromised renal system; product is excreted slowly in poor renal system function; toxicity may occur rapidly; BUN, creatinine
- Serum levels: peak 1 hr after 1 hr inf 25-40 mg/ml, trough prior to next dose 5-10 mg/ml
- C&S
- Auditory function during, after treatment
- B/P during administration; sudden drop may indicate red man syndrome
- Hearing loss, ringing, roaring in ears; product should be discontinued
- Skin eruptions
- Respiratory status: rate, character, wheezing, tightness in chest
- Allergies before treatment, reaction of each medication

Administer:

- Use only for susceptible organisms to prevent product-resistant bacteria
- Antihistamine if red man syndrome occurs: decreased B/P, flushing of neck, face
- Dose based on serum concentration

IT route

- Use preservative-free 0.9% NaCl (2-5 mg/ml final conc)

Intermittent IV route

- After reconstitution with 10 ml sterile water for injection (500 mg/10 ml); further dilution is needed for IV, 500 mg/100 ml 0.9% NaCl, D_5W given as int inf over 1 hr; decrease rate of infusion if red man syndrome occurs

CONT IV INF route

- May infuse 1-2 g in volume to give over 24 hr if intermittent IV route cannot be used

Y-site compatibilities: Acyclovir, allopurinol, amifostine, amiodarone, amsacrine, atracurium, cisatracurium, cyclophosphamide, diltiazem, DOXOrubicin liposome, enalaprilat, esmolol, filgrastim, fluconazole, fludarabine, gallium, granisetron, hydromorphone, insulin (regular), labetalol, lorazepam, magnesium sulfate, melphalan, meperidine, meropenem, midazolam, morphine, ondansetron, paclitaxel, pancuronium, perphenazine, propofol, remifentanil, sodium bicarbonate, tacrolimus, teniposide, theophylline, thiotepa, tolazoline, vecuronium, vinorelbine, warfarin, zidovudine

Perform/provide:
- Storage at room temperature for up to 2 wk after reconstitution
- epinephrine, suction, tracheostomy set, endotracheal intubation equipment on unit; anaphylaxis may occur
- Adequate intake of fluids (2 L/day) to prevent nephrotoxicity

Evaluate:
- Therapeutic response: absence of fever, sore throat; negative culture

Teach patient/family:
- All aspects of product therapy: need to complete entire course of medication to ensure organism death (7-10 days); culture may be taken after completed course of medication
- To report sore throat, fever, fatigue; could indicate superinfection
- That product must be taken in equal intervals around clock to maintain blood levels

vardenafil (℞)
(var-den'a-fil)
Levitra
Func. class.: Impotence agent
Chem. class.: Phosphodiesterase type 5 inhibitor

Action: Inhibits phosphodiesterase type 5 (PDE5), enhances erectile function by increasing the amount of cGMP, which in turn causes smooth muscle relaxation and increased blood flow into the corpus cavernosum

Uses: Treatment of erectile dysfunction

DOSAGE AND ROUTES
- *Adult:* **PO** 10 mg taken 1 hr before sexual activity; dose may be reduced to 5 mg or increased to a max of 20 mg; max dosing frequency is once daily
- *Geriatric >65 yr:* **PO** 5 mg initially, titrated as needed/tolerated

Hepatic dose
- *Adult:* **PO** (Child-Pugh B) 5 mg, max 10 mg/day

Concomitant medications
- Ritonavir, max 2.5 mg q72hr; for indinavir, ketoconazole 400 mg/day and itraconazole 400 mg/day, max 2.5 mg/day; for ketoconazole 200 mg/day, itraconazole 200 mg/day and erythromycin max 5 mg/day

Available forms: Tabs 2.5, 5, 10, 20 mg

SIDE EFFECTS
CNS: Headache, flushing, dizziness, insomnia, **seizures,** transient global amnesia

CV: Hypertension, **MI, CV collapse,** chest pain

EENT: Conjunctivitis, tinnitus, photophobia, diminished vision, glaucoma, hearing loss

GU: Abnormal ejaculation, priapism

MISC: Rash, GERD, GGTP increased, **NAION (nonarteritic ischemic optic neuropathy),** dyspepsia

MS: Myalgia, arthralgia, neck pain

RESP: Rhinitis, sinusitis, dyspnea, pharyngitis, epistaxis

Contraindications: Hypersensitivity, coadministration of α-blockers or nitrates, renal failure, congenital or acquired QT prolongation

Precautions: Pregnancy (B); not indicated for women, children, or newborns; hepatic impairment, retinitis pigmentosa, anatomical penile deformities, sickle cell anemia, leukemia, multiple myeloma, bleeding disorders, active peptic ulceration, CV/renal disease

PHARMACOKINETICS
Rapidly absorbed, bioavailability 15%, protein binding 95%, metabolized by liver, terminal half-life 4-5 hr, onset 20 min, peak ½-1½ hr, duration <5 hr, reduced absorption with high-fat meal, primarily excreted in feces (91%-95%)

INTERACTIONS
⚠ Do not use with nitrates because of unsafe decrease in B/P, which could result in MI or stroke

V

⚠ Serious dysrhythmias: class IA/III antiarrhythmics, clarithromycin, droperidol, procainamide, quinidine, quinolones; do not use concurrently

Increase: hypotension—α-blockers, protease inhibitors, metoprolol, NIFEdipine, alcohol, amlodipine, angiotensin II receptor blockers; do not use concurrently

Increase: vardenafil levels—erythromycin, azole antifungals (ketoconazole intraconazole), cimetidine, antiretroviral protease inhibitors

NURSING CONSIDERATIONS

Assess:

- For any severe loss of vision occurs while taking this or any similar products, these products should not be used
- For use of organic nitrates that should not be used with this product

Administer:

- Approximately 1 hr before sexual activity; do not use more than once a day
- Do not use with nitrates in any form

Teach patient/family:

- That product does not protect against STDs, including HIV
- That product absorption is reduced with a high-fat meal
- That product should not be used with nitrates in any form
- That product has no effect in the absence of sexual stimulation
- That patient should seek immediate medical attention if erections last for more than 4 hr
- To inform physician of all medications being taken
- To notify prescriber immediately and stop taking product if vision loss occurs

varenicline (℞)

(var-e-ni′kleen)

Chantix

Func. class.: Smoking cessation agent

Action: Partial agonist for nicotine receptors; partially activates receptors to help curb cravings; occupies receptors to prevent nicotine binding

Uses: Smoking deterrent

DOSAGE AND ROUTES

- *Adult:* **PO** Therapy should begin 1 week prior to smoking stop date (i.e., take product plus tobacco for 7 days); titrate for 1 wk, days 1 through 3, 0.5 mg/day; days 4 through 7, 0.5 mg bid; day 8 through end of treatment 1 mg bid; treatment is 12 wk and may repeat for another 12 wk

Available forms: Tabs 0.5, 1 mg

SIDE EFFECTS

CNS: Headache, agitation, dizziness, insomnia, abnormal dreams, fatigue, malaise, behavior changes, depression, suicidal ideation, **suicide,** amnesia, hallucinations, hostility, mania, psychosis, tremor

CV: Dysrhythmias, hypo/hypertension, palpitations, tachycardia, angina, **MI**

EENT: ***Blurred vision,*** tinnitus

GI: ***Nausea, vomiting,*** anorexia, ***dry mouth,*** increased/decreased appetite, ***constipation,*** flatulence, GERD

GU: Erectile dysfunction, urinary frequency, menstrual irregularities

INTEG: Rash, pruritus, **angioedema, Stevens-Johnson syndrome**

MISC: Weight loss or gain

RESP: Dyspnea, rhinorrhea

Contraindications: Hypersensitivity, eating disorders

Precautions: Pregnancy (C), breastfeeding, children <18 yr, geriatric patients, renal disease, recent MI

Black Box Warning: Bipolar disorder, depression, schizophrenia, suicidal ideation

PHARMACOKINETICS

Elimination half-life 24 hr; metabolism is minimal, 92% excreted unchanged in urine; steady state 4 days

NURSING CONSIDERATIONS

Assess:

- Renal function in geriatric patients
- For smoking cessation after 12 wk; if progress has not been made, product may be used for an additional 12 wk
- Neuropsychiatric symptoms: mood, sensorium, affect; behavior changes, agitation, depression, suicidal ideation; suicide has occurred

Administer:

- Do not break, crush, or chew tabs
- Increased fluids, bulk in diet if constipation occurs
- After eating with a full glass of water
- Sugarless gum, hard candy, or frequent sips of water for dry mouth

Evaluate:

- Therapeutic response: smoking cessation

Teach patient/family:

- That treatment for smoking cessation lasts 12 wk and another 12 wk may be required
- To use caution in driving, other activities requiring alertness; blurred vision may occur
- To set a date to quit smoking and initiate treatment 1 wk prior to that date
- How to titrate product
- Not to use with nicotine patches unless directed by prescriber; may increase B/P
- To notify prescriber if pregnancy is suspected or planned
- Common side effects to be expected

vasopressin (℞)

(vay-soe-press′in)

Pitressin, Pressyn ✦

Func. class.: Pituitary hormone

Chem. class.: Lysine vasopressin

Action: Promotes reabsorption of water by action on renal tubular epithelium; causes vasoconstriction

Uses: Diabetes insipidus (nonnephrogenic/nonpsychogenic), abdominal distention postoperatively, bleeding esophageal varices

DOSAGE AND ROUTES

Diabetes insipidus

- *Adult:* **IM/SUBCUT** 5-10 units bid-qid as needed; **CONT IV INF** 0.0005 units/kg/hr (0.05 milliunit/kg/hr), double dose q30min as needed
- *Child:* **IM/SUBCUT** 2.5-10 units bid-qid as needed; **IM/SUBCUT** 1.25-2.5 units q2-3days (Pitressin Tannate) for chronic therapy

Abdominal distention

- *Adult:* **IM** 5 units, then q3-4hr, increasing to 10 units if needed (aqueous)

Available forms: Inj 20, 5 units/ml (tannate)

SIDE EFFECTS

CNS: Drowsiness, headache, lethargy, flushing, vertigo

CV: Increased B/P, dysrhythmias, **cardiac arrest, shock**, chest pain, **MI**

EENT: Nasal irritation, congestion, rhinitis

GI: Nausea, heartburn, cramps, vomiting, flatus

GU: Vulval pain, uterine cramping

MISC: Tremor, sweating, vertigo, urticaria, bronchial constriction

Contraindications: Hypersensitivity, chronic nephritis

Precautions: Pregnancy (C), breastfeeding, CAD, asthma, vascular/renal disease, migraines, seizures

PHARMACOKINETICS

Nasal: Onset 1 hr; duration 3-8 hr; half-life 15 min; metabolized in liver, kidneys; excreted in urine

INTERACTIONS

Increase: antidiuretic effect—tricyclics, carbamazepine, chloropromide, fludrocortisone, clofibrate, urea

Decrease: antidiuretic effect—lithium, demeclocycline

NURSING CONSIDERATIONS

Assess:

• Pulse, B/P, when giving product IV or IM

• I&O ratio, weight daily, fluid/electrolyte balance; check for edema in extremities; if water retention is severe, diuretic may be prescribed

• H_2O intoxication: lethargy, behavioral changes, disorientation, neuromuscular excitability

• Small doses may precipitate coronary adverse effects, keep emergency equipment nearby

Evaluate:

• Therapeutic response: absence of severe thirst, decreased urine output, osmolality

Teach patient/family:

• To measure and record I&O

• To avoid alcohol, all OTC medications unless approved by prescriber

⚠ High Alert

vecuronium (℞)

(vek-yoo-roe′nee-um)

Func. class.: Neuromuscular blocker, nondepolarizing

Chem. class.: Monoquaternary analog of pancuronium

Action: Inhibits transmission of nerve impulses by binding with cholinergic receptor sites, antagonizing action of acetylcholine

Uses: Facilitation of endotracheal intubation, skeletal muscle relaxation during mechanical ventilation, surgery, general anesthesia

DOSAGE AND ROUTES

• *Adult and child >1 yr:* **IV** Initially 0.08-0.1 mg/kg or 0.04-0.06 mg/kg if given with succinylcholine, maintenance 0.01-0.015 mg/kg 25-40 min after initial dose, then 0.01-0.015 mg/kg q12-15min

• *Infant 7 wk-1 yr:* **IV** 0.08-0.1 mg/kg, maintenance 0.05-0.1 mg/kg q60min as needed

• *Neonate:* **IV** 0.1 mg/kg/dose, maintenance 0.03-0.15 mg/kg/dose q1-2hr as needed

Available forms: 10 mg/5-ml vial

SIDE EFFECTS

CNS: Skeletal muscle weakness or paralysis (rare)

INTEG: Urticaria, flushing

MISC: Myopathy, hypotension

RESP: **Prolonged apnea, possible respiratory paralysis,** bronchospasm, tachycardia, dyspnea

SYST: **Anaphylaxis**

Contraindications: Hypersensitivity

Precautions: Pregnancy (C), breastfeeding, children <2 yr, electrolyte imbalances, dehydration, hepatic/cardiac/neuromuscular disease

Black Box Warning: Respiratory disease

PHARMACOKINETICS

IV: Onset 2-3 min, peak 3-5 min, duration 15-25 (recovery index) min, half-life 65-75 min, not metabolized, excreted in urine/feces, crosses placenta

INTERACTIONS

• Dysrhythmias: theophylline

Increase: neuromuscular blockade—aminoglycosides, amphotericin B, clindamycin, lincomycin, quinidine, local anesthetics, polymyxin antibiotics, lithium, opioid analgesics, phenytoin, piperacillin, thiazides, enflurane, isoflurane, succinylcholine, verapamil

NURSING CONSIDERATIONS

Assess:

• VS (B/P, pulse, respirations, airway) q15min until fully recovered; rate, depth, pattern of respirations, strength of hand grip

• I&O ratio; check for urinary retention, frequency, hesitancy

• Recovery: decreased paralysis of face, diaphragm, leg, arm, rest of body; allow to recover fully before completing neurologic assessment
• Allergic reactions: rash, fever, respiratory distress, pruritus; product should be discontinued

Administer:
• With diazepam or morphine when used for therapeutic paralysis; provides no sedation alone
• Using nerve stimulator by anesthesiologist to determine neuromuscular blockade
• Anticholinesterase to reverse neuromuscular blockade
• IV after diluting with diluent provided; give by direct IV over 1 min; may give as continuous inf 10-20 mg/100 ml; titrate to patient response (only by qualified person)

Y-site compatibilities: Aminophylline, cefazolin, cefuroxime, cimetidine, diltiazem, DOBUTamine, DOPamine, epinephrine, esmolol, fentanyl, fluconazole, gentamicin, heparin, hydrocortisone, hydromorphone, isoproterenol, labetalol, lorazepam, midazolam, milrinone, morphine, niCARdipine, nitroglycerin, norepinephrine, propofol, ranitidine, sodium nitroprusside, trimethoprim-sulfamethoxazole, vancomycin

Perform/provide:
• Storage in refrigerator; discard in 24 hr
• Reassurance if communication is difficult during recovery from neuromuscular blockade

Evaluate:
• Therapeutic response: paralysis of jaw, eyelid, head, neck, rest of body

Treatment of overdose: Edrophonium or neostigmine, atropine, monitor VS; may require mechanical ventilation

venlafaxine (℞)
(ven-la-fax′een)
Effexor, Effexor XR
Func. class.: Antidepressant—miscellaneous

Action: Potent inhibitor of neuronal serotonin and norepinephrine uptake, weak inhibitor of DOPamine; no muscarinic, histaminergic, or α-adrenergic receptors in vitro

Uses: Prevention/treatment of major depression, to treat depression at end of life; long-term treatment of general anxiety disorder, panic disorder, social anxiety disorder (Effexor XR only)

Unlabeled uses: Hot flashes, premenstrual dysphoric disorder (PMDD), headache, neuropathic pain

DOSAGE AND ROUTES

Depression
• *Adult:* **PO** 75 mg/day in 2 or 3 divided doses; taken with food, may be increased to 150 mg/day; if needed, may be further increased to 225 mg/day; increments of 75 mg/day at intervals of no less than 4 days; some hospitalized patients may require up to 375 mg/day in 3 divided doses; **EXT REL** 37.5-75 mg PO daily, max 225 mg/day; give XR daily

Anxiety disorders
• *Adult:* **PO** 75 mg/day or 37.5 mg/day × 4-7 days initially, max 225 mg/day

Renal dose
• *Adult:* **PO** CCr 10-70 ml/min reduce dose by 25%-50%; CCr <10 ml/min reduce dose by 50%

Hepatic dose
• *Adult:* **PO** Moderate impairment, 50% of dose

Hot flashes (unlabeled)
• *Adult (male, prostate cancer):* **PO** 12.5 mg bid × 4 wk

Available forms: Tabs scored (Effexor) 25, 37.5, 50, 75, 100 mg; ext rel cap (Effexor XR) 37.5, 75, 150, 225 mg

SIDE EFFECTS

CNS: Emotional lability, vertigo, apathy, ataxia, CNS stimulation, euphoria, hallucinations, hostility, increased libido, hypertonia, hypotonia, psychosis, insomnia, anxiety, **suicidal ideation in children/adolescents, seizures, neuroleptic malignant syndrome–like reaction**

CV: Migraine, angina pectoris, hypertension, **sustained hypertension, change in QTc interval,** increased pulse, increased cholesterol, extrasystoles, postural hypotension, syncope, thrombophlebitis

EENT: Abnormal vision, taste, *ear pain,* cataract, conjunctivitis, corneal lesions, dry eyes, otitis media, photophobia

GI: Dysphagia, eructation, nausea, anorexia, dry mouth, colitis, gastritis, gingivitis, **rectal hemorrhage,** stomatitis, stomach and mouth ulceration

GU: Anorgasmia, abnormal ejaculation, *dysuria, hematuria, metrorrhagia, vaginitis, impaired urination,* albuminuria, amenorrhea, kidney calculus, cystitis, nocturia, breast and bladder pain, polyuria, **uterine hemorrhage, vaginal hemorrhage,** moniliasis

HEMA: **Agranulocytosis, aplastic anemia, neutropenia, pancytopenia, abnormal bleeding**

INTEG: Ecchymosis, acne, alopecia, brittle nails, dry skin, photosensitivity, sweating

META: Peripheral edema, weight loss or gain, diabetes mellitus, edema, glycosuria, hyperlipemia, hypokalemia

MS: Arthritis, bone pain, bursitis, myasthenia, tenosynovitis, arthralgia

RESP: Bronchitis, dyspnea, asthma, chest congestion, epistaxis, hyperventilation, laryngitis

SYST: Malaise, neck pain, enlarged abdomen, cyst, facial edema, hangover, hernia

Contraindications: Hypersensitivity, bipolar disorder, interstitial lung disease

Precautions: Pregnancy (C), breastfeeding, geriatric patients, mania, hypertension, seizure disorder, recent MI, cardiac/renal/hepatic disease, eosinophilic pneumonia

Black Box Warning: Children, suicidal ideation

PHARMACOKINETICS

Well absorbed; extensively metabolized in the liver to an active metabolite; 87% of product recovered in urine; 27% protein binding; half-life 5, 11 hr (active metabolite) respectively

INTERACTIONS

⚠ Hyperthermia, rigidity, rapid fluctuations of vital signs, mental status changes, neuroleptic malignant syndrome: MAOIs

Increase: venlafaxine effect—cimetidine

Increase: CNS depression—alcohol, opioids, antihistamines, sedative/hypnotics

Increase: levels of clozapine, desipramine, haloperidol, warfarin

Increase: serotonin syndrome—sibutramine, sumatriptan, trazadone

Decrease: effect of indinavir

Decrease: venlafaxine effect—cyproheptadine

Drug/Herb

- Serotonin syndrome: SAM-e, St. John's wort

Increase: CNS depression—chamomile, hops, kava, lavender, skullcap, valerian

Increase: anticholinergic effect—corkwood, jimsonweed

Increase: hypertension—yohimbe

Drug/Lab Test

Increase: alk phos, bilirubin, AST, ALT, BUN, creatinine, serum cholesterol, CPK, LDH

NURSING CONSIDERATIONS

Assess:

- Mental status: mood, sensorium, affect, increase in psychiatric symptoms; depression, panic; assess for suicidal ideation in children/adolescents
- B/P lying, standing; pulse q4hr; if systolic B/P drops 20 mm Hg, hold product, notify prescriber; take VS q4hr in patients with CV disease

• Electrolytes: Hypo/hyperkalemia, hypo/hyperphosphatemia, hyponatremia, hyperuricemia, hypo/hyperglycemia can occur
• Blood studies: CBC, differential, leukocytes, cardiac enzymes if patient is receiving long-term therapy
• Hepatic studies: AST, ALT, bilirubin
• Weight q wk; weight loss or gain; appetite may increase; peripheral edema may occur
• Withdrawal symptoms: headache, nervousness, agitation, nausea, vomiting, muscle pain, weakness; not usual unless product is discontinued abruptly
⚠ For neuroleptic malignant syndrome–like reactions

Administer:
• With food, milk for GI symptoms
• Sugarless gum, hard candy, frequent sips of water for dry mouth
• Avoid use with CNS depressants
• In small amounts because of suicide potential, especially in the beginning of therapy

Perform/provide:
• Storage in tight container at room temperature; do not freeze
• Assistance with ambulation during beginning therapy, since drowsiness, dizziness occur
• Checking to see if PO medication swallowed

Evaluate:
• Therapeutic response: decreased depression, anxiety; increased well-being

Teach patient/family:
• To notify prescriber of rash, hives, or allergic reactions
• To use with caution when driving or other activities requiring alertness because of drowsiness, dizziness, blurred vision
• That worsening of symptoms, suicidal thoughts/behavior may occur in children, young adults
• To avoid alcohol ingestion
• Not to discontinue medication abruptly after long-term use; may cause nausea, headache, malaise
• To wear sunscreen or large hat, since photosensitivity occurs
• To avoid pregnancy or breastfeeding while taking this product
• To monitor B/P in hypertension

Treatment of overdose: ECG monitoring; lavage, activated charcoal; administer anticonvulsant, may need whole bowel irrigation for ER product

verapamil (℞)
(ver-ap'a-mill)
Apo-Verap ✤, Calan, Calan SR, Covera-HS, Isoptin, Isoptin SR, Novo-Verapamil ✤, Nu-Verap ✤, verapamil HCl, verapamil HCl SR, Verelan PM

Func. class.: Calcium channel blocker; antihypertensive; antianginal, antidysrhythmic (class IV)
Chem. class.: Diphenylalkylamine

Action: Inhibits calcium ion influx across cell membrane during cardiac depolarization; produces relaxation of coronary vascular smooth muscle; dilates coronary arteries; decreases SA/AV node conduction; dilates peripheral arteries

Uses: Chronic stable, vasospastic, unstable angina; dysrhythmias, hypertension, supraventricular tachycardia, atrial flutter or fibrillation

Unlabeled uses: Prevention of migraine headaches, claudication, mania

DOSAGE AND ROUTES

Angina
• *Adult:* **PO** 80-120 mg tid, increase q wk

Dysrhythmias
• *Adult:* **PO** 240-320 mg/day in 3-4 divided doses in digitalized patients
• *Adult:* **IV BOL** 5-10 mg (0.075-0.15 mg/kg) over 2 min, may repeat 10 mg (0.15 mg/kg) ½ hr after 1st dose
• *Child 1-15 yr:* **IV BOL** 0.1-0.3 mg/kg over 2 min or more, repeat in 30 min, max 5 mg in a single dose
• *Child 0-1 yr:* **IV BOL** 0.1-0.2 mg/kg over ≥2 min, may repeat after 30 min

Hypertension

• *Adult:* **PO** 80 mg tid, may titrate upward; **EXT REL** 120-240 mg/day as a single dose, may increase to 240-480 mg/day

Hepatic disease/geriatric patients/compromised ventricular function

• *Adult:* **PO** 40 mg tid initially, increase as tolerated

Claudication due to PVD (unlabeled)

• *Adult:* **PO** 120-480 mg/day in divided doses

Mania (unlabeled)

• *Adult:* **PO** 160-320 mg/day in divided doses, may be given with lithium

Migraine prophylaxis (unlabeled)

• *Adult:* **PO** 80 mg tid

Available forms: Tabs 40, 80, 120 mg; ext rel tabs 120, 180, 240 mg; inj 2.5 mg/ml in ampules, syringes, vials; ext rel caps 100, 200, 240, 300 mg

SIDE EFFECTS

CNS: *Headache, drowsiness,* dizziness, anxiety, depression, weakness, insomnia, confusion, light-headedness, asthenia, fatigue

CV: *Edema,* **CHF,** bradycardia, hypotension, palpitations, AV block, **dysrhythmias**

GI: *Nausea,* diarrhea, gastric upset, *constipation,* increased LFTs

GU: Impotence, gynecomastia, nocturia, polyuria

HEMA: Bruising, petechiae, bleeding

INTEG: Rash, bruising

MISC: Gingival hyperplasia

SYST: **Stevens-Johnson syndrome**

Contraindications: Sick sinus syndrome, 2nd-/3rd-degree heart block, hypotension <90 mm Hg systolic, cardiogenic shock, severe CHF

Precautions: Pregnancy (C), breastfeeding, children, geriatric patients, CHF, hypotension, hepatic injury, renal disease, concomitant β-blocker therapy

PHARMACOKINETICS

Metabolized by liver, excreted in urine (70% as metabolites)

PO: Onset variable; peak 3-4 hr; duration 17-24 hr; half-life (biphasic) 4 min, 3-7 hr (terminal)

IV: Onset 3 min, peak 3-5 min, duration 10-20 min

INTERACTIONS

Increase: hypotension—prazosin, quinidine, fentanyl, other antihypertensives, nitrates

Increase: effects of verapamil—β-blockers, cimetidine, telithromycin

Increase: levels of digoxin, theophylline, cycloSPORINE, carbamazepine, nondepolarizing muscle relaxants

Decrease: effects of lithium

Decrease: antihypertensive effects—NSAIDs

Drug/Herb

Increase: effect—barberry, betel palm, burdock, goldenseal, khat, lily of the valley, plantain

Decrease: effect—yohimbe

Drug/Food

Increase: hypotensive effects—grapefruit juice

Drug/Lab Test

Increase: AST, ALT, alk phos, BUN, creatinine, serum cholesterol

NURSING CONSIDERATIONS

Assess:

• Cardiac status: B/P, pulse, respiration, ECG intervals (PR, QRS, QT); notify prescriber if <50 bpm, systolic B/P <90 mm Hg

⚠ I&O ratios, weight daily; CHF: crackles, weight gain, dyspnea, jugular vein distention

• Renal, hepatic studies during long-term treatment, serum potassium periodically

Administer:

PO route

• Do not crush or chew ext rel products; caps may be opened and contents sprinkled on food; do not dissolve chew cap contents

• Before meals, at bedtime; give ext rel with food

IV route

• Undiluted through Y-tube or 3-way stopcock of compatible sol; give over 2 min, or 3 min geriatric patients, discard unused solution

Additive compatibilities: Amikacin, amiodarone, ascorbic acid, atropine, bretylium, calcium chloride, calcium gluconate, cefazolin, cefotaxime, cefoxitin, cephapirin, chloramphenicol, cimetidine, clindamycin, dexamethasone, diazepam, digoxin, DOPamine, epinephrine, erythromycin, gentamicin, heparin, hydrocortisone sodium phosphate, hydrocortisone, hydromorphone, insulin (regular), isoproterenol, lidocaine, magnesium sulfate, mannitol, meperidine, metaraminol, methicillin, methyldopate, methylPREDNISolone, metoclopramide, mezlocillin, morphine, moxalactam, multivitamins, naloxone, nitroglycerin, norepinephrine, oxytocin, pancuronium, penicillin G potassium, penicillin G sodium, pentobarbital, phenobarbital, phentolamine, phenytoin, piperacillin, potassium chloride, potassium phosphates, procainamide, propranolol, protamine, quinidine, sodium bicarbonate, sodium nitroprusside, theophylline, ticarcillin, tobramycin, tolazoline, vancomycin, vasopressin, vit B/C

Syringe compatibilities: Inamrinone, heparin, milrinone

Y-site compatibilities: Inamrinone, ciprofloxacin, DOBUTamine, DOPamine, famotidine, hydrALAZINE, meperidine, methicillin, milrinone, penicillin G potassium, piperacillin, propofol, ticarcillin

Evaluate:

• Therapeutic response: decreased anginal pain, decreased B/P, dysrhythmias

Teach patient/family:

• To increase fluids/fiber to counteract constipation
• How to take pulse, B/P before taking product; to keep record or graph
• To avoid hazardous activities until stabilized on product, dizziness no longer a problem
• To limit caffeine consumption; no alcohol products
• To avoid OTC or grapefruit products unless directed by prescriber
• To comply with all areas of medical regimen: diet, exercise, stress reduction, product therapy
• To change positions slowly to prevent syncope
• Not to discontinue abruptly; chest pain may occur
• To report chest pain, palpitations, irregular heart beats, swelling of extremities, skin irritation, rash, tremors, weakness

Treatment of overdose: Defibrillation, atropine for AV block, vasopressor for hypotension, IV calcium

vidarabine ophthalmic

See Appendix B

vigabatrin

See Appendix A—Selected New Drugs

⚠ High Alert

*vinBLAStine (VLB) (℞)

(vin-blast'een)

Velbe ✦, vinblastine sulfate

Func. class.: Antineoplastic

Chem. class.: Vinca rosea alkaloid

Do not confuse:

vinBLAStine/vinCRIStine

Action: Inhibits mitotic activity, arrests cell cycle at metaphase; inhibits RNA synthesis, blocks cellular use of glutamic acid needed for purine synthesis; a vesicant

Uses: Breast, testicular cancer, lymphomas, neuroblastoma; Hodgkin's, non-Hodgkin's lymphomas; mycosis fungoides, histiocytosis, Kaposi's sarcoma, Langerhans cell histiocytosis

Unlabeled uses: Lung, bladder, prostate cancer, desmoid tumor, malignant melanoma

V

DOSAGE AND ROUTES

- *Adult:* **IV** 0.1 mg/kg or 3-6 mg/m^2 q wk or q2wk, max 0.5 mg/kg or 18.5 mg/m^2 q wk
- *Child:* 2.5 mg/m^2 then 3.75, 5, 6.25, 7.5 at 7-day intervals

Available forms: Inj, powder 10 mg for 10 ml IV; sol for inj 1 mg/ml

SIDE EFFECTS

CNS: Paresthesias, peripheral neuropathy, depression, headache, **seizures,** malaise

CV: Tachycardia, orthostatic hypo/hypertension

GI: *Nausea, vomiting,* ileus, *anorexia, stomatitis, constipation,* abdominal pain, **GI/rectal bleeding, hepatotoxicity,** pharyngitis

GU: Urinary retention, **renal failure,** hyperuricemia

HEMA: **Thrombocytopenia, leukopenia, myelosuppression,** agranulocytosis, granulocytosis, aplastic anemia, neutropenia, pancytopenia

INTEG: *Rash, alopecia,* photosensitivity, **extravasation, tissue necrosis**

META: SIADH

RESP: **Fibrosis, pulmonary infiltrate, bronchospasm**

SYST: **Tumor lysis syndrome (TLS)**

Contraindications: Pregnancy (D), breastfeeding, infants, hypersensitivity, leukopenia, granulocytopenia, bone marrow suppression, infection

Black Box Warning: Intrathecal use

Precautions: Renal/hepatic disease, tumor lysis syndrome

Black Box Warning: Extravasation

PHARMACOKINETICS

Half-life (triphasic) <5 min, 50-155 min, 23-85 hr; metabolized in liver, excreted in urine, feces; crosses blood-brain barrier

INTERACTIONS

- Synergism: bleomycin
- Bronchospasm: mitomycin
- Do not use with radiation

Increase: bleeding risk—NSAIDs, anticoagulants

Increase: toxicity, bone marrow suppression—antineoplastics

Increase: action of methotrexate

Increase: adverse reactions—live virus vaccines

Increase: toxicity—CYP3A4 inhibitors (aprepitant, antiretroviral protease inhibitors, clarithromycin, danazol, delavirdine, diltiazem, erythromycin, fluconazole, fluoxetine, fluvoxamine, imatinib, ketoconazole, mibefradil, nefazodone, telithromycin, voriconazole)

Decrease: vinBLAStine effect—CYP3A4 inducers (barbiturates, bosentan, carbamazepine, efavirenz, phenytoins, nevirapine, rifabutin, rifampin)

Drug/Herb

- Avoid use with St. John's wort

NURSING CONSIDERATIONS

Assess:

⚠ CBC, differential, platelet count q wk; withhold product if WBC is <2000/mm^3 or platelet count is <75,000/mm^3; notify prescriber; RBC, Hct, Hgb may be decreased

- Pulmonary function tests, chest x-ray studies before, during therapy; chest x-ray film should be obtained q2wk during treatment
- Neurologic status: sensory-vibratory evaluation if side effects occur
- Renal studies: BUN, serum uric acid, urine CCr, electrolytes before, during therapy; I&O ratio; report fall in urine output of 30 ml/hr
- Monitor temp; may indicate beginning infection
- Hepatic studies before, during therapy (bilirubin, AST, ALT, LDH) as needed or qmo
- Bleeding: hematuria, guaiac, bruising or petechiae, mucosa of orifices
- Dyspnea, crackles, unproductive cough, chest pain, tachypnea, fatigue, increased pulse, pallor, lethargy
- Effects of alopecia on body image; discuss feelings about body changes

• Sensitivity of feet/hands, which precedes neuropathy
• Jaundiced skin, sclera; dark urine, clay-colored stools, itchy skin, abdominal pain, fever, diarrhea
• Buccal cavity q8hr for dryness, sores or ulceration, white patches, oral pain, bleeding, dysphagia
• Local irritation, pain, burning, discoloration at inj site, extravasation
• Symptoms indicating severe allergic reaction: rash, pruritus, urticaria, purpuric skin lesions, itching, flushing
• Frequency of stools and characteristics: cramping; acidosis; signs of dehydration: rapid respirations, poor skin turgor, decreased urine output, dry skin, restlessness, weakness
• For gout, joint pain, swelling, increased uric acid; allopurinol or other treatment may be used

Administer:
• Antiemetic 30-60 min before giving product and prn to prevent vomiting
• Hyaluronidase 150 units/ml in 1 ml NaCl, warm compress for extravasation for vesicant activity treatment

IV inj route
• After diluting 10 mg/10 ml NaCl; give through Y-tube or 3-way stopcock or directly over 1 min

Intermittent IV INF route
• Further dilute in 50-100 ml of NS, infuse over 15-30 min

Additive compatibilities: Bleomycin

Syringe compatibilities: Bleomycin, cisplatin, cyclophosphamide, droperidol, fluorouracil, leucovorin, methotrexate, metoclopramide, mitomycin, vinCRIStine

Y-site compatibilities: Allopurinol, amifostine, amphotericin B cholesteryl, aztreonam, bleomycin, cisplatin, cyclophosphamide, DOXOrubicin, DOXOrubicin liposome, droperidol, filgrastim, fludarabine, fluorouracil, granisetron, heparin, leucovorin, melphalan, methotrexate, metoclopramide, mitomycin, ondansetron, paclitaxel, piperacillin/tazobactam, sargramostim, teniposide, thiotepa, vinCRIStine, vinorelbine

Perform/provide:
• Liquid diet: cola, Jell-O; dry toast or crackers may be added if patient is not nauseated or vomiting
• Increase fluid intake to 2-3 L/day to prevent urate deposits, calculi formation
• Rinsing of mouth tid-qid with water
• Brushing of teeth bid-tid with soft brush or cotton-tipped applicators for stomatitis; use unwaxed dental floss
• Nutritious diet with iron, vitamin supplements

Evaluate:
• Therapeutic response: decreased tumor size, spread of malignancy

Teach patient/family:
• To report any complaints or side effects to nurse or prescriber
• To report any changes in breathing or coughing; to avoid exposure to persons with infection
• That hair may be lost during treatment, a wig or hairpiece may make patient feel better; tell patient that new hair may be different in color, texture
• To report change in gait or numbness in extremities; may indicate neuropathy
• To avoid foods with citric acid, hot or rough texture
• To report any bleeding, white spots or ulcerations in mouth to prescriber; to examine mouth daily
• To wear sunscreen, protective clothing, sunglasses
• To avoid receiving vaccinations
• To use effective contraception, avoid breastfeeding; may cause male infertility

⚠ High Alert

*vinCRIStine (VCR) (℞)

(vin-kris'teen)

Oncovin, Vincasar PFS, vincristine sulfate

Func. class.: Antineoplastic—miscellaneous

Chem. class.: Vinca alkaloid

Do not confuse:
vinCRIStine/vinBLAStine

Action: Inhibits mitotic activity, arrests

cell cycle at metaphase; inhibits RNA synthesis, blocks cellular use of glutamic acid needed for purine synthesis; a vesicant

Uses: Lymphomas, neuroblastoma, Hodgkin's disease, acute lymphoblastic and other leukemias, rhabdomyosarcoma, Wilms' tumor, non-Hodgkin's lymphoma, malignant glioma, soft tissue sarcoma

Unlabeled uses: Lung, breast, colorectal, head/neck, osteogenic sarcomas, small cell lung cancer, trophoblastic disease

DOSAGE AND ROUTES

- *Adult:* **IV** 0.4-1.4 mg/m^2/wk, max 2 mg
- *Child:* **IV** 1-2 mg/m^2/wk, max 2 mg

Available forms: Inj 1 mg/ml; powder for inj 5 mg/vial

SIDE EFFECTS

CNS: Decreased reflexes, numbness, weakness, motor difficulties, CNS depression, cranial nerve paralysis, **seizures,** peripheral neuropathy

CV: Orthostatic hypotension

EENT: Diplopia

GI: Nausea, vomiting, anorexia, stomatitis, constipation, **paralytic ileus,** *abdominal pain,* **hepatotoxicity**

GU: **Renal tubular obstruction**

HEMA: **Thrombocytopenia, leukopenia, myelosuppression, anemia**

INTEG: Alopecia, extravasation

SYST: **Tumor lysis syndrome (TLS)**

Contraindications: Pregnancy (D), breastfeeding, infants, hypersensitivity, radiation therapy

Black Box Warning: Intrathecal use

Precautions: Renal/hepatic disease, hypertension, neuromuscular disease

Black Box Warning: Extravasation

PHARMACOKINETICS

Half-life (triphasic) <5 min, 50-155 min, 23-85 hr; metabolized in liver; excreted in bile, feces; crosses placental barrier, blood-brain barrier

INTERACTIONS

- Neurotoxicity: peripheral nervous system products
- Do not use with radiation
- Acute pulmonary reactions: mitomycin-c

Increase: toxicity—CYP3A4 inhibitors (aprepitant, antiretroviral protease inhibitors, clarithromycin, danazol, delavirdine, diltiazem, erythromycin, fluconazole, fluoxetine, fluvoxamine, imatinib, ketoconazole, mibefradil, nefazodone, telithromycin, voriconazole)

Decrease: immune response—vaccines/toxoids

Decrease: digoxin level—digoxin

Decrease: vinCRIStine effect—CYP3A4 inducers (barbiturates, bosentan, carbamazepine, efavirenz, phenytoins, nevirapine, rifabutin, rifampin)

Drug/Herb

- Avoid use with St. John's wort

NURSING CONSIDERATIONS

Assess:

- CBC, differential, platelet count q wk; withhold product if WBC is <4000/mm^3 or platelet count is <75,000/mm^3; notify prescriber; RBC, Hct, Hgb; may be decreased
- Renal studies: BUN, serum uric acid, urine CCr, electrolytes before, during therapy; I&O ratio, report fall in urine output of 30 ml/hr
- Monitor temp q4hr; may indicate beginning infection
- Hepatic studies before, during therapy (bilirubin, AST, ALT, LDH) as needed or monthly
- Deep tendon reflexes; product is neurotoxic
- Sensitivity of feet/hands, which precedes neuropathy
- Bleeding: hematuria, guaiac, bruising or petechiae, mucosa of orifices q8hr
- Effects of alopecia on body image, discuss feelings about body changes
- Jaundiced skin, sclera; dark urine, clay-colored stools, itchy skin, abdominal pain, fever, diarrhea

• Buccal cavity q8hr for dryness, sores or ulceration, white patches, oral pain, bleeding, dysphagia
• Symptoms indicating severe allergic reaction: rash, pruritus, urticaria, purpuric skin lesions, itching, flushing
• Frequency of stools, characteristics: cramping, acidosis; signs of dehydration: rapid respirations, poor skin turgor, decreased urine output, dry skin, restlessness, weakness

Administer:
• Antiemetic 30-60 min before giving product and prn
• Antispasmodic for GI symptoms
⚠ Do not give intrathecally, fatal

IV route
• After diluting with diluent provided or 1 mg/10 ml of sterile H_2O or NaCl; give through Y-tube or 3-way stopcock or directly over 1 min
• Hyaluronidase 150 units/ml in 1 ml NaCl; apply warm compress for extravasation

Additive compatibilities: Bleomycin, cytarabine, fluorouracil, methotrexate

Syringe compatibilities: Bleomycin, cisplatin, cyclophosphamide, doxapram, DOXOrubicin, droperidol, fluorouracil, heparin, leucovorin, methotrexate, metoclopramide, mitomycin, vinBLAStine

Y-site compatibilities: Allopurinol, amifostine, amphotericin B cholesteryl, aztreonam, bleomycin, cisplatin, cladribine, cyclophosphamide, DOXOrubicin, DOXOrubicin liposome, droperidol, filgrastim, fludarabine, fluorouracil, granisetron, heparin, leucovorin, melphalan, methotrexate, metoclopramide, mitomycin, ondansetron, paclitaxel, piperacillin/tazobactam, sargramostim, teniposide, thiotepa, vinBLAStine, vinorelbine

Perform/provide:
• Liquid diet: cola, Jell-O; dry toast or crackers may be added if patient is not nauseated or vomiting
• Rinsing of mouth tid-qid with water
• Brushing of teeth bid-tid with soft brush or cotton-tipped applicators for stomatitis; use unwaxed dental floss
• Nutritious diet with iron, vitamin supplements

Evaluate:
• Therapeutic response: decreased tumor size, spread of malignancy

Teach patient/family:
• To report change in gait or numbness in extremities; may indicate neuropathy
• To report any complaints or side effects to nurse or prescriber
• To report any bleeding, white spots or ulcerations in mouth to prescriber; to examine mouth daily
• To increase bulk, fluids, exercise to prevent constipation
• To avoid persons with infections
• To avoid vaccinations
• That hair may be lost; hair will grow back but different texture, color
• To use effective contraception during and 2 mo posttherapy, avoid breastfeeding

⚠ High Alert

vinorelbine (℞)

(vi-nor′el-bine)
Navelbine
Func. class.: Antineoplastic—miscellaneous
Chem. class.: Semisynthetic vinca alkaloid

Action: Inhibits mitotic spindle activity, arrests cell cycle at metaphase; inhibits RNA synthesis, blocks cellular use of glutamic acid needed for purine synthesis; a vesicant

Uses: Unresectable advanced non–small cell lung cancer (NSCLC) stage IV; may be used alone or in combination with cisplatin for stage III or IV NSCLC

Unlabeled uses: Hodgkin's disease, breast/ovarian/head/neck cancer, desmoid tumor

V

DOSAGE AND ROUTES

• *Adult:* **IV** 30 mg/m^2 q wk
• *ANC 1000-1499:* Give 50% of dose; <1000, hold dose; <1000 × 3 wk, discontinue

Hepatic dose
• *Adult:* **IV** Total bilirubin 2.1-3 mg/dl 15 mg/m^2 q wk; total bilirubin ≥3 mg/dl 7.5 mg/m^2/day
Available forms: Inj 10 mg/ml

SIDE EFFECTS

CNS: Paresthesias, peripheral neuropathy, depression, headache, **seizures,** weakness, jaw pain, asthenia
CV: Chest pain
GI: Nausea, vomiting, ileus, *anorexia, stomatitis,* constipation, abdominal pain, *diarrhea,* **hepatotoxicity, GI obstruction/perforation**
HEMA: **Neutropenia, anemia, thrombocytopenia, granulocytopenia**
INTEG: Rash, alopecia, photosensitivity, inj site reaction, necrosis
META: SIADH
MS: Myalgia
RESP: Shortness of breath
Contraindications: Pregnancy (D), breastfeeding, infants, hypersensitivity, granulocyte count <1000 cells/mm^3 pretreatment

Black Box Warning: Severe neutropenia, intrathecal administration

Precautions: Children, geriatric patients, renal/hepatic/pulmonary/neurologic disease, anemia, bone marrow suppression

Black Box Warning: Extravasation

PHARMACOKINETICS

Half-life 27-43 hr; peak 1-2 hr; highly bound to platelets, lymphocytes; metabolized in liver; excreted in feces; small amount unchanged in kidneys

INTERACTIONS

Increase: bleeding risk—NSAIDs, anticoagulants
Increase: toxicity—CYP3A4 inhibitors (aprepitant, antiretroviral protease inhibitors, clarithromycin, danazol, delavirdine, diltiazem, erythromycin, fluconazole, fluoxetine, fluvoxamine, imatinib, ketoconazole, mibefradil, nefazodone, telithromycin, voriconazole)
Decrease: vinorelbine effect—CYP3A4 inducers (barbiturates, bosentan, carbamazepine, efavirenz, phenytoins, nevirapine, rifabutin, rifampin)
Drug/Herb
• Avoid use with St. John's wort

NURSING CONSIDERATIONS

Assess:
• B/P (baseline and q15min) during administration
• CBC, differential, platelet count weekly; withhold product if WBC is <4000/mm^3 or platelet count is <75,000/mm^3; notify prescriber of results, recovery will take 3 wk
• Respiratory status: dyspnea, crackles, unproductive cough, chest pain, tachypnea
• Renal studies: BUN, serum uric acid, urine CCr before, during therapy; I&O ratio; report fall in urine output to <30 ml/hr; for decreased hyperuricemia
• For infection, cold, fever, sore throat; notify prescriber if these occur; effects of alopecia on body image
• For bleeding: hematuria, guaiac, bruising or petechiae, mucosa or orifices, no rectal temps; avoid IM inj; use pressure to venipuncture sites
• Nutritional status: an antiemetic may be needed
• Hepatic function tests: AST, ALT, bilirubin, LDH
⚠ For symptoms of severe allergic reactions: rash, pruritus, urticaria, itching, flushing, bronchospasm, hypotension, epinephrine and crash cart should be nearby
• Neurologic status: numbness, pain, tingling, loss of Achilles reflex, weakness, palsies
• For gout: pain, swelling, increased uric acid levels
Administer:
⚠ Do not give intrathecally, fatal
• Antiemetic 30-60 min before giving product and prn to prevent vomiting

Intermittent IV INF route
• Dilute to 0.5-2 mg/ml with 0.9% NaCl, 0.45% NaCl, D_5W, D_5/0.45% NaCl, LR, Ringer's, give over 6-10 min into Y-site or central line, flush line
• Hyaluronidase 150 units/ml in 1 ml NaCl, warm compress for extravasation for vesicant activity treatment

CONT IV INF route
• 40 mg/m² q3wk after an IV bol of 8 mg/m²; may be given in combination with DOXOrubicin, fluorouracil, cisplatin

Y-site compatibilities: Amikacin, aztreonam, bleomycin, bumetanide, buprenorphine, butorphanol, calcium gluconate, carboplatin, carmustine, cefotaxime, ceftazidime, ceftizoxime, chlorproMAZINE, cimetidine, cisplatin, clindamycin, cyclophosphamide, cytarabine, dacarbazine, dactinomycin, DAUNOrubicin, dexamethasone, diphenhydrAMINE, DOXOrubicin, DOXOrubicin liposome, doxycycline, droperidol, enalaprilat, etoposide, famotidine, filgrastim, floxuridine, fluconazole, fludarabine, gallium, gentamicin, granisetron, haloperidol, heparin, hydrocortisone, hydromorphone, hydrOXYzine, idarubicin, ifosfamide, imipenem-cilastatin, lorazepam, mannitol, mechlorethamine, melphalan, meperidine, mesna, methotrexate, metoclopramide, metronidazole, minocycline, mitoxantrone, morphine, nalbuphine, netilmicin, ondansetron, plicamycin, streptozocin, teniposide, ticarcillin, ticarcillin/clavulanate, tobramycin, vancomycin, vinBLAStine, vinCRIStine, zidovudine

Perform/provide:
• Liquid diet: cola, Jell-O; dry toast or crackers if patient not nauseated or vomiting
• Brushing of teeth bid-tid with soft brush or cotton-tipped applicators for stomatitis; unwaxed dental floss
• Nutritious diet with iron, vitamin supplements; avoid herbals

Evaluate:
• Therapeutic response: decreased tumor size, spread of malignancy

Teach patient/family:
• To report change in gait or numbness in extremities, continuing constipation; may indicate neurotoxicity
• To report any complaints or side effects to nurse or prescriber
• To examine mouth daily for bleeding, white spots, ulcerations; notify prescriber
• To avoid crowds, people with infections, vaccinations, OTC products
• To use effective contraception during and for ≥2 mo after product is discontinued; avoid breastfeeding
• That hair may be lost; hair will grow back, but different texture, color

vitamin A (℞, OTC)

Aquasol A, Del-Vi-A, Vitamin A
Func. class.: Vitamin, fat soluble
Chem. class.: Retinol

Action: Needed for normal bone, tooth development, visual dark adaptation, skin disease, mucosa tissue repair, assists in production of adrenal steroids, cholesterol, RNA
Uses: Vit A deficiency

DOSAGE AND ROUTES

• *Adult and child >8 yr:* **PO** 100,000-500,000 international units/day × 3 days, then 50,000/day × 2 wk; dose based on severity of deficiency; maintenance 10,000-20,000 international units for 2 mo
• *Child 1-8 yr:* **IM** 5000-15,000 international units/day × 10 days
• *Infant <1 yr:* **IM** 5000-15,000 international units × 10 days

Maintenance
• *Child 4-8 yr:* **IM** 15,000 international units/day × 2 mo
• *Child <4 yr:* **IM** 10,000 international units/day × 2 mo

Available forms: Caps 10,000, 25,000, 50,000 international units; drops 5000 international units; inj 50,000 international units/ml; tabs 10,000, 25,000, 50,000 international units

SIDE EFFECTS

CNS: Headache, **increased intracranial pressure, intracranial hypertension,** lethargy, malaise
EENT: Gingivitis, papilledema, exophthalmos, inflammation of tongue and lips
GI: Nausea, vomiting, anorexia, abdominal pain, **jaundice**
INTEG: Drying of skin, pruritus, increased pigmentation, night sweats, alopecia
META: Hypomenorrhea, hypercalcemia
MS: Arthralgia, retarded growth, hard areas on bone

Contraindications: Pregnancy (X), hypersensitivity to vit A, malabsorption syndrome, hypervitaminosis A, parenteral, IV administration

Precautions: Pregnancy (C) (PO), breastfeeding, impaired renal function, children, hepatic disease, infants, alcoholism, hepatitis

PHARMACOKINETICS

Stored in liver, kidneys, fat; excreted (metabolites) in urine, feces

INTERACTIONS

Increase: levels of vit A—corticosteroids, oral contraceptives
Decrease: absorption of vit A—mineral oil, cholestyramine, colestipol

Drug/Lab Test
False increase: bilirubin, serum cholesterol

NURSING CONSIDERATIONS

Assess:
- Nutritional status: yellow and dark green vegetables, yellow/orange fruits, vit A–fortified foods, liver, egg yolks
- Vit A deficiency: decreased growth; night blindness; dry, brittle nails; hair loss; urinary stones; increased infection; hyperkeratosis of skin; drying of cornea

Administer:

PO route
- With food (PO) for better absorption
- Do not administer IV because of risk of anaphylactic shock; IM only
- Oral preparations are not indicated for vit A deficiency in those with malabsorption syndrome

IM route
- Give deep in large muscle mass; do not use deltoid muscle for administration of >1 ml

Perform/provide:
- Storage in tight, light-resistant container

Evaluate:
- Therapeutic response: increased growth rate, weight; absence of dry skin and mucous membranes, night blindness

Teach patient/family:
- That if dose is missed, it should be omitted
- That ophthalmic exams may be required periodically throughout therapy
- Not to use mineral oil while taking this product
- To notify prescriber of nausea, vomiting, lip cracking, loss of hair, headache
- Not to take more than the prescribed amount

Treatment of overdose: Discontinue product

vitamin E (OTC)

Amino-Opti-E, Aquasol E, Daltose ♣, E-Complex-600, E-Ferol, E-Vitamin Succinate, E-200 I.U. Softgels, Gordo-Vite E, Tocopherol, Vita-Plus E Softgels, Vitec
Func. class.: Vit E
Chem. class.: Fat soluble

Action: Needed for digestion and metabolism of polyunsaturated fats, decreases platelet aggregation, decreases blood clot formation, promotes normal growth and development of muscle tissue, prostaglandin synthesis

Uses: Vit E deficiency, impaired fat absorption, hemolytic anemia in premature neonates, prevention of retrolental fibroplasia, sickle cell anemia, supplement in malabsorption syndrome

DOSAGE AND ROUTES

Deficiency

• *Adult:* **PO** 60-75 international units/day

• *Child:* **PO** 1 international units/kg (malabsorption)

Prevention of deficiency

• *Adult:* **PO** 30 international units/day; **TOP** apply to affected areas

• *Infant:* **PO** 5 international units/day

Available forms: Caps 100, 200, 400, 500, 600, 1000 international units; tabs 100, 200, 400 international units; drops 50 mg/ml; chew tabs 400 units; ointment; cream; lotion; oil

SIDE EFFECTS

CNS: Headache, fatigue
CV: Increased risk of thrombophlebitis
EENT: Blurred vision
GI: Nausea, cramps, diarrhea
GU: Gonadal dysfunction
INTEG: Sterile abscess, contact dermatitis
META: Altered metabolism of hormones (thyroid, pituitary, adrenal), altered immunity
MS: Weakness

Contraindications: IV use in infants

Precautions: Pregnancy (A), anemia, breastfeeding, hypoprothrombinemia

PHARMACOKINETICS

PO: Metabolized in liver, excreted in bile

INTERACTIONS

Increase: action of oral anticoagulants

Decrease: absorption—cholestyramine, colestipol, mineral oil, sucralfate

NURSING CONSIDERATIONS

Assess:

• Nutritional status: wheat germ; dark green, leafy vegetables; nuts; eggs; liver; vegetable oils; dairy products; cereals

Administer:

PO route

• Administer with or after meals
• Chew chewable tabs well
• Sol may be dropped in mouth or mixed with food

Topical route

• To moisturize dry skin

Perform/provide:

• Storage in tight, light-resistant container

Evaluate:

• Therapeutic response: absence of hemolytic anemia, adequate vit E levels, improvement in skin lesions, decreased edema

Teach patient/family:

• The necessary foods in diet
• To omit if dose is missed
• To avoid vitamin supplements unless directed by prescriber

voriconazole (℞)

(vohr-i-kahn′a-zol)
Vfend
Func. class.: Antifungal, systemic
Chem. class.: Triazole derivative

Action: Inhibits fungal CYP 450-mediation demethylation, needed for biosynthesis

Uses: Invasive aspergillosis, serious fungal infections (*Candida* sp., *Scedosporium apiospermum, Fusarium* sp., *Monosporium, Apiospermum*)

Unlabeled uses: *Acremonium sp., Blastomyces dermatitidis, Coccidioides immitis, Cryptococcus neoformans,* febrile neutropenia, fungal keratitis, *Histoplasma capsulatum,* oropharyngeal candidiasis, *Rhodotorula sp., Scedosporium sp.,* cutaneous aspergillosis, candidemia (premature neonates), fungal infections in children ≥12 yr

DOSAGE AND ROUTES

• *Adult/geriatric/child ≥12 yr:* **PO** Give 1 hr before or after meals; ≥40 kg, loading dose 400 mg q12hr on day 1, then 200 mg q12hr; <40 kg, loading dose 200 mg q12hr on day 1, then 100 mg q12hr

• *Adult/geriatric/child ≥12 yr:* **IV INF** Loading dose 6 mg/kg q12hr × 2 dose, then 4 mg/kg q12hr; may switch to oral dosing

CNS blastomycosis/blastomycosis meningitis (unlabeled)
• *Adult:* **PO** 200-400 mg bid × at least 12 mo and until resolution of CSF abnormalities

Renal dose
• *Adult:* **PO** CCr <50 ml/min; use orally only

Hepatic dose
• *Adult:* **PO** 6 mg/kg q12hr × 2 doses, then 2 mg/kg q12hr or 100 mg q12hr if >40 kg; 50 mg q12hr if <40 kg

Available forms: Tabs 50, 200 mg; powder for inj, lyophilized 200 mg voriconazole, powder for oral susp 45 g (40 mg/ml after reconstitution)

SIDE EFFECTS

CNS: *Headache,* paresthesias, peripheral neuropathy, hallucinations, psychosis, EPS, depression, Guillain-Barré syndrome, insomnia, suicidal ideation, dizziness

CV: **Tachycardia,** hypo/hypertension, vasodilation, **atrial arrhythmias, atrial fibrillation, AV block, bradycardia, CHF, MI, QT prolongation, torsade de pointes**

EENT: Blurred vision, eye hemorrhage

GI: *Nausea, vomiting, anorexia,* diarrhea, cramps, **hemorrhagic gastroenteritis, acute hepatic failure, hepatitis, intestinal perforation, pancreatitis**

GU: *Hypokalemia,* azotemia, **renal tubular necrosis, permanent renal impairment, anuria, oliguria**

HEMA: Anemia, **eosinophilia,** hypomagnesemia, **thrombocytopenia, leukopenia, pancytopenia**

INTEG: *Burning, irritation,* pain, necrosis at inj site with extravasation, dermatitis, rash, photosensitivity

MISC: Respiratory disorder

SYST: **Stevens-Johnson syndrome, toxic epidermal necrolysis, sepsis**

Contraindications: Pregnancy (D), breastfeeding, children, hypersensitivity, severe bone marrow depression, severe hepatic disease

Precautions: Renal disease (IV)

PHARMACOKINETICS

By CYP3A4, CYP2C9 enzymes, protein binding 58%; max serum conc 1-2 hr after dosing; eliminated via hepatic metabolism

INTERACTIONS

Increase: effects of benzodiazepines, calcium channel blockers, cycloSPORINE, ergots, HMG-CoA reductase inhibitors, pimozide, quinidine, prednisoLONE, sirolimus, sulfonylureas, tacrolimus, vinca alkaloids, warfarin, rifabutin, proton pump inhibitors, NNRTIs, protease inhibitors, phenytoin

Increase: nephrotoxicity—other nephrotoxic antibiotics (aminoglycosides, cisplatin, vancomycin, cycloSPORINE, polymyxin B)

Increase: hypokalemia—corticosteroids, digoxin, skeletal muscle relaxants, thiazides

Increase: QT prolongation—other drugs that prolong QT

Drug/Herb
• Do not use with St. John's wort

Increase: possibility of nephrotoxicity—gossypol

Drug/Food
• Avoid use with high-fat meals

NURSING CONSIDERATIONS

Assess:
• VS q15-30min during first infusion; note changes in pulse, B/P
• I&O ratio; watch for decreasing urinary output, change in specific gravity; discontinue product to prevent permanent damage to renal tubules
• Blood studies: CBC, K, Na, Ca, Mg q2wk, BUN, creatinine weekly
• Weight weekly; if weight increases over 2 lb/wk, edema is present; renal damage should be considered
▲ For renal toxicity: increasing BUN, serum creatinine; if BUN is >40 mg/dl or if serum creatinine >3 mg/dl, product may be discontinued or dosage reduced
▲ For hepatotoxicity: increasing AST, ALT, alk phos, bilirubin

• For allergic reaction: dermatitis, rash; product should be discontinued, antihistamines (mild reaction) or epinephrine (severe reaction) administered
• For hypokalemia: anorexia, drowsiness, weakness, decreased reflexes, dizziness, increased urinary output, increased thirst, paresthesias
• For ototoxicity: tinnitus (ringing, roaring in ears), vertigo, loss of hearing (rare); visual disturbance

Administer:

PO route

• Oral susp: tap bottle; add 46 ml of water to bottle; shake well; remove cap; push bottle adaptor into neck of bottle; replace cap; write expiration date (14 days); shake well before each use; administer using only oral dispenser supplied
• 1 hr before or after meals

IV route

• Product only after C&S confirms organism, product needed to treat condition; make sure product is used in life-threatening infections
• Reconstitute powder with 19 ml water for inj to 10 mg/ml, shake until dissolved; infuse over 1-2 hr at a conc of 5 mg/ml or less; do not admix with other products, 4.2% sodium bicarbonate inf
• Store at room temperature (powder, tabs)

Evaluate:

• Therapeutic response: decreased fever, malaise, rash, negative C&S for infecting organism

Teach patient/family:

• That long-term therapy may be needed to clear infection (2 wk-3 mo depending on type of infection)
• To notify prescriber of bleeding, bruising, or soft tissue swelling
• Take 1 hr before or after meal
• Do not drive at night because of vision changes
• Avoid strong, direct sunlight
• Women of childbearing age should use effective contraceptive

⚠ High Alert

warfarin (℞)

(war′far-in)

Coumadin, Jantoven, warfarin sodium, Warfilone ✤

Func. class.: Anticoagulant

Do not confuse:

Coumadin/Cardura/Compazine

Action: Interferes with blood clotting by indirect means; depresses hepatic synthesis of vit K–dependent coagulation factors (II, VII, IX, X)

Uses: Antiphospholipid antibody syndrome, arterial thromboembolism prophylaxis, DVT, MI prophylaxis, post MI, stroke prophylaxis, thrombosis prophylaxis

Unlabeled uses: Angina, mural thrombosis, unstable angina

DOSAGE AND ROUTES

• *Adult:* **PO/IV** 2.5-10 mg/day × 3 days, then titrated to INR
• *Geriatric:* **PO/IV** 2-10 mg/day
• *Child:* **PO/IV** 0.2 mg/kg/day titrated to INR

Available forms: Tabs 1, 2, 2.5, 3, 4, 5, 6, 7.5, 10 mg; inj 5.4 mg powder for inj

SIDE EFFECTS

CNS: Fever, dizziness, fatigue, headache, lethargy

CV: Angina, chest pain, edema, hypotension, syncope

GI: Diarrhea, nausea, vomiting, anorexia, stomatitis, cramps, **hepatitis,** cholestatic jaundice

GU: **Hematuria**

HEMA: **Hemorrhage, agranulocytosis, leukopenia, eosinophilia,** anemia, ecchymosis, petechiae

INTEG: Rash, dermatitis, urticaria, alopecia, pruritus

MISC: Epistaxis, hemoptysis, mouth ulcers, taste disturbances, priapism, dyspnea

MS: Bone fractures

SYST: **Anaphylaxis,** coma, cholesterol, microembolism, **exfoliative dermatitis, purple toe syndrome**

Contraindications: Pregnancy (X), breastfeeding, hypersensitivity, hemophilia, leukemia with bleeding, peptic ulcer disease, thrombocytopenic purpura, hepatic disease (severe), malignant hypertension, subacute bacterial endocarditis, acute nephritis, blood dyscrasias, eclampsia, preeclampsia, hemorrhagic tendencies; surgery of CNS, eye; traumatic surgery with large open surface, bleeding tendencies of GI/GU/respiratory, stroke, aneurysms, pericardial effusion, spinal puncture, major regional/lumbar block anesthesia

Black Box Warning: Bleeding

Precautions: Geriatric patients, alcoholism, CHF, debilitated patients, trauma, indwelling catheters, severe hypertension, active infections, protein C deficiency, polycythemia vera, vasculitis, severe diabetes

PHARMACOKINETICS

PO: Onset 12-24 hr, peak 1½-4 days, duration 3-5 days, effective half-life 20-60 hr; metabolized in liver, excreted in urine/feces (active/inactive metabolites), crosses placenta, 99% bound to plasma proteins

INTERACTIONS

Increase: warfarin action—allopurinol, amiodarone, chloral hydrate, chloramphenicol, cimetidine, clofibrate, cotrimoxazole, COX-2 selective inhibitors, dextrothyroxine, diflunisal, disulfiram, erythromycin, ethacrynic acids, furosemide, glucagon, heparin, HMG-CoA reductase inhibitors, indomethacin, isoniazid, mefenamic acid, metronidazole, mifepristone, NSAIDs, oxyphenbutazones, penicillins, phenylbutazone, quinidine, quinolone antiinfectives, RU-486, salicylates, sulfinpyrazone, sulfonamides, sulindac, SSRIs, steroids, thrombolytic agents, thyroid, tricyclics

Increase: toxicity—oral sulfonylureas, phenytoin

Decrease: warfarin action—aprepitant, azathioprine, barbiturates, bile acid sequestrants, bosentan, carbamazepine, dicloxacillin, estrogens, ethchlorvynol, factor IX/VIIa, griseofulvin, nafcillin, oral contraceptives, phenytoin, rifampin, sucralfate, sulfasalazine, thyroid, vit K, vit K foods

Drug/Herb

Increase: risk of bleeding—agrimony, angelica, anise, basil, bay, bilberry, black currant, black haw, bogbean, bromelain, buchu, cat's claw, chamomile, chondroitin, cinchona bark, cranberry, danshen, devil's claw, dong quai, evening primrose, fenugreek, feverfew, garlic, ginger, ginkgo, ginseng, horse chestnut, Irish moss, kava, kelp, kelpware, khella, licorice, lovage, lungwort, meadowsweet, melatonin, motherwort, mugwort, nettle, papaya, parsley (large amts), pau d'arco, pineapple, poplar, prickly ash, red clover, red yeast rice, safflower, saw palmetto, skullcap, tonka bean, turmeric, wintergreen, yarrow

Decrease: anticoagulant effect—alfalfa, coenzyme Q10, flax, glucomannan, goldenseal, guar gum, St. John's wort, hypericum perforatum

Drug/Lab Test

Increase: T_3 uptake, LFTs

Decrease: uric acid

NURSING CONSIDERATIONS

Assess:

- Blood studies (Hct, platelets, occult blood in stools) q3mo
- INR: In hospital daily after 2nd or 3rd dose; once in therapeutic range for 2 consecutive days, monitor 2-3× wk for 1-2 wk, then less frequently depending on stability of INR results; *Outpatient:* monitor every few days until stable dose, then periodically thereafter depending on stability of INR results

⚠ Bleeding gums, petechiae, ecchymosis, black tarry stools, hematuria; fatal hemorrhage can occur

⚠ Fever, skin rash, urticaria

Administer:

- At same time each day to maintain steady blood levels
- Tabs whole or crushed
- Avoiding all IM inj that may cause bleeding

IV route

- Reconstitute with 2.7 ml of sterile water for inj; do not use solution that is discolored or has particulates
- Give over 1-2 min into peripheral vein

Y-site compatibilities: Amikacin, cefazolin, ceftriaxone, DOPamine, heparin, lidocaine, morphine, nitroglycerin, potassium chloride, ranitidine

Perform/provide:

- Storage in tight container

Evaluate:

- Therapeutic response: decrease of deep vein thrombosis

Teach patient/family:

- To avoid OTC preparations that may cause serious product interactions unless directed by prescriber
- To use soft-bristle toothbrush to avoid bleeding gums, and to use electric razor
- To carry emergency ID identifying product taken
- The importance of compliance
- To report any signs of bleeding: gums, under skin, urine, stools
- To avoid hazardous activities (football, hockey, skiing), dangerous work
- The importance of avoiding unusual changes in vitamin intake, diet, or lifestyle
- To inform dentists and other physicians of anticoagulant intake

Treatment of overdose: Administer vit K

xylometazoline nasal agent

See Appendix B

zafirlukast (℞)

(za-feer′loo-cast)

Accolate

Func. class.: Bronchodilator

Chem. class.: Leukotriene receptor antagonist

Action: Antagonizes the contractile action of leukotrienes (LTC_4, LTD_4, LTE_4) in airway smooth muscle; inhibits bronchoconstriction caused by antigens

Uses: Prophylaxis and chronic treatment of asthma in adults/children >5 yr

Unlabeled uses: Chronic urticaria

DOSAGE AND ROUTES

- *Adult and child ≥12 yr:* **PO** 20 mg bid, take 1 hr before or 2 hr after meals
- *Child 5-11 yr:* **PO** 10 mg bid

Available forms: Tabs 10, 20 mg

SIDE EFFECTS

CNS: Headache, dizziness, **suicidal ideation,** insomnia, fever

GI: Nausea, diarrhea, abdominal pain, vomiting, dyspepsia, **hepatic failure, hepatitis**

HEMA: **Agranulocytosis**

OTHER: Infections, pain, asthenia, myalgia, fever, increased ALT, urticaria, rash, **angioedema**

Contraindications: Hypersensitivity

Precautions: Pregnancy (B), breastfeeding, children, geriatric patients, hepatic disease

PHARMACOKINETICS

Rapidly absorbed, peak 3 hr, 99% protein binding (albumin), extensively metabolized, inhibits CYP4502C9 and 3A4 enzyme systems; excreted in feces, clearance is reduced in the geriatric patient, hepatic impairment, half-life 10 hr

INTERACTIONS

Increase: plasma levels of zafirlukast—aspirin

Increase: PT—warfarin

Decrease: plasma levels of zafirlukast—erythromycin, theophylline

Drug/Herb

Increase: effect—green tea (large amounts), guarana

Drug/Food

Decrease: bioavailability

NURSING CONSIDERATIONS

Assess:

⚠ Adult patients carefully for symptoms of Churg-Strauss syndrome (rare), including eosinophilia, vasculitic rash, worsening pulmonary symptoms, cardiac complications, and/or neuropathy

- Respiratory rate, rhythm, depth; auscultate lung fields bilaterally; notify prescriber of abnormalities

Administer:

- 1 hr before or 2 hr after meals; absorption may be decreased if given with food
- With water if GI upset occurs

Evaluate:

- Therapeutic response: ability to breathe more easily

Teach patient/family:

- To check OTC medications, current prescription medications, which will increase stimulation
- To avoid hazardous activities; dizziness may occur
- That if GI upset occurs, to take product with 8 oz water; avoid food if possible, absorption may be decreased
- To notify prescriber of nausea, vomiting, diarrhea, abdominal pain, fatigue, jaundice, anorexia, flulike symptoms (hepatic dysfunction)
- Not to use for acute asthma episodes
- Not to take if breastfeeding
- To take even if symptom free

zaleplon (℞)

(zal'eh-plon)

Sonata

Func. class.: Sedative/hypnotic, nonbarbiturate

Chem. class.: Pyrazolopyrimidine

Controlled Substance Schedule IV

Action: Binds selectively to omega-1 receptor of the $GABA_A$ receptor complex; results are sedation, hypnosis, skeletal muscle relaxation, anticonvulsant activity, anxiolytic action

Uses: Insomnia

DOSAGE AND ROUTES

- *Adult:* **PO** 10 mg at bedtime; may increase dose to 20 mg at bedtime if needed; 5 mg may be used in low-weight persons
- *Geriatric:* **PO** 5 mg at bedtime; may increase if needed

Available forms: Caps 5, 10 mg

SIDE EFFECTS

CNS: Lethargy, drowsiness, daytime sedation, dizziness, confusion, anxiety, amnesia, depersonalization, hallucinations, hyperesthesia, paresthesia, somnolence, tremor, vertigo, complex sleep related reactions: sleep driving, sleep eating

EENT: Vision change, ear/eye pain, hyperacusis, parosmia

GI: Nausea, abdominal pain, constipation, anorexia, colitis, dyspepsia, dry mouth

MISC: Asthenia, fever, headache, myalgia, dysmenorrhea

SYST: **Severe allergic reactions**

Contraindications: Hypersensitivity, severe hepatic disease

Precautions: Pregnancy (C), breastfeeding, children <15 yr, geriatric patients, respiratory/renal/hepatic disease, psychosis, angioedema, depression, sleep-related behaviors (sleep walking)

PHARMACOKINETICS

Rapid onset, metabolized by liver extensively, excreted by kidneys (inactive metabolites), half-life 1 hr

INTERACTIONS

Increase: effects of zaleplon—cimetidine
Decrease: effect of zaleplon—rifampin
Increase and decrease: zaleplon levels—CYP3A4 inhibitors/inducers

Drug/Herb

Increase: CNS depression—catnip, chamomile, clary, cowslip, hops, kava, lavender, mistletoe, nettle, pokeweed, poppy, Queen Anne's lace, senega, skullcap, valerian
Increase: hypotension—black cohosh

Drug/Food

- Prolonged absorption, sleep onset reduced: high-fat/heavy meal

NURSING CONSIDERATIONS

Assess:

- Mental status: mood, sensorium, affect, memory (long, short), excessive sedation, impaired coordination
- Type of sleep problem: falling asleep, staying asleep

Administer:

- After removal of cigarettes to prevent fires
- After trying conservative measures for insomnia
- Immediately before bedtime for sleeplessness
- On empty stomach for fast onset
- Avoid use with CNS depressants

Perform/provide:

- Assistance with ambulation after receiving dose
- Safety measure: night-light, call bell within easy reach
- Checking to see if PO medication has been swallowed
- Storage in tight container in cool environment

Evaluate:

- Therapeutic response: ability to sleep at night, decreased amount of early morning awakening

Teach patient/family:

- To avoid driving or other activities requiring alertness until product is stabilized
- To avoid alcohol ingestion
- Alternative measures to improve sleep: reading, exercise several hours before bedtime, warm bath, warm milk, TV, self-hypnosis, deep breathing
- That product may cause memory problems, dependence (if used for longer periods of time), changes in behavior/thinking, complex sleep-related behaviors (sleep eating/driving)
- That product is for short-term use only
- To take immediately before going to bed
- Not to ingest a high-fat/heavy meal before taking

zanamivir (℞)

(zan'ah-mih-veer)
Relenza
Func. class.: Antiviral
Chem. class.: Neuramidase inhibitor

Action: Inhibits neuramidase enzyme needed for influenza virus replication
Uses: Treatment of influenza types A and B for those that have been symptomatic for no more than 2 days
Unlabeled uses: Prophylaxis against influenza and biinfections; swine flu (H1N1)

DOSAGE AND ROUTES

- *Adult and child >7 yr:* **INH** 2 inhalations (two 5 mg blisters) q12hr × 5 days, on the 1st day 2 doses should be taken with at least 2 hr between doses

H1N1 (swine flu) (unlabeled)

- *Adult/adolescent/child ≥7 yr:* **INH** 2 bid × 5 days

Available forms: Blisters of powder for inhalation: 5 mg

SIDE EFFECTS

CNS: Headache, dizziness, **seizures,** fatigue; self-injury, delirium (child)
EENT: Ear, nose, throat infections

Z

GI: Nausea, vomiting, diarrhea
RESP: Nasal symptoms, cough, sinusitis, bronchitis, **bronchospasm**
SYST: **Angioedema**
Contraindications: Hypersensitivity
Precautions: Pregnancy (C), breastfeeding, children <7 yr, geriatric patients, respiratory disease, angioedema, milk protein hypersensitivity, Reye's syndrome

PHARMACOKINETICS

Half-life 2½-5 hr, not metabolized, excreted in urine unchanged

INTERACTIONS

• May decrease intranasal influenzae vaccine; separate by ≥48 hr, do not restart antiviral products for ≥2 wk

NURSING CONSIDERATIONS

Assess:
• Bowel pattern before, during treatment
• Skin eruptions, photosensitivity after administration of product
• Respiratory status: rate, character, wheezing, tightness in chest
• Allergies before initiation of treatment, reaction of each medication
• Signs of infection
Administer:
• Within 2 days of symptoms of influenza; continue for 5 days
• Give patient "Patient's Instruction for Use" and review all points before using delivery system
Perform/provide:
• Storage in tight, dry container
Evaluate:
• Therapeutic response: absence of fever, malaise, cough, dyspnea in infection
Teach patient/family:
• That this product does not reduce transmission risk of influenza to others
• Patients with asthma or COPD to carry a fast-acting inhaled bronchodilator since bronchospasm may occur; to use scheduled inhaled bronchodilators before using this product
• To avoid hazardous activities if dizziness occurs
• To take product exactly as prescribed

zidovudine (℞)
(zye-doe'-vue-deen)
Apo-Zidovudine ♣, Azidothymidine, AZT, Novo-AZT ♣, Retrovir
Func. class.: Antiretroviral
Chem. class.: Nucleoside reverse transcriptase inhibitor (NRTI)

Action: Inhibits replication of HIV-1 virus by incorporating into cellular DNA by viral reverse transcriptase, thereby terminating the cellular DNA chain
Uses: Used in combination with other antiretrovirals for HIV-1 infection, human T-lymphotropic virus type I (HILV-I)
Unlabeled uses: Epstein Barr, hepatitis B, T-cell leukemia/lymphoma, thrombocytopenia

DOSAGE AND ROUTES

• *Adult:* **PO** 600 mg/day in divided doses, either 200 mg tid or 300 mg bid in combination with other antiretrovirals; **IV** 1-2 mg/kg q4hr, initiate **PO** as soon as possible up to 1000 mg
• *Child 6 wk-12 yr:* **PO** 160 mg/m^2 q8hr (480 mg/m^2/day, max 200 mg q8hr) in combination with other antiretrovirals; **IV** same as adult
• *Neonate:* **PO** 2-3 mg/kg/dose q6hr; **IV** 1.5 mg/kg infused over 30 min q6hr
Treatment of HIV in combination with other antiretrovirals
• *Adult/adolescent/child ≥30 kg:* **PO** 300 mg bid or 200 mg tid
• *Neonate and infant <6 wk (unlabeled):* **PO** 2 mg/kg q6hr
• *Premature neonate (unlabeled):* **PO** 2 mg/kg q12hr, increase to 2 mg/kg q8hr at 2 wk for neonates ≥30 wk gestation or at 4 wk for neonates <30 wk gestation
Perinatal transmission prophylaxis
• *Full term neonate:* **PO** 2 mg/kg or **IV** 1.5 mg/kg q6h starting 12 hr after birth, continue up to 6 wk of age
• *Preterm neonate:* **PO** 2 mg/kg or **IV** 1.5 mg/kg q12hr; if >30 wk gestation at birth, advance to q8hr at 2 wk of age; if

<30 wk gestation at birth, advance to q8hr at 4 wk of age

Prevention of maternal-fetal HIV transmission

• *Neonatal:* **PO** 2 mg/kg/dose q6hr × 6 wk beginning 8-12 hr after birth; **IV** 1.5 mg/kg/dose over 30 min q6hr until able to take **PO**

• *Maternal (>14 wk gestation):* **PO** 100 mg 5×/day until start of labor, then during labor/delivery **IV** 2 mg/kg over 1 hr followed by **IV INF** 1 mg/kg/hr until umbilical cord clamped

Symptomatic HIV infection

• *Adult:* **PO** 100 mg q4hr; **IV** 1-2 mg/kg over 1 hr q4hr

• *Child 3 mo to 12 yr:* **PO** 90-180 mg/m^2 q6hr (max 200 mg q6hr); **IV** 1-2 mg/kg over 1 hr q4hr

Prevention of HIV following needlestick

• *Adult:* **PO** 200 mg tid plus lamivudine 150 mg bid, plus a protease inhibitor for high-risk exposure; begin within 2 hr of exposure

Thrombocytopenia associated with HIV infection (unlabeled)

• *Adult:* **PO** 500 mg qid × 2 wk, then 250 mg qid × 6 wk

T-cell leukemia/lymphoma in combination with interferon-alfa in patients infected with T-lymphotropic virus type I (HTLV-I) (unlabeled)

• *Adult:* **PO** 200 mg q4hr while awake, continue for ≥4 wk after remission, adjust for hematologic toxicity

Available forms: Caps 100; tabs 300 mg; inj 200 mg/20 ml; oral syr 50 mg/5 ml

SIDE EFFECTS

CNS: Fever, headache, malaise, diaphoresis, *dizziness, insomnia,* paresthesia, somnolence, chills, tremor, twitching, anxiety, confusion, depression, lability, vertigo, loss of mental acuity, **seizures,** malaise

EENT: Taste change, hearing loss, photophobia

GI: Nausea, vomiting, diarrhea, anorexia, cramps, *dyspepsia, constipation,* dysphagia, *flatulence,* rectal bleeding, mouth ulcer, abdominal pain, hepatomegaly

GU: Dysuria, polyuria, urinary frequency, hesitancy

HEMA: **Granulocytopenia, anemia**

INTEG: Rash, acne, pruritus, urticaria

MS: Myalgia, arthralgia, muscle spasm

RESP: Dyspnea

SYST: **Lactic acidosis**

Contraindications: Hypersensitivity

Precautions: Pregnancy (C), breastfeeding, children, granulocyte count <1000/mm^3 or Hgb <9.5 g/dl, severe renal disease, obesity

Black Box Warning: Impaired hepatic function, anemia, lactic acidosis, myopathy, neutropenia

PHARMACOKINETICS

PO: Rapidly absorbed from GI tract, peak ½-1½ hr, metabolized in liver (inactive metabolites), excreted by kidneys, protein binding 38%, terminal half-life ½-3 hr

INTERACTIONS

• Toxicity: probenecid, fluconazole

Increase: bone marrow depression—antineoplastics, radiation, ganciclovir, valganciclovir, trimethoprim-sulfamethoxazole

Increase: zidovudine level—methadone

NURSING CONSIDERATIONS

Assess:

• Blood counts q2wk; watch for decreasing granulocytes, Hgb; if low, therapy may have to be discontinued and restarted after hematologic recovery; blood transfusions may be required; viral load, CD4 counts, LFTs, plasma HIV RNA, serum creatinine/BUN baseline and throughout

Administer:

• By mouth; capsules should be swallowed whole

• Bid or tid

• Trimethoprim-sulfamethoxazole, pyrimethamine, or acyclovir as ordered to

Z

prevent opportunistic infections; if these products are given, watch for neurotoxicity

IV route

• After diluting each 1 mg/0.25 ml or more D_5W to 4 mg/ml or less; give over 1 hr

Y-site compatibilities: Acyclovir, allopurinol, amifostine, amikacin, amphotericin B, amphotericin B cholesteryl, aztreonam, cefepime, ceftazidime, ceftriaxone, cimetidine, cisatracurium, clindamycin, dexamethasone, DOBUTamine, DOPamine, DOXOrubicin liposome, erythromycin, filgrastim, fluconazole, fludarabine, gentamicin, granisetron, heparin, imipenem/cilastatin, lorazepam, melphalan, metoclopramide, morphine, nafcillin, ondansetron, oxacillin, paclitaxel, pentamidine, phenylephrine, piperacillin, piperacillin/tazobactam, potassium chloride, ranitidine, remifentanil, sargramostim, teniposide, thiotepa, tobramycin, trimethoprim-sulfamethoxazole, trimetrexate, vancomycin, vinorelbine

Perform/provide:

• Storage in cool environment; protect from light

Evaluate:

• Blood dyscrasias (anemia, granulocytopenia): bruising, fatigue, bleeding, poor healing

Teach patient/family:

• That GI complaints and insomnia resolve after 3-4 wk of treatment
• That product is not cure for AIDS but will control symptoms
• To notify prescriber of sore throat, swollen lymph nodes, malaise, fever; other infections may occur
• That patient is still infective, may pass AIDS virus on to others
• That follow-up visits must be continued since serious toxicity may occur; blood counts must be done q2wk
• That product must be taken bid or tid
• That serious product interactions may occur if OTC products are ingested; check with prescriber before taking aspirin, acetaminophen, indomethacin
• That other products may be necessary to prevent other infections
• That product may cause fainting or dizziness

zinc (℞, OTC)

Orazinc, PMS Egozinc ♣, Verazinc, Zinca-Pak, Zincate, Zinc 15, Zinc-220, zinc sulfate

Func. class.: Trace element; nutritional supplement

Action: Needed for adequate healing, bone and joint development (23% zinc)

Uses: Prevention of zinc deficiency, adjunct to vit A therapy

Unlabeled uses: Wound healing

DOSAGE AND ROUTES

Dietary supplement (elemental zinc)

• *Adult/adolescent/pregnant females:* **PO** 11-13 mg/day
• *Adult and lactating females:* **PO** 12-14 mg/day × 12 mo
• *Adult and adolescent males ≥14 yr:* **PO** 11 mg/day
• *Adult females ≥19 yr:* **PO** 8 mg/day
• *Adolescent females ≥14 yr:* **PO** 9 mg/day
• *Child 9-13 yr:* **PO** 8 mg/day
• *Child 4-8 yr:* **PO** 5 mg/day
• *Child 1-3 yr:* **PO** 3 mg/day
• *Infant 7-12 mo:* **PO** 3 mg/day
• *Infant birth to 6 mo:* **PO** 2 mg/day (adequate intake)

Nutritional supplement (IV)

• *Adult:* **IV** 2.5-4 mg/day; may increase by 2 mg/day if needed
• *Child 1-5 yr:* **IV** 50 mcg/kg/day

Wound healing

Adult: **PO** 50 mg tid until healed (elemental zinc)

Available forms: Tabs 66, 110 mg; caps 220 mg; inj 1 mg, 5 mg/ml

SIDE EFFECTS

GI: Nausea, vomiting, cramps, heartburn, ulcer formation

OVERDOSE: Diarrhea, rash, dehydration, restlessness
Precautions: Pregnancy (C) parenteral; breastfeeding, neonates, hypocupremia, neonatal prematurity, renal disease

INTERACTIONS

Decrease: absorption of fluoroquinolones tetracyclines

NURSING CONSIDERATIONS

Assess:
- Zinc levels during treatment

Administer:
- With meals to decrease gastric upset; avoid dairy products

Evaluate:
- Therapeutic response: absence of zinc deficiency

Teach patient/family:
- That element must be taken for 2-3 mo to be effective
- To report immediately nausea, diarrhea, rash, severe vomiting, restlessness, abdominal pain, tarry stools

ziprasidone (℞)

(zi-praz'ih-dohn)
Geodon, Zeldox ♣
Func. class.: Antipsychotic/neuroleptic
Chem. class.: Benzisoxazole derivative

Action: Unknown; may be mediated through both DOPamine type 2 (D_2) and serotonin type 2 ($5\text{-}HT_2$) antagonism
Uses: Schizophrenia, acute agitation, acute psychosis, bipolar disorder, mania, psychotic depression
Unlabeled uses: Tourette's syndrome

DOSAGE AND ROUTES

- *Adult:* **PO** 20 mg bid with food, adjust dosage every 2 days upward to max of 80 mg bid; **IM** 10-20 mg; may give 10 mg q2hr; doses of 20 mg may be given q4hr; max 40 mg/day

Tourette's syndrome (unlabeled)
- *Adolescent and child ≥7 yr:* **PO** 5 mg/day, may increase in divided doses to 20 mg bid

Available forms: Caps 20, 40, 60, 80 mg; inj 20 mg/ml

SIDE EFFECTS

CNS: EPS, pseudoparkinsonism, akathisia, dystonia, tardive dyskinesia; drowsiness, insomnia, agitation, anxiety, headache, **seizures, neuroleptic malignant syndrome,** dizziness, tremor, facial droop
CV: Orthostatic hypotension, **tachycardia, prolonged QT/QTc,** hypertension; **sudden death, heart failure (geriatric patients), torsade de pointes**
EENT: Blurred vision, diplopia
ENDO: Metabolic changes
GI: Nausea, vomiting, *anorexia, constipation,* jaundice, weight gain, diarrhea, dry mouth, abdominal pain
GU: Enuresis, urinary incontinence, gynecomastia, impotence, priapism
RESP: Rhinitis, dyspnea, infection, cough
Contraindications: Breastfeeding, hypersensitivity, acute MI, heart failure, QT prolongation
Precautions: Pregnancy (C), children, geriatric patients, cardiac/renal/hepatic disease, breast cancer, diabetes, seizure disorders, AV block, CNS depression

Black Box Warning: Dementia

PHARMACOKINETICS

PO: Extensively metabolized by liver to a major active metabolite, plasma protein binding 90%, peak 6-8 hr, terminal half-life 7 hr

INTERACTIONS

⚠ ***Increase:*** QT prolongation—class IA/III antidysrhythmics, some phenothiazines, β-agonists, local anesthetics, tricyclics, bepridil, haloperidol, methadone, chloroquine, clarithromycin, droperidol, erythromycin, grepafloxacin, halofantrine, pentamidine, probucol, sparfloxacin, moxifloxacin

Increase: sedation—other CNS depressants, alcohol
Increase: EPS—other antipsychotics, lithium
Increase: ziprasidone excretion—carbamazepine
Increase: ziprasidone level—ketoconazole
Increase: hypotension—antihypertensives

Drug/Herb
Increase: CNS depression—chamomile, hops, kava, skullcap, valerian
Increase: EPS—betel palm, kava
Increase: action—cola tree, hops, nettle, nutmeg

NURSING CONSIDERATIONS

Assess:
• Mental status before initial administration
⚠ Geriatric closely; heart failure, sudden death have occured
• Swallowing of PO medication; check for hoarding or giving of medication to other patients
• I&O ratio; palpate bladder if urinary output is low
• Bilirubin, CBC, LFTs, fasting blood glucose q mo
• Urinalysis before, during prolonged therapy
• Affect, orientation, LOC, reflexes, gait, coordination, sleep pattern disturbances
• B/P standing and lying; also pulse, respirations; take these q4hr during initial treatment; establish baseline before starting treatment; report drops of 30 mm Hg; watch for ECG changes; QT prolongation may occur
• Dizziness, faintness, palpitations, tachycardia on rising, metabolic changes, weight gain
• EPS, including akathisia (inability to sit still, no pattern to movements), tardive dyskinesia (bizarre movements of the jaw, mouth, tongue, extremities), pseudoparkinsonism (rigidity, tremors, pill rolling, shuffling gait)
⚠ For neuroleptic malignant syndrome: hyperthermia, increased CPK, altered mental status, muscle rigidity
• Skin turgor daily
• Constipation, urinary retention daily; if these occur, increase bulk and water in diet

Administer:

PO route
• Reduced dose in geriatric patients
• Anticholinergic agent on order from prescriber, to be used for EPS
• Avoid use with CNS depressants
• With food, increases absorption

IM route
• Add 1.2 ml sterile water for inj to vial; shake vigorously until product is dissolved; do not admix; give only IM

Perform/provide:
• Decreased stimulus by dimming lights, avoiding loud noises
• Supervised ambulation until patient is stabilized on medication; do not involve in strenuous exercise program because fainting is possible; patient should not stand still for a long time
• Increased fluids to prevent constipation
• Sips of water, candy, gum for dry mouth
• Storage in tight, light-resistant container

Evaluate:
• Therapeutic response: decrease in emotional excitement, hallucinations, delusions, paranoia; reorganization of patterns of thought, speech

Teach patient/family:
• That orthostatic hypotension may occur and to rise from sitting or lying position gradually
• To avoid hot tubs, hot showers, tub baths; hypotension may occur
• To avoid abrupt withdrawal of this product; EPS may result; product should be withdrawn slowly
• To avoid OTC preparations (cough, hay fever, cold) unless approved by prescriber, since serious product interactions may occur; avoid use with alcohol; increased drowsiness may occur

• To avoid hazardous activities if drowsy or dizzy
• Compliance with product regimen
• To report impaired vision, tremors, muscle twitching
• In hot weather, that heat stroke may occur; take extra precautions to stay cool

Treatment of overdose: Lavage if orally ingested; provide airway; *do not induce vomiting*

zoledronic acid (℞)

(zoh'leh-drah'nick ass'id)

Reclast, Zometa

Func. class.: Bone-resorption inhibitor

Chem. class.: Bisphosphonate

Action: Potent inhibitor of osteoclastic bone resorption; inhibits osteoclastic activity, inhibits skeletal calcium release caused by stimulating factors released by tumors; reduction of abnormal bone resorption is responsible for therapeutic effect in hypercalcemia; may directly block dissolution of hydroxyapatite bone crystals

Uses: Moderate to severe hypercalcemia associated with malignancy; multiple myeloma; bone metastases from solid tumors (used with antineoplastics); active Paget's disease; osteoporosis, glucocorticoid-induced osteoporosis, osteoporosis prophylaxis in postmenopausal women

DOSAGE AND ROUTES

Hypercalcemia of malignancy

• *Adult:* **IV INF** 4 mg, given as a single infusion over ≥15 min; may re-treat with 4 mg if serum calcium does not return to normal within 1 wk

Multiple myeloma/metastatic bone lesions

• *Adult:* **IV INF** 4 mg, give over 15 min q3-4wk

Osteoporosis

• *Adult:* **IV INF** 5 mg over ≥15 min or more q12mo

Active Paget's disease

• *Adult:* **IV INF** 5 mg over ≥15 min or more

Osteoporosis prophylaxis (Reclast), postmenopausal women

• *Adult:* **IV INF** 5 mg every other year

Osteoporosis prophylaxis (Reclast) when taking systemic glucocorticoids

• *Adult:* **IV** 5 mg qyr

Available forms: (Zometa) sol for inj 4 mg/5 ml; (Reclast) inj 5 mg/100 ml

SIDE EFFECTS

CNS: Dizziness, headache, anxiety, confusion, insomnia, agitation

CV: Hypotension, leg edema, **atrial fibrillation,** chest pain

GI: Abdominal pain, anorexia, constipation, nausea, diarrhea, vomiting, taste change

GU: UTI, possible reduced renal function, **renal damage**

META: Anemia, hypokalemia, hypomagnesemia, hypophosphatemia, hypocalcemia, increased serum creatinine

MISC: Fever, chills, flulike symptoms

MS: Severe bone pain, *arthralgias, myalgias,* osteonecrosis of the jaw

Contraindications: Pregnancy (D), breastfeeding, hypersensitivity to this product or bisphosphonates, hypocalcemia

Precautions: Children, geriatric patients, renal dysfunction, aspirin sensitive asthma, asthmatic patients, acute bronchospasm, anemia, chemotherapy, coagulopathy, dehydration, dental disease, diabetes mellitus, renal disease, electrolyte imbalance, hypertension, hypomagnesemia, hypophosphatemia, hypovolemia, infection, multiple myeloma, phosphate hypersensitivity

PHARMACOKINETICS

Rapidly cleared from circulation and taken up mainly by bones, not metabolized, eliminated primarily by kidneys, approximately 50% is eliminated in urine within 24 hr of administration, max effect 7 days; terminal half-life 167 hr, protein binding 22%

INTERACTIONS

• Hypomagnesemia, hypokalemia: digoxin
• Do not mix with calcium-containing infusion sol such as lactated Ringer's sol
Increase: nephrotoxicity—aminoglycosides, NSAIDs, radiopaque contrast agents
Decrease: effect of zoledronic acid—calcium, vit D
Decrease: serum calcium, aminoglycosides, loop diuretics

NURSING CONSIDERATIONS

Assess:

• Renal tests and Ca, PO_4, Mg, K; creatinine, BUN; if creatinine is elevated hold treatment
• For hypocalcemia: paresthesia, twitching, laryngospasm; Chvostek's, Trousseau's signs
• Dental status; cover with antiinfectives for dental extraction
• For atrial fibrillation

Administer:

• Saline hydration must be performed before administration; urine output should be 2 L/day during treatment, do not overhydrate

IV route

Zometa

• Administer after reconstituting by adding 5 ml of sterile water for inj to each vial, then add to ≥100 ml of sterile 0.9% NaCl, D_5W; run over ≥15 min
• Administer in separate IV line from all other products

Reclast

• No further dilution required
• Infuse over ≥15 min at constant rate; max 5 mg

Perform/provide:

• Sol reconstituted with sterile water may be stored under refrigeration for up to 24 hr
• Acetaminophen before and for 72 hr after to decrease pain

Evaluate:

• Therapeutic response: decreased calcium levels, increased bone density

Teach patient/family:

• To report hypercalcemic relapse: nausea, vomiting, bone pain, thirst
• To continue with dietary recommendations including calcium and vit D; take a multiple vitamin daily, 500 mg of calcium, 400 international units vit D in multiple myeloma
• If nausea/vomiting occur, eat small frequent meals, use lozenges or chewing gum
• If bone pain occurs, notify prescriber to obtain analgesics
• Avoid use in pregnancy
• Continue good oral hygiene

zolmitriptan (℞)

(zole-mih-trip'tan)
Zomig, Zomig-ZMT
Func. class.: Migraine agent, abortive
Chem. class.: $5\text{-HT}_{1B}/5\text{HT}_{1D}$ receptor agonist (triptan)

Action: Binds selectively to the vascular $5\text{-HT}_{1B}/5\text{HT}_{1D}$ receptor subtype, exerts antimigraine effect; causes vasoconstriction in cranial arteries
Uses: Acute treatment of migraine with or without aura

DOSAGE AND ROUTES

• *Adult:* **PO** Start on 2.5 mg or lower (tab may be broken), may repeat after 2 hr, max 10 mg/24 hr; **NASAL** 1 spray in one nostril at onset of migraine, repeat in 2 hr if no relief

Available forms: Tabs 2.5, 5 mg; orally disintegrating tabs 2.5, 5 mg; nasal spray 5 mg

SIDE EFFECTS

CNS: Tingling, hot sensation, burning, feeling of pressure, tightness, numbness, dizziness, sedation
CV: Palpitations, chest pain
GI: Abdominal discomfort, nausea, dry mouth, dyspepsia, dysphagia
MISC: Odd taste (spray)

MS: *Weakness, neck stiffness,* myalgia
RESP: Chest tightness, pressure

Contraindications: Angina pectoris, history of MI, documented silent ischemia, ischemic heart disease, concurrent ergotamine-containing preparations, uncontrolled hypertension, hypersensitivity, basilar or hemiplegic migraine, risk of CV events

Precautions: Pregnancy (C), breastfeeding, children, postmenopausal women, men >40 yr, geriatric patients, risk factors for CAD, hypercholesterolemia, obesity, diabetes, impaired renal/hepatic function

PHARMACOKINETICS

Duration 2-3½ hr; 25% plasma protein binding; half-life 3-3½ hr; metabolized in the liver (metabolite); excreted in urine (60%-80%), feces (20%-40%)

INTERACTIONS

⚠ Extended vasospastic effects: ergot, ergot derivatives

⚠ Do not use within 2 wk of MAOIs

⚠ Weakness, hyperreflexia, incoordination: SSRIs (fluoxetine, fluvoxamine, paroxetine, sertraline)

Increase: half-life of zolmitriptan—cimetidine, oral contraceptives

Increase: zolimitriptan levels—sibutramine

Drug/Herb

- Serotonin syndrome: SAM-e, St. John's wort

Increase: effect—butterbur, feverfew

NURSING CONSIDERATIONS

Assess:

- Tingling, hot sensation, burning, feeling of pressure, numbness, flushing
- For stress level, activity, recreation, coping mechanisms
- Neurologic status: LOC, blurring vision, nausea, vomiting, tingling in extremities preceding headache
- Ingestion of tyramine foods (pickled products, beer, wine, aged cheese), food additives, preservatives, colorings, artificial sweeteners, chocolate, caffeine, which may precipitate these types of headaches
- For serotonin syndrome, if also taking an SSRI
- Kidney function, urine output

Administer:

- Take with fluids as soon as symptoms of migraine occur

Perform/provide:

- Quiet, calm environment with decreased stimulation for noise, bright light, excessive talking

Evaluate:

- Therapeutic response: decrease in frequency, severity of headache

Teach patient/family:

- To report any side effects to prescriber
- To use contraception while taking product
- That product does not prevent or reduce the number of migraines

zolpidem (℞)

(zole'pih-dem)

Ambien, Ambien CR, Edluar, Zolpimist

Func. class.: Sedative-hypnotic
Chem. class.: Nonbenzodiazepine of imidazopyridine class

Controlled Substance Schedule IV

Action: Produces CNS depression at limbic, thalamic, hypothalamic levels of CNS; may be mediated by neurotransmitter γ-aminobutyric acid (GABA); results are sedation, hypnosis, skeletal muscle relaxation, anticonvulsant activity, anxiolytic action

Uses: Insomnia, short-term treatment; insomnia with difficulty of sleep onset/maintenance (ext rel)

DOSAGE AND ROUTES

- *Adult:* **PO** 10 mg at bedtime × 7-10 days only; total max dose 10 mg; **EXT REL** 12.5 mg immediately before bedtime, may be useful for up to 24 wk in people 18-64 yr with primary insomnia; oral spray (zolpimist) 10 mg (2 sprays) immediately before bedtime, max 10 mg/

Z

day; **SL** (Edluar) 10 mg just before bedtime

• *Geriatric:* **PO** 5 mg at bedtime; **EXT REL** 6.25 mg

Available forms: Tabs 5, 10 mg; ext rel tabs 6.25, 12.5 mg; orally disintegrating tabs 5, 10 mg; oral spray 5 mg/spray

SIDE EFFECTS

CNS: Headache, lethargy, drowsiness, daytime sedation, dizziness, confusion, lightheadedness, anxiety, irritability, amnesia, poor coordination, complex sleep related reactions (sleep driving, sleep eating), depression, somnolence, **suicidal ideation,** abnormal thinking/behavioral changes

CV: Chest pain, palpitation

GI: Nausea, vomiting, diarrhea, heartburn, abdominal pain, constipation

HEMA: **Leukopenia, granulocytopenia (rare)**

MISC: Myalgia

SYST: **Severe allergic reactions**

Contraindications: Hypersensitivity to benzodiazepines

Precautions: Pregnancy (C), breastfeeding, children <18 yr, geriatric patients, anemia, renal/hepatic disease, suicidal individuals, drug abuse, psychosis, seizure disorders, angioedema, depression, respiratory disease, sleep apnea, sleep-related behaviors (sleepwalking), myasthenia gravis

PHARMACOKINETICS

PO: Onset up to 1.5 hr, metabolized by liver, excreted by kidneys (inactive metabolites), crosses placenta, excreted in breast milk, half-life 2-3 hr

INTERACTIONS

Increase: action of both products—alcohol, CNS depressants

Increase and decrease: zolpidem levels—CYP3A4 inhibitors/inducers

Drug/Herb

Increase: CNS depression—chamomile, hops, kava, skullcap, valerian

Drug/Lab Test

Increase: ALT, AST, serum bilirubin

Decrease: RAI uptake

False increase: urinary 17-OHCS

NURSING CONSIDERATIONS

Assess:

• Mental status: mood, sensorium, affect, memory (long, short), excessive sedation, impaired coordination

• Blood dyscrasias: fever, sore throat, bruising, rash, jaundice, epistaxis (rare)

• Type of sleep problem: falling asleep, staying asleep

Administer:

• Do not break, crush, or chew ext rel

• After trying conservative measures for insomnia

• ½-1 hr before bedtime (PO); right before retiring (ext rel)

• On empty stomach for fast onset but may be taken with food if GI symptoms occur

• Do not use spray with or after a meal

• Avoid use with CNS depressants; serious CNS depression may result

Perform/provide:

• Assistance with ambulation after receiving dose

• Storage in tight container in cool environment

Evaluate:

• Therapeutic response: ability to sleep at night, decreased amount of early morning awakening if taking product for insomnia

Teach patient/family:

• That dependence is possible after long-term use

• That complex sleep-related behaviors may occur (sleep driving/eating)

• To avoid driving or other activities requiring alertness until product is stabilized

• To avoid alcohol ingestion

• That effects may take 2 nights for benefits to be noticed

• Alternative measures to improve sleep: reading, exercise several hours before bedtime, warm bath, warm milk, TV, self-hypnosis, deep breathing

• That hangover is common in geriatric patients but less common than with barbiturates; rebound insomnia may occur for 1-2 nights after discontinuing product; do not discontinue abruptly, taper
Treatment of overdose: Lavage, activated charcoal; monitor electrolytes, VS

zonisamide (℞)
(zone-is′a-mide)
Zonegran
Func. class.: Anticonvulsant
Chem. class.: Sulfonamides

Action: May act through action at sodium and calcium channels, but exact action is unknown; serotonergic action
Uses: Epilepsy, adjunctive therapy of partial seizures
Unlabeled uses: Bipolar disorder (mania)

DOSAGE AND ROUTES
• *Adult and child >16 yr:* 100 mg/day, may increase after 2 wk to 200 mg/day, may increase q2wk, max dose 400 mg/day
Mania (unlabeled)
• *Adult:* **PO** 100-200 mg/day, max 600 mg/day
Available forms: Caps 25, 50, 100 mg

SIDE EFFECTS
CNS: Dizziness, insomnia, paresthesias, depression, fatigue, headache, confusion, somnolence, agitation, irritability, speech disturbance, **suicidal ideation**
EENT: Diplopia, verbal difficulty, speech abnormalities, taste perversion
GI: Nausea, constipation, anorexia, weight loss, diarrhea, dyspepsia
HEMA: **Aplastic anemia, granulocytopenia** (rare)
INTEG: Rash
SYST: **Stevens-Johnson syndrome**, metabolic acidosis
Contraindications: Hypersensitivity to this product or sulfonamides, psychiatric condition, hepatic failure
Precautions: Pregnancy (C), breastfeeding, children <16 yr, geriatric patients, allergies, renal/hepatic disease

PHARMACOKINETICS
Peak 2-6 hr, half-life 63 hr, metabolized by liver, excreted by kidneys, protein binding 40%

INTERACTIONS
Decrease: half-life of zonisamide—products inducing CYP450 enzymes (carbamazepine, phenytoin, phenobarbital)
Increase: CNS depression—alcohol
Drug/Herb
Increase: effect of this product—St. John's wort
Drug/Food
• Do not use with grapefruit

NURSING CONSIDERATIONS
Assess:
• For seizures: duration, type, intensity precipitating factors
• Renal function: albumin conc, BUN, creatinine; serum bicarbonate baseline and periodically
⚠ Mental status: mood, sensorium, affect, memory (long, short), suicidal thoughts/behaviors
• For rash, hypersensitivity reactions
Evaluate:
• Therapeutic response: decrease in severity of seizures
Teach patient/family:
• Not to discontinue product abruptly; seizures may occur
• To avoid hazardous activities until stabilized on product
• To carry emergency ID stating product use
• To notify prescriber of rash immediately; also, back pain, abdominal pain, blood in urine, increase fluid intake to reduce risk of kidney stones
• To notify prescriber if pregnancy is planned or suspected
• To take adequate fluids, not to use grapefruit

Appendix a

Selected new drugs

abobotulinumtoxinA
See page 80

asenapine
See page 164

canakinumab
See page 230

dexlansoprazole
See page 370

dronedarone
See page 423

eltrombopag
See page 434

everolimus
See page 477

febuxostat
See page 487

fenofibric acid
See page 491

ferumoxytol
See page 498

fibrinogen, concentrate, human
See page 501

⚠ High Alert

fospropofol (℞)
(fos-proe′poe-fol)
Lusedra
Func. class.: General anesthetic

Action: Produces dose-dependent CNS depression by activation of GABA receptor

Uses: Induction or maintenance of anesthesia as part of balanced anesthetic technique; sedation in mechanically ventilated patients

DOSAGE AND ROUTES

Induction/Maintenance

- *Adult <65 (healthy) >90 kg:* 577.5 **IV BOL,** may give supplemental doses up to max of 140 mg, give no more frequently than q4min; 61-89 kg 6.5 mg/kg (max 577.5 mg) **IV BOL** may give supplemental doses up to 1.6 mg/kg/dose (max 140 mg/dose; give no more frequently than q4min); <60 kg 385 mg **IV BOL,** may give supplemental doses up to max 105 mg/dose, give no more frequently than q4min
- *Adult: <65 yr (severe systemic disease) ≥90 kg* 437.5 mg **IV BOL,** give supplemental doses up to max 105 mg/dose, give no more frequently than q4min; 61-89 kg 4.875 mg/kg (max 437.5 mg) give supplemental doses of 75% of stan-

dard dose/up to 1.2 mg/kg/dose (max 105 mg/dose) give no more frequently than q4min; <60 kg 297.5 **IV BOL,** give supplemental doses up to max 70 mg/dose, give no more frequently than q4min • *Geriatric ≥90 kg:* **IV BOL** 437.5, then supplemental doses up to max 105 mg; give no more frequently than q4min; 61-89 kg, **IV BOL** give 75% standard dosing regimen (4.875 mg/kg) give no more frequently than q4min (max 105 mg/dose)

Available forms: Inj 1050 mg/30 ml

SIDE EFFECTS

CNS: Involuntary movement, headache, jerking, fever, dizziness, shivering, tremor, confusion, somnolence, paresthesia, agitation, abnormal dreams, euphoria, fatigue, **increased intracranial pressure, impaired cerebral flow, seizures**

CV: *Bradycardia, hypotension,* hypertension, PVC, PAC, tachycardia, abnormal ECG, ST segment depression, **asystole, bradydysrhythmias**

EENT: Blurred vision, tinnitus, eye pain, strange taste, diplopia

GI: *Nausea, vomiting, abdominal cramping,* dry mouth, swallowing, hypersalivation, **pancreatitis**

GU: Urine retention, green urine, cloudy urine, oliguria

INTEG: *Flushing, phlebitis, hives, burning/stinging at inj site,* rash, pain of extremities

MS: Myalgia

RESP: **Apnea,** *cough, hiccups,* dyspnea, hypoventilation, sneezing, wheezing, tachypnea, hypoxia, respiratory acidosis

Contraindications: Hypersensitivity to product or soybean oil, egg, benzyl alcohol (some products)

Precautions: Pregnancy (B), breastfeeding, children, geriatric patients, respiratory depression, severe respiratory disorders, cardiac dysrhythmias, labor and delivery, renal disease, hyperlipidemia

PHARMACOKINETICS

Onset 15-30 sec, rapid distribution, half-life 1-8 min, terminal half-life .81-.88 hr; 70% excreted in urine; metabolized in liver by conjugation to inactive metabolites, 95%-99% protein binding

INTERACTIONS

• Do not use within 10 days of MAOIs

Increase: CNS depression—alcohol, opioids, sedative/hypnotics, antipsychotics, skeletal muscle relaxants, inhalational anesthetics

Drug/Herb

Increase: fospropofol effect—St. John's wort

NURSING CONSIDERATIONS

Assess:

• Inj site: phlebitis, burning, stinging

• ECG for changes: PVC, PAC, ST segment changes; monitor VS

• CNS changes: movement, jerking, tremors, dizziness, LOC, pupil reaction

• Allergic reactions: hives

• Respiratory dysfunction: respiratory depression, character, rate, rhythm; notify prescriber if respirations are <10/min

Administer:

IV Bolus route

• Visually inspect for particulate matter and discoloration

• Each vial is single patient/single use

• Draw from vial, discard unused portion

• Do not mix with other drugs prior to use

• Give by IV Bolus, in free-flowing peripheral IV line of D_5W, 5% Dextrose/0.2% NaCl, 5% Dextrose/0.45% NaCl D_5LR, LR, 0.45% NaCl, NS, 5% Dextrose/0.45% NaCl/20 mEq KCl, do not mix with other fluids, flush line with NS before and after administration

• No filtration needed

• Only with resuscitative equipment available

• Only by qualified persons trained in anesthesia

Perform/provide:

- Storage at room temperature of unopened vials

Evaluate:

- Therapeutic response: induction of anesthesia

Teach patient/family:

- That this medication will cause dizziness, drowsiness, sedation

Treatment of overdose: Discontinue product; administer vasopressor agents or anticholinergics, artificial ventilation

golimumab
See page 563

hylan G-F 20
See page 588

iloperidone
See page 599

pitavastatin
See page 911

plerixafor (℞)

(pler-ix'a-fore)

Mozobil

Func. class.: Biologic modifier

Chem. class.: Colony-stimulating factor

Action: Competitively inhibits the binding of Stromal-derived factors, allowing hematopoietic stem cells to mobilize into peripheral blood

Uses: For peripheral blood stem cell (PBSC) mobilization for collection and autologous transplant in non-Hodgkin's lymphoma, multiple myeloma; used with a granulocyte colony stimulating factor (G-CSF)

DOSAGE AND ROUTES

- *Adult:* **SUBCUT** 0.24 mg/kg daily about 11 hr prior to initiation of apheresis, give up to 4 consecutive days; give filgrastim 10 mcg/kg; **SUBCUT** daily each AM beginning 4 days prior to the 1st evening dose of plerixafor and on each day of apheresis; give filgrastim before procedure

Available forms: Inj 300 mcg/ml, 480 mcg/1.6 ml, 480 mcg/0.8 ml, 3000 mcg/0.5 ml

SIDE EFFECTS

CNS: Syncope, dizziness, fatigue, headache, insomnia, malaise, paresthesias

GI: Nausea, vomiting, diarrhea, abdominal pain, constipation

HEMA: **Thrombocytopenia,** leukocytosis

INTEG: Rash, skin irritation, pruritus, inj site reaction, erythema, urticaria

MS: Musculoskeletal pain

RESP: Dyspnea, hypoxia

Contraindications: Hypersensitivity, breastfeeding

Precautions: Pregnancy (D), children, renal disease, thrombocytopenia

PHARMACOKINETICS

SUBCUT: 30-60 min, peak mobilization 6-9 hr, 58% protein binding, 70% excreted via kidneys (parent drug), terminal half-life 3-5 hr

INTERACTIONS

Increase: adverse reactions—do not use this product concomitantly with lithium, may increase leukocytosis

NURSING CONSIDERATIONS

Assess:

- Blood studies: CBC/differential
- B/P, respirations, pulse before and during therapy
- Bone pain, give mild analgesics

Administer:

- Each single use vial contains 24 mg of plerixafor (1.2 ml of 20 mg/ml sol) the volume is calculated by multiplying 0.012 by the actual body wt (kg)

- Give 11 hr before apheresis
- Max 40 mg/day, or 27 mg/day in renal disease

Perform/provide:
- Storage at room temperature

Evaluate:
- Therapeutic response: collection of stem cells

Teach patient/family:
- Reason for use and expected results

pralatrexate
See page 919

prasugrel
See page 923

saxagliptin
See page 1016

tapentadol
See page 1066

telavancin
See page 1068

tolvaptan
See page 1119

ustekinumab
See page 1152

vigabatrin (℞)
(vye-ga'ba-trin)
Sabril
Func. class.: Anticonvulsant

Action: May inhibit reuptake and metabolism of GABA, may increase seizure threshold; structurally similar to GABA
Uses: Adjunct treatment of partial seizures in adults and children ≥12 yr, infantile spasm

DOSAGE AND ROUTES

Partial seizures
- *Adult:* **PO** 500 mg bid, titrate in 500-mg increments at weekly intervals, up to 1.5 g bid

Infantile spasm
- *Infant >1 mo, child ≤2 yr:* **PO** 50 mg/kg/day in 2 divided doses titrate in 25-50 mg/kg/day increments q3days, max 150 mg/kg/day

Renal dose
- *Adult:* **PO** CCr 50-80 ml/min, reduce dose by 25%
- *Adult:* **PO** CCr 30-50 ml/min, reduce dose by 50%
- *Adult:* **PO** CCr 10-30 ml/min, reduce dose by 75%

Available forms: Powder for solution; tabs 500 mg

SIDE EFFECTS

CNS: *Dizziness,* irritability, lethargy, **malignant hyperthermia,** insomnia
CV: Edema
EENT: **Visual impairment**
GI: Nausea, vomiting, diarrhea, increased appetite, abdominal pain, GI bleeding, hemorrhoids, weight gain, constipation
HEMA: Anemia
INTEG: Pruritus, rash
RESP: Coughing, **respiratory depression, pulmonary embolism**
Contraindications: Hypersensitivity to this product
Precautions: Pregnancy (C), breast-feeding, children <2 yr, geriatric patients,

renal/hepatic disease, suicidal ideation/ behavior, abrupt discontinuation

Black Box Warning: Visual disturbance

PHARMACOKINETICS

Absorption >95%, no protein binding, widely distributed, not metabolized excretion urine 80% parent drug, excretion slowed in renal disease peak 2 hr, half-life 7.5 hr

INTERACTIONS

Increase: CNS depression—CNS depressants

- Serious ophthalmic effects (glaucoma, retinopathy): azathioprine, chloroquine, corticosteroids, deferoxamine, ethambutol, hydroxychloroquine, interferons, loxapine, mecasermin, rh-IGF-1, pentostatin, phenothiazine, phosphodiesterase inhibitors, tamoxifen, thiothixene, avoid concurrent use

NURSING CONSIDERATIONS

Assess:

- Renal studies: urinalysis, BUN, urine creatinine q3mo
- Hepatic studies: ALT, AST, bilirubin
- Description of seizures: location, duration, presence of aura
- Mental status: mood, sensorium, affect, behavioral changes; if mental status changes, notify prescriber

Administer:

PO route (tab)

- Give without regard to meals

PO route oral solution

- Reconstitute immediately before using
- Empty contents into a clean cup
- For each packet, dissolve 10 ml of water, conc 50 mg/ml, do not use other liquids
- Stir until dissolved, solution should be clear
- Use calibrated oral syringe to measure correct dosage
- Discard any unused solution

Perform/provide:

- Storage at room temperature
- Assistance with ambulation during early part of treatment; dizziness occurs
- Seizure precautions: padded side rails; move objects that may harm patient

Evaluate:

- Therapeutic response: decreased seizure activity; document on patient's chart

Teach patient/family:

- To carry emergency ID stating patient's name, products taken, condition, prescriber's name and phone number
- To avoid driving, other activities that require alertness
- Not to discontinue medication quickly after long-term use

Treatment of overdose: Lavage, VS

Appendix b

Ophthalmic, otic, nasal, and topical products

OPHTHALMIC PRODUCTS

α-ADRENERGIC BLOCKER

dapiprazole (℞)
(da-pip'ra-zole)
Rev-Eyes

ANESTHETICS

lidocaine (℞)
Akten

proparacaine (℞)
(proe-par'a-kane)
Alcaine, Diocaine ♣, Ophthaine, Ophthetic

tetracaine (℞)
(tet'ra-kane)
Minims Tetracaine ♣, Pontocaine, Tetracaine

ANTIHISTAMINES

azelastine (℞)
(ay-zell'ah-steen)
Optivar

emedastine (℞)
(ee-med'ah-steen)
Emadine

epinastine (℞)
(ep-een'as-teen)
Elestat

ketotifen (℞, OTC)
(kee-toh-tif'en)
Zaditor

levocabastine (℞)
(lee-voh-cab'ah-steen)
Livostin

olopatadine (℞)
(oh-loh-pat'ah-deen)
Patanol

ANTIINFECTIVES

azithromycin (℞)
(ay-zi-thro-my'sin)
AzaSite

besifloxacin (℞)
(be'si-flox'a-sin)
Besivance

chloramphenicol (℞)
(klor-am-fen'i-kole)
AK-Chlor, Chloramphenicol, Chloromycetin Ophthalmic, Chloroptic, Chloroptic S.O.P., Fenicol ♣, Isopto Fenicol ♣, Pentamycin ♣

ciprofloxacin (℞)
(sip-ro-floks'a-sin)
Ciloxan

erythromycin (℞)
(er-ith-roe-mye'sin)
Erythromycin, Ilotycin

ganciclovir (℞)
(gan-sye'kloe-vir)
Virgan

gatifloxacin (℞)
(gat-i-flox'a-sin)
Zymar

gentamicin (℞)
(jen-ta-mye'sin)
Garamycin Ophthalmic, Genoptic Ophthalmic, Genoptic S.O.P., Gentacidin, Gentamicin Ophthalmic, Gentak

levofloxacin (℞)
(lee-voh-floks'a-sin)
Quixin

moxifloxacin (℞)
(mox-i-flox'a-sin)
Vigamox

natamycin (℞)
(nat-a-mye'sin)
Natacyn

norfloxacin (℞)
(nor-floks'a-sin)
Chibroxin

ofloxacin (℞)
(oh-flox'a-sin)
Ocuflox

silver nitrate 1% (℞)
silver nitrate

sulfacetamide sodium (℞)
(sul-fa-seet'a-mide)
AK-Sulf, Bleph-10, Bleph-10 S.O.P., Cetamide, Isopto Cetamide, Ocusulf-10, Sodium Sulamyd, Sodium Sulfacetamide, Storzsulf, Sulf-10, Sulster

tobramycin (℞)
(toe-bra-mye'sin)
AKTob, Defy, Tobrex

trifluridine (℞)
(trye-floor'i-deen)
Viroptic

vidarabine (℞)
(vye-dare'a-been)
Vira-A

β-ADRENERGIC BLOCKERS

betaxolol (℞)
(beh-tax'oh-lole)
Betoptic, Betoptic S

carteolol (℞)
(kar-tee'oh-lole)
Carteolol HCl, Ocupress

levobetaxolol (℞)
(lee-voh-beh-tax'oh-lole)
Betaxon

levobunolol (℞)
(lee-voe-byoo'no-lole)
AKBeta, Betagen

metipranolol (℞)
(met-ee-pran'oh-lole)
OptiPranolol

timolol (℞)
(tye'moe-lole)
Apo-Timop ♣, Betimol, Timoptic, Timoptic-XE

CARBONIC ANHYDRASE INHIBITORS

brinzolamide (℞)
(brin-zoh'la-mide)
Azopt

dorzolamide (℞)
(dor-zol'a-mide)
Trusopt

CHOLINERGICS

(Direct-acting)

acetylcholine (℞)
(ah-see-til-koe'leen)
Miochol-E

carbachol (℞)
(kar'ba-kole)
Carbastat, Carboptic, Isopto Carbachol, Miostat

pilocarpine (℞)
(pye-loe-kar'peen)
Adsorbocarpine, Akarpine, Isopto Carpine, Ocu-Carpine, Ocusert Pilo-20, Ocusert Pilo-40, Pilagan, Pilocar, pilocarpine, Pilopine HS, Piloptic-½, Piloptic-1, Piloptic-2, Piloptic-3, Piloptic-4, Piloptic-6, Pilostat, Pilopto-Carpine

CHOLINESTERASE INHIBITORS

demecarium (℞)
(dem-e-kare′ee-um)
Humorsol

echothiophate (℞)
(ek-oh-thye′eh-fate)
Phospholine Iodide

isoflurophate (℞)
(i-se-flur′e-fate)
Floropryl

physostigmine (℞)
(fi-zoe-stig′meen)
Eserine Salicylate, Isopto Eserine

CORTICOSTEROIDS

dexamethasone (℞)
(dex-a-meth′a-sone)
AK-Dex, Decadron Phosphate, Dexamethasone Ophthalmic Suspension, Maxidex, Ozurdex

difluprednate (℞)
(dye′floo-pred′nate)
Durezol

fluocinolone (℞)
(floo-oh-sin′oh-lone)
Retisert

fluorometholone (℞)
(flure-oh-meth′oh-lone)
Flarex, Fluor-Op, FML, FML Forte, FML S.O.P.

loteprednol (℞)
(loe-tee-pred′nole)
Alrex, Lotemax

medrysone (℞)
(me′dri-sone)
HMS

* **prednisoLONE** (℞)
(pred-niss′oh-lone)
Econopred, Econopred Plus, AK-Pred, Inflamase Forte, Inflamase Mild, Pred-Forte

rimexolone (℞)
(ri-mex′a-lone)
Vexol

triamcinolone (℞)
(trye-am-sin′oh-lone)
Triesence

MYDRIATICS

atropine (℞)
(a′troe-peen)
Atropine-1, Atropine Care, Atropine Sulfate Ophthalmic, Atropisol, Isopto Atropine

cyclopentolate (℞)
(sye-kloe-pen′toe-late)
AK-Pentolate, Cyclogyl, Cyclopentolate HCl

homatropine (℞)
(home-a′troe-peen)
Homatrine HBr, Isopto Homatropine, Minims Homatropine ♣

phenylephrine (OTC)
(fen-ill-ef′rin)
AK-Dilate, AK-Nefrin, Isopto Frin, Neo-Synephrine 2.5%, Neo-Synephrine 10%, phenylephrine HCl, 2.5% Mydfrin, Phenoptic Relief, Prefrin

scopolamine (℞)
(skoe-pol′a-meen)
Isopto Hyoscine

tropicamide (℞)
(troe-pik′a-mide)
Mydriacyl, Opticyl, Tropicacyl, Tropicamide

NONSTEROIDAL ANTIINFLAMMATORIES

bromfenac (℞)
(brome′fen-ak)
Xibrom

diclofenac (℞)
(dye-kloe'fen-ak)
Voltaren

flurbiprofen (℞)
(flure-bih-proh'fen)
Ocufen

ketorolac (℞)
(kee-toe'role-ak)
Acular, Acurail

nepafenac (℞)
(ne-pa-fen'ak)
Nevanac

suprofen (℞)
(soo-proe'fen)
Profenal

SYMPATHOMIMETICS

apraclonidine (℞)
(a-pra-klon'i-deen)
Iopidine

brimonidine (℞)
(brih-moh'nih-deen)
Alphagan, Alphagan P

dipivefrin (℞)
(dye-pi'vef-rin)
Propine, AKPro

epinephrine/ epinephryl borate (℞)
(ep-i-nef'rin)
Epifrin, Glaucon/Epinal, Eppy ✤

OPHTHALMIC DECONGESTANTS/ VASOCONSTRICTORS

lodoxamide
(loe-dox'a-mide)
Alomide

naphazoline (OTC, ℞)
(naf-az'oh-leen)
20/20 Eye Drops, Allergy Drops, AK-Con, Albalon, Allerest Eye Drops, Clear Eyes, Clear Eyes ACR, Comfort Eye Drops, Degest 2, Maximum Strength Allergy Drops, Nafazair, naphazoline HCl, Naphcon, Naphcon Forte, Opcon, Vasoclear, Vasocon Regular

oxymetazoline (℞)
(ox-i-meth'oh-lone)
OcuClear, Visine L.R.

tetrahydrozoline (OTC)
(tet-ra-hye-dro'zoe-leen)
Collyrium Fresh, Eyesine, Geneye, Geneye Extra, Mallazine Eye Drops, Murine Plus, Optigene 3, tetrahydrozoline HCl, Tetrasine, Tetrasine Extra, Visine Moisturizing

MISCELLANEOUS OPHTHALMICS

bimatoprost (℞)
(bih-mat'o-prost)
Latisse, Lumigan

latanoprost (℞)
(la-tan'oh-prost)
Xalatan

travoprost (℞)
(tra'voe-prost)
Travatan

unoprostone (℞)
(un-oh-proe'stone)
Rescula

β-Adrenergic blockers

Action: Reduces production of aqueous humor by unknown mechanism

Uses: Ocular hypertension, chronic open-angle glaucoma

Anesthetics

Action: Decreases ion permeability by stabilizing neuronal membrane

Uses: Cataract extraction, tonometry, gonioscopy, removal of foreign objects, corneal suture removal, glaucoma surgery (ophthalmic); pruritus, sunburn, toothache, sore throat, cold sores, oral pain, rectal pain and irritation, control of gagging (topical)

Antiinfectives
Action: Inhibits folic acid synthesis by preventing PABA use, which is necessary for bacterial growth
Uses: Conjunctivitis, superficial eye infections, corneal ulcers, prophylaxis against infection after removal of foreign matter from the eye
Antiinflammatories
Action: Decreases inflammation, resulting in decreased pain, photophobia, hyperemia, cellular infiltration
Uses: Inflammation of eye, eyelids, conjunctiva, cornea; uveitis, iridocyclitis, allergic conditions, burns, foreign bodies, postoperatively in cataract
Carbonic anhydrase inhibitor
Action: Converted to epinephrine, which decreases aqueous production and increases outflow
Uses: Open-angle glaucoma, ocular hypertension
Direct-acting miotic
Action: Acts directly on cholinergic receptor sites; induces miosis, spasm of accommodation, fall in intraocular pressure, caused by stimulation of ciliary, pupillary sphincter muscles, which leads to pulling away of iris from filtration angle, resulting in increased outflow of aqueous humor
Uses: Primary glaucoma, early stages of wide-angle glaucoma (less useful in advanced stages), chronic open-angle glaucoma, acute closed-angle glaucoma before emergency surgery; also neutralizes mydriatics used during eye exam; may be used alternately with mydriatics to break adhesions between iris and lens

SIDE EFFECTS

CNS: Headache
CV: Hypertension, tachycardia, dysrhythmias
EENT: Burning, stinging
GI: Bitter taste
Contraindications: Hypersensitivity
Precautions: Pregnancy, breastfeeding, children, aphakia, hypersensitivity to carbonic anhydrase inhibitors, sulfonamides, thiazide diuretics, ocular inhibitors, hepatic/renal insufficiency

NURSING CONSIDERATIONS

Assess:
- Ophth exams and intraocular pressure readings
- Blood counts; hepatic, renal function tests and serum electrolytes during long-term treatment

Perform/provide:
- Storage at room temperature away from light

Evaluate:
- Positive therapeutic response
- Absence of increased intraocular pressure

Teach patient/family:
- How to instill drops
- That product may cause burning, itching, blurring, dryness of eye area

NASAL AGENTS

NASAL ANTIHISTAMINES

olopatadine (℞)
(oh-low-pat′uh-deen)
Patanase

NASAL DECONGESTANTS

azelastine (℞)
(ay-zell′ah-steen)
Astelin, Astepro

desoxyephedrine (OTC)
(des-oxy-e-fed′rin)
Vicks Vapor Inhaler

ephedrine (OTC)
(e-fed′rin)
Pretz-D

epinephrine (OTC)
(ep-i-neff′rin)
Adrenalin

naphazoline (OTC)
(naff-a-zoe′leen)
Privine

oxymetazoline (OTC)
(ox-i-met-az′oh-leen)
12-Hour Nasal, Afrin 12-Hour Original, Afrin 12-Hour Original Pump Mist, Afrin Severe Congestion with Menthol, Afrin Sinus with Vapornase, Afrin No-Drip 12-Hour, Afrin No-Drip 12-Hour Extra Moisturizing, Dristan, Duramist Plus, Duration, Genasal, Nafrine ♣, Nasal Relief, Neo-Synephrine 12-Hour, Nostrilla, oxymetazoline HCl, Nasal Decongestant Maximum Strength, Vicks Sinex 12-Hour Long-Acting, Vicks Sinex 12-Hour Ultra Fine Mist for Sinus Relief

phenylephrine (OTC)
(fen-ill-eff′rin)
Alconefrin 12, Children's Nostril, Neo-Synephrine, Sinex

propylhexadrine (OTC)
(proe-pil-hex′a-dreen)
Benzedrex Inhaler

pseudoephedrine (℞, OTC)
(soo-doe-e-fed′rin)
Cenafed, Decofed, Dimetapp, Genaphed, Sudafed, Triaminic

tetrahydrozoline (OTC)
(tet-ra-hye-dro′zoe-leen)
Tyzine, Tyzine Pediatric

xylometazoline (OTC)
(zye-loh-meh-tazz′oh-leen)
Natru-vent, Otrivin, Otrivin Pediatric Nasal

NASAL STEROIDS

beclomethasone (℞)
(be-kloe-meth′a-sone)
Beconase AQ Nasal, Beconase Inhalation, Vancenase AQ Nasal, Vancenase Pocket Inhaler

budesonide (℞)
(byoo-des′oh-nide)
Rhinocort, Rhinocort Aqua

flunisolide (℞)
(floo-niss′oh-lide)
Nasalide, Nasarel

fluticasone (℞)
(floo-tic′a-son)
Flonase, Veramyst

triamcinolone (℞)
(trye-am-sin′oh-lone)
Nasacort AQ

Action: Produces vasoconstriction (rapid, long acting) of arterioles, thereby decreasing fluid exudation, mucosal engorgement by stimulation of α-adrenergic receptors in vascular smooth muscle
Uses: Nasal congestion

DOSAGE AND ROUTES

Desoxyephedrine
- *Adult and child >6 yr:* 1-2 **INH** in each nostril q2hr or less

Ephedrine
- *Adult:* Fill dropper to the level marked, then use in each nostril q4hr or less

Epinephrine
- *Adult and child >6 yr:* Apply with swab, drops, spray prn

Naphazoline
- *Adult and child >6 yr:* 1-2 drops/spray q6hr or less

Oxymetazoline
- *Adult and child >6 yr:* **INSTILL** 2-3 gtt or sprays to each nostril bid
- *Child 2-6 yr:* **INSTILL** 2-3 gtt or sprays 0.025 sol bid, max 3 days

Phenylephrine
- *Adult and child >12 yr:* 2-3 drops/spray (0.25-0.5) in each nostril q3-4hr or less; or 2-3 drops/spray (1%) in each nostril q4hr or less
- *Child 6-12 yr:* 2-3 drops/spray (0.25%) in each nostril q3-4hr
- *Infant >6 mo:* 1-2 drops (0.16%) in each nostril q3hr

Propylhexadrine
- *Adult and child >6 yr:* 1-2 **INH** in each nostril q2hr or less

Tetrahydrozoline
- *Adult and child >6 yr:* 2-4 drops (0.1%) q3-4hr prn or 3-4 sprays in each nostril q4hr prn
- *Child 2-6 yr:* 2-3 drops (0.05%) in each nostril q4-6hr prn

Xylometazoline
- *Adult and child >12 yr:* 2-3 drops/spray (0.1%) in each nostril q8-10hr
- *Child 2-12 yr:* 2-3 drops (0.05%) in each nostril q8-10hr

Available forms: Nasal sol 0.025%, 0.05%

SIDE EFFECTS

CNS: Anxiety, restlessness, tremors, weakness, insomnia, dizziness, fever, headache
EENT: Irritation, burning, sneezing, stinging, dryness, rebound congestion
GI: Nausea, vomiting, anorexia
INTEG: Contact dermatitis

Contraindications: Hypersensitivity to sympathomimetic amines

Precautions: Pregnancy (C), children <6 yr, geriatric, diabetes, CV disease, hypertension, hyperthyroidism, increased intracranial pressure, prostatic hypertrophy, glaucoma

NURSING CONSIDERATIONS

Assess:
- For redness, swelling, pain in nasal passages before and during treatment
- For systemic absorption; hypertension, tachycardia; notify prescriber; systemic absorption occurs at high doses or after prolonged use

Administer:
- Having patient tilt head back, squeeze bulb to create a vacuum, and draw correct amount of sol into dropper; insert 2 gtt of sol into nostril; repeat in other nostril
- Store in light-resistant container; do not expose to high temperature or let sol come into contact with aluminum
- For <4 consecutive days
- Environmental humidification to decrease nasal congestion, dryness

Evaluate:
- Therapeutic response: decreased nasal congestion

Teach patient/family:
- That stinging may occur for several applications; drying of mucosa may be decreased by environmental humidification
- To notify prescriber if irregular pulse, insomnia, dizziness, or tremors occur
- Proper administration to avoid systemic absorption
- To rinse dropper with very hot water to prevent contamination

TOPICAL GLUCOCORTICOIDS

betamethasone (℞)
(bay-ta-meth'a-sone)
Alphatrex, Beben ♣, Betacort ♣, Betatrex, Beta-Val, Betnovate ♣, Celestoderm ♣, Diprosone, Ectosone ♣, Luxiq, Maxivate, Metaderm ♣, Psorion, Valisone

betamethasone (augmented) (℞)
(bay-ta-meth'a-sone)
Diprolene, Diprolene AF

clobetasol (℞)
(kloe-bay'ta-sol)
Clobex, Cormax, Dermovate ♣, Embeline E 0.05%, Temovate

desonide (℞)
(dess'oh-nide)
Verdeso Foam

desoximetasone (℞)
(dess-ox-i-met'a-sone)
Topicort, Topicort LP

dexamethasone (℞)
(dex-a-meth'a-sone)
Aeroseb-Dex, Decaspray

fluocinolone (℞)

(floo-oh-sin'oh-lone)

Derma-Smoothe/FSoil, Fluocin, Licon, Lidemol ♣, Lidex, Lyderm ♣, Topsyn ♣, Vasoderm

flurandrenolide (℞)

(flure-an-dren'oh-lide)

Cordran, Cordran SP, Drenison 1/4 ♣, Drenison Tape ♣

fluticasone (℞)

(floo-tik'a-sone)

Cutivate

halcinonide (℞)

(hal-sin'oh-nide)

Halog, Halog-E

hydrocortisone (℞)

(hye-droe-kor'ti-sone)

Acticort, Aeroseb-HC, Ala-Cort, Allercort, Alphaderm, Anusol HC, Bactine, Barriere-HC ♣, Calde-CORT Anti-Itch, Carmol HC, Cetacort, Cortacet ♣, Cortaid, Cortalo, Cortate ♣, Cort-Dome, Cortef ♣, Corticaine, Corticreme ♣, Cortifair, Corti-zone, Cortoderm ♣, Cortril, Delcort, Dermacort, DemiCort, Dermtex HC, Emo-Cort, Epifoam, FoilleCort, Gly-Cort, Gynecort, Hi-Cor, Hycort, Hyderm ♣, Hydro-Tex, Hytone, Lacti-Care-HC, Lanacort, Lemoderm, Locoid, Locoid Lotion, My Cort, Novohydrocort ♣, Nutracort Pharm, Pharmacort, Pentacort, Rederm, Rhulicort S-T Cort, Synacort, Sarna HC ♣, Texa-Cort, Unicort ♣, Westcort

triamcinolone (℞)

(trye-am-sin'oh-lone)

Aristocort, Delta-Tritex, Flutex, Kenac, Kenalog, Kenonel, Triaderm, Trianide ♣, Triderm, Trymex

Action: Antipruritic, antiinflammatory

Uses: Psoriasis, eczema, contact dermatitis, pruritus; usually reserved for severe dermatoses that have not responded to less potent formulation

DOSAGE AND ROUTES

- *Adult and child:* Apply to affected area

SIDE EFFECTS

INTEG: Acne, atrophy, epidermal thinning, purpura, striae

Contraindications: Hypersensitivity, viral infections, fungal infections

Precautions: Pregnancy (C)

NURSING CONSIDERATIONS

Assess:

- Temp; if fever develops, product should be discontinued
- For systemic absorption, increased temp, inflammation, irritation

Administer:

- Only to affected areas; do not get in eyes
- Leaving site uncovered or lightly covered; occlusive dressing is not recommended—systemic absorption may occur
- Use only on dermatoses; do not use on weeping, denuded, or infected area
- Cleansing before application of product
- Continuing treatment for a few days after area has cleared
- Store at room temperature

Evaluate:

- Therapeutic response: absence of severe itching, patches on skin, flaking

Teach patient/family:

- To avoid sunlight on affected area, burns may occur
- To limit treatment to 14 days

TOPICAL ANTIFUNGALS

clotrimazole (OTC)
(kloe-trye′ma-zole)
Canestew ♣, Clotrimaderm ♣, Clotrimazole, Cruex, Desenex, Lotrimin AF, Myclo ♣, Neozol ♣

econazole (OTC)
(ee-kon′a-zole)
Spectazole

ketoconazole (OTC)
(kee-toe-kon′a-zole)
Nizoral, Xolegel

miconazole (OTC)
(mye-kon′a-zole)
Absorbine Antifungal Foot Powder, Breeze Mist Antifungal, Fungoid Tincture, Lotrimin AF, Maximum Strength Desenex Antifungal, Micatin, Monistat-Derm, Ony-clear, Tetterine, Zeasorb-AF

nystatin (OTC)
(nye-stat′in)
Mycostatin, Nadostine ♣, Nilstat, Nyaderm ♣, Nystex

selenium (OTC)
(see-leen′ee-um)
Exsel, Head and Shoulders Intensive Treatment, Selenium Sulfide, Selsun, Selsun Blue

terbinafine (OTC)
(ter-bin′a-feen)
Lamisil

tolnaftate (OTC)
(tole-naf′tate)
Absorbine Athlete's Foot Cream, Aftate for Athlete's Foot, Aftate for Jock Itch, Genaspor, Quinsana Plus, Tinactin, Ting, tolnaftate

undecylenic acid (OTC)
(un-deh-sih-len′ik)
Blis-To-Sol, Breeze Mist, Caldesene, Cruex, Decylenes, Desenex, Desenex Maximum Strength, Pedi-Pro, Phicon F, Protectol

Action: Interferes with fungal cell membrane permeability

Uses: Tinea cruris, tinea pedis, diaper rash, minor skin irritations; amphotericin B is used for candida infections

DOSAGE AND ROUTES

- Massage into affected area, surrounding area daily or bid, continue for 7-14 days, not to exceed 4 wk

SIDE EFFECTS

INTEG: Burning, stinging, dryness, itching, local irritation

Contraindications: Hypersensitivity

Precautions: Pregnancy (B), breastfeeding, children

NURSING CONSIDERATIONS

Assess:
- Skin for fungal infections; peeling, dryness, itching before and throughout treatment
- For continuing infection; increased size, number of lesions

Administer:

Topical route
- To affected area, surrounding area; do not cover with occlusive dressings
- Store below 30° C (86° F)

Evaluate:
- Therapeutic response: decrease in size, number of lesions

Teach patient/family:
- To apply with glove to prevent further infection; not to cover with occlusive dressings
- That long-term therapy may be needed to clear infection (2 wk-6 mo depending on organism); compliance is needed even after feeling better

• Proper hygiene; hand-washing technique, nail care, use of concomitant top agents if prescribed
• To avoid use of OTC creams, ointments, lotions unless directed by prescriber
• To use medical asepsis (hand washing) before, after each application; to change socks and shoes once a day during treatment of tinea pedis
• To report to health care prescriber if infection persists or recurs; if blisters, burning, oozing, swelling occur
• To avoid alcohol because nausea, vomiting, hypertension may occur
• To use sunscreen or avoid direct sunlight to prevent photosensitivity
• To notify health care prescriber of sore throat, fever, skin rash, which may indicate overgrowth of organisms

TOPICAL ANTIINFECTIVES

azelaic acid (℞)
(a-zuh-lay′ic)
Azelex, Finacen

bacitracin (OTC)
(bass-i-tray′sin)
Bacitin ♣, Bacitracin

clindamycin (℞)
(klin-da-my′sin)
Cleocin T, Clindagel, ClindaMax, Clindets

erythromycin (℞, OTC)
(er-ith-roe-mye′sin)
A/T/S, Akne-Mycin, Eryderm, Erygel, Erythromycin, Staticin, T-Stat

gentamicin (℞)
(jen-ta-mye′sin)
Gentamicin

mafenide (℞)
(ma′fe-nide)
Sulfamylon

metronidazole (℞)
(met-roh-nye′da-zole)
MetroGel, MetroCream, MetroLotion, Noritate

mupirocin (℞)
(myoo-peer′oh-sin)
Bactroban

neomycin (OTC)
(nee-oh-mye′sin)
Neomycin Sulfate

nitrofurazone (℞)
(nye-troe-fyoor′a-zone)
Furacin, Nitrofurazone

retapamulin (℞)
(re-tap′a-mue′lin)
Altabax

salicylic acid (℞)
(sal′i-sil′ik)
Salitop

***silver sulfADIAZINE** (℞)
(sul-fa-dye′a-zeen)
Flamazine ♣, Silvadene, SSD, SSD AF, Thermazene

tretinoin (℞)
(treh′tih-noyn)
Atralin

Action: Interferes with bacterial protein synthesis
Uses: Skin infections, minor burns, wounds, skin grafts, primary pyodermas, otitis externa

SIDE EFFECTS

INTEG: Rash, urticaria, scaling, redness
Contraindications: Hypersensitivity, large areas, burns, ulcerations
Precautions: Pregnancy (C), breastfeeding, impaired renal function, external ear or perforated eardrum

NURSING CONSIDERATIONS

Assess:
• Allergic reaction: burning, stinging, swelling, redness
• For signs of nephrotoxicity or ototoxicity
Administer:
• Enough medication to cover lesions completely
• After cleansing with soap, water before each application; dry well
• To less than 20% of body surface area when patient has impaired renal function

Perform/provide:
• Storage at room temperature in dry place
Evaluate:
• Therapeutic response: decrease in size, number of lesions

TOPICAL ANTIVIRALS

acyclovir (℞)
(ay-sye'kloe-ver)
Zovirax
penciclovir (℞)
(pen-sye'kloe-ver)
Denavir

Action: Interferes with viral DNA replication
Uses: Simple mucocutaneous herpes simplex, in immunocompromised clients with initial herpes genitalis

SIDE EFFECTS

INTEG: Rash, urticaria, stinging, burning, pruritus, vulvitis
Contraindications: Hypersensitivity
Precautions: Pregnancy (C), breastfeeding

NURSING CONSIDERATIONS

Assess:
• Allergic reaction: burning, stinging, swelling, redness, rash, vulvitis, pruritus
Administer:
• Using finger cot or rubber glove to prevent further infection
• Enough medication to cover lesions completely
• After cleansing with soap, water before each application; dry well
Perform/provide:
• Storage at room temperature in dry place
Evaluate:
• Therapeutic response: decrease in size, number of lesions
Teach patient/family:
• Not to use in eyes or when there is no evidence of infection
• To apply with glove to prevent further infection
• To avoid use of OTC creams, ointments, lotions unless directed by prescriber
• To use medical asepsis (hand washing) before, after each application and avoid contact with eyes
• To adhere strictly to prescribed regimen to maximize successful treatment outcome
• To begin taking product when symptoms arise

TOPICAL ANESTHETICS

benzocaine (OTC)
(ben'zoe-kane)
Americaine Anesthetic, Anbesol Maximum Strength, Baby Anbesol, Biozene, Boil-Ease, Children's Chloraseptic, Dermoplast, Foille, Foille Plus, Hurricaine, Lanacane, Medamint, Orabase, Oracin, Ora-Jel
dibucaine (OTC)
(dye'byoo-kane)
Dibucaine, Nupercainal
lidocaine (℞, OTC)
(lye'doe-kane)
Anestacon, Burn-O-Jel, Derma Flex, Dentipatch, ELA-Max, Lidocaine HCl Topical, Lidocaine Viscous, Numby Stuff, Solarcaine Aloe Extra Burn Relief, Xylocaine, Xylocaine 10% oral, Xylocaine Viscous, Zilactin-L
pramoxine (OTC)
(pra-mox'een)
Itch-X, PrameGel, Prax, Tronothane
tetracaine (℞, OTC)
(tet'ra-cane)
Pontocaine, Viractin

Action: Inhibits conduction of nerve impulses from sensory nerves

Uses: Oral irritation, sore throat, toothache, cold sore, canker sore, sunburn, minor cuts, insect bites, pain, itching

DOSAGE AND ROUTES

• *Adult and child:* **TOP** apply qid as needed; **RECT** insert tid and after each BM

SIDE EFFECTS

INTEG: Rash, irritation, sensitization

Contraindications: Hypersensitivity, infants <1 yr, application to large areas

Precautions: Pregnancy (C), children <6 yr, sepsis, denuded skin

NURSING CONSIDERATIONS

Assess:

• Pain: location, duration, characteristics before and after administration

• For infection: redness, drainage, inflammation; this product should not be used until infection is treated

Perform/provide:

• Storage in tight, light-resistant container; do not freeze, puncture, or incinerate aerosol container

Evaluate:

• Therapeutic response: decreased redness, swelling, pain

Teach patient/family:

• To avoid contact with eyes

• Not to use for prolonged periods: use for <1 wk; if condition remains, prescriber should be contacted

TOPICAL MISCELLANEOUS

docosanol (OTC)
(doe-koe′san-ole)
Abreva

pimecrolimus (℞)
(pim-eh-croh′lim-us)
Elidel

Action: Docosanol unknown; pimecrolimus may bind with macrophilin and inhibit calcium-dependent phosphatase

Uses: Docosanol applied to fever blisters to promote more rapid healing; pimecrolimus used to treat mild to moderate atopic dermatitis in nonimmunocompromised patients ≥2 yr who are unresponsive to other treatment

DOSAGE AND ROUTES

Docosanol

• *Adult:* **TOP** Rub into blisters 5×/day until healing occurs

Pimecrolimus

• *Adult and child ≥2 yr:* **TOP** Apply thin layer 2×/day and rub in, use as long as needed

SIDE EFFECTS

Pimecrolimus

INTEG: Burning

Contraindications: Hypersensitivity

Precautions: Pregnancy (C), breastfeeding, dermal infections

NURSING CONSIDERATIONS

Assess:

• Skin condition (color, pain, inflammation) before and after administration

• For signs and symptoms of skin infections (redness, draining lesions); if present, avoid use of product (pimecrolimus)

Administer:

• To skin, rub in gently

Evaluate:

• Therapeutic response: decreased inflammation, redness

Teach patient/family:

• To avoid contact between medication and eyes

• To discontinue use of product when condition clears

VAGINAL ANTIFUNGALS

butoconazole (OTC)
(byoo-toh-kone'ah-zole)
Femstat-3, Gynazol-1, Mycelex-3

clotrimazole (OTC)
(kloe-trye'ma-zole)
Canesten ✦, Clotrimazole, Gyne-Lotrimin 3, Gyne-Lotrimin 7, Mycelex 7, Myclo ✦

miconazole (OTC)
(mye-kon'a-zole)
Femizole-M, Monistat, Monistat 3, Monistat 7, Monistat Dual Pak, M-Zole 7 Dual Pack

nystatin (OTC)
(nye-stat'in)
Nystatin

terconazole (OTC)
(ter-kone'ah-zole)
Terazol 7, Terazol 3

tioconazole (OTC)
(tye-oh-kone'ah-zole)
Gyne-Trosyd ✦, Monistat 1, Vagistat-1

Action: Interferes with fungal DNA replication; binds sterols in fungal cell membranes, which increases permeability, leaking of nutrients

Uses: Vaginal, vulval, vulvovaginal candidiasis (moniliasis)

DOSAGE AND ROUTES

Butoconazole
- *Adult:* **VAG** 5 g (1 applicator) at bedtime × 3-6 days

Clotrimazole
- *Adult:* 100 mg (1 vag tab, 100 mg) at bedtime × 1 wk, or 200 mg (2 vag tab, 100 mg) at bedtime × 3 nights, or 500 mg (1 vag tab, 500 mg); or 5 g (1 applicator) at bedtime × 1-2 wk

Miconazole
- *Adult:* 200 mg supp at bedtime × 3 days or 100 mg supp × 1 wk

Nystatin
- *Adult:* 100,000 units daily × 2 wk

Terconazole
- *Adult:* **VAG** 5 g (1 applicator) at bedtime × 7 days

Tioconazole
- *Adult:* 1 applicator at bedtime × 1 wk

SIDE EFFECTS

GU: Vulvovaginal burning, itching, pelvic cramps
INTEG: Rash, urticaria, stinging, burning
MISC: Headache, body pain

Contraindications: Hypersensitivity
Precautions: Pregnancy, breastfeeding, children <2 yr

NURSING CONSIDERATIONS

Assess:
- For allergic reaction: burning, stinging, itching, discharge, soreness

Administer:

Topical route
- One full applicator every night high into the vagina
- Store at room temperature in dry place

Evaluate:
- Therapeutic outcome: decrease in itching or white discharge (vaginal)

Teach patient/family:
- About asepsis (hand washing) before, after each application
- To apply with applicator only; to avoid use of any other vaginal product unless directed by prescriber; sanitary napkin may prevent soiling of undergarments
- To abstain from sexual intercourse until treatment is completed; reinfection and irritation may occur
- To notify prescriber if symptoms persist

OTIC ANTIINFECTIVES

boric acid (OTC)
(bor′ik as′id)
Auro-Dri, Dri/Ear, Ear Dry
chloramphenicol (℞)
(klor-am-fen′i-kole)
Chloromycetin Otic
ciprofloxacin (℞)
Cetraxel

Action: Inhibits protein synthesis in susceptible microorganisms
Uses: Ear infection (external), short-term use

SIDE EFFECTS

EENT: Itching, irritation in ear
INTEG: Rash, urticaria
Contraindications: Hypersensitivity, perforated eardrum
Precautions: Pregnancy (C)

NURSING CONSIDERATIONS

Assess:
- For redness, swelling, fever, pain in ear, which indicates superinfection

Administer:
- After removing impacted cerumen by irrigation
- After cleaning stopper with alcohol
- After restraining child if necessary
- After warming sol to body temp

Evaluate:
- Therapeutic response: decreased ear pain

Teach patient/family:
- The correct method of instillation using aseptic technique, including not touching dropper to ear
- That dizziness may occur after instillation

Appendix c Vaccines and toxoids

GENERIC NAME	TRADE NAME	USES	DOSAGE AND ROUTES	CONTRAINDICATIONS
avian influenza A (H5N1) virus vaccine		Prophylaxis	Adult: IM 1 ml (90 mcg) 2 doses, 28 days apart	IV
anthrax vaccine	BioThrax	Pre-/postexposure prophylaxis	**Preexposure** Adult: SUBCUT 0.5 ml at 0, 2, 4 wk, then 0.5 ml at 6, 12, 18 mo **Postexposure** Adult: SUBCUT 0.5 ml 0, 2, 4 wk, with antibiotics	Hypersensitivity
BCG vaccine	TICE BCG	TB exposure	Adult and child >1 mo: 0.2-0.3 ml Child <1 mo: Reduce dose by 50% using 2 ml of sterile water after reconstituting	Hypersensitivity, hypogammaglobulinemia, positive TB test, burns
cholera vaccine	No trade name	Immunization for cholera outside the United States	Adult and child >10 yr: IM/SUBCUT 2× of 0.5 ml, 7-30 days before traveling to cholera areas Booster is used q6mo 0.5 ml prn	Hypersensitivity, acute febrile illness
diphtheria and tetanus toxoids, adsorbed	No trade name	Induces antitoxins to provide immunity to diphtheria and tetanus	Adult and child ≥7 yr: IM (adult strength) 0.5 ml q4-8wk × 2 doses, then 3rd dose 6-12 mo after 2nd dose, booster IM 0.5 ml q10yr Child 1-6 yr: IM (pediatric strength) 0.5 ml q4wk × 2 doses, booster 6-12 mo after 2nd dose Infant 6 wk-1 yr: IM (pediatric strength) 0.5 ml q4wk × 3 doses, booster 6-12 mo after 3rd dose	Hypersensitivity to mercury, thimerosal; immunocompromised patients; radiation; corticosteroids; acute illness
diphtheria and tetanus toxoids and whole-cell pertussis vaccine (DPT, DTP)	DTwP, Tr-Immunol	Prevention of diphtheria, tetanus, pertussis	Adult: Booster dose q10yr Child >6 wk-6 yr: IM 0.5 ml at 2, 4, 6 mo, 1½ yr; booster needed 0.5 ml at age 6	Hypersensitivity, active infection, poliomyelitis outbreak, immunosuppression, febrile illness
diphtheria and tetanus toxoids and acellular pertussis vaccine	Acel-Imune, DTaP, Tripedia			

Continued

Appendix c Vaccines and toxoids—cont'd

GENERIC NAME	TRADE NAME	USES	DOSAGE AND ROUTES	CONTRAINDICATIONS
diphtheria, tetanus, pertussis, haemophilus, polio IPV	Pentacel	Immunity to diphtheria, tetanus, pertussis, haemophilus, polio IPV	Infant >6 wk and child ≤5 yr: IM 0.5 ml at 2, 4, 6, and 15-18 mo	Hypersensitivity, polio outbreak, acute infection, immunosuppression
diphtheria, tetanus, pertussis, polio vaccine IPV	Kinrix	Immunity to diphtheria, tetanus, pertussis, polio vaccine IPV	Child: IM 0.5 ml	Hypersensitivity, polio outbreak, acute infection, immunosuppression
H1N1 influenza A (swine flu) virus vaccine	Influenza A (H1N1)	Immunity to H1N1	Adult <50 yr, adolescent, child ≥2 yr: Intranasal 1 dose (roughly 0.1 ml) into each nostril; child 2-9 repeat dose ≥4 wk later Adult, adolescent, child ≥3 yr: IM 0.5 ml as a single dose; child 3-9 yr repeat dose ≥4 wk later (Sanofi) (CSL); child 4-9 yr repeat dose ≥4 wk later (Novartis); infants ≥6 mo-child <36 mo: IM 0.25 ml, repeat in 4 wk (Sanofi) Adult: IM 0.5 ml as a single dose (GSK)	
haemophilus b conjugate vaccine, diphtheria CRM_{197} protein conjugate (HbOC)	HibTITER	Polysaccharide immunization of children 2-6 yr against *H. influenzae* b, conjugate	**HibTITER (IM only)** Child: IM 0.5 ml Child 2-6 mo: 0.5 ml q2mo × 3 inj	Hypersensitivity, febrile illness, active infection
haemophilus b conjugate vaccine, meningococcal protein conjugate (PRP-OMP)	PedvaxHIB	Immunization of child 2, 4, 6 mo	Child 7-11 mo: Previously unvaccinated 0.5 ml q2mo inj Child 12-14 mo: Previously unvaccinated 0.5 ml × 1 inj **PedvaxHIB (IM only)** Child 2-14 mo: 0.5 ml × 2 inj at 2, 4 mo of age (6 mo dose not needed), then booster at 12-18 mo against invasive disease Child ≥15 mo: Previously unvaccinated 0.5 ml inj	

hepatitis A vaccine, inactivated	Havrix, VAQTA	Active immunization against hepatitis A virus	Adult: IM 1440 EL units (Havrix) or 50 units (VAQTA) as a single dose; booster dose is the same given at 6, 12 mo Child 2-18 yr: IM 720 EL units (Havrix) or 25 units (VAQTA) as a single dose, booster dose is the same given at 6, 12 mo	Hypersensitivity
hepatitis B vaccine, recombinant	Engerix-B, Recombivax HB	Immunization against all subtypes of hepatitis B virus	Varies widely	Hypersensitivity to this vaccine or yeast
herpes zoster virus vaccine	Zostavax	Prevention of herpes zoster	Adult ≥60 yr: SUBCUT 0.65 ml	<60 yr, child, infant, AIDS, IM/IV, leukemia, lymphoma, pregnancy
human papillomavirus recombinant vaccine, quadrivalent	Gardasil	Prevention of HPV types 6, 11, 16, 18, cervical cancer, genital warts, precancerous dysplasic lesions	Adult up to 26 yr and child >9 yr to 26 yr: IM give as 3 separate doses; 1st dose as elected; 2nd dose 2 mo after 1st dose; 3rd dose 6 mo after 1st dose	Child <9 yr, pregnancy, breastfeeding, geriatric, active disease, hypersensitivity
influenza virus vaccine	Afluria, FluMist, Fluogen, Flu-Shield, Fluviral*, Fluvirin, Fluzone, influenza virus vaccine, trivalent	Prevention of Russian, Chilean, Philippine influenza	Adult and child >12 yr: IM 0.5 ml in 1 dose Child 3-12 yr: IM 0.5 ml, repeat in 1 mo (split) unless 1978-1985 vaccine was given; also given nasal Child 6 mo to 3 yr: IM 0.25 ml, repeat in 1 mo (split) unless 1978-1985 vaccine was given; also given nasal child ≤2 yr	Hypersensitivity, active infection, chicken egg allergy, Guillain-Barré syndrome, active neurologic disorders
Japanese encephalitis virus vaccine, inactivated	JE-VAX	Active immunity against Japanese encephalitis (JE)	Adult and child ≥3 yr: SUBCUT 1 ml, days 0, 7, 30; booster SUBCUT 1 ml 2 yr after last dose Child 1-3 yr: SUBCUT 0.5 ml, days 0, 7, 30; booster SUBCUT 0.5 ml 2 yr after last dose	Hypersensitivity to murine, thimerosal; allergic reactions to previous dose
Lyme disease vaccine (recombinant OspA)	LYMErix	Immunization against Lyme disease	Adult and adolescent 15-70 yr: IM 30 mcg in deltoid, repeat at 1, 12 mo after first dose	Hypersensitivity, antibiotic refractory Lyme arthritis
measles and rubella virus vaccine, live attenuated	M-R-Vax II	Immunity to measles and rubella by antibody production	Adult and child ≥15 mo: SUBCUT 0.5 ml (1000 units)	Hypersensitivity, immunocompromised patients, active untreated TB, cancer, blood dyscrasias, radiation, corticosteroids, pregnancy; allergic reactions to neomycin, eggs

*Canada only.

Continued

Appendix c Vaccines and toxoids—cont'd

GENERIC NAME	TRADE NAME	USES	DOSAGE AND ROUTES	CONTRAINDICATIONS
measles, mumps, and rubella vaccine, live	M-M-R-II	Prevention of measles, mumps, rubella	Adult: SUBCUT 1 vial; 2 vials separated by 1 mo, in person born after 1957 Child >15 mo and adult: SUBCUT 0.5 ml	Hypersensitivity, blood dyscrasias, anemia, active infection, immunosuppression; egg, chicken allergy; pregnancy, febrile illness, neomycin allergy, neoplasms
measles, mumps, rubella, varicella	ProQuad	Immunity to measles, mumps, rubella, varicella	Child: SUBCUT 0.5 ml	Hypersensitivity to eggs, neomycin, cancer, radiation, corticosteroids, blood dyscrasias, active untreated TB
measles virus vaccine, live attenuated	Attenuvax	Immunity to measles by antibody production	Adult and child ≥15 mo: SUBCUT 0.5 ml (1000 units), 1 dose 15 mo, 2nd dose age 4-6 or 11, or 12	Hypersensitivity to eggs, neomycin; cancer, radiation, corticosteroids, pregnancy, immunocompromised patients, blood dyscrasias, active untreated TB
meningococcal polysaccharide vaccine	Menomune-A/C/Y/W-135, Menactra	Prophylaxis to meningococcal meningitis	Adult and child >2 yr: SUBCUT 0.5 ml	Hypersensitivity to thimerosal, pregnancy, acute illness
mumps virus vaccine, live	Mumpsvax	Active immunity to mumps	Adult and child ≥1 yr: SUBCUT 0.5 ml (20,000 units)	Hypersensitivity to eggs, neomycin; cancer, radiation, corticosteroids, pregnancy, immunocompromised patients, blood dyscrasias, active untreated TB
plague vaccine	No trade name	Active immunity to *Yersinia pestis* plague	Adult: IM 1 ml, then 0.2 ml in 4-12 wk, then 0.2 ml 5-6 mo after 2nd dose; booster 0.1-0.2 ml q6mo when in plague area	Hypersensitivity to phenol, sulfites, formaldehyde, beef, soy, casein; pregnancy, coagulation disorders
pneumococcal 7-valent conjugate vaccine	Prevnar	Immunity against *Streptococcus pneumoniae*	Child: IM 0.5 ml × 3 doses (7-11 mo); × 2 doses (12-23 mo); × 1 dose >2-9 yr	Hypersensitivity to diphtheria toxoid or this product
pneumococcal vaccine, polyvalent	Pneumovax 23, Pnu-Imune 23	Pneumococcal immunization	Adult and child >2 yr: IM/SUBCUT 0.5 ml	Hypersensitivity, Hodgkin's disease, ARDS

poliovirus vaccine, live, oral, trivalent (TOPV) poliovirus vaccine (IPV)	Orimune, IPOL	Prevention of polio	Adult and child >2 yr: PO 0.5 ml, given q8wk × 2 doses, then 0.5 ml ½-1 yr after dose 2 Infant: PO 0.5 ml at 2, 4, 18 mo; booster at 4-6 yr; may also be given: IPV at 2, 4 mo, then TOPV at 12-18 mo, booster at 4-6 yr	Hypersensitivity, active infection, allergy to neomycin/streptomycin, immunosuppression, vomiting, diarrhea
rabies vaccine, adsorbed	No trade name	Active immunity to rabies	**Preexposure** Adult and child: IM 1 ml day 0, 7, 21, or 28 days (total 3 doses); booster IM 1 ml prn q2-5yr **Postexposure** Adult and child not vaccinated: IM 20 international units/kg of human rabies immune globulin (HRIG), give 5 total doses of 1-ml inj of rabies vaccine on days 0, 3, 7, 14, 28	Severe hypersensitivity to previous inj of vaccine, thimerosol
rabies vaccine, human diploid cell (HDCV)	Imovax Rabies, Imovax Rabies I.D.	Active immunity to rabies	**Preexposure** Adult and child: IM 1 ml day 0, 7, 21, or 28 (total 4 doses) **Postexposure** Adult and child: IM 1 ml on day 0, 3, 7, 14, 28 (total 5 doses)	No contraindications
rotovirus	RotaTeq	Prevents rotovirus	Infant: PO 3 doses given between 6 and 32 wk of age; 1st dose between 6-12 wk of age; 2nd and 3rd doses q4-10wk	Hypersensitivity, immunocompromised, blood products given within 6 wk, lymphatic disorders
rubella and mumps virus vaccine, live	Biavax II	Immunity to rubella and mumps by antibody production	Adult and child ≥1 yr: SUBCUT 0.5 ml	Hypersensitivity to eggs, neomycin; cancer, radiation, corticosteroids, pregnancy, immunocompromised patients, blood dyscrasias, active untreated TB
rubella virus vaccine, live attenuated (RA 27/3)	Meruvax II	Immunity to rubella by antibody production	Adult and child ≥1 yr: SUBCUT 0.5 ml (1000 units)	Hypersensitivity to eggs, neomycin; cancer, radiation, corticosteroids

Continued

Appendix c Vaccines and toxoids—cont'd

GENERIC NAME	TRADE NAME	USES	DOSAGE AND ROUTES	CONTRAINDICATIONS
smallpox vaccine	ACAM 2000, Dry Vax	Prevention of smallpox	See package insert	No contraindications
tetanus toxoid, adsorbed/ tetanus toxoid	No trade name	Tetanus toxoid: Used for prophylactic treatment of wounds	Adult and child: IM 0.5 ml q4-6wk × 2 doses, then 0.5 ml 1 yr after dose 2 (adsorbed); SUBCUT/IM 0.5 ml q4-8wk × 3 doses, then 0.5 ml ½-1 yr after dose 3, booster dose 0.5 ml q10yr	Hypersensitivity, active infection, poliomyelitis outbreak, immunosuppression
typhoid vaccine, parenteral typhoid vaccine, oral	No trade name Vivotif Berna Vaccine	Active immunity to typhoid fever	Adult: PO 1 cap 1 hr before meals × 4 doses, booster q5yr Adult and child >10 yr: SUBCUT 0.5 ml, repeat in 4 wk, booster q3yr Child 6 mo-10 yr: SUBCUT 0.25 ml, repeat in 4 wk, booster q3yr	Parenteral: Systemic or allergic reaction, acute respiratory or other acute infection, intensive physical exercise in high temperatures Oral: Hypersensitivity, acute febrile illness, suppressive or antibiotic products
typhoid Vi polysaccharide vaccine	Typhim Vi	Active immunity to typhoid fever	Adult and child ≥2 yr: IM 0.5 ml as a single dose, reimmunize q2yr 0.5 ml IM, if needed	Hypersensitivity, chronic typhoid carriers
varicella virus vaccine	Varivax	Prevention of varicella-zoster (chickenpox)	Adult and child ≥13 yr: SUBCUT 0.5 ml, 2nd dose SUBCUT 0.5 ml 4-8 wk later	Hypersensitivity to neomycin; blood dyscrasias, immunosuppression, active untreated TB, acute illness, prenancy, diseases of lymphatic system
yellow fever vaccine	YF-Vax	Active immunity to yellow fever	Adult and child ≥9 mo: SUBCUT 0.5 ml deeply, booster q10yr Child 6-9 mo: same as above if exposed	Hypersensitivity to egg or chicken embryo protein, pregnancy, child <6 mo, immunodeficiency
zoster vaccine, live	Zostavax	Herpes zoster prevention	Reconstitute immediately after removing from freezer; give SUBCUT as a single dose; inject total amount of single-dose vial	Immunosuppression; neomycin, gelatin allergy; children, TB, pregnancy (C)

Appendix d Antitoxins and antivenins

GENERIC NAME	TRADE NAME	USE	DOSAGE AND ROUTES	CONTRAINDICATIONS
Black widow spider antivenin *(Lactrodectus mactans)*	No trade name	Black widow spider bite	Adult and child: IM 2.5 ml, 2nd dose may be given if severe; give in anterolateral thigh, obtain test for sensitivity before inj	Hypersensitivity to this product or horse serum
Crotalidae antivenom, polyvalent	No trade name	Rattlesnake bite	Adult and child: IV 20-150 ml depending on seriousness of bite, may give additional doses based on response	Hypersensitivity
Diphtheria antitoxin, equine	No trade name	Diphtheria	Adult and child: IM/slow IV 20,000-120,000 units, may give additional doses after 24 hr	Hypersensitivity
Micrurus fulvius antivenin	No trade name	East/Texas coral snake bite	Adult and child: IV 30-50 ml, give through running IV line of normal saline, give 1st 1-2 ml over 4-5 min, watch for allergic reaction	Hypersensitivity

Appendix e

Selected combination products

A-200 Lice Killing Shampoo:
0.33% pyrethrins
4% piperonyl butoxide
Uses: Scabicide, pediculicide
Accuretic 10/12.5:
quinapril 10 mg
hydrochlorthiazide 12.5 mg
Uses: Antihypertensive
Accuretic 20/12.5:
quinapril 20 mg
hydrochlorthiazide 12.5 mg
Uses: Antihypertensive
Accuretic 20/25:
quinapril 20 mg
hydrochlorthiazide 25 mg
Uses: Antihypertensive
Aceta-Gesic:
acetaminophen 325 mg
phenyltoloxamine 30 mg
Uses: Pain
Activella Tablets:
estriol 1 mg
norethindrone 0.5 mg
Uses: Vasomotor symptoms (menopause)
Actonel with Calcium:
calcium carbonate 1250 mg
risedronate 35 mg
Uses: Osteoporosis
Actoplus Met:
pioglitazone 15 mg
metformin 500 mg
pioglitazone 15 mg
metformin 850 mg
Uses: Type 2 diabetes
Adderall 5 mg:
dextroamphetamine sulfate 1.25 mg
dextroamphetamine saccharate 1.25 mg
amphetamine sulfate 1.25 mg
amphetamine aspartate 1.25 mg
Uses: CNS stimulant
Adderall 7.5 mg:
dextroamphetamine sulfate 1.875 mg
dextroamphetamine saccharate 1.875 mg
dextroamphetamine aspartate 1.875 mg
amphetamine sulfate 1.875 mg
Uses: CNS stimulant
Adderall 10 mg:
dextroamphetamine sulfate 5 mg
dextroamphetamine saccharate 2.5 mg
amphetamine sulfate 2.5 mg
amphetamine aspartate 2.5 mg
Uses: CNS stimulant
Adderall 12.5 mg:
dextroamphetamine sulfate 3.125 mg
dextroamphetamine saccharate 3.125 mg
dextroamphetamine aspartate 3.125 mg
amphetamine sulfate 3.125 mg
Uses: CNS stimulant
Adderall 15 mg:
dextroamphetamine sulfate 3.75 mg
dextroamphetamine saccharate 3.75 mg
dextroamphetamine aspartate 3.75 mg
amphetamine sulfate 3.75 mg
Uses: CNS stimulant
Adderall 20 mg:
dextroamphetamine sulfate 5 mg
dextroamphetamine saccharate 5 mg
amphetamine sulfate 5 mg
amphetamine aspartate 5 mg
Uses: CNS stimulant
Adderall 30 mg:
dextroamphetamine sulfate 7.5 mg
dextroamphetamine saccharate 7.5 mg
amphetamine sulfate 7.5 mg
amphetamine aspartate 7.5 mg
Uses: CNS stimulant

Adderall XR 5 mg:
dextroamphetamine sulfate 1.25 mg
dextroamphetamine saccharate 1.25 mg
amphetamine sulfate 1.25 mg
amphetamine aspartate 1.25 mg
Uses: CNS stimulant

Adderall XR 10 mg:
dextroamphetamine sulfate 2.5 mg
dextroamphetamine saccharate 2.5 mg
amphetamine sulfate 2.5 mg
amphetamine aspartate 2.5 mg
Uses: CNS stimulant

Adderall XR 15 mg:
dextroamphetamine sulfate 3.75 mg
dextroamphetamine saccharate 3.75 mg
amphetamine sulfate 3.75 mg
amphetamine aspartate 3.75 mg
Uses: CNS stimulant

Adderall XR 20 mg:
dextroamphetamine sulfate 5 mg
dextroamphetamine saccharate 5 mg
amphetamine sulfate 5 mg
amphetamine aspartate 5 mg
Uses: CNS stimulant

Adderall XR 25 mg:
dextroamphetamine sulfate 6.25 mg
dextroamphetamine saccharate 6.25 mg
amphetamine sulfate 6.25 mg
Uses: CNS stimulant

Adderall XR 30 mg:
dextroamphetamine sulfate 7.5 mg
dextroamphetamine saccharate 7.5 mg
amphetamine sulfate 7.5 mg
amphetamine aspartate 7.5 mg
Uses: CNS stimulant

Advair Diskus 100:
fluticasone 100 mcg
salmeterol 50 mcg
Uses: Corticosteroid, bronchodilator

Advair Diskus 250:
fluticasone 250 mcg
salmeterol 50 mcg
Uses: Corticosteroid, bronchodilator

Advair Diskus 500:
fluticasone 500 mcg
salmeterol 50 mcg
Uses: Corticosteroid, bronchodilator

Advicor 500:
niacin 500 mg
lovastatin 20 mg
Uses: Antilipidemic

Advicor 750:
niacin 750 mg
lovastatin 20 mg
Uses: Antilipidemic

Advicor 1000:
niacin 1000 mg
lovastatin 20 mg
niacin 1000 mg
lovastatin 40 mg
Uses: Antilipidemic

Advil Cold and Sinus Caplets:
pseudoephedrine 30 mg
ibuprofen 200 mg
Uses: Decongestant

Aggrenox:
200 mg ext rel dipyridamole
25 mg aspirin
Uses: Antiplatelet

AK-Cide Ophthalmic Suspension/ Ointment:
10% sulfacetamide sodium
0.5% prednisoLONE acetate
Uses: Ophthalmic antiinfective, antiinflammatory

Aldactazide 25/25:
spironolactone 25 mg
hydrochlorothiazide 25 mg
Uses: Diuretic

Aldactazide 50/50:
spironolactone 50 mg
hydrochlorothiazide 50 mg
Uses: Diuretic

Aldoril 15:
methyldopa 250 mg
hydrochlorothiazide 15 mg
Uses: Antihypertensive

Aldoril 25:
methyldopa 250 mg
hydrochlorothiazide 25 mg
Uses: Antihypertensive

Aldoril D30:
methyldopa 500 mg
hydrochlorothiazide 30 mg
Uses: Antihypertensive

Aldoril D50:
methyldopa 500 mg
hydrochlorothiazide 50 mg
Uses: Antihypertensive

Aleve Cold and Sinus:
naproxen 200 mg
ER pseudoephedrine 120 mg
Uses: Analgesic, adrenergic

Aleve Sinus and Headache:
naproxen 220 mg
ER pseudoephedrine 120 mg
Uses: Analgesic, adrenergic

Alka-Seltzer:
sodium bicarbonate 1916 mg
citric acid 1000 mg
aspirin 325 mg
Uses: Antacid, adsorbent, antiflatulent

Alka-Seltzer Plus Cold:
acetaminophen 250 mg
chlorpheniramine 2 mg
phenylephrine 5 mg
Uses: Decongestant, analgesic, antihistamine

Alka-Seltzer Plus Night-Time Cold Liqui-Gels:
doxylamine 6.25 mg
dextromethorphan 10 mg
pseudoephedrine 30 mg
acetaminophen 325 mg
Uses: Antitussive, decongestant, antihistamine, analgesic

Allegra-D:
fexofenadine 60 mg
pseudoephedrine 120 mg
Uses: Antihistamine, adrenergic

Allercon Tablets:
triprolidine 2.5 mg
pseudoephedrine 60 mg
Uses: Antihistamine, adrenergic

Allerest Maximum Strength:
pseudoephedrine 30 mg
chlorpheniramine 2 mg
Uses: Decongestant, antihistamine

Allerfrim Syrup:
Per 5 ml:
triprolidine 1.25 mg
pseudoephedrine 30 mg
Uses: Antihistamine, adrenergic

Allerfrim Tablets:
triprolidine 2.5 mg
pseudoephedrine 60 mg
Uses: Antihistamine, adrenergic

All-Nite Cold:
Per 15 ml:
pseudoephedrine 30 mg
doxylamine 6.25 mg
dextromethorphan 15 mg
acetaminophen 500 mg
Uses: Decongestant, antihistamine, analgesic

Alor 5/500:
hydrocodone 5 mg
aspirin 500 mg
Uses: Analgesic

Amaphen:
acetaminophen 325 mg
butalbital 50 mg
caffeine 40 mg
Uses: analgesic, barbiturates

Ambenyl Cough Syrup:
Per 5 ml:
bromodiphenhydramine 12.5 mg
codeine 10 mg
5% alcohol
Uses: Antihistamine, opioid analgesic

Anacin:
aspirin 400 mg
caffeine 32 mg
Uses: Analgesic

Anacin Maximum Strength:
aspirin 500 mg
caffeine 32 mg
Uses: Analgesic

Anacin PM Aspirin Free:
diphenhydrAMINE 25 mg
acetaminophen 500 mg
Uses: Analgesic

Anaplex DM:
Per 5 ml:
brompheniramine 4 mg
dextromethorphan 30 mg
pseudoephedrine 60 mg
Uses: Decongestant, antitussive, antihistamine

Anaplex DMX:
Per 5 ml:
brompheniramine 8 mg
dextromethorphan 60 mg
pseudoephedrine 90 mg
Uses: Decongestant, antitussive, antihistamine

Anaplex HD Oral Solution:
Per 5 ml:
hydrocodone 1.7 mg
brompheniramine 2 mg
pseudoephedrine 30 mg
Uses: Antihistamine, decongestant, analgesic

Angeliq:
drospirenone 0.5 mg
estradiol 1 mg
Uses: Vasomotor symptoms (menopause)

Apresazide 25/25:
hydrALAZINE 25 mg
hydrochlorothiazide 25 mg
Uses: Antihypertensive

Apresazide 50/50:
hydrALAZINE 50 mg
hydrochlorothiazide 50 mg
Uses: Antihypertensive

Apri 28-Day:
desorgestrel 0.15 mg
ethinyl estradiol 30 mcg
Uses: Estrogen, progestin

Arthrotec:
diclofenac 50 or 75 mg
misoprostol 200 mcg
Uses: NSAID, gastric protectant

Ascriptin:
aspirin 325 mg
magnesium hydroxide 50 mg
aluminum hydroxide 50 mg
calcium carbonate 50 mg
Uses: Nonopioid analgesic, antipyretic

Ascriptin A/D:
aspirin 325 mg
aluminum hydroxide 75 mg
magnesium hydroxide 75 mg
calcium carbonate 75 mg
Uses: Analgesic

Aspirin-Free Bayer Select Allergy Sinus:
pseudoephedrine 30 mg
chlorpheniramine 2 mg
acetaminophen 500 mg
Uses: Adrenergic, antihistamine, analgesic

Aspirin Free Excedrin:
acetaminophen 500 mg
caffeine 65 mg
Uses: Analgesic

Aspirin Free Excedrin Dual:
acetaminophen 500 mg
calcium carbonate 111 mg
magnesium carbonate 64 mg
magnesium oxide 30 mg
Uses: Analgesic, antacid

Atacand HCT 16:
candesartan 16 mg
hydrochlorthiazide 12.5 mg
Uses: Antihypertensive

Atacand HCT 32:
candesartan 32 mg
hydrochlorthiazide 12.5 mg
Uses: Antihypertensive

Atripla:
efavirenz 600 mg
emtricitabine 200 mg
tenofovir 300 mg
Uses: HIV

Augmentin 250:
amoxicillin 250 mg
clavulanic acid 125 mg
Uses: Antiinfective

Augmentin 500:
amoxicillin 500 mg
clavulanic acid 125 mg
Uses: Antiinfective

Augmentin 875:
amoxicillin 875 mg
clavulanic acid 125 mg
Uses: Antiinfective
Augmentin 125 Chewable:
amoxicillin 125 mg
clavulanic acid 31.25 mg
Uses: Antiinfective
Augmentin 200 Chewable:
amoxicillin 200 mg
clavulanic acid 28.5 mg
Uses: Antiinfective
Augmentin 250 Chewable:
amoxicillin 250 mg
clavulanic acid 62.5 mg
Uses: Antiinfective
Augmentin 125 mg/5 ml Suspension:
Per 5 ml:
amoxicillin 125 mg
clavulanic acid 31.25 mg
Uses: Antiinfective
Augmentin 200 mg/5 ml Suspension:
Per 5 ml:
amoxicillin 200 mg
clavulanic acid 28.5 mg
Uses: Antiinfective
Augmentin 250 mg/5 ml Suspension:
Per 5 ml:
amoxicillin 250 mg
clavulanic acid 62.5 mg
Uses: Antiinfective
Augmentin 400 mg/5 ml Suspension:
Per 5 ml:
amoxicillin 400 mg
clavulanic acid 57 mg
Uses: Antiinfective
Auralgan Otic Solution:
5.4% antipyrine
1.4% benzocaine
Uses: Otic analgesic
Avalide:
hydrochlorthiazide 12.5 mg
irbesartan 150 mg
Uses: Antihypertensive
Avalide 300:
hydrochlorthiazide 12.5 mg
irbesartan 300 mg
Uses: Antihypertensive
Avandamet:
rosiglitazone/metformin
1 mg/500 mg
2 mg/500 mg
2 mg/1000 mg
4 mg/500 mg
4 mg/1000 mg
Uses: Diabetes mellitus
Avandaryl 4/1:
rosiglitazone 4 mg
glimepiride 1 mg
Uses: Antidiabetic
Avandaryl 4/2:
rosiglitazone 4 mg
glimepiride 2 mg
Uses: Antidiabetic
Avandaryl 4/4:
rosiglitazone 4 mg
glimepiride 4 mg
Uses: Antidiabetic
Azor:
amlodipine 5 mg
olmesartan 20 mg
amlodipine 10 mg
olmesartan 20 mg
amlodipine 5 mg
olmesartan 40 mg
amlodipine 10 mg
olmesartan 40 mg
Uses: Hypertension
Bactrim:
trimethoprim 80 mg
sulfamethoxazole 400 mg
Uses: Antiinfective
Bactrim DS:
trimethoprim 160 mg
sulfamethoxazole 800 mg
Uses: Antiinfective
Bancap HC:
acetaminophen 500 mg
hydrocodone 5 mg
Uses: Analgesic
Bellatal:
phenobarbital 16.2 mg

hyoscyamine sulfate 0.1037 mg
atropine sulfate 0.0194 mg
scopolamine hydrobromide 0.0065 mg
Uses: Barbiturate, anticholinergic

Bellergal-S:
ergotamine 0.6 mg
belladonna alkaloids 0.2 mg
phenobarbital 40 mg
Uses: α-Adrenergic blocker, anticholinergic, barbiturate

Bel-Phen-Ergot-SR:
phenobarbital 40 mg
ergotamine tartrate 0.6 mg
belladonna alkaloids 0.2 mg
Uses: α-Adrenergic blocker, anticholinergic, barbiturate

Benadryl Allergy Decongestant Liquid:
Per 5 ml:
diphenhydrAMINE 12.5 mg
pseudoephedrine 30 mg
Uses: Antihistamine, adrenergic

Benadryl Allergy/Sinus Headache Caplets:
diphenhydrAMINE 12.5 mg
pseudoephedrine 30 mg
acetaminophen 500 mg
Uses: Antihistamine, adrenergic, analgesic

Benadryl Decongestant Allergy:
pseudoephedrine 60 mg
diphenhydrAMINE 25 mg
Uses: Adrenergic, antihistamine

Benylin Expectorant Liquid:
Per 5 ml:
dextromethorphan 5 mg
guaifenesin 100 mg
5% alcohol
Uses: Expectorant, antitussive

Benylin Multi-Symptom Liquid:
Per 5 ml:
dextromethorphan 5 mg
pseudoephedrine 15 mg
guaifenesin 100 mg
Uses: Antitussive, adrenergic, expectorant

BenzaClin:
clindamycin 10%
benzoyl peroxide 5%
Uses: Antiinfective

Benzamycin:
benzoyl peroxide 5%
erythromycin 3%
Uses: Antiinfective

Beta Tan Suspension:
Per 5 ml:
carbetapentane 30 mg
brompheniramine 4 mg
phenylephrine 7.5 mg
Uses: Antitussive

BiDil:
isosorbide 20 mg
hydrALAZINE 37.5 mg
Uses: Vasodilator

Blephamide Ophthalmic Suspension/ Ointment:
0.2% prednisoLONE
10% sodium sulfacetamide
Uses: Ophthalmic antiinfective, antiinflammatory

Butibel:
belladonna extract 15 mg
butabarbital 15 mg
Uses: Anticholinergic, barbiturate

Cafatine PB:
ergotamine 1 mg
caffeine 100 mg
belladonna alkaloids 0.125 mg
pentobarbital 30 mg
Uses: Migraine agent

Cafergot:
ergotamine 1 mg
caffeine 100 mg
Uses: Adrenergic blocker

Cafergot Suppositories:
ergotamine 2 mg
caffeine 100 mg
Uses: Adrenergic blocker

Caladryl:
8% calamine, camphor
2.2% alcohol
1% pramoxine
Uses: Topical antihistamine

Calcet:
calcium 152.8 mg
vitamin D 100 international units
Uses: Supplement

Caltrate 600+D:
vitamin D 200 international units
calcium 600 mg
Uses: Supplement

Cama Arthritis Pain Reliever:
aspirin 500 mg
magnesium oxide 150 mg
aluminum hydroxide 125 mg
Uses: Nonopioid analgesic, antacid

Capital w/Codeine:
Per 5 ml:
acetaminophen 120 mg
codeine 12 mg
Uses: Opioid analgesic

Capozide 25/15:
captopril 25 mg
hydrochlorothiazide 15 mg
Uses: Antihypertensive

Capozide 25/25:
captopril 25 mg
hydrochorothiazide 25 mg
Uses: Antihypertensive

Capozide 50/15:
captopril 50 mg
hydrochlorothiazide 15 mg
Uses: Antihypertensive

Capozide 50/25:
captopril 50 mg
hydrochlorothiazide 25 mg
Uses: Antihypertensive

Cardec DM Syrup:
Per 5 ml:
pseudoephedrine 60 mg
carbinoxamine 4 mg
dextromethorphan 15 mg
Uses: Adrenergic, antitussive

Cenafed Plus Tablets:
triprolidine 2.5 mg
pseudoephedrine 60 mg
Uses: Antihistamine, adrenergic

Cetapred Ophthalmic Ointment:
0.25% prednisoLONE
10% sodium sulfacetamide
Uses: Ophthalmic antiinfective, antiinflammatory

Cheracol Cough Syrup:
Per 5 ml:
codeine 10 mg
guaifenesin 100 mg
Uses: Analgesic, expectorant

Cheracol Syrup:
Per 5 ml:
codeine 10 mg
guaifenesin 100 mg
Uses: Analgesic, expectorant

Chromagen:
ferrous fumarate 66 mg
vitamin B_{12} 10 mcg
vitamin C 250 mg
intrinsic factor 100 mg
Uses: Supplement

Cipro HC Otic:
Per 1 ml:
ciprofloxacin 2 mg
hydrocortisone 10 mg
Uses: Antiinfective/antiinflammatory

Citracal+D:
calcium 315 mg
cholecalciferol 200 international units
Uses: Osteoporosis

Claritin-D 12 Hour:
loratidine 5 mg
pseudoephedrine 120 mg
Uses: Antihistamine, adrenergic

Claritin-D 24-Hour:
loratidine 10 mg
pseudoephedrine 240 mg
Uses: Antihistamine, adrenergic

Climara Pro (transdermal)
estradiol 0.045 mg
levonorgestrel 0.015 mg
Uses: Vasomotor symptoms (menopause)

Clindex:
chlordiazepoxide 5 mg
clidinium 2.5 mg
Uses: Antianxiety, anticholinergic

Clomycin Ointment:
bacitracin 500 units
neomycin sulfate 3.5 g
polymyxin B sulfate 500 units
lidocaine 40 mg
Uses: Antiinfective, local anesthetic

Co-Apap:
pseudoephedrine 30 mg
chlorpheniramine 2 mg
dextromethorphan 15 mg
acetaminophen 325 mg
Uses: Adrenergic, antihistamine, antitussive, analgesic

Co-Gesic:
acetaminophen 500 mg
hydrocodone 5 mg
Uses: Analgesic

Codeprex Extended Release Suspension:
Per 5 ml:
codeine 20 mg
chlorpheniramine 4 mg
Uses: Cough, rhinitis

Codiclear DH Syrup:
Per 5 ml:
hydrocodone 5 mg
guaifenesin 100 mg
Uses: Analgesic, expectorant

Codimal DH Syrup:
Per 5 ml:
hydrocodone 1.66 mg
phenylephrine 5 mg
pyrilamine 8.33 mg
Uses: Analgesic, adrenergic

Codimal DM Syrup:
Per 5 ml:
phenylephrine 5 mg
pyrilamine 8.33 mg
dextromethorphan 10 mg
Uses: Adrenergic, antitussive

ColBenemid:
probenecid 500 mg
colchicine 0.5 mg
Uses: Antigout agent

Coldrine:
pseudoephedrine 30 mg
acetaminophen 500 mg
Uses: Decongestant, nonopioid analgesic

Col-Probenecid:
probenecid 500 mg
colchicine 0.5 mg
Uses: Antigout

Coly-Mycin S Otic Suspension:
1% hydrocortisone
neomycin base 3.3 mg/ml
colistin 3 mg/ml
0.05% thonzonium bromide
Uses: Otic antiinfective

Combigan:
brimonidine 0.2%
timolol 0.5%
Uses: Glaucoma

CombiPatch 0.05/0.14:
estradiol 0.05 mg/day
norethindrone 0.14 mg/day
Uses: Hypoestrogenism

CombiPatch 0.05/0.25:
estradiol 0.05 mg/day
norethindrone 0.25 mg/day
Uses: Hypoestrogenism

Combivent:
ipratropium bromide 18 mcg
albuterol 103 mcg/actuation
Uses: Bronchodilator

Combivir:
lamivudine 150 mg
zidovudine 300 mg
Uses: HIV

Comvax:
Per 0.5 ml:
haeomophilus B conjugate 7.5 mcg
meningococcal protein 125 mcg
hepatitis B recombinant 5 mcg
Uses: Vaccine

Congestac:
guaifenesin 400 mg
pseudoephedrine 60 mg
Uses: Expectorant, decongestant

Contac Severe Cold & Flu:
chlorpheniramine 2 mg
acetaminophen 500 mg
pseudoephedrine 30 mg

dextromethorphan 15 mg
18.5% alcohol
Uses: Decongestant, antihistamine, antitussive, analgesic

Cortisporin Ophthalmic/Otic Suspension:
0.35% neomycin polymyxin B 10,000 units/ml
1% hydrocortisone
Uses: Ophthalmic antiinfective, antiinflammatory

Cortisporin Topical Cream:
0.5% neomycin sulfate
polymyxin B 10,000 units
0.5% hydrocortisone
Uses: Topical antiinfective

Cortisporin Topical Ointment:
0.5% neomycin sulfate
bacitracin 400 units
polymyxin B 5000 units
1% hydrocortisone
Uses: Topical antiinfective

Corzide 40/5:
nadolol 40 mg
bendroflumethiazide 5 mg
Uses: Antihypertensive

Corzide 80/5:
nadolol 80 mg
bendroflumethiazide 5 mg
Uses: Antihypertensive

Cosopt:
dorzolamide 2%
timolol 0.5%
Uses: Antihypertensive

Cough-X:
dextromethorphan 5 mg
benzocaine 2 mg
Uses: Antitussive, local anesthetic

Creon:
lipase 8000 units
amylase 30,000 units
protease 13,000 units
pancreatin 300 mg
Uses: Digestive enzyme

Cyclomydril Ophthalmic Solution:
0.2% cyclopentolate
1% phenylephrine
Uses: Mydriatic

Dallergy Tablets:
chlorpheniramine 4 mg
phenylephrine 10 mg
methscopolamine 1.25 mg
Uses: Antihistamine, adrenergic

Damason-P:
hydrocodone 5 mg
aspirin 500 mg
Uses: Analgesic

Darvocet-N 100:
propoxyphene-N 100 mg
acetaminophen 650 mg
Uses: Analgesic

Darvon Compound-65:
propoxyphene 65 mg
aspirin 389 mg
caffeine 32.4 mg
Uses: Analgesic

🍁 Darvon-N Compound:
aspirin 375 mg
propoxyphene 100 mg
caffeine 30 mg
Uses: Analgesic

🍁 Darvon-N w/A.S.A.:
aspirin 325 mg
propoxyphene 100 mg
Uses: Analgesic

Decadron Phosphate with Xylocaine:
Per ml:
dexamethasone 4 mg
lidocaine 10 mg
Uses: Local anesthetic

Deconamine:
pseudoephedrine 60 mg
chlorpheniramine 4 mg
Uses: Antihistamine, decongestant

Deconamine SR:
pseudoephedrine 120 mg
chlorpheniramine 8 mg
Uses: Antihistamine, decongestant

Deconamine Syrup:
Per 5 ml:
pseudoephedrine 30 mg

chlorpheniramine 2 mg
Uses: Antihistamine, decongestant

Demi-Regroton:
chlorthalidone 25 mg
reserpine 0.125 mg
Uses: Antihypertensive

Demulen 1/35:
ethinyl estradiol 35 mcg
ethynodiol diacetate 1 mg
Uses: Oral contraceptive

Demulen 1/50:
ethinyl estradiol 50 mcg
ethynodiol diacetate 1 mg
Uses: Oral contraceptive

Desogen:
ethinyl estradiol 30 mcg
desorgestrel 0.15 mg
Uses: Estrogen, progestin

Dexacidin Ophthalmic Ointment/ Suspension:
Per ml:
0.1% dexamethasone
0.35% neomycin
polymyxin B 10,000 units/g
Uses: Ophthalmic, antiinfective/ antiinflammatory

Dexasporin Ophthalmic Ointment:
Per gram:
0.1% dexamethasone
0.35% neomycin
polymyxin B 10,000 units
Uses: Ophthalmic, antiinfective/ antiinflammatory

DHC Plus:
dihydrocodeine 16 mg
acetaminophen 356.4 mg
caffeine 30 mg
Uses: Analgesic

Di-Gel Liquid:
Per 5 ml:
aluminum hydroxide 200 mg
magnesium hydroxide 200 mg
simethicone 20 mg
Uses: Antacid, adsorbent, antiflatulent

Dihistine DH Liquid:
Per 5 ml:
pseudoephedrine 30 mg
chlorpheniramine 2 mg
codeine 10 mg
Uses: Decongestant, antihistamine, analgesic

Dilaudid Cough Syrup:
Per 5 ml:
guaifenesin 100 mg
hydromorphone 1 mg
5% alcohol
Uses: Expectorant, analgesic

Diovan 80 HCT:
valsartan 80 mg
hydrochlorthiazide 12.5 mg
Uses: Antihypertensive

Diovan 160 HCT:
valsartan 160 mg
hydrochlorthiazide 12.5 mg
Uses: Antihypertensive

Diurigen w/Reserpine:
chlorothiazide 250 mg
reserpine 0.125 mg
Uses: Antihypertensive

Diutensen-R:
methylclothiazide 2.5 mg
reserpine 0.1 mg
Uses: Antihypertensive

Doan's PM Extra Strength:
magnesium salicylate 500 mg
diphenhydrAMINE 25 mg
Uses: Analgesic, antihistamine

Dolacet:
hydrocodone 5 mg
acetaminophen 500 mg
Uses: Analgesic

Donnatal:
phenobarbital 16.2 mg
hyoscyamine 0.1037 mg
atropine 0.0194 mg
scopolamine 0.0065 mg
Uses: Anticholinergic, barbiturate

Donnatal Elixir:
Per 5 ml:
phenobarbital 16.2 mg

hyoscyamine 0.1037 mg
atropine 0.0194 mg
scopolamine 0.0065 mg
23% alcohol
Uses: Anticholinergic, barbiturate

Donnatal Extentabs:
phenobarbital 48.6 mg
hyoscyamine 0.3111 mg
atropine 0.0582 mg
scopolamine 0.0195 mg
Uses: Anticholinergic, barbiturate

Donnazyme:
pancreatin 500 mg
lipase 1000 units
protease 12,500 units
amylase 12,500 units
Uses: Pancreatic enzymes

Dristan Cold Non-Drowsy:
pseudoephedrine 30 mg
acetaminophen 500 mg
Uses: Decongestant, analgesic

Dristan Cold Multi-Symptom Formula:
acetaminophen 325 mg
phenylephrine 5 mg
chlorpheniramine 2 mg
Uses: Analgesic, adrenergic, antihistamine

Drixoral Cold & Allergy:
pseudoephedrine 120 mg
dexbrompheniramine 6 mg
Uses: Decongestant, antihistamine

DT:
Per 5 ml:
diphtheria toxoid 2 LfU
tetanus toxoid 5 LfU
Uses: Vaccine

DTP:
Per 0.5 ml:
diphtheria toxoid 6.5 LfU
tetanus toxoid 5 LfU
pertussis 4 LfU
Uses: Vaccine

Duac:
benzoyl peroxide 5%
clindamycin 300 mg bulk powder
Uses: Antiinfective, topical

Duetact:
glimepiride 2 mg
pioglitazone 30 mg
glimepiride 4 mg
pioglitazone 30 mg
Uses: Antidiabetic

DuoDote:
atropine 21 mg
pralidoxine 0.7 ml
atropine 600 mg
pralidoxine 2 ml
Uses: Organophate toxicity

DuoNeb:
Per 3 ml:
albuterol 3 mg
ipratroprium 0.5 mg
Uses: Bronchodilator

Dura-Vent/DA:
phenylephrine 20 mg
chlorpheniramine 8 mg
methscopolamine 2.5 mg
Uses: Adrenergic, antihistamine

Durabac Forte:
acetaminophen 500 mg
caffeine 50 mg
magnesium salicylate 500 mg
phenyltoloxamine 20 mg
Uses: Analgesic, antihistamine

Duratuss AC 12:
Per 5 ml:
dextromethorphan 15 mg
diphenhydrAMINE 12.5 mg
phenylephrine 15 mg
Uses: Allergic rhinitis, common cold, flu

Dyazide:
hydrochlorothiazide 25 mg
triamterene 37.5 mg
Uses: Diuretic

Dylline-GG Tablets:
dyphylline 200 mg
guaifenesin 200 mg
Uses: Bronchodilator, expectorant

Dynafed Asthma Relief:
ephedrine 25 mg
guaifenesin 200 mg
Uses: Adrenergic, expectorant

Dynafed Plus Maximum Strength:
pseudoephedrine 30 mg
acetaminophen 500 mg
Uses: Decongestant, analgesic

Dynex 12:
Per 5 ml:
carbetapentane 22.5 mg
phenylephrine 9 mg
Uses: Antitussive, nasal decongestant

Dyphylline GG:
dyphylline 200 mg
guaifenesin 200 mg
Uses: Bronchodilator, expectorant

Elase Ointment:
Per gram:
fibrinolysin 1 unit
desoxyribonuclease 666.6 units
Uses: Enzyme

Elixophyllin GG Liquid:
Per 5 ml:
theophylline 100 mg
guaifenesin 100 mg
Uses: Expectorant, bronchodilator

Embeda:
morphine/naltrexone
100 mg/4 mg
80 mg/3.2 mg
60 mg/2.4 mg
50 mg/2 mg
30 mg/1.2 mg
20 mg/0.8 mg

EMLA Cream:
lidocaine 2.5 mg
prilocaine 2.5 mg
Uses: Local anesthetic

Empirin w/Codeine #3:
aspirin 325 mg
codeine phosphate 30 mg
Uses: Analgesic

Empirin w/Codeine #4:
aspirin 325 mg
codeine phosphate 60 mg
Uses: Analgesic

🍁 **Empracet-60:**
acetaminophen 300 mg
codeine 60 mg
Uses: Analgesic

Endocet:
acetaminophen 325 mg
oxycodone 5 mg
Uses: Analgesic

🍁 **Endodan:**
aspirin 325 mg
oxycodone 5 mg
Uses: Analgesic

Entex PSE:
pseudoephedrine 120 mg
guaifenesin 600 mg
Uses: Adrenergic, expectorant

Epifoam Aerosol Foam:
1% hydrocortisone
1% pramoxine
Uses: Topical corticosteroid

Epzicom:
abacavir 600 mg
lamivudine 300 mg
Uses: HIV infection

Eryzole:
Per 5 ml:
erythromycin 200 mg
sulfisoxazole 600 mg
Uses: Macrolide antiinfective

Esgic-Plus:
butalbital 50 mg
acetaminophen 500 mg
caffeine 40 mg
Uses: Barbiturate, analgesic

Esimil:
guanethidine 10 mg
hydrochlorothiazide 25 mg
Uses: Antihypertensive

Estratest:
esterified estrogens 1.25 mg
methyltestosterone 2.5 mg
Uses: Vasomotor symptoms (menopause)

Estratest HS:
esterified estrogens 1.25 mg
methyltestosterone 2.5 mg
Uses: Vasomotor symptoms (menopause)

Excedrin Extra Strength:
acetaminophen 250 mg

aspirin 250 mg
caffeine 65 mg
Uses: Analgesic

Excedrin Migraine:
aspirin 250 mg
acetaminophen 250 mg
caffeine 65 mg
Uses: Migraine agent

Excedrin P.M.:
acetaminophen 500 mg
diphenhydrAMINE citrate 38 mg
Uses: Analgesic, antihistamine

Exforge:
amlodipine 5 mg
valsartan 160 mg
amlodipine 5 mg
valsartan 320 mg
amlodipine 10 mg
valsartan 160 mg
amlodipine 10 mg
valsartan 320 mg
Uses: Hypertension

Extra Strength Alka-Seltzer:
aspirin 500 mg
citric acid 1000 mg
sodium bicarbonate 1985 mg
Uses: Analgesic

Fansidar:
sulfidoxine 500 mg
pyrimethamine 25 mg
Uses: Antimalarial

Fem-1:
acetaminophen 500 mg
pamabrom 25 mg
Uses: Nonopioid analgesic

Femhrt 1/5:
norethindrone 1 mg
ethinyl estradiol 5 mcg
norethindrone 1 mg
ethinyl estradiol 5 mcg
Uses: Vasomotor symptoms (menopause)

Ferro-Sequels:
docusate sodium 100 mg
ferrous fumarate 150 mg
Uses: Laxative, hematinic

Fioricet:
acetaminophen 325 mg
caffeine 40 mg
butalbital 50 mg
Uses: Analgesic, barbiturate

Fioricet w/Codeine:
acetaminophen 325 mg
caffeine 40 mg
butalbital 50 mg
codeine 30 mg
Uses: Analgesic, barbiturate

Fiorinal:
aspirin 325 mg
caffeine 40 mg
butalbital 50 mg
Uses: Analgesic, barbiturate

Fiorinal w/Codeine:
aspirin 325 mg
caffeine 40 mg
butalbital 50 mg
codeine 30 mg
Uses: Analgesic, barbiturate

FML-S Ophthalmic Suspension:
0.1% fluorometholone
10% sulfacetamide
Uses: Ophthalmic, antiinfective/antiinflammatory

Gas-Ban:
calcium carbonate 500 mg
simethicone 40 mg
Uses: Antiflatulent, antacid

Gaviscon:
magnesium trisilicate 20 mg
aluminum hydroxide 80 mg
Uses: Antacid, adsorbent, antiflatulent

Gaviscon Liquid:
Per 5 ml:
aluminum hydroxide 31.7 mg
magnesium carbonate 119.3 mg
Uses: Antacid, adsorbent, antiflatulent

Gelusil:
aluminum hydroxide 200 mg
magnesium hydroxide 200 mg
simethicone 25 mg
Uses: Antacid, adsorbent, antiflatulent

Genac Tablets:
triprolidine 2.5 mg
pseudoephedrine 60 mg
Uses: Antihistamine
Genatuss DM Syrup:
Per 5 ml:
guaifenesin 100 mg
dextromethorphan 10 mg
Uses: Expectorant, antitussive
Glucovance 1.25:
glyBURIDE: 1.25 mg
metformin: 250 mg
Uses: Antidiabetic
Glucovance 2.50:
glyBURIDE: 2.5 mg
metformin: 500 mg
Uses: Antidiabetic
Glucovance 5:
glyBURIDE: 5 mg
metformin: 500 mg
Uses: Antidiabetic
Guaifenex PSE 60:
pseudoephedrine 60 mg
guaifenesin 600 mg
Uses: Decongestant, expectorant
Guaifenex PSE 120:
pseudoephedrine 120 mg
guaifenesin 600 mg
Uses: Decongestant, expectorant
Guiatuss AC:
Per 5 ml:
codeine 10 mg
guafenesin 100 mg
Uses: Analgesic, expectorant
Haley's M-O Liquid:
Per 15 ml:
magnesium hydroxide 900 mg
mineral oil 3.75 ml
Uses: Laxative
Halotussin-DM Sugar Free Liquid:
Per 5 ml:
guaifenesin 100 mg
dextromethorphan 10 mg
Uses: Expectorant, antitussive
Helidac:
In a compliance package:
bismuth subsalicylate 262.4-mg tabs
metronidazole 250-mg tabs
tetracycline 500-mg caps
Uses: Antiinfective
Humalog KwikPen Mix 50/50:
Per 1 ml:
insulin lispro protamine 50 units
insulin lispro 50 units
Uses: Antidiabetic
Humalog KwikPen Mix 75/25:
Per 1 ml:
insulin lispro protamine 75 units
insulin lispro 25 units
Uses: Antidiabetic
Humalog Mix 50/50:
insulin lispro protamine 50 units
insulin lispro (rDNA) 50 units
Uses: Antidiabetic
Humalog Mix 75/25:
insulin lispro protamine 75 units
insulin lispro (rDNA) 25 units
Uses: Antidiabetic
Humibid DM Pediatric:
dextromethorphan 15 mg
guaifenesin 300 mg
Uses: Expectorant, antitussive
Humibid DM Tablets:
dextromethorphan 30 mg
guaifenesin 600 mg
Uses: Expectorant, antitussive
HycoClear Tuss:
Per 5 ml:
hydrocodone 5 mg
guaifenesin 100 mg
Uses: Analgesic, expectorant
Hycodan:
hydrocodone 5 mg
homatropine 1.5 mg
Uses: Analgesic, mydriatic
Hycodan Syrup:
Per 5 ml:
hydrocodone 5 mg
homatropine 1.5 mg
Uses: Analgesic, mydriatic
Hycomine Compound:
chlorpheniramine 2 mg

acetaminophen 250 mg
phenylephrine 10 mg
hydrocodone 5 mg
caffeine 30 mg
Uses: Antihistamine, analgesic, adrenergic

Hycotuss Expectorant Syrup:
Per 5 ml:
guaifenesin 100 mg
hydrocodone 5 mg
10% alcohol
Uses: Expectorant

Hydrocet:
hydrocodone 5 mg
acetaminophen 500 mg
Uses: Opioid analgesic

Hydrogesic:
hydrocodone 5 mg
acetaminophen 500 mg
Uses: Opioid analgesic

Hydropres-50:
hydrochlorothiazide 50 mg
reserpine 0.125 mg
Uses: Antihypertensive

Hyzaar:
losartan potassium 50 mg
hydrochlorothiazide 12.5 mg
potassium 4.24 mg
Uses: Antihypertensive

Ibudone:
ibuprofen 200 mg
hydrocodone 10 mg
ibuprofen 200 mg
hydrocodone 5 mg
Uses: Analgesic

Imodium Advanced:
loperamide 2 mg
simethicone 125 mg
Uses: Antidiarrheal, antiflatulent

Innovar:
Per ml:
droperidol 2.5 mg
fentanyl 0.05 mg
Uses: Opioid analgesic, general anesthetic

Iofed:
brompheniramine 12 mg
pseudoephedrine 120 mg
Uses: Antihistamine, adrenergic

Iofed PD:
brompheniramine 6 mg
pseudoephedrine 60 mg
Uses: Antihistamine, adrenergic

Janumet:
metformin 500 mg
sitagliptan 50 mg
metformin 1000 mg
sitagliptan 50 mg
Uses: Antidiabetic

Kaletra Capsules:
lopinavir 133.3 mg
ritonavir 33.3 mg
Uses: HIV

Kaletra Solution:
Per 1 ml:
lopinavir 80 mg
ritonavir 20 mg
Uses: HIV

Kaletra Tablets
lopinavir 200 mg
ritonavir 50 mg
Uses: HIV

Lactinex:
Mixed culture of:
Lactobacillus acidophilus and
Lactobacillus bulgaricus
Uses: Supplement

Levell 12.5 ml Suspension:
carbetapentane 30 mg
phenylephrine 30 mg
Uses: Antitussive

Levlite:
levonorgestrel 0.100 mg
ethinyl estradiol 20 mcg
Uses: Estrogen, progestin

Levsin PB Drops:
Per ml:
hyoscyamine 0.125 mg
phenobarbital 15 mg
5% alcohol
Uses: Anticholinergic, barbiturate

Levsin w/Phenobarbital:
hyoscyamine 0.125 mg

phenobarbital 15 mg
Uses: Anticholinergic, barbiturate

Lexxel 1:
enalapril 5 mg
felodipine 5 mg
Uses: Antihypertensive

Lexxel 2:
enalapril 5 mg
felodipine 2.5 mg
Uses: Antihypertensive

Librax:
chlordiazepoxide 5 mg
clidinium 2.5 mg
Uses: Antianxiety, anticholinergic

Lida-Mantel-HC-Cream:
0.5% hydrocortisone
3% lidocaine
Uses: Antiinflammatory, analgesic

Limbitrol DS 10-25:
chlordiazepoxide 10 mg
amitriptyline 25 mg
Uses: Antidepressant, antianxiety

Lobac:
salicylamide 200 mg
phenyltoloxamine 20 mg
acetaminophen 300 mg
Uses: Skeletal muscle relaxant, analgesic

Loestrin Fe 1/20:
norethindrone acetate 1 mg/tablet
ethinyl estradiol 20 mcg/tablet
with 7 tablets of ferrous fumarate
75 mg/container
Uses: Oral contraceptive

Loestrin Fe 1.5/30:
norethindrone acetate 1.5 mg
ethinyl estradiol 30 mcg
Uses: Oral contraceptive

Lomotil:
diphenoxylate 2.5 mg
atropine 0.025 mg
Uses: Antidiarrheal, anticholinergic

Lomotil Liquid:
Per 5 ml:
diphenoxylate 2.5 mg
atropine 0.025 mg
Uses: Antidiarrheal, anticholinergic

Lo Ovral:
ethinyl estradiol 30 mcg
norgestrel 0.3 mg
Uses: Oral contraceptive

Lopressor HCT 50/25:
metoprolol 50 mg
hydrochlorothiazide 25 mg
Uses: Antihypertensive

Lopressor HCT 100/25:
metoprolol 100 mg
hydrochlorothiazide 25 mg
Uses: Antihypertensive

Lopressor HCT 100/50:
metoprolol 100 mg
hydrochlorothiazide 50 mg
Uses: Antihypertensive

Lorcet 10/650:
acetaminophen 650 mg
hydrocodone 10 mg
Uses: Analgesic

Lorcet-HD:
hydrocodone 10 mg
acetaminophen 300 mg
Uses: Analgesic

Lorcet Plus:
acetaminophen 650 mg
hydrocodone 7.5 mg
Uses: Analgesic

Lortab 2.5/500:
hydrocodone 2.5 mg
acetaminophen 500 mg
Uses: Analgesic

Lortab 5/500:
hydrocodone 5 mg
acetaminophen 500 mg
Uses: Analgesic

Lortab 7.5/500:
hydrocodone 7.5 mg
acetaminophen 500 mg
Uses: Analgesic

Lortab 10/500:
hydrocodone 10 mg
acetaminophen 500 mg
Uses: Analgesic

Lortab Oral Sol:
Per 15 ml:
hydrocodone 7.5 mg
acetaminophen 500 mg
Uses: Analgesic
LoSeasonique:
ethinyl estradiol 0.02 mg
levonorgestrel 0.1 mg
Uses: Oral contraceptive
Losec 1-2-3A ✦:
omeprazole 20 mg
clarithromycin 500 mg
amoxicillin 1 g
Uses: Antiinfective
Losec 1-2-3M ✦:
omeprazole 20 mg
clarithromycin 250 mg
metronidazole 500 mg
Uses: Antiinfective
Lotrel 10/20:
amlopidine 10 mg
benazepril 20 mg
Uses: Antihypertensive
Lotrel 10/40:
amlopidine 10 mg
benazepril 40 mg
Uses: Antihypertensive
Lotrisone Topical:
0.05% betamethasone
1% clotrimazole
Uses: Local antiinfective, antiinflammatory
Lufyllin-EPG Elixir:
Per 5 ml:
dyphylline 150 mg
ephedrine 24 mg
guaifenesin 300 mg
phenobarbital 24 mg
Uses: Bronchodilator, expectorant
Lufyllin-GG:
dyphylline 200 mg
guaifenesin 200 mg
Uses: Bronchodilator, expectorant
Lunelle Monthly Contraceptive Injection:
25 mg medroxyprogesterone
5 mg estradiol/0.5 ml
Uses: Contraceptive
Lybrel:
ethinyl estridiol 20 mcg
levonorgestrel 90 mcg
Uses: Continuous contraceptive
M-M-R-II:
measles
mumps
rubella
Uses: Vaccine, toxoid
Maalox:
aluminum hydroxide 200 mg
magnesium hydroxide 200 mg
Uses: Antacid, adsorbent, antiflatulent
Maalox Extra Strength Suspension:
Per 5 ml:
aluminum hydroxide 500 mg
magnesium hydroxide 450 mg
simethicone 40 mg
Uses: Antacid, adsorbent, antiflatulent
Maalox Plus:
aluminum hydroxide 200 mg
magnesium hydroxide 200 mg
simethicone 25 mg
Uses: Antacid, adsorbent, antiflatulent
Maalox Suspension:
Per 5 ml:
aluminum hydroxide 225 mg
magnesium hydroxide 200 mg
Uses: Antacid, adsorbent, antiflatulent
Macrobid:
nitrofurantoin macrocrystals 25 mg
nitrofurantoin monohydrate 75 mg
Uses: Antiinfective
Malarone:
250 mg atovaquone
100 mg proguanil
Uses: Malaria
Malarone Pediatric:
62.5 mg atovaquone
25 mg proguanil
Uses: Malaria
Mapap Cold Formula:
acetaminophen 325 mg
chlorpheniramine 2 mg

pseudoephedrine 30 mg
dextromethorphan 15 mg
Uses: Bronchodilator, expectorant

Maxitrol Ophthalmic Suspension/ Ointment:
Per ml:
0.35% neomycin
0.1% dexamethasone
polymyxin B 10,000 units
Uses: Ophthalmic antiinfective, antiinflammatory

Maxzide:
hydrochlorothiazide 50 mg
triamterene 75 mg
Uses: Antihypertensive, diuretic

Maxzide-25 MG:
hydrochlorothiazide 25 mg
triamterene 37.5 mg
Uses: Diuretic

Medigesic:
acetaminophen 325 mg
caffeine 40 mg
butalbital 50 mg
Uses: Nonopioid analgesic

Mepergan Fortis:
meperidine 50 mg
promethazine 25 mg
Uses: Analgesic, antihistamine

Mepergan Injection:
meperidine 25 mg
promethazine 25 mg
Uses: Analgesic

Metaglip 2.5:
glipiZIDE/metformin 2.5 mg/250 mg, 2.5 mg/500 mg, 5 mg/500 mg
Uses: Diabetes mellitus

Metimyd Ophthalmic Suspension/ Ointment:
0.5% prednisoLONE
10% sodium sulfacetamide
Uses: Ophthalmic antiinfective, antiinflammatory

Micardis HCT 40/12.5:
telmesartan 40 mg
hydrochlorthiazide 12.5 mg
Uses: Antihypertensive

Micardis HCT 80/12.5:
telmesartan 80 mg
hydrochlorthiazide 12.5 mg
Uses: Antihypertensive

Micardis HCT 80/25:
telmesartan 80 mg
hydrochlorothiazide 25 mg
Uses: Antihypertensive

Microgestin Fe 1/20:
norethindrone 1 mg
ethinyl estradiol 20 mcg
ferrous fumarate 75 mg in container
Uses: Estrogen, progestin

Microgestin Fe 1.5/30:
norethindrone 1.5 mg
ethinyl estradiol 30 mcg
ferrous fumarate 75 mg in container
Uses: Estrogen, progestin

Midol Multi-Symptom Menstrual Complete:
acetaminophen 500 mg
pyrilamine 15 mg
caffeine 60 mg
Uses: Analgesic

Midol PMS:
acetaminophen 500 mg
pyrilamine 15 mg
pamabrom 25 mg
Uses: Analgesic

Midol, Teen:
acetaminophen 400 mg
pamabrom 25 mg
Uses: Analgesic

Midrin:
isometheptene 65 mg
acetaminophen 325 mg
dichloralphenazone 100 mg
Uses: Analgesic

Moduretic:
hydrochlorothiazide 50 mg
amiloride 5 mg
Uses: Diuretic

Monopril-HCT 10:
fosinopril 10 mg
hydrochlorthiazine 12.5 mg
Uses: Antihypertensive

Monopril-HCT 20:
fosinopril 20 mg
hydrochlorthiazine 12.5 mg
Uses: Antihypertensive

Motrin Children's Cold Suspension:
Per 5 ml:
ibuprofen 100 mg
pseudoephedrine 15 mg
Uses: Nonopioid analgesic, decongestant

Motrin Sinus Headache:
pseudoephedrine 30 mg
ibuprofen 200 mg
Uses: Adrenergic, analgesic

Mucinex D:
guaifenesin/pseudoephedrine 1200 mg/120 mg, 600 mg/60 mg
Uses: Expectorant, decongestant

Mucinex DM:
dextromethorphan 30 mg
guaifenesin 600 mg
Uses: Antitussive, expectorant

Murocoll-2 Ophthalmic Drops:
0.3% scopolamine
10% phenylephrine
Uses: Ophthalmic anticholinergic, mydriatic

Mycolog II Topical:
Per gram:
0.1% triamcinolone acetonide
nystatin 100,000 units
Uses: Local antiinfective, antiinflammatory

Mylanta:
aluminum hydroxide 200 mg
magnesium hydroxide 200 mg
simethicone 20 mg
Uses: Antacid, adsorbent, antiflatulent

Mylanta Double Strength Liquid:
Per 5 ml:
aluminum hydroxide 400 mg
magnesium hydroxide 400 mg
simethicone 40 mg
Uses: Antacid, adsorbent, antiflatulent

Mylanta Gelcaps:
calcium carbonate 311 mg
magnesium carbonate 232 mg
Uses: Antacid, adsorbent, antiflatulent

Naphcon-A Ophthalmic Solution:
0.25% naphazoline
0.3% pheniramine
Uses: Ophthalmic vasoconstrictor

Nasatab LA:
guaifenesin 500 mg
pseudoephedrine 120 mg
Uses: Expectorant, decongestant

NeoDecadron Ophthalmic Ointment:
0.35% neomycin
0.05% dexamethasone
Uses: Ophthalmic antiinfective, antiinflammatory

NeoDecadron Ophthalmic Solution:
0.35% neomycin
0.1% dexamethasone
Uses: Ophthalmic antiinfective, antiinflammatory

Neosporin Cream:
Per gram:
polymyxin B 10,000 units
neomycin 3.5 mg
Uses: Topical antiinfective

Neosporin G.U. Irrigant:
Per ml:
neomycin 40 mg
polymyxin B 200,000 units
Uses: Antiinfective

Neosporin Ophthalmic Ointment:
Per gram:
neomycin 3.5 mg
polymyxin B 10,000 units
bacitracin zinc 400 units
Uses: Ophthalmic antiinfective

Neosporin Ophthalmic Solution:
Per ml:
neomycin 1.75 mg
polymyxin B 10,000 units
gramicidin 0.025 mg
Uses: Ophthalmic antiinfective

Neosporin Plus Cream:
polymyxin B 10,000 units
neomycin 3.5 mg
lidocaine 40 mg
Uses: Topical antiinfective

Neosporin Topical Ointment:
Per gram:
polymyxin B 5000 units
bacitracin zinc 400 units
neomycin 3.5 mg
Uses: Topical antiinfective

Niferex-150 Forte:
ferrous sulfate 150 mg
vitamin B_{12} 25 mcg
folic acid 1 mg
Uses: Supplement

Norco:
hydrocodone 10 mg
acetaminophen 325 mg
Uses: Analgesic, opioid, nonopioid

Norco 5/325:
hydrocodone 5 mg
acetaminophen 325 mg
Uses: Analgesic, opioid, nonopioid

Norgesic:
orphenadrine 25 mg
aspirin 385 mg
caffeine 30 mg
Uses: Skeletal muscle relaxant, analgesic

Norgesic Forte:
orphenadrine 50 mg
aspirin 770 mg
caffeine 60 mg
Uses: Skeletal muscle relaxant, analgesic

Novacet Lotion:
sodium sulfacetamine 10%
sulfur 5%
Uses: Acne agent

Novafed A:
pseudoephedrine 120 mg
chlorpheniramine 8 mg
Uses: Adrenergic, antihistamine

Novo-Gesic ✤C8:
acetaminophen 300 mg
codeine 8 mg
caffeine 15 mg
Uses: Analgesic

Novolog Mix 50/50:
insulin aspart 500 mg/1 ml
insulin aspart protamine 500 mg/1 ml
Uses: Antidiabetic

NuLytely:
PEG 3350/420 g
sodium bicarbonate 5.72 g
sodium chloride 11.2 g
potassium chloride 1.48 g
Uses: Laxative

NuvaRing:
ethinyl estradiol 0.015 mg/24 hr
etonogestrel 0.12 mg/24 hr
Uses: Contraceptive

Octicair Otic Suspension:
1% hydrocortisone
neomycin 5 mg/ml
polymyxin B 10,000 units/ml
Uses: Otic antiinflammatory, antiinfective

Opcon-A Ophthalmic Solution:
0.027% naphazoline
0.315% pheniramine
Uses: Ophthalmic vasoconstrictor

Ornade Spansules:
phenylpropanolamine 75 mg
chlorpheniramine 12 mg
Uses: Antihistamine, decongestant

Ornex:
pseudoephedrine 30 mg
acetaminophen 500 mg
Uses: Adrenergic, analgesic

Ornex No Drowsiness Caplets:
acetaminophen 325 mg
pseudoephedrine 30 mg
Uses: Adrenergic, analgesic

Orphengesic:
orphenadrine 25 mg
aspirin 385 mg
caffeine 30 mg
Uses: Analgesic

Orphengesic Forte:
orphenadrine 50 mg
aspirin 770 mg
caffeine 60 mg
Uses: Analgesic

Ortho-cept:
ethinyl estradiol 30 mcg
desogestrel 0.15 mg
Uses: Oral contraceptive

Ortho-cyclen:
ethinyl estradiol 35 mcg
norgestimate 0.25 mg
Uses: Oral contraceptive

Ortho-Prefest:
estradiol 1 mg (15)
norgestimate 0.09 mg (15)
Uses: Vasomotor symptoms (menopause)

Ovcon-50:
ethinyl estradiol 50 mcg
norethindrone 1 mg
Uses: Oral contraceptive

🍁 **Oxycocet:**
acetaminophen 325 mg
oxycodone 5 mg
Uses: Analgesic

P-A-C Analgesic:
aspirin 400 mg
caffeine 32 mg
Uses: Nonopioid analgesic

Pain-X Topical:
0.05% capsaicin
5% menthol
4% camphor
Uses: Topical analgesic

Pamprin Cramp:
acetaminophen 250 mg
pamabrom 25 mg
magnesium salicylate 250 mg
Uses: Analgesic

Pamprin Multi-Symptom:
acetaminophen 500 mg
pamabrom 25 mg
pyrilamine 15 mg
Uses: Analgesic

Panacet 5/500:
hydrocodone 5 mg
acetaminophen 500 mg
Uses: Analgesic

Panasal 5/500:
hydrocodone 5 mg
aspirin 500 mg
Uses: Analgesic

Pancrease Capsules:
amylase 20,000 units
protease 25,000 units
lipase 4500 units (microspheres)
Uses: Digestive enzyme

Pedia Care NightRest Cough-Cold Liquid:
Per 5 ml:
pseudoephedrine 15 mg
chlorpheniramine 1 mg
dextromethorphan 7.5 mg
Uses: Adrenergic, antihistamine, antitussive

Pediazole Suspension:
Per 5 ml:
erythromycin 200 mg
sulfiSOXAZOLE 600 mg
Uses: Antiinfective

Pepcid Complete:
calcium carbonate 800 mg
magnesium hydroxide 165 mg
famotidine 10 mg
Uses: Antiulcer agent

Percocet 2.5/325:
oxycodone 2.5 mg
acetaminophen 325 mg
Uses: Analgesic

Percocet 5/325:
oxycodone 5 mg
acetaminophen 325 mg
Uses: Analgesic

Percocet 7.5/500:
oxycodone 7.5 mg
acetaminophen 500 mg
Uses: Analgesic

Percocet 10/650:
oxycodone 10 mg
acetaminophen 650 mg
Uses: Analgesic

Percodan:
oxycodone 4.88 mg
aspirin 325 mg
Uses: Analgesic

Percogesic:
phenyltoloxamine 30 mg
acetaminophen 325 mg
Uses: Analgesic

Perdiem Granules:
Per teaspoon:
senna 0.74 g
psyllium 3.25 g
sodium 1.8 mg
potassium 35.5 mg
Uses: Laxative

Peri-Colace:
docusate sodium 100 mg
casanthranol 30 mg
Uses: Laxative

Peri-Colace Syrup:
Per 15 ml:
docusate sodium 60 mg
casanthranol 30 mg
Uses: Laxative

Phenerbel-S:
ergotamine tartrate 0.6 mg
belladonna alkaloids 0.2 mg
phenobarbital 40 mg
Uses: α-Adrenergic blocker, anticholinergic

Phenergan VC Syrup:
Per 5 ml:
phenylephrine 5 mg
promethazine 6.25 mg
Uses: Adrenergic, antihistamine

Phenergan VC w/Codeine Syrup:
Per 5 ml:
phenylephrine 5 mg
promethazine 6.25 mg
codeine 10 mg
Uses: Adrenergic, antihistamine, opioid analgesic

Phenergan w/Codeine Syrup:
Per 5 ml:
promethazine 6.25 mg
codeine 10 mg
Uses: Antihistamine, analgesic

Phenflu G:
acetaminophen 500 mg
dextromethorphan 30 mg
guaifenesin 600 mg
phenylephrine 15 mg
Uses: Analgesic, antitussive, expectorant, decongestant

Polaramine Expectorant Liquid:
Per 5 ml:
guaifenesin 100 mg
dexchlorpheniramine 2 mg
pseudoephedrine 20 mg
7.5% alcohol
Uses: Expectorant

Polycitra Syrup:
Per 5 ml:
potassium citrate 550 mg
sodium citrate 500 mg
citric acid 334 mg
Uses: Laxative

Poly-Histine Elixir:
Per 5 ml:
pheniramine 4 mg
pyrilamine 4 mg
phenyltoloxamine 4 mg
4% alcohol
Uses: Antihistamine

Polysporin Ophthalmic Ointment:
Per gram:
polymyxin B 10,000 units
bacitracin zinc 500 units
Uses: Ophthalmic antiinfective

Polysporin Topical Ointment:
Per gram:
polymyxin B 10,000 units
bacitracin zinc 500 units
Uses: Topical antiinfective

Polytrim Ophthalmic Solution:
Per ml:
trimethoprim 1 mg
polymyxin B 10,000 units
Uses: Ophthalmic antiinfective

PrandiMet:
metformin 500 mg
repaglinide 1 mg
metformin 500 mg
repaglinide 2 mg
Uses: Antidiabetic

Pravigard PAC:
aspirin 81 mg
pravastatin 20, 40, 80 mg
aspirin 325 mg

pravastatin 20, 40, 80 mg
Uses: Antihyperlipidemic, antithrombotic

Prefest:
estradiol 1 mg
norgestimate 0.09 mg
Uses: Vasomotor symptoms (menopause)

Premphase:
In a compliance package:
conjugated estrogens 0.625 mg
medroxyPROGESTERone 5 mg
Uses: Vasomotor symptoms (menopause)

Prempro:
In a compliance package:
conjugated estrogens 0.3 mg
medroxyPROGESTERone 1.5 mg
conjugated estrogens 0.45 mg
medroxyPROGESTERone 1.5 mg
conjugated estrogens 0.625 mg
medroxyPROGESTERone 2.5 mg
conjugated estrogens 0.625 mg
medroxyPROGESTERone 5 mg
Uses: Vasomotor symptoms (menopause)

Premsyn PMS:
acetaminophen 500 mg
pamabrom 25 mg
pyrilamine 15 mg
Uses: Analgesic

Prevpac:
In a compliance package:
amoxicillin 500-mg caps
clarithromycin 500-mg tabs
lansoprazole 30-mg caps
Uses: Antiinfective

Primaxin 250 mg IV for Injection:
imipenem 250 mg
cilastatin sodium 250 mg
Uses: Antiinfective

Primaxin 500 mg IV for Injection:
imipenem 500 mg
cilastatin sodium 500 mg
Uses: Antiinfective

Prinzide 10-12.5:
lisinopril 10 mg
hydrochlorothiazide 12.5 mg
Uses: Antihypertensive

Prinzide 20-12.5:
lisinopril 20 mg
hydrochlorothiazide 12.5 mg
Uses: Antihypertensive

Prinzide 20-25:
lisinopril 20 mg
hydrochlorothiazide 25 mg
Uses: Antihypertensive

Proben-C:
colchicine 0.5 mg
probenecid 500 mg
Uses: Antigout agent

Proctofoam-HC Aerosol Foam:
1% hydrocortisone
1% pramoxine
Uses: Topical corticosteroid

Pronto Plus Lice Killing Shampoo:
piperonyl butoxide 4%
pyrethrum extract 0.33%
Uses: Lice

Propacet 100:
propoxyphene-N 100 mg
acetaminophen 650 mg
Uses: Analgesic

Pseudo-Chlor:
pseudoephedrine 120 mg
chlorpheniramine 8 mg
Uses: Antihistamine

Pseudo-Gest Plus:
pseudoephedrine 60 mg
chlorpheniramine 4 mg
Uses: Antihistamine

Pylera:
bismuth subcitrate potassium 140 mg
metronidazole 125 mg
tetracycline 125 mg
Uses: Helicobacter pylori

Pyrlex CB:
Suspension per 5 ml:
carbetapentane 22.5 mg
pyrilamine 12 mg
Uses: Cough

Quadrinal:
ephedrine 24 mg
theophylline 65 mg
potassium iodide 320 mg

phenobarbital 24 mg
Uses: Adrenergic, bronchodilator, barbiturate

Quibron-300:
theophylline 300 mg
guaifenesin 180 mg
Uses: Bronchodilator, expectorant

Rebetron:
interferon alfa-2b 3 million units/0.5 ml
ribavirin, PO 200 mg
Uses: Biologic response modifier, antiviral

Regulace:
docusate sodium 100 mg
casanthranol 30 mg
Uses: Laxative

Renese-R:
polythiazide 2 mg
reserpine 0.25 mg
Uses: Diuretic, antihypertensive

Respahist:
pseudoephedrine 60 mg
brompheniramine 6 mg
Uses: Adrenergic, antihistamine

Respaire-60:
guaifenesin 200 mg
pseudoephedrine 60 mg
Uses: Expectorant, adrenergic

Respi-TANN:
Per 5 ml:
carbetapentane 20 mg
pseudoephedrine 30 mg
Uses: Cough suppressant, decongestant

Respi-TANN Pd:
Per 5 ml:
carbetapentane 7.5 mg
pseudoephedrine 30 mg
Uses: Cough suppressant, decongestant

Rifamate:
isoniazid 150 mg
rifampin 300 mg
Uses: Antitubercular, antileprotic

Rifater:
rifampin 120 mg
isoniazid 50 mg
pyrazinamide 300 mg
Uses: Antitubercular

Riopan Plus Suspension:
Per 5 ml:
magaldrate 540 mg
simethicone 40 mg
Uses: Antacid, adsorbent, antiflatulent

Robaxisal:
methocarbamol 400 mg
aspirin 325 mg
Uses: Skeletal muscle relaxant, analgesic

Robitussin-DM Liquid:
Per 5 ml:
guaifenesin 100 mg
dextromethorphan 10 mg
Uses: Expectorant, antitussive

Rolaids Calcium Rich:
magnesium hydroxide 80 mg
calcium carbonate 412 mg
Uses: Antacid, adsorbent, antiflatulent

Rondec:
pseudoephedrine 60 mg
carbinoxamine 4 mg
Uses: Adrenergic

Rondec DM Drops:
Per ml:
pseudoephedrine 25 mg
carbinoxamine 2 mg
dextromethorphan 4 mg
Uses: Adrenergic, antitussive

Rondec DM Syrup:
Per 5 ml:
pseudoephedrine 60 mg
carbinoxamine 4 mg
dextromethorphan 15 mg
Uses: Adrenergic, antitussive

Rondec Oral Drops:
Per 5 ml:
pseudoephedrine 25 mg
carbinoxamine 2 mg
Uses: Adrenergic

Roxicet 5/325:
acetaminophen 325 mg
oxycodone 5 mg
Uses: Opioid analgesic

Roxicet 5/500:
oxycodone 5 mg
acetaminophen 500 mg
Uses: Opioid analgesic

Roxicet Oral Solution:
Per 5 ml:
acetaminophen 325 mg
oxycodone 5 mg
Uses: Analgesic

Roxiprin:
aspirin 325 mg
oxycodone HCl 4.5 mg
oxycodone terephthalate 0.38 mg
Uses: Analgesic

Salutensin Demi:
hydroflumethiazide 25 mg
reserpine 0.125 mg
Uses: Antihypertensive

Sedapap-10:
acetaminophen 650 mg
butalbital 50 mg
Uses: Analgesic, barbiturate

Semprex-D:
acrivastine 8 mg
pseudoephedrine 60 mg
Uses: Adrenergic, bronchodilator

Senokot-S:
docusate 50 mg
senna concentrate 187 mg
Uses: Laxative

Septra:
sulfamethoxazole 400 mg
trimethroprim 80 mg
Uses: Antiinfective

Septra DS:
sulfamethoxazole 800 mg
trimethroprim 160 mg
Uses: Antiinfective

Ser-Ap-Es:
hydrochlorothiazide 15 mg
reserpine 0.1 mg
hydrALAZINE 25 mg
Uses: Diuretic, antihypertensive

Silafed Syrup:
Per 5 ml:
pseudoephedrine 30 mg
triprolidine 1.25 mg
Uses: Adrenergic, antihistamine

Silaminic Cold Syrup:
Per 5 ml:
phenylpropanolamine 12.5 mg
chlorpheniramine 2 mg
Uses: Antihistamine, decongestant

Simcor:
niacin 500 mg
simvastatin 20 mg
niacin 750 mg
simvastatin 20 mg
niacin 1000 mg
simvastatin 20 mg
Uses: Hypercholesterolemia

Sinemet 10/100:
carbidopa 10 mg
levodopa 100 mg
Uses: Antiparkinsonian

Sinemet 25/100:
carbidopa 25 mg
levodopa 100 mg
Uses: Antiparkinsonian

Sinemet 25/250:
carbidopa 25 mg
levodopa 250 mg
Uses: Antiparkinsonian

Sinemet CR 25-100:
carbidopa 25 mg
levodopa 100 mg
Uses: Antiparkinsonian

Sinemet CR 50-200:
carbidopa 50 mg
levodopa 200 mg
Uses: Antiparkinsonian

Slo-Phyllin GG Syrup:
theophylline 150 mg
guaifenesin 90 mg
Uses: Bronchodilator, expectorant

Slow-Salt-K:
sodium chloride 410 mg
potassium chloride 15 mg
Uses: Potassium, sodium supplement

Solage:
mequinol 2%
tretinoin 0.01%
Uses: Antineoplastic

Soma Compound:
carisoprodol 200 mg
aspirin 325 mg
Uses: Skeletal muscle relaxant

Spec-T Lozenge:
dextromethorphan 10 mg
benzocaine 10 mg
Uses: Antitussive, topical anesthetic

Stalevo 50:
carbidopa 12.5 mg
levodopa 50 mg
entacapone 200 mg
Uses: Parkinsonism

Stalevo 100:
carbidopa 25 mg
levodopa 100 mg
entacapone 200 mg
Uses: Parkinsonism

Stalevo 150:
carbidopa 37.5 mg
levodopa 150 mg
entacapone 200 mg
Uses: Parkinsonism

Sudafed Sinus & Cold:
pseudoephedrine 30 mg
acetaminophen 325 mg
Uses: Adrenergic, analgesic

Sudal 60/500:
pseudoephedrine 60 mg
guaifenesin 500 mg
Uses: Adrenergic, expectorant

Sudal 120/600:
pseudoephedrine 120 mg
guaifenesin 600 mg
Uses: Adrenergic, expectorant

Sultrin Triple Sulfa Vaginal Cream:
3.42% sulfathiazole
2.86% sulfacetamine
3.7% sulfabenzamide
Uses: Antiinfective

Sultrin Triple Sulfa Vaginal Tablets:
sulfathiazole 172.5 mg
sulfacetamide 143.75 mg
sulfabenzamide 184 mg
Uses: Antiinfective

Symbicort:
budesonide 80 mcg
formoterol 4.5 mcg
budesonide 160 mcg
formoterol 4.5 mcg
Uses: Asthma

Symbyax:
olanzapine 6 mg
fluoxetine 25 mg
olanzapine 6 mg
fluoxetine 50 mg
olanzapine 12 mg
fluoxetine 25 mg
olanzapine 12 mg
fluoxetine 50 mg
Uses: Bipolar disorder

Synalgos-DC:
aspirin 356.4 mg
caffeine 30 mg
dihydrocodeine 16 mg
Uses: Analgesic

Synercid:
quinupristin 150 mg
dalfopristin 350 mg
Uses: Antiinfective

Syntest H.S.:
esterified estrogens 0.625 mg
methylTESTOSTERone 1.25 mg
Uses: Vasomotor symptoms (menopause)

Taclonex:
betamethasone 0.064%
calcipotriene 0.005%
Uses: Plaque psoriasis

Talacen:
acetaminophen 650 mg
pentazocine 25 mg
Uses: Analgesic

Talwin Compound:
aspirin 325 mg
pentazocine 12.5 mg
Uses: Analgesic

Talwin NX:
pentazocine 50 mg
naloxone 0.5 mg
Uses: Analgesic, opioid antagonist
Tarka 182:
trandolapril 2 mg (immed rel)
verapamil 180 mg (sus rel)
Uses: Antihypertensive, calcium channel blocker
Tarka 241:
trandolapril 1 mg (immed rel)
verapamil 240 mg (sus rel)
Uses: Antihypertensive, calcium channel blocker
Tarka 242:
trandolapril 2 mg (immed rel)
verapamil 240 mg (sus rel)
Uses: Antihypertensive, calcium channel blocker
Tarka 244:
trandolapril 4 mg (immed rel)
verapamil 240 mg (sus rel)
Uses: Antihypertensive, calcium channel blocker
🍁 Tecnal:
aspirin 330 mg
caffeine 40 mg
butalbital 50 mg
Uses: Nonopioid analgesic
Teczem:
enalapril 5 mg (extended release)
diltiazem 180 mg (extended release)
Uses: Antihypertensive, calcium channel blocker
Tegrin-LT Shampoo:
0.33% pyrethrins
3.15% piperonyl butoxide
Uses: Scabicide, pediculicide
Tekturna HCT:
aliskiren 150 mg
hydrochlorothiazide 12.5 mg
aliskiren 150 mg
hydrochlorothiazide 25 mg
aliskiren 300 mg
hydrochlorothiazide 12.5 mg
aliskiren 300 mg
hydrochlorothiazide 25 mg
Uses: Hypertension
Tenoretic 50:
atenolol 50 mg
chlorthalidone 25 mg
Uses: Antihypertensive
Tenoretic 100:
atenolol 100 mg
chlorthalidone 25 mg
Uses: Antihypertensive
Terra-Cortril Ophthalmic Suspension:
1.5% hydrocortisone acetate
0.5% oxytetracycline
Uses: Ophthalmic antiinflammatory, antiinfective
Terramycin w/Polymycin B Sulfate Ophthalmic Ointment:
Per gram:
polymyxin B 10,000 units
oxytetracycline 5 mg
Uses: Ophthalmic antiinfective
T-Gesic:
hydrocodone 5 mg
acetaminophen 500 mg
Uses: Analgesic
Timentin for Injection:
Per 3.1-g vial:
ticarcillin 3 g
clavulanic acid 0.1 g
Uses: Antiinfective
Timolide 10/25:
timolol 10 mg
hydrochlorothiazide 25 mg
Uses: Antihypertensive
Titralac Plus:
calcium carbonate 420 mg
simethicone 21 mg
Uses: Antacid, adsorbent, antiflatulent
Tobra Dex Ophthalmic Suspension/Ointment:
tobramycin 0.3%
dexamethasone 0.1%
Uses: Ophthalmic antiinfective, antiinflammatory

Treximet:
naproxen 500 mg
sumatriptan 85 mg
Uses: Antimigraine

Triacin-C Cough Syrup:
Per 5 ml:
codeine 10 mg
pseudoephedrine 30 mg
triprolidine 1.25 mg
Uses: Analgesic, adrenergic, antihistamine

Tri-Hydroserpine:
hydrALAZINE 25 mg
hydrochlorothiazide 15 mg
reserpine 0.1 mg
Uses: Antihypertensive

Trinalin Repetabs:
azatadine maleate 1 mg
pseudoephedrine 120 mg
Uses: Antihistamine

TriOxin:
Per ml:
benzocaine 15 mg
chloroxylenol 1 mg
hydrocortisone 10 mg

Triple Antibiotic Ophthalmic Ointment:
Per gram:
polymyxin B 10,000 units
neomycin 3.5 mg
bacitracin 400 units
Uses: Antiinfective

Triprolidine/Pseudoephedrine Syrup (generic):
Per 5 ml
triprolidine 1.25 mg
pseudoephedrine 50 mg
Uses: Antihistamine, decongestant

Triprolidine/Pseudoephedrine Tablets (generic):
triprolidine 2.5 mg
pseudoephedrine 60 mg
Uses: Antihistamine, decongestant

Trizivir:
300 mg abacavir
150 mg lamivudine
300 mg zidovudine
Uses: HIV

Tusibron-DM Syrup:
Per 5 ml:
guaifenesin 100 mg
dextromethorphan 15 mg
Uses: Expectorant, antitussive

Tussionex:
Per 5 ml:
chlorpheniramine 8 mg
hydrocodone 10 mg
Uses: Cold, cough

Tylenol Allergy Complete Multi-Symptom:
acetaminophen 500 mg
chlorpheniramine 2 mg
pseudoephedrine 30 mg
Uses: Antihistamine, adrenergic, analgesic

Tylenol Children's Cold:
acetaminophen 80 mg
chlorpheniramine 0.5 mg
pseudoephedrine 7.5 mg
Uses: Antihistamine, adrenergic, analgesic

Tylenol Cold & Flu Severe Daytime:
Per 30 ml:
dextromethorphan 30 mg
pseudoephedrine 60 mg
acetaminophen 1000 mg
Uses: Antitussive, decongestant, analgesic

Tylenol Cold Multi-Symptom Nighttime Tablets:
acetaminophen 325 mg
chlorpheniramine 2 mg
phenylephrine 5 mg
dextromethorphan 10 mg
Uses: Antihistamine, adrenergic, analgesic

Tylenol Cold Severe Congestion Daytime Non-Drowsy Tablets:
dextromethorphan 10 mg
guaifenesin 200 mg

phenylephrine 5 mg
acetaminophen 325 mg
Uses: Antitussive, expectorant, decongestant, analgesic

Tylenol Cough & Sore Throat Daytime Liquid:
Per 30 ml:
dextromethorphan 30 mg
acetaminophen 1000 mg
Uses: Antitussive, analgesic

Tylenol Flu Nighttime Gelcaps:
diphenhydrAMINE 25 mg
pseudoephedrine 30 mg
acetaminophen 500 mg
Uses: Antihistamine, decongestant, analgesic

Tylenol PM, Extra Strength:
Per 30 ml:
acetaminophen 1000 mg
diphenhydrAMINE 50 mg
Uses: Analgesic, antihistamine

Tylenol Severe Allergy:
diphenhydrAMINE 12.5 mg
acetaminophen 500 mg
Uses: Analgesic, antihistamine

Tylenol w/Codeine No. 3:
acetaminophen 300 mg
codeine 30 mg
Uses: Analgesic

Tylenol w/Codeine No. 4:
acetaminophen 300 mg
codeine 60 mg
Uses: Analgesic

Tylox:
oxycodone 5 mg
acetaminophen 500 mg
Uses: Analgesic

Ultracet:
tramadol 37.5 mg
acetaminophen 325 mg
Uses: Analgesic

Unasyn for Injection 3 g:
ampicillin 2 g
sulbactam 1 g
Uses: Antiinfective

Uniretic:
moexipril 7.5 mg
hydrochlorothiazide 12.5 mg
moexipril 15 mg
hydrochlorothiazide 25 mg
Uses: Antihypertensive, diuretic

Urised:
methenamine 40.8 mg
phenylsalicylate 18.1 mg
atropine 0.03 mg
hyoscyamine 0.03 mg
benzoic acid 4.5 mg
methylene blue 5.4 mg
Uses: Antiinfective

Vanquish:
aspirin 227 mg
acetaminophen 194 mg
caffeine 33 mg
aluminum hydroxide 25 mg
magnesium hydroxide 50 mg
Uses: Nonopioid analgesic

Vaseretic 5-12.5:
enalapril 5 mg
hydrochlorthiazide 12.5 mg
Uses: Antihypertensive diuretic

Vaseretic 10-25:
enalapril 10 mg
hydrochlorothiazide 25 mg
Uses: Antihypertensive, diuretic

Vasocidin Ophthalmic Ointment:
sulfacetamide 10%
prednisoLONE 0.5%
Uses: Ophthalmic antiinfective, antiinflammatory

Vasocidin Ophthalmic Solution:
sulfacetamide 10%
prednisoLONE 0.25%
Uses: Ophthalmic antiinfective, antiinflammatory

Vasocon-A Ophthalmic Solution:
naphazoline 0.05%
antazoline 0.5%
Uses: Ophthalmic vasoconstrictor

Vicks 44D Cough & Head Congestion Relief:
Per 15 ml:
dextromethorphan 30 mg
pseudoephedrine 60 mg
Uses: Antitussive, adrenergic

Vicks 44E Liquid:
Per 5 ml:
dextromethorphan 6.7 mg
guaifenesin 66.7 mg
Uses: Antitussive, expectorant

Vicks 44M Cough, Cold, & Flu Relief:
Per 5 ml:
dextromethorphan 7.5 mg
pseudoephedrine 15 mg
chlorpheniramine 1 mg
acetaminophen 162.5 mg
Uses: Antitussive, adrenergic, antihistamine, analgesic

Vicks 44M Pediatric Cough and Cold Relief Syrup:
Per 15 ml:
pseudoephedrine 30 mg
chlorpheniramine 2 mg
dextromethorphan 15 mg
Uses: Adrenergic, antihistamine, antitussive

Vicks DayQuil Pressure & Pain Caplet:
pseudoephedrine 30 mg
ibuprofen 200 mg
Uses: Adrenergic, analgesic

Vicks NyQuil LiquiCaps:
pseudoephedrine 30 mg
doxylamine 6.25 mg
dextromethorphan 10 mg
acetaminophen 250 mg
Uses: Adrenergic, antihistamine, antitussive, analgesic

Vicks NyQuil Multi-Symptom Cold Flu Relief Liquid:
pseudoephedrine 10 mg
doxylamine 2.1 mg
dextromethorphan 5 mg
acetaminophen 167 mg
Uses: Adrenergic, antihistamine, antitussive, analgesic

Vicodin:
acetaminophen 500 mg
hydrocodone 5 mg
Uses: Analgesic

Vicodin ES:
acetaminophen 750 mg
hydrocodone 7.5 mg
Uses: Analgesic

Vicodin HP:
acetaminophen 660 mg
hydrocodone 10 mg
Uses: Analgesic

Vicodin Tuss:
Per 5 ml:
hydrocodone 5 mg
guaifenesin 100 mg
Uses: Analgesic, expectorant

Vicoprofen:
hydrocodone 7.5 mg
ibuprofen 200 mg
Uses: Analgesic

Vytorin:
ezetimibe: 10, 10, 10, 10 mg
simvastatin: 10, 20, 40, 80 mg
Uses: Antihyperlipidemic

Yasmin 28:
ethinyl estadiol 30 mcg
dropirenone 3 mg
Uses: Oral contraceptive

YAZ:
prospirenone 3 mg
ethinyl estradiol 0.02 mg
Uses: Vasomotor symptoms (menopause)

Zegerid Capsules:
omeprazole 20 mg
sodium bicarbonate 1100 mg
omeprazole 40 mg
sodium bicarbonate 1100 mg
Uses: Gastric ulcer, GERD

Zegerid Powder (Oral Solution):
omeprazole 20 mg
sodium bicarbonate 1680 mg,
omeprazole 40 mg
sodium bicarbonate 1680 mg
Uses: Gastric ulcer, GERD

Zestoretic 10/12.5:
lisinopril 10 mg
hydrochlorothiazide 12.5 mg
Uses: Antihypertensive

Zestoretic 20/12.5:
lisinopril 20 mg
hydrochlorothiazide 12.5 mg
Uses: Antihypertensive

Zestoretic 20/25:
lisinopril 20 mg
hydrochlorothiazide 25 mg
Uses: Antihypertensive

Ziac 2.5:
bisoprolol 2.5 mg
hydrochlorothiazide 6.25 mg
Uses: Antihypertensive

Ziac 5:
bisoprolol 5 mg
hydrochlorothiazide 6.25 mg
Uses: Antihypertensive

Ziac 10:
bisoprolol 10 mg
hydrochlorothiazide 6.25 mg
Uses: Antihypertensive

Ziana:
clindamycin 1.2%
tretinoin 0.025%
Uses: Acne vulgaris

Zydone:
hydrocodone 5 mg
acetaminophen 500 mg
Uses: Analgesic

Zypram:
hydrocortisone 2.35%
pramoxine 1%
Uses: Antiinflammatory

Zyrtec-D:
cetirizine 5 mg
pseudoephedrine 120 mg
Uses: Antihistamine, decongestant

Appendix f

FDA pregnancy categories

A No risk demonstrated to the fetus in any trimester

B No adverse effects in animals; no human studies available

C Only given after risks to the fetus are considered; animal studies have shown adverse reactions, no human studies available

D Definite fetal risks, may be given in spite of risks if needed in life-threatening conditions

X Absolute fetal abnormalities; not to be used at any time during pregnancy

Note: **UK** = Unknown fetal risk (used in this text but not an official FDA pregnancy category).

Appendix g

Abbreviations

ABG arterial blood gas
ADA American Diabetes Association
ADH antidiuretic hormone
ALT alanine aminotransferase
ANA antinuclear antibody
APLA antiphospholipid antibody syndrome
APTT activated partial thromboplastin time
ASA acetylsalicylic acid, aspirin
AST aspartate aminotransferase (SGOT)
AV atrioventricular
bid twice a day
BPH benign prostatic hypertrophy
BPM beats per minute
BUN blood urea nitrogen
CAD coronary artery disease
CBC complete blood cell count
CCr creatinine clearance
CHF congestive heart failure
CNS central nervous system
CONT continuous
COPD chronic obstructive pulmonary disease
CPAP continuous positive airway pressure
CPK creatine phosphokinase
CPS carbamoyl phosphate synthetase
C&S culture and sensitivity
CSF cerebrospinal fluid
CTCL cutaneous T-cell lymphoma
CV cardiovascular
CVA cerebrovascular accident
CVP central venous pressure
D&C dilatation and curettage
DIC diffuse intravascular coagulation
DIR INF direct infusion
D_5W 5% glucose in distilled water
DVT deep vein thrombosis
ECG electrocardiogram (EKG)
EDTA ethylenediamine tetraacetic acid
EEG electroencephalogram
EPS extrapyramidal symptom
ESR erythrocyte sedimentation rate
EXT REL extended release
FBS fasting blood sugar
FHT fetal heart tones
FSH follicle-stimulating hormone
GABA γ-aminobutyric acid
GPC giant papillary conjunctivitis
gr grain
GT glucose tolerance test
GU genitourinary
GVHD graft-versus-host disease
H_2 histamine$_2$
hCG human chorionic gonadotropin
Hct hematocrit
HDCV human diploid cell rabies vaccine
Hgb hemoglobin
H & H hematocrit and hemoglobin
5-HIAA 5-hydroxyindoleacetic acid
HIV human immunodeficiency virus (AIDS)
HR heart rate
IBD inflammatory bowel disease
IC intracardiac
ICP intracranial pressure
ID intradermal
IgG immunoglobulin G
IM intramuscular
INF infusion
INH inhalation
inj injection
I&O intake and output
INT intermittent
IPPB intermittent positive-pressure breathing
IT intrathecal
ITP idiopathic thrombocytopenic purpura
IUD intrauterine device
IV intravenous
IVP intravenous pyelogram
K potassium
LDH lactic dehydrogenase
LE lupus erythematosus
LFT liver function test

LH luteinizing hormone
LOC level of consciousness
LR lactated Ringer's solution
LT leukotriene
m minim
m² square meter
MAC monitored anesthesia care
MAOI monoamine oxidase inhibitor
mcg microgram
mEq milliequivalent
mg milligram
MI myocardial infarction
ml milliliter
mm millimeter
mo month
Na sodium
ng nanogram
NGU non-gonococcal urethritis
NHL non-Hodgkin's lymphoma
NPO nothing by mouth (Lat. *nulla per os*)
NS normal saline
OBS organic brain syndrome
OTC over-the-counter
P56 plasma-lyte 56
$PaCO_2$ arterial carbon dioxide tension (pressure)
PaO_2 arterial oxygen tension (pressure)
PAT paroxysmal atrial tachycardia
PBI protein-bound iodine
PCI percutaneous coronary intervention
PCWP pulmonary capillary wedge pressure
PEEP positive end-expiratory pressure
pH hydrogen ion concentration
PO by mouth
PP postprandial
PPHN persistent pulmonary hypertension of the newborn
prn as required
PT prothrombin time
PTT partial thromboplastin time
PVC premature ventricular contraction
pwd powder
qAM every morning
qhr every hour
q2hr every 2 hours
q3hr every 3 hours
q4hr every 4 hours
q6hr every 6 hours
q12hr every 12 hours
qid four times daily
qPM every night
RAIU radioactive iodine uptake
RBC red blood cell count or red blood cell
RECT rectal
ROM range of motion
SARS severe acute respiratory syndrome
SCr serum creatinine
SIMV synchronous intermittent mandatory ventilation
SL sublingual
SLE systemic lupus erythematosus
sol solution
STD sexually transmitted disease
SUBCUT subcutaneous
supp suppository
SUS REL sustained release
syr syrup
TD transdermal
tid three times daily
tinc tincture
TPN total parenteral nutrition
TSH thyroid-stimulating hormone
TT thrombin time
UA urinalysis
UTI urinary tract infection
UV ultraviolet
VMA vanillylmandelic acid
VS vital sign
WBC white blood cell count

- For a list of the Institute for Safe Medicine Practices (ISMP) error-prone abbreviations, symbols and dose designations, please see http://www.ismp.org/tools/errorproneabbreviations.pdf.
- For 2010 National Patient Safety Goals, please visit The Joint Commission website at http://www.jointcommission.org/PatientSafety/NationalPatientSafetyGoals.

Index

Entries can be identified as follows: *Combination Products,* DISEASES/DISORDERS, *DRUG CATEGORIES,* generic names, Trade Names.

Entries can be identified as follows: *Combination Products,* DISEASES/DISORDERS, *DRUG CATEGORIES,* generic names, Trade Names.

Entries can be identified as follows: *Combination Products,* DISEASES/DISORDERS, *DRUG CATEGORIES,* generic names, Trade Names.

Entries can be identified as follows: *Combination Products,* DISEASES/DISORDERS, *DRUG CATEGORIES,* generic names, Trade Names.

Entries can be identified as follows: *Combination Products,* DISEASES/DISORDERS, *DRUG CATEGORIES,* generic names, Trade Names.

Entries can be identified as follows: *Combination Products,* DISEASES/DISORDERS, *DRUG CATEGORIES,* generic names, Trade Names.

Entries can be identified as follows: *Combination Products,* DISEASES/DISORDERS, *DRUG CATEGORIES,* generic names, Trade Names.

Entries can be identified as follows: *Combination Products,* DISEASES/DISORDERS, *DRUG CATEGORIES,* generic names, Trade Names.

Entries can be identified as follows: *Combination Products,* DISEASES/DISORDERS, *DRUG CATEGORIES,* generic names, Trade Names.

Entries can be identified as follows: *Combination Products,* DISEASES/DISORDERS, *DRUG CATEGORIES,* generic names, Trade Names.

Mosby's 2011 Nursing Drug Reference Companion CD-ROM

Use *Mosby's 2011 Nursing Drug Reference Companion CD-ROM* to find drug information fast! This six-in-one CD-ROM provides you with profiles of the top 100 prescribed drugs in the United States, patient teaching guides, normal laboratory values, English-to-Spanish translations, calculators, and Canadian resources.

This Companion CD-ROM includes:

- **Top 100 Drugs**
  Complete, printable information on the 100 most commonly prescribed drugs in the United States.
- **Patient Teaching Guides**
  Select up-to-date English and Spanish patient teaching guides for the top 100 drugs.
- **Normal Laboratory Values**
  Features hundreds of normal reference values.
- **English-to-Spanish Translations**
  Provides Spanish translations and pronunciations for common drug phrases and terms.
- **Calculators**
  Contains 30 handy clinical calculators, including several IV and PO dosage calculators, and an IV dose rate calculator.
- **Canadian Resources**
  Includes high-alert medications, a controlled substance chart, and immunization schedules for infants and children.

Contact Us

For further information, visit us at http://www.us.elsevierhealth.com or call us at (800) 545-2522.

Mini CD-ROM

This mini CD-ROM will work in your CD-ROM drive. Place it on the inner ring of the tray, as shown, and follow the on-screen installation instructions.

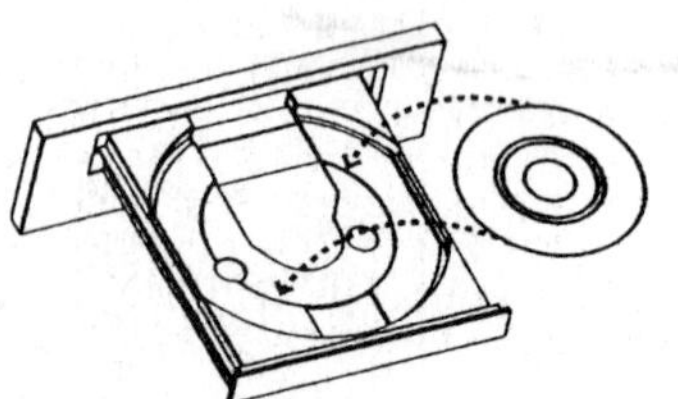

This mini-CD does not work in:
- Floppy Drives
- Slot Drives
- Zip Drives
- Stereos

Insert this mini-CD into your CD-ROM drive as shown at left.

Important

No credit or refund will be issued on this book if the CD envelope has been opened, torn, or otherwise tampered with.

Companion CD-ROM to accompany *Mosby's 2011 Nursing Drug Reference*

MINIMUM SYSTEM REQUIREMENTS

Windows®
XP or higher
200 MHz processor or faster
64 MB or more of installed RAM
30 MB free hard disk space
2× or faster CD-ROM drive
800 × 600 monitor or larger
256 Colors

Macintosh®
OS X or greater
Power Macintosh
At least 64 MB RAM recommended
1 GHz+ PowerPC G4
10 MB free hard disk space
48× or faster CD-ROM drive
800 × 600 monitor with millions of colors

Software Requirement
This product was designed to work with Internet Explorer 6.0 or higher, or Firefox 2.0 or higher. Other browsers may work; however, if problems occur, your first step should be to make sure the product is running Internet Explorer 6.0.

INSTALLATION INSTRUCTIONS

If the autorun feature is on, the program will automatically start after the CD is inserted into the CD-ROM drive. If the program does not launch automatically, follow these steps.
1. Start Microsoft Windows® and insert the CD-ROM.
2. Click the *Start* button from the Taskbar and select the *Run* option.
3. Type d:\Skidmore.exe (where "d:\" is your CD-ROM drive) and press *Enter*.
4. Follow the on-screen instructions for installation.

TECHNICAL SUPPORT

Technical support for this product is available between 7:30 AM and 7 PM CST, Monday through Friday. Before calling, make sure that your computer meets the minimum system requirements to run this software. Inside the United States, call (800) 692-9010. Outside the United States, call (314) 997-1176. You may also fax your questions to (314) 523-4932.

You may also contact Technical Support via e-mail at:
technical.support@elsevier.com

Copyright © 2011, Mosby, Inc., an affiliate of Elsevier Inc. All rights reserved.

No part of this product may be reproduced or transmitted in any form or by any means, electronic, or mechanical, including input into or storage in any information system, without permission in writing from the publisher.

Produced in the United States of America.

Part number: 9996074331

Windows and Macintosh are registered trademarks.

IV Drug/Solution Compatibility Chart

			D_5					
	D_5	D_{10}	½S	S	NS	R	LR	OTHER
AcetaZOLAMIDE	C	C	C	C	C	C	C	
Acyclovir	C							
$Alpha_1$-proteinase inhibitor								Sterile water for inj
Alprostadil	C	C			C			
Alteplase								Sterile water for inj
Amikacin	C				C			
Aminocaproic acid			C	C	C	C		D in distilled water
Ammonium Cl					C			May add KCl to solution
Amphotericin B	C							
Ampicillin	C				C			
Antithrombin III	C				C			Sterile water for inj
Ascorbic acid	C				C	C	C	Sodium lactate
Atenolol	C				C			0.45% saline
Azlocillin	C		C		C			
Aztreonam	C	C			C	C	C	Normosol-R
Cefazolin	C				C			
Cefotetan	C				C			
Cefoxitin	C	C			C	C	C	Aminosol
Ceftazidime	C		C	C	C	C	C	M/G Sodium lactate

This chart is not inclusive and is based on manufacturers' recommendations.

Key

C = Compatible
D_5 = Dextrose 5%
D_{10} = Dextrose 10%
D_5½S = Dextrose 5% in saline 0.45%
D_5S = Dextrose 5% in saline 0.9%
NS = Sodium chloride 0.9% (normal saline)
R = Ringer's solution
LR = Lactated Ringer's solution

	D_5	D_{10}	D_5		NS	R	LR	OTHER
			½S	S				
Ceftriaxone	C				C			
Cefuroxime	C		C	C		C		M/G Sodium lactate
Ciprofloxacin	C				C			
CycloSPORINE	C				C			Use only glass containers
DOBUTamine	C				C			Sodium lactate
DOPamine	C		C	C	C		C	M/G Sodium lactate
Doxycycline	C	C			C			Invert sugar 10%
Edetate Na	C							Isotonic saline
Ganciclovir	C				C	C	C	
Gentamicin	C	C			C			Normosol-R
Heparin Na	C				C	C		
Ifosfamide	C				C		C	Sterile water for inj
Inamrinone lactate					C			0.45% saline
Kanamycin	C				C			
Metaraminol	C			C	C	C	C	Normosol-R
Methicillin	C			C				
Metoclopramide	C	C		C		C	C	
Mezlocillin	C	C	C	C	C	C	C	Fructose 5%
Nitroglycerin	C	C			C			
Norepinephrine	C			C			C	
Piperacillin	C			C	C		C	
Ritodrine	C							
Ticarcillin	C				C		C	
Tobramycin	C	C			C			
Vidarabine	C				C			

Syringe Compatibility

	Atropine	Buprenorphine	Butorphanol	ChlorproMAZINE	Codeine	Diazepam	DimenhyDRINATE	DiphenhydrAMINE	Droperidol	Fentanyl	Glycopyrrolate	Heparin
Atropine			C	C		I	C	C	C	C	C	
Buprenorphine												
Butorphanol	C			C		I	I	C	C	C		
ChlorproMAZINE	C		C			I	I	C	C	C	C	C
Codeine						I						
Diazepam	I		I	I	I		I	I	I	I	I	
DimenhyDRINATE	C		I	I		I		C	C	C	I	
DiphenhydrAMINE	C		C	C		I	C		C	C	C	
Droperidol	C		C	C		I	C	C		C	C	I
Fentanyl	C		C	C		I	C	C	C		C	
Glycopyrrolate	C			C		I	I	C	C	C		
Heparin			I	C		I			I			
HydrOXYzine	C		C	C		I	I	C	C	C	C	
Meperidine	C		C	C		I	C	C	C	C	C	I
Metoclopramide	C		C	C		I	C	C	C	C		
Midazolam	C		C	C			I	C	C	C	C	
Morphine	C		C	C		I	C	C	C	C	C	I
Nalbuphine	C					I			C			
Pentazocine	C		C	C		I	C	C	C	C	I	I
Pentobarbital	C		I	I	I	I	I	I	I	I	I	
Perphenazine	C		C	C		I	C	C	C	C		
Prochlorperazine	C		C	C		I	I	C	C	C	C	
Promazine	C			C		I	I	C	C	C	C	
Promethazine	C		C	C		I	I	C	C	C	C	
Ranitidine	C			C			C	C		C	C	
Scopolamine Hbr	C		C	C		I	C	C	C	C	C	
Secobarbital	I		I	I	I	I	I	I	I	I	I	
Thiethylperazine			C			I						

Developed by Providence Memorial Hospital, El Paso, Texas.

NOTE: Give within 15 minutes of mixing.

C = compatible; I = incompatible; ☐ = no documented information.

* = compatibility depends on manufacturer; Wyeth and DuPont forms are incompatible.